CURRENT CLINICAL PATHOLOGY

ANTONIO GIORDANO, MD, PhD

SERIES EDITOR

DIRECTOR, SBARRO INSTITUTE FOR CANCER RESEARCH
AND MOLECULAR MEDICINE AND CENTER FOR BIOTECHNOLOGY
TEMPLE UNIVERSITY
PHILADELPHIA, PA, USA

For further volumes:
http://www.springer.com/series/7632

Mauro Bologna
Editor

Biotargets of Cancer in Current Clinical Practice

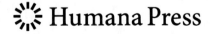

Editor
Mauro Bologna, M.D.
Department of Experimental Medicine
University of L'Aquila
L'Aquila, Italy

ISBN 978-1-61779-614-2   e-ISBN 978-1-61779-615-9
DOI 10.1007/978-1-61779-615-9
Springer New York Dordrecht Heidelberg London

Library of Congress Control Number: 2012934059

© Springer Science+Business Media, LLC 2012
All rights reserved. This work may not be translated or copied in whole or in part without the written permission of the publisher (Humana Press, c/o Springer Science+Business Media, LLC, 233 Spring Street, New York, NY 10013, USA), except for brief excerpts in connection with reviews or scholarly analysis. Use in connection with any form of information storage and retrieval, electronic adaptation, computer software, or by similar or dissimilar methodology now known or hereafter developed is forbidden.
The use in this publication of trade names, trademarks, service marks, and similar terms, even if they are not identified as such, is not to be taken as an expression of opinion as to whether or not they are subject to proprietary rights.
While the advice and information in this book are believed to be true and accurate at the date of going to press, neither the authors nor the editors nor the publisher can accept any legal responsibility for any errors or omissions that may be made. The publisher makes no warranty, express or implied, with respect to the material contained herein.

Printed on acid-free paper

Humana Press is part of Springer Science+Business Media (www.springer.com)

I dedicate this work to all those from whom I learned, during my professional education path, but mostly to

Pietro Ubaldo Angeletti, M.D., Professor of General Pathology at the University of L'Aquila Medical School in the 1970s and 1980s and coworker of Rita Levi Montalcini in the Nerve Growth Factor discovery, who had me in his laboratory at the beginning of my career (since 1977), as Assistant Fellow and later Professor; I learnt many fundamental aspects of research from him; I am especially in debt to him, since he acted also as my supportive mentor in following times, until his premature passing away in 1992 at age 59.

Renato Dulbecco, M.D., Nobel Prize winner for Medicine, who accepted me in his laboratory for about 3 years at the Salk Institute (La Jolla, CA, USA), first when I was awarded a fellowship from Accademia dei Lincei (Rome, Italy, 1979) and later in quality of visiting research associate. I absorbed a great deal of methodology, scientific deduction and character from him. His beautiful mind passed away in february 2012 at age 98.

Moreover, I dedicate this work to my family and, in particular, to my wife, Donatella, who always supported me lovingly and magnificently, and by doing so made (and still makes) all my productive efforts possible.

Preface

Biotargets of cancer are continuously evolving. Clinically valuable Biotargets are a subcategory of Biomarkers, molecules of note in the field, with their time variations in different physiological and pathological situations. Today, biomarkers are essential for diagnosis, prognosis, and prediction of therapeutic response. Biotargets are essential for an updated therapeutic approach in oncology.

Every week, in this very fertile moment of biomolecular research in all fields of life sciences, there is news in the literature concerning new molecules, new levels of already known molecular actors, new interactions of the complex biochemical pathways network of the eukaryotic cells and of the tumor cells, which may arise in multicellular live beings as an aggressive, disturbing, and deadly subpopulation of body components. Humans are at the forefront in this pathological area, since many mutagens are introduced in the environment by human activities and by human ignorance of biological equilibria.

Cancer is a genetic disease of somatic cells, with relevant geographic epidemiological variations and hundreds of different genetic mutations identified so far, due to the repeated mutagenic insults in time on the same subject, leading to the final result of aggressive, invasive neoplastic disease.

The clinical work of oncologists, the physicians who are called to provide assistance to the tumor patients, is today impossible without a good knowledge of basic science, since many new drugs act on specific biological pathways, and the current trend to ensure "personalized" therapy to each patient involves deeper and deeper knowledge, not only of clinical aspects of care but also of biochemical pathways and pharmacological interactions of molecules (basic constituents of the cells and synthetic interactors which are used therapeutically).

For the reasons just summarized, an update on biotargets of cancer is felt necessary by many professionals in oncology. It is to them that this book is addressed.

With a truly international team of coworkers, this book includes, for each major cancer type, a comprehensive although concise discussion of epidemiology, affirmed and innovative biomarkers for diagnosis, description of the relevant genes for prognosis, and (potentially individualized) therapy through biotarget-specific new molecules, with the latest information on the validation status of each novel biomarker. The last two chapters deal with topics of very general interest: tumor metastasis and miRNA interference on gene expression, a very promising and highly selective new approach for cancer research and therapy.

The target readers of the book are clinicians in the field (oncologists, pathologists, interns) and medical students.

I feel it is necessary to stress that the emerging evidence in most tumors points to two main novelties: the necessity of personalized treatments (since many similar tumors have peculiar molecular variants, that is, different subcategories of molecular profiles) and the necessity of multitargeted therapies (since single tumors easily develop resistance to monotherapies).

These two principles are becoming more and more verified in many current basic and clinical research efforts, both at the experimental and the clinical levels. After all, nature is very redundant in its physiological patterns of growth control and growth-stimulation mechanisms: a wise strategy in medicine is to mimic nature; therefore, a good approach in cancer control should be the redundant inhibition of cancer cell proliferation through multitargeted therapies. Ideally, multiple, synergic drugs should be used at the lowest effective dosage, minimizing the possible side effects of each molecule.

Therefore, the future of clinical oncology is based on deeper and deeper molecular knowledge concerning a wide variety of biomarkers and a numerous series of druggable and approachable biotargets. A totally new category of targets is composed by fusion proteins, actively searched, studied, and possibly targeted by specifically engineered drugs.

Far from being exhaustive in covering the necessary knowledge, this book attempts, however, to provide a wide spectrum of current scientific information about cancer clinical management based on such molecular aspects, with many insights toward future — not yet validated, but currently investigated — clinical applications.

We hope that the readers will find this book useful for their daily practice, at least through the principle of a better patient selection based on tumor molecular profiles, and for their professional update.

L'Aquila, Italy   Mauro Bologna, M.D.

Acknowledgments

The expert and the very professional collaboration of Michael D. Sova, Developmental Editor at Springer/Humana Press is gratefully acknowledged.

Contents

1 Central Nervous System Tumors 1
Paolo Aloisi, Francesco Martella, Davide Cerone,
and Giampiero Porzio

2 Head and Neck Tumours 19
Keith D. Hunter and Robert Bolt

3 Thyroid Cancer 61
Laura D. Locati, Angela Greco, Maria Grazia Borrello,
Maria Luisa Carcangiu, Paolo Bossi, Roberta Granata,
and Lisa Licitra

4 Targeted Therapies for Non-small-Cell Lung Cancer 93
Giulio Metro and Lucio Crinò

5 Non-Hodgkin's Lymphomas 115
Roberta Zappasodi and Massimo Di Nicola

6 Leukemias 159
Lia Ginaldi and Massimo De Martinis

7 Breast Cancer 195
Nadia Rucci, Luca Ventura, and Anna Teti

8 Oesophago-Gastric Cancer 221
Alex M. Reece-Smith, Simon L. Parsons,
and Sue A. Watson

9 Colorectal Cancer 245
David N. Church, Rachel Susannah Midgley,
and David J. Kerr

10 Hepatocellular Carcinoma 273
Yasunori Minami and Masatoshi Kudo

**11 Biomarkers for Prognosis and Molecularly Targeted
Therapy in Renal Cell Carcinoma** 289
Laura S. Schmidt

12 Bladder Cancer 325
Andrea Tubaro, Daniele Santini, Cosimo De Nunzio,
Alice Zoccoli, and Michele Iuliano

13 Biomarkers in Prostate Cancer 355
Mauro Bologna and Carlo Vicentini

14 Ovarian Cancer 381
Jessica Wangui Oribabor, Allison Ambrosio,
Cesar M. Castro, and Michael J. Birrer

**15 Uterine Cancer: The Influence of Genetics
and Environment on Cell Cycling Pathways in Cancer** 403
Annekathryn Goodman, Leslie S. Bradford,
and Leslie A. Garrett

**16 Biotargets in Sarcomas: The Past, Present, and a Look
into the Future** 419
Vivek Subbiah and Razelle Kurzrock

17 Melanoma and Other Skin Cancers 439
Kim H.T. Paraiso, Jobin K. John, and Keiran S.M. Smalley

**18 Molecular Pathology of Cancer Metastasis: Suggestions
for Future Therapy** 469
Adriano Angelucci and Edoardo Alesse

**19 Current and Future Developments in Cancer Therapy
Research: miRNAs as New Promising Targets or Tools** 517
Marilena V. Iorio, Patrizia Casalini, Claudia Piovan,
Luca Braccioli, and Elda Tagliabue

Index 547

Contributors

Edoardo Alesse, M.D., Ph.D. Department of Experimental Medicine, University of L'Aquila, L'Aquila, Italy

Paolo Aloisi, M.D. Department of Neurosciences, San Salvatore Hospital, Via Lorenzo Natali, Coppito, L'Aquila, Italy

Allison Ambrosio, B.A. Gillette Center for Women's Cancers, Massachusetts General Hospital, Boston, MA, USA

Adriano Angelucci, Ph.D. Department of Experimental Medicine, University of L'Aquila, L'Aquila, Italy

Michael J. Birrer, M.D., Ph.D. Gillette Center for Women's Cancers, Massachusetts General Hospital, Boston, MA, USA

Mauro Bologna, M.D. Department of Experimental Medicine, University of L'Aquila, L'Aquila, Italy

Robert Bolt, B.D.S., M.F.D.S., M.B.Ch.B. Department of Oral Surgery, Charles Clifford Dental School, Sheffield, South Yorkshire, UK

Maria Grazia Borrello, Ph.D. Department of Experimental Oncology and Molecular Medicine, Fondazione IRCCS Istituto Nazionale dei Tumori, Milan, Italy

Paolo Bossi, M.D. Head and Neck Medical Oncology Unit, Fondazione IRCCS Istituto Nazionale dei Tumori, Milan, Italy

Luca Braccioli, Ph.D. Department of Experimental Oncology, Fondazione IRCCS Istituto Nazionale dei Tumori, Milan, Italy

Leslie S. Bradford, M.D. Division of Gynecologic Oncology, Massachusetts General Hospital, Boston, MA, USA

Maria Luisa Carcangiu, M.D. Department of Pathology, Fondazione IRCCS Istituto Nazionale dei Tumori, Milan, Italy

Patrizia Casalini, Ph.D. Department of Experimental Oncology, Fondazione IRCCS Istituto Nazionale dei Tumori, Milan, Italy

Cesar M. Castro, M.D., M.M.Sc. Department of Medicine, Massachusetts General Hospital, Boston, MA, USA

Davide Cerone, M.D. Department of Neuroscience, San Salvatore Hospital, Via Lorenzo Natali, L'Aquila, Italy

David N. Church, M.B.Ch.B., M.R.C.P., D.Phil. University Department of Medical Oncology, Churchill Hospital, Oxford, Oxfordshire, UK

Lucio Crinò, M.D. Santa Maria della Misericordia Hospital, Medical Oncology, Azienda Ospedaliera di Perugia, Perugia, Italy

Massimo De Martinis, M.D. Department of Internal Medicine and Public Health, University of L'Aquila, Coppito, L'Aquila, Italy

Cosimo De Nunzio, M.D. Department of Urology, Sant'Andrea Hospital, Rome, Italy

Massimo Di Nicola, M.D. "C. Gandini" Bone Marrow Transplantation Unit, Department of Medical Oncology, Fondazione IRCCS Istituto Nazionale dei Tumori, Milan, Italy

Leslie A. Garrett, M.D. Department of Obstetrics and Gynecology, Massachusetts General Hospital, Boston, MA, USA

Lia Ginaldi, M.D. Department of Internal Medicine and Public Health, University of L'Aquila, Coppito, L'Aquila, Italy

Annekathryn Goodman, M.D. Department of Obstetrics and Gynecology, Massachusetts General Hospital, Boston, MA, USA

Roberta Granata, M.D. Head and Neck Medical Oncology Unit, Fondazione IRCCS Istituto Nazionale dei Tumori, Milan, Italy

Angela Greco, Ph.D. Department of Experimental Oncology and Molecular Medicine, Fondazione IRCCS Istituto Nazionale dei Tumori, Milan, Italy

Keith D. Hunter, B.Sc., B.D.S., F.D.S.R.C.S.Ed., Ph.D., F.R.C.Path. Unit of Oral and Maxillofacial Pathology, School of Clinical Dentistry, University of Sheffield, Sheffield, South Yorkshire, UK

Marilena V. Iorio, Ph.D. Department of Experimental Oncology, Fondazione IRCCS Istituto Nazionale dei Tumori, Milan, Italy

Michele Iuliano, M.D. Department of Medical Oncology, Campus Bio-Medico University, Rome, Italy

Jobin K. John, M.D. Department of Molecular Oncology, The Moffitt Cancer Center, Tampa, FL, USA

David J. Kerr, M.A., M.D., D.Sc., F.R.C.P., F.Med.Sci., C.B.E. Nuffield Department of Clinical and Laboratory Sciences, University of Oxford, Oxford, Oxfordshire, UK

Masatoshi Kudo, M.D., Ph.D. Department of Gastroenterology and Hepatology, Kinki University School of Medicine, Osaka-Sayama, Osaka, Japan

Razelle Kurzrock, M.D. Department of Investigational Cancer Therapeutics, MD Anderson Cancer Center, Houston, TX, USA

Lisa Licitra, M.D. Head and Neck Oncology Unit, Fondazione IRCCS Istituto Nazionale dei Tumori, Milan, Italy

Laura D. Locati, M.D. Head and Neck Medical Oncology Unit, Fondazione IRCCS Istituto Nazionale dei Tumori, Milan, Italy

Francesco Martella, Ph.D. Home Care Unit: L'Aquila per la Vita, Via Rocco, Carabba, L'Aquila, Italy

Giulio Metro, M.D. Santa Maria della Misericordia Hospital, Medical Oncology, Azienda Ospedaliera di Perugia, Perugia, Italy

Rachel Susannah Midgley, M.B.Ch.B., F.R.C.P., Ph.D. Department of Oncology, Churchill Hospital, Oxford, Oxfordshire, UK

Yasunori Minami, M.D. Department of Gastroenterology and Hepatology, Kinki University School of Medicine, Osaka-Sayama, Osaka, Japan

Jessica Wangui Oribabor, B.S. Gillette Center for Women's Cancers, Massachusetts General Hospital, Boston, MA, USA

Kim H.T. Paraiso, M.S. Department of Molecular Oncology, The Moffitt Cancer Center, Tampa, FL, USA

Simon L. Parsons, D.M., F.R.C.S. Oesophago-gastric surgery, Nottingham University Hospitals NHS Trust, Nottingham, Nottinghamshire, UK

Claudia Piovan, Ph.D. Department of Experimental Oncology, Fondazione IRCCS Istituto Nazionale dei Tumori, Milan, Italy

Giampiero Porzio, Ph.D. Department of Experimental Medicine, University of L'Aquila, Via Vetoio, Coppito, L'Aquila, Italy

Alex M. Reece-Smith, M.B.B.S., M.R.C.S. Division of Pre-Clinical Oncology, PRECOS Ltd, School of Clinical Sciences, University of Nottingham, Queen's Medical Centre, Nottingham, UK

Nadia Rucci, Ph.D. Department of Experimental Medicine, University of L'Aquila, L'Aquila, Italy

Daniele Santini, M.D. Department of Medical Oncology, Campus Bio-Medico University, Rome, Italy

Laura S. Schmidt, Ph.D. Urologic Oncology Branch, National Cancer Institute, National Institutes of Health, Bethesda, MD, USA

Basic Science Program, SAIC-Frederick, Inc., NCI-Frederick, Frederick, MD, USA

Keiran S.M. Smalley, Ph.D. Department of Molecular Oncology, The Moffitt Cancer Center, Tampa, FL, USA

Vivek Subbiah, M.D. Division of Cancer Medicine, The University of Texas MD Anderson Cancer Center, Houston, TX, USA

Elda Tagliabue, Ph.D. Department of Experimental Oncology, Fondazione IRCCS Istituto Nazionale dei Tumori, Milan, Italy

Anna Teti, Ph.D. Department of Experimental Medicine, University of L'Aquila, L'Aquila, Italy

Andrea Tubaro, M.D., F.E.B.U. Department of Urology, Sant'Andrea Hospital, "La Sapienza" University of Rome, Rome, Italy

Luca Ventura, M.D. Department of Pathology, San Salvatore Hospital, L'Aquila, Italy

Carlo Vicentini, M.D. Department of Urology, University Hospital of Teramo, L'Aquila, Italy

Sue A. Watson, Ph.D. Division of Pre-Clinical Oncology, School of Clinical Sciences, University of Nottingham, Queen's Medical Centre, Nottingham, UK

Roberta Zappasodi, Ph.D. "C. Gandini" Bone Marrow Transplantation Unit, Department of Medical Oncology, Fondazione IRCCS Istituto Nazionale dei Tumori, Milan, Italy

Alice Zoccoli, M.D. Department of Medical Oncology, Campus Bio-Medico University, Rome, Italy

Central Nervous System Tumors

1

Paolo Aloisi, Francesco Martella, Davide Cerone, and Giampiero Porzio

Introduction

Each year, there are about 7.5 million deaths for cancer worldwide [1, 2]. Among these, primary central nervous system (CNS) cancer mortality seems to be relatively small. Due to a restricted number of patients, CNS cancers have been an orphan disease with a quite limited funding to study. Nevertheless, these malignancies constitute a vital important chapter in neurology, because they can produce many different neurological symptoms, like CNS tissue disruption and displacement, increasing intracranial pressure and, the most important thing, they are often lethal. In fact, on account of all causes of intracranial disease, the CNS cancers constitute the second cause of death, exceeded in frequency only by stroke. On the other hand, it is interesting to observe that, in children, primary CNS cancers are the most common solid neoplasm, and they are second only to leukemia [2].

P. Aloisi, M.D. (✉) • D. Cerone, M.D.
Department of Neurosciences, San Salvatore Hospital, Via Lorenzo Natali, Coppito, L'Aquila 67100, Italy
e-mail: neurofisiopatologia@asl1abruzzo.it

F. Martella, Ph.D.
Home Care Unit: L'Aquila per la Vita,
Via Rocco, Carabba, L'Aquila 67100, Italy
e-mail: martella_francesco@yahoo.it

G. Porzio, Ph.D.
Department of Experimental Medicine,
University of L'Aquila, Via Vetoio, Coppito,
L'Aquila 67100, Italy
e-mail: porzio@sctf.it

Incidence and Mortality

It is quite difficult to obtain accurate and exhaustive data regarding different types of CNS tumors. Most part of data is obtained from specialized neurosurgical centers, causing possible bias since they often examine the most easily diagnosed and treatable forms; even data coming from other sources as autopsy statistics are often unclear and show very wide range. For example, data related to the amount of metastatic forms obtained from autopsy of municipal hospitals vary from 20% to 42% of all CNS tumors [3, 4], whereas considering different data, resumed in previous works, should greatly exceed primary tumors [5–8]. More reliable data can be provided from national cancer registry program which resume a large number of population-based data [9].

The overall incidence for primary CNS tumors is about 19.34/100,000 person-years, with higher rates in women than in men (20.67 vs. 17.88/100,000 person-years) [9–11]. Men generally have higher rates of primary malignant CNS tumors, whereas women have higher rates of nonmalignant forms, such as meningiomas (Table 1.1). The overall incidence rate is lower in children (4.84 and 4.69/100,000 person-years for 0–19 and 0–15 years of age, respectively) than adults (25.17/100,000 person-years for age ≥20 years). Many data support differences in the epidemiology of CNS tumors between children and adults. For example, in Sweden, the most common types of tumors in children aged <15 result to be medulloblastoma and low-grade

M. Bologna (ed.), *Biotargets of Cancer in Current Clinical Practice*, Current Clinical Pathology,
DOI 10.1007/978-1-61779-615-9_1, © Springer Science+Business Media, LLC 2012

Table 1.1 Distribution and incidence ratesa of primary CNS tumors by major histology groupings and sex

Histology	Percentage of all reported CNS tumors	Incidence rate[a] (both sexes)	Incidence rate[a] in men	Incidence rate[a] in women
Tumors of neuroepithelial tissue	33.7	6.55	7.72	5.55
Pilocytic astrocytoma	1.6	0.33	0.34	0.32
Protoplasmic and fibrillary astrocytoma	0.5	0.11	0.13	0.09
Anaplastic astrocytoma	2.1	0.41	0.48	0.35
Unique astrocytoma variants	0.5	0.10	0.12	0.07
Astrocytoma, NOS	2.3	0.45	0.51	0.40
Glioblastoma	16.7	3.19	3.99	2.53
Oligodendroglioma	1.4	0.28	0.31	0.24
Anaplastic oligodendroglioma	0.6	0.12	0.14	0.10
Ependymoma/anaplastic ependymoma	1.3	0.26	0.27	0.25
Ependymoma variants	0.5	0.10	0.11	0.08
Mixed glioma	1.0	0.20	0.23	0.16
Glioma malignant, NOS	2.2	0.43	0.47	0.41
Choroid plexus	0.2	0.05	0.05	0.05
Neuroepithelial	0.1	0.02	0.02	0.02
Nonmalignant and malignant neuronal/glial	1.4	0.28	0.30	0.26
Pineal parenchymal	0.2	0.04	0.03	0.04
Embryonal/primitive/medulloblastoma	1.0	0.20	0.23	0.18
Tumors of cranial and spinal nerves	8.6	1.66	1.66	1.66
Nerve sheath, nonmalignant and malignant	8.6	1.66	1.66	1.66
Tumors of meninges	35.5	6.81	4.16	9.07
Meningioma	34.4	6.59	3.91	8.87
Other mesenchymal, nonmalignant and malignant	0.3	0.06	0.06	0.05
Hemangioblastoma	0.8	0.16	0.19	0.14
Lymphomas and hematopoietic neoplasms	2.4	0.46	0.54	0.39
Lymphoma	2.4	0.46	0.54	0.39
Germ cell tumors and cysts	0.5	0.10	0.13	0.06
Germ cell tumors, cysts, and heterotopias	0.5	0.10	0.13	0.06
Tumors of sellar region	13.8	2.70	2.58	2.89
Pituitary	13.1	2.56	2.44	2.75
Craniopharyngioma	0.7	0.14	0.14	0.14
Local extensions from regional tumors	0.1	0.02	0.02	0.02
Chordoma/chondrosarcoma	0.1	0.02	0.02	0.02
Unclassified tumors	5.4	1.05	1.06	1.04
Hemangioma	0.8	0.16	0.14	0.17
Neoplasm, unspecified	4.6	0.88	0.91	0.86
All other	0.1	0.01	0.02	0.01
Total[b]	100.0	19.34	17.88	20.67

Modified from CBTRUS [9]

[a]Rates per 100,000 person-years adjusted to the 2000 US standard population

[b]All brain tumors including histologies not reported in this table

glioma (23.5% and 31.7%, respectively), while in adult patients, high-grade glioma (30.5%) and meningioma (29.4%) are the most common types (data from Swedish Cancer Registry). Similar data are reported also for the population of the USA, as shown in Table 1.2. Valid data on the incidence rate and proportion of different histology characterization can be gathered from the Central Brain Tumor Registry of the USA, which can be considered representative of a wide and

1 Central Nervous System Tumors

Table 1.2 Number of childhood (ages 0–19) brain and CNS tumors by major histology groupings, histology, and age at diagnosis

Histology	0–14 years	0–19 years
Tumors of neuroepithelial tissue	8,525	10,732
Pilocytic astrocytoma	2,034	2,529
Protoplasmic and fibrillary astrocytoma	109	149
Anaplastic astrocytoma	179	256
Unique astrocytoma variants	232	334
Astrocytoma, NOS	531	699
Glioblastoma	292	440
Oligodendroglioma	112	203
Anaplastic oligodendroglioma	23	49
Ependymoma/anaplastic ependymoma	628	776
Ependymoma variants	52	116
Mixed glioma	67	111
Glioma malignant, NOS	1,561	1,746
Choroid plexus	255	284
Neuroepithelial	<16	40
Nonmalignant and malignant neuronal/glial	895	1,268
Pineal parenchymal	99	128
Embryonal/primitive/medulloblastoma	1,429	1,604
Tumors of cranial and spinal nerves	521	802
Nerve sheath, nonmalignant and malignant	521	802
Tumors of meninges	297	574
Meningioma	206	391
Other mesenchymal, nonmalignant and malignant	58	79
Hemangioblastoma	33	104
Lymphomas and hematopoietic neoplasms	34	60
Germ cell tumors and cysts	420	638
Tumors of sellar region	729	1,762
Pituitary	359	1,286
Craniopharyngioma	370	476
Local extensions from regional tumors	<16	16
Unclassified tumors	468	711
Hemangioma	102	172
Neoplasm, unspecified	351	519
Total	11,004	15,295

Modified from CBTRUS [9]

heterogeneous population (Table 1.1). As showed in the table, the most common types of CNS tumors are meningiomas and glioblastomas. Meningiomas account for more than 34%, and it is reported that 98% of these tumors have a nonmalignant behavior. Meningiomas are more common in female than in male population, and their incidence increases with aging, peaking after 65 year. Also the glioblastomas show a remarkable frequency, accounting for 17% of all primary CNS tumors and representing the most common malignancy.

These tumors are more common in men and in older adults, and their incidence rises with age, peaking in the 75–84 years old. It should be remarked that incidence rate of primary CNS lymphoma, representing about 2.4% of all CNS tumors, has raised prominently over the last decades, and some specialized centers report that incidence has more than tripled [12–14]. This increase could be related to immunosuppressed individuals, but it also seems to be present in patients with ostensibly normal immune function.

Table 1.3 One-, five-, and ten-year relative survival rates[a] for selected malignant brain and central nervous system tumors

Histology	1-year (%)	5-year (%)	10-year (%)
Pilocytic astrocytoma	97.79	94.40	92.10
Protoplasmic and fibrillary astrocytoma	74.30	48.10	36.35
Anaplastic astrocytoma	60.32	27.36	21.87
Astrocytoma, NOS	70.01	48.16	39.10
Glioblastoma	34.60	4.75	2.80
Oligodendroglioma	94.17	79.48	63.58
Anaplastic oligodendroglioma	79.91	49.40	34.95
Ependymoma/anaplastic ependymoma	94.00	82.41	76.22
Mixed glioma	87.52	57.32	46.37
Glioma malignant, NOS	60.40	43.27	39.54
Neuroepithelial	54.10	33.02	28.74
Malignant neuronal/glial, neuronal, and mixed	88.48	70.66	58.93
Embryonal/primitive/medulloblastoma	82.42	61.71	55.05
Lymphoma	47.48	28.52	21.61
Total: all brain and CNS[b]	57.21	35.47	31.73

Modified from CBTRUS [9]

[a]Rates are an estimate of the percentage of patients alive at 1-, 5-, and 10-year, respectively

[b]Includes histologies not listed in this table

Worldwide, age-standardized mortality for primary CNS tumors is about 2.5/100,000 person-years, it is higher in men (3.0/100,000) than in women (2.2/100,000) [2]. Like incidence rate, also the estimated mortality is higher in the most developed countries than in the least ones, with a crude mortality rate of 6.1/100,000 vs. 2.1/100,000 respectively; this difference subsists also after standardization even if less wide (2.6 vs. 2.1, respectively) [2]. Data from the USA show a standardized rate for primary malignant CNS tumors of 3.6/100,000 in women and 5.4/100,000 in men [15]. The 5-year and 10-year survival rates in the USA for selected malignant CNS tumors are listed in Table 1.3; these rates differ significantly because of histology. Less than 5% of the patients with glioblastoma survived 5 years postdiagnosis, and only 2.8% of these patients reached 10-year survival, even if it should be remarked that survival estimates are higher for patients diagnosed under age 20 [9]. Differently, the 5-year survival rate for meningioma is about 69% (70% for benign and 55% for malignant) [16]. Furthermore, it seems clear that some histological types present a quite benign outcome. It is the case of pilocytic astrocytoma, characterized by a 10-year survival rate of 92.1%, due to the low grade of replication and to the possibility of complete recovery after radical surgical removal.

Variations in survival rates related to race/ethnicity are reported in different reports [17–21]. Caucasians had a 5-year relative survival rate of 33.5% and African-Americans of 37%. Data from the Surveillance, Epidemiology, and End Results Program (SEER) indicate that African-Americans had a similar or poorer survival than Caucasians [19], but after statistical adjustment, we observe that African-Americans had 13% higher risk of death for primary malignant CNS tumors and 40% higher risk for low-grade tumors [18].

Clinical Presentation

CNS tumors may manifest themselves in a very subtle way. At onset, slowness in comprehension and loss of capacity to sustain mental activity could be the only deviation as regard to normal. Otherwise, in some patients, there is an early beginning of focal cerebral signs. Generally, it is useful for clinicians to subdivide these patients into three principal groups: patients with focal cerebral signs and impairment of cerebral functions, patients with evidence of increased intracranial pressure, and patients with specific intracranial tumor syndromes.

First group patients are difficult to diagnose until the advent of modern neuroimaging procedures. Many different histological types of CNS tumors such as high-grade gliomas, astrocytoma, meningioma, oligodendroglioma, sarcomas of the brain, and CNS lymphoma, but also ependymoma and many others, can occur with this clinical pattern. Most common symptoms are changes in mental function (i.e., irritability, emotional lability, indifference to common social practice, and apathy that conduce to a clinical pattern named "psychomotor asthenia"), headache (representing an early symptom in about one-quarter of patients variable in nature and intensity), vomiting/dizziness (frequent in tumors located in the posterior fossa), and seizures. Seizures are, together with changes in mental functions, the major manifestation of CNS tumors, and they are often reported as the most common initial symptom. Seizures due to CNS tumors have often a focal onset (that can have a localizing meaning) and then become generalized. Finally, all patients with CNS tumors can develop focal cerebral signs, but nearly always those signs are at first slight and subtle, and frequently, neuroimaging will have disclosed the presence of CNS tumor before focal cerebral signs become prominent.

As primary clinical sign or among other symptoms, CNS tumors are able to raise intracranial pressure. Malignancies which most likely present themselves in such way are medulloblastoma, ependymoma of the fourth ventricle, hemangioblastoma of the cerebellum, pinealoma, colloid cyst of third ventricle, and even craniopharyngioma and high spinal cord tumors. The typical symptoms begin with a periodic bifrontal and bioccipital headache that awakes the patients; afterwards, patients can usually present projectile vomiting, unsteady gait, sphincteric incontinence, and mental torpor. Examination of fundus oculi shows papilledema. Most of these symptoms related to increase of intracranial pressure are usually the result of hydrocephalus, and this clinical pattern can evolve to coma.

The third group includes all CNS tumors with special clinical syndromes, related to intracranial localization, useful to localize and diagnose the lesion coming from neurologic findings. CNS tumors producing more often unique clinical syndromes are acoustic neuroma (and tumors of cerebellopontine angle), craniopharyngioma, pituitary adenomas, meningiomas of the sphenoid ridge and olfactory groove, glioma of the optic nerve and chiasm, pontine glioma, chordoma, and a number of other tumors at the base of the skull. The diagnosis will be made on the basis of neurological deficit (i.e., loss of hearing and balance disorders in acoustic neuroma or bilateral vision field defects in glioma of optic nerves and chiasm) or on more complex clinical syndromes (i.e., amenorrhea–galactorrhea syndrome or Cushing disease that can be related to pituitary adenomas); investigation by CT, MRI, and other special studies will confirm the clinical hypothesis.

Biotargets in Central Nervous System Cancer

The development of new molecular analysis techniques targeting specific cancer pathways allowed finding new specific gene or protein useful to predict cancer behavior or drug sensibility.

These biomarkers are useful tools able to characterize cancer aggressiveness and response to the standard radio- or chemotherapy treatment; moreover, these studies lead to the development of new drug able to switch off specific genetic pathway involved in cancerogenesis.

Between all the CNS cancers, glioblastoma multiforme (GBM) is the most studied form, due to its high incidence and mortality; studies involving other CNS cancers are very few, and they are not relevant in this discussion.

Glioblastoma Multiforme

Among the primary brain malignancies, in clinical practice, tumors arising from glial cells are the most frequent, aggressive, and studied [22]. In fact, besides an appropriate surgery, GBM treatment requires a specific chemotherapy and radiotherapy approach; the term "multiforme" illustrates the heterogeneity exhibited by this tumor in every aspect, including clinical presentation, pathology, genetic signature, and response to different therapies [23]. GBM accounts for 12–15% of all brain tumors and 50–60% of astrocytomas; the incidence is less than 10–100,000, with a median overall survival (OS) of 1 year. The incidence is fairly constant worldwide, leading to the logical inference that environmental, geographical, and nutritional factors probably do not play a major role in this cancer, whereas genetics is more likely to tip the scale of etiology. Peak of incidence is included between 45 and 70 years; only 8.8% of children with CNS tumors had GBM, while congenital cases are extremely rare [24]. It is slightly more common in men, with a male-to-female ratio of 1.5:1. Black population incidence is lower than other ethnic groups like whites, latinos, and Asians. GBMs appear to be sporadic, although several genetic disorders are associated with increased incidence, including tuberous sclerosis, neurofibromatosis types 1 and 2, von Hippel–Lindau disease, and Turcot and Li–Fraumeni syndromes [23]. There is a proven association between GBM and exposure to ionizing radiation or polyvinyl chloride (a polymer commonly used in construction), but no links have been found between GBM and smoking, diet, cellular phones, or electromagnetic fields [25].

GBM Pathology

GBMs preferentially have a supratentorially location; more often, they are in the cerebral hemispheres, preferably in the frontal lobes rather than the temporal lobes or basal ganglia (although a combined frontotemporal mass is particularly typical of GBM). Although tumor cells are considered to be already disseminated at time of diagnosis far in the surrounding parenchyma, they are generally a single mass, while true multifocal glioblastoma usually has distinct histo-

logical appearance and is most likely polyclonal, usually presenting as simultaneous infra- and supratentorial masses (incidence 2.5%) [26, 27]. GBMs are typically unilateral or involve the *corpus callosum* crossing the midline ("butterfly" appearance). Grossly, it appears topographically diffuse with a poorly delineated mass with no capsule, with areas of old and recent hemorrhage, necrosis, and cystic areas. Microscopically, characteristic histopathological features include cellular and nuclear polymorphism, nuclear atypia, high mitotic activity, vascular thrombosis, microvascular proliferation, and necrosis, with regions of pseudopalisading. The presence of necrosis is linked with the aggressiveness of the cells, and it is a sine qua non diagnostic criterion to histopathologically "upgrade" an anaplastic astrocytoma to GBM. Another important diagnostic clue is the presence of secondary structures such as *perineuronal and perivascular satellitosis*, resulting from the glioma cells and host brain structures interaction. Histological tumor variants, which do not alter the prognosis of the tumor, include giant cell glioblastoma, gliosarcoma, and gliomatosis cerebri. Extension within and along perivascular spaces is common, but invasion of the vessel lumen seems to occur infrequently, correlating with a very low incidence of hematogenous spread to extraneural tissues. Metastatic spread of GBM occurs in less than 5% of cases, late in the illness course, and it was almost unheard of before the adjuvant therapy.

Treatment

Several factors concur to make GBM treatment notoriously difficult:
- GBM tumor cells, despite their rapid cycle, are quite resistant to conventional therapies.
- Brain has a limited capacity to repair itself, and any damage may be definitive.
- Adequate penetration of the blood–brain barrier (BBB) by chemotherapeutical agents could not be achieved without dose-limiting systemic side effects.

Nowadays, the mainstay of therapy consists of surgery, radiation, and chemotherapy.

Surgery

The extent of an appropriate surgical resection depends on location and tumor size; however, surgery is often an incomplete debulking. The margin considered for a radical resection should not be less than 2 cm. Whether aggressive "radical" surgery prolongs survival, it is still debatable, but several studies suggest a close inverse correlation between survival and the amount of residual tumor observed on postoperative MRI scans [28]. Radical resection maintains several advantages, such as reversal of some neurologic deficits, lowering seizure incidence, or even abolishing them, a definitive pathology diagnosis and the assumption that a "more cytoreductive" surgery may facilitate adjuvant treatment modalities and ultimately improve survival. Arguments against radical resection arise from the inherent invasiveness of GBM, which cannot be totally resected anyway, the potential to facilitating tumor cells migration, and the possibility of surgical complications and new neurological deficits.

Radiotherapy

Radiotherapy (RT) can be started 4–6 weeks after surgery and administered in a standard fractionated regimen over 6–7 weeks [29]. The standard dose of external beam RT is 60 Gy in single daily fractions of 1.7–2 Gy, five times a week, applied to a limited field that includes the enhancing volume on CT scans with a 2–3 cm margin or 2 cm on MR images. Whole brain RT does not improve survival when compared to the more precise and targeted three-dimensional conformal RT.

New variants of RT have been introduced in clinical practice, like *Gamma Knife*, the *Leksell Perfexion*, and the *CyberKnife* or *LINAC*. Stereotactic brachytherapy involves using stereotactic techniques to accurately place radioactive isotopes. Typically, brachytherapy delivers an additional 50–60 Gy of radiation, bringing the total dose of radiation up to 110–120 Gy. This is indicated in patients with unifocal, well-defined, supratentorial tumors less than 5 cm in diameter not involving the corpus callosum, brain stem, or ependymal surfaces, currently as a salvage modality, in recurrent GBM after repeat resection of the tumor. Boron neutron capture therapy (BNCT) is an experimental form of RT where the damage occurs through the interaction between a beam of thermally slowed neutrons with boron 10, which is injected to a patient and preferentially binds to tumor cells. Still investigational and costly, this is a treatment modality with great promise.

The mean survival after optimal surgery and adjuvant RT is about 12.1 months [29]. There are several limitations to RT that make adjuvant chemotherapy a must: the infiltrative nature of GBM, the risk of radiation necrosis and radiation-induced permanent neuronal damage (radiation encephalopathy), as well as intrinsic or acquired radioresistance.

Chemotherapy

Among many chemotherapeutic agents tested to improve GBM overall survival, alkylating agents have demonstrated some benefit; either chloroethylating drugs such as carmustine (BCNU) and lomustine (CCNU) or methylating agents such as temozolomide (TMZ) are used in the majority of GBM clinical protocols.

Chloroethylating agents are able to penetrate into the BBB due to high hydrophobicity, and they can also be administered orally [30]. Forming O6-chloroethylguanine lesions, they lead to G-C interstrand cross-links and trigger apoptosis in a tumor, as well as in a normal cell. However, an aggressive regimen with these agents causes considerable side effects, leading to dose reductions and corresponding decrease in therapeutic efficacy.

Methylating agents such as TMZ show reduced toxicity toward normal cells and are much better tolerated. Oral administration of TMZ, either concomitant with radiotherapy followed by adjuvant TMZ or as adjuvant TMZ alone after completion of radiation, is increasingly becoming standard of care for GBM patients [31]. The use of TMZ has been significantly increased as a result of a phase III trial that showed survival advantage to newly diagnosed GBM patients receiving TMZ with standard radiotherapy [29].

Second-line cytotoxic agents include carboplatin, etoposide, oxaliplatin, and irinotecan. Sometimes, procarbazine and vincristine may be added to CCNU as the PCV regimen, which used to be a first-line approach before the supremacy of TMZ.

GBM Genomics and New Prognostic Factors

The overall survival of GBM is about 1 year on average; this survival pattern has not improved in some time, although radiation and chemotherapy appear to extend the life of the patient. Most common drug handling to treat GBM often has minimal effect, and doctors usually have time to try only one or two treatments before the disease causes severe impairment.

Nowadays, several studies, due to the development of new molecular analysis technique, like microarray technology, show that GBMs have many genetic variations able to influence chemo- and radiosensibility. This chapter will try to describe these genetic alterations, allowing to distinguish which patients are the most likely to benefit from specific drugs or using gene mutations as prognostic and predictive factors.

Loss of Heterozygosity

Loss of heterozygosity (LOH) is the loss of normal function of one allele of a gene in which the other allele was already inactivated. In oncology, LOH occurs when the remaining functional allele in a somatic cell of the offspring becomes inactivated by mutation. This could cause a normal tumor suppressor to no longer be produced which could result in tumorigenesis.

LOH is the most frequent genetic alteration in GBM. A study performed on 220 primary GBMs showed 75% of LOH on 10q, 47% on 9p, 29% on 19q, and 19% on 1p [32]. It should be noted that 10q contains PTEN gene and other potential tumor-suppressor genes, such as MXI1, which suggests that loss of this region may contribute to the development or malignant progression of GBM. A recent study, correlating LOH with survival of patients with GBM, showed that LOH 1p was associated with longer survival (hazard ratio [HR] 0.7; 95% confidence interval [CI], 0.5–1.0), whereas LOH 10q was associated with shorter

survival (HR 1.4; 95% CI, 1.0–1.8) of patients with glioblastoma [33].

In addition, oligodendroglioma with 1p/19q deletions shows particular sensitivity to radiotherapy and chemotherapy; it may have practical importance to identify the subset of GBMs with recognizable oligodendroglial features [34].

EGFR (Epidermal Growth Factor Receptor)

The epidermal growth factor receptor (EGFR) (with a gene located on chromosome 7p12) belongs to the ErbB family of tyrosine kinase receptors; it has been detected in abnormal forms or in enhanced expression in a series of tumors like glioma, breast, colon–rectal, bladder, ovary, and oral cavity cancer. EGFR has three key nuclear functions: gene regulation, kinase function leading to tyrosine phosphorylation of target proteins, and protein–protein interactions leading to DNA repair. As a transcription cofactor with a functional transactivation domain, nuclear EGFR activates expression of a number of genes, including cyclin D1, inducible nitric oxide synthase (iNOS), B-Myb, aurora A, and cyclooxygenase-2 (COX-2). Consistent with the fact that EGFR lacks a DNA-binding domain, nuclear EGFR interacts with DNA-binding transcription factors to activate gene transcription. In this context, nuclear EGFR cooperates with signal transducer and activator of transcription-3 (STAT3) to upregulate expression of iNOS and COX-2 genes, with E2F1 to activate B-Myb gene expression, and with STAT5 to enhance aurora A gene expression. Another mechanism underlying nuclear EGFR-mediated gene regulation could be attributed to its interaction with mucin 1 (MUC1). This interaction may promote the accumulation of chromatin-bound EGFR and significant colocalization of EGFR with phosphorylated RNA polymerase II. In addition to transcriptional regulation, nuclear EGFR retains its tyrosine kinase activity and phosphorylates proliferating cell nuclear antigen (PCNA) to promote cell proliferation and DNA repair. Chromatin-bound PCNA protein is phosphorylated on the Tyr211 amino acid residue by nuclear EGFR, leading to increased PCNA stability. This important finding raised the possibility that additional nuclear proteins may be phosphorylated by nuclear EGFR and their functions, stability, and/or subcellular localization altered as a consequence of tyrosine phosphorylation [35].

Amplification of the EGFR gene occurs in 34–50% of GBM; EGFR overexpression is also more common gene alteration in primary GBM (>60%). All primary GBMs with EGFR amplification show EGFR overexpression, and 70–90% of those with EGFR overexpression have EGFR amplification [32, 36, 37]. EGFR rearrangements or aberrant protein expression is also common in GBM. Five common variants that harbor exon or N- or C-terminal deletion, and a small number of variants consisting of a variety of tandem duplications of exons, as well as missense and insertion mutations, have been identified, of which the variant 3 (EGFRvIII) containing an in-frame deletion of exons 2–7 within the extracellular ligand-binding domain is the most frequent type. The joining of exons 1–8 creates a novel tertiary conformation of the extracellular domain that lacks ligand-binding ability. As a result, EGFRvIII is not activated by its ligand; however, it is constitutively activated, thus leading to constitutive long-term signaling. Aberrant activation of EGFR-mediated signal-transduction pathways has been found in GBM, which may be caused by the genetic alterations and contribute to the induction of glial transformation and progression. For example, in the absence of ligand binding, the constitutively active EGFRvIII causes the activation of downstream lipid kinase PI3K/Akt and MAPK pathways [38, 39] conferring cell proliferation advantages and increasing cell survival by inhibiting apoptosis. An in vitro assay has shown that expression of extracellular matrix components and metalloproteases was enhanced in EGFRvIII-expressing GBM cells, and the authors confirmed that the mutant EGFR did make GBM cells both more motile and invasive [40].

The presence of EGFRvIII, a specific variant of the EGFR lacking exons 2–7, is an independent predictor of poor survival in patients with primary GBM [32]. A different study revealed that EGFRvIII overexpression in the presence of EGFR amplification is the strongest indicator of a poor survival prognosis ($P=0.0044$, HR $=2.71$) [41].

In a phase I clinical trial conducted at the University of California, San Francisco, glioma patients were treated with erlotinib either alone or in combination with TMZ. Eight of these patients responded to erlotinib, and response was independent of TMZ administration. Response to erlotinib was associated with both EGFR overexpression and EGFR amplification. In addition, response to erlotinib was highly dependent on the phosphorylation status of PKB/Akt. Of 22 tumors with high levels of phosphorylated PKB/Akt, none responded to erlotinib, whereas 8 of 18 tumors with low levels of phosphorylated PKB/Akt responded. In addition to radiographic response, time to progression (TTP) highly correlated with phospho-PKB/Akt levels [42].

PTEN (Phosphatase and Tensin Homolog)

The tumor-suppressor gene PTEN function (located at 10q23.3) is frequently lost in GBM due to LOH or mutations (15–40%) [43]. The PTEN protein is a phosphatase, and one of its primary cellular targets is the phosphatidylinositol-3,4,5-trisphosphate, a plasma membrane lipid that is produced during cellular signaling events by the action of PI3K. PTEN removes the phosphate group on the D3 position of the inositol, the same position where PI3K deposits a phosphate group after it is activated. Thus, PTEN serves as a negative regulator of the PI3K pathway, and loss of PTEN function results in constitutive activation of the PI3K pathway.

PTEN loss has been correlated with higher activated Akt levels in glioma cells. The protein phosphatase activity of PTEN is involved in cell migration, a malignant phenotypic change that contributes to the morbidity and mortality of the advanced glioma. A very recent study suggests that PTEN regulates glioma cell migration through its control of FYN and RAC GTPase downstream of $\alpha v \beta 3$ integrin engagement in a PI3K/Akt-independent manner [44]. While PTEN has been assigned a tumor-suppressor function, a recent study showed that it has tumor-promoting properties in the setting of gain-of-function p53 mutations [45]. PTEN restoration to GBM cells harboring gain-of-function p53 mutations leads to induction of cell proliferation and inhibition of cell death, possibly via inhibition of mut-p53 degradation by murine double minute (MDM2) and direct stabilization of mut-p53 protein. Conversely, inhibition of endogenous PTEN in glioma cells expressing mut p53 leads to inhibition of cell proliferation and inhibition of in vivo tumor growth.

Nowadays, some studies show that PTEN mutation remained a powerful prognostic factor correlated to glioma survival [46, 47].

p53/MDM2/p14^{ARF}

The p53 tumor-suppressor gene is active in response to diverse stresses, including DNA damage, overexpressed oncogenes, and various metabolic limitations, and can induce either cell cycle arrest or apoptosis. After stress, the activity of p53 is blocked by its crucial negative regulator, MDM2, via ubiquitin-dependent degradation, while reaccumulation and activation of p53 is achieved through the inactivation of MDM2 by the binding of p14^{ARF}. This switch system for the p53 signaling pathway is disrupted in many tumors, including GBM, due to p53 mutation, MDM2 amplification, or overexpression or loss of expression of p14^{ARF}, thus, blocking p53 activity and leading to uncontrolled cell proliferation and tumor formation.

The p53 mutations occur in two-thirds of secondary GBM, while a lower frequency of p53 mutations (<30%) is seen in primary GBM [36]. Amplification and overexpression of MDM2 occurs in 6–12% of GBM. GBM also has frequent p14^{ARF} deletion or methylation (36–58%) and loss of p14^{ARF} expression (76%) [32, 48].

There is growing evidence that GBMs may be generated and maintained by a small subset of cancer stem cells, and these stem cells display some features of normal neural stem cells, such as the potential for self-renewal. Meletis et al. showed that p53 is expressed in the neural stem cell lineage in the adult brain, and knockdown of p53 led to increased self-renewal of neural stem cells by increasing cell proliferation and decreasing apoptotic cell death, implicating p53 as a suppressor of tissue and cancer stem cell self-renewal. Further evidence for the role of p53 in stem cell differentiation was provided by Lin et al. who demonstrated that p53 induced differentiation of mouse embryonic stem cells by downregulation of a gene involved in self-renewal [49, 50].

Many studies show a p53 role as prognostic factor; in fact, Li et al. showed that low expression of p53 is a significant independent favorable prognostic factor for progression-free survival (PFS) ($P=0.017$) [51]. In addition, primary GBM tumors showing simultaneous EGFR and p53 alterations were significantly associated with shorter survival ($P<0.01$) [52].

Epigenetic Changes

A better understanding of the epigenetic changes that occur within GBM has added to the available chemotherapeutic agents employed in the treatment of the disease. TMZ, an oral alkylating agent, has demonstrated a benefit in the treatment of a subset of GBM patients.

The mechanism of action of TMZ involves the alkylation of the O-6 position of guanine within DNA strands producing interstrand cytotoxic cross-links, leading to apoptosis. The adducts created by TMZ are reversible through the action of the DNA repair enzyme, O-6-methylguanine DNA methyltransferase (MGMT). The presence of MGMT leads to a decrease in the effectiveness of TMZ. Conversely, a decrease in the expression of MGMT is beneficial for the action of TMZ. A decrease in MGMT expression occurs through hypermethylation of CpG islands in the promoter region of the MGMT gene, leading to silencing of transcription and a decrease in the amount of gene product. In one study, methylation of the MGMT promoter region was present within 47.7%.

Several clinical trials have demonstrated the benefit of TMZ in patients with GBM. The largest study, a multi-institutional randomized trial encompassing 573 patients, demonstrated an improved median survival of 14.6 months when TMZ was added to the treatment regimen, compared with a median survival of 12.1 months without the medication. A separate subset analysis of this trial examined the survival of those in whom the methylation status of the MGMT promoter could be determined; those patients with a methylated MGMT promoter had a significantly

1 Central Nervous System Tumors

better median survival when they received TMZ compared with those that did not (21.7 vs. 15.3 months) [53].

New Targeted Therapies

Nowadays, conventional protocols in GBM treatment include maximally safe surgical resection followed by fractioned RT and systemic chemotherapy with alkylating compounds. The efficacy of alkylating drugs, however, such as nitrosoureas or TMZ, is fairly limited due to the existence of alternative pathways like epigenetic inactivation of the DNA repair enzyme methylguanine methyltransferase, the DNA mismatch repair, and the base excision repair pathways able to confer a chemoresistance to alkylating agents.

Altered expression or specific mutation of receptors and intracellular downstream effectors has been observed in malignant glioma (MG). These pathways are regulated by several growth factors linked to tyrosine kinase, such as the EGFR, insulin-like growth factor receptor (IGFR), platelet-derived growth factor receptor (PDGFR), and vascular endothelial growth factor receptor (VEGFR). Specific targeting of these signaling pathways that lead to uncontrolled cellular proliferation and cell migration and invasion could provide new molecularly targeted treatment options for MG.

EGFRs

Treatment options that target EGFRs include *gefitinib* (ZD-1839) and *erlotinib* (OSI-774). However, efficacy of these agents is modest in CNS tumors.

Gefitinib was evaluated in an open-label phase II clinical trial in patients with first recurrence of a GBM. Each patient initially received 500 mg/die of gefitinib, and the dose was escalated up to 1,000 mg in patients receiving enzyme-inducing antiepileptic drugs or dexamethasone. Quantification of gefitinib efficacy was assessed by 6-month progression-free survival (PFS-6) and brain magnetic resonance imaging (MRI) quantification of tumor response. The study population had a PFS-6 of 13% and a median OS time from treatment initiation of 39.4 weeks, but no radiographic response was observed [54].

In a multicenter, open-label, and single-arm phase II clinical trial of gefitinib in patients with recurrent MG after surgery plus radiotherapy and first-line chemotherapy, overall median TTP was 8.4 weeks, PFS-6 was 14.3%, and median OS was 24.6 weeks. None of the patients presented objective radiographic response [55], and it was concluded that gefitinib demonstrated limited efficacy against GBM, in comparison with the standard Stupp regimen [29].

In several phase I/II clinical trials, OS rates for erlotinib and gefitinib treatment were similar, but erlotinib was more effective than gefitinib treatment in terms of objective radiographic responses. A multicenter, open-label phase I clinical trial evaluated the efficacy of erlotinib plus RT in patients with GBM. With a median follow-up of 52 weeks, progression was assessed in 16 patients, and 13 deaths occurred. Median TTP was 26 weeks, and median OS was 55 weeks [56]. Additionally, in an open-label phase I dose escalation clinical trial, patients with stable or progressive malignant primary gliomas received erlotinib alone or combined with TMZ [57]. Of the patients assessed, eight patients demonstrated a PR, and six patients demonstrated a median PFS of greater than 6 months, which included four patients with a PR [57]. Erlotinib treatment was equally as effective as the standard Stupp regimen [29].

The favorable tolerability profile and evidence of antitumor activity suggest that additional evaluation of erlotinib treatment is warranted. However, it should also be noted that responders to drugs targeting EGFR usually have intact PTEN and EGFRvIII and no phospho-Akt [58, 59].

Cetuximab treatment alone or in combination with RT or chemotherapy was assessed in vivo. Treated mice with cetuximab significantly increased median OS compared with the control (65 days vs. 24 days) [60].

PDGFR

The PDGFR regulates angiogenesis and is overexpressed in approximately 75% of MGs. Administration of imatinib (STI-571), a PDGFR inhibitor, either as monotherapy or in combination (hydroxyurea or radiotherapy), has been associated with modest activity in CNS tumors.

An open-label phase II trial of imatinib monotherapy (400 mg, once a day) in patients with anaplastic glioma or GBM demonstrated minimal efficacy. Radiographic response was <6% for both types of brain tumors; in patients with GBM, two patients (6%) demonstrated partial responses (PR) and six patients (18%) demonstrated stable disease (SD), but there were no complete responses (CR). Among the patients with anaplastic glioma, there were no CR or PR, and five patients had SD response. The PFS-6 was 10% in patients with anaplastic glioma, and PFS-6 was just 3% in patients with GBM [61].

In an open-label, single-arm phase II clinical trial, patients with recurrent GBM received imatinib mesylate (500 mg, twice a day) plus orally hydroxyurea on a continuous daily schedule. At a median follow-up of 58 weeks, 27% of patients were progression free at 6 months, with a median PFS of 14.4 weeks. Radiographic responses were observed in three patients (9%), 14 (42%) achieved stable disease, and the median OS rates were 48.9 weeks [62]. In all cases, the responses observed in these clinical trials in patients with recurrent GBM were inferior to those observed with the standard Stupp regimen (PFS-6, 53.9%; median, PFS 6.9 months; overall response rate 38.7%, including 7 [11.3%] CR and 17 [27.4%] PR) [29, 63].

VEGFR

GBMs, depending to an adequate blood supply, are highly vascularized. New blood vessels formation is coordinated by the complex interaction of many angiogenic factors, including vascular endothelial growth factor (VEGF), basic fibroblast growth factor (bFGF), and PDGF. Therefore, targeting factors and pathways implicated in angiogenesis may represent potential approaches to the treatment of this disease. Because VEGF represents a major stimulatory factor for the initiation of angiogenesis, the inhibition of VEGFRs is a promising treatment for malignant gliomas.

A phase II clinical trial in patients with recurrent GBM used a series of MRI protocols to assess the efficacy of *cediranib* (AZD-2171; AstraZeneca), a rapid-onset, reversible, and orally administered VEGFR tyrosine kinase inhibitor. Permeability was measured by using dynamic contrast-enhanced MRI techniques, and in addition, correlations between temporal changes in these parameters and molecular markers in blood (angiogenic cytokines) and cellular biomarkers of vascular response were assessed. Cediranib treatment normalized tumor blood vessels in patients with recurrent GBM and alleviated edema. Moreover, relative tumor vessel size significantly decreased as early as 1 day after the onset of AZD-2171 treatment ($P<0.05$) and remained decreased at day 28. At day 56, the relative vessel size reversed (day 56 vs. day 28; $P<0.05$) toward abnormal values [64].

An open-label phase II trial in patients ($n=23$) with MG assessed the efficacy of bevacizumab (10 mg/kg every 21 days), a humanized mAb antibody against VEGF, and irinotecan (CPT-11). A response rate of 63%, a median PFS time of 23 weeks, and a PFS-6 of 38% were observed [65].

The synergistic beneficial effect was confirmed by the same researchers in a second phase II clinical trial in patients with recurrent GBM. Two cohorts of patients were included. The initial cohort of patients received bevacizumab (10 mg/kg) plus irinotecan every 2 weeks. After this regimen was deemed safe and effective, the irinotecan schedule was changed to a regimen of four doses in 6 weeks. The second cohort of patients ($n=12$) received bevacizumab (15 mg/kg) every 21 days and irinotecan on days 1, 8, 22, and 29. Each cycle was 6-week long. Patients in the second cohort ($n=35$) demonstrated a PFS-6 of 46% and a 6-month OS of 77%, and PR were observed in 57% of patients [66].

Overall, regimens consisting of bevacizumab plus irinotecan demonstrated similar survival and progression rates compared with the standard Stupp regimen [29]. Of note, however, is that trials assessing the efficacy of bevacizumab plus irinotecan enrolled a relatively small number of patients and therefore were not powered adequately to provide more significant results.

Vatalanib (PTK-787; ZK-222584; Novartis AG, Basel, Switzerland), an oral controlled-release

PDGF/VEGF-receptor tyrosine kinase angiogenesis inhibitor, was assessed in preclinical models for efficacy against VEGF-dependent glioma vascularization and growth. Vatalanib significantly limited VEGF-mediated glioma growth, thereby providing a promising new treatment option for MGs. Vatalanib was evaluated in patients with recurrent MG in a open-label, nonrandomized phase I/II clinical trial as a monotherapy [67] as well as in a similarly designed phase I/II clinical trial with temozolomide or lomustine [68]. Preliminary results showed that vatalanib monotherapy (1,200 or 1,500 mg/day) led to 2 patients (4%) with PR, 31 patients (56%) with SD, and 14 patients (25%) with disease progression, compared with the standard Stupp regimen (overall response rate of 38.7%, including 11.3% CR and 27.4% PR) [29]. However, final results from these trials are awaited to potentially support the significance of using vatalanib because disappointing efficacy data were obtained in other clinical trials in patients with primary and recurrent MG.

Mammalian Target of Rapamycin

Signaling mammalian target of rapamycin (mTOR) is a critical downstream kinase in the PI3K/Akt/mTOR pathway. Combination therapy of AEE-788 (Novartis AG), an EGFR/VEGFR-2 inhibitor, and everolimus (RAD-001), an inhibitor of mTOR, inhibited the tumor growth of GBM during in vitro study. The combination of AEE-788 and RAD-001 increased rates of cell cycle arrest and apoptosis and reduced proliferation more than either agent alone. In a single-arm, open-label phase II clinical trial in patients with GBM, temsirolimus (CCI-779; 250 mg weekly) demonstrated modest efficacy, with 20 patients (36%) showing radiographic improvement, the PFS-6 was 7.8%, and the median OS was 4.4 months [69]. Similarly, in another open-label, nonrandomized phase II clinical trial to determine the efficacy of temsirolimus in patients with recurrent GBM, one patient remained progression free at 6 months, and of the patients assessable for response, two PR were observed, and 20 patients had SD. In addition, the median time to progression was 9 weeks [70]; therefore, compared with the standard Stupp regimen (PFS-6 = 53.9, median OS = 58 weeks, median PFS = 6.9 months; overall response rate = 38.7%), there was no evidence of an improved response to temsirolimus treatment in patients with recurrent GBM. Overall, temsirolimus treatment appears to be less effective than the standard Stupp regimen.

RAS

MGs often show increased RAS activity because of mutation or amplification of upstream growth factor receptors. Farnesyltransferases are part of the RAS signal-transduction pathway, and farnesyltransferase inhibitors, including *tipifarnib* (R-115777; Johnson & Johnson Pharmaceutical Research and Development, Brunswick, NJ, USA) and *lonafarnib* (Sch-66336), have been assessed and shown to have modest survival benefits in phase I and II clinical trials in patients with recurrent MGs. In an open-label, nonrandomized, phase II clinical trial to determine the efficacy and safety of tipifarnib in patients ($n = 67$) with recurrent GBM, eight patients (11.9%) had a PFS of >6 months [71]. In addition, a PFS-6 of 33% was observed in a nonrandomized phase I clinical trial of temozolomide and lonafarnib in patients with recurrent GBM [72]. However, PFS rates following administration of tipifarnib or TMZ plus lonafarnib were inferior to those observed after administration of the standard Stupp regimen [29].

Protein Kinase C

Enzastaurin (LY-317615; Eli Lilly, Indianapolis, IN, USA), a selective inhibitor of activated protein kinase C (PKC)β, suppressed tumor cell proliferation. In addition, enzastaurin treatment suppressed the phosphorylation of glycogen synthase kinase 3β (GSK3β), a serine/threonine PK, in GBM xenograft tumor tissues. Enzastaurin also limited the growth of human GBM xenografts. These effects are supported by data from a preclinical study that investigated the effects of enzastaurin and radiotherapy in vitro and in vivo compared with either treatment alone. This study demonstrated that combining cerebral irradiation with enzastaurin decreased the following parameters: tumor volume, irradiation-induced tumor satellite formation, upregulation of VEGF expression in vitro and in vivo, and enhanced microvessel density in vivo [73]. However, in an open-label, multicenter phase III clinical trial that compared enzastaurin with lomustine treatment in patients ($n=266$) with recurrent GBM, treatment effects were modest. Median PFS, OS, and PFS-6 rates were not significantly different between treatment arms, and therefore, enzastaurin was not superior to lomustine in patients with recurrent GBM [74].

Ligand–Toxin Conjugates

The Her1/EGFR-expressing tumors can be targeted by radioisotopes or toxic compounds conjugated to Her1/EGFR-specific antibodies or ligands, including 125iodine (I)-MAb 425, TP-38, and DAB389-EGF. Regional administration of radiolabeled mAbs targeting tumor-specific antigens expressed by MG has demonstrated encouraging antitumor activity and acceptable toxicity in clinical trials. The 125I-MAb 425 binds to the external domain of human EGFRs, is internalized upon binding target, and downregulates EGFR expression without stimulating receptor tyrosine kinase activity.

In an open-label, nonrandomized phase I/II clinical trial, adjuvant administration of 125I-MAb 425 in MG patients significantly increased median survival compared with controls receiving radiotherapy alone. The OS range for GBM and AA patients was 4–150 months and 4–270 months, respectively [75].

A similar study investigated the benefits of teleradiotherapy and 125I-MAb 425 radioimmunotherapy administered after neurosurgery in high-grade gliomas compared with teleradiotherapy alone. A median OS of 14 months for both treatment groups was observed, with no improvement in disease-free survival or OS in either treatment group after neurosurgery. Therefore, radiotherapy and radioimmunotherapy with anti-EGFR 125I-MAb 425 was not beneficial compared with radiotherapy alone for the adjuvant treatment of high-grade gliomas following neurosurgery [76]. Therefore, compared with the standard Stupp regimen (OS range for GBM was 13.2–16.8 months) [29], 125I-MAb 425 greatly increased the OS range.

In addition, mAb-806 (Life Science Pharmaceuticals) and 3C10 mAb are mAbs directed against EGFRvIII with conjugated toxins or radioisotopes and may represent other targeted treatment options for MG. The administration of the mAb against tenascin-C, an extracellular matrix glycoprotein ubiquitously expressed by malignant gliomas, has also been evaluated in clinical trials. In a nonrandomized, phase II, dose–response clinical trial in patients with primary MG, 131I-81C6 (Bradmer Pharmaceuticals, Toronto, Canada), a radiolabeled mAb targeting tenascin (an extracellular matrix protein present in MG, but not in normal brain tissue), was injected directly into surgically created cavities followed by conventional external beam radiotherapy and chemotherapy. This treatment strategy demonstrated a median survival of 86 weeks for patients with anaplastic astrocytomas. In patients with GBM, a median OS of 79 weeks was observed. Therefore, 131I-81C6 increased the median survival of GBM patients compared with the standard Stubb regimen [77].

Furthermore, histopathological analyses were conducted in patients treated with combined external beam radiotherapy and a brachytherapy consisting of 131I-81C6 injected into surgically created cavities during brain tumor resections. Histological tissue classification outcomes included "proliferative glioma," "quiescent glioma," and "negative for neoplasm." Median survival with tissue classified as proliferative glioma, quiescent glioma, and negative for neoplasm was 3.5, 15, and 27.5 months, respectively. Median survival in patients receiving a total radiation dose greater than 86 Gy was 19 months, compared with 7 months for those receiving less than 86 Gy, thus suggesting that the total dose of radiotherapy was a significant predictor of survival ($P<0.002$) [78].

Therefore, additional clinical trials are warranted to determine the effectiveness of 131I-81C6 for the treatment of MG. TP-38 is a recombinant chimeric protein composed of transforming growth factor α combined with a mutated form of Pseudomonas exotoxin. Binding specificity of TP-38 for cells in the brain was demonstrated by the ability of nonradiolabeled TP-38 to block the binding of 125I-EGF to EGFR-expressing non-small-cell lung cancer cell lines. TP-38 has also demonstrated toxicity to human glioma cell lines [79]. However, in a pilot phase I clinical trial, TP-38 was associated with an inferior clinical response, compared with the Stupp regimen. Efficacy results of this pilot study [80] showed that after TP-38 administration, the median OS of patients with recurrent malignant brain tumors was 23 weeks. Median OS for patients with residual disease at the time of TP-38 therapy was 18.7 weeks, whereas for those without radiographic evidence of residual disease, median survival was 32.9 weeks. Overall, 14% of patients show residual disease at the time of therapy-induced and radiographically confirmed responses. One patient (7%) had CR, and another (7%) had a PR with >50% tumor shrinkage 34 weeks after TP-38 therapy [80]. However, interpretation of data from trials, such as those described above, is challenging because of methodological problems, mainly consisting of the small sample sizes enrolled and the open-label study design.

Integrins
Integrins are cell surface receptors that play important roles in tumor invasion. *Cilengitide* (a synthetic molecule able to interfere with integrin function essential in angiogenesis) has demonstrated some efficacy against MG in both a preclinical study and in a nonrandomized phase I clinical trial. Cilengitide at dose 2,400 mg/m^2 was used for treating 51 patients with MG, including 37 with GBM [81]. Among the evaluable patients, 4% showed a CR, 6% a PR, and 8% a SD. Considering these preliminary results, cilengitide appears to be a promising new agent against MG, and therefore, the final results of this study are awaited before definite conclusions can be drawn.

Histone Deacetylase Inhibitors
Epigenetic changes to the genome, through DNA methylation and covalent modification of the histones that form the nucleosome, are key to maintenance of the differentiated state of the cell. Thus, inhibition of deacetylation, which is controlled by histone deacetylases, may lead to chromatin remodeling, upregulation of key tumor repressor genes, differentiation, or apoptosis. Histone deacetylase inhibitors, by altering functional epigenetic modifications, are additional potential anticancer agents for the treatment of MGs. Structurally diverse histone deacetylase inhibitors, including *vorinostat* and *romidepsin* (FK-228; Gloucester Pharmaceuticals, Cambridge, MA, USA), have demonstrated their ability to inhibit proliferation and induce differentiation and/or apoptosis of tumor cells in culture and in animal models, suggesting that treatment with vorinostat may enhance radiation-induced cytotoxicity in MG [82].

Conclusion

Among CNS tumors, GBM is one of the most aggressive. Conventional protocols in GBM treatment include surgical resection followed by RT and systemic chemotherapy with alkylating compounds. The overall survival of GBM is about 1 year on average, and the drug efficacy is fairly limited due to the existence of alternative genetic or epigenetic pathways able to confer a strong chemoresistance. Nowadays, several studies show that GBM cases have many genetic variations (LOH, EGFR, PTEN, p53, or MGMT) able to predict cancer behavior; despite encouraging data obtained from these studies, it is difficult to introduce in clinical practice the genetic mutation as prognostic or predictive factor in lack of large phase 3 study including genetic validation and uniformity in molecular analysis technique.

Furthermore, in the last years, genetic studies led to the development of new drugs able to target and switch off specific genetic pathways involved in cancerogenesis. Nevertheless, these new drugs often failed to demonstrate a significant survival benefit; therefore, more effective therapies may be those that target multiple signaling pathways simultaneously by multitargeted kinase inhibitors or combinations of kinase inhibitors that target single kinases. Additional clinical trials are required to elucidate whether multitargeting strategies will improve survival rates in patients with MG. Important areas for additional research may include the assessment of serum or tissue biomarkers; moreover, biological endpoints should be included in the design of clinical trials aiming at the objective evaluation of standard or novel targeted therapies against MG.

References

1. World Health Organization. The global burden of disease: 2004 update. World Health Organization, Geneva. 2008. http://www.who.int/evidence/bod. Accessed April 2011.
2. Ferlay J, Shin HR, Bray F, Forman D, Mathers C, Parkin DM. GLOBOCAN 2008, Cancer incidence and mortality worldwide: IARC CancerBase No. 10 [Internet]. Lyon, France: International Agency for Research on Cancer; 2010. http://globocan.iarc.fr. Accessed April 2011.
3. Rubinstein LJ. Tumors of the central nervous system, Atlas of tumor pathology, 2nd series, Fasc 6. Washington, DC: Armed Forces Institute of Pathology; 1972.
4. Russell DS. Cellular changes and patterns of neoplasia. In: Haymaker W, Adams RD, editors. Histology and histopathology of the nervous system. Springfield, IL: Charles C Thomas; 1982. p. 1493–515.
5. Posner JB. Neurologic complications of cancer. F.A. Davis: Philadelphia; 1995.
6. Olivecrona H. The surgical treatment of intracranial tumors, Handbuch der Neurochirurgie, vol. IV. Berlin: Springer; 1967. p. 1–300.
7. Zimmerman HM. Brain tumors: their incidence and classification in man and their experimental production. Ann N Y Acad Sci. 1969;159:337.
8. Zulch KJ. Brain tumors, their biology and pathology. 3rd ed. New York: Springer; 1986.
9. CBTRUS. CBTRUS statistical report: primary brain and central nervous system tumors diagnosed in the United States in 2004–2007. Hinsdale, IL: Central Brain Tumor Registry of the United States; 2011. www.cbtrus.org.
10. Central Brain Tumor Registry of the United States (CBTRUS). Statistical report: primary brain tumors in the United States, 2000–2004. Hinsdale, IL: Central Brain Tumor Registry of the United States; 2008.
11. Bondy ML, Scheurer ME, Malmer B, Barnholtz-Sloan JS, Davis FG, Il'yasova D, Kruchko C, McCarthy BJ, Rajaraman P, Schwartzbaum JA, Sadetzki S, Schlehofer B, Tihan T, Wiemels JL, Wrensch M, Buffler PA, Brain Tumor Epidemiology Consortium. Brain tumor epidemiology: consensus from the Brain Tumor Epidemiology Consortium. Cancer. 2008;113(7 Suppl):1953–68.
12. Posner JB. Primary lymphoma of the CNS. Neurol Alert. 1987;5:21.
13. De Angelis LM. Primary central nervous system lymphoma: a new clinical challenge. Neurology. 1991; 41:619.
14. De Angelis LM. Current management of primary central nervous system lymphoma. Oncology. 1995;9:63.
15. Copeland G, Lake A, Firth R, Bayakly R, Wu XC, Stroup A, Russell C, Boyuk K, Niu X, Schymura MJ, Hofferkamp J, Kohler B. Cancer incidence in North America, 2003–2007, Vol 3, Section IV; 2010. p. 2.
16. McCarthy BJ, Davis FG, Freels S, Surawicz TS, Damek DM, Grutsch J, Menck HR, Laws Jr ER. Factors associated with survival in patients with meningioma. J Neurosurg. 1998;88:831–9.
17. Ries LAG, Eisner MP, Kosary CL, et al. SEER cancer statistics review, 1975–2002. Bethesda, MD: National Cancer Institute; 2005.
18. Claus EB, Black PM. Survival rates and patterns of care for patients diagnosed with supratentorial low-grade gliomas: data from the SEER Program, 1973–2001. Cancer. 2006;106:1358–63.
19. Barnholtz-Sloan JS, Sloan AE, Schwartz AG. Relative survival rates and patterns of diagnosis analyzed by time period for individuals with primary malignant brain tumor, 1973–1997. J Neurosurg. 2003;99:458–66.
20. Barnholtz-Sloan JS, Sloan AE, Schwartz AG. Racial differences in survival after diagnosis with primary malignant brain tumor. Cancer. 2003;98:603–9.
21. Robertson JT, Gunter BC, Somes GW. Racial differences in the incidence of gliomas: a retrospective study from Memphis, Tennessee. Br J Neurosurg. 2002;16:562–6.
22. Kitange GJ, Templeton KL, Jenkins RB. Recent advances in the molecular genetics of primary gliomas. Curr Opin Oncol. 2003;15(3):197–203.
23. Iacob G, Dinca EB. Current data and strategy in glioblastoma multiforme. J Med Life. 2009; 2(4): 386–93.
24. Dohrmann D, Farwell RJ, Flannery JT. Glioblastoma multiforme in children. J Neurosurg. 1976;44(4): 442–8.
25. Inskip PD, Hatch EE. Cellular-telephone use and brain tumors. N Engl J Med. 2001;344:79–86.
26. Batzdorf U, Malamud N. The problem of multicentric gliomas. J Neurosurg. 1963;20:122–36.
27. Russell SJ, Rubinstein LJ. Pathology of tumors of the nervous system. 4th ed. Baltimore: Williams and Wilkins; 1977. p. 240–1.
28. Lacroix M. A multivariate analysis of 416 patients with glioblastoma multiforme: prognosis, extent of resection and survival. J Neurosurg. 2001;95:190–8.
29. Stupp R, et al. Radiotherapy plus concomitant and adjuvant temozolomide for glioblastoma. N Engl J Med. 2005;352(10):987–96.
30. Ostermann S, et al. Plasma and cerebrospinal fluid population pharmacokinetics of temozolomide in malignant glioma patients. Clin Cancer Res. 2004;10(11):3728–36.
31. Lonardi S, Tosoni A. Adjuvant chemotherapy in the treatment of high grade gliomas. Cancer Treat Rev. 2005;31(2):79–89.
32. Houillier C, Lejeune J, Benouaich-Amiel A, et al. Prognostic impact of molecular markers in a series of 220 primary glioblastomas. Cancer. 2006;106(10): 2218–23.

33. Homma T, Fukushima T, Vaccarella S, et al. Correlation among pathology, genotype, and patient outcomes in glioblastoma. J Neuropathol Exp Neurol. 2006;65(9):846–54.
34. Stupp R, Hegi ME, van den Bent MJ, et al. Changing paradigms—an update on the multidisciplinary management of malignant glioma. Oncologist. 2006;11(2):165–80.
35. Lo HW, et al. Nuclear mode of the EGFR signaling network: biology, prognostic value, and therapeutic implications. Discov Med. 2010;10(50):44–51.
36. Ohgaki H, Kleihues P. Genetic pathways to primary and secondary glioblastoma. Am J Pathol. 2007; 170(5):1445–53.
37. Ruano Y, Mollejo M, Ribalta T, et al. Identification of novel candidate target genes in amplicons of glioblastoma multiforme tumors detected by expression and CGH microarray profiling. Mol Cancer. 2006;5:39.
38. Li B, Yuan M, Kim IA, Chang CM, Bernhard EJ, Shu HK. Mutant epidermal growth factor receptor displays increased signaling through the phosphatidylinositol-3 kinase/AKT pathway and promotes radioresistance in cells of astrocytic origin. Oncogene. 2004;23(26):4594–602.
39. Narita Y, Nagane M, Mishima K, Huang HJ, Furnari FB, Cavenee WK. Mutant epidermal growth factor receptor signaling down-regulates p27 through activation of the phosphatidylinositol 3 kinase/Akt pathway in glioblastomas. Cancer Res. 2002;62(22): 6764–9.
40. Lal A, Glazer CA, Martinson HM, et al. Mutant epidermal growth factor receptor up-regulates molecular effectors of tumor invasion. Cancer Res. 2002;62(12):3335–9.
41. Shinojima N, Tada K, Shiraishi S, Kamiryo T, Kochi M, Nakamura H, Makino K, Saya H, Hirano H, Kuratsu J, Oka K, Ishimaru Y, Ushio Y. Prognostic value of epidermal growth factor receptor in patients with glioblastoma multiforme. Cancer Res. 2003; 63(20):6962–70.
42. Haas-Kogan DA, Prados MD, Lamborn KR, Tihan T, Berger MS, Stokoe D. Biomarkers to predict response to epidermal growth factor receptor inhibitors. Cell Cycle. 2005;4(10):1369–72.
43. Knobbe CB, Merlo A, Reifenberger G. Pten signaling in gliomas. Neuro Oncol. 2002;4(3):196–211.
44. Dey N, Crosswell HE, De P, et al. The protein phosphatase activity of PTEN regulates SRC family kinases and controls glioma migration. Cancer Res. 2008;68(6):1862–71.
45. Li Y, Guessous F, Kwon S, et al. PTEN has tumor-promoting properties in the setting of gain-of function p53 mutations. Cancer Res. 2008;68(6):1723–31.
46. Smith JS, Tachibana I, Passe SM, Huntley BK, Borell TJ, Iturria N, O'Fallon JR, Schaefer PL, Scheithauer BW, James CD, Buckner JC, Jenkins RB. PTEN mutation, EGFR amplification, and outcome in patients with anaplastic astrocytoma and glioblastoma multiforme. J Natl Cancer Inst. 2001;93(16): 1246–56.
47. Ang C, Guiot MC, Ramanakumar AV, Roberge D, Kavan P. Clinical significance of molecular biomarkers in glioblastoma. Can J Neurol Sci. 2010;37(5): 625–30.
48. Nakamura M, Watanabe T, Klangby U, et al. p14[ARF] deletion and methylation in genetic pathways to glioblastomas. Brain Pathol. 2001;11(2):159–68.
49. Meletis K, Wirta V, Hede SM, et al. p53 suppresses the self-renewal of adult neural stem cells. Development. 2006;133(2):363–9.
50. Lin T, Chao C, Saito S, et al. p53 induces differentiation of mouse embryonic stem cells by suppressing Nanog expression. Nat Cell Biol. 2005;7(2):165–71.
51. Li S, Zhang W, Chen B, Jiang T, Wang Z. Prognostic and predictive value of p53 in low MGMT expressing glioblastoma treated with surgery, radiation and adjuvant temozolomide chemotherapy. Neurol Res. 2010;32(7):690–4.
52. Ruano Y, Ribalta T, de Lope AR, Campos-Martín Y, Fiaño C, Pérez-Magán E, Hernández-Moneo JL, Mollejo M, Meléndez B. Worse outcome in primary glioblastoma multiforme with concurrent epidermal growth factor receptor and p53 alteration. Am J Clin Pathol. 2009;131(2):257–63.
53. Hegi ME, Diserens AC, Gorlia T, et al. MGMT gene silencing and benefit from temozolomide in glioblastoma. N Engl J Med. 2005;352(10):997–1003.
54. Rich JN, et al. Phase II trial of gefitinib in recurrent glioblastoma. J Clin Oncol. 2004;22:133–42.
55. Franceschi E, et al. Gefitinib in patients with progressive high-grade gliomas: a multicentre phase II study by Gruppo Italiano Cooperativo di Neuro-Oncologia (GICNO). Br J Cancer. 2007;96:1047–51.
56. Krishnan S, et al. Phase I trial of erlotinib with radiation therapy in patients with glioblastoma multiforme: results of North Central Cancer Treatment Group protocol N0177. Int J Radiat Oncol Biol Phys. 2006;65: 1192–9.
57. Prados MD, et al. Phase 1 study of erlotinib HCl alone and combined with temozolomide in patients with stable or recurrent malignant glioma. Neuro Oncol. 2006;8:67–78.
58. Mellinghoff IK, et al. Molecular determinants of the response of glioblastomas to EGFR kinase inhibitors. N Engl J Med. 2005;353:2012–24.
59. Haas-Kogan DA, et al. Epidermal growth factor receptor, protein kinase B/Akt, and glioma response to erlotinib. J Natl Cancer Inst. 2005;97:880–7.
60. Eller JL, et al. Anti-epidermal growth factor receptor monoclonal antibody cetuximab augments radiation effects in glioblastoma multiforme in vitro and in vivo. Neurosurgery. 2005;56:155–62.
61. Wen PY, et al. Phase I/II study of Imatinib mesylate for recurrent malignant gliomas: North American Brain Tumor Consortium Study 99–08. Clin Cancer Res. 2006;12:4899–907.
62. Reardon DA, et al. Phase II study of Imatinib mesylate plus hydroxyurea in adults with recurrent glioblastoma multiforme. J Clin Oncol. 2005;23: 9359–68.

63. Yaman E, et al. Temozolomide in newly diagnosed malignant gliomas: administered concomitantly with radiotherapy, and thereafter as consolidation treatment. Onkologie. 2008;31:309–13.

64. Batchelor TT, et al. AZD2171, a pan-VEGF receptor tyrosine kinase inhibitor, normalizes tumor vasculature and alleviates edema in glioblastoma patients. Cancer Cell. 2007;11:83–95.

65. Vredenburgh JJ, et al. Phase II trial of bevacizumab and irinotecan in recurrent malignant glioma. Clin Cancer Res. 2007;13:1253–9.

66. Vredenburgh JJ, et al. Bevacizumab plus irinotecan in recurrent glioblastoma multiforme. J Clin Oncol. 2007;25:4722–9.

67. Conrad C, et al. A phase I/II trial of single-agent PTK787/ZK222584, a novel oral angiogenesis inhibitor, in patients with recurrent GBM. http://meeting.ascopubs.org/cgi/content/abstract/22/14_suppl/1512?sid=dfd9ea4d-7472-4576-bf8b-8cda81fd260e.

68. Reardon D, Friedman H, Yung WKA. A phase I/II trial of PTK787/ZK222584 (PTK/ZK), a novel oral angiogenesis inhibitor, in combination with either temozolomide or lomustine for patients with recurrent glioblastoma multiforme. Proc Am Soc Clin Oncol. 2004;23:110.

69. Galanis E, et al. Phase II trial of temsirolimus (CCI-779) in recurrent glioblastoma multiforme: a North Central Cancer Treatment Group Study. J Clin Oncol. 2005;23:5294–304.

70. Chang SM, et al. Phase II study of CCI-779 in patients with recurrent glioblastoma multiforme. Invest New Drugs. 2005;23:357–61.

71. Cloughesy TF, et al. Phase II trial of tipifarnib in patients with recurrent malignant glioma either receiving or not receiving enzyme inducing antiepileptic drugs: a North American Brain Tumor Consortium Study. J Clin Oncol. 2006;24:3651–6.

72. Gilbert MR, et al. A phase I study of temozolomide (TMZ) and the farnesyltransferase inhibitor (FTI), lonafarnib (Sarasar, SCH66336) in recurrent glioblastoma. Proc Am Soc Clin Oncol. 2006;24:1556.

73. Tabatabai G, et al. Synergistic antiglioma activity of radiotherapy and enzastaurin. Ann Neurol. 2007;61:153–61.

74. Fine HA, et al. Enzastaurin (ENZ) versus lomustine (CCNU) in the treatment of recurrent, intracranial glioblastoma multiforme (GBM): a phase III study. http://meeting.ascopubs.org/cgi/content/abstract/26/15_suppl/2005?sid=b1d59689-ffac-4576-b48e-ad1aa6ff7872.

75. Quang TS, Brady LW. Radioimmunotherapy as a novel treatment regimen: 125I-labeled monoclonal antibody 425 in the treatment of high-grade brain gliomas. Int J Radiat Oncol Biol Phys. 2004;58:972–5.

76. Wygoda Z, et al. Use of monoclonal anti- EGFR antibody in the radioimmunotherapy of malignant gliomas in the context of EGFR expression in grade III and IV tumors. Hybridoma (Larchmt). 2006;25:125–32.

77. Akabani G, et al. Dosimetry and radiographic analysis of 131I-labeled anti-tenascin 81C6 murine monoclonal antibody in newly diagnosed patients with malignant gliomas: a phase II study. J Nucl Med. 2005;46:1042–51.

78. McLendon RE, et al. Tumor resection cavity administered iodine-131-labeled antitenascin 81C6 radioimmunotherapy in patients with malignant glioma: neuropathology aspects. Nucl Med Biol. 2007;34:405–13.

79. Pastan I, Chaudhary V, FitzGerald DJ. Recombinant toxins as novel therapeutic agents. Annu Rev Biochem. 1992;61:331–54.

80. Sampson JH, et al. Progress report of a Phase I study of the intracerebral microinfusion of a recombinant chimeric protein composed of transforming growth factor (TGF)-β and a mutated form of the Pseudomonas exotoxin termed PE-38 (TP-38) for the treatment of malignant brain tumors. J Neurooncol. 2003;65:27–35.

81. Nabors LB, et al. A phase I trial of EMD 121974 for treatment of patients with recurrent malignant gliomas. Neuro Oncol. 2004;6:379.

82. Chinnaiyan P, Vallabhaneni G, Armstrong E, Huang SM, Harari PM. Modulation of radiation response by histone deacetylase inhibition. Int J Radiat Oncol Biol Phys. 2005;62:223–9.

Head and Neck Tumours

2

Keith D. Hunter and Robert Bolt

Introduction

The term "head and neck tumours" encompasses a wide range of heterogeneous histologically defined entities which arise from the tissues of the head and neck region. In excess of 90% of these are squamous cell carcinomas (SCC) which most commonly arise from the mucosa of the oral cavity, pharynx and larynx. By necessity, this chapter will concentrate on these. Consideration of these tumours is very timely: there are important changes afoot in the epidemiology of these diseases, the most significant of these being the increasing role of human papillomavirus (HPV) in the aetiology of SCC in certain sub-sites of the head and neck. Furthermore, the recognition of distinct molecular features of tumours at various sites in the upper aero-digestive tract reinforces the concept that there is wide heterogeneity in tumours of the head and neck. This poses a challenge in the development of diagnostic and therapeutic biomarkers, yet this provides a great

K.D. Hunter, B.Sc., B.D.S., F.D.S.R.C.S.Ed., Ph.D., F.R.C.Path. (✉)
Unit of Oral and Maxillofacial Pathology, School of Clinical Dentistry, University of Sheffield, Claremont Crescent, Sheffield, South Yorkshire, S10 2TA, UK
e-mail: k.hunter@sheffield.ac.uk

R. Bolt, B.D.S., M.F.D.S., M.B.Ch.B.
Department of Oral Surgery, Charles Clifford Dental School, Sheffield, South Yorkshire, UK

opportunity for the individualisation of care for patients.

It is also important to include other groups of tumours which are unique to the head and neck region, such as malignant salivary gland tumours and odontogenic tumours. Whilst much less common, many of these have significant potential for application of molecular diagnostics and therapeutics, albeit with developments proceeding at a slower pace. Other tumours, such as soft tissue tumours and malignancies of the skin of the head and neck, will be covered in other chapters.

Epidemiology

Head and Neck Squamous Cell Carcinoma

The incidence of head and neck squamous cell carcinoma (HNSCC) as reported by IARC is divided by sub-site of the head and neck, namely, lip and oral cavity, larynx, pharynx and nasopharynx, covering the ICD10 codes C01–C14. As with all global cancer data, much of the incidence is estimated due to the lack of complete data available from many parts of the world. The most recent estimated age standardised incidence figures are seen in Table 2.1. Cumulatively, HNSCC (across all 4 sub-sites) is the sixth most common cancer worldwide, but this headline figure obscures large variations across the world. Less recent data demonstrated marked differences in the incidence in developed and developing parts of the world,

Table 2.1 The worldwide incidence of HNSCC, divided by region and tumour site

Site	Region	Numbers	ASR
Lip, oral cavity	World	170,496	5.3
	Africa	8,361	3.0
	Asia	91,327	4.7
	Europe	40,026	7.4
	Latin America	11,569	4.6
	North America	17,201	7.1
	Oceania	2,012	9.5
Nasopharynx	World	57,852	1.7
	Africa	5,957	1.9
	Asia	46,496	2.3
	Europe	2,811	0.6
	Latin America	928	0.4
	North America	1,524	0.7
	Oceania	136	0.7
Other pharynx	World	108,588	3.4
	Africa	3,585	1.3
	Asia	62,003	3.3
	Europe	26,731	5.1
	Latin America	6,808	2.8
	North America	8,847	3.8
	Oceania	614	2.9
Larynx	World	129,651	4.1
	Africa	7,594	3.0
	Asia	61,739	3.3
	Europe	36,573	6.7
	Latin America	12,597	5.2
	North America	10,508	4.3
	Oceania	640	2.9

ASR: weighted age-standardised rate per 100,000
Based on data from GLOBOCAN 2008. Cancer Incidence and Mortality Worldwide in 2008. http://globocan.iarc.fr

with HNSCC placed sixth in men in developing countries [1]. The reported estimated age standardised incidence varied from 2.2/100,000 per annum (Western Africa) to 33.6/100,000 per annum (Melanesia). In many areas, the high incidence reported can be attributed to one or a small number of particular aetiological factors, such as habits of betel/areca nut chewing.

In general, HNSCC occurs in patients in the sixth decade of life and older and is more common in males. For most patients, this represents the cumulative effects of decades of tobacco smoking and alcohol intake, both of which still tend to be higher in males. However, the marked male predominance is reducing as more female patients develop HNSCC [2]. In some countries, such as the USA, recent data indicate that the incidence of oral cavity cancer is stable and may even be in slow decline [3]. This may, in part,

parallel the reduction in lung cancer as smoking rates have dropped [4]. Other populations, such as Japan and the UK, do not mirror such changes and report increases in incidence and/or mortality [5, 6]. In the USA, there appears to be a slow and steady increase in overall survival [7, 8].

Recent Changes of Note

A rise in the number of patients younger than 40 years has been reported over the past two to three decades [9–12]. Many of these patients do exhibit a similar risk factor profile to older patients, albeit over a generally shorter timescale [12]. However, a significant number of young patients do not report the traditional risk factors of tobacco usage and alcohol intake [10, 11, 13, 14]. This indicates that other factors may have an important role in the development of HNSCC. One such explanation for the most dramatic change in the epidemiology of HNSCC over the past two decades has been the increase in the incidence of tumours of the oropharynx (mainly tonsil and base of tongue [15]) which have been associated with infection by HPV [16–18]. This will be discussed in detail later in this chapter. An increase in oral tongue cancer, particularly in young white patients, has also been reported [19]. The reasons for this are unclear, but smokeless tobacco, marijuana and HPV have been suggested as possible aetiological factors.

These recent changes in the incidence and distribution of HNSCC present new challenges in diagnosis and treatment. The increasing number of younger patients, who present with a much lower burden of co-morbidities, may allow for more aggressive treatment of disease. Conversely, as will be discussed later, the involvement of HPV in a number of HNSCCs has opened the possibility for reduced intensity of therapy.

Tumours of the Sinonasal Tract and Nasopharynx (ICD10 C31 and C11)

Malignant sinonasal tumours are rare and account for 3% of all head and neck malignancies [20]. Most arise in the maxillary sinus, and incidence is relatively stable, with the exception of Japan and China, in which higher rates have been recorded.

Nasopharyngeal carcinoma encompasses a number of histological entities and demonstrates a clear racial and geographical distribution. The incidence is relatively high in Chinese, Southeast Asian populations and some North Africans, but is rare in most other parts of the world [21]. The incidence is declining in some high incidence populations [22].

Malignant Salivary Gland Tumours (ICD10 C07–08)

Malignant tumours of the salivary glands are rare, comprising approximately 4–6% of all head and neck tumours [23]. The most recent WHO classification identifies 20 distinct histological sub-types, and, despite this, a significant number of tumours are still not easily classified [24]. The most recent SEER data demonstrate a small but significant increase in overall incidence of salivary gland carcinoma in the USA over the period 1975–2007 [25]. Much of the data on the relative incidence of sub-types come from large case series. AFIP data indicate that the most common malignant salivary gland tumour in the population of the USA is mucoepidermoid carcinoma, followed by adenoid cystic carcinoma [26]; however, data from other countries, including Brazil [27] and the UK [28], show adenoid cystic carcinoma is the most common tumour. Some analyses have indicated a high frequency of squamous cell carcinoma, but as primary SCC of salivary gland is rare, it appears likely that this represents a cohort of lesions that include metastases from the upper aero-digestive tract or skin of the face and scalp [29]. The epidemiology of the individual histological sub-types of malignant salivary gland tumours is insufficiently documented to comment on changes in incidence.

Malignant Odontogenic Tumours

Odontogenic malignancies are exceedingly rare, and cancer registry data are not readily available. In general, odontogenic carcinomas are much more common than odontogenic sarcomas

[30, 31]. Ameloblastic carcinoma and malignant/metastasising ameloblastoma account for most of the carcinomas, and these tend to follow an aggressive clinical course [32]. The true incidence of the tumours is unknown.

Biomarkers for Diagnosis

HNSCC

The mainstay for diagnosis in HNSCC is a good biopsy, but this depends on the identification (or at least suspicion) of a lesion which prompted the biopsy. In many cases, the diagnosis can be established from the biopsy material by morphology alone. However, some borderline cases prove challenging, and the drive for screening and early detection means biomarkers in smaller samples, such as cytological preparations from brush biopsies, are eagerly sought. A very large number of genetic alterations, from whole genome, chromosome, allelic imbalance and mutation of individual genes, have been described in HNSCC. However, the vast majority of these appear to have found very little routine diagnostic application to date. This is an ongoing concern in a number of smoking-related malignancies, and potential approaches and applications have been reviewed by Hu et al. [33].

Tissue Biomarkers (Including Cytology)

One key area for development of diagnostic use of biomarkers is in the analysis of material from brush biopsies of the mucosa of the upper aero-digestive tract. Brush biopsies may form part of a strategy for screening in high-risk individuals and allow for the sampling of mucosa without the need for a formal biopsy. Comparisons between cytological features and molecular analysis for the detection of head and neck squamous cell carcinoma have been made using oesophageo-pharyngeal and laryngeal brush samples. Initial studies were rather inconclusive [34], but later investigation of microsatellite instability (MSI) and p16 methylation demonstrated a good match between the abnormalities found in the brush sample and tumour [35]. Both, however, emphasise the importance of identification of more robust biomarkers to increase sensitivity of the test. In other studies, allelic imbalance (AI) at loci 3p, 9p, 11q and 17p in brush biopsy samples was investigated. The assay was validated against the biopsy results of the leukoplakia lesions, yielding an estimated sensitivity of 78% and a positive predictive value of 100%, albeit in a small sample size [36]. Fluorescence in situ hybridisation (FISH) has also been applied to brush specimens in order to detect genetically aberrant cells in brush specimens. The presence of genetic alterations in >5% of cells correlated well with cytological features suspicious of malignancy [37]. The logistics of implementing such genetic-based tests in a diagnostic service may prove prohibitive. However, as FISH is already used in the diagnosis of other malignancies, it may be possible to develop an appropriately specific, sensitive and inexpensive test using this technology. The addition of DNA cytometric analysis to cytology in the assessment of brush biopsies may be useful [38]. This is reported to increase the sensitivity of such assays to close to 100% and may be a more easily implemented test in the clinical care pathway [39].

Other approaches include identification of transcriptomic signatures in tissues or cytological specimens. However, numerous studies comparing expression patterns in normal and SCC tissues have been published which demonstrate marked heterogeneity and lack of agreement. The possible reasons for this are beyond the scope of this chapter, but are discussed elsewhere [40]. In bringing together the large number of microarray studies, Lallemant and co-workers selected 9 genes from 23 published HNSCC transcriptome studies [41]. They suggested a panel of 3 markers for diagnosis. None correlated with histopathological features or prognosis. The panel requires further validation and may find its application in salivary profiling for diagnosis, rather than in tissues. Other investigators have used principle component analysis of gene expression data, trained with known HNSCC transcription data to identify unknown samples [42]. It is not clear, however, how this can be applied in routine

diagnosis, but various suggestions have been made in recent reviews [43, 44].

Signatures associated with microRNA or proteomic changes have also been demonstrated. Novel and established proteomic biomarkers have been recently reviewed [45], and proteomic biomarkers do find extensive use in diagnosis of HNSCC and other malignancies. Differential immunohistochemical expression of cytokeratins has been used for many years in the diagnosis of poorly differentiated or basaloid tumours [46], and this is particularly valuable if there is an occult primary tumour [47–49]. Whilst this technique is easily applied in clinical practice, some authors have suggested that quantitative reverse transcriptase PCR (RTPCR) may be more sensitive, particularly for use in sentinel lymph nodes [50]. Other methods of proteomic analysis have identified successive alterations in protein expression in normal, tumour adjacent and invasive HNSCC by application of SELDI-TOF mass spectrometry [51]. This method for identification of novel biomarkers looks promising, and several other candidates have been suggested (reviewed by Rezende et al. [45]). All of these potential new biomarkers need to be assessed in larger prospective studies to determine their utility in HNSCC diagnosis.

Salivary Biomarkers

Saliva is a very attractive medium for diagnostic use due to ease of collection in a non-invasive manner [52]. In addition to its role in maintaining oral health, saliva contains many markers related to systemic disease. These markers include not only proteins but also genomic and transcriptomic biomarkers which may be of use in the diagnosis of a number of local (such as HNSCC) and systemic diseases, such as cancer and HIV infection. The potential uses of saliva in cancer diagnostics are now beginning to be realised.

Genomic Biomarkers in Saliva

The detection of tumour-associated mutations was demonstrated in 1994 by Boyle and co-workers

2 Head and Neck Tumours

Table 2.2 Selected biomarkers in HNSCC which have demonstrated promoter methylation

Gene	Function	References
CDKN2A/p16	Cell cycle	[61, 62]
P14ARF	Cell cycle	[63]
CDKN2B/p15	Cell cycle	[64]
Cyclin A1	Cell cycle	[65]
DBC1	Cell cycle	[66]
ATM	Cell cycle	[67]
FHIT	Apoptosis/cell cycle	[68]
TP73	Apoptosis/cell cycle	[68]
RASSF1	Apoptosis/cell cycle	[69]
DCC	Apoptosis	[70]
DAPK1	Apoptosis	[63, 68, 69]
RARβ	Differentiation	[65, 71]
MLH1	Mismatch repair	[72]
SERPINB5	Tumour suppressor	[73]
TIMP-3	Matrix remodelling	[68]
E-cadherin	Cell–cell interactions	[74]

Based on data from Ref. [75]

who found an identical p53 mutation in 71% of patients with HNSCC when comparing tumour and saliva [53]. Despite recent advances in sequencing technology, the potentially laborious nature of this investigation has limited its application in clinical practice. Assessment of microsatellite instability and DNA content in the saliva of patients with HNSCC demonstrated good sensitivity and specificity in distinguishing known cancer patients from normal controls [52, 54, 55]. Others have demonstrated significant genetic heterogeneity between the saliva and primary tumour, which may reduce sensitivity [56].

More recently, there has been interest in aberrant patterns of gene promoter methylation. A large number of genes which demonstrate abnormal promoter methylation have been suggested for such an analysis (Table 2.2) [57–60]. Many of these have already been demonstrated in primary tumours, but the sensitivity and specificity of these analyses in saliva for primary diagnoses is a matter of debate. The level of detection of methylated genes in the published series is often much less than in primary tumours, and as such, its use as a primary screening tool is questionable unless more sensitive biomarkers can be identified [59]. It has been suggested that salivary monitoring

for recurrence may be possible, and indeed, the small studies published so far look promising, but much larger cohorts are required [58].

Mitochondrial DNA (mtDNA) is a further biomarker which has been detected in saliva, with mutated mtDNA in particular being readily detectable [76]. An increase in mtDNA in saliva has been reported in HNSCC patients [77]. Other authors have demonstrated a link between increased mtDNA and smoking in general [78], but in the study by Jiang and co-workers, mtDNA levels were independently associated with HNSCC [77]. A decrease in mtDNA has also been demonstrated in post-treatment salivary rinses in HNSCC patients, raising the possibility of longitudinal testing as a monitoring tool for recurrence [79].

Transcriptomic and Proteomic Biomarkers in Saliva

The identification of RNA and microRNA of sufficient quality for analysis in saliva has opened the full remit of RNA analyses in material derived from saliva [80–82]. Using RNA from the saliva of HNSCC patients, Li and co-workers identified 8 potential markers to distinguish HNSCC from normal patients, with combined specificity and sensitivity in excess of 90% [83], whilst others found detection of MMP1 mRNA in saliva was 100% specific for detection of HNSCC (although sensitivity was very low) [41]. This type of analysis appears to have great potential, but no large-scale prospective trials using this technology have been published.

Analysis of the salivary proteome has demonstrated that up to 40% of candidate serum proteomic biomarkers for a number of diseases can be identified in saliva [84–86]. Potential applications in cancer diagnosis/biomarker discovery have been reported, again with promising sensitivity and specificity, but only in a retrospective study population [87]. Considerable investigation is still required before salivary diagnostics become a viable part of routine chair-side testing for head and neck cancer.

Serum Markers

Analysis of circulating biomarkers is being applied to a number of tumours. The particular analyte is varied, with sources such as genomic and proteomic markers widely studied. More recently, serum microRNA profiles have shown promise of clinical utility [88].

Genomic Biomarkers in Serum

Analysis of the patterns of LoH and AI in tissues and serum in HNSCC patients has demonstrated good agreement of the pattern of changes in tumour and serum [89]. A number of groups have also demonstrated in DNA retrieved from serum that identification of patterns of MSI matched to the primary tumour was a marker of advanced disease and poor prognosis [90–92]. Furthermore, there is potential for application in monitoring of recurrence as one study has shown that AI positive serum samples at 4 weeks post-operation were a marker of poor prognosis [89].

Serum analysis of gene promoter methylation demonstrated the same pattern in the tumours in 42% of patients. The difference in metastatic rate seen in patients with methylation in serum versus those without was not significant [93]. Other small studies have demonstrated p16 promoter methylation in the serum of oral cancer patients [94]. More recently, larger studies with an extended panel of genes demonstrated the added benefit of a larger panel of biomarkers, but the specificity was still disappointing [60].

Proteomic Biomarkers in Serum

A number of studies have reported on the use of various forms of mass spectrometry (SELDI-TPF, MALDI-TOF) in the discrimination of normal from HNSCC patients and also in the monitoring of recurrence. So far, all of these cohorts use known HNSCC patients and report high sensitivity and specificity in discriminating these patients from normal controls [95–98]. In one of the largest studies, Linkov et al. assessed a 60 marker panel, including HB-EGF, EGFR and multiple cytokines in sera from cohorts of active HNSCC patients, successfully treated patients, and 117 smoker controls with no evidence of HNSCC [99]. In the marker panel, the greatest predictive power was found with a smaller 25 marker panel which identified patients in the active disease group with a sensitivity of 84.5% and specificity of 98%. Similar results have been demonstrated by other groups, showing changes in the serum biomarkers post-treatment and also longitudinally at the time of recurrence [100–102].

Human Papillomavirus

As indicated in the introduction, one of the most important biomarkers which have been demonstrated over the past decade is the presence of human papillomavirus (HPV) in a sub-set of tumours of the head and neck. HPV is a non-enveloped, double-stranded DNA virus that is strictly epitheliotropic [103]. HPV is very slow to evolve due to its stable, DNA-based genome, but an estimated 200 HPV "types" exist [104]. The resultant variation in biological activity between types has led to different pathogenic effects. However, only a handful of HPV types have been implicated in carcinogenesis and are therefore referred to as "high risk". Whereas most HPV-related carcinomas have been linked to a number of high-risk viral types, oropharyngeal carcinoma has been consistently linked to HPV 16 [104, 105]. This relationship is not exclusive, but accounts for at least 90% HPV-positive oropharyngeal tumours. The reasons for this are not known, although it is recognised that the affinity of its oncoproteins to host tumour suppressor proteins is higher than in other viral types [106].

The Role of HPV in Carcinogenesis

HPV-related carcinogenesis is linked to viral integration into the host genome. Under normal circumstances, HPV remains episomal throughout its life cycle and has relatively low expression

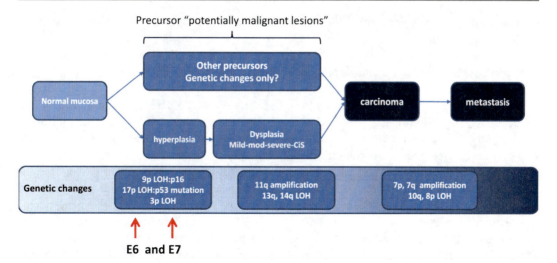

Fig. 2.1 Mutational events seen in the multistep process of head and neck cancer formation. In many patients, the presence of a clinically or even histopathologically evident, precancerous lesion is unclear. Whilst the precise sequence of molecular events in the development of HNSCC is not entirely clear, the patterns of LOH and amplification as shown in the diagram are now well established. In HPV infection, E6 and E7 inactivate p53 and pRb, respectively; thus, the early changes are often not present [110]. (Modified from [111, 222])

of its two oncoproteins, E6 and E7 [107, 108]. Integration requires a break in the circular viral DNA sequence which tends to disrupt the E2 gene, rendering it inactive and thereby allowing E6/E7 transcription to continue unsuppressed [109]. Unlike the multistep process of cumulative mutations and chromosomal losses classically described in non-HPV head and neck cancer, HPV-related carcinogenesis involves fewer alterations in genetic material [110]. It appears that important steps in the pathway of head and neck carcinogenesis as proposed by Califano et al. (Fig. 2.1 [111]) are bypassed due to the effect of viral oncoproteins E6 and E7.

E6 and E7 act to deregulate host cell cycle control [112]. Although both E6 and E7 have effects on multiple intra-cellular signalling pathways, their major actions are on the tumour suppressor proteins p53 and pRb, respectively [113]. E6 complexes with E6AP (E6-associated protein), which then binds p53 and induces ubiquitin-mediated degradation [103, 114]. E7 binds to hypophosphorylated pRb [104]. The interaction between E7 and pRb leads to the release of E2F, a factor that promotes DNA synthesis and cell cycle progression when in its free form [115]. An important consequence of virally induced free E2F is the activation of a feedback loop which increases the expression of p16 [116]. As this feedback loop has no effect on the actions of E7, p16 will continue to be over-expressed during viral infection, a feature that can be utilised in immunohistochemistry as a surrogate marker of HPV infection within pathological specimens. This is in contrast to non-HPV head and neck cancer, which tends to involve promoter methylation, deletion or mutation of p16 (chromosomal locus 9p21, Fig. 2.1) that leads to loss of expression [110].

HPV in Head and Neck Tumours

The reported prevalence of HPV in head and neck cancer varies considerably, with findings of between 0 and 100% of all head and neck tumours testing positive [117]. Several variables influence the proportion of tumour specimens testing positive for HPV, notably anatomical sub-site, method used to detect HPV, study date and geographic location. HPV is thought to have site specificity within the head and neck region, with a predilection for tumours in the tonsil and base of tongue regions. Even when taking this into account, the reported prevalence of HPV-positive oropharyngeal carcinoma varies widely [118, 119]. A recent systematic review found overall HPV prevalence to be 35.6% and suggested a higher prevalence in North America and Asia (47.0 and 46.3%, respectively) and a lower prevalence in Europe (28.2%) [117].

There is a general consensus that HPV-positive oropharyngeal carcinoma is becoming more common and accounts for the 3–4% per year rise in incidence rate of oropharyngeal carcinomas seen recently [4, 120, 121]. These temporal changes will undoubtedly have an effect on the prevalence of HPV-positive specimens noted in studies conducted over different periods. Indeed, Nasman et al. found such a change in tonsillar specimens collected between 1970 and 2007 [121]. HPV-positive oropharyngeal carcinoma has generally been found to occur in a younger cohort than for HPV-negative counterparts, although this relationship has not been consistently demonstrated [122–126]. In those studies demonstrating an age difference, patients are around 3–5 years younger than HPV-negative cases. As with HPV-negative oropharyngeal carcinoma, a significant male predominance is seen [122, 123].

HPV Detection Methods

There is currently no accepted standard test for the detection of HPV in head and neck cancer specimens [127]. Possible methods are outlined in Table 2.3. No single method is available that can be applied to both frozen and formalin-fixed paraffin-embedded (FFPE) specimens, with 100% sensitivity and specificity. Proxy measures of HPV infection, such as serum analysis of antibodies to E6, E7 and L1, are poorly specific due to the potential for HPV infection at other sites [128]. No other systemic markers of HPV exist, as there is no blood-borne phase of HPV infection [16].

RTPCR amplification of viral E6/E7 mRNA is now considered as "gold standard" for the detection of clinically significant HPV infection within tumour specimens [129, 130]. However, the method is only reliable when applied to fresh frozen specimens, with an estimated 50% reduction in sensitivity when applied to FFPE samples [131].

PCR amplification of viral DNA is a highly sensitive method of HPV detection and either can be applied to a single HPV type by amplification of a sequence specific to that type or can be used less specifically to assess presence of multiple HPV types by use of a consensus primer. Despite this, there are significant limitations of the method due to its inability to distinguish clinically relevant HPV infection. Presence of latent virus leads to false-positive results due to the ability of PCR to detect just a few copies of HPV DNA per cell. Attempts have been made to resolve this issue through the use of real-time PCR, which provides a quantitative analysis of viral load. However, a criticism of this method is that it still provides no direct evidence of viral integration or oncogene expression. Furthermore, sensitivity is estimated at 92% and specificity 97% when using a cut-off viral load of >0.5 copies per cell; false positives and false negatives therefore still exist [132].

In situ hybridisation (ISH) may overcome some of the limitations of PCR by detecting only clinically relevant infection. Nuclear hybridisation signals can be visually inspected for punctuate or diffuse staining, representing integrated and episomal viral DNA, respectively [133]. Presence of a punctuate hybridisation signal, either alone or in combination with diffuse nuclear signals, therefore reflects clinically relevant HPV infection. Although specificity of this method is high (100%), sensitivity is not ideal (83%) [132]. It has been estimated that around 10 copies of virus per cell must be present in order for ISH to detect HPV, although newer ISH kits are thought to be more sensitive [131].

p16 immunohistochemistry has become an established marker of HPV infection, as discussed earlier. However, there are a number of HPV-negative tumours that also over-express p16, leading to false positives [131]. Although sensitivity is quoted as high (100%), Weinberger et al. have reported a sub-set of HPV-positive tumours which do not over-express p16, inferring a sensitivity of less than 100% [134]. However,

2 Head and Neck Tumours

Table 2.3 A summary of methods of detection of HPV in HNSCC

Method	Advantages	Disadvantages
p16 immunohistochemistry: use of monoclonal antibody raised against p16 to assess for over-expression	High sensitivity Accessible to most laboratories Easily applied to FFPE tissue Implies presence of transcriptionally active virus through marker of host cell feedback mechanism	Surrogate marker; limited face validity Sensitivity may be less than published data suggests due to existence of HPV-positive, non-p16 over-expressing sub-type Specificity not ideal
Consensus PCR: general primer used to assess for presence of viral DNA Several available primers, including GP5+/6+, SPF10 and PGMY09/11	High sensitivity Assesses for papillomaviridae other than HPV16 SPF10 primers capable of amplifying highly degraded DNA samples	Low specificity; false positives relating to incidental detection of virus not involved in tumourigenesis Provides no quantitative measure of viral load No confirmation of transcriptionally active virus Full spectrum of sequence amplification not published
Type-specific PCR: single HPV genotype targeted for PCR (usually HPV16)	Can be used as a technique specific to HPV16 Avoids false positives relating to non-HPV16 viral types	Lower sensitivity compared to consensus primers due to type specificity Similar issues to consensus PCR with respect to specificity, viral load and transcriptional activity
Quantitative PCR: real-time PCR technique used to estimate HPV16 DNA copy number (viral copies per cell)	Quantitative measure of viral load Improved specificity	Labour intensive Improved specificity is at the expense of sensitivity
In situ hybridisation: labelled, HPV type-specific complimentary DNA sequence used to produce hybridisation signal	Allows distinction between episomal and integrated virus Can distinguish a single viral copy per cell High specificity	Overall sensitivity not ideal Not available to every laboratory
E6/E7 mRNA: RT-PCR used to amplify E6/E7 mRNA sequence	"Gold standard" for frozen specimens Confirmation of transcriptionally active virus	Poor sensitivity in FFPE specimens
HPV16 serology: detection of serum antibodies to L1 capsid protein Detection of serum antibodies to E6 and E7 (can be used in combination with L1)	Useful test when applied to epidemiological studies Does not require biopsy	Very poor specificity due to HPV infection at other anatomical sites Not all exposed individuals develop antibody response L1 cross-reactivity from low-risk HPV, further reducing specificity

Weinberger used real-time PCR as conclusive evidence of HPV infection, with a lower cut-off of 1 viral copy per 10 cell genomes' worth of DNA [135]. This work would therefore almost certainly include a number of false positives. However, Weist et al. also reported HPV E6/E7 positive, p16 negative tumours, albeit with a lower prevalence than that seen by Weinberger et al. (14% vs. 37%) [136]. Irrespective of the existence of a non-p16 over-expressing sub-set, p16 immunohistochemistry is not an ideal test in isolation due to its low specificity (79%) [132].

In the absence of a single, ideal method of HPV detection, some authors have applied a combination of tests to improve reliability [132, 137, 138]. Smeets et al. recommended p16 immunostaining, followed by GP5+/6+ PCR (general primer consensus PCR) in those samples p16 positive [132]. Their rationale for using this method was based on data suggesting 100% sensitivity and specificity when compared to an E6 mRNA gold standard. However, it should be noted that there were independently several false positives for both p16 immunohistochemistry and GP5+/6+ PCR, and the size of the study (48 samples) makes interpretation difficult, as the absence of simultaneous false-positive results for p16/general primer analysis may have occurred by chance. The authors acknowledged this and calculated a likely 2% chance of concurrent false positives when using the technique.

The combination of two tests considered 100% sensitive should improve specificity with no detriment to sensitivity. As discussed, p16 immunohistochemistry is not necessarily 100% sensitive, and one must therefore consider the potential for false negatives in using this technique. Despite this, p16 immunohistochemistry is perhaps the most appropriate marker to use in combination with another test, as it assesses a very different parameter to other available techniques. HPV16 PCR, GP5+/6+ PCR and ISH all assess for presence of viral DNA; combining such tests is therefore of questionable value.

It therefore follows that many authors have adopted a PCR-based technique in combination with p16 immunohistochemistry to identify HPV-positive tumours. Whilst E6/E7 mRNA detection remains the gold standard, its limitations with FFPE specimens have thus far precluded the technique from becoming universally adopted. ISH is therefore an appropriate test for research in which sensitivity is not of paramount concern.

Other Mucosal Head and Neck Tumours

Due to their relative inaccessibility, many sinonasal and nasopharyngeal tumours often present at an advanced clinical stage. Thus, the identification of biomarkers, particularly in high-risk populations, has great potential use in diagnosis.

Epstein–Barr Virus

Epstein–Barr virus (EBV) is a DNA virus of the herpes group which is strongly linked to undifferentiated carcinoma of the nasopharynx (nasopharyngeal carcinoma, NPC). It has also been associated with sinonasal undifferentiated carcinoma (SNUC) in Asian patients and lymphoepithelial carcinoma of the salivary glands. EBV is primarily B lymphotropic but also infects epithelial cells. A number of viral genes have been shown to be oncogenic, and the pattern of gene expression seen in latent-type EBV infection is also pro-oncogenic, due to aberrant expression of genes such as bcl-2 and fos/jun [139, 140].

EBV Detection in the Diagnosis of Nasopharyngeal Carcinoma

EBV detection is possible in tissue sections and in cytological specimens from suspicious lesions. Additional information to the cytology finding was provided by EBV PCR which improved sensitivity to 90% and specificity to 99% [141]. In a study of 517 patients, 156 of whom had NPC, Chang and co-workers demonstrated that serum testing for antibodies to EBV nuclear antigen-1 and early antigen predicted NPC in patients with specificity as high as 99.2% [142]. This may be used in endemic areas as part of a screening programme. Furthermore, EBV DNA load was associated with N stage and overall stage, thus raising the potential for use in post-treatment monitoring. Serum markers of EBV infection, such as IgA against VCA-p18, or detection of circulating EBV DNA may also be useful, particularly in the monitoring of recurrences [143, 144]. Serum proteomic analysis has also demonstrated a number of NPC metastasis-specific markers which need prospective validation [145].

Salivary Gland Tumours

The large range of possible diagnoses and the often overlapping histological features mean that salivary gland tumours often provide a diagnostic challenge. The search for diagnostic markers has resulted in the identification of a number of tumour-specific chromosomal translocations in malignant salivary tumours. The MECT1–MAML2 fusion transcript has been identified in over half of all mucoepidermoid carcinomas (MEC), whilst the MYB–NFIB fusion has been described in a sub-set of adenoid cystic carcinomas (AdCC) [146, 147]. Recent investigation has complicated the issue by suggesting that MECT1–MAML2 fusion-negative MECs should be categorised as another tumour type [148]. This uncertainty indicates that the identification of specific chromosome rearrangements is not yet appropriate for routine diagnostic use.

Investigation of other potential biomarkers has largely pursued proteomic targets, either by tissue immunohistochemistry or by more sophisticated techniques such as 2D-mass spectrometry. Some markers, such as SPKH-1 and Ki-67, have been applied to all tumours regardless of type, as overall markers of poor outcome [149, 150]. Proteomic analysis of AdCC identified a number of potential biomarkers for diagnosis, but none other than c-kit has demonstrated any real promise as a diagnostic, prognostic and therapeutic biomarker, albeit its specificity has been called into question [151, 152]. Promoter methylation has been demonstrated in a number of salivary gland tumours, including AdCC [153] and carcinoma arising in pleomorphic adenoma [154], but

this analysis has not been translated into routine clinical use.

Odontogenic Tumours

The rarity of these tumours means no robust diagnostic biomarkers have been identified. The observation that CD56 (NCAM) is expressed by a number of odontogenic tumours may be useful in differentiating odontogenic tumours from mucosal SCC [155]; however, this has not been clearly demonstrated in a large cohort.

Validation Status

Many potential diagnostic biomarkers in HNSCC have been very slow to translate from lab to the clinic. In particular, despite a number of interesting gene expression profiles, there has been a distinct lack of large studies to test the gene signatures identified. It is undoubtedly true that the technology exists to implement chair-side molecular testing, but very few sufficiently robust biomarkers have been identified. Tests for HPV and EBV are standard of care in sub-populations of patients which can also be applied to identification of the primary tumour site in cases where the patient presents with a lymph node metastasis, but an unknown primary.

If non-invasive testing using validated biomarkers can be developed for use in screening, this will be of great benefit to patients with this disease, particularly in terms of early detection. Otherwise, the real use is in prognosis and individualisation of therapy, and it is to these issues we now turn.

Genes for Prognosis

HNSCC

The present prognostic scheme in HNSCC is largely centred on the importance of staging (using TNM) and a number of other histopathological features. These include the pattern at the invasive front, the presence of perineural or lymphovascular invasion and the margin status [156]. There are very few biomarkers currently being used in routine clinical practice. This most likely reflects the complexity of HNSCC development, which is reflected in the variable specificity and sensitivity of many suggested markers. At present, identification of HPV infection and over-expression of EGFR are the only molecular biomarkers which are routinely used in assessment of prognosis. However, there are a large number of other markers and methodologies which merit brief discussion if only to underline their potential uses.

One of the main barriers to the translation of molecular markers for prognosis in HNSCC is the lack of appropriately powered longitudinal studies. A number of these are underway, but are lengthy studies [particularly related to oral potentially malignant lesion (OPMLs) progression]. The consistent and systematic collection of clinical and follow-up data relating to cohorts has been prioritised, and this should translate into prospective validation of many of these markers in years to come. Undoubtedly, many will not make the step into routine clinical use.

Prognosis of Oral Potentially Malignant Lesions

The presence and severity of epithelial dysplasia are currently used in the prediction of malignant transformation of potentially malignant lesions in the upper aero-digestive tract. It has long been recognised that assessment of dysplasia is a subjective process with poor inter- and intra-examiner reproducibility [157]. This limits the predictive power of severity of epithelial dysplasia in these lesions, reinforcing the need for biomarkers of risk of malignant transformation.

The identification of consistent patterns in microsatellite analysis of LoH in OPMLs suggested that LoH at particular chromosomal loci may be useful clinically (Fig. 2.1) [158]. Mao et al. identified LoH at 9p21 and 3p14 in 51% of patients. Of the patients who had alteration at both loci, 37% developed oral SCC [159].

Assessment in a larger cohort of patients over 10 years allowed development of a hazard model including 3 factors (chromosomal polysomy, p53 protein expression and loss of heterozygosity at chromosome 3p or 9p) which indicated elevated risk of OPML progression. Further chemoprevention trials have added LoH at 17q and p53 mutations as possible biomarkers [160], and other refinements demonstrate certain patterns of LoH are associated with up to a 33-fold increase in relative cancer risk [161]. More recently, LoH has been combined with a morphometric "nuclear phenotype score" [162].

Despite much initial promise, testing for patterns of LoH has not found its way into the clinic. The large prospective trials evaluating its use (largely chemoprevention trials) have not yet reported. A recent systematic review highlighted that validation of these markers in large cohorts of patients is urgently required [163]. Technology and affordability in routine use may also be a barrier to widespread clinical application. Other components of the diagnostic models outlined above, such as p53 expression and mutations, have some limited use in predicting the behaviour of OPMLs, largely in conjunction with standard histological parameters [164].

The potential for the use of morphometric analysis of DNA content has been indicated above. Abnormal DNA content is an indicator of gross chromosomal abnormalities. The presence of a modal chromosome content which is not an exact multiple of the modal number is termed aneuploidy, and this has been shown to be a predictor of progression of pre-malignant disease at a number of sites, including oesophagus and oral cavity [165]. These systems allow for the assessment of ploidy using the optical density of the stained nuclei in tissues as a surrogate for DNA content. Several authors have shown that aneuploidy is associated with progression of OPMLs to OSCC [166–168]. Sensitivity and specificity are such that it is unlikely to be suitable for use if divorced from histopathological assessment of the tissue, and other authors have raised the problem of tissue heterogeneity and appropriate sampling [166]. Aneuploidy appears much less sensitive than assessment of LOH [169].

Table 2.4 Selected biomarkers in HNSCC in which relation to prognosis has been demonstrated

Cellular function	Examples	References
Signalling pathways	EGF receptor	[176–178]
	cerbB2	[176, 178]
	IL13 receptor α2	[179]
	Phosphatidylinositol-3 kinase catalytic alpha polypeptide	[180]
Cell cycle/apoptosis	cdc2	[181]
	p53 mutation	[182–185]
	p16^{INK4A}	[185, 186]
	p14^{ARF}	[187]
	Cyclin D1	[184, 186]
	Polo-like kinase 1	[188]
	Survivin	[189]
		[190]
Adhesion/motility	E-cadherin	[191–193]
	S100 Ca^{++} regulated protein A4	[194]
	CD44	[195]
	Hyaluronan	[196]
	Metalloproteinase (MMP)-9	[197]
	Tissue inhibitor of MMPs (TIMPs)1/2/3	[197]
	Moesin	[198]
	DCC	[187]
	Integrin αVβ6	[199]
Angiogenesis	VEGF	[200, 201]
	HIF-1α	[202]
Transcription	HMGA2	[203]
	SCC-related oncogene	[180]
Chemokines and inflammation	CXCR4 receptor	[204]
	COX2	[205]
Immortalisation	Telomerase	[206]
Others	MINT1 and MINT 31	[187]
	Haem oxygenase	[207]
	Coractin	[208]
	HPV infection	[209]

Nevertheless, DNA image cytometry is available as a test in some centres, to guide assessment of the behaviour of these lesions. One advantage of such image analysis techniques is that they can be done on brush samples [170], and their ultimate use may be in determining when and where biopsies are required.

Other Potentially Malignant Lesions

In schneiderian papillomas, severe dysplasia and p53 protein expression were strongly associated with malignant progression [171]. An association between HPV infection and malignant transformation has been demonstrated in up to a third of patients [171].

Individual Biomarkers in HNSCC

Alterations in large numbers of individual biomarkers have been linked to the prognosis of HNSCC, mostly by univariate analysis [172]. Many of these are reviewed in Hunter et al. (Table 2.4). There are far too many to discuss in the present context and, in any event, very few are used in clinical practice. Recent studies have suggested prognostic biomarkers as varied as S100A7 [173], microRNA-210 [174] and NBS1 [175], amongst many others, and have demonstrated a relationship to clinical outcome in retrospective cohorts of patients. The longitudinal prospective studies required to establish any of these markers for routine clinical use, as yet, have not been published. It is difficult, in the face of a

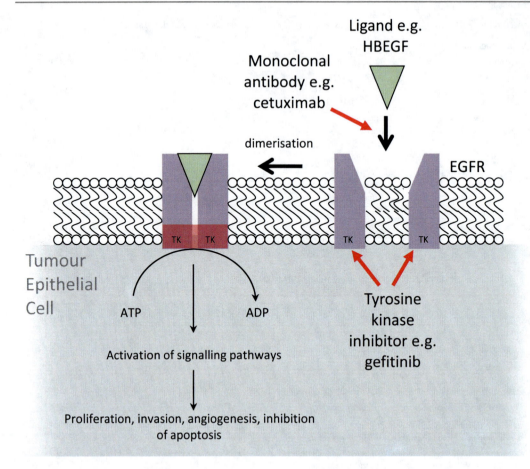

Fig. 2.2 EGFR signalling and the action of anti-EGFR agents. EGF receptors on the cell membrane dimerise in response to ligand binding, activating the intra-cellular tyrosine kinase (TK) domains. ATP-dependent phosphorylation of intra-cellular proteins then acts as a signalling pathway, ultimately leading to a number of different phenotypic responses. The diagram also indicates the site of action of the two main classes of anti-EGFR agent: monoclonal antibodies and tyrosine kinase inhibitors

vast number of potentially useful markers, to determine which are related to fundamental processes in tumour development and which may merely be surrogate markers or by-products of the progression of the tumour. Whilst this distinction is important in our understanding of the biology of HNSCC and in the search for novel targets for therapeutic intervention, it could be argued that this is not necessarily the case for prognostic markers: all that is required is a sensitive, specific and reproducible test which will accurately represent the prognosis for an individual patient. However, other than for EGFR and HPV, this appears elusive in HNSCC.

EGFR

The epidermal growth factor receptor is a cell surface receptor of the ErbB family which binds a number of ligands including HB-EGF, TGFα and amphiregulin [210]. EGFR is involved in control of proliferation and differentiation in squamous and other epithelia and has been associated with invasion and metastasis in a number of cancers (Fig. 2.2). Over-expression of EGFR has been reported in a number of malignancies, including HNSCC [211]. Initial reports of studies using IHC indicated that elevated levels of EGFR expression were associated with poor disease-specific and cause-specific survival [212].

Poor correlation between the level of EGFR protein expression and clinical response to anti-EGFR biological agents has prompted further investigations of the biology of EGFR. This has demonstrated that EGFR gene amplification is also associated with poor prognosis [213], although perhaps less than a third of patients show evidence of amplification [214, 215]. Mutations in EGFR are rare in HNSCC [216], but EGFR phosphorylation, particularly on a background of no mutations, is a marker of early relapse [217]. Furthermore, one recent paper demonstrated that high EGFR copy number is associated with an increased risk of OPML progression to HNSCC, particularly if associated with high EGFR expression [218].

As indicated above, there are numerous assays for EGFR. A number of recent reviews have highlighted concerns about assessment of EGFR expression by immunohistochemistry, given the lack of standardisation of assays and the wide variation in reported over-expression [219, 220]. Amplification and mutation appear to be relatively infrequent events, and there are a number of controversies and unanswered questions with regard to EGFR biology [221]. Nevertheless, EGFR is now established as an oncogene in HNSCC [222].

HPV and Prognosis

The favourable prognosis of HPV-positive oropharyngeal carcinoma is well documented (Table 2.5) [223]. It was initially thought that this improvement in outcome was a function of tumour radiosensitivity. Although HPV-positive oropharyngeal carcinomas are indeed more responsive to radiotherapy, the improved outcome of these tumours appears to also be translated to surgery [124, 224]. A more comprehensive effect of viral carcinogenesis must therefore be responsible for tumour behaviour. Persistence of wild-type TP53 and RB1 genes may very well underpin the altered behaviour seen in HPV-positive oropharyngeal carcinoma. It has been proposed that the cellular insult sustained as a result of radiotherapy may send the cell beyond a critical threshold necessary to overcome the effects of viral oncogenes, allowing p53 and pRb expression to become re-established.

Immunomodulation is also potentially important—radiotherapy may cause an increased immune response through many possible pathways. These pathways include increased antigen presentation as a result of uptake of necrotic, viral-loaded cells; improved penetrance of immune cells into tumour as a result of reduced cellular adhesion post-radiotherapy; upregulation of MHC class I; and induction of pro-inflammatory cytokines such as TNF, which may act to reverse viral tolerance [225]. Alterations in viral antigenicity as a response to therapy may also explain improvements in outcome seen in the surgical management of HPV-positive cancer. Local inflammatory response to the trauma of tissue excision, in addition to the release of cellular contents at incomplete surgical margins, may also have an influence on immunity.

One must also consider the potential for a phenotypically less aggressive tumour which is more responsive to treatment, irrespective of the therapeutic modality chosen. Lack of field cancerisation is well recognised in HPV-positive tumours and may contribute in part to the improved outcome seen [226]. The true cause of the improved behaviour will have implications on providing targeted treatment for HPV-positive oropharyngeal carcinoma, as HPV infection may ultimately be a non-manipulable prognostic factor. However, early reports on HPV-targeted therapy are encouraging.

Global Markers/Patterns of Expression

The advent of high-throughput technologies has brought unprecedented opportunities and challenges in the search for predictive molecular signature in HNSCC.

Comparative Genomic Hybridisation

Using comparative genomic hybridisation (CGH), Smeets and co-workers demonstrated 3 groups of

Table 2.5 A summary of recent clinical studies of HPV infection in HNSCC

References	n	Method	Measures	Treatment	HPV+	HPV−	Conclusions
Snijders [370]	63	C-PCR	OS, RR	S	–	–	No difference[a]
Paz [371]	167	C-PCR	OS	Not stated	43.1 (3)	48.8 (3)	No difference[a]
Pintos [372]	117	C-PCR	OS, DFS	Not stated	66.7 (5)	58.3 (5)	No difference[a]
Gillison [18]	253	C-PCR, TS-PCR, ISH	DSS	S/RT/CRT	91 (3)	79 (3)	Favourable
Mellin [373]	60	C-PCR	SR, CSMR	RT	53.5 (5)	31.5 (5)	Favourable
Friesland [374]	40	C-PCR	OS	RT	30 (5)	19 (5)	Favourable
Ringstrom [125]	89	C-PCR	DSS	Not stated	94.1 (5)	54 (5)	Favourable
Klussmann [375]	34	C-PCR, p16	OS, DFS	S±CRT	62 (4)	33 (4)	Favourable
Li [376]	86	C-PCR, TS-PCR, p16	DSS	S/RT/SRT	89 (5)	65 (5)	Favourable
Ritchie [122]	139	C-PCR	SR	S/RT/CRT	71 (5)	49 (5)	Favourable
Baez [377]	118	TS-PCR	OS, DFS	Not stated	50 (3)	31.8 (3)	No difference[a]
Wittekindt [378]	34	C-PCR, p16	DFS, RR	Not stated	72 (4)	23 (4)	Favourable
Licitra [124]	90	RT-PCR	OS	S±RT	79[b] (5)	46 (5)	Favourable
Weinberger [135]	79	RT-PCR, p16	OS, DFS	SRT/RT	79 (5)	20 (5)	Favourable
Badaracco [379]	115	TS-PCR	DFS, OS	S	66.1 (2)	53.2 (2)	No difference[a]
Reimers [380]	106	C-PCR, p16	OS, DFS	S±RT/CRT	84 (5)	49 (5)	Favourable
Na [381]	108	C-PCR	SR	S/RT±C	100 (5)	44 (5)	Favourable
Fahkry [382]	96	C-PCR, ISH	OS, RR	CRT	95 (2)	62 (2)	Favourable
Klozar [383]	81	C-PCR	OS, DSS	S±RT	73 (3)	35 (3)	Favourable
Smith [384]	294	C-PCR	DSS, RFS	S/RT/SRT	58 (5)	15 (5)	Favourable
Chung [385]	46	RT-PCR, ISH	OS, LRR, MFS	CRT	86 (5)	35 (5)	Favourable
Kong [386]	82	C-PCR	OS	Not stated	79 (5)	50 (5)	Favourable
Lassen [387]	195	ISH, p16	OS, DSS, LRR	RT	62 (5)	26 (5)	Favourable
Shi [129]	111	RT-PCR, ISH, p16	OS, DFS	RT±C	88 (3)	67 (3)	Favourable
Hafkamp [388]	77	PCR, ISH, p16	DSS	Not stated	69 (5)	31 (5)	Favourable
Rischin [389]	172	ISH, p16, PCR	OS, FFS	CRT	91 (2)	74 (2)	Favourable
Hannisdal [390]	137	C-PCR	CS	S±RT	54 (5)	33 (5)	Favourable
Fischer [224]	365	p16	OS	S/CRT	76.7 (5)	41.5 (5)	Favourable
Ang [391]	323	ISH, p16	OS	CRT	82.4 (3)	57.1 (3)	Favourable
Fischer [392]	102	p16	OS	S/RT±C	59.3 (5)	24.5 (5)	Favourable
Smith [393]	237	C-PCR, p16	OS, DSS	Not stated	83[b] (2)	54 (2)	Favourable
Lewis [394]	239	ISH, C-PCR, p16	OS, DFS, DSS	S/S+RT/S+C	86.2 (2)	44.2 (2)	Favourable

OS overall survival, *PFS* progression-free survival, *DHR* death hazard ratio, *CS* cumulative survival, *DSS* disease-specific survival, *DR* disease recurrence, *FFS* failure-free survival, *SR* survival rate, *CSMR* cause-specific mortality risk, *RFS* recurrence-free survival, *RR* response rate, *LRR* loco-regional recurrence, *MFS* metastasis-free survival

Techniques: *TS-PCR* type-specific PCR, *C-PCR* consensus PCR, *RT-PCR* real-time PCR, *ISH* in situ hybridisation, *p16* p16 immunohistochemistry, *SAb* serum antibodies

[a] Majority of samples not oropharyngeal

[b] Survival rate quoted is for specifically those HPV positive cancers also p53 positive

HNSCC with differing extents of chromosomal aberration which correlated with clinical outcome [138]. A number of other chromosomal aberrations have been associated with outcome, including amplification at 11q13, gain of 12q24 and losses at 5q11, 6q14 and 21q11 [227, 228].

Gene Expression Profiling

Gene expression microarrays bind labelled nucleic acid, allowing inference of level of expression by measurement of the extent of binding. Such studies have identified sub-groups of HNSCCs with gene expression profiles that correlate with different aspects of prognosis, including recurrence, risk of lymph node metastasis and overall survival [229–234]. However, few have attempted to validate their predictive gene expression signature in an independent dataset.

One barrier to extrapolation of these gene expression signatures into a clinically useful test is the lack of agreement between these prognostic expression signatures, both in terms of content and size. These discrepancies have prompted scathing critiques of the prognostic usefulness of expression profiling [235] although variables such as differences in site within the upper aero-digestive tract, differences in sample preparation and differences in the platform used for hybridisation and analysis have been cited in explanation. Another issue is whether it is preferable to use pure epithelial cell material (obtained by laser capture microdissection) or fresh biopsy material (which introduces heterogeneity into the samples due to the content of stromal and immune cells). Both approaches have their value, given recent work in other models indicating that gene expression changes occur in both tumour stroma and epithelial compartments of epithelial cancers and together facilitate cancer development (reviewed in [236–238]). Recent studies have further highlighted the importance of the extracellular matrix and the pattern of the immune response in the prognosis of HNSCC [239, 240]. The gene expression pathways identified outperformed all standard methods of assessment of prognosis, and the power of this analysis was demonstrated by reproduction of the prognostic signature in an independent dataset [239].

Thus, the ability to map a particular gene expression signal consistently to clinical outcome or response to therapy is still elusive [241]. Prospective studies which test the clinical predictive power of these gene expression profiles are still lacking, and it is uncertain if any of these expression profiles will complete the translation into the clinic.

Surgical Margin Analysis and Minimal Residual Cancer

One of the key parameters in the excision of HNSCC and limitation of recurrence is the status of the surgical margin [242]. Given the concept of field cancerisation, the area of genetically abnormal epithelium may extend some distance beyond clinically or histopathologically evident abnormality. The potential for molecular analysis of surgical margin to predict prognosis (local recurrence) and/or to prompt further treatment is clear. For example, Graveland et al. demonstrated that the combination of LOH at 9p and/or a large p53 positive field is predictive of local recurrence, whilst the presence and grade of dysplasia were not [243]. Numerous individual biomarkers in the surgical margin have been linked to local recurrence of HNSCC including hLy-6D and eIF4E [244, 245]. Assessment of keratin 4 and cornulin expression by immunohistochemistry (IHC) outperforms histological assessment in prediction of recurrence [246].

The presence of p53 mutations in the surgical margin has been associated with a 7.1× relative risk of local recurrence if identified in the surgical margin [247–249]. Further investigations by Partridge indicated that the presence of clonal p53 mutations in deep tissues may be a more important cause of treatment failure than mutations within the epithelium at the surgical margins [250]. Despite compelling evidence of the usefulness of such analyses, none of these is used in routine clinical practice.

Molecular Analysis for Occult Metastases in Lymph Nodes and Bone Marrow

The assessment of lymph nodes for staging purposes is largely done by histological assessment, with all the inherent sampling issues which that entails. Given that the presence of lymph node metastases is a vitally important element in the assessment of prognosis for a patient, application of molecular techniques to lymph nodes may yield further useful information. The use of immunohistochemical analysis of cytokeratin expression in the assessment of light microscopy metastasis-negative sentinel nodes is well established, and this forms part of the recently published European guideline [251].

Ferris et al. used real-time PCR for pemphigus vulgaris antigen (PVA) and another 4 markers in sentinel lymph nodes [252]. PVA discriminated the positive from negative nodes with 100% accuracy, and they demonstrated application of this in an automated testing system. Nieuwenhuis et al. demonstrated E48 (Ly-6D) expression in lymph node aspirates which improved diagnosis over cytology alone [253]. E48 expression in aspirates from bone marrow in patients with lymph node metastases correlated with a poor distant metastasis-free survival [254]. These refinements of molecular testing for metastases still require further validation in larger prospective patient cohorts.

Molecular Markers of Response to Standard Therapies

Many new molecular markers have been described which can be used to predict response to chemotherapy or radiotherapy regimens in HNSCC [255]. Some of these have emerged as surrogate markers in larger clinical trials of standard therapy (mostly cisplatin-based chemotherapy). These studies have identified gene expression profiles which predict loco-regional control after chemoradiation therapy [256] and altered expression of individual markers such as bcl-2, ERCC1, HIF1α, MRP2 and Rb which correlate with clinical outcome in multivariate analysis [255, 257–259]. In each case, the markers described still require validation in large independent patient groups.

Validation Status

The presence of HPV is an established biomarker of improved prognosis in HNSCC in patients who are not smokers. Other biomarkers of prognosis are insufficiently validated for routine clinical use and decision-making.

Table 2.6 The main biological targeted agents in use/under investigation in HNSCC

Agent	Target	Current status
Monoclonal antibodies		
Cetuximab	EGFR	Approved
Matuzumab	EGFR	Phase II
Nimotuzumab	EGFR	Phase II
Zalutumumab	EGFR	Phase III
Panitumumab	EGFR	Phase III
Bevacizumab	VEGFR	Phase III
Kinase inhibitors		
Gefitinib	EGFR	Phase III
Erlotinib	EGFR	Phase III
Lapatinib	EGFR/HER2	Phase III
Vandetanib	EGFR/VEGFR	Phase II
Sorafenib	VEGFR, PDGFR, RAF	Phase II

Biomarkers for Therapy

Anti-EGFR Therapies

The deregulation of EGFR and its signalling pathways was introduced in an earlier part of the chapter. The link between over-expression and poor prognosis has resulted in a number of therapeutic strategies aimed at disruption of EGFR function and signalling. Two main structural classes of agents have been developed (Fig. 2.2): monoclonal antibodies directed against the receptor or small molecule tyrosine kinase inhibitors (TKIs). Many individual agents have been tested in clinical trials in HNSCC, but to date, only one has gained regulatory approval.

Antibodies

The main predicted action of anti-EGFR monoclonal antibodies is high affinity interference with ligand binding, thus preventing receptor activation [260]. Other effects, such as antibody-directed cellular cytotoxicity (ADCC) and depletion of receptors from the cell surface by various mechanisms, have also been reported [261, 262]. The observation that cetuximab may block nuclear import of EGFR is particularly relevant as this may inhibit DNA repair mechanisms activated after chemotherapy or radiotherapy [263, 264]. The EGFR-targeting monoclonal antibodies in clinical studies in HNSCC are shown in Table 2.6.

2 Head and Neck Tumours

Table 2.7 Selected phase II/III published clinical studies of anti-EGFR therapy in HNSCC

Agent	Drug type	Setting	Phase	Regimen	Outcome	References
Cetuximab	mAb	LAD	III	Radiotherapy ± cetuximab	OS 49mo vs.	[272]
		RMD	III	Platinum/5FU ± cetuximab	29.3mo	[275]
		RMD	III	Cisplatin ± cetuximab	OS 10.1mo	[276]
		P-Ref	II	Cetuximab monotherapy	vs. 7.4 mo	[265]
		P-Ref	II	Pt plus cetuximab	OS 9.2 mo	[270]
		Induction	II	Carboplatin + paclitaxel + cetuximab, followed by RT ± surgery or chemo	vs. 8 mo RR 13% RR 10% ORR 96%	[277]
Gefitinib	TKI	RMD	III	Methotrexate ± gefitinib	No	[278]
		RMD	III	Docetaxel ± gefitinib	improvement	Argiris et al. 2009
		LANPC	II	Monotherapy	in survival	JCO (abstract)
		pre-treated	II	Gefitinib plus induction	No	[279]
		LAD	II	chemotherapy, followed by	improvement	Doss et al. 2006
		RMD		chemoRT	in survival	JCO (abstract)
				Monotherapy	No response 32% CR, 53% PR OR 8%	[280]
Erlotinib	TKI	RMD	I/II	Cisplatin, radiotherapy and	OR 74%	[281]
		RMD	II	erlotinib Cisplatin plus erlotinib		[282]
Lapatinib	Dual TKI	RMD	II	Monotherapy	OR 0%	[283]
Combination		RMD	II	Erlotinib + bevacizumab	ORR 15%	[284]

mAb monoclonal antibody, *TKI* tyrosine kinase inhibitor, *LAD* locally advanced disease, *RMD* relapsed/metastatic disease, *P-Ref* platinum refractory, *OS* overall survival, *RR* response rate, *OR* overall response, *CR* complete response, *PR* partial response

Cetuximab

Cetuximab is a human-mouse chimeric IgG1 monoclonal antibody which has been extensively studied in pre-clinical and clinical evaluation. Early-stage clinical trials indicated efficacy in combination with radiotherapy or chemotherapy. The use of cetuximab as monotherapy has also found some success, and it is active and well tolerated in patients who had progressed on platinum-based therapy [265, 266].

In combination with other treatment regimen, cetuximab showed good indication of efficacy in a number of pre-clinical and early-stage clinical trials in locally advanced disease [267–271]. A summary of selected clinical trials is presented in Table 2.7. In a randomised phase III clinical trial, Bonner et al. reported the addition of cetuximab to radiotherapy in locally advanced disease resulted in improvement in loco-regional control and survival (progression-free and overall), with no increase in the acute toxicity of therapy

[272]. There was no reduction in the rate of distant metastases, and post hoc analyses have demonstrated differences in efficacy between sub-sites, with most effect in the oropharynx (but interestingly, no investigation of the possible influence of HPV) [273]. Similar findings have been found in other phase III trials [274]. There is interest in the combination of cetuximab and platinum therapy combined with irradiation and an exploratory phase II study initially showed promising efficacy [269]. However, adverse events resulted in early termination of this study. A large phase III trial studying the role of cetuximab with increasing treatment intensity has recently closed for patient enrolment (RTOG 0522).

A further use of cetuximab is in relapsed or metastatic disease (RMD) in addition to chemotherapy, which has been the subject of a recent review [285]. Burtness demonstrated improved response rates upon addition of cetuximab

(26% vs. 10% for placebo) [276]. Further phase II/III trials have demonstrated improved overall and progression-free survival when cetuximab was added to a first-line chemotherapy regimen [275, 286]. Sub-set analysis demonstrated greater efficacy in young and fit patients and in those who received cisplatin. A number of questions relating to the sequence of drugs in the regime and the possibility of cross resistance have been raised by other authors, and these issues will be addressed in future randomised studies [287]. Phase II trials of cetuximab with other agents, such as pacli-taxel, have commenced, as this combination has been investigated in NSCLC [288].

A number of studies are underway in patients with advanced disease to assess the efficacy of the addition of cetuximab to induction regimens in locally advanced disease [274, 289]. The use of cetuximab monotherapy prior to cetuximab plus concurrent chemoradiotherapy resulted in good disease control [290]. Other phase II studies have used cetuximab with other chemotherapeutic agents in the induction setting (either doublet or triplet) [277]. The initial data from these trials are encouraging, but further investigation is needed to determine the safety and efficacy of cetuximab in combination with induction chemotherapy.

Toxicity Profile

The toxicity profile of cetuximab includes the characteristic skin toxicities, namely, rash, hair and nail changes [291]. Other side effects include asthenia, pain, fever and weight loss [268, 292]. Occasional allergic reactions have been reported [293, 294]. Whilst many trials have reported no increase in acute toxicity in combination therapy, late toxicities may yet emerge, and some investi-gators have suggested that cetuximab toxicity may have been underestimated [295].

Validation Status

Cetuximab has proven benefit in the treatment of locally advanced HNSCC, treatment of incurable relapsed/metastatic disease and as second-line treatment after failure of platinum-based therapy. Regulatory approval has been obtained for primary therapy, with radiotherapy, in locally

advanced HNSCC. Clinical trials for use in refractory disease in combination with other drug regimen are ongoing.

Other Anti-EGFR Antibodies

A number of other monoclonal antibodies are in clinical studies in HNSCC. These are listed in Table 2.6 and include zalutumumab, panitu-mumab, matuzumab and nimotuzumab [296].

Zalutumumab is a completely human IgG1 antibody against human EGFR. As it has no murine component, it is predicted to be much less immunogenic, with consequent reduction in hypersensitivity reactions [297]. Zalutumumab has shown promise for use in recurrent/metastatic HNSCC in phase I/II studies, with one such study reporting partial response or disease stability in 9/11 patient with the highest dose [297]. Other phase I/II studies in locally advanced disease with chemoradiotherapy or with radiotherapy in patients who are not able to receive platinum-based chemotherapy are underway as are a number of phase III trials (including DEHANCA 19, in combination with radiotherapy as primary treatment). One phase III trial has demonstrated extension of progression-free survival (but not overall survival) in HNSCC patients who had failed platinum-based therapy [298].

Panitumumab has demonstrated safety and effi-cacy in combination with carboplatin and radio-therapy in pre-clinical and phase I clinical studies in advanced HNSCC [299, 300]. A number of clinical studies (mostly phase II) are currently underway to assess the use of panitumumab in locally advanced or recurrent/metastatic disease. Nimotuzumab similarly shows some promise in treatment naïve HNSCC [301]. Matuzumab is yet another monoclonal antibody, but has a markedly extended half-life which allows for reduction in frequency of administration [302]. It is currently in early-stage clinical studies in HNSCC.

Validation Status

Other monoclonal antibodies show promise for use in locally advanced or recurrent HNSCC. Phase II and III clinical trials are currently underway.

Tyrosine Kinase Inhibitors

Ligand binding to EGFR results in receptor dimerisation and the activation of tyrosine kinase domains in the cytoplasmic region of the receptor. A number of small molecule inhibitors of the EGFR tyrosine kinase have been developed. These inhibit the phosphorylation of tyrosine residues of EGFR in a selective and reversible manner. Agents with this activity which are presently undergoing clinical evaluation include gefitinib, erlotinib and lapatinib (Tables 2.6 and 2.7).

A number of phase I/II trials have reported the use of gefitinib in relapsed/metastatic HNSCC as first- or second-line treatment [278, 303, 304] and also in locally advanced disease [305–309]. These reveal a response rate of 8–10%, with disease control varying from 36 to 53% [304]. Initial studies of gefitinib with chemoradiotherapy showed promising response rates with acceptable toxicity, but a number of phase III trials have demonstrated little or no improvement in survival [278]. The main toxicities reported in the clinical trials of gefitinib have been skin rash and gastrointestinal effects [310].

Erlotinib has also been studied in cohorts of patients with relapsed/metastatic HNSCC. Several phase I/II trials have demonstrated clinical benefit, some in combination with other targeted therapies [281, 282, 284]. However, some phase III investigations have been terminated early. Lapatinib shows dual specificity for EGFR and Her2 tyrosine kinase [311]. In phase I studies in HNSCC, lapatinib was well tolerated, and a number of phase II studies are underway [312].

Validation Status

TKIs have demonstrated some clinical efficacy and a good safety profile for use in clinical trials in HNSCC. None have been approved for use in HNSCC.

Markers of Response to Anti-EGFR Therapy

The identification of molecular markers to both predict and reflect the action of anti-EGFR therapies has proved problematic.

- Clinical markers: the development of the characteristic "acneiform" rash on the face and torso has been reported after the use of a number of both monoclonal antibodies and TKIs. This affects approximately 60% of patients and usually develops within the first 3 weeks of treatment. A number of studies have demonstrated higher response rate and improvement in survival in patients who develop this skin toxicity [273].

- EGFR protein expression: the correlation between EGFR expression and response to anti-EGFR therapy is poor, as seen in other cancers [313]. A number of explanations have been mooted including variation in laboratory techniques or in assessment of the staining [221, 314]. Recent attempts to standardise assessment are more promising [315].

- EGFR gene amplification: the rate of amplification of EGFR varies greatly between studies (10–58%) [214, 316–318]. No study has definitively identified an association between gene amplification and response to anti-EGFR therapy in HNSCC nor has a convincing association between amplification and expression been demonstrated [315, 316]. Many factors may play a part in such marked variation, including differences in sub-site or method of analysis.

- Several EGFR polymorphisms have been shown to be associated with variation in response to anti-EGFR therapy in a number of cancers, including NSCLC [319, 320]. This has not, as yet, been convincingly demonstrated in HNSCC.

- Mutations: the incidence of mutations in the kinase domain is low in HNSCC when compared to other cancers, such as NSCLC [216, 321]. Mutations in K-RAS in colorectal carcinoma and NSCLC predict resistance to EGFR therapy, but these are also very rare in HNSCC [322].

- Others: many other possible markers for predication of response to EGFR-targeted therapy in HNSCC have been suggested. These include activation of the MAPK pathway, PI3K, AKT, STAT 3/5 and crosstalk with IGF-1R [323–325].

Anti-angiogenic Therapy

The control of tumour vascularisation involves a number of both pro- and anti-angiogenic factors. Perhaps, the most noteworthy of these is VEGF, a

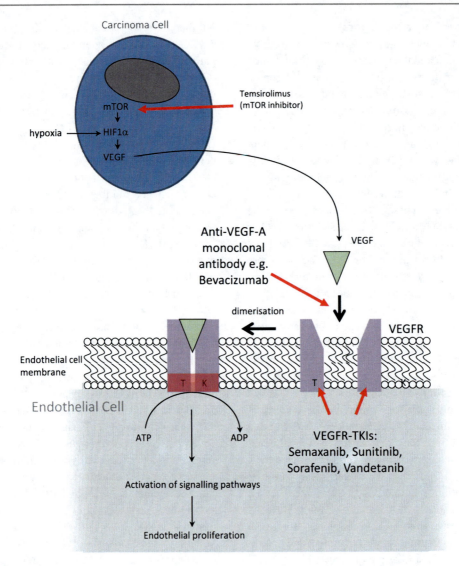

Fig. 2.3 VEGF signalling and the action of anti-angiogenic agents. In the tumour cells, one method of VEGF production is via mTOR. mTOR stimulates hypoxia inducible factor 1α (HIF-1α) synthesis. In hypoxic conditions, persistence of HIF-1α leads to release of VEGF. VEGF receptors on endothelial cell membrane dimerise in response to ligand binding, activating intra-cellular tyrosine kinase (TK) activity. ATP-dependent phosphorylation of intra-cellular proteins then acts as a signalling pathway, ultimately leading to endothelial activation and proliferation. The diagram also indicates the site of action of the two main classes of anti-VEGFR agent: monoclonal antibodies and tyrosine kinase inhibitors

pro-angiogenic growth factor known to be expressed by approximately 60% of all human cancer types, including cancers of the head and neck region [326, 327]. Significant attention has therefore been paid to the development of drugs which either inhibit the action of VEGF directly or influence the subsequent signalling cascades triggered by receptor binding. The actions of VEGF, along with targets of anti-angiogenic agents, are summarised in Fig. 2.3 [328–330].

Inhibition of VEGF Function

VEGF belongs to the platelet-derived growth factor superfamily and can be sub-classified into types A to E, plus PlGF (placental growth factor) [327]. VEGF-A is by far the most important of these sub-types with respect to angiogenesis; other sub-types are generally less influential or have more specialist roles, such as the promotion of lymphangiogenesis and embryonic angiogenesis. Ligand binding leads to receptor dimerisation, thereby activating an intra-cellular tyrosine kinase domain responsible for catalysing ATP-dependent protein phosphorylation.

To date, only a single anti-VEGFR antibody (bevacizumab) has FDA approval for the management of certain metastatic cancers, namely, colon, NSCLC and breast [331]. In a similar manner to anti-EGFR therapy, there is an apparent lack of validated biomarkers to predict or reflect response to bevacizumab [332]. A number of small molecules have been developed which inhibit VEGFR tyrosine kinase, although for many, their clinical efficacy is yet to be fully determined. Sunitinib, one such tyrosine kinase inhibitor, has gained FDA approval for use in renal cell carcinoma and gastrointestinal stromal tumours and European Commission approval for use in advanced pancreatic neuroendocrine tumours [333].

Clinical Application of Anti-angiogenic Agents

The application of anti-angiogenic agents in head and neck cancer has so far been limited to early clinical trials, for which promising results have been reported when used as adjuvant therapy [334]. Single-agent therapy has largely been unsuccessful, illustrated by the early trial closure of sunitinib monotherapy following interim analysis demonstrating low efficacy [335]. The majority of available data for head and neck cancer relate to phase II trials with a number of anti-angiogenic agents (Table 2.8), although phase III trials are ongoing. It should be noted that studies have largely targeted locally advanced, recurrent or metastatic disease, and the value of anti-angiogenic agents in early head and neck cancer has yet to be determined.

Efficacy of VEGF/VEGFR inhibition is now established in the management of a number of cancers outside the head and neck region. In most cases, a moderate improvement in life expectancy

is seen, as tumours ultimately develop resistance to therapy. These modest benefits have led researchers to consider more widespread inhibition of growth factor pathways in an attempt to improve outcome further. An intuitive "next step" has been to assess the value of dual inhibition of VEGF and EGF pathways [284]. Agents, such as vandetanib, are dual TKIs and will inhibit both EGF and VEGF. Use of these agents in HNSCC is largely at pre-clinical stage, but the early results have been encouraging [343].

Other Anti-angiogenic Agents

VEGF Trap is a novel molecule which comprises a VEGF receptor decoy fused to the Fc region of human IgG1. As its receptor domain is derived from human VEGFRs 1 and 2, its affinity for VEGF is greater than that of bevacizumab. It is capable of binding all isoforms of VEGF A, B and PlGF and is therefore a potent inhibitor of the VEGF pathway. VEGF Trap is currently in phase II/III trials for colonic cancer, NSCLC and prostatic cancer, amongst others [344]. No studies are currently underway for the management of head and neck cancer, and the prospect of such trials is likely to rely on the success of this drug in the management of cancers elsewhere.

As VEGF is just one of many signalling molecules that influence angiogenesis, tumour resistance to VEGF blockade occurs through the activation of alternative, secondary pathways of angiogenesis, which are now gaining interest in the attempt to control such resistance. Another area of interest lies in the production of vascular disrupting agents: these agents aim to completely deprive the tumour of a blood supply, leading to widespread cell death. Assessment of vascular disrupting agents has so far been limited to phase II trials, and little data outside of laboratory studies are available on their effect in head and neck cancer. It is beyond the scope of this chapter to discuss vascular disrupting agents in detail, although they have been reviewed elsewhere [345].

Management of HPV-Positive Oropharyngeal Carcinoma

The ultimate goal in the management of HPV-positive cancer is the application of a tailored

Table 2.8 Selected clinical studies with anti-angiogenic agents

Agent(s)	Setting	Phase	Outcome	Reference
Semaxanib	RMD	II	Single partial response, single minor response	[336]
Sorafenib	RMD	II	Sorafenib well tolerated: modest activity comparable to monotherapy with other targeted agents	[337]
Bevacizumab and pemetrexed	RMD	II	ORR 36%. Bleeding complications implicated with therapy, but encouraging efficacy	Feinstein et al. 2008, J Clin Oncol (abstract)
Bevacizumab and docetaxel	LAD	II	89% 1-year survival: No episodes of severe bleeding noted	Savvides et al. 2008, J Clin Oncol (abstract)
Bevacizumab and erlotinib	RMD	II	15% RR, 4 CR. High ratio of phosphorylated: total VEGFR2 in pre-treatment biopsies associated with response	[284]
Cediranib monotherapy	RMD	II	Cediranib monotherapy has anti-tumour activity — 19% PRR	Saura et al, 2009, J Clin Oncol (abstract)
Bevacizumab plus 5-fluorouracil	Intermed stage	II	RR 92% no increase in bleeding complications	Choong et al. 2009, J Clin Oncol (abstract)
Bevacizumab plus cisplatin	LAD	II	100% loco-regional control rate	Pfister et al, 2009, J Clin Oncol (abstract)
Bevacizumab and erlotinib	LAD	II	87% 18-month overall survival	Meluch et al, 2009, J Clin Oncol (abstract)
Vandetanib plus radiotherapy ± cisplatin	LAD	II	2 patients completed 24-month follow-up: trial ongoing	Papadimitrakopoulou et al, 2009, J Clin Oncol (Abstract)
Sorafenib	LAD/RMD	II	2% response probability: well tolerated	[338]
Sunitinib monotherapy	Palliative	II	4 grade 5 head and neck bleeds Modest activity in palliative head and neck cancer	[339]
Sunitinib monotherapy	RMD	II	Low single-agent activity, leading to early closure of trial	[335]
Sunitinib monotherapy	RMD	II	Early closure of trial due to futility 10 bleeding complications in 7 patients	[340]
Bevacizumab in combination with pemetrexed	RMD	II	Overall response rate 30%: 5% complete response rate. 15% grade 3–5 bleeding events	[341]
Sunitinib	Irradiated nasopharyngeal carcinoma	II	64% of cases developed haemorrhagic complications: 2 fatal haemorrhages	[342]

ORR overall response rate, *RR* response rate, *CR* complete response, *PRR* partial response rate

therapeutic measure that will beneficially influence outcome. This may take many guises, from the alteration of currently utilised modalities (i.e. radiotherapy, chemotherapy, surgery), to account for the less aggressive course of disease, to the use of adjuvants that act to improve survival. Primary prevention, namely the inclusion of males in current HPV vaccination programmes, is also a potential, yet widely disputed option; the cost of such a public health measure is currently regarded as excessive [346, 347].

The Potential Role of Gene Therapy in HPV-Positive OPC

Sima et al. used small hairpin RNA (shRNA) to deliver small interfering RNA (siRNA) targeting the HPV16 E7 oncogene in HPV-positive cervical cancer cell lines [348]. E6 and E7 expression was found to be suppressed, allowing intra-cellular accumulation of p53 and p21, ultimately leading to massive apoptotic cell death. The authors concluded that use of RNA interference may have gene therapy potential for HPV16-related cancers. Similar findings have also been documented with the use of adenovirus to deliver anti-sense RNA transcripts of E6 and E7 in cervical cancer cell lines [349]. As yet, no clinical trials have taken place for HPV-targeted gene therapy.

Therapeutic Vaccination in HPV-Positive OPC

To date, the application of the two commercially available HPV vaccines (Gardasil and Cervarix) is limited to prophylaxis [128]. There is no therapeutic benefit of these vaccines, as they have no influence on established infection, as demonstrated in a large, randomised trial [350]. The vaccines act by inducing an immune response to viral capsid proteins L1 and L2; lack of therapeutic effect is due to these proteins not being expressed by already-infected basal cells [112]. The therapeutic shortcomings of L1/L2-based vaccines have led to the recent development of further vaccines which utilise other viral antigens. Obvious targets are E6 and E7, due to their intimate relationship with disease progression. Current interest lies in DNA-based vaccines due to their safety and stability, although they have been found to be poorly immunogenic [112].

Other Therapies

A number of other therapies are under early-stage clinical investigation for use in HNSCC. Agents which target various elements of the intra-cellular signalling pathways have been developed. In HNSCC, much interest has centred on the PI3K/AKT/mTOR pathway. Potent inhibitors of mTOR such as everolimus are currently in early-stage clinical studies in HNSCC [351]. Alterations in this pathway are not ubiquitous in HNSCC; thus, sensitive molecular markers are needed to guide therapy.

The family of Src kinases are activated in response to EGFR stimulation. Activation of these kinases has been associated with epithelial–mesenchymal transition (EMT) in HNSCC and thus with the promotion of invasion [352]. A number of Src targeting agents have been developed, including dasatinib and AZD0530, both of which are being used in phase II studies in HNSCC [353]. The possibility of combination with anti-EGFR therapy is also being explored [354].

Targeting the tumour microenvironment is a large area of development of new anti-cancer therapies. Cancer-associated inflammation plays a key role in the development of many tumours including HNSCC. Cyclooxygenase 2 is a pro-inflammatory mediator which promotes a number of other cell functions, many of which are pro-tumourigenic in an appropriate environment. Recent phase I/II trials of COX2 inhibition showed benefit in combination with erlotinib [355]. The use of COX2 inhibitors has also been suggested as a chemopreventive strategy in potentially malignant lesions [356]. Other components of the cancer-associated inflammatory/immune response also prove to be promising targets for molecular therapy, for example, chemokine receptors such as CXCR4 [357].

Identification of the key events in the control of tumours invasion has also provided a number of interesting targets for novel therapies. For the most part, these are still in pre-clinical development, but modulation of integrin function, for example, of integrin $\alpha V\beta 6$, is a promising area of development [199, 358].

Recombinant pro-apoptotic receptor ligands are being used to enhance pro-apoptotic signalling in a number of cancers. Studies of TRAIL receptor antibodies are underway in a number of cancers, including HNSCC [359]. A number of other pro-apoptotic agents are being developed.

Validation Status

All other therapies are at a pre-clinical or early phase clinical study.

Other Tumour Types

Sinonasal and Nasopharynx

The potential of anti-EGFR therapy in nasopharyngeal carcinoma has been investigated in a number of phase II trials. Results of the use of gefitinib in relapsed/metastatic disease showed no evidence of response [279, 360]. However, the addition of cetuximab to platinum-based therapy demonstrated a 12% overall response rate [361]. In locally advanced disease, cetuximab has been added to platinum-based chemoradiotherapy with encouraging early results, but the full report is still awaited.

Salivary Gland

Despite expression of CD117 (c-kit) in up to 80% of cases of ADCC, the use of imatinib has been disappointing [362–364]. There is, to date, no evidence of an improved overall response rate. Studies using sunitinib have proved similarly disappointing as have those using cetuximab, gefitinib or other agents such as bortezomib [365, 366]. However, all of these studies reported some amount of disease stabilisation whilst on therapy.

The role of molecular targeted therapy in other salivary gland carcinomas has been the subject of very limited investigation. Phase II trials of gefitinib, trastuzumab and lapatinib and other agents have included non-ADCC salivary carcinomas and demonstrate variable disease stabilisation, but no increase in overall response rate [366–369].

Odontogenic Carcinomas

There have been no clinical trials of targeted therapy in odontogenic malignant tumours.

Validation Status

The potential for use of targeted therapy is being explored in a number of other histologically defined head and neck tumours. All are in early-stage clinical studies, and none are approved for routine clinical use.

Conclusion

There is great potential for the use of biologically targeted therapy in head and neck tumours, particularly given the rather dismal prognosis of many HNSCC patients. Many agents are now undergoing phase III clinical assessment, and although only one (cetuximab) has received approval, it appears likely that others will follow. For some, toxicities may limit use; thus, it is vital that new agents are identified with validated pharmacodynamic and pharmacokinetic markers. However, progress is hampered by a lack of well-validated markers for diagnosis, prognostication and assessment of overall response to targeted therapy. In rarer head and neck tumours, such as those of the nasopharynx, sinonasal region and salivary glands, there has been much less investigation, but there is some promise that targeted therapy may find a place in the management of these tumours.

References

1. Parkin DM, Bray F, Ferlay J, Pisani P. Global cancer statistics, 2002. CA Cancer J Clin. 2005;55(2):74–108.
2. Kruse AL, Bredell M, Grätz KW. Oral cancer in men and women: are there differences? Oral Maxillofac Surg. 2011;15(1):51–5.
3. Fast Stats: An interactive tool for access to SEER cancer statistics. Surveillance Research Program, National Cancer Institute. http://seer.cancer.gov/faststats. (Accessed 17 Feb 2011).
4. Sturgis EM, Cinciripini PM. Trends in head and neck cancer incidence in relation to smoking prevalence: an emerging epidemic of human papillomavirus-associated cancers? Cancer. 2007;110(7): 1429–35.
5. Tanaka S, Sobue T. Comparison of oral and pharyngeal cancer mortality in five countries: France, Italy, Japan, UK and USA from the WHO Mortality Database (1960–2000). Jpn J Clin Oncol. 2005;35(8): 488–91.

6. Conway DI, Stockton DL, Warnakulasuriya KA, Ogden G, Macpherson LM. Incidence of oral and oropharyngeal cancer in United Kingdom (1990–1999)—recent trends and regional variation. Oral Oncol. 2006;42(6):586–92.

7. Jemal A, Center MM, DeSantis C, Ward EM. Global patterns of cancer incidence and mortality rates and trends. Cancer Epidemiol Biomarkers Prev. 2010; 19(8):1893–907.

8. Jemal A, Siegel R, Xu J, Ward E. Cancer statistics, 2010. CA Cancer J Clin. 2010;60(5):277–300.

9. Toner M, O'Regan EM. Head and neck squamous cell carcinoma in the young: a spectrum or a distinct group? Part 2. Head Neck Pathol. 2009;3(3): 249–51.

10. Toner M, O'Regan EM. Head and neck squamous cell carcinoma in the young: a spectrum or a distinct group? Part 1. Head Neck Pathol. 2009;3(3):246–8.

11. Llewellyn CD, Linklater K, Bell J, Johnson NW, Warnakulasuriya KA. Squamous cell carcinoma of the oral cavity in patients aged 45 years and under: a descriptive analysis of 116 cases diagnosed in the South East of England from 1990 to 1997. Oral Oncol. 2003;39(2):106–14.

12. Llewellyn CD, Linklater K, Bell J, Johnson NW, Warnakulasuriya S. An analysis of risk factors for oral cancer in young people: a case-control study. Oral Oncol. 2004;40(3):304–13.

13. Shiboski CH, Shiboski SC, Silverman Jr S. Trends in oral cancer rates in the United States, 1973–1996. Community Dent Oral Epidemiol. 2000;28(4): 249–56.

14. Harris SL, Kimple RJ, Hayes DN, Couch ME, Rosenman JG. Never-smokers, never-drinkers: unique clinical subgroup of young patients with head and neck squamous cell cancers. Head Neck. 2010;32(4):499–503.

15. Shiboski CH, Schmidt BL, Jordan RC. Tongue and tonsil carcinoma: increasing trends in the U.S. population ages 20–44 years. Cancer. 2005;103(9): 1843–9.

16. Adelstein DJ, Ridge JA, Gillison ML, Chaturvedi AK, D'Souza G, Gravitt PE, et al. Head and neck squamous cell cancer and the human papillomavirus: summary of a National Cancer Institute State of the Science Meeting, November 9–10, 2008, Washington, DC. Head Neck. 2009;31(11):1393–422.

17. D'Souza G, Kreimer AR, Viscidi R, Pawlita M, Fakhry C, Koch WM, et al. Case-control study of human papillomavirus and oropharyngeal cancer. N Engl J Med. 2007;356(19):1944–56.

18. Gillison ML, Koch WM, Capone RB, Spafford M, Westra WH, Wu L, et al. Evidence for a causal association between human papillomavirus and a subset of head and neck cancers. J Natl Cancer Inst. 2000; 92(9):709–20.

19. Schantz SP, Yu GP. Head and neck cancer incidence trends in young Americans, 1973–1997, with a special analysis for tongue cancer. Arch Otolaryngol Head Neck Surg. 2002;128(3):268–74.

20. Batsakis JG, Rice DH, Solomon AR. The pathology of head and neck tumors: squamous and mucous-gland carcinomas of the nasal cavity, paranasal sinuses, and larynx, part 6. Head Neck Surg. 1980; 2(6):497–508.

21. O'Sullivan EM. International variation in the incidence of oral and pharyngeal cancer. Community Dent Health. 2008;25(3):148–53.

22. Parkin DM, S.L. W, Ferlay J, Teppo L, Thomas DB. Cancer incidence in five continents, vols. V-VIII: IARC Scientific Publication; 2003

23. Spiro RH. Salivary neoplasms: overview of a 35-year experience with 2,807 patients. Head Neck Surg. 1986;8(3):177–84.

24. Barnes L, Eveson J, Reichart P, Sidransky DE. Pathology and genetics of head and neck tumours. Lyon: IARC Press; 2005.

25. Altekruse SF, Kosary CL, Krapcho M, Neyman N, Aminou R, Waldron W, et al. SEER cancer statistics review, 1975–2007, National Cancer Institute. Bethesda, MD, http://seer.cancer.gov/csr/1975_2007/, based on November 2009 SEER data submission, posted to the SEER web site, 2010

26. Goode RK, Auclair PL, Ellis GL. Mucoepidermoid carcinoma of the major salivary glands: clinical and histopathologic analysis of 234 cases with evaluation of grading criteria. Cancer. 1998;82(7): 1217–24.

27. de Oliveira FA, Duarte EC, Taveira CT, Maximo AA, de Aquino EC, Alencar Rde C, et al. Salivary gland tumor: a review of 599 cases in a Brazilian population. Head Neck Pathol. 2009;3(4):271–5.

28. Eveson JW, Cawson RA. Salivary gland tumours. A review of 2410 cases with particular reference to histological types, site, age and sex distribution. J Pathol. 1985;146(1):51–8.

29. Boukheris H, Curtis RE, Land CE, Dores GM. Incidence of carcinoma of the major salivary glands according to the WHO classification, 1992 to 2006: a population-based study in the United States. Cancer Epidemiol Biomarkers Prev. 2009;18(11): 2899–906.

30. Mosqueda-Taylor A, Ledesma-Montes C, Caballero-Sandoval S, Portilla-Robertson J, Ruiz-Godoy Rivera LM, Meneses-Garcia A. Odontogenic tumors in Mexico: a collaborative retrospective study of 349 cases. Oral Surg Oral Med Oral Pathol Oral Radiol Endod. 1997;84(6):672–5.

31. Buchner A, Merrell PW, Carpenter WM. Relative frequency of central odontogenic tumors: a study of 1,088 cases from Northern California and comparison to studies from other parts of the world. J Oral Maxillofac Surg. 2006;64(9):1343–52.

32. Hall JM, Weathers DR, Unni KK. Ameloblastic carcinoma: an analysis of 14 cases. Oral Surg Oral Med Oral Pathol Oral Radiol Endod. 2007;103(6): 799–807.

33. Hu YC, Sidransky D, Ahrendt SA. Molecular detection approaches for smoking associated tumors. Oncogene. 2002;21(48):7289–97.

34. Temam S, Trassard M, Leroux G, Bosq J, Luboinski B, Lenoir G, et al. Cytology vs molecular analysis for the detection of head and neck squamous cell carcinoma in oesopharyngeal brush samples: a prospective study in 56 patients. Br J Cancer. 2003; 88(11):1740–5.

35. Temam S, Benard J, Dugas C, Trassard M, Gormally E, Soria JC, et al. Molecular detection of early-stage laryngopharyngeal squamous cell carcinomas. Clin Cancer Res. 2005;11(7):2547–51.

36. Bremmer JF, Graveland AP, Brink A, Braakhuis BJ, Kuik DJ, Leemans CR, et al. Screening for oral precancer with noninvasive genetic cytology. Cancer Prev Res (Phila). 2009;2(2):128–33.

37. Veltman JA, Hopman AH, Bot FJ, Ramaekers FC, Manni JJ. Detection of chromosomal aberrations in cytologic brush specimens from head and neck squamous cell carcinoma. Cancer. 1997;81(5):309–14.

38. Bocking A, Sproll C, Stocklein N, Naujoks C, Depprich R, Kubler NR, et al. Role of brush biopsy and DNA cytometry for prevention, diagnosis, therapy, and followup care of oral cancer. J Oncol. 2011:875959

39. Remmerbach TW, Meyer-Ebrecht D, Aach T, Wurflinger T, Bell AA, Schneider TE, et al. Toward a multimodal cell analysis of brush biopsies for the early detection of oral cancer. Cancer Cytopathol. 2009;117(3):228–35.

40. Roepman P, Holstege FCP. Tumor profiling turmoil. Cell Cycle (Georgetown, Tex). 2005;4(5):659–60.

41. Lallemant B, Evrard A, Combescure C, Chapuis H, Chambon G, Raynal C, et al. Clinical relevance of nine transcriptional molecular markers for the diagnosis of head and neck squamous cell carcinoma in tissue and saliva rinse. BMC Cancer. 2009;9:370.

42. Whipple ME, Mendez E, Farwell DG, Agoff SN, Chen C. A genomic predictor of oral squamous cell carcinoma. Laryngoscope. 2004;114(8):1346–54.

43. Roepman P. The future of diagnostic gene-expression microarrays: bridging the gap between bench and bedside. Bioanalysis. 2010;2(2):249–62.

44. Lallemant B, Evrard A, Chambon G, Sabra O, Kacha S, Lallemant JG, et al. Gene expression profiling in head and neck squamous cell carcinoma: Clinical perspectives. Head Neck. 2010;32(12):1712–9.

45. Rezende TM, de Souza Freire M, Franco OL. Head and neck cancer: proteomic advances and biomarker achievements. Cancer. 2010;116(21):4914–25.

46. Winters RD, Naud S, Evans MF, Trotman WE, Kasznica P, Elhosseiny A. Ber-EP4, CK1, CK7 and CK14 are useful markers for identifying basaloid squamous carcinoma. A study of 45 cases. Lab Invest. 2008;88:243a–44a.

47. Suo Z, Holm R, Nesland JM. Squamous cell carcinomas. An immunohistochemical study of cytokeratins and involucrin in primary and metastatic tumours. Histopathology. 1993;23(1):45–54.

48. Suo Z, Qvist H, Su W, Holm R, Giercksky KE, Nesland JM. Undifferentiated carcinoma: an immunohistochemical and ultrastructural study. Anticancer Res. 1993;13(3):643–9.

49. Park JM, Jung CK, Choi YJ, Lee KY, Kang JH, Kim MS, et al. The use of an immunohistochemical diagnostic panel to determine the primary site of cervical lymph node metastases of occult squamous cell carcinoma. Hum Pathol. 2010;41(3):431–7.

50. Garrel R, Dromard M, Costes V, Barbotte E, Comte F, Gardiner Q, et al. The diagnostic accuracy of reverse transcription-PCR quantification of cytokeratin mRNA in the detection of sentinel lymph node invasion in oral and oropharyngeal squamous cell carcinoma: a comparison with immunohistochemistry. Clin Cancer Res. 2006;12(8):2498–505.

51. Roesch-Ely M, Nees M, Karsai S, Ruess A, Bogumil R, Warnken U, et al. Proteomic analysis reveals successive aberrations in protein expression from healthy mucosa to invasive head and neck cancer. Oncogene. 2007;26(1):54–64.

52. Sethi S, Benninger MS, Lu M, Havard S, Worsham MJ. Noninvasive molecular detection of head and neck squamous cell carcinoma: an exploratory analysis. Diagn Mol Pathol. 2009;18(2):81–7.

53. Boyle JO, Mao L, Brennan JA, Koch WM, Eisele DW, Saunders JR, et al. Gene mutations in saliva as molecular markers for head and neck squamous cell carcinomas. Am J Surg. 1994;168(5):429–32.

54. Spafford MF, Koch WM, Reed AL, Califano JA, Xu LH, Eisenberger CF, et al. Detection of head and neck squamous cell carcinoma among exfoliated oral mucosal cells by microsatellite analysis. Clin Cancer Res. 2001;7(3):607–12.

55. Okami K, Imate Y, Hashimoto Y, Kamada T, Takahashi M. Molecular detection of cancer cells in saliva from oral and pharyngeal cancer patients. Tokai J Exp Clin Med. 2002;27(3):85–9.

56. El-Naggar AK, Mao L, Staerkel G, Coombes MM, Tucker SL, Luna MA, et al. Genetic heterogeneity in saliva from patients with oral squamous carcinomas: implications in molecular diagnosis and screening. J Mol Diagn. 2001;3(4):164–70.

57. Rosas SL, Koch W, da Costa Carvalho MG, Wu L, Califano J, Westra W, et al. Promoter hypermethylation patterns of p16, O6-methylguanine-DNA-methyltransferase, and death-associated protein kinase in tumors and saliva of head and neck cancer patients. Cancer Res. 2001;61(3):939–42.

58. Righini CA, de Fraipont F, Timsit JF, Faure C, Brambilla E, Reyt E, et al. Tumor-specific methylation in saliva: a promising biomarker for early detection of head and neck cancer recurrence. Clin Cancer Res. 2007;13(4):1179–85. ·

59. Demokan S, Chang X, Chuang A, Mydlarz WK, Kaur J, Huang P, et al. KIF1A and EDNRB are differentially methylated in primary HNSCC and salivary rinses. Int J Cancer. 2010;127(10):2351–9.

60. Carvalho AL, Jeronimo C, Kim MM, Henrique R, Zhang Z, Hoque MO, et al. Evaluation of promoter hypermethylation detection in body fluids as a screening/diagnosis tool for head and neck squamous cell carcinoma. Clin Cancer Res. 2008;14(1):97–107.

61. Yakushiji T, Noma H, Shibahara T, Arai K, Yamamoto N, Tanaka C, et al. Analysis of a role for

p16/CDKN2 expression and methylation patterns in human oral squamous cell carcinoma. Bull Tokyo Dent Coll. 2001;42(3):159–68.

62. Nakahara Y, Shintani S, Mihara M, Ueyama Y, Matsumura T. High frequency of homozygous deletion and methylation of p16(INK4A) gene in oral squamous cell carcinomas. Cancer Lett. 2001;163(2):221–8.

63. Calmon MF, Colombo J, Carvalho F, Souza FP, Filho JF, Fukuyama EE, et al. Methylation profile of genes CDKN2A (p14 and p16), DAPK1, CDH1, and ADAM23 in head and neck cancer. Cancer Genet Cytogenet. 2007;173(1):31–7.

64. Wong TS, Man MWL, Lam AKY, Wei WI, Kwong YL, Yuen APW. The study of p16 and p15 gene methylation in head and neck squamous cell carcinoma and their quantitative evaluation in plasma by real-time PCR. Eur J Cancer. 2003;39(13):1881–87.

65. Shaw RJ, Liloglou T, Rogers SN, Brown JS, Vaughan ED, Lowe D, et al. Promoter methylation of P16, RAR beta, E-cadherin, cyclin A1 and cytoglobin in oral cancer: quantitative evaluation using pyrosequencing. Br J Cancer. 2006;94(4):561–68.

66. Gao S, Worm J, Guldberg P, Eiberg H, Krogdahl A, Sorensen JA, et al. Loss of heterozygosity at 9q33 and hypermethylation of the DBCCR1 gene in oral squamous cell carcinoma. Br J Cancer. 2004;91(4):760–64.

67. Bolt J, Vo QN, Kim WJ, McWhorter AJ, Thomson J, Hagensee ME, et al. The ATM/p53 pathway is commonly targeted for inactivation in squamous cell carcinoma of the head and neck (SCCHN) by multiple molecular mechanisms. Oral Oncol. 2005;41(10):1013–20.

68. Worsham MJ, Chen KM, Meduri V, Nygren AO, Errami A, Schouten JP, et al. Epigenetic events of disease progression in head and neck squamous cell carcinoma. Arch Otolaryngol Head Neck Surg. 2006;132(6):668–77.

69. Laytragoon-Lewin N, Chen F, Castro J, Elmberger G, Rutqvist LE, Lewin F, et al. DNA content and methylation of p16, DAPK and RASSF1A gene in tumour and distant, normal mucosal tissue of head and neck squamous cell carcinoma patients. Anticancer Res. 2010;30(11):4643–8.

70. Kaur J, Demokan S, Tripathi SC, Macha MA, Begum S, Califano JA, et al. Promoter hypermethylation in Indian primary oral squamous cell carcinoma. Int J Cancer. 2010;127(10):2367–73.

71. McGregor F, Wagner E, Felix D, Soutar D, Parkinson K, Harrison PR. Inappropriate retinoic acid receptor-beta expression in oral dysplasias: correlation with acquisition of the immortal phenotype. Cancer Res. 1997;57(18):3886–9.

72. Smigiel R, Stembalska-Kozlowska A, Mirghomizadeh F, Krecicki T, Zatonski T, Ramsey D, et al. Correlation among loss of heterozygosity, promoter methylation and protein expression of MLH1 in larynx cancer. Oncol Rep. 2004;11(3):707–10.

73. Murakami J, Asaumi J, Maki Y, Tsujigiwa H, Kuroda M, Nagai N, et al. Effects of demethylating agent 5-aza-2('-)-deoxycytidine and histone deacetylase

inhibitor FR901228 on maspin gene expression in oral cancer cell lines. Oral Oncol. 2004;40(6):597–603.

74. Nakayama S, Sasaki A, Mese H, Alcalde RE, Tsuji T, Matsumura T. The E-cadherin gene is silenced by CpG methylation in human oral squamous cell carcinomas. Int J Cancer. 2001;93(5):667–73.

75. Ha PK, Califano JA. Promoter methylation and inactivation of tumour-suppressor genes in oral squamous-cell carcinoma. Lancet Oncol. 2006;7(1):77–82.

76. Fliss MS, Usadel H, Caballero OL, Wu L, Buta MR, Eleff SM, et al. Facile detection of mitochondrial DNA mutations in tumors and bodily fluids. Science. 2000;287(5460):2017–9.

77. Jiang WW, Masayesva B, Zahurak M, Carvalho AL, Rosenbaum E, Mambo E, et al. Increased mitochondrial DNA content in saliva associated with head and neck cancer. Clin Cancer Res. 2005;11(7):2486–91.

78. Masayesva BG, Mambo E, Taylor RJ, Goloubeva OG, Zhou S, Cohen Y, et al. Mitochondrial DNA content increase in response to cigarette smoking. Cancer Epidemiol Biomarkers Prev. 2006;15(1):19–24.

79. Jiang WW, Rosenbaum E, Mambo E, Zahurak M, Masayesva B, Carvalho AL, et al. Decreased mitochondrial DNA content in posttreatment salivary rinses from head and neck cancer patients. Clin Cancer Res. 2006;12(5):1564–9.

80. Palanisamy V, Wong DT. Transcriptomic analyses of saliva. Methods Mol Biol. 2010;666:43–51.

81. Li Y, Zhou X, St John MA, Wong DT. RNA profiling of cell-free saliva using microarray technology. J Dent Res. 2004;83(3):199–203.

82. Park NJ, Zhou H, Elashoff D, Henson BS, Kastratovic DA, Abemayor E, et al. Salivary microRNA: discovery, characterization, and clinical utility for oral cancer detection. Clin Cancer Res. 2009;15(17):5473–7.

83. Li Y, St John MA, Zhou X, Kim Y, Sinha U, Jordan RC, et al. Salivary transcriptome diagnostics for oral cancer detection. Clin Cancer Res. 2004;10(24):8442–50.

84. Loo JA, Yan W, Ramachandran P, Wong DT. Comparative human salivary and plasma proteomes. J Dent Res. 2010;89(10):1016–23.

85. Hu S, Loo JA, Wong DT. Human saliva proteome analysis and disease biomarker discovery. Expert Rev Proteomics. 2007;4(4):531–8.

86. Hu S, Loo JA, Wong DT. Human saliva proteome analysis. Ann N Y Acad Sci. 2007;1098:323–9.

87. Hu S, Arellano M, Boontheung P, Wang J, Zhou H, Jiang J, et al. Salivary proteomics for oral cancer biomarker discovery. Clin Cancer Res. 2008;14(19):6246–52.

88. Wittmann J, Jack H-M. Serum microRNAs as powerful cancer biomarkers. Biochimica et Biophysica Acta. 2010;1806(2):200–7.

89. Hamana K, Uzawa K, Ogawara K, Shiiba M, Bukawa H, Yokoe H, et al. Monitoring of circulating tumour-associated DNA as a prognostic tool for oral

squamous cell carcinoma. Br J Cancer. 2005;92(12): 2181–4.

90. Nawroz H, Koch W, Anker P, Stroun M, Sidransky D. Microsatellite alterations in serum DNA of head and neck cancer patients. Nat Med. 1996;2(9):1035–7.

91. Kakimoto Y, Yamamoto N, Shibahara T. Microsatellite analysis of serum DNA in patients with oral squamous cell carcinoma. Oncol Rep. 2008;20(5):1195–200.

92. Nawroz-Danish H, Eisenberger CF, Yoo GH, Wu L, Koch W, Black C, et al. Microsatellite analysis of serum DNA in patients with head and neck cancer. Int J Cancer. 2004;111(1):96–100.

93. Sanchez-Cespedes M, Esteller M, Wu L, Nawroz-Danish H, Yoo GH, Koch WM, et al. Gene promoter hypermethylation in tumors and serum of head and neck cancer patients. Cancer Res. 2000;60(4):892–5.

94. Nakahara Y, Shintani S, Mihara M, Hino S, Hamakawa H. Detection of p16 promoter methylation in the serum of oral cancer patients. Int J Oral Maxillofac Surg. 2006;35(4):362–5.

95. Wadsworth JT, Somers KD, Cazares LH, Malik G, Adam BL, Stack Jr BC, et al. Serum protein profiles to identify head and neck cancer. Clin Cancer Res. 2004;10(5):1625–32.

96. Wadsworth JT, Somers KD, Stack Jr BC, Cazares L, Malik G, Adam BL, et al. Identification of patients with head and neck cancer using serum protein profiles. Arch Otolaryngol Head Neck Surg. 2004; 130(1):98–104.

97. Gourin CG, Xia ZS, Han Y, French AM, O'Rourke AK, Terris DJ, et al. Serum protein profile analysis in patients with head and neck squamous cell carcinoma. Arch Otolaryngol Head Neck Surg. 2006; 132(4):390–7.

98. Sidransky D, Irizarry R, Califano JA, Li X, Ren H, Benoit N, et al. Serum protein MALDI profiling to distinguish upper aerodigestive tract cancer patients from control subjects. J Natl Cancer Inst. 2003; 95(22):1711–7.

99. Linkov F, Lisovich A, Yurkovetsky Z, Marrangoni A, Velikokhatnaya L, Nolen B, et al. Early detection of head and neck cancer: development of a novel screening tool using multiplexed immunobead-based biomarker profiling. Cancer Epidemiol Biomarkers Prev. 2007;16(1):102–7.

100. Gourin CG, Zhi W, Adam BL. Proteomic identification of serum biomarkers for head and neck cancer surveillance. Laryngoscope. 2009;119(7): 1291–302.

101. Gourin CG, Moretz 3rd WH, Weinberger PM, Xia ZS, Liu Z, Terris DJ, et al. Serum protein profile analysis following definitive treatment in patients with head and neck squamous cell carcinoma. Arch Otolaryngol Head Neck Surg. 2007;133(11): 1125–30.

102. Freed GL, Cazares LH, Fichandler CE, Fuller TW, Sawyer CA, Stack Jr BC, et al. Differential capture of serum proteins for expression profiling and biomarker discovery in pre- and posttreatment head and

neck cancer samples. Laryngoscope. 2008;118(1): 61–8.

103. zur Hausen H. Papillomaviruses causing cancer: evasion from host-cell control in early events in carcinogenesis. J Natl Cancer Inst 2000;92(9):690–8.

104. Lizano M, Berumen J, Garcia-Carranca A. HPV-related carcinogenesis: basic concepts, viral types and variants. Arch Med Res. 2009;40(6):428–34.

105. Scully C. Oral cancer; the evidence for sexual transmission. Br Dent J. 2005;199(4):203–7.

106. Gage JR, Meyers C, Wettstein FO. The E7 proteins of the nononcogenic human papillomavirus type 6b (HPV-6b) and of the oncogenic HPV-16 differ in retinoblastoma protein binding and other properties. J Virol. 1990;64(2):723–30.

107. Chow LT, Broker TR, Steinberg BM. The natural history of human papillomavirus infections of the mucosal epithelia. APMIS. 2010;118(6–7):422–49.

108. Wentzensen N, Vinokurova S, von Knebel Doeberitz M. Systematic review of genomic integration sites of human papillomavirus genomes in epithelial dysplasia and invasive cancer of the female lower genital tract. Cancer Res. 2004;64(11):3878–84.

109. zur Hausen H. Papillomaviruses and cancer: from basic studies to clinical application. Nat Rev Cancer. 2002;2(5):342–50.

110. Braakhuis BJ, Snijders PJ, Keune WJ, Meijer CJ, Ruijter-Schippers HJ, Leemans CR, et al. Genetic patterns in head and neck cancers that contain or lack transcriptionally active human papillomavirus. J Natl Cancer Inst. 2004;96(13):998–1006.

111. Califano J, van der Riet P, Westra W, Nawroz H, Clayman G, Piantadosi S, et al. Genetic progression model for head and neck cancer: implications for field cancerization. Cancer Res. 1996;56(11): 2488–92.

112. Huang CF, Monie A, Weng WH, Wu T. DNA vaccines for cervical cancer. Am J Transl Res. 2010;2(1):75–87.

113. Ganguly N, Parihar SP. Human papillomavirus E6 and E7 oncoproteins as risk factors for tumorigenesis. J Biosci. 2009;34(1):113–23.

114. Lazo PA. The molecular genetics of cervical carcinoma. Br J Cancer. 1999;80(12):2008–18.

115. McKaig RG, Baric RS, Olshan AF. Human papillomavirus and head and neck cancer: epidemiology and molecular biology. Head Neck. 1998;20(3): 250–65.

116. Li Y, Nichols MA, Shay JW, Xiong Y. Transcriptional repression of the D-type cyclin-dependent kinase inhibitor p16 by the retinoblastoma susceptibility gene product pRb. Cancer Res. 1994;54(23):6078–82.

117. Kreimer AR, Clifford GM, Boyle P, Franceschi S. Human papillomavirus types in head and neck squamous cell carcinomas worldwide: a systematic review. Cancer Epidemiol Biomarkers Prev. 2005;14(2):467–75.

118. Szkaradkiewicz A, Kruk-Zagajewska A, Wal M, Jopek A, Wierzbicka M, Kuch A. Epstein-Barr virus and human papillomavirus infections and

119. Koskinen WJ, Chen RW, Leivo I, Makitie A, Back L, Kontio R, et al. Prevalence and physical status of human papillomavirus in squamous cell carcinomas of the head and neck. Int J Cancer. 2003;107(3): 401–6.

120. Marur S, D'Souza G, Westra WH, Forastiere AA. HPV-associated head and neck cancer: a virus-related cancer epidemic. Lancet Oncol. 2010;11(8): 781–9.

121. Nasman A, Attner P, Hammarstedt L, Du J, Eriksson M, Giraud G, et al. Incidence of human papillomavirus (HPV) positive tonsillar carcinoma in Stockholm, Sweden: an epidemic of viral-induced carcinoma? Int J Cancer. 2009;125(2):362–6.

122. Ritchie JM, Smith EM, Summersgill KF, Hoffman HT, Wang D, Klussmann JP, et al. Human papillomavirus infection as a prognostic factor in carcinomas of the oral cavity and oropharynx. Int J Cancer. 2003;104(3):336–44.

123. Worden FP, Kumar B, Lee JS, Wolf GT, Cordell KG, Taylor JM, et al. Chemoselection as a strategy for organ preservation in advanced oropharynx cancer: response and survival positively associated with HPV16 copy number. J Clin Oncol. 2008;26(19): 3138–46.

124. Licitra L, Perrone F, Bossi P, Suardi S, Mariani L, Artusi R, et al. High-risk human papillomavirus affects prognosis in patients with surgically treated oropharyngeal squamous cell carcinoma. J Clin Oncol. 2006;24(36):5630–6.

125. Ringstrom E, Peters E, Hasegawa M, Posner M, Liu M, Kelsey KT. Human papillomavirus type 16 and squamous cell carcinoma of the head and neck. Clin Cancer Res. 2002;8(10):3187–92.

126. Sisk EA, Bradford CR, Jacob A, Yian CH, Staton KM, Tang G, et al. Human papillomavirus infection in "young" versus "old" patients with squamous cell carcinoma of the head and neck. Head Neck. 2000;22(7):649–57.

127. Singhi AD, Westra WH. Comparison of human papillomavirus in situ hybridization and p16 immunohistochemistry in the detection of human papillomavirus-associated head and neck cancer based on a prospective clinical experience. Cancer. 2010; 116(9):2166–73.

128. Gillespie MB, Rubinchik S, Hoel B, Sutkowski N. Human papillomavirus and oropharyngeal cancer: what you need to know in 2009. Curr Treat Options Oncol. 2009;10(5–6):296–307.

129. Shi W, Kato H, Perez-Ordonez B, Pintilie M, Huang S, Hui A, et al. Comparative prognostic value of HPV16 E6 mRNA compared with in situ hybridization for human oropharyngeal squamous carcinoma. J Clin Oncol. 2009;27(36):6213–21.

130. Gillison ML. Human papillomavirus and prognosis of oropharyngeal squamous cell carcinoma: implications for clinical research in head and neck cancers. J Clin Oncol. 2006;24(36):5623–5.

131. Allen CT, Lewis Jr JS, El-Mofty SK, Haughey BH, Nussenbaum B. Human papillomavirus and oropharynx cancer: biology, detection and clinical implications. Laryngoscope. 2010;120(9):1756–72.

132. Smeets SJ, Hesselink AT, Speel EJ, Haesevoets A, Snijders PJ, Pawlita M, et al. A novel algorithm for reliable detection of human papillomavirus in paraffin embedded head and neck cancer specimen. Int J Cancer. 2007;121(11):2465–72.

133. Cooper K, Herrington CS, Stickland JE, Evans MF, McGee JO. Episomal and integrated human papillomavirus in cervical neoplasia shown by non-isotopic in situ hybridisation. J Clin Pathol. 1991;44(12): 990–6.

134. Weinberger PM, Yu Z, Kountourakis P, Sasaki C, Haffty BG, Kowalski D, et al. Defining molecular phenotypes of human papillomavirus-associated oropharyngeal squamous cell carcinoma: validation of three-class hypothesis. Otolaryngol Head Neck Surg. 2009;141(3):382–9.

135. Weinberger PM, Yu Z, Haffty BG, Kowalski D, Harigopal M, Brandsma J, et al. Molecular classification identifies a subset of human papillomavirus–associated oropharyngeal cancers with favorable prognosis. J Clin Oncol. 2006;24(5):736–47.

136. Wiest T, Schwarz E, Enders C, Flechtenmacher C, Bosch FX. Involvement of intact HPV16 E6/E7 gene expression in head and neck cancers with unaltered p53 status and perturbed pRb cell cycle control. Oncogene. 2002;21(10):1510–7.

137. Thavaraj S, Stokes A, Guerra E, Bible J, Halligan E, Long A, et al. Evaluation of human papillomavirus testing for squamous cell carcinoma of the tonsil in clinical practice. J Clin Pathol. 2011;64(4):308–12.

138. Smeets SJ, Brakenhoff RH, Ylstra B, van Wieringen WN, van de Wiel MA, Leemans CR, et al. Genetic classification of oral and oropharyngeal carcinomas identifies subgroups with a different prognosis. Cell Oncol. 2009;31(4):291–300.

139. Watanabe A, Maruo S, Ito T, Ito M, Katsumura KR, Takada K. Epstein-Barr virus-encoded Bcl-2 homologue functions as a survival factor in Wp-restricted Burkitt lymphoma cell line P3HR-1. J Virol. 2010;84(6):2893–901.

140. Vaysberg M, Hatton O, Lambert SL, Snow AL, Wong B, Krams SM, et al. Tumor-derived variants of Epstein-Barr virus latent membrane protein 1 induce sustained Erk activation and c-Fos. J Biol Chem. 2008;283(52):36573–85.

141. Tune CE, Liavaag PG, Freeman JL, van den Brekel MW, Shpitzer T, Kerrebijn JD, et al. Nasopharyngeal brush biopsies and detection of nasopharyngeal cancer in a high-risk population. J Natl Cancer Inst. 1999;91(9):796–800.

142. Chang KP, Hsu CL, Chang YL, Tsang NM, Chen CK, Lee TJ, et al. Complementary serum test of antibodies to Epstein-Barr virus nuclear antigen-1 and early antigen: a possible alternative for primary screening of nasopharyngeal carcinoma. Oral Oncol. 2008;44(8):784–92.

143. Chan KC, Zhang J, Chan AT, Lei KI, Leung SF, Chan LY, et al. Molecular characterization of circulating EBV DNA in the plasma of nasopharyngeal carcinoma and lymphoma patients. Cancer Res. 2003;63(9):2028–32.
144. Fachiroh J, Stevens SJ, Haryana SM, Middeldorp JM. Combination of Epstein-Barr virus scaffold (BdRF1/VCA-p40) and small capsid protein (BFRF3/VCA-p18) into a single molecule for improved serodiagnosis of acute and malignant EBV-driven disease. J Virol Methods. 2010;169(1): 79–86.
145. Liao Q, Zhao L, Chen X, Deng Y, Ding Y. Serum proteome analysis for profiling protein markers associated with carcinogenesis and lymph node metastasis in nasopharyngeal carcinoma. Clin Exp Metastasis. 2008;25(4):465–76.
146. Bhaijee F, Pepper DJ, Pitman KT, Bell D. New developments in the molecular pathogenesis of head and neck tumors: a review of tumor-specific fusion oncogenes in mucoepidermoid carcinoma, adenoid cystic carcinoma, and NUT midline carcinoma. Ann Diagn Pathol. 2011;15(1):69–77.
147. Mitani Y, Li J, Rao PH, Zhao YJ, Bell D, Lippman SM, et al. Comprehensive analysis of the MYB-NFIB gene fusion in salivary adenoid cystic carcinoma: Incidence, variability, and clinicopathologic significance. Clin Cancer Res. 2010;16(19):4722–31.
148. Seethala RR, Dacic S, Cieply K, Kelly LM, Nikiforova MN. A reappraisal of the MECT1/MAML2 translocation in salivary mucoepidermoid carcinomas. Am J Surg Pathol. 2010;34(8):1106–21.
149. Liu G, Zheng H, Zhang Z, Wu Z, Xiong H, Li J, et al. Overexpression of sphingosine kinase 1 is associated with salivary gland carcinoma progression and might be a novel predictive marker for adjuvant therapy. BMC Cancer. 2010;10:495.
150. Vacchi-Suzzi M, Bocciolini C, Bertarelli C, Dall'Olio D. Ki-67 Proliferation rate as a prognostic marker in major salivary gland carcinomas. Ann Oto Rhinol Laryn. 2010;119(10):677–83.
151. Bell D, Roberts D, Kies M, Rao P, Weber RS, El-Naggar AK. Cell type-dependent biomarker expression in adenoid cystic carcinoma: biologic and therapeutic implications. Cancer. 2010;116(24): 5749–56.
152. Andreadis D, Epivatianos A, Poulopoulos A, Nomikos A, Papazoglou G, Antoniades D, et al. Detection of C-KIT (CD117) molecule in benign and malignant salivary gland tumours. Oral Oncol. 2006;42(1):57–65.
153. Bell A, Bell D, Weber RS, El-Naggar AK. CpG island methylation profiling in human salivary gland adenoid cystic carcinoma. Cancer. 2011;117(13):
154. Schache AG, Hall G, Woolgar JA, Nikolaidis G, Triantafyllou A, Lowe D, et al. Quantitative promoter methylation differentiates carcinoma ex pleomorphic adenoma from pleomorphic salivary adenoma. Br J Cancer. 2010;103(12):1846–51.
155. Cairns L, Naidu A, Robinson CM, Sloan P, Wright JM, Hunter KD. CD56 (NCAM) expression in ameloblastomas and other odontogenic lesions. Histopathology. 2010;57(4):544–8.
156. Woolgar JA, Hall GL. Determinants of outcome following surgery for oral squamous cell carcinoma. Future Oncol. 2009;5(1):51–61.
157. Abbey L, Kaugars G, Gunsolley JC, Burns J, Page D, Svirsky J, et al. Intraexaminer and interexaminer reliability in the diagnosis of oral epithelial dysplasia. Oral Surg, Oral Med, Oral Pathol, Oral Radiol Endod. 1995;80:188–91.
158. Zhang L, Rosin MP. Loss of heterozygosity: a potential tool in management of oral premalignant lesions? J Oral Pathol Med. 2001;30(9):513–20.
159. Mao L, Lee J, Fan Y, Ro J, Batsakis J, Lippman S, et al. Frequent microsatelite alterations at chromosomes 9p21 and 3p14 in oral premalignant lesions and their value in cancer risk assessment. Nat Med. 1996;2(6):682–85.
160. Papadimitrakopoulou VA, Liu DD, Mao L, Shin DM, El-Naggar A, Ibarguen H, et al. Biologic correlates of a biochemoprevention trial in advanced upper aerodigestive tract premalignant lesions. Cancer Epidemiol Biomarkers Prev. 2002;11(12):1605–10.
161. Rosin MP, Cheng X, Poh C, Lam WL, Huang Y, Lovas J, et al. Use of allelic loss to predict malignant risk for low-grade oral epithelial dysplasia. Clin Cancer Res. 2000;6(2):357–62.
162. Guillaud M, Zhang L, Poh C, Rosin MP, MacAulay C. Potential use of quantitative tissue phenotype to predict malignant risk for oral premalignant lesions. Cancer Res. 2008;68(9):3099–107.
163. Smith J, Rattay T, McConkey C, Helliwell T, Mehanna H. Biomarkers in dysplasia of the oral cavity: a systematic review. Oral Oncol. 2009;45(8):647–53.
164. Cruz I, Snijders P, Meijer C, Braakhuis B, Snow G, Walboomers J, et al. p53 expression above the basal layer in oral mucosa is an early event of malignant transformation and has predictive value for developing oral squamous cell carcinoma. J Pathol. 1998;184:360–68.
165. Hittelman WN. Genetic instability in epithelial tissues at risk for cancer. Ann N Y Acad Sci. 2001;952:1–12.
166. Diwakar N, Sperandio M, Sherriff M, Brown A, Odell EW. Heterogeneity, histological features and DNA ploidy in oral carcinoma by image-based analysis. Oral Oncol. 2005;41(4):416–22.
167. Torres-Rendon A, Stewart R, Craig GT, Wells M, Speight PM. DNA ploidy analysis by image cytometry helps to identify oral epithelial dysplasias with a high risk of malignant progression. Oral Oncol. 2009;45(6):468–73.
168. Klanrit P, Sperandio M, Brown AL, Shirlaw PJ, Challacombe SJ, Morgan PR, et al. DNA ploidy in proliferative verrucous leukoplakia. Oral Oncol. 2007;43(3):310–6.
169. Bremmer JF, Braakhuis BJ, Brink A, Broeckaert MA, Belien JA, Meijer GA, et al. Comparative evaluation of genetic assays to identify oral precancerous fields. J Oral Pathol Med. 2008;37(10): 599–606.

170. Pektas ZO, Keskin A, Gunhan O, Karslioglu Y. Evaluation of nuclear morphometry and DNA ploidy status for detection of malignant and premalignant oral lesions: quantitative cytologic assessment and review of methods for cytomorphometric measurements. J Oral Maxillofac Surg. 2006;64(4):628–35.

171. Cheung FM, Lau TW, Cheung LK, Li AS, Chow SK, Lo AW. Schneiderian papillomas and carcinomas: a retrospective study with special reference to p53 and p16 tumor suppressor gene expression and association with HPV. Ear Nose Throat J. 2010;89(10):E5–E12.

172. Hunter KD, Parkinson EK, Harrison PR. Opinion: profiling early head and neck cancer. Nat Rev Cancer. 2005;5(2):127–35.

173. Tripathi SC, Matta A, Kaur J, Grigull J, Chauhan SS, Thakar A, et al. Nuclear S100A7 is associated with poor prognosis in head and neck cancer. PLoS One. 2010;5(8):e11939.

174. Gee HE, Camps C, Buffa FM, Patiar S, Winter SC, Betts G, et al. hsa-mir-210 is a marker of tumor hypoxia and a prognostic factor in head and neck cancer. Cancer. 2010;116(9):2148–58.

175. Hsu DS, Chang SY, Liu CJ, Tzeng CH, Wu KJ, Kao JY, et al. Identification of increased NBS1 expression as a prognostic marker of squamous cell carcinoma of the oral cavity. Cancer Sci. 2010;101(4):1029–37.

176. Ulanovski D, Stern Y, Roizman P, Shpitzer T, Popovtzer A, Feinmesser R. Expression of EGFR and Cerb-B2 as prognostic factors in cancer of the tongue. Oral Oncol. 2004;40(5):532–7.

177. Ang KK, Berkey BA, Tu X, Zhang HZ, Katz R, Hammond EH, et al. Impact of epidermal growth factor receptor expression on survival and pattern of relapse in patients with advanced head and neck carcinoma. Cancer Res. 2002;62(24):7350–6.

178. Chen IH, Chang JT, Liao CT, Wang HM, Hsieh LL, Cheng AJ. Prognostic significance of EGFR and Her-2 in oral cavity cancer in betel quid prevalent area cancer prognosis. Br J Cancer. 2003;89(4):681–6.

179. Kawakami M, Kawakami K, Kasperbauer JL, Hinkley LL, Tsukuda M, Strome SE, et al. Interleukin-13 receptor alpha2 chain in human head and neck cancer serves as a unique diagnostic marker. Clin Cancer Res. 2003;9(17):6381–8.

180. Estilo CL, O-Charoenrat P, Ngai I, Patel SG, Reddy PG, Dao S, et al. The role of novel oncogenes squamous cell carcinoma-related oncogene and phosphatidylinositol 3-kinase p110alpha in squamous cell carcinoma of the oral tongue. Clin Cancer Res. 2003;9(6):2300–6.

181. Wada S, Yue L, Furuta I. Prognostic significance of p34cdc2 expression in tongue squamous cell carcinoma. Oral Oncol. 2004;40(2):164–9.

182. Mineta H, Borg A, Dictor M, Wahlberg P, Akervall J, Wennerberg J. p53 mutation, but not p53 overexpression, correlates with survival in head and neck squamous cell carcinoma. Br J Cancer. 1998;78(8):1084–90.

183. Nathan CA, Sanders K, Abreo FW, Nassar R, Glass J. Correlation of p53 and the proto-oncogene eIF4E in larynx cancers: prognostic implications. Cancer Res. 2000;60(13):3599–604.

184. Nogueira CP, Dolan RW, Gooey J, Byahatti S, Vaughan CW, Fuleihan NS, et al. Inactivation of p53 and amplification of cyclin D1 correlate with clinical outcome in head and neck cancer. Laryngoscope. 1998;108(3):345–50.

185. Geisler SA, Olshan AF, Weissler MC, Cai J, Funkhouser WK, Smith J, et al. p16 and p53 Protein expression as prognostic indicators of survival and disease recurrence from head and neck cancer. Clin Cancer Res. 2002;8(11):3445–53.

186. Bova R, Quinn D, Nankervis J, Cole I, Sheridan B, Jensen M, et al. Cyclin D1 and p16INK4a expression predict reduced survival in carcinoma of the anterior tongue. Clin Cancer Res. 1999;5:2810–19.

187. Ogi K, Toyota M, Ohe-Toyota M, Tanaka N, Noguchi M, Sonoda T, et al. Aberrant methylation of multiple genes and clinicopathological features in oral squamous cell carcinoma. Clin Cancer Res. 2002;8(10):3164–71.

188. Knecht R, Elez R, Oechler M, Solbach C, von Ilberg C, Strebhardt K. Prognostic significance of Polo-like kinase expression in squamous cell carcinomas of the head and neck. Cancer Res. 1999;59:2794–97.

189. Lo Muzio L, Pannone G, Staibano S, Mignogna MD, Rubini C, Mariggio MA, et al. Survivin expression in oral squamous cell carcinoma. Br J Cancer. 2003;89(12):2244–8.

190. Su L, Wang Y, Xiao M, Lin Y, Yu L. Up-regulation of survivin in oral squamous cell carcinoma correlates with poor prognosis and chemoresistance. Oral Surg Oral Med Oral Pathol Oral Radiol Endod. 2010;110(4):484–91.

191. Chang HW, Chow V, Lam KY, Wei WI, Yuen A. Loss of E-cadherin expression resulting from promoter hypermethylation in oral tongue carcinoma and its prognostic significance. Cancer. 2002;94(2):386–92.

192. Lim SC, Zhang S, Ishii G, Endoh Y, Kodama K, Miyamoto S, et al. Predictive markers for late cervical metastasis in stage I and II invasive squamous cell carcinoma of the oral tongue. Clin Cancer Res. 2004;10(1 Pt 1):166–72.

193. Chow V, Yuen AP, Lam KY, Tsao GS, Ho WK, Wei WI. A comparative study of the clinicopathological significance of E-cadherin and catenins (alpha, beta, gamma) expression in the surgical management of oral tongue carcinoma. J Cancer Res Clin Oncol. 2001;127(1):59–63.

194. Moriyama-Kita M, Endo Y, Yonemura Y, Heizmann CW, Schafer BW, Sasaki T, et al. Correlation of S100A4 expression with invasion and metastasis in oral squamous cell carcinoma. Oral Oncol. 2004;40(5):496–500.

195. Gonzalez-Moles MA, Bravo M, Ruiz-Avila I, Esteban F, Rodriguez-Archilla A, Gonzalez-Moles S, et al. Adhesion molecule CD44 as a prognostic factor in tongue cancer. Anticancer Res. 2003;23(6D):5197–202.

196. Kosunen A, Ropponen K, Kellokoski J, Pukkila M, Virtaniemi J, Valtonen H, et al. Reduced expression of hyaluronan is a strong indicator of poor survival in oral squamous cell carcinoma. Oral Oncol. 2004;40(3):257–63.

197. Katayama A, Bandoh N, Kishibe K, Takahara M, Ogino T, Nonaka S, et al. Expressions of matrix metalloproteinases in early-stage oral squamous cell carcinoma as predictive indicators for tumor metastases and prognosis. Clin Cancer Res. 2004; 10(2):634–40.

198. Kobayashi H, Sagara J, Kurita H, Morifuji M, Ohishi M, Kurashina K, et al. Clinical significance of cellular distribution of moesin in patients with oral squamous cell carcinoma. Clin Cancer Res. 2004;10(2):572–80.

199. Thomas GJ, Nystrom ML, Marshall JF. Alphavbeta6 integrin in wound healing and cancer of the oral cavity. J Oral Pathol Med. 2006;35(1):1–10.

200. Uehara M, Sano K, Ikeda H, Sekine J, Irie A, Yokota T, et al. Expression of vascular endothelial growth factor and prognosis of oral squamous cell carcinoma. Oral Oncol. 2004;40(3):321–5.

201. Shintani S, Li C, Ishikawa T, Mihara M, Nakashiro K, Hamakawa H. Expression of vascular endothelial growth factor A, B, C, and D in oral squamous cell carcinoma. Oral Oncol. 2004;40(1):13–20.

202. Beasley NJ, Leek R, Alam M, Turley H, Cox GJ, Gatter K, et al. Hypoxia-inducible factors HIF-1alpha and HIF-2alpha in head and neck cancer: relationship to tumor biology and treatment outcome in surgically resected patients. Cancer Res. 2002; 62(9):2493–7.

203. Miyazawa J, Mitoro A, Kawashiri S, Chada KK, Imai K. Expression of mesenchyme-specific gene HMGA2 in squamous cell carcinomas of the oral cavity. Cancer Res. 2004;64(6):2024–9.

204. Delilbasi CB, Okura M, Iida S, Kogo M. Investigation of CXCR4 in squamous cell carcinoma of the tongue. Oral Oncol. 2004;40(2):154–7.

205. Chang BW, Kim DH, Kowalski DP, Burleson JA, Son YH, Wilson LD, et al. Prognostic significance of cyclooxygenase-2 in oropharyngeal squamous cell carcinoma. Clin Cancer Res. 2004;10(5):1678–84.

206. Liao CT, Tung-Chieh Chang J, Wang HM, Chen IH, Lin CY, Chen TM, et al. Telomerase as an independent prognostic factor in head and neck squamous cell carcinoma. Head Neck. 2004;26(6):504–12.

207. Yanagawa T, Omura K, Harada H, Nakaso K, Iwasa S, Koyama Y, et al. Heme oxygenase-1 expression predicts cervical lymph node metastasis of tongue squamous cell carcinomas. Oral Oncol. 2004; 40(1):21–7.

208. Hofman P, Butori C, Havet K, Hofman V, Selva E, Guevara N, et al. Prognostic significance of cortactin levels in head and neck squamous cell carcinoma: comparison with epidermal growth factor receptor status. Br J Cancer. 2008;98(5):956–64.

209. Ang KK, Harris J, Wheeler R, Weber R, Rosenthal DI, Nguyen-Tan PF, et al. Human papillomavirus and survival of patients with oropharyngeal cancer. N Engl J Med. 2010;363(1):24–35.

210. Prigent SA, Lemoine NR. The type 1 (EGFR-related) family of growth factor receptors and their ligands. Prog Growth Factor Res. 1992;4(1):1–24.

211. Ozanne B, Richards CS, Hendler F, Burns D, Gusterson B. Over-expression of the EGF receptor is a hallmark of squamous cell carcinoma. J Pathol. 1986;149(1):9–14.

212. Rubin Grandis J, Melhem M, Gooding W, Day R, Holst V, Wagener M, et al. Levels of TGFa and EGFR protein in head and neck squamous cell carcinoma and patients survival. J Natl Cancer Inst. 1998;90(11):824–32.

213. Chung CH, Ely K, McGavran L, Varella-Garcia M, Parker J, Parker N, et al. Increased epidermal growth factor receptor gene copy number is associated with poor prognosis in head and neck squamous cell carcinomas. J Clin Oncol. 2006;24(25):4170–76.

214. Temam S, Kawaguchi H, El-Naggar AK, Jelinek J, Tang H, Liu DD, et al. Epidermal growth factor receptor copy number alterations correlate with poor clinical outcome in patients with head and neck squamous cancer. J Clin Oncol. 2007;25(16):2164–70.

215. Sheu JJ, Hua CH, Wan L, Lin YJ, Lai MT, Tseng HC, et al. Functional genomic analysis identified epidermal growth factor receptor activation as the most common genetic event in oral squamous cell carcinoma. Cancer Res. 2009;69(6):2568–76.

216. Loeffler-Ragg J, Witsch-Baumgartner M, Tzankov A, Hilbe W, Schwentner I, Sprinzl GM, et al. Low incidence of mutations in EGFR kinase domain in Caucasian patients with head and neck squamous cell carcinoma. Eur J Cancer. 2006;42(1):109–11.

217. Hama T, Yuza Y, Saito Y, Ou J, Kondo S, Okabe M, et al. Prognostic significance of epidermal growth factor receptor phosphorylation and mutation in head and neck squamous cell carcinoma. Oncologist. 2009;14(9):900–8.

218. Taoudi Benchekroun M, Saintigny P, Thomas SM, El-Naggar AK, Papadimitrakopoulou V, Ren H, et al. Epidermal growth factor receptor expression and gene copy number in the risk of oral cancer. Cancer Prev Res (Phila). 2010;3(7):800–9.

219. Dei Tos AP. The biology of epidermal growth factor receptor and its value as a prognostic/predictive factor. Int J Biol Markers. 2007;22(1 Suppl 4):S3–9.

220. Eberhard DA, Giaccone G, Johnson BE. Biomarkers of response to epidermal growth factor receptor inhibitors in Non-Small-Cell Lung Cancer Working Group: standardization for use in the clinical trial setting. J Clin Oncol. 2008;26(6):983–94.

221. Gusterson B, Hunter K. Should we be surprised at the paucity of response to EGFR inhibitors? Lancet Oncol. 2009;10(5):522–7.

222. Leemans CR, Braakhuis BJ, Brakenhoff RH. The molecular biology of head and neck cancer. Nat Rev Cancer. 2011;11(1):9–22.

223. Ragin CC, Taioli E. Survival of squamous cell carcinoma of the head and neck in relation to human

papillomavirus infection: review and meta-analysis. Int J Cancer. 2007;121(8):1813–20.

224. Fischer CA, Zlobec I, Green E, Probst S, Storck C, Lugli A, et al. Is the improved prognosis of p16 positive oropharyngeal squamous cell carcinoma dependent of the treatment modality? Int J Cancer. 2010;126(5):1256–62.

225. Vu HL, Sikora AG, Fu S, Kao J. HPV-induced oropharyngeal cancer, immune response and response to therapy. Cancer Lett. 2010;288(2): 149–55.

226. Klozar J, Tachezy R, Rotnaglova E, Koslabova E, Salakova M, Hamsikova E. Human papillomavirus in head and neck tumors: epidemiological, molecular and clinical aspects. Wien Med Wochenschr. 2010;160(11–12):305–9.

227. Wreesmann VB, Shi W, Thaler HT, Poluri A, Kraus DH, Pfister D, et al. Identification of novel prognosticators of outcome in squamous cell carcinoma of the head and neck. J Clin Oncol. 2004;22(19): 3965–72.

228. Wreesmann VB, Wang D, Goberdhan A, Prasad M, Ngai I, Schnaser EA, et al. Genetic abnormalities associated with nodal metastasis in head and neck cancer. Head Neck. 2004;26(1):10–5.

229. Ginos MA, Page GP, Michalowicz BS, Patel KJ, Volker SE, Pambuccian SE, et al. Identification of a gene expression signature associated with recurrent disease in squamous cell carcinoma of the head and neck. Cancer Res. 2004;64(1):55–63.

230. Chung CH, Parker JS, Karaca G, Wu J, Funkhouser WK, Moore D, et al. Molecular classification of head and neck squamous cell carcinomas using patterns of gene expression. Cancer Cell. 2004;5(5): 489–500.

231. Roepman P, Kemmeren P, Wessels LF, Slootweg PJ, Holstege FC. Multiple robust signatures for detecting lymph node metastasis in head and neck cancer. Cancer Res. 2006;66(4):2361–6.

232. Roepman P, Wessels LF, Kettelarij N, Kemmeren P, Miles AJ, Lijnzaad P, et al. An expression profile for diagnosis of lymph node metastases from primary head and neck squamous cell carcinomas. Nat Genet. 2005;37(2):182–6.

233. Cromer A, Carles A, Millon R, Ganguli G, Chalmel F, Lemaire F, et al. Identification of genes associated with tumorigenesis and metastatic potential of hypopharyngeal cancer by microarray analysis. Oncogene. 2004;23(14):2484–98.

234. Braakhuis BJ, Senft A, de Bree R, de Vries J, Ylstra B, Cloos J, et al. Expression profiling and prediction of distant metastases in head and neck squamous cell carcinoma. J Clin Pathol. 2006;59(12):1254–60.

235. Michiels S, Koscielny S, Hill C. Prediction of cancer outcome with microarrays: a multiple random validation strategy. Lancet. 2005;365(9458):488–92.

236. Mueller MM, Fusenig NE. Tumor-stroma interactions directing phenotype and progression of epithelial skin tumor cells. Differentiation. 2002;70(9–10): 486–97.

237. Park CC, Bissell MJ, Barcellos-Hoff MH. The influence of the microenvironment on the malignant phenotype. Mol Med Today. 2000;6(8):324–9.

238. Tlsty TD, Hein PW. Know thy neighbor: stromal cells can contribute oncogenic signals. Curr Opin Genet Dev. 2001;11(1):54–9.

239. Thurlow JK, Pena Murillo CL, Hunter KD, Buffa FM, Patiar S, Betts G, et al. Spectral clustering of microarray data elucidates the roles of microenvironment remodeling and immune responses in survival of head and neck squamous cell carcinoma. J Clin Oncol. 2010;28(17):2881–8.

240. Marsh D, Suchak K, Moutasim KA, Vallath S, Hopper C, Jerjes W, et al. Stromal features are predictive of disease mortality in oral cancer patients. J Pathol. 2011;223(4):470–81.

241. Braakhuis BJ, Brakenhoff RH, Leemans CR. Gene expression profiling in head and neck squamous cell carcinoma. Curr Opin Otolaryngol Head Neck Surg. 2010;18(2):67–71.

242. Sutton DN, Brown JS, Rogers SN, Vaughan ED, Woolgar JA. The prognostic implications of the surgical margin in oral squamous cell carcinoma. Int J Oral Maxillofac Surg. 2003;32(1):30–4.

243. Graveland AP, Golusinski PJ, Buijze M, Douma R, Sons N, Kuik DJ, et al. Loss of heterozygosity at 9p and p53 immunopositivity in surgical margins predict local relapse in head and neck squamous cell carcinoma. Int J Cancer. 2011;128(8):1852–9.

244. Graveland AP, de Maaker M, Braakhuis BJ, de Bree R, Eerenstein SE, Bloemena E, et al. Molecular detection of minimal residual cancer in surgical margins of head and neck cancer patients. Cell Oncol. 2009;31(4):317–28.

245. Nathan CO, Amirghahri N, Rice C, Abreo FW, Shi R, Stucker FJ. Molecular analysis of surgical margins in head and neck squamous cell carcinoma patients. Laryngoscope. 2002;112(12):2129–40.

246. Schaaij-Visser TB, Bremmer JF, Braakhuis BJ, Heck AJ, Slijper M, van der Waal I, et al. Evaluation of cornulin, keratin 4, keratin 13 expression and grade of dysplasia for predicting malignant progression of oral leukoplakia. Oral Oncol. 2010;46(2): 123–7.

247. Brennan JA, Boyle JO, Koch WM, Goodman SN, Hruban RH, Eby YJ, et al. Association between cigarette smoking and mutation of the p53 gene in squamous-cell carcinoma of the head and neck. N Engl J Med. 1995;332(11):712–7.

248. Partridge M, Pateromichelakis S, Phillips E, Emilion G, A'Hern R, Langdon J. A case-control study confirms that microsatelite assay can identify patients at risk of developing oral squamous cell carcinoma within a field of cancerization. Cancer Res. 2000; 60:3893–98.

249. van Houten VM, Leemans CR, Kummer JA, Dijkstra J, Kuik DJ, van den Brekel MW, et al. Molecular diagnosis of surgical margins and local recurrence in head and neck cancer patients: a prospective study. Clin Cancer Res. 2004;10(11):3614–20.

250. Partridge M, Costea DE, Huang X. The changing face of p53 in head and neck cancer. Int J Oral Maxillofac Surg. 2007;36(12):1123–38.

251. Alkureishi LW, Burak Z, Alvarez JA, Ballinger J, Bilde A, Britten AJ, et al. Joint practice guidelines for radionuclide lymphoscintigraphy for sentinel node localization in oral/oropharyngeal squamous cell carcinoma. Eur J Nucl Med Mol Imaging. 2009;36(11):1915–36.

252. Ferris RL, Xi L, Raja S, Hunt JL, Wang J, Gooding WE, et al. Molecular staging of cervical lymph nodes in squamous cell carcinoma of the head and neck. Cancer Res. 2005;65(6):2147–56.

253. Nieuwenhuis EJ, Jaspars LH, Castelijns JA, Bakker B, Wishaupt RG, Denkers F, et al. Quantitative molecular detection of minimal residual head and neck cancer in lymph node aspirates. Clin Cancer Res. 2003;9(2):755–61.

254. Colnot DR, Nieuwenhuis EJ, Kuik DJ, Leemans CR, Dijkstra J, Snow GB, et al. Clinical significance of micrometastatic cells detected by E48 (Ly-6D) reverse transcription-polymerase chain reaction in bone marrow of head and neck cancer patients. Clin Cancer Res. 2004;10(23):7827–33.

255. van den Broek GB, Wildeman M, Rasch CR, Armstrong N, Schuuring E, Begg AC, et al. Molecular markers predict outcome in squamous cell carcinoma of the head and neck after concomitant cisplatin-based chemoradiation. Int J Cancer. 2009;124(11):2643–50.

256. Pramana J, Van den Brekel MW, van Velthuysen ML, Wessels LF, Nuyten DS, Hofland I, et al. Gene expression profiling to predict outcome after chemoradiation in head and neck cancer. Int J Radiat Oncol Biol Phys. 2007;69(5):1544–52.

257. Michaud WA, Nichols AC, Mroz EA, Faquin WC, Clark JR, Begum S, et al. Bcl-2 blocks cisplatin-induced apoptosis and predicts poor outcome following chemoradiation treatment in advanced oropharyngeal squamous cell carcinoma. Clin Cancer Res. 2009;15(5):1645–54.

258. De Castro Jr G, Pasini FS, Siqueira SA, Ferraz AR, Villar RC, Snitcovsky IM, et al. ERCC1 protein, mRNA expression and T19007C polymorphism as prognostic markers in head and neck squamous cell carcinoma patients treated with surgery and adjuvant cisplatin-based chemoradiation. Oncol Rep. 2011;25(3):693–9.

259. Silva P, Slevin NJ, Sloan P, Valentine H, Cresswell J, Ryder D, et al. Prognostic significance of tumor hypoxia inducible factor-1alpha expression for outcome after radiotherapy in oropharyngeal cancer. Int J Radiat Oncol Biol Phys. 2008;72(5): 1551–9.

260. Li S, Schmitz KR, Jeffrey PD, Wiltzius JJ, Kussie P, Ferguson KM. Structural basis for inhibition of the epidermal growth factor receptor by cetuximab. Cancer Cell. 2005;7(4):301–11.

261. Kurai J, Chikumi H, Hashimoto K, Yamaguchi K, Yamasaki A, Sako T, et al. Antibody-dependent cellular cytotoxicity mediated by cetuximab against lung cancer cell lines. Clin Cancer Res. 2007;13(5): 1552–61.

262. Sigismund S, Woelk T, Puri C, Maspero E, Tacchetti C, Transidico P, et al. Clathrin-independent endocytosis of ubiquitinated cargos. Proc Natl Acad Sci U S A. 2005;102(8):2760–5.

263. Dittmann K, Mayer C, Rodemann HP. Inhibition of radiation-induced EGFR nuclear import by C225 (Cetuximab) suppresses DNA-PK activity. Radiother Oncol. 2005;76(2):157–61.

264. Li C, Iida M, Dunn EF, Ghia AJ, Wheeler DL. Nuclear EGFR contributes to acquired resistance to cetuximab. Oncogene. 2009;28(43):3801–13.

265. Vermorken JB, Trigo J, Hitt R, Koralewski P, Diaz-Rubio E, Rolland F, et al. Open-label, uncontrolled, multicenter phase II study to evaluate the efficacy and toxicity of cetuximab as a single agent in patients with recurrent and/or metastatic squamous cell carcinoma of the head and neck who failed to respond to platinum-based therapy. J Clin Oncol. 2007; 25(16):2171–7.

266. Vermorken JB, Herbst RS, Leon X, Amellal N, Baselga J. Overview of the efficacy of cetuximab in recurrent and/or metastatic squamous cell carcinoma of the head and neck in patients who previously failed platinum-based therapies. Cancer. 2008; 112(12):2710–9.

267. Robert F, Ezekiel MP, Spencer SA, Meredith RF, Bonner JA, Khazaeli MB, et al. Phase I study of anti-epidermal growth factor receptor antibody cetuximab in combination with radiation therapy in patients with advanced head and neck cancer. J Clin Oncol. 2001;19(13):3234–43.

268. Bourhis J, Rivera F, Mesia R, Awada A, Geoffrois L, Borel C, et al. Phase I/II study of cetuximab in combination with cisplatin or carboplatin and fluorouracil in patients with recurrent or metastatic squamous cell carcinoma of the head and neck. J Clin Oncol. 2006;24(18):2866–72.

269. Pfister DG, Su YB, Kraus DH, Wolden SL, Lis E, Aliff TB, et al. Concurrent cetuximab, cisplatin, and concomitant boost radiotherapy for locoregionally advanced, squamous cell head and neck cancer: a pilot phase II study of a new combined-modality paradigm. J Clin Oncol. 2006;24(7): 1072–8.

270. Baselga J, Trigo JM, Bourhis J, Tortochaux J, Cortes-Funes H, Hitt R, et al. Phase II multicenter study of the antiepidermal growth factor receptor monoclonal antibody cetuximab in combination with platinum-based chemotherapy in patients with platinum-refractory metastatic and/or recurrent squamous cell carcinoma of the head and neck. J Clin Oncol. 2005;23(24):5568–77.

271. Merlano M, Russi E, Benasso M, Corvo R, Colantonio I, Vigna-Taglianti R, et al. Cisplatin-based chemoradiation plus cetuximab in locally advanced head and neck cancer: a phase II clinical study. Ann Oncol. 2011;22(3):712–7.

272. Bonner JA, Harari PM, Giralt J, Azarnia N, Shin DM, Cohen RB, et al. Radiotherapy plus cetuximab for squamous-cell carcinoma of the head and neck. N Engl J Med. 2006;354(6):567–78.

273. Bonner JA, Harari PM, Giralt J, Cohen RB, Jones CU, Sur RK, et al. Radiotherapy plus cetuximab for locoregionally advanced head and neck cancer: 5-year survival data from a phase 3 randomised trial, and relation between cetuximab-induced rash and survival. Lancet Oncol. 2010;11(1):21–8.

274. Argiris A, Heron DE, Smith RP, Kim S, Gibson MK, Lai SY, et al. Induction docetaxel, cisplatin, and cetuximab followed by concurrent radiotherapy, cisplatin, and cetuximab and maintenance cetuximab in patients with locally advanced head and neck cancer. J Clin Oncol. 2010;28(36):5294–300.

275. Vermorken JB, Mesia R, Rivera F, Remenar E, Kawecki A, Rottey S, et al. Platinum-based chemotherapy plus cetuximab in head and neck cancer. N Engl J Med. 2008;359(11):1116–27.

276. Burtness B, Goldwasser MA, Flood W, Mattar B, Forastiere AA. Phase III randomized trial of cisplatin plus placebo compared with cisplatin plus cetuximab in metastatic/recurrent head and neck cancer: an Eastern Cooperative Oncology Group study. J Clin Oncol. 2005;23(34):8646–54.

277. Kies MS, Holsinger FC, Lee JJ, William Jr WN, Glisson BS, Lin HY, et al. Induction chemotherapy and cetuximab for locally advanced squamous cell carcinoma of the head and neck: results from a phase II prospective trial. J Clin Oncol. 2010; 28(1):8–14.

278. Stewart JS, Cohen EE, Licitra L, Van Herpen CM, Khorprasert C, Soulieres D, et al. Phase III study of gefitinib compared with intravenous methotrexate for recurrent squamous cell carcinoma of the head and neck [corrected]. J Clin Oncol. 2009;27(11): 1864–71.

279. Chua DT, Wei WI, Wong MP, Sham JS, Nicholls J, Au GK. Phase II study of gefitinib for the treatment of recurrent and metastatic nasopharyngeal carcinoma. Head Neck. 2008;30(7):863–7.

280. Kirby AM, A'Hern RP, D'Ambrosio C, Tanay M, Syrigos KN, Rogers SJ, et al. Gefitinib (ZD1839, Iressa(TM)) as palliative treatment in recurrent or metastatic head and neck cancer. Br J Cancer. 2006; 94(5):631–36.

281. Herchenhorn D, Dias FL, Viegas CM, Federico MH, Araujo CM, Small I, et al. Phase I/II study of erlotinib combined with cisplatin and radiotherapy in patients with locally advanced squamous cell carcinoma of the head and neck. Int J Radiat Oncol Biol Phys. 2010;78(3):696–702.

282. Siu LL, Soulieres D, Chen EX, Pond GR, Chin SF, Francis P, et al. Phase I/II trial of erlotinib and cisplatin in patients with recurrent or metastatic squamous cell carcinoma of the head and neck: a Princess Margaret Hospital phase II consortium and National Cancer Institute of Canada Clinical Trials Group Study. J Clin Oncol. 2007;25(16):2178–83.

283. Abidoye OO, Cohen EE, Wong SJ, Kozloff MF, Nattam SR, Stenson KM, et al. A phase II study of lapatinib (GW572016) in recurrent/metastatic (RIM) squamous cell carcinoma of the head and neck (SCCHN). J Clin Oncol. 2006;24(18):297s–97s.

284. Cohen EE, Davis DW, Karrison TG, Seiwert TY, Wong SJ, Nattam S, et al. Erlotinib and bevacizumab in patients with recurrent or metastatic squamous-cell carcinoma of the head and neck: a phase I/II study. Lancet Oncol. 2009;10(3):247–57.

285. Vermorken JB, Specenier P. Optimal treatment for recurrent/metastatic head and neck cancer. Ann Oncol. 2010;21((Suppl 7)):vii252–vii61.

286. Herbst RS, Arquette M, Shin DM, Dicke K, Vokes EE, Azarnia N, et al. Phase II multicenter study of the epidermal growth factor receptor antibody cetuximab and cisplatin for recurrent and refractory squamous cell carcinoma of the head and neck. J Clin Oncol. 2005;23(24):5578–87.

287. Boshoff C, Posner M. Targeting EGFR in head and neck cancer: a decade of progress. Nat Clin Pract Oncol. 2009;6(3):123.

288. Herbst RS, Kelly K, Chansky K, Mack PC, Franklin WA, Hirsch FR, et al. Phase II selection design trial of concurrent chemotherapy and cetuximab versus chemotherapy followed by cetuximab in advanced-stage non-small-cell lung cancer: Southwest Oncology Group study S0342. J Clin Oncol. 2010; 28(31):4747–54.

289. Argiris A, Karamouzis MV. Empowering induction therapy for locally advanced head and neck cancer. Ann Oncol. 2011;22(4):773–81.

290. Bourhis J, Lefebvre JL, Vermorken JB. Cetuximab in the management of locoregionally advanced head and neck cancer: expanding the treatment options? Eur J Cancer. 2010;46(11):1979–89.

291. Li T, Perez-Soler R. Skin toxicities associated with epidermal growth factor receptor inhibitors. Target Oncol. 2009;4(2):107–19.

292. Walsh L, Gillham C, Dunne M, Fraser I, Hollywood D, Armstrong J, et al. Toxicity of cetuximab versus cisplatin concurrent with radiotherapy in locally advanced head and neck squamous cell cancer (LAHNSCC). Radiother Oncol. 2011;98(1): 38–41.

293. Kuhnt T, Sandner A, Wendt T, Engenhart-Cabillic R, Lammering G, Flentje M, et al. Phase I trial of dose-escalated cisplatin with concomitant cetuximab and hyperfractionated-accelerated radiotherapy in locally advanced squamous cell carcinoma of the head and neck. Ann Oncol. 2010;21(11): 2284–9.

294. Hansen NL, Chandiramani DV, Morse MA, Wei D, Hedrick NE, Hansen RA. Incidence and predictors of cetuximab hypersensitivity reactions in a North Carolina academic medical center. J Oncol Pharm Pract. 2011;17(2):125–30.

295. Lord HK, Junor E, Ironside J. Cetuximab is effective, but more toxic than reported in the Bonner trial. Clin Oncol (R Coll Radiol). 2008;20(1):96.

296. Rivera F, Vega-Villegas ME, Lopez-Brea MF, Marquez R. Current situation of Panitumumab, Matuzumab, Nimotuzumab and Zalutumumab. Acta Oncol. 2008;47(1):9–19.

297. Rivera F, Salcedo M, Vega N, Blanco Y, Lopez C. Current situation of zalutumumab. Expert Opin Biol Ther. 2009;9(5):667–74.

298. Machiels JP, Subramanian S, Ruzsa A, Repassy G, Lifirenko I, Flygare A, et al. Zalutumumab plus best supportive care versus best supportive care alone in patients with recurrent or metastatic squamous-cell carcinoma of the head and neck after failure of platinum-based chemotherapy: an open-label, randomised phase 3 trial. Lancet Oncol. 2011;12(4):333–43.

299. Liu Z, Liu Y, Jia B, Zhao H, Jin X, Li F, et al. Epidermal growth factor receptor-targeted radioimmunotherapy of human head and neck cancer xenografts using 90Y-labeled fully human antibody panitumumab. Mol Cancer Ther. 2010;9(8): 2297–308.

300. Wirth LJ, Allen AM, Posner MR, Haddad RI, Li Y, Clark JR, et al. Phase I dose-finding study of paclitaxel with panitumumab, carboplatin and intensity-modulated radiotherapy in patients with locally advanced squamous cell cancer of the head and neck. Ann Oncol. 2010;21(2):342–7.

301. Basavaraj C, Sierra P, Shivu J, Melarkode R, Montero E, Nair P. Nimotuzumab with chemoradiation confers a survival advantage in treatment-naive head and neck tumors over expressing EGFR. Cancer Biol Ther. 2010;10(7):673–81.

302. Schiller JH. Developments in epidermal growth factor receptor-targeting therapy for solid tumors: focus on matuzumab (EMD 72000). Cancer Invest. 2008; 26(1):81–95.

303. Cohen EEW, Kane MA, List MA, Brockstein BE, Mehrotra B, Huo DZ, et al. Phase II trial of gefitinib 250 mg daily in patients with recurrent and/or metastatic squamous cell carcinoma of the head and neck. Clin Cancer Res. 2005;11(23):8418–24.

304. Cohen EE, Rosen F, Stadler WM, Recant W, Stenson K, Huo D, et al. Phase II trial of ZD1839 in recurrent or metastatic squamous cell carcinoma of the head and neck. J Clin Oncol. 2003;21(10):1980–7.

305. Saarilahti K, Bono P, Kajanti M, Back L, Leivo I, Joensuu T, et al. Phase II prospective trial of gefitinib given concurrently with cisplatin and radiotherapy in patients with locally advanced head and neck cancer. J Otolaryngol Head Neck Surg. 2010;39(3):269–76.

306. Cohen EE, Haraf DJ, Kunnavakkam R, Stenson KM, Blair EA, Brockstein B, et al. Epidermal growth factor receptor inhibitor gefitinib added to chemoradiotherapy in locally advanced head and neck cancer. J Clin Oncol. 2010;28(20):3336–43.

307. Hainsworth JD, Spigel DR, Burris 3rd HA, Markus TM, Shipley D, Kuzur M, et al. Neoadjuvant chemotherapy/gefitinib followed by concurrent chemotherapy/radiation therapy/gefitinib for patients with locally advanced squamous carcinoma of the head and neck. Cancer. 2009;115(10):2138–46.

308. Chen C, Kane M, Song J, Campana J, Raben A, Hu K, et al. Phase I trial of gefitinib in combination with radiation or chemoradiation for patients with locally advanced squamous cell head and neck cancer. J Clin Oncol. 2007;25(31):4880–6.

309. Caponigro F, Romano C, Milano A, Solla R, Franchin G, Adamo V, et al. A phase I/II trial of gefitinib and radiotherapy in patients with locally advanced inoperable squamous cell carcinoma of the head and neck. Anticancer Drugs. 2008;19(7):739–44.

310. Herbst RS, LoRusso PM, Purdom M, Ward D. Dermatologic side effects associated with gefitinib therapy: clinical experience and management. Clin Lung Cancer. 2003;4(6):366–9.

311. Montemurro F, Valabrega G, Aglietta M. Lapatinib: a dual inhibitor of EGFR and HER2 tyrosine kinase activity. Expert Opin Biol Ther. 2007;7(2):257–68.

312. Harrington KJ, El-Hariry IA, Holford CS, Lusinchi A, Nutting CM, Rosine D, et al. Phase I study of lapatinib in combination with chemoradiation in patients with locally advanced squamous cell carcinoma of the head and neck. J Clin Oncol. 2009;27(7):1100–7.

313. Chung KY, Shia J, Kemeny NE, Shah M, Schwartz GK, Tse A, et al. Cetuximab shows activity in colorectal cancer patients with tumors that do not express the epidermal growth factor receptor by immunohistochemistry. J Clin Oncol. 2005;23(9): 1803–10.

314. Ciardiello F, Tortora G. Epidermal growth factor receptor (EGFR) as a target in cancer therapy: understanding the role of receptor expression and other molecular determinants that could influence the response to anti-EGFR drugs. Eur J Cancer. 2003; 39(10):1348–54.

315. Pectasides E, Rampias T, Kountourakis P, Sasaki C, Kowalski D, Fountzilas G, et al. Comparative prognostic value of epidermal growth factor quantitative protein expression compared with FISH for head and neck squamous cell carcinoma. Clin Cancer Res. 2011;17(9):2947–54.

316. Licitra L, Mesia R, Rivera F, Remenár E, Hitt R, Erfán J, et al. Evaluation of EGFR gene copy number as a predictive biomarker for the efficacy of cetuximab in combination with chemotherapy in the first-line treatment of recurrent and/or metastatic squamous cell carcinoma of the head and neck: EXTREME study. Ann Oncol. 2011;22(5):1078–87.

317. Chau NG, Perez-Ordonez B, Zhang K, Pham NA, Ho J, Zhang T, et al. The association between EGFR variant III, HPV, p16, c-MET, EGFR gene copy number and response to EGFR inhibitors in patients with recurrent or metastatic squamous cell carcinoma of the head and neck. Head Neck Oncol. 2011;27(3):11.

318. Ryott M, Wangsa D, Heselmeyer-Haddad K, Lindholm J, Elmberger G, Auer G, et al. EGFR protein overexpression and gene copy number increases in oral tongue squamous cell carcinoma. Eur J Cancer. 2009;45(9):1700–8.

319. Giovannetti E, Erdem L, Olcay E, Leon LG, Peters GJ. Influence of polymorphisms on EGFR targeted therapy in non-small-cell lung cancer. Front Biosci. 2011;16:116–30.

320. Klinghammer K, Knodler M, Schmittel A, Budach V, Keilholz U, Tinhofer I. Association of epidermal growth factor receptor polymorphism, skin toxicity, and outcome in patients with squamous cell carcinoma of the head and neck receiving cetuximab-docetaxel treatment. Clin Cancer Res. 2010;16(1):304–10.

321. Murray S, Bobos M, Angouridakis N, Nikolaou A, Linardou H, Razis E, et al. Screening for EGFR mutations in patients with head and neck cancer treated with gefitinib on a compassionate-use program: A Hellenic Cooperative Oncology Group Study. J Oncol. 2010;2010:709678.

322. Weber A, Langhanki L, Sommerer F, Markwarth A, Wittekind C, Tannapfel A. Mutations of the BRAF gene in squamous cell carcinoma of the head and neck. Oncogene. 2003;22(30):4757–9.

323. Yamatodani T, Ekblad L, Kjellen E, Johnsson A, Mineta H, Wennerberg J. Epidermal growth factor receptor status and persistent activation of Akt and p44/42 MAPK pathways correlate with the effect of cetuximab in head and neck and colon cancer cell lines. J Cancer Res Clin Oncol. 2009;135(3): 395–402.

324. Park JH, Han SW, Oh DY, Im SA, Jeong SY, Park KJ, et al. Analysis of KRAS, BRAF, PTEN, IGF1R, EGFR intron 1 CA status in both primary tumors and paired metastases in determining benefit from cetuximab therapy in colon cancer. Cancer Chemother Pharmacol. 2011;68(4):1045–55.

325. Barnes CJ, Ohshiro K, Rayala SK, El-Naggar AK, Kumar R. Insulin-like growth factor receptor as a therapeutic target in head and neck cancer. Clin Cancer Res. 2007;13(14):4291–99.

326. Folkman J. Angiogenesis. Annu Rev Med. 2006;57: 1–18.

327. Christopoulos A, Ahn SM, Klein JD, Kim S. Biology of vascular endothelial growth factor and its receptors in head and neck cancer: beyond angiogenesis. Head Neck. 2011;33(8):1220–9.

328. Wan X, Shen N, Mendoza A, Khanna C, Helman LJ. CCI-779 inhibits rhabdomyosarcoma xenograft growth by an antiangiogenic mechanism linked to the targeting of mTOR/Hif-1alpha/VEGF signaling. Neoplasia. 2006;8(5):394–401.

329. Hay N, Sonenberg N. Upstream and downstream of mTOR. Genes Dev. 2004;18(16):1926–45.

330. Holmes K, Roberts OL, Thomas AM, Cross MJ. Vascular endothelial growth factor receptor-2: structure, function, intracellular signalling and therapeutic inhibition. Cell Signal. 2007;19(10):2003–12.

331. Van Meter ME, Kim ES. Bevacizumab: current updates in treatment. Curr Opin Oncol. 2010;22(6): 586–91.

332. Jubb AM, Harris AL. Biomarkers to predict the clinical efficacy of bevacizumab in cancer. Lancet Oncol. 2010;11(12):1172–83.

333. Goodman VL, Rock EP, Dagher R, Ramchandani RP, Abraham S, Gobburu JV, et al. Approval summary: sunitinib for the treatment of imatinib refractory or intolerant gastrointestinal stromal tumors and advanced renal cell carcinoma. Clin Cancer Res. 2007;13(5):1367–73.

334. Seiwert TY, Cohen EE. Targeting angiogenesis in head and neck cancer. Semin Oncol. 2008;35(3): 274–85.

335. Choong NW, Kozloff M, Taber D, Hu HS, Wade 3rd J, Ivy P, et al. Phase II study of sunitinib malate in head and neck squamous cell carcinoma. Invest New Drugs. 2010;28(5):677–83.

336. Fury MG, Zahalsky A, Wong R, Venkatraman E, Lis E, Hann L, et al. A Phase II study of SU5416 in patients with advanced or recurrent head and neck cancers. Invest New Drugs. 2007;25(2):165–72.

337. Elser C, Siu LL, Winquist E, Agulnik M, Pond GR, Chin SF, et al. Phase II trial of sorafenib in patients with recurrent or metastatic squamous cell carcinoma of the head and neck or nasopharyngeal carcinoma. J Clin Oncol. 2007;25(24):3766–73.

338. Williamson SK, Moon J, Huang CH, Guaglianone PP, LeBlanc M, Wolf GT, et al. Phase II evaluation of sorafenib in advanced and metastatic squamous cell carcinoma of the head and neck: Southwest Oncology Group Study S0420. J Clin Oncol. 2010;28(20):3330–5.

339. Machiels JP, Henry S, Zanetta S, Kaminsky MC, Michoux N, Rommel D, et al. Phase II study of sunitinib in recurrent or metastatic squamous cell carcinoma of the head and neck: GORTEC 2006–01. J Clin Oncol. 2010;28(1):21–8.

340. Fountzilas G, Fragkoulidi A, Kalogera-Fountzila A, Nikolaidou M, Bobos M, Calderaro J, et al. A phase II study of sunitinib in patients with recurrent and/or metastatic non-nasopharyngeal head and neck cancer. Cancer Chemoth Pharm. 2010;65(4): 649–60.

341. Argiris A, Karamouzis MV, Gooding WE, Branstetter BF, Zhong S, Raez LE, et al Phase II trial of pemetrexed and bevacizumab in patients with recurrent or metastatic head and neck cancer. J Clin Oncol. 2011;29(9):1140–5.

342. Hui EP, Ma BB, King AD, Mo F, Chan SL, Kam MK, et al. Hemorrhagic complications in a phase II study of sunitinib in patients of nasopharyngeal carcinoma who has previously received high-dose radiation. Ann Oncol. 2011;22(6):1280–7.

343. Sano D, Matsumoto F, Valdecanas DR, Zhao M, Molkentine DP, Takahashi Y, et al. Vandetanib restores head and neck squamous cell carcinoma cells' sensitivity to cisplatin and radiation in vivo and in vitro. Clin Cancer Res. 2011;17(7):1815–27. Epub 2011 Feb 24.

344. Twardowski P, Stadler WM, Frankel P, Lara PN, Ruel C, Chatta G, et al. Phase II study of Aflibercept (VEGF-Trap) in patients with recurrent or metastatic urothelial cancer, a California Cancer Consortium Trial. Urology. 2010;76(4):923–6.

345. Lippert 3rd JW. Vascular disrupting agents. Bioorg Med Chem. 2007;15(2):605–15.
346. Kim JJ, Goldie SJ. Cost effectiveness analysis of including boys in a human papillomavirus vaccination programme in the United States. BMJ. 2009;339: b3884.
347. Jit M, Choi YH, Edmunds WJ. Economic evaluation of human papillomavirus vaccination in the United Kingdom. BMJ. 2008;337:a769.
348. Sima N, Wang W, Kong D, Deng D, Xu Q, Zhou J, et al. RNA interference against HPV16 E7 oncogene leads to viral E6 and E7 suppression in cervical cancer cells and apoptosis via upregulation of Rb and p53. Apoptosis. 2008;13(2):273–81.
349. Hamada K, Shirakawa T, Gotoh A, Roth JA, Follen M. Adenovirus-mediated transfer of human papillomavirus 16 E6/E7 antisense RNA and induction of apoptosis in cervical cancer. Gynecol Oncol. 2006; 103(3):820–30.
350. Hildesheim A, Herrero R, Wacholder S, Rodriguez AC, Solomon D, Bratti MC, et al. Effect of human papillomavirus 16/18L1 viruslike particle vaccine among young women with preexisting infection: a randomized trial. JAMA. 2007;298(7):743–53.
351. Nathan CO, Amirghahari N, Rong X, Giordano T, Sibley D, Nordberg M, et al. Mammalian target of rapamycin inhibitors as possible adjuvant therapy for microscopic residual disease in head and neck squamous cell cancer. Cancer Res. 2007;67(5): 2160–8.
352. Mandal M, Myers JN, Lippman SM, Johnson FM, Williams MD, Rayala S, et al. Epithelial to mesenchymal transition in head and neck squamous carcinoma: association of Src activation with E-cadherin down-regulation, vimentin expression, and aggressive tumor features. Cancer. 2008;112(9):2088–100.
353. Brooks HD, Glisson BS, Bekele BN, Ginsberg LE, El-Naggar A, Culotta KS, et al Phase 2 study of dasatinib in the treatment of head and neck squamous cell carcinoma. Cancer. 2011;117(10):2112–9.
354. Egloff AM, Grandis JR. Improving response rates to EGFR-targeted therapies for head and neck squamous cell carcinoma: candidate predictive biomarkers and combination treatment with Src inhibitors. J Oncol. 2009;2009:896407.
355. Kao J, Genden EM, Chen CT, Rivera M, Tong CC, Misiukiewicz K, et al. Cancer. Phase 1 trial of concurrent erlotinib, celecoxib, and reirradiation for recurrent head and neck cancer. 2011;117(14):3173–81.
356. Wirth LJ, Krane JF, Li Y, Othus M, Moran AE, Dorfman DM, et al. A pilot surrogate endpoint biomarker study of celecoxib in oral premalignant lesions. Cancer Prev Res (Phila). 2008;1(5):339–48.
357. Yu T, Wu Y, Helman JI, Wen Y, Wang C, Li L. CXCR4 promotes oral squamous cell carcinoma migration and invasion through inducing expression of MMP-9 and MMP-13 via the ERK signaling pathway. Mol Cancer Res. 2011;9(2).161–72.
358. Hsiao JR, Chang Y, Chen YL, Hsieh SH, Hsu KF, Wang CF, et al. Cyclic alphavbeta6-targeting peptide

selected from biopanning with clinical potential for head and neck squamous cell carcinoma. Head Neck. 2010;32(2):160–72.
359. Harrington KJ, Kazi R, Bhide SA, Newbold K, Nutting CM. Novel therapeutic approaches to squamous cell carcinoma of the head and neck using biologically targeted agents. Indian J Cancer. 2010;47(3):248–59.
360. Ma B, Hui EP, King A, To KF, Mo F, Leung SF, et al. A phase II study of patients with metastatic or locoregionally recurrent nasopharyngeal carcinoma and evaluation of plasma Epstein-Barr virus DNA as a biomarker of efficacy. Cancer Chemother Pharmacol. 2008;62(1):59–64.
361. Chan AT, Hsu MM, Goh BC, Hui EP, Liu TW, Millward MJ, et al. Multicenter, phase II study of cetuximab in combination with carboplatin in patients with recurrent or metastatic nasopharyngeal carcinoma. J Clin Oncol. 2005;23(15):3568–76.
362. Hotte SJ, Winquist EW, Lamont E, MacKenzie M, Vokes E, Chen EX, et al. Imatinib mesylate in patients with adenoid cystic cancers of the salivary glands expressing c-kit: A Princess Margaret Hospital phase II consortium study. J Clin Oncol. 2005;23(3):585–90.
363. Pfeffer MR, Talmi Y, Catane R, Symon Z, Yosepovitch A, Levitt M. A phase II study of imatinib for advanced adenoid cystic carcinoma of head and neck salivary glands. Oral Oncol. 2007;43(1):33–6.
364. Ghosal N, Mais K, Shenjere P, Julyan P, Hastings D, Ward T, et al. Phase II study of cisplatin and imatinib in advanced salivary adenoid cystic carcinoma. Br J Oral Maxillofac Surg. 2011;49(7):510–5.
365. Argiris A, Ghebremichael M, Burtness B, Axelrod RS, Deconti RC, Forastiere AA. A phase 2 trial of bortezomib followed by the addition of doxorubicin at progression in patients with recurrent or metastatic adenoid cystic carcinoma of the head and neck: a trial of the Eastern Cooperative Oncology Group (E1303). Cancer. 2011;117(15):3374–82.
366. Agulnik M, Cohen EWE, Cohen RB, Chen EX, Vokes EE, Hotte SJ, et al. Phase II study of lapatinib in recurrent or metastatic epidermal growth factor receptor and/or erbB2 expressing adenoid cystic carcinoma and non-adenoid cystic carcinoma malignant tumors of the salivary glands. J Clin Oncol. 2007;25(25):3978–84.
367. Haddad R, Posner MR. Palliative chemotherapy in patients with salivary gland neoplasms and preliminary reports of 2 recent phase II studies with trastuzumab and gemcitabine. Clin Adv Hematol Oncol. 2003;1(4):226–8.
368. Haddad R, Colevas AD, Krane JF, Cooper D, Glisson B, Amrein PC, et al. Herceptin in patients with advanced or metastatic salivary gland carcinomas. A phase II study. Oral Oncol. 2003;39(7):724–7.
369. Locati LD, Bossi P, Perrone F, Potepan P, Crippa F, Mariani L, et al. Cetuximab in recurrent and/or metastatic salivary gland carcinomas: a phase II study. Oral Oncol. 2009;45(7):574–78.

370. Snijders PJ, Scholes AG, Hart CA, Jones AS, Vaughan ED, Woolgar JA, et al. Prevalence of mucosotropic human papillomaviruses in squamous-cell carcinoma of the head and neck. Int J Cancer. 1996;66(4):464–9.

371. Paz IB, Cook N, Odom-Maryon T, Xie Y, Wilczynski SP. Human papillomavirus (HPV) in head and neck cancer. An association of HPV 16 with squamous cell carcinoma of Waldeyer's tonsillar ring. Cancer. 1997;79(3):595–604.

372. Pintos J, Franco EL, Black MJ, Bergeron J, Arella M. Human papillomavirus and prognoses of patients with cancers of the upper aerodigestive tract. Cancer. 1999;85(9):1903–9.

373. Mellin H, Friesland S, Lewensohn R, Dalianis T, Munck-Wikland E. Human papillomavirus (HPV) DNA in tonsillar cancer: clinical correlates, risk of relapse, and survival. Int J Cancer. 2000;89(3): 300–4.

374. Friesland S, Mellin H, Munck-Wikland E, Nilsson A, Lindholm J, Dalianis T, et al. Human papilloma virus (HPV) and p53 immunostaining in advanced tonsillar carcinoma–relation to radiotherapy response and survival. Anticancer Res. 2001;21(1B):529–34.

375. Klussmann JP, Gultekin E, Weissenborn SJ, Wieland U, Dries V, Dienes HP, et al. Expression of p16 protein identifies a distinct entity of tonsillar carcinomas associated with human papillomavirus. Am J Pathol. 2003;162(3):747–53.

376. Li W, Thompson CH, O'Brien CJ, McNeil EB, Scolyer RA, Cossart YE, et al. Human papillomavirus positivity predicts favourable outcome for squamous carcinoma of the tonsil. Int J Cancer. 2003;106(4):553–8.

377. Baez A, Almodovar JI, Cantor A, Celestin F, Cruz-Cruz L, Fonseca S, et al. High frequency of HPV16-associated head and neck squamous cell carcinoma in the Puerto Rican population. Head Neck. 2004; 26(9):778–84.

378. Wittekindt C, Gultekin E, Weissenborn SJ, Dienes HP, Pfister HJ, Klussmann JP. Expression of p16 protein is associated with human papillomavirus status in tonsillar carcinomas and has implications on survival. Adv Otorhinolaryngol. 2005;62:72–80.

379. Badaracco G, Rizzo C, Mafera B, Pichi B, Giannarelli D, Rahimi SS, et al. Molecular analyses and prognostic relevance of HPV in head and neck tumours. Oncol Rep. 2007;17(4):931–9.

380. Reimers N, Kasper HU, Weissenborn SJ, Stutzer H, Preuss SF, Hoffmann TK, et al. Combined analysis of HPV-DNA, p16 and EGFR expression to predict prognosis in oropharyngeal cancer. Int J Cancer. 2007;120(8):1731–8.

381. Na, II, Kang HJ, Cho SY, Koh JS, Lee JK, Lee BC, et al. EGFR mutations and human papillomavirus in squamous cell carcinoma of tongue and tonsil. Eur J Cancer. 2007;43(3):520–6.

382. Fakhry C, Westra WH, Li S, Cmelak A, Ridge JA, Pinto H, et al. Improved survival of patients with human papillomavirus-positive head and neck squamous cell carcinoma in a prospective clinical trial. J Natl Cancer Inst. 2008;100(4):261–9.

383. Klozar J, Kratochvil V, Salakova M, Smahelova J, Vesela E, Hamsikova E, et al. HPV status and regional metastasis in the prognosis of oral and oropharyngeal cancer. Eur Arch Otorhinolaryngol. 2008;265 Suppl 1:S75–82.

384. Smith EM, Wang D, Rubenstein LM, Morris WA, Turek LP, Haugen TH. Association between p53 and human papillomavirus in head and neck cancer survival. Cancer Epidemiol Biomarkers Prev. 2008; 17(2):421–7.

385. Chung YL, Lee MY, Horng CF, Jian JJ, Cheng SH, Tsai SY, et al. Use of combined molecular biomarkers for prediction of clinical outcomes in locally advanced tonsillar cancers treated with chemoradiotherapy alone. Head Neck. 2009;31(1):9–20.

386. Kong CS, Narasimhan B, Cao H, Kwok S, Erickson JP, Koong A, et al. The relationship between human papillomavirus status and other molecular prognostic markers in head and neck squamous cell carcinomas. Int J Radiat Oncol Biol Phys. 2009;74(2):553–61.

387. Lassen P, Eriksen JG, Hamilton-Dutoit S, Tramm T, Alsner J, Overgaard J. Effect of HPV-associated p16INK4A expression on response to radiotherapy and survival in squamous cell carcinoma of the head and neck. J Clin Oncol. 2009;27(12):1992–8.

388. Hafkamp HC, Mooren JJ, Claessen SM, Klingenberg B, Voogd AC, Bot FJ, et al. P21 Cip1/WAF1 expression is strongly associated with HPV-positive tonsillar carcinoma and a favorable prognosis. Mod Pathol. 2009;22(5):686–98.

389. Rischin D, Young RJ, Fisher R, Fox SB, Le QT, Peters LJ, et al. Prognostic significance of p16INK4A and human papillomavirus in patients with oropharyngeal cancer treated on TROG 02.02 phase III trial. J Clin Oncol. 2010;28(27):4142–8.

390. Hannisdal K, Schjolberg A, De Angelis PM, Boysen M, Clausen OP. Human papillomavirus (HPV)-positive tonsillar carcinomas are frequent and have a favourable prognosis in males in Norway. Acta Otolaryngol. 2010;130(2):293–9.

391. Ang KK, Harris J, Wheeler R, Weber R, Rosenthal DI, Nguyen-Tan PF, et al. Human papillomavirus and survival of patients with oropharyngeal cancer. N Engl J Med. 2010;363(1):24–35.

392. Fischer CA, Kampmann M, Zlobec I, Green E, Tornillo L, Lugli A, et al. p16 expression in oropharyngeal cancer: its impact on staging and prognosis compared with the conventional clinical staging parameters. Ann Oncol. 2010;21(10):1961–6.

393. Smith EM, Rubenstein LM, Hoffman H, Haugen TH, Turek LP. Human papillomavirus, p16 and p53 expression associated with survival of head and neck cancer. Infect Agent Cancer. 2010;5:4.

394. Lewis JS, Jr., Thorstad WL, Chernock RD, Haughey BH, Yip JH, Zhang Q, et al. p16 positive oropharyngeal squamous cell carcinoma: an entity with a favorable prognosis regardless of tumor HPV status. Am J Surg Pathol. 2010;34(8):1088–96.

Thyroid Cancer

3

Laura D. Locati, Angela Greco, Maria Grazia Borrello, Maria Luisa Carcangiu, Paolo Bossi, Roberta Granata, and Lisa Licitra

Introduction

Although thyroid cancer (TC) is considered a rare tumor, representing only 1.7% of the total estimated new cancer cases around the world in 2008 [1], it is, however, the most common tumor of the endocrine system, accounting for more than 95% of all endocrine cancers in the USA [2]. The incidence of this cancer has risen worldwide in the last decades [3–7] doubling since the seventies, and for women, it is the cancer with the fastest-growing number of new cases. A huge increase in the incidence of this cancer has been recorded also in Italy, where in the 2-year period 2003–2005 thyroid was the second most common cancer after breast tumor among women under the age of 44 years and the fifth most common

L.D. Locati, M.D. • R. Granata, M.D.
• L. Licitra, M.D. • P. Bossi, M.D. (✉)
Head and Neck Medical Oncology Unit,
Fondazione IRCCS Istituto Nazionale dei Tumori,
via Venezian 1, Milan 20133, Italy
e-mail: laura.locati@istitutotumori.mi.it

A. Greco, Ph.D. • M.G. Borrello, Ph.D.
Department of Experimental Oncology and Molecular
Medicine, Fondazione IRCCS Istituto Nazionale dei
Tumori, via Venezian 1, Milan 20133, Italy

M.L. Carcangiu, M.D.
Department of Pathology, Fondazione IRCCS
Istituto Nazionale dei Tumori, via Venezian 1,
Milan 20133, Italy

among men [8]. Virtually, the entire increase is attributable to a raise in incidence of papillary thyroid cancer, which in the USA has increased from 2.7 to 7.7 per 100,000 — a 2.9-fold increase (95% CI, 2.6–3.2; $P<0.001$). No significant change has been observed in the incidence of the less common histological types follicular, medullary, and anaplastic ($P>0.20$) [9]. It has not yet been clarified if the rise in incidence rates is a true biological issue or if it is a result of the improvement in the diagnostic tools, such as ultrasound and fine-needle biopsy. Small papillary thyroid carcinomas (<1 cm, defined as microcarcinoma) are the most common contributors to this incidence increase [10], supporting the correlation with the improvement in diagnostic detection. However, this would not explain the rising number of larger tumors in all age groups [11] which suggests, on the contrary, the involvement of multiple contributing factors. Exposure to radiation during medical procedures [12], obesity [13], as well as the increase in pathological detection of incidental papillary thyroid cancer [14] are some possible explanations. Mortality rates, in contrast to incidence rates, are stable or decreasing both in the USA [9] and in Europe [15]. The 10-year relative survival rate is commonly very good, ranging from 90% in differentiated thyroid cancer [16] to 74% in medullary thyroid cancer while it is dramatically short (<1 year) in case of anaplastic thyroid cancer which

M. Bologna (ed.), *Biotargets of Cancer in Current Clinical Practice*, Current Clinical Pathology,
DOI 10.1007/978-1-61779-615-9_3, © Springer Science+Business Media, LLC 2012

represents one of the most aggressive malignant tumors in humans.

Surgery remains the cornerstone of the management of thyroid tumors. TSH suppression and radioactive iodine (RAI) follow surgery as adjuvant treatments in differentiated thyroid cancers, while they play no curative role in medullary thyroid cancer. In anaplastic thyroid cancer, surgery is not often technically feasible due to the local extension and invasion of the contiguous anatomic structures.

Metastatic disease is a rare event, occurring in about 20% of patients with differentiated thyroid cancer [17]. The 10-year survival rate is 42% for metastatic differentiated thyroid cancer patients [18] while it decreases to 24% in case of medullary thyroid cancer. Prolonged survival of metastatic patients is a peculiar characteristic that distinguishes these cancers from the great part of advanced malignant tumors. Anaplastic cancer is an exception: median survival is commonly less than 1 year. RAI is the most employed systemic treatment in metastatic differentiated thyroid carcinomas with curative role only in still ^{131}I-avid cases (<50%). A large tumor burden, bone metastases, an older age, and a poorly differentiated histology characterize a group of patients with high probability of no or low ^{131}I uptake [17]. The 10-year overall survival in case of RAI-resistant disease falls to 10%. Doxorubicin was the only treatment approved by Food and Drug Administration (FDA) for metastatic TCs until 2011. Doxorubicin alone or combined with other drugs administered in RAI-resistant patients obtained poor results [19]. Several chemotherapeutic agents have been attempted in MTC with discouraging results. Chemotherapy is not recommended as first choice for advanced medullary thyroid cancer due to the low response rates. Reports on radiolabeled molecules such as ^{90}Yttrium-DOTA-TOC, ^{111}In-Octreoscan, and ^{131}I-MIBG have been published, but only a modest activity was observed together with no impact on survival [20].

In recent years, major advances in understanding TC have been made, with a great improvement in the field of molecular biology. TC represents a unique and fascinating model that includes several histotypes characterized by peculiar biological and clinical characteristics. Molecular markers involved in TC pathogenesis and progression have been extensively investigated in the recent years, becoming the biological base for the delivery of tailored treatments. At present, these latter have found their practical application in advanced and/or metastatic RAI-resistant differentiated, medullary and anaplastic carcinomas.

In the next paragraphs, we will provide a brief characterization of the peculiar clinical features of each main TC histotype; a detailed description on molecular markers and signals pathways involved in TCs pathogenesis and progression and, finally, a wide overview on the clinical applications deriving from the translational research.

Histological Classification and Clinical Overview

According to the cell of origin, TCs are divided into those derived from follicular cells and those originated in C cells. The first ones, which are by far the most common, comprise papillary carcinoma (about 80% of the cases), follicular carcinoma (10%), poorly differentiated carcinoma (4–6%) Hürthle cell (oxyphil) tumors (3%), and anaplastic carcinoma (2–5%). The second ones, originating in the C cells, are known as medullary carcinomas (5–10%) (Fig. 3.1).

Papillary cancer, follicular carcinoma, and their variants are commonly grouped under the name of differentiated thyroid cancer. Poorly differentiated carcinoma, medullary carcinoma, and anaplastic carcinomas are much less common.

According to the latest WHO classification [21], malignant thyroid tumors are classified as reported in Table 3.1. For the purpose of this chapter, we will focus our attention on differentiated, poorly differentiated, anaplastic, and medullary thyroid cancers. We will not discuss the characteristics of rare thyroid tumors such as squamous, mucoepidermoid, and other exceptional subtypes.

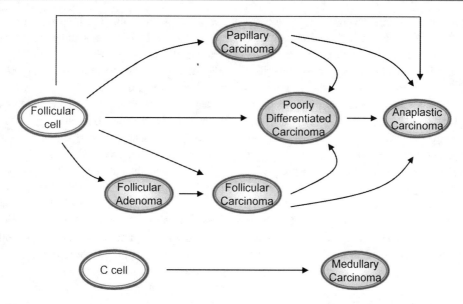

Fig. 3.1 Schematic representation of thyroid carcinogenesis

Table 3.1 Classification of thyroid carcinomas

Papillary carcinoma	8260/3[a]
Follicular carcinoma	8330/3
Poorly differentiated carcinoma	
Undifferentiated (anaplastic) carcinoma	8020/3
Squamous cell carcinoma	8070/3
Mucoepidermoid carcinoma	8430/3
Sclerosing mucoepidermoid carcinoma with eosinophilia	8430/3
Mucinous carcinoma	8480/3
Medullary carcinoma	8345/3
Mixed medullary and follicular cell carcinoma	8346/3
Spindle cell tumor with thymus-like differentiation	8588/3
Carcinoma showing thymus-like differentiation	8589/3

[a]Morphology code of the international classification of disease for oncology (ICD-0) and the systematized nomenclature of medicine

Papillary Thyroid Carcinoma

PTC is the most frequent epithelial thyroid cancer (80% of the cases). It is most commonly seen in adults aged 20–50, and the female to male ratio is 4:1. PTC is also the most common pediatric thyroid malignancy. Radiation exposure is recognized as the main cause for PTC development. The tumor presents as an enlarged solid node in more than half of patients, being multifocal in one lobe at least in 50% of cases and bilateral in up to 30%. Microcarcinoma is rare in childhood but very common in the general population (present in up to 33% of individuals in autopsy series). It has a very good prognosis, not significantly different from that of people lacking this abnormality, except in cases of lymph node metastases and/or extrathyroid extension.

Lymphatic vessels are the main pathway of diffusion of PTC, and cervical lymph node metastases are very frequent at the time of diagnosis.

"Classical" PTC is microscopically characterized by a papillary architecture and a population of follicular cells with "ground glass" nuclei and irregularities of nuclear contours, including grooves and nuclear pseudoinclusions. Psammoma bodies, which represent a typical PTC feature, are found in at least 50% of cases: they are rounded and concentrically laminated calcifications which can be present within the tumor stroma, in the tip of the papillae or in lymphatic spaces. PTC is immunoreactive for cytokeratins, thyroglobulin, and thyroid transcription factor-1 (TTF-1). Metastatic PTCs express TTF-1 and thyroglobulin, while pulmonary adenocarcinomas express TTF-1 but not thyroglobulin, for a feature of value in the differential diagnosis.

Histological variants account for 15–20% of PTCs. The most common histological PTC variants are follicular, oncocytic, clear cell, diffuse sclerosing, tall cell, columnar cell, solid, and cribriform. For most of these variants, the prognosis is similar to classic PTC, whereas in some histotypes such as tall cell, columnar cell, and solid variants, the outcome is worse. These rare variants are characterized by an aggressive behavior, with the primary tumor often presenting with extrathyroid extension and vascular invasion. The prognosis of classic PTC is excellent and influenced by patient age, tumor size, extrathyroid extension, completeness of surgery, and presence of distant metastases.

Follicular Thyroid Carcinoma

Follicular carcinoma is more common in women over 50. It is rare in children and more prevalent in iodine-deficient areas. FTC is usually encapsulated and solitary. It is composed of epithelial cells with follicular differentiation lacking the above described nuclear features of PTC. Frequently it grows as an asymptomatic and enlarged thyroid mass. Hematogenous diffusion is more frequent than lymphatic spread. Compared to PTC, cervical lymph node involvement is less common at diagnosis while distant metastases can be found in 20% of the cases, lung and bone being the most involved sites. Invasiveness of the capsule (defined as tumor full penetration through the capsule at a location other than the previous biopsy site) and vascular invasion are the microscopic characteristics that distinguish FTC from follicular adenoma (FA) from which FTC may develop. The risk of metastatic spread is higher in those cases with widespread vascular invasion. FTC cells are commonly immunoreactive for thyroglobulin, TTF-1, and low molecular weight cytokeratin.

Hürthle cell carcinoma (HCC) or "oncocytic or oxyphilic" variant is a rare variant of follicular or (less commonly) of papillary carcinoma. Oncocytic FTC differs from conventional FTCs on biological and clinical grounds, leading some groups to regard HCCs as a distinct pathologic entity. HCCs are defined as tumors composed of 75% or greater Hürthle cells and exhibiting complete capsular and/or vascular invasion. The tumor cells are typically characterized by an abundant granular, eosinophilic cytoplasm derived from the presence of a large number of mitochondria. In contrast to the typical FTC behavior, HCC presents with cervical node involvement in 30% of the cases, and distant metastases can also occur.

Fifty percent of patients with a widely invasive FTC die of their disease, whereas patients with a minimally invasive FTC have a survival expectance similar to that of a normal population matched for age and sex. This is true both for FTC and HCC, although the latter is generally associated with a more aggressive behavior with respect to conventional FTC, in the form of higher frequency of loco-regional relapse and distant metastases.

Poorly Differentiated Thyroid Carcinoma

PDTC is a rare and controversial entity, more commonly seen in women and patients over 50. The etiology is unknown. It can be the terminal stage of the dedifferentiation process of PTC or FTC or can grow ex novo [22]. At presentation, it can appear as a unique thyroid mass, often rapidly growing, with or without cervical node involvement. Distant metastases can be also present. Three different histological patterns have been described: insular, trabecular, and solid [23]. Infiltrative pattern of growth, necrosis, and vascular invasion along with the identification of the patterns described above should allow its recognition. Immunoreactivity for TTF-1 and thyroglobulin is common. The mean 5-year survival is less than 50% [24, 25].

Anaplastic Thyroid Carcinoma

ATC is one of the most malignant tumors in humans. It occurs more commonly in the elderly, only a quarter of patients being under 60 years old. As PDTC, it can derive from DTCs or can arise ex novo. All ATCs are by definition T4 tumors in the AJCC classification [26]. ATC is composed of undifferentiated cells that show immunohistochemical features of epithelial differentiation. Cytokeratin is the most expressed epithelial marker, TTF-1 and thyroglobulin are generally negative, while there is strong positivity for TP53. At the clinical level, a large thyroid mass, rapidly growing and infiltrating surrounding tissues and muscles, characterizes ATC. The larynx (15%), laryngeal nerve (30%), esophagus (45%), and trachea (50%) are frequently involved [27]. The clinical course of the disease can be so rapid that surgical procedures performed as supportive care (e.g., tracheotomy and gastrostomy) are often useless. In addition, a tracheotomy could sometimes be technically impossible to perform due to the tumor mass encasing carotid and trachea. Diffuse distant spread is present in more than 50% of patients at diagnosis. Five-year survival ranges from 0% to 14% [27–29].

Medullary Thyroid Cancer

MTC is a neuroendocrine tumor which is sporadic in about 75% of the cases. In the other 25%, it occurs as a component of the autosomal dominant familial multiple endocrine neoplasia type 2 (MEN 2) syndrome. MEN 2, first described by Sipple [30], includes three disorders: MEN 2A, MEN 2B, and familial MTC (FMTC) [31–33]. Activating rearranged during transfection (RET) mutations are present in more than 95% of FMTCs and in 20–50% of sporadic MTCs. Nests or trabeculae of polygonal, round, or spindle cells, separated by fibrovascular stroma, characterize MTC. Tumor cells are immunoreactive for calcitonin, a polypeptide almost exclusively produced by MTC, carcinoembryonic antigen (CEA), and other neuroendocrine markers such as chromogranin A and synaptophysin. TTF-1 and low molecular weight keratins can be also expressed. The median age at presentation is 50. MTC is typically located in the middle third of the lobe (where C cells are most represented) and can be unilateral in case of sporadic tumors or multiple and bilateral in FMTC, and commonly

not capsulated. Tumor diameter can vary from less than 1 cm to a larger mass. Up to 50% of the patients present with cervical node involvement, and up to 15% with distant metastases. Calcitonin has a diagnostic [34] and prognostic value at diagnosis [35]. Occult distant metastases after thyroidectomy and neck dissection are responsible for the persistence of high levels of calcitonin. Sometimes diarrhea and flushing can be associated with advanced disease.

Five- and 10-year survival rates are 83 and 74%. Some clinical features are related to a lower survival. These include older age, male gender, extent of local tumor, and presence of distant metastases [36].

Molecular Genetics of Thyroid Carcinoma

PTC

The last two decades have been marked by significant expansion in the understanding of the molecular basis of PTC. It is now apparent that this tumor type is characterized by genetic lesions leading to the activation of the mitogen-activated protein kinase (MAPK) signaling pathway [37] (Fig. 3.2). In fact, chromosomal rearrangements involving *RET* or *TRK* (Table 3.2), or activating point mutations of *BRAF* or *RAS* genes, account for about 70% of PTC. PTC-associated genetic lesions are generally mutually exclusive.

Discordant patterns of *BRAF* mutation have been found in about 40% of the multifocal PTCs as well as in 50% of the cases in which multiple foci of different histopathologic variants were present [38]. Moreover, simultaneous presence of different RET/PTC and BRAF mutations have been reported [39, 40].

PTC was the first, and for a long time the only, epithelial tumor in which an acquired chromosomal rearrangement had generated a transforming fusion gene. Despite the high frequency of chromosomal rearrangements in PTC, the molecular bases underlying the predisposition of thyrocytes to undergo chromosomal rearrangements are not completely understood. Spatial genome

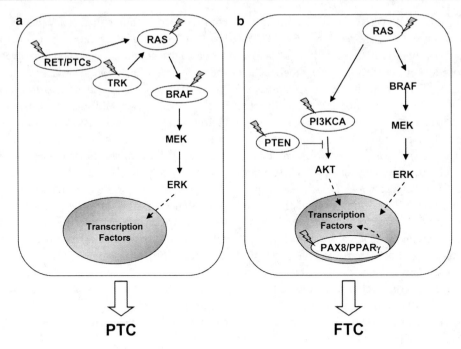

Fig. 3.2 Molecular alterations in papillary and follicular thyroid carcinomas. (**a**) In PTC, rearrangements involving RET or *NTRK1* and point mutation of *RAS* or *BRAF* genes lead to alterations of the MAPK pathway. (**b**) In FTC, alterations of the MAPK and the PI3K/AKT pathway result from rearrangements involving *PPARγ* or deregulation of *RAS, PI3KCA,* or *PTEN*

Table 3.2 Fusion oncogenes in papillary thyroid carcinomas

Oncogene	Donor gene
RET/PTC1	CCDC6 (coiled-coil domain containing 6) /H4/D10S170
RET/PTC2	PRKAR1A (protein kinase, cCAMP-dependent, regulatory, type I, alpha)
RET/PTC3	NCOA4 (nuclear coactivator 4)/RFG/ ELE1/ARA70
RET/PTC4	NCOA4 (nuclear coactivator 4)/RFG/ ELE1/ARA70
RET/PTC5	GOLGA5 (golgin subfamily a, 5)/ RFG5/RET-II
RET/PTC6	TRIM24 (tripartite motif-containing 24) /TIF1/TIF1A
RET/PTC7	TRIM33 (tripartite motif-containing 33) /RFG7/TIF1G
RET/PTC8	KTN1 (kinectin 1)/CG1
RET/PTC9	RFG9
ELKS-RET	ELKS/RAB6IP2/KIAA1081
PCM1-RET	PCM1 (pericentriolar material 1)
RFP-RET	TRIM27 (tripartite motif-containing 27) /RFP
HOOK3-RET	HOOK3 (homo sapiens hook homolog 3) /HK3
TRK	TPM3 (tropomyosin3)
TRK-T1, TRK-T2	TPR (translocated promoter region)
TRK-T3	TFG (TRK-fused gene)
AKAP9-BRAF	AKAP9 (A-kinase anchor protein 9)

topology has been proposed as a contributing factor in the formation of PTC-associated chromosomal translocations, based on the evidence of proximity between rearranging gene pairs such as *RET* and *H4* and *NTRK1* and *TPR* in interphase thyrocytes. On the other hand, the high proneness of thyroid epithelium to chromosomal rearrangements might reflect a peculiar sensitivity of thyrocytes to ionizing radiations, as well as the intrinsic capacity of a cell to repair DNA double-strand breaks induced by ionizing radiation [37].

RET/PTC and *TRK* oncoproteins contain the receptor tyrosine kinase (TK) domain fused to sequences from different donor genes which confer the following features: (1) ectopic expression in thyrocytes; (2) cytoplasmic localization; and (3) constitutive dimerization, mediated by coiled-coil domains, resulting in constitutive kinase activity [41].

RET/PTC Oncogenes

Oncogenic *RET* rearrangements, designated *RET/PTCs*, were the first genetic lesion identified in PTC more than 20 years ago [42]. *RET* proto-oncogene, located at chromosome 10q11.2, encodes a receptor type TK, an orphan receptor when *RET/PTC* oncogenes were identified. *RET* is now known to be the signaling component of a multimolecular complex that includes the glial cell line-derived neurotrophic factor (GDNF) and co-receptors α (GFRα1-4). Upon interaction with one of the four GFRα co-receptors, RET binds with high affinity to the GDNF family of peptides including GDNF, neurturin, persephin, and artemin [43]. Ontogenetically, the *RET* gene is essential for the development of the sympathetic, parasympathetic, and enteric neurons, kidney, and male germ cells [44]. Germ line loss of function mutations of *RET* causes impaired formation of the enteric nervous system and congenital aganglionosis of the colon (Hirschsprung's disease), while germ line activating point mutations are causally related to the hereditary forms of MTC, MEN 2A, MEN 2B, and FMTC [44].

In a significant fraction (20–30%) of PTCs, *RET* is subjected to chromosomal rearrangements leading to in-frame fusion of intracellular domains (including the TK and the C-terminal tail) to the 5′ end of heterologous genes (donor genes). The resulting fusion genes are named *RET/PTCs* and are listed in Table 3.2. *RET/PTC1* and *RET/PTC3* oncogenes are the most frequent, accounting together for more than 90% of all the rearrangements. The donor gene for *RET/PTC1* is the coiled coil containing domain 6 (*CCDC6*, formerly *H4* and *D10S170*). *RET/PTC3* donor gene is the nuclear receptor coactivating gene (*NCOA4*, formerly RFG, ELE, *ARA70*). *CCDC6* and *NCOA4*, as well as *RET*, map on the long arm of chromosome 10 so that a paracentric inversion of chromosome 10 creates *RET/PTC1* and *RET/PTC3* oncogenes. The majority of the other infrequent *RET* donor genes are located on different chromosomes, and the corresponding oncogenes derive from interchromosomal rearrangements. Several lines of evidence indicate that *RET/PTC* oncogenes are an early event in the pathogenesis of PTC: (1) *RET/PTC* expression has been detected in microscopic and occult PTCs [45]; (2) in in vitro models, *RET/PTC* oncogene expression in human normal primary thyrocytes causes PTC-diagnostic alteration in the nuclear envelope and chromatin structure [46]; and (3) induce morphological transformation of PC-Cl3 rat thyroid epithelial cells [47].

PTCs harboring RET/PTC rearrangements display predominantly the classical papillary variant. Patients have a high rate of lymph node metastases and possibly a more favorable prognosis, especially when RET/PTC1 oncogene is present [48].

RET/PTC incidence is higher in tumors from pediatric patients and from patients with a history of therapeutic as well as accidental (as in the case of Chernobyl accident) radiation exposure. The majority of post-Chernobyl PTCs carry *RET/PTC3* and are associated with the solid/follicular variant of PTC, while the less frequent *RET/PTC1* is associated with the classical and diffuse sclerosing variant [49].

It appears evident that deregulated RET signaling may have a major role in thyroid carcinogenesis. Constitutive dimerization of RET/PTC oncoproteins results in constitutive autophosphorylation and signaling. The crucial RET tyrosine residues identified include (1) Y900 and Y905, the latter being docking site for Grb7 and SH2B1β; (2) Y1015, docking site for PLCγ; (3) the major RET docking site Y1062, binding multiple proteins including Shc, ShcC, Irs1/2, Frs2, Dok1/4/5, and Enigma. Downstream to the cited adaptor proteins, RET activates Ras/ERK and PI3K/AKT pathways, as well as NFκB pathway [44, 50, 51]. Moreover, *RET/PTC1* induces nuclear translocation of β-catenin in thyrocytes as well as in a PTC cell line, suggesting a crucial role for β-catenin in RET neoplastic signaling in PTC [52, 53]. Besides proximal signaling relying on already available signaling molecules, RET activates a transcriptional program [54] including the transcription of inflammatory molecules (see below) and of other RTK proteins, as *MET/HGFR*. It was recently shown that *RET/PTC1* cross talks with Met at transcriptional and signaling levels to drive thyrocyte neoplastic transformation [52].

TRK Oncogenes

TRK oncogenes arise from rearrangements of the *NTRK1* gene (also known as *TRKA*, encoding the high-affinity receptor for NGF [41] on chromosome 1). *NTRK1* was originally isolated from a human colon carcinoma as a transforming oncogene activated by a somatic rearrangement that fused TPM3 (nonmuscle tropomyosin) gene to the kinase domain of a novel TK receptor. Cloning of the full-length gene and identification of the NGF as a ligand occurred few years later [55].

Several *TRK* oncogenes differing in the activating portions have been isolated from thyroid tumors (Table 3.2). The most frequent oncogene is *TRK* [56], identical to that first isolated from colon carcinoma, and containing sequences from the TPM3 gene on chromosome 1q22-23. *TRK-T1* and *TRK-T2* derive both from rearrangement between *NTRK1* and *TPR* gene on chromosome 1q25 but display different structure. *TRK-T3* is activated by *TFG*, a novel gene on chromosome 3q11-12, first identified in this rearranged version [57]. All TRK oncoproteins retain the five tyrosine residues crucial for *NTRK1* activity and mediate their effects through activation of PLCγ, SHC, FRS2, FRS3, IRS1, and IRS2 [58].

Somatic rearrangements of the *NTRK1* gene in PTC are less common than those involving *RET* gene; their frequency does not exceed 12%. The association of *NTRK1* rearrangements with radiation is not clearly defined, as their frequency in PTCs associated to therapeutic or accidental (Chernobyl) radiations was similar to that of sporadic tumors [59, 60]. Analysis of correlation between *NTRK1* rearrangements with clinical and pathological features did not produce unequivocal data. This is related to the limited number of PTCs carrying *TRK* oncogenes so far identified, also because in some studies the genotyping of PTCs is restricted to *RET* rearrangements and *BRAF* mutation analysis.

Experimental evidence suggests that *TRK* oncogenes exert a direct role and represent an early event in the process of thyroid carcinogenesis. Transgenic mice carrying *TRK-T1* oncogene under the control of thyroglobulin promoter (Tg-*TRK-T1* mice) develop thyroid hyperplasia and papillary carcinoma [61]. Crossing of Tg-*TRK-T1* mice with *p27^kip1*-deficient mice increased the penetrance of thyroid cancer and shortens the latency period of tumor incidence, indicating that TRK-T1 needs the cooperation with oncosuppressor genes to transform thyroid epithelium [62].

BRAF Oncogenes

BRAF is one of three mammalian isoforms of serine-threonine Raf kinase family, which upon activation by Ras binding and recruitment to the cell membrane generates a cascade of events leading to activation of MAPK signaling pathways [63]. *BRAF* gene is frequently mutated in a wide range of human cancers [64]. The prevalent mutation is a valine-to-glutamate substitution at residue 600 (V600E) which increases the BRAF basal kinase activity, resulting in constitutive activation and continuous phosphorylation of downstream effectors of the MAPK pathway [65]. *BRAF*V600E mutation is the most common genetic lesion in PTC, being detected in about 29–69% of cases [66, 67], and is highly prevalent in PTC with classical histology and in tall cell variant tumors [65, 67–69]. Many studies have reported association of *BRAF* mutation with aggressive tumor features, advanced tumor stage at presentation, tumor recurrence, and metastasis. *BRAF*V600E has been proposed as an independent predictor of tumor recurrence [70]. PTC carrying *BRAF*V600E mutation exhibit decreased expression of genes involved in thyroid hormone biosynthesis, including sodium-iodide symporter (NIS), decreased ability to trap radioiodine, and consequent treatment failure [71, 72]. *BRAF* mutations are present in microscopic PTCs, suggesting that they can occur early in tumor development [48]. In addition to PTC, *BRAF*V600E mutation is also present in PDTC and ATC [71, 73, 74]. Transgenic mice with thyroid-specific expression of *BRAF*V600E developed

PTC closely recapitulating those seen in human tumors [75], thus supporting the role of mutant *BRAF* in tumor initiation and differentiation, as well as its correlation with tumor characteristics. It has been recently demonstrated that BRAFV600E localizes to mitochondria and exerts an antiapoptotic effect, independent from kinase activity, which is not abrogated by BRAF inhibitors [76]. Other and rare mechanisms, alternative to *BRAF*V600E, contribute to *BRAF* oncogenic activation in PTC. These include (1) the K601E point mutation, small in-frame insertions or deletions surrounding codon 600 [77, 78], and (2) the AKAP9-BRAF fusion protein. This latter is produced by a paracentric inversion on chromosome 7q and detected in 11% of radiation-induced PTCs, showing elevated kinase activity and transforming activity comparable with the BRAFV600E oncoprotein [79].

RAS Oncogenes

The *RAS* genes *HRAS, KRAS,* and *NRAS* encode highly related small G proteins located at the inner surface of the plasma membrane, playing a central role in intracellular signaling. In their inactive state, Ras proteins are bound to GDP; upon activation, they bind GTP and become quickly inactive due to their intrinsic GTPase activity. Point mutations at codons 12, 13, or 61 result in mutant proteins permanently switched in the active status and constitutively activating their downstream targets.

Mutations of all the three *RAS* genes have been detected in about 10–20% of PTCs, almost exclusively in the follicular, and not in classical variant. Active *RAS* may promote thyroid tumorigenesis through the classic MAP kinase pathway (Ras → Raf → MEK → ERK) or through interaction with the PI3K/AKT pathway.

FTC

FTCs can develop in an adenoma-carcinoma sequence or directly, bypassing the stage of FA. Frequent genetic alterations in FTCs are *RAS* mutations, *PAX8/PPARγ* rearrangement, and PI3K/AKT pathway deregulation. *PAX8/PPARγ*

rearrangement has been proposed to be prevalent in patients with a history of radiation exposure [80].

RAS Oncogenes

Oncogenic mutations of *RAS* gene family members are among the first genetic lesions identified in tumors originating from the thyroid follicular epithelium. Some discrepancies related to the overall frequency of *RAS* mutations and their prevalence in specific thyroid tumors may be ascribed to the mutation screening methods and to the selection of patients. However, it has been reported that *RAS* mutations occur in up to 50% of FTCs, 25% of HCCs, and also in 10–20% of PTCs belonging to the follicular variant. *RAS* mutations are also present at a high frequency in PDTC and ATC (reviewed in [81]). *RAS* mutations are also reported in 40% of FAs, suggesting that RAS activation could be an early step in thyroid carcinogenesis. This hypothesis is supported by studies in transgenic mice showing that expression of NRAS-Q61K in thyrocytes can drive the formation of tumors that undergo differentiation and neoplastic progression [82]. Accordingly, a significant correlation between *RAS* mutations, metastases, and poor prognosis has been found in patients [83, 84]. It is conceivable that *RAS* activation may be insufficient to induce malignant growth but may predispose to acquire further genetic or epigenetic alterations that lead to a fully transformed phenotype. This is consistent with the observation that *RAS* mutations may affect chromosomal stability in vitro [85]. As *RAS* mutations are a marker for aggressive thyroid cancer behavior and poor outcome, surgical resection of *RAS*-positive adenomas might be proposed to prevent progression to carcinoma [81].

PAX8/PPARγ Rearrangement

PAX8/PPARγ rearrangement is a result of the translocation t(2;3)(q13;p25) that fuses the DNA binding domain of thyroid-specific *PAX8* transcription factor to the peroxisome proliferator-activated receptor *PPARγ*, expressed at low level in normal thyroid and has no known function in this organ (reviewed in [81]). *PAX8/PPARγ* has the highest incidence in FTCs (up to 60%);

it has also been described in approximately 8% of FA and in a small fractions of HCCs (reviewed in [86]. A novel *CREB3L2/PPARγ* fusion generated by t(3;7)(q34;p25) rearrangement has been detected in <3% of FTCs [87]. It has been reported that both PAX8/PPARγ and CREB3L2/PPARγ fusion proteins have oncogenic properties in normal human thyroid cells, but their mechanisms of action are still unclear [88]. With respect to the mechanisms activated by *PAX8/PPARγ*, both gain and loss of function activities have been suggested. Specifically, deregulation of *PAX8* and *PPARγ* normal functions and unique transcriptional activities of the fusion oncoprotein have been reported [81, 88]. It has been proposed that *PAX8/PPARγ*-stimulated growth could depend at least in part on loss of PPARγ functions caused by inhibition of wild-type protein [81]. This is consistent with the concept that PPARγ downregulation or inhibition may be a key event in thyroid carcinogenesis [86], as also suggested by the evidence that *PPARγ* is downregulated in translocation-negative papillary or follicular thyroid tumors, and a further reduction of its expression has been associated with dedifferentiation at later stages of tumor development and progression [89, 90]. Of note, *PAX8/PPARγ* rearrangement and *RAS* mutations rarely overlap in FTC, and it has been proposed that they lead to tumor development through distinct pathways [91]. In keeping with this, analyses of gene expression profiles of *PAX8/PPARγ*-positive FTCs have confirmed that these carcinomas have a distinct transcriptional signature [81, 87]. Based on its presence in both benign and malignant lesions, the diagnostic, preoperative value of *PPARγ* rearrangement is debated; nevertheless, it is plausible that benign nodules carrying the translocation may be considered at risk for progression.

The use of *PAX8/PPARγ* rearrangement as novel therapeutic target for FTC was being hampered by the nonexhaustive knowledge of *PAX8/PPARγ*-mediated carcinogenesis. Some clinical studies with PPARγ agonists, alone or combined with other chemotherapeutic agents, are currently ongoing [86], taking advantage of the availability of a number of approved modulators of the PPARγ used in the treatment of type 2 diabetes.

PI3K/AKT Pathway Mutations

The phosphatidylinositol 3-kinase (PI3K)/AKT pathway plays a central role in many cellular events, including growth, proliferation, and apoptosis, and it is frequently activated in cancer [92, 93]. Enhanced signaling by this pathway can be achieved through several mechanisms, including (1) mutations or amplification of the *PI3KCA* gene, encoding the catalytic subunit of PI3K [94, 95]; (2) decreased expression or inactivation of its negative regulator *PTEN* [96–98] ; and (3) activation by constitutively active *RAS* oncogenes [93]. *PTEN* reduction through epigenetic and posttranslational mechanisms or *PI3KCA* amplification have been detected in a significant fraction of FTCs, whereas *PTEN* or *PI3KCA* mutations seem to be relatively uncommon [98]. Analysis of a large series of thyroid tumors for the presence of *PI3KCA* copy gain or *PI3KCA*, *RAS*, and *PTEN* mutations showed a high additive prevalence of genetic alterations in the PIK3/AKT pathway and their mutual exclusivity in adenomas and in differentiated tumors. These findings have supported the concept of an independent role of *RAS* mutations in thyroid tumorigenesis through the PI3K/AKT pathway and have suggested that each of these genetic alterations may be individually sufficient to play a significant oncogenic role in thyroid cancerogenesis. The occurrence of some of these genetic alterations, e.g., *PI3KCA* copy gain and *RAS* mutations, even in FAs has suggested that the PI3K/AKT pathway plays a role at an early stage of thyroid tumorigenesis. Of note, the mutual exclusivity of these genetic alterations has not been observed in ATCs, implying a role of the PI3K/AKT pathway in progression of FTC to ATC [99]. To date, several drugs targeting the PI3K/AKT pathway have been developed; their therapeutic potential for the treatment of cancer is currently evaluated in various clinical trials [100].

PDTC and ATC

PDTC is a rare thyroid tumor and is characterized by a partial loss of thyroid differentiation and less favorable prognosis compared to well differentiated carcinomas. ATC represents the most undifferentiated thyroid tumor; it is characterized by poor prognosis, chemoresistance, local invasion, and distant metastases. Overall, ATC and PDTC are responsible for more than half of thyroid cancer patient deaths in spite of their low incidence [81].

There is evidence that PDTC and ATC may arise from well-differentiated precursor lesions: in thyroidectomy samples of PDTC and ATC, areas of well-differentiated and conventional follicular and oncocytic carcinomas are often found. Moreover, genetic lesions found in well-differentiated carcinomas, such as *BRAF* and *RAS* mutations, considered as early events in thyroid carcinogenesis, are found also in ATC and PDTC [81]. In this respect, the aggressive phenotype of PDTC would be conferred by additional mutations acquired during progression.

Inactivating mutations of *TP53* tumor suppressor gene represent the most common mutations in human cancer and a late event in tumorigenesis. *TP53* mutations have been found in 80% of ATC and 30% of PDTC (very rarely in well DTCs) (reviewed in [81]). Such mutations are associated with cell proliferation and loss of differentiation, as restoration of p53 function in ATC cell lines drives to reduction of proliferation rate, reexpression of thyroid-specific genes, and responsiveness to TSH stimulation [101, 102].

Point mutations of *CTNNB1* gene (encoding β-catenin) have been found in 25% of PDTC and 66% of ATC (and not in DTCs) [103, 104]. These mutations lead to increased stability and nuclear localization of β-catenin protein, which is associated to deregulated β-catenin signal and leads to increased cell proliferation [105].

Point mutations of the *RAS* genes have been found in PDTC and ATC in 18–27% and 50–60% of cases, respectively. It is likely that *RAS* mutants lead to genomic instability in the affected cells and predispose them to additional genetic alterations.

BRAF mutations are found in both PDTC (15%) and ATC (20%), often in tumors containing also well-differentiated areas. Mutations are detectable on both differentiated and undifferentiated areas suggesting their early occurrence in thyroid tumorigenesis [73, 74, 106]. Mutations affecting the PI3K pathway have been found in ATC, involving the *PIK3CA* and *PTEN* genes with frequencies of 20 and 15%, respectively [107].

Deregulation of PI3K/AKT pathway in ATC may occur concomitantly with other alterations, underlying their role in tumor progression [99].

MTC

RET gene is crucial in MTC being mutated in more than 95% of MEN 2 families and in 30–50% of sporadic MTCs. *RET* gene encodes a TK receptor with a crucial role in development. It comprises 21 exons and generates a transcript subjected to alternative splicing leading to two main isoforms. The RET receptor system also comprises the GFRα1-4 alternative co-receptors and GDNF family ligands, including GDNF, neurturin, persephin, and artemin (reviewed in [44]). Physiologically, RET, GFRα4, and persephin appear necessary for migration of neural crest calcitonin-producing cells into developing thyroid gland: a markedly diminished parafollicular C cells are present in RET$^{-/-}$ mice [108, 109].

A spectrum of RET mutations has been identified in MEN 2 families. In 98% of MEN 2A, the mutations affect one of the five cysteines in the extracellular cysteine-rich domain of RET: codons 609, 611, 618, 629 (exon 10), and 634 (exon 11) [110]. These "gain-of-function" mutations result in receptor dimerization and constitutive activation. Codon 634 is the most commonly affected codon (mutated in 65% of MEN 2A cases) [111]. In FMTC, mutations affect either the already described extracellular cysteines or the intracellular domain of RET (codons 768, 790, 791, 804, 806, and 891 are mainly involved) [33, 112, 113]. Most MEN 2B patients (95% of cases) carry the M918T mutation in *RET* kinase domain, causing receptor autophosphorylation and activation, resulting in a shift in substrate specificity [114]; the remaining fraction harbors the A883F substitution or other rare mutations. Altered RET signaling is responsible for the more aggressive MTC and the other pathological features associated with MEN 2B [114, 115]. Rarely, more than one mutation in RET can be associated with MTC. The MEN 2 RET database (www.arup.utah.edu/database/MEN2) will serve as a repository for MEN-2-associated *RET* sequence variation and reference for *RET* genotype/MEN 2 phenotype correlations.

The presence of a known MEN-2-associated *RET* mutation in the germ line of a MTC patient identifies hereditary MTC disease, thus allowing preclinical identification of family members at risk for MTC, as well as providing information about the risk for the patient to develop other tumors associated to MEN 2 syndromes. Moreover, the *RET* mutation type, assessed by *RET* genetic testing, guides clinical decision, as different *RET* mutants have been associated to different risk profiles. Consequently, prophylactic thyroidectomy for asymptomatic mutation carriers is recommended at early ages (from first months of life to 5 years) for higher risk mutations (codons 883/918 and 634, respectively), whereas for milder mutation carriers, surgery may be delayed [116].

Besides *RET* mutations, other genetic alterations must occur at the somatic level and act in concert with *RET* mutations for the tumor to develop, as suggested by the fact that in FMTC patients displaying germ line *RET* mutation, tumors are monoclonal [117]. Moreover, few MEN 2 families negative for *RET* mutations have been described, thus suggesting the existence of rare loci predisposing to MEN 2 additional to *RET* locus [118].

RET oncogenes are able to drive MTC formation, as demonstrated by transgenic mice models. Mice expressing *RET-C634R* (MEN 2A mutant) or *RET-M918T* (MEN 2B mutant), but not *RET-wt* under the control of calcitonin gene promoter, developed MTC [119, 120]. However, knock-in of the M918T mutation into mouse endogenous *RET* gene caused CCH but not MTC, suggesting that additional genetic alterations are required for development of MTC [121]. A secondary genetic event may target *RET* gene itself: duplication of the mutant allele or deletion of wt allele have been reported [122]. In addition, secondary events may involve chromosome deletion and amplification, as exemplified by the deletion in chromosome lp [123, 124].

In summary, hereditary MTC is a model of genetically determined cancer in which both diagnostic and therapeutic strategies rely on the identification of specific mutations.

Nonetheless, a variable phenotypic expression within and between families for the same mutation has been reported, suggesting the existence of modifier genes, which may act directly on RET signaling as well as on other aspects. The existence of modifier genes is also suggested by transgenic mice experiments showing that genetic background may strongly affect the MTC phenotype with tumor penetrance varying from 0 to 98% in different mouse strains [125].

The genetic lesions associated with sporadic MTC are less defined. *RET* gene activation is again involved: approximately 50% of sporadic MTCs harbor an activating mutation of *RET* detected in 12–100% depending on the reported series. Importantly, the presence of a codon 918 somatic *RET* mutation, the same associated to MEN 2B and the most frequent RET mutation in sporadic form, is associated with aggressive disease [126].

The involvement of *RAS* mutations in sporadic MTCs is less established. Recently, however, *RAS* mutations, specifically *HRAS* and *KRAS* mutations at codon 61, have been found in 68% (17 of 25) of the *RET*-negative fraction of MTC. The fact that only 2.5% of the *RET*-positive MTCs harbor *RAS* mutation suggests that activation of the proto-oncogenes *RAS* and *RET* represents alternative genetic events in sporadic MTC tumorigenesis [127] The involvement of *TP53* gene, by mutation or deletion, and of *CDKN2C* gene, by loss of function mutations, has been suggested to have a role in MTC [128–130] but need further analysis in larger cases collections.

Other Gene Defects Involved in TCs

Other molecular abnormalities, considered as secondary events to primary oncogenic activation, have also been observed in thyroid tumors.

The importance of VEGFR2 and angiogenesis in thyroid cancer tumor progression is well established. The first evidence is provided by the observation that thyroid cancers are highly vascular, showing high tumor microvessel density. Increased VEGF expression has been reported in well-differentiated thyroid cancer, and this was linked with shortened disease-free survival and risk for the development of metastatic disease [131, 132].

Furthermore, VEGF expression in thyroid cells has been linked with tumorigenic potential, and VEGFR overexpression was associated with *BRAF*V600E [133] as well as with ATC [45].

Overexpression of c-Met and EGFR and their cognate ligands have been observed in thyroid tumors, and experimental studies support their role in triggering thyroid carcinogenesis.

Met is overexpressed in most PTCs, whereas it is not present in the normal thyroid follicle [134]. Experimental and clinical data point to Met deregulation as a key event in tumor invasive growth and metastatic spreading [135] possibly by modulating cell motility and invasiveness and promoting angiogenesis [136, 137]. Such molecular network, promoting disease initiation and acquisition of a proinvasive phenotype, highlights new options to design multitarget therapeutic strategies for PTCs. Of note, RET oncoproteins were recently shown to establish cross talks with Met at transcriptional and signaling levels, thus driving thyrocyte neoplastic transformation [52].

EGFR is expressed in TCs [138, 139]. A functional TGFA/EGFR autocrine signaling loop has been shown to sustain the proliferation of PTC cells, contributing to PI3K/AKT activation. TGFA/EGFR was common in PTC cells harboring BRAF and RET/PTC mutations. Other signal pathways have been demonstrated to function in tandem with EGFR pathway; therefore, targeting EGFR alone in this context could be inadequate [140].

Aurora kinases (A, B, and C) are serine/threonine kinases overexpressed in several malignant tumors, including TCs [141]. Aurora kinases A and B are key regulators of mitosis, chromosome segregation, and cytokinesis and are associated with the MAP kinase pathway [142, 143]. Preclinical data deriving from MLN8054, an inhibitor of Aurora kinases, demonstrated a decrease of cell growth along with induction of apoptosis in ATC cell lines; moreover, reduction of tumor growth and vascularization was observed in vivo [144].

Biological Targets and Treatment Implications

The better understanding of the biological characteristics of TCs in the past few years has permitted the use of experimental compounds targeting molecular cancer profiles.

Two main pathways are involved in TC pathogenesis and progression: the deregulation of TC genes such as *BRAF, RAS,* and *RET* and the angiogenesis, both signal through MAPK and PI3K/AKT pathways. VEGFR2 is the principal mediator of angiogenesis both in thyroid tumor cells and in the microenvironment.

The main strategy to block the signal transduction is to target kinases involved in cancer growth and angiogenesis with the aim of inhibiting the tumor proliferation. Tyrosine kinase inhibitors (TKIs) are small molecules, which can be taken orally, that compete with ATP for the binding to the catalytic pocket of TK. Several compounds such as sorafenib, sunitinib, motesanib, axitinib, and pazopanib belong to this class and inhibit both pathways. Sorafenib and sunitinib have already been approved by the FDA and European Medicines Agency (EMA) for other type of advanced malignant tumors (sorafenib for hepatocellular cancer, sunitinib for gastrointestinal stromal tumor and pancreatic neuroendocrine tumors, and both agents for renal cell cancer).

Another therapeutic approach consists in the use of compounds targeting molecules other than TKs. Some agents such as demethylating and redifferentiating agents act by interfering with the epigenetic mechanisms involved in thyroid cancer pathogenesis while other compounds exert their action through the inhibition of angiogenesis (e.g., thalidomide, lenalidomide, and combretastatin A4 phosphate).

TKIs and Thyroid Cancer: Activity of the Compounds and Current Issues

TKIs are the most investigated compounds in TCs. This type of therapeutic approach has grown very fast in the last few years, and dozens of new compounds are already primed to begin clinical studies. An updated list of all clinical trials with TKIs in TCs is provided in Table 3.3.

At present, patients with advanced TCs, not suitable for surgery and with evidence of progression of disease according to RECIST within a range of 12–14 months, are candidated to receive a TKI. In case of DTCs, besides the characteristics previously described, RAI-refractoriness is required.

Table 3.3 TKIs and clinical trials

Author, year	Drug	Phase	Target	Histology	ORR%	Median PFS, months	Median duration of response, mo	Comments
DTC								
Sherman SI, 2008 [145]	Motesanib	II	VEGFR1–3 PDGFR RET KIT	PTC 57 HCC 17 FTC 15 Other 4	14	9.2	8	G4 event in 5 pts, 2 pts died of bleeding
Kloos RT, 2009 [146]	Sorafenib	IIR	BRAF, CRAF VEGFR1–3 PDGFRβ RET KIT FLT3	Arm A: chemonaïve PTC (N=19) Arm B: previously treated PTC = 22, other = 15	Arm A 15 Arm B 13 in PTC, 0 in other	Arm A: 16, Arm B: PTC 10, Other 4.5	Arm A: 9, Arm B: 6	52% required a dose reduction
Leboulleux S, 2010 [147]	Vandetanib vs. placebo	IIR	VEGFR2–3 RET EGFR	DTC 145	8.3 vs. 5.5	11* vs. 5.8	nr	*Statistically significant; dose reduction in 22% of pts
Bible KC, 2010 [148]	Pazopanib	II	VEGFR1–3 PDGFR KIT	PTC 15 HCC 11 FTC 11	49	11.7	nr	Two bleeding events ≥ G3, 2 G5 cases: 1 myocardial infarction and 1 acute complications of cholecystitis
Lucas AS. 2010 [149]	AZD6244	II	MEK1-2	PTC 32	3	13.5	nr	
Sherman S, 2011 [150]	E7080	II	VEGFR1–3 FGFR1 RET KIT PDGFRβ	DTC 58	50	12.6	nr	Phase III study has been already planned
Ongoing study	Sorafenib	III	BRAF, CRAF VEGFR1–3 PDGFRβ RET KIT FLT3					Enrolment completed

3 Thyroid Cancer

MTC								
de Groot JW, 2007 [151]	Imatinib	II	KIT Bcr-Abl RET PDGFRalpha PDGFRβ	15	0	nr	na	20% of patients stopped imatinib due to toxicity; 20% of pts had ≥G3 TSH
Frank-Raue K, 2007 [152]	Imatinib	II	KIT Bcr-Abl RET PDGFRalpha PDGFRβ	9	0	6	na	
Schlumberger MJ, 2009 [153]	Motesanib	II	VEGFR 1–3 PDGFR RET KIT	91	2	12	nr	Gallbladder G3 toxicity in 4% of patients
Lam ET, 2010 [154]	Sorafenib	II	BRAF, CRAF VEGFR 1–3 PDGFRβ RET KIT FLT3	Arm A FMTC: 5 Arm B sporadic: 16	6	17.9	nr	1 G5 toxicity (hemorrhagic and necrotic segment of small bowel at autopsy); all *RET* 918 mutation patients had PD within 12 months of study entry
Robinson BG, 2010 [155]	Vandetanib 100 mg	II	RET VEGFR2–3 EGFR	19 FMTC	16			21% required dose reduction or interruption; G3-G4 toxicities in 5%; G3 QTc prolongation in 5%
Wells SA, 2010 (ZETA trial) [156]	Vandetanib 300 mg vs. placebo	III	RET VEGFR2–3 EGFR	331 12% and 5% in the treatment and placebo arm were FMTC	45* vs. 13	Not reached* vs. 19.3	Not reached	*Statistically significant; 12% of patients discontinued vandetanib due to toxicity; diarrhea was the worst grade 3 + toxicity in 11% of patients; 5 deaths in the vandetanib arm RR was greater in RET918 mutated cases; 12% of patients discontinued vandetanib due to toxicity; diarrhea was the worst grade 3+ toxicity in 11% of cases; G3+ QTc prolongation 8%; 5 deaths in the vandetanib arm

(continued)

Table 3.3 (continued)

Author year	Drug	Phase	Target	Histology	ORR%	Median PFS, months	Median duration of response, mo	Comments
Wells SA, 2010 [157]	Vandetanib 300 mg	II	RET VEGFR2–3 EGFR	30 FMTC	20	27.9	10.2	80% of the patients required a dose reduction; G1-G2 toxicities >50%; G3 QTc prolongation 20%
MTC								
De Souza JA, 2010 [158]	Sunitinib 50 mg at a 4/2-week schedule	II	PDGFR VEGFR1–3 KIT RET FLT3 CSF-1R	25	35		9	Evidence of PR or SD ≥ 24 weeks in 7 of 9 MTC patients with RET918 mutation
Ongoing study	Cabozantinib (XL184)	III	c-MET RET VEGFR1–2	330				Enrolment completed; crossover not permitted in case of PD
Ongoing study	E7080	II	VEGFR1–3 FGFR1 RET KIT PDGFRβ	59				Enrolment completed
Mixed histology								
Cohen EE, 2008 [159]	Axitinib	II	VEGFR1–3 PDGF KIT	PTC 30 HCC 11 FTC 15 ATC 2 Other 2 MTC 11	31 18	18.1	Not still reached	13% discontinued due to adverse events; G1-G3 events in 32%; G4 in 5%
Ongoing study	Axitinib	II	VEGFR1–3 PDGF KIT					Enrollment completed

Study	Drug	Phase	Targets	Histology				Comments
Gupta-Abramson V, 2008 [160]	Sorafenib	II	BRAF, CRAF VEGFR1–3 PDGFRβ RET KIT FLT3	PTC 18 FTC/HCC 9 PDTC/ATC 2 MTC 1	23	19.3	nr	63% required drug holiday; 1 patient died of hepatic failure
Pennel NA, 2008 [161]	Gefitinib	II	EGFR	PTC 11 FTC/HCC 7 ATC 5 MTC 4	0	3.7 <3	na	32% had a tumor reduction that did not reach the PR according to RECIST; grade 3 toxicity in 11% of patients
Cohen EE, 2009 [162]	Sunitinib 50 mg at a 4/2-week schedule	II	PDGFR VEGFR1–3 KIT RET FLT3 CSF-1R	DTC 37 (31 evaluable) MTC 6	13 0			Grade 3–4 toxicity: neutropenia 26%; trombocytopenia 16%; hypertension 16%; fatigue 14%; palmar-plantar erythrodysesthesia 14%, and gastrointestinal events 14%
Carr LL, 2010 [163]	Sunitinib 37.5 mg	II	PDGFR VEGFR1–3 KIT RET FLT3 CSF-1R	PTC 18 FTC/HCC 10 MTC 7	28 43	12.8	8	60% required dose reduction; 1 death due to gastrointestinal bleeding
ATC								
Nagaiah G, 2009 6058 [164]	Sorafenib	II	BRAF, CRAF VEGFR1–3 PDGFRβ RET KIT FLT3	15	13	1.9	5.1	ATC patients in progression to chemotherapy

nr not reported

Sorafenib (Nexavar®) is one of the most investigated agent in TCs, due to its inhibiting activity on BRAF, RET, and VEGFR (Table 3.3). In DTCs, the response rate (RR) in two phase II trials ranges from 13–15% [146] to 23% [160]. Kloos and colleagues reported also a stable disease (SD) that lasted more than 6 months in 23 patients while no response has been demonstrated in patients with tumors other than PTCs. *BRAF* analysis was performed in 22 cases: 17 tumors (77%) harbored a *BRAF* mutation, being V600E in 14 cases and K601E in 3 cases. Based on the sorafenib activity in the prior studies, a phase III trial comparing sorafenib to placebo with the possibility of crossover is ongoing in patients with advanced and RAI-resistant DTCs.

Sorafenib has been investigated in a phase II trial in FMTC (arm A) and sporadic MTC (arm B). Arm A was prematurely stopped due to the lack of accrual. In arm B, one out of 16 enrolled patients had a partial response (6%) while 14 patients (87.5%) experienced an SD [154].

Sorafenib demonstrated its activity also in ATC: in a phase II trial including 15 patients, disease control was 40% with 13% of partial remissions [164].

Sunitinib (Sutent®) has been investigated both in DTCs and MTC at two different dose levels. In DTCs, response rate varied from 13% obtained in a phase II trial with a dose of 50 mg at 4 weeks on and 2 weeks off (a 4/2 week schedule) [162] to 28% in a phase II study at the continuous dose of 37.5 mg daily [163]. In MTC, RR ranged from 0 to 35% at the dose of 50 mg at a 4/2-week schedule [158, 162]. Three out of seven MTC patients had a PR with a dose of sunitinib of 37.5 mg/day [163]. Median duration of response was similar in DTC and MTC patients independently from the dose, 8 months with the lower dose of 37.5 mg/day in MTC [163] and 9 months with 50 mg at 4/2 weeks in DTCs and MTC [158].

A phase II study with axitinib, a potent inhibitor of VEGFR1–3, enrolled 60 patients with all TC histotypes. Partial response (PR) was reported in 17 patients (28%): 14 DTCs (8 PTCs and 6 FTCs), 2 MTCs, and 1 ATC underlying the activity of axitinib in each TC histotype. Notably, axitinib was associated with a prolonged progression-free survival (PFS) (median PFS 18.1 months) [159]. Another phase II study with axitinib involving DTC and MTC patients is currently under way.

Motesanib (AMG706), a multikinase inhibitor, was investigated in 93 patients with DTCs, obtaining a 14% confirmed PR by the RECIST criteria, 10% of unconfirmed PR, 67% of SD, and 35% of which longer than 6 months with a median PFS of 10 months [145]. A response rate of 2% and an SD of 81% along with a PFS of 48 weeks was observed in 91 patients with MTC treated with motesanib [153]. Tumor genotype was assessed in 47 subjects: *RET* mutation was found in 33 cases (70%). Motesanib did not inhibit mutant *RET*; thus, the probability of response in sporadic MTC and FMTC carrying *RET* mutation was very low [165, 166].

Pazopanib (Votrient®) and E7080 are two potent antiangiogenic agents with very promising effects in cases of DTCs. In a phase II trial with 37 patients with aggressive DTCs (disease progression within 6 months at study entry was required), pazopanib obtained an RR of 49% with a PFS of 11.7 months [148]. Comparable results were gained with E7080 in a phase II study: 58 DTC patients were enrolled obtaining an RR of 50% with a PFS of 12.6 months [150]. A phase II study with E7080 in MTC is ongoing.

Cabozantinib (XL184) is a potent inhibitor of MET, VEGFR2, and RET. A phase I study was conducted, enrolling 85 patients, 35 of which had MTC. Ten (29%) out of 35 MTC patients with measurable disease had a confirmed PR [166]. Cabozantinib at the dose of 175 mg (the maximum-tolerated dose found in the phase I study) is currently being studied in MTC patients in a randomized placebo-controlled trial (crossover is not allowed).

Vandetanib (Zactima®) targets VEGFR2–3, EGFR, and RET and, for this pattern of inhibition, it was considered as a very promising agent in MTC. A phase II study accrued 30 FMTC patients with *RET* mutation: vandetanib at the dose of 300 mg demonstrated a PR in 6 subjects (20%) and an SD in other 9 cases [157]. Vandetanib at the dose of 100 mg was investigated in a phase II trial in 19 FMTC patients (79% of whom with confirmed *RET* mutation) with a PR of 16%. Treatment-related adverse events profile was similar in the two previous studies, although the incidence of serious adverse events was lower at the dose of 100 mg (Table 3.3).

Vandetanib is the first TKI agent to have demonstrated a PFS increase over placebo in two randomized studies in DTCs [147] as well as in MTC [156]. Leboullex and colleagues compared vandetanib at the dose of 300 mg to placebo in 145 DTC patients in a randomized phase II study [147]. The response rate was similar among the two arms (8.3% vs. 5.5%; $p=0.501$) while median PFS was significantly in favor of the vandetanib arm (11 months vs. 5.8 months; $p=0.008$).

ZETA trial was a large, randomized, double-blind phase III trial where vandetanib was employed at the dose of 300 mg for FMTC and sporadic MTC patients. The response rate as well as the median PFS (still not reached in the vandetanib arm at the time of publication) were significantly in favor of vandetanib in respect of a placebo. Serious adverse events higher or equal to G3 were common, involving more than 55% of the patients in the vandetanib arm (Table 3.3). Based on the results derived from the ZETA trial [156], FDA approved vandetanib at the daily dose of 300 mg in April 2011 for advanced MTC patients, becoming the first target agent licensed in TC. However, due to the high rate of adverse events reported, it has been recommended for patients with symptomatic or progressive, unresectable or metastatic MTC.

The use of TKIs is recommended within clinical trials, although guidelines from the National Comprehensive Cancer Network (NCCN) and the American Thyroid Association (ATA) suggest the use of sorafenib and sunitinib in TC subjects with the characteristics described above, also in cases where the patients are not able to participate in a clinical trial.

The Target

The rationale for the employment of target therapy is to block off known aberrancies involved in TC pathogenesis (e.g., *RAF, RAS, RET*) (Fig. 3.3) [167], but till now none of the genetic defects have been identified as clearly linked to the activity of the experimental compounds, probably because more than one pathway could be activated in

signaling transduction in the tumor cells, in addition to the targeted molecules.

However, translation researches conducted within clinical trials looked for targets on primary thyroid tumors. The peculiar clinical behavior of metastatic TC could introduce potential pitfalls in the use of primary cancer specimens. Since the diagnosis of a primary tumor can precede the appearance of metastases by several years, mostly in DTCs, we cannot exclude that the long period between the primary diagnosis and the appearance of metastasis could have changed the molecular profile of the tumor, acquiring or losing genetic defects able to confer a more aggressive phenotype. Biological data seem to confirm this hypothesis: RAI-resistant DTC metastasis during cancer progression can acquire *PI3K/AKT* mutations [168] that are particularly common in aggressive tumors such as PDTC and ATC. This means that in advanced RAI-resistant DTCs, we probably need to block more than one target, combining different TKIs.

Among the molecular targets, only *BRAF* status seems to be the most related to TKI activity. In fact, in a phase II study with sorafenib, a selective *BRAF* inhibitor, a trend to a prolonged PFS was observed in cases of *BRAF*V600E tumor compared to wild-type *BRAF* (84 weeks vs. 54 weeks; $p=0.028$), suggesting that patients with *BRAF*V600E may be more likely to benefit from sorafenib [169]. PX4032 [170] and XL281 are TKIs selective for *BRAF*V600E kinase. Three patients with PTC *BRAF*V600E tumors have been enrolled in a phase I trial with PX4032 obtaining one partial lung response and two prolonged disease stabilizations [171]. PX4032 is currently under investigation in phase II in *BRAF*V600E PTCs. In another phase I trial with XL281, a pan RAF inhibitor targeting *BRAF*, *BRAF*V600E, and *CRAF*, no responses were seen. However, 2 out of 6 PTCs with *BRAF*V600E tumor (no tissue samples were available for the other 4 PTCs) have remained in study for a prolonged time, experiencing a stable disease up to 84 weeks [172].

The Activity of TKIs

The activity of TKIs can be influenced by several factors including the histotype and the genetic

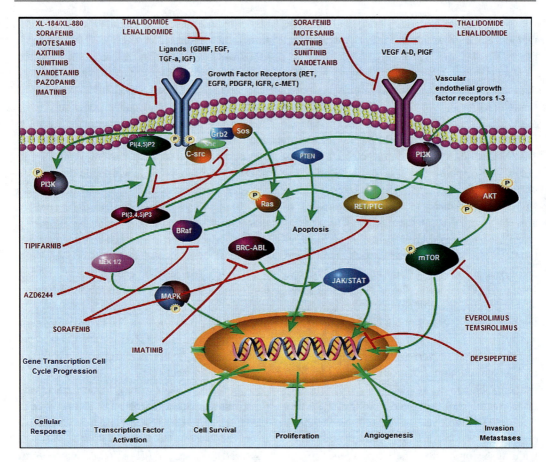

Fig. 3.3 Molecular markers and pathways involved in thyroid cancer and tailored drugs. [From Capdevila J et al. New Approaches in the Management of Radioiodine-refractory Thyroid Cancer: The Molecular Targeted Therapy Era. *Discovery Medicine* 9(45):153–162, 2010. With permission from *Discovery Medicine*]

susceptibility of the subject. In the pazopanib study, a higher response rate (73% vs. 33%) along with a prolonged disease control longer than 1 year has been described in FTC in respect of PTC [148], suggesting that genetic differences existing among the DTC histotypes could potentially influence also the responsiveness to the drug. Nevertheless, PTC is characterized by genetic heterogeneity, and this feature may be an issue for tailored therapies.

Mutations in the kinase domain could also alter the TKIs activity. For example, RET kinase inhibition depends on the RET genotype and on the type of TKI [173]. V804L, a mutation at the putative *RET* gatekeeper residue, has demonstrated resistance to several TKIs in vitro: substitution of *RET*V804L with bulkier residues appears to cause a steric hindrance with the possible loss of fundamental interactions with the drugs [174].

An organ-specific activity of TKIs has been supposed since bone, pleura, and lymph node metastases seem to be less sensitive to sorafenib than lung metastases [175]. It is not clear whether it could depend on different drug levels in the tissue or different expression levels of the targets or due to a specific metastatization pattern according to tumor heterogeneity. However, this finding has not been reported in other trials and needs to be further investigated.

The clinical response also correlates with the agent exposure. Response was higher in patients with a maximum pazopanib plasma concentration in the phase II study [148]. In the case of motesanib maximum and trough plasma concentrations in MTC, patients were lower than those reported in DTCs, probably contributing to the low response rate (2%) [153]. In the future, dose adjustment might be hypothesized during treatments, based on pharmacogenomic and pharmacogenetic data.

Unfortunately, we are still not able to predict in advance which TC patients will (or will not) obtain a benefit from TKIs. To this end, biological predictive factors potentially associated with response were investigated. High concentrations of IL-8 and TGF-β2 were found in the serum of metastatic MTC patients. Both serum markers were downregulated by sunitinib, suggesting their potential role as surrogate biomarkers [176]. In the pazopanib trial, changes in plasma levels of IL-6, IL-8, hepatocyte growth factor, E-selectin, VEGF, and PDGF did not correlate with response to the agent [148].

Changes in the levels of circulating biomarkers such as placental growth factor (PlGF), sVEGF2, and caspase-3/7 activity correlate significantly with response to motesanib in DTC or MTC patients [177]. However, these exploratory analyses are investigational, and none of these biomarkers have been approved for routine use.

Neither thyroglobulin nor calcitonin serum levels are useful in monitoring response. Thyroglobulin and calcitonin serum levels commonly decrease during TKI intake without any significant correlation with response [146, 161, 163] except in a motesanib study where a significant correlation was described between PR and the decrease of thyroglobulin of 50% or more from baseline [145]. A preclinical study suggests that *RET* kinase inhibitors may inhibit tumor growth in a manner dissociated from inhibition of calcitonin gene transcription and protein secretion [178]; thus, we can hypothesize that decreases in serum level of calcitonin will simply provide indirect evidence that *RET* kinase is effectively inhibited.

Improvement of TKI Activity

The response of TCs to TKIs is followed almost inevitably by progression. Interestingly, no cross resistance has been observed among TKIs. In a phase II trial with E7080 in DTCs, pretreated patients experienced an RR ranging from 41 to 54% according to prior exposure to anti-VEGFR or not [150]. This suggests that (1) the acquired resistance to a TKI can be overcome by switching to another TKI agent and (2) the employment of TKIs in sequence is feasible also in TCs, although in this latter case it is yet to be proven which is the best TKI sequence.

Efforts to improve the activity of the TKIs are under way and include the combination of agents with different mechanisms of action in the attempt to find a synergistic effect. A phase I trial combining bortezomib, a proteasome inhibitor approved for the treatment of multiple myeloma, and sunitinib has included seven TCs (2 MTCs, 3 PTCs, and 2 HCCs): 2 out of 6 evaluable patients experienced a PR, while 4 had a stable disease with a median PFS of 12 months [179]. Preclinical evidence showed that bortezomib enhanced the vandetanib activity against MTC cell lines, and a phase I/II trial combining bortezomib and vandetanib is ongoing. The phase I part was completed, and 5 out of 17 MTC patients enrolled showed a PR (29%) [180]. Tipifarnib, a farnesyltransferase inhibitor, has been tested in combination with sorafenib in a phase I trial. The combination of a farnesyltransferase inhibitor with a RAF kinase inhibitor might have a synergic or additive inhibiting effect on the RAS/RAF/MEK/ERK pathways. Among 76 enrolled patients, 35 were TC patients (13 MTCs and 22 DTCs) and 80% of them were previously treated. This combination has demonstrated different PRs according to the histotype: 5% in DTCs and 38% in MTCs with a similar PFS of 20 and 15 months, respectively [181]. In MTC, the combination seems to be more promising than sorafenib alone [154].

Everolimus inhibits a protein kinase called mTOR ("mammalian target of rapamycin") involved in a pathway which is aberrantly activated in around half of human tumors including TCs. In patients with advanced renal cell cancer, the use of everolimus after a sorafenib or sunitinib failure versus placebo demonstrated a PFS improvement of more than double (4.9 months vs. 1.9 months) [182]. A phase II trial with everolimus in combination with sorafenib is ongoing in patients with advanced DTC progressed with sorafenib (http://www.cancer.gov/clinicaltrials).

The Toxicities

Toxicities derived from TKIs in TCs are not negligible. According to the National Cancer Institute Common Terminology Criteria for Adverse Events (CTCAEs), events grade below or equal to 2 are very common, affecting at least 50% of patients, while adverse events grade above or equal to 3 are less frequent, generally involving about 15–20% of the patients, although in rare cases a higher percentage has been reported (Table 3.3). TKIs are commonly administered as continuous daily therapy. In this context, persistent grade 1 and 2 toxicities could result in a poor compliance that includes frequent dose interruption and titration, suggesting the necessity of modifying the CTCAEs for TKIs treatment to better capture treatment side effects duration [183]. Dose reduction and drug interruption are commonly described during TKI treatments (Table 3.3). During antiangiogenic treatment, drug interruption is particularly important as angiogenesis can rapidly restart after agent withdrawal. In case of axitinib, for example, data in vitro have demonstrated that neoangiogenesis appeared as early as 1 day after the withdrawal of the compound, and the tumor became revascularized within 7 days [184].

Toxicities are very similar among the different compounds due to the targeting similarities for various kinases of most of these agents. Cardiovascular toxicity, common during antiangiogenic therapy, includes hypertension, QTc prolongation, bleeding, and myocardial infarction. Other toxicities comprise skin toxicity such as hand–foot syndrome, skin rash particularly in the case of vandetanib, alopecia almost always related with sorafenib, hair and skin hypopigmentation, and gastrointestinal problems such as stomatitis, diarrhea, dysgeusia (loss of taste), acute cholecystitis (motesanib), dysphonia, nephrotic syndrome, and hypothyroidism. This latter is worth noting and suggests a monitoring of TSH level and subsequent levothyroxine dose

adjustment. Bone marrow toxicities (neutropenia, anemia, thrombocytopenia, etc.) are rarely reported although are more frequent in the case of sunitinib and vandetanib. Fatigue is commonly reported among different TKI trials while cutaneous squamocellular cancers are restricted almost exclusively to RAF-selective compounds, ranging from 27% with sorafenib [175] to 2% with XL281 [172].

We would add that tumor lesions previously treated with external beam radiotherapy require a close clinical and radiological monitoring as they potentially have an increased risk of local complication during antiangiogenic therapy (e.g., bleeding) [185].

Among these toxicities, only hypertension seems to correlate with response and outcome. Hypertension was already described in other reports as a surrogate marker of antiangiogenic treatment efficacy [186–192]. In a multivariate analysis performed on 230 patients enrolled in axitinib trials (including TC patients), a diastolic blood pressure ≥ 90 mmHg was significantly linked with the RR and the outcome [193].

Toxicity might be related to the genetic makeup of the patients. A link between VEGFR polymorphisms and sorafenib-related toxicity has been demonstrated. Blood samples from 47 patients on sorafenib were analyzed for the following VEGFR polymorphisms: −460, −1,154, −1,947, and −2,578. Polymorphisms −460, −1,947, and −2,578 resulted closely related to the incidence of the hand–foot skin reaction and hand–foot pain, not to hypertension. Likewise, no association was found between each of the four VEGF polymorphisms and the grade of the toxicities [194]. Genetic information could have a direct impact in the early recognition and prompt management of these expected toxicities, allowing as many patients as possible to continue on therapy for as long as they have a clinical benefit.

In most of the cases, a careful use of supportive care allows us to manage side effects (e.g., loperamide in the case of diarrhea; topical skin cream for hand–foot syndrome and skin rash) without dose reduction or interruption of treatment.

Agents with Mechanism of Action Other than TKIs

Antiangiogenic Agents

Thalidomide, a glutamic acid derivative, has in the past been demonstrated to be a potent teratogen by inhibiting vasculogenesis [195]. Its precise mechanism of action is not yet clarified, although it combines many properties such as immunomodulatory, anti-inflammatory, and antiangiogenic. A phase II trial in TCs with mixed histologies has been conducted with a starting dose of 200 mg daily with a progressive dose titration up to a median daily dose of 600 mg. Despite the activity demonstrated in 28 evaluable patients (18% of PR and 32% of SD), expected toxicities (constipation, neuropathy, somnolence, fatigue, etc.) were dose limiting in most of the patients [196]. Based on the activity of this compound, a phase II trial was conducted using lenalidomide, a thalidomide derivate which is supposed to be less toxic. The trial was started in DTC progressive and RAI-refractory patients, obtaining in 18 evaluable patients a PR of 22% and SD of 44% (RECIST criteria were not employed to assess response). Despite the activity, the median overall survival (OS) was less than 11 months [197].

Combretastatin A-4 phosphate is a reversible tubulin-binding tumor vascular-disrupting agent which causes cancer cell death by stopping tumor blood supply. In a phase II study in 18 metastatic ATC patients, no response was obtained with a median survival of 4.7 months together with 34 and 23% of patients still alive at 6 and 12 months, respectively [198]. A phase III study in ATC comparing carboplatin AUC 6 in combination with paclitaxel 200 mg/m^2 triweekly with or without combretastatin 60 mg/mq weekly has been conducted. Enrolment was stopped at 80 patients due to the scarce accrual. One-year survival was 23% for patients treated with combretastatin plus chemotherapy compared to 9% for patients who received chemotherapy only (Hazard Ratio 0.71; 95% CI 0.42, 1.22). The survival advantage was more remarkable in the combined arm in patients aged under 60 (10.9 months of median survival in the combined arm and 3.1 months in the chemotherapy arm) and in cases of tumor diameter greater than 6 cm (median survival was 5.7 months in the combined arm vs. 3.9 months in the chemotherapy arm) [199].

Redifferentiating Agents

Treatment of DTC with RAI relies on the ability of the malignant cells to accumulate iodine in the same way as normal thyroid epithelial cells. However, due to loss of differentiation, some thyroid cancers lose their capability to concentrate RAI.

The histone deacetylation is one of the mechanisms implicated in thyroid cancer progression, in particular in the loss of RAI avidity. Vorinostat is a small orally taken molecule that inhibits the histone deacetylase (HDAC). No response has been observed in 19 patients (16 DTC and 3 MTC) in a phase II study, and adverse events were frequent and caused most of the treatment interruptions [200]. Romidepsin, approved by FDA for cutaneous T cell lymphoma, selectively inhibits four isotypes of HDAC. Romidepsin increased the expression of the thyroglobulin and the Na^+/I^- symporter (NIS), improving the ability of the cells to accumulate ^{125}I potentially reversing the radioactive iodine resistance [201]. No response has been observed in 20 patients enrolled in a phase II trial. In two cases, a restoration of iodine uptake was obtained. However, an excessive number of vascular events were described [202]. Also valproic acid, a weak inhibitor of several isotypes of HDCA, has been investigated in vivo in anaplastic cell lines where it was able to induce apoptosis [203]. In addition, similar to romidepsin, valproic acid increased the NIS gene expression and radioiodine uptake in TC cell lines [204]. Valproic acid was combined with 5-azacytidine in a phase I trial, and one patient with PTC had an SD for 12 months [205]. A phase II study with valproic acid in monotherapy is under way. Other agents employed in the past to reinduce the susceptibility to ^{131}I were retinoids [206–208], rosiglitazone, a compound triggering PPARγ [209], and lithium carbonate [210].

Other Agents

Bortezomib is a proteasome inhibitor approved by the FDA and EMA for the treatment of multiple myeloma and mantle cell lymphoma. Bortezomib was active on MTC and ATC cell lines, at the opposite papillary and follicular cell lines were less sensitive to bortezomib. In addition, bortezomib combined with doxorubicin had a synergistic effect in all thyroid cancer cell lines [211]. The efficacy of bortezomib alone and in combination is under evaluation in clinical trials, as we have already discussed in the previous paragraph.

17-Allylamino-17-demethoxygeldanamycin (17-AAG) is a molecule under study in patients with advanced TCs. It is able to induce the inhibition of heat shock protein 90 (HSP90), a molecular chaperone necessary for the activity of oncogenic protein kinases. Similar to romidepsin and valproic acid, 17-AGG increased radioiodine accumulation in thyroid cells [212, 213]. In vitro, the biology of thyroid cells with rearranged RET is altered by the inhibition of HSP90 [212]. In preclinical studies, 17-AGG inhibits the growth of thyroid cancer cells: its cytotoxicity is related to HSP90 levels rather than the histotype [214].

Conclusions

Thyroid cancer is a rare and challenging tumor. Until a few years ago, RAI-resistant DTC and MTC patients with advanced disease did not receive any efficacious systemic therapy. Molecular biology has been fundamental in providing the input to conduct clinical investigations with tailored treatments. At present, several new compounds are under investigation in TCs. In this context, TKIs with antiangiogenic properties are the most promising treatment strategy for advanced TCs, and vandetanib is the first TKI to have been approved by the FDA in advanced MTC patients.

Several clinical issues regarding TKI therapy are still open, such as the selection of patients, the lack of predictive markers of response, the toxicity profile, the length of time of TKI administration, the overcoming of drug resistance, the optimal sequence of drug administration, the optimal trials design, the endpoints of clinical trials (OS vs. PFS), and so on.

Further analyses are required to improve the obtained results, in particular to ameliorate the activity of the compound sparing the toxicity. Blood and tumor biomarkers could be useful in the future to achieve these objectives.

References

1. Ferlay J, Shin HR, Bray F, et al. Estimates of worldwide burden of cancer in 2008: GLOBOCAN 2008. Int J Cancer. 2010;127:2893–917.
2. American Cancer Society. Cancer facts and figures 2009. Available at: http://www.cancer.org. Accessed 10 Apr 2011.
3. Liu S, Semenciw R, Ugnat AM, et al. Increasing thyroid cancer incidence in Canada, 1970–1996: time trends and age-period-cohort effects. Br J Cancer. 2001;85:1335–9.
4. Lubina A, Cohen O, Barchana M, et al. Time trends of incidence rates of thyroid cancer in Israel: what might explain the sharp increase. Thyroid. 2006;16:1033–40.
5. Akslen LA, Haldorsen T, Thoresen SO, et al. Incidence pattern of thyroid cancer in Norway: influence of birth cohort and time period. Int J Cancer. 1993;53:183–7.
6. Reynolds RM, Weir J, Stockton DL, et al. Changing trends in incidence and mortality of thyroid cancer in Scotland. Clin Endocrinol. 2005;62:156–62.
7. Levi F, Randimbison L, Te VC, La Vecchia C. Thyroid cancer in Vaud, Switzerland: an update. Thyroid. 2002;12:163–8.
8. Italian Association of Cancer Registries. http://www.registri-tumori.it/. Accessed 10 Apr 2011.
9. Davies L, Welch HG. Increasing incidence of thyroid cancer in the United States, 1973–2002. JAMA. 2006;295:2164–7.
10. Hughes DT, Haymart MR, Miller BS, et al. The most commonly occurring papillary thyroid cancer in the United States is now a microcarcinoma in a patient older than 45 years. Thyroid. 2011;21:231–6.
11. Chen AY, Jemal A, Ward EM. Increasing incidence of differentiated thyroid cancer in the United States, 1988–2005. Cancer. 2009;115:3801–7.
12. Mettler Jr FA, Bhargavan M, Faulkner K, et al. Radiologic and nuclear medicine studies in the United States and worldwide: frequency, radiation dose, and comparison with other radiation sources–1950–2007. Radiology. 2009;253:520–31.
13. Kitahara CM, Platz EA, Freeman LE, et al. Obesity and thyroid cancer risk among U.S. men and women: a pooled analysis of five prospective studies. Cancer Epidemiol Biomarkers Prev. 2011;20:464–72.
14. Grodski S, Brown T, Sidhu S, et al. Increasing incidence of thyroid cancer is due to increased

pathologic detection. Surgery. 2008;144:1038–43. discussion 1043.

15. La Vecchia C, Bosetti C, Lucchini F, et al. Cancer mortality in Europe, 2000–2004, and an overview of trends since 1975. Ann Oncol. 2010;21:1323–60.

16. Hundahl SA, Fleming ID, Fremgen AM, et al. A National Cancer Data Base report on 53,856 cases of thyroid carcinoma treated in the U.S., 1985–1995. Cancer. 1998;83:2638–48.

17. Durante C, Haddy N, Baudin E, et al. Long-term outcome of 444 patients with distant metastases from papillary and follicular thyroid carcinoma: benefits and limits of radioiodine therapy. J Clin Endocrinol Metab. 2006;91:2892–9.

18. Haq M, Harmer C. Differentiated thyroid carcinoma with distant metastases at presentation: prognostic factors and outcome. Clin Endocrinol. 2005;63:87–93.

19. Bossi P, Locati LD. Role of chemotherapy in thyroid cancer. In Thyroid cancer: from emergent biotechnologies to clinical practice guidelines. Carpi A, Mechanick ed. CRC Press, 2011: 313–318.

20. American Thyroid Association (ATA) Guidelines Task Force. Medullary thyroid cancer: management guidelines of the American Thyroid Association. Thyroid. 2009;19:565–612. Review. Erratum in: Thyroid. 2009;19:1295.

21. DeLellis RA, Lloyd RV, Heitz PU, Eng C (eds.): World Health Organisation Classification of Tumours. Pathology and Genetics of Tumours of Endocrine Organs. Tumors of the thyroid and parathyroid: 49–133; IARC Press: Lyon 2004.

22. Pilotti S, Collini P, Mariani L, et al. Insular carcinoma. A distinct de novo entity among follicular carcinomas of the thyroid gland. Am J Surg Pathol. 1997;21:1466–73.

23. Sobrinho-Simoes M. Poorly differentiated carcinomas of the thyroid. Endocr Pathol. 1996;7:99–102.

24. Sobrinho-Simoes M. Tumor of the thyroid: a brief overview with emphasis on the most controversial issues. Curr Diagn Pathol. 1995;2:15–22.

25. Sobrinho-Simoes M, Sambade C, Fonseca E, et al. Poorly differentiated carcinomas of the thyroid gland: a review of the clinicopathologic features of a series of 28 cases of a heterogeneous, clinically aggressive group of thyroid tumors. Int J Surg Pathol. 2002;10:123–31.

26. Green FL, Page DL, Fleming ID, et al. AJCC cancer staging handbook from the AJCC cancer system manual. 7th ed. New York: Springer; 2009.

27. McIver B, Hay ID, Giuffrida DF, et al. Anaplastic thyroid carcinoma: a 50-year experience at a single institution. Surgery. 2001;130:1028–34.

28. Sugitani I, Kasai N, Fujimoto Y, et al. Prognostic factors and therapeutic strategy for anaplastic carcinoma of the thyroid. World J Surg. 2001;25:617–22.

29. Voutilainen PE, Multanen M, Haapiainen RK, et al. Anaplastic thyroid carcinoma survival. World J Surg. 1999;23:975–8. discussion 978–9.

30. Sipple JH. The association of pheochromocytoma with carcinoma of the thyroid gland. Am J Med. 1961;31:163–6.

31. Marx SJ. Molecular genetics of multiple endocrine neoplasia types 1 and 2. Nature Reviews. Nat Rev Cancer. 2005;5:367–75. Review. Erratum in: Nat Rev Cancer. 2005;5:663.

32. Elisei R, Romei C, Cosci B, et al. RET genetic screening inpatients with medullary thyroid cancer and their relatives: experience with 807 individuals at one center. J Clin Endocrinol Metab. 2007;92:4725–9.

33. Zbuk KM, Eng C. Cancer phenomics: RET and PTEN as illustrative models. Nat Rev Cancer. 2007;7:35–45.

34. Elisei R. Routine serum calcitonin measurement in the evaluation of thyroid nodules. Best Pract Res Clin Endocrinol Metab. 2008;22:941–53.

35. Pacini F, Castagna MG, Cipri C, et al. Medullary thyroid carcinoma. Clin Oncol (R Coll Radiol). 2010;22:475–85. Review.

36. Bhattacharyya N. A population-based analysis of survival factors in differentiated and medullary thyroid carcinoma. Otolaryngol Head Neck Surg. 2003;128:115–23.

37. Greco A, Borrello MG, Miranda C, et al. Molecular pathology of differentiated thyroid cancer. Q J Nucl Med Mol Imaging. 2009;53:440–53.

38. Giannini R, Ugolini C, Lupi C, et al. The heterogeneous distribution of BRAF mutation supports the independent clonal origin of distinct tumor foci in multifocal papillary thyroid carcinoma. J Clin Endocrinol Metab. 2007;92:3511–6.

39. Romei C, Ciampi R, Faviana P, et al. BRAFV600E mutation, but not RET/PTC rearrangements, is correlated with a lower expression of both thyroperoxidase and sodium iodide symporter genes in papillary thyroid cancer. Endocr Relat Cancer. 2008;15:511–20.

40. Muzza M, Degl'Innocenti D, Colombo C, et al. The tight relationship between papillary thyroid cancer, autoimmunity and inflammation: clinical and molecular studies. Clin Endocrinol (Oxf). 2010;72:702–8.

41. Alberti L, Carniti C, Miranda C, et al. RET and NTRK1 proto-oncogenes in human diseases. J Cell Physiol. 2003;195:168–86.

42. Fusco A, Grieco M, Santoro M, et al. A new oncogene in human papillary thyroid carcinomas and their lymph-nodal metastases. Nature. 1987;328:170–2.

43. Airaksinen MS, Saarma M. The GDNF family: signalling, biological functions and therapeutic value. Nat Rev Neurosci. 2002;3:383–94.

44. Arighi E, Borrello MG, Sariola H. RET tyrosine kinase signaling in development and cancer. Cytokine Growth Factor Rev. 2005;16:441–67.

45. Viglietto G, Chiappetta G, Martinez-Tello FJ, et al. RET/PTC oncogene activation is an early event in thyroid carcinogenesis. Oncogene. 1995;11:1207–10.

46. Fischer AH, Bond JA, Taysavang P, et al. Papillary thyroid carcinoma oncogene (RET/PTC) alters the

nuclear envelope and chromatin structure. Am J Pathol. 1998;153:1443–50.

47. Jhiang SM, Sagartz JE, Tong Q, et al. Targeted expression of the RET/PTC1 oncogene induces papillary thyroid carcinomas. Endocrinology. 1996;137:375–8.

48. Adeniran AJ, Zhu Z, Gandhi M, et al. Correlation between genetic alterations and microscopic features, clinical manifestations, and prognostic characteristics of thyroid papillary carcinomas. Am J Surg Pathol. 2006;30:216–22.

49. Nikiforov YE. Radiation-induced thyroid cancer: what we have learned from Chernobyl. Endocr Pathol. 2006;17:307–17.

50. Asai N, Jijiwa M, Enomoto A, et al. Ret receptor signaling: dysfunction in thyroid cancer and Hirschsprung's disease. Pathol Int. 2006;56:164–72.

51. Castellone MD, Santoro M. Dysregulated RET signaling in thyroid cancer. Endocrinol Metab Clin North Am. 2008;37:363–74.

52. Cassinelli G, Favini E, Degl'Innocenti D, et al. RET/PTC1-driven neoplastic transformation and proinvasive phenotype of human thyrocytes involve Met induction and beta-catenin nuclear translocation. Neoplasia. 2009;11:10–21.

53. Castellone MD, De Falco V, Rao DM, et al. The {beta}-catenin axis integrates multiple signals downstream from RET/papillary thyroid carcinoma leading to cell proliferation. Cancer Res. 2009;69:1867–76.

54. Borrello MG, Alberti L, Fischer A, et al. Induction of a proinflammatory programme in normal human thyrocytes by the RET/PTC1 oncogene. Proc Natl Acad Sci U S A. 2005;102:14825–30.

55. Kaplan DR, Miller FD. Neurotrophin signal transduction in the nervous system. Curr Opin Neurobiol. 2000;10:381–91.

56. Butti MG, Bongarzone I, Ferraresi G, et al. A sequence analysis of the genomic regions involved in the rearrangements between TPM3 and NTRK1 genes producing TRK oncogenes in papillary thyroid carcinomas. Genomics. 1995;28:15–24.

57. Greco A, Roccato E, Pierotti MA. TRK oncogenes in papillary thyroid carcinoma. In: Farid NR, editor. Molecular basis of thyroid cancer. Ith ed. Boston: Kluwer; 2004. p. 207–19.

58. Pierotti MA, Greco A. Oncogenic rearrangements of the NTRK1/NGF receptor. Cancer Lett. 2006;232: 90–8.

59. Bounacer A, Schlumberger M, Wicker R, et al. Search for NTRK1 proto-oncogene rearrangements in human thyroid tumours originated after therapeutic radiation. Br J Cancer. 2000;82:308–14.

60. Rabes HM, Demidchik EP, Sidorow JD, et al. Pattern of radiation-induced RET and NTRK1 rearrangements in 191 post-Chernobyl papillary thyroid carcinomas: biological, phenotypic, and clinical implications. Clin Cancer Res. 2000;6:1093–103.

61. Russell JP, Powell DJ, Cunnane M, et al. The TRK-T1 fusion protein induces neoplastic transformation of thyroid epithelium. Oncogene. 2000;19:5729–35.

62. Fedele M, Palmieri D, Chiappetta G, et al. Impairment of the p27kip1 function enhances thyroid carcinogenesis in TRK-T1 transgenic mice. Endocr Relat Cancer. 2009;16:483–90.

63. Wellbrock C, Karasarides M, Marais R. The RAF proteins take centre stage. Nat Rev Mol Cell Biol. 2004;5:875–85.

64. Davies H, Bignell GR, Cox C, et al. Mutations of the BRAF gene in human cancer. Nature. 2002;417: 949–54.

65. Wan PT, Garnett MJ, Roe SM, et al. Mechanism of activation of the RAF-ERK signaling pathway by oncogenic mutations of B-RAF. Cell. 2004;116: 855–67.

66. Kimura ET, Nikiforova MN, Zhu Z, et al. High prevalence of BRAF mutations in thyroid cancer: gene evidence for constitutive activation of RET/PTC-RAS-BRAF signaling pathway in papillary thyroid carcinoma. Cancer Res. 2003;63:1454–7.

67. Frattini M, Ferrario C, Bressan P, et al. Alternative mutations of BRAF, RET and NTRK1 are associated with similar but distinct gene expression patterns in papillary thyroid cancer. Oncogene. 2004;23: 7436–40.

68. Xing M. BRAF mutation in thyroid cancer. Endocr Relat Cancer. 2005;12:245–62.

69. Cohen Y, Xing M, Mambo E, et al. BRAF mutation in papillary thyroid carcinoma. J Natl Cancer Inst. 2003;95:625–7.

70. Xing M. BRAF mutation in papillary thyroid cancer: pathogenic role, molecular bases, and clinical implications. Endocr Rev. 2007;28:742–62.

71. Xing M, Westra WH, Tufano RP, et al. BRAF mutation predicts a poorer clinical prognosis for papillary thyroid cancer. J Clin Endocrinol Metab. 2005;90: 6373–9.

72. Riesco-Eizaguirre G, Gutierrez-Martinez P, Garcia-Cabezas MA, et al. The oncogene BRAF V600E is associated with a high risk of recurrence and less differentiated papillary thyroid carcinoma due to the impairment of Na+/I- targeting to the membrane. Endocr Relat Cancer. 2006;13:257–69.

73. Namba H, Nakashima M, Hayashi T, et al. Clinical implication of hot spot BRAF mutation, V599E, in papillary thyroid cancers. J Clin Endocrinol Metab. 2003;88:4393–7.

74. Begum S, Rosenbaum E, Henrique R, et al. BRAF mutations in anaplastic thyroid carcinoma: implications for tumor origin, diagnosis and treatment. Mod Pathol. 2004;17:1359–63.

75. Knauf JA, Ma X, Smith EP, et al. Targeted expression of BRAFV600E in thyroid cells of transgenic mice results in papillary thyroid cancers that undergo dedifferentiation. Cancer Res. 2005;65:4238–45.

76. Lee MH, Lee SE, Kim DW, et al. Mitochondrial localization and regulation of BRAFV600E in thyroid cancer: a clinically used RAF inhibitor is unable to block the mitochondrial activities of BRAFV600E. J Clin Endocrinol Metab. 2011;96:E19–30.

77. Trovisco V, Vieira de Castro I, Soares P, et al. BRAF mutations are associated with some histological types of papillary thyroid carcinoma. J Pathol. 2004;202:247–51.
78. Hou P, Liu D, Xing M. Functional characterization of the T1799-1801del and A1799-1816ins BRAF mutations in papillary thyroid cancer. Cell Cycle. 2007;6:377–9.
79. Ciampi R, Knauf JA, Kerler R, et al. Oncogenic AKAP9-BRAF fusion is a novel mechanism of MAPK pathway activation in thyroid cancer. J Clin Invest. 2005;115:94–101.
80. Nikiforova MN, Biddinger PW, Caudill CM, et al. PAX8-PPARgamma rearrangement in thyroid tumors: RT-PCR and immunohistochemical analyses. Am J Surg Pathol. 2002;26:1016–23.
81. Nikiforova MN, Nikiforov YE. Molecular genetics of thyroid cancer: implications for diagnosis, treatment and prognosis. Expert Rev Mol Diagn. 2008;8:83–95.
82. Vitagliano D, Portella G, Troncone G, et al. Thyroid targeting of the N-ras(Gln61Lys) oncogene in transgenic mice results in follicular tumors that progress to poorly differentiated carcinomas. Oncogene. 2006;25:5467–74.
83. Manenti G, Pilotti S, Re FC, et al. Selective activation of ras oncogenes in follicular and undifferentiated thyroid carcinomas. Eur J Cancer. 1994;30:987–93.
84. Garcia-Rostan G, Zhao H, Camp RL, et al. Ras mutations are associated with aggressive tumor phenotypes and poor prognosis in thyroid cancer. J Clin Oncol. 2003;21:3226–35.
85. Saavedra HI, Knauf JA, Shirokawa JM, et al. The RAS oncogene induces genomic instability in thyroid PCCL3 cells via the MAPK pathway. Oncogene. 2000;19:3948–54.
86. Placzkowski KA, Reddi HV, Grebe SK, et al. The role of the PAX8/PPARgamma fusion oncogene in thyroid cancer. PPAR Res. 2008;29:672829.
87. Lui WO, Zeng L, Rehrmann V, Deshpande S, et al. CREB3L2-PPARgamma fusion mutation identifies a thyroid signaling pathway regulated by intramembrane proteolysis. Cancer Res. 2008;68:7156–64.
88. Lui WO, Foukakis T, Liden J, et al. Expression profiling reveals a distinct transcription signature in follicular thyroid carcinomas with a PAX8-PPAR(gamma) fusion oncogene. Oncogene. 2005;24:1467–76.
89. Aldred MA, Morrison C, Gimm O, et al. Peroxisome proliferator-activated receptor gamma is frequently downregulated in a diversity of sporadic nonmedullary thyroid carcinomas. Oncogene. 2003;22:3412–6.
90. Marques AR, Espadinha C, Frias MJ, et al. Underexpression of peroxisome proliferator-activated receptor (PPAR)gamma in PAX8/PPARgamma-negative thyroid tumours. Br J Cancer. 2004;91:732–8.
91. Nikiforova MN, Lynch RA, Biddinger PW, et al. RAS point mutations and PAX8-PPAR gamma rearrangement in thyroid tumors: evidence for distinct molecular pathways in thyroid follicular carcinoma. J Clin Endocrinol Metab. 2003;88:2318–26.
92. Ringel MD, Hayre N, Saito J, et al. Overexpression and overactivation of Akt in thyroid carcinoma. Cancer Res. 2001;61:6105–11.
93. Vasko V, Saji M, Hardy E, et al. Akt activation and localisation correlate with tumour invasion and oncogene expression in thyroid cancer. J Med Genet. 2004;41:161–70.
94. Wu G, Mambo E, Guo Z, et al. Uncommon mutation, but common amplifications, of the PIK3CA gene in thyroid tumors. J Clin Endocrinol Metab. 2005;90:4688–93.
95. Wang Y, Hou P, Yu H, et al. High prevalence and mutual exclusivity of genetic alterations in the phosphatidylinositol-3-kinase/akt pathway in thyroid tumors. J Clin Endocrinol Metab. 2007;92:2387–90.
96. Dahia PL, Marsh DJ, Zheng Z, et al. Somatic deletions and mutations in the Cowden disease gene, PTEN, in sporadic thyroid tumors. Cancer Res. 1997;57:4710–3.
97. Bruni P, Boccia A, Baldassarre G, et al. PTEN expression is reduced in a subset of sporadic thyroid carcinomas: evidence that PTEN-growth suppressing activity in thyroid cancer cells mediated by p27kip1. Oncogene. 2000;19:3146–55.
98. Paes JE, Ringel MD. Dysregulation of the phosphatidylinositol 3-kinase pathway in thyroid neoplasia. Endocrinol Metab Clin North Am. 2008;37:375–9.
99. Hou P, Liu D, Shan Y, et al. Genetic alterations and their relationship in the phosphatidylinositol 3-kinase/Akt pathway. Clin Cancer Res. 2007;13:1161–70.
100. Liu P, Cheng H, Roberts TM, et al. Targeting the phosphoinositide 3-kinase pathway in cancer. Nat Rev Drug Discov. 2009;8:627–44.
101. Fagin JA, Tang SH, Zeki K, et al. Reexpression of thyroid peroxidase in a derivative of an undifferentiated thyroid carcinoma cell line by introduction of wild-type p53. Cancer Res. 1996;56:765–71.
102. Moretti F, Farsetti A, Soddu S, et al. A p53 re-expression inhibits proliferation and restores differentiation of human thyroid anaplastic carcinoma cells. Oncogene. 1997;14:729–40.
103. Garcia-Rostan G, Camp RL, Herrero A, et al. Beta-catenin dysregulation in thyroid neoplasms: downregulation, aberrant nuclear expression, and CTNNB1 exon 3 mutations are markers for aggressive tumor phenotypes and poor prognosis. Am J Pathol. 2001;158:987–96.
104. Miyake N, Maeta H, Horie S, et al. Absence of mutations in the beta-catenin and adenomatous polyposis coli genes in papillary and follicular thyroid carcinomas. Pathol Int. 2001;51:680–5.
105. Tauriello DVF, Maurice MM. The various roles of ubiquitin in Wnt pathway regulation. Cell Cycle. 2010;9:3700–9.

106. Nikiforova MN, Kimura ET, Gandhi M, et al. BRAF mutations in thyroid tumors are restricted to papillary carcinomas and anaplastic or poorly differentiated carcinomas arising from papillary carcinomas. J Clin Endocrinol Metab. 2003;88:5399–404.

107. Garcia-Rostan G, Costa AM, Pereira-Castro I, et al. Mutation of the PIK3CA gene in anaplastic thyroid cancer. Cancer Res. 2005;65:10199–207.

108. Lindahl M, Timmusk T, Rossi J, et al. Expression and alternative splicing of mouse Gfra4 suggest roles in endocrine cell development. Mol Cell Neurosci. 2000;15:522–33.

109. Lindfors PH, Lindahl M, Rossi J, et al. Ablation of persephin receptor glial cell line derived neurotrophic factor family receptor alpha4 impairs thyroid calcitonin production in young mice. Endocrinology. 2006;147:2237–44.

110. Eng C, Clayton D, Schuffenecker I, et al. The relationship between specific RET proto-oncogene mutations and disease phenotype in MEN type 2. International RET mutation consortium analysis. JAMA. 1996;276:1575–9.

111. Machens A, Niccoli-Sire P, Hoegel J, et al. Early malignant progression of hereditary medullary thyroid cancer. NEJM. 2003;349:1517–25.

112. Niccoli-Sire P, Murat A, Rohmer V, et al. Familial medullary thyroid carcinoma with noncysteine ret mutations: phenotype–genotype relationship in a large series of patients. J Clin Endocrinol Metab. 2001;86:3746–53.

113. Kouvaraki MA, Shapiro SE, Perrier ND, et al. RET proto-oncogene: a review and update of genotype-phenotype correlations in hereditary medullary thyroid cancer and associated endocrine tumors. Thyroid. 2005;15:531–44.

114. Hansford JR, Mulligan LM. Multiple endocrine neoplasia type 2 and RET: from neoplasia to neurogenesis. J Med Genet. 2000;37:817–27.

115. Santoro M, Carlomagno F, Romano A, et al. Activation of RET as a dominant transforming gene by germline mutations of MEN2A and MEN2B. Science. 1995;267:381–3.

116. Frank-Raue K, Rondot S, Raue F. Molecular genetics and phenomics of RET mutations: impact on prognosis of MTC. Mol Cell Endocrinol. 2010; 322(1–2):2–7.

117. Gagel FR, Marx SJ. Multiple endocrine neoplasia. In: Larsen PR, editor. Williams textbook of endocrinology. 10th ed. Philadelphia: Saunders; 2003. p. 1717–62.

118. Montero-Conde C, Ruiz-Llorente S, Gonza'lez-Albarran O, et al. Identification of a candidate chromosomal region using a SNP linkage panel suggests a second locus responsible for non-RET MEN2 families. Hor Res. 2007;68:6–7.

119. Michiels FM, Chappuis S, Caillou B, et al. Development of medullary thyroid carcinoma in transgenic mice expressing the RET protooncogene altered by a multiple endocrine neoplasia type 2A mutation. PNAS. 1997;94:3330–5.

120. Acton DS, Velthuyzen D, Lips CJ, et al. Multiple endocrine neoplasia type 2B mutation in human RET oncogene induces medullary thyroid carcinoma in transgenic mice. Oncogene. 2000;19:3121–5.

121. Smith-Hicks CL, Sizer KC, Powers JF, et al. C-cell hyperplasia, pheochromocytoma and sympathoadrenal malformation in a mouse model of multiple endocrine neoplasia type 2B. EMBO J. 2000;19:612–22.

122. Huang SC, Torres-Cruz J, Pack SD, et al. Amplification and overexpression of mutant RET in multiple endocrine neoplasia type 2-associated medullary thyroid carcinoma. J Clin Endocrin Metab. 2003;88:459–63.

123. Mathew CG, Smith BA, Thorpe K, et al. Deletion of genes on chromosome 1 in endocrine neoplasia. Nature. 1987;328:524–6.

124. Ye L, Santarpia L, Cote GJ, et al. High resolution array-comparative genomic hybridization profiling reveals deoxyribonucleic acid copy number alterations associated with medullary thyroid carcinoma. J Clin Endocrin Metab. 2008;93:4367–72.

125. Cranston AN, Ponder BA. Modulation of medullary thyroid carcinoma penetrance suggests the presence of modifier genes in a RET transgenic mouse model. Cancer Res. 2003;63:4777–80.

126. Zedenius J. Is somatic RET mutation a prognostic factor for sporadic medullary thyroid carcinoma? Nat Clin Pract Endocrinol Metab. 2008;4:432–3.

127. Moura MM, Cavaco BM, Pinto AE, et al. High prevalence of RAS mutations in RET-negative sporadic medullary thyroid carcinomas. J Clin Endocrinol Metab. 2011;96:E863.

128. Pavelic K, Dedivitis RA, Kapitanovic S, et al. Molecular genetic alterations of FHIT and p53 genes in benign and malignant thyroid gland lesions. Mutat Res. 2006;599:45–57.

129. Sheikh HA, Tometsko M, Niehouse L, et al. Molecular genotyping of medullary thyroid carcinoma can predict tumor recurrence. Am J Surg Pathol. 2004;28:101–6.

130. van Veelen W, van Gasteren CJ, Acton DS, et al. Synergistic effect of oncogenic RET and loss of p18 on medullary thyroid carcinoma development. Cancer Res. 2008;68:1329–37.

131. Fenton C, Patel A, Dinauer C, et al. The expression of vascular endothelial growth factor and the type 1 vascular endothelial growth factor receptor correlate with the size of papillary thyroid carcinoma in children and young adults. Thyroid. 2000;10:349–57.

132. Dhar DK, Kubota H, Kotoh T, et al. Tumor vascularity predicts recurrence in differentiated thyroid carcinoma. Am J Surg. 1998;176:442–7.

133. Espinosa AV, Porchia L, Ringel MD. Targeting BRAF in thyroid cancer. Br J Cancer. 2007;96:16–20.

134. Di Renzo MF, Olivero M, Ferro S, et al. Overexpression of the c-MET/HGF receptor gene in human thyroid carcinomas. Oncogene. 1992;7:2549–53.

135. Gentile A, Trusolino L, Comoglio PM. The Met tyrosine kinase receptor in development and cancer. Cancer Metastasis Rev. 2008;27:85–94.

136. Ruco LP, Stoppacciaro A, Ballarini F, et al. Met protein and hepatocyte growth factor (HGF) in papillary carcinoma of the thyroid: evidence for a pathogenic role in tumourigenesis. J Pathol. 2001;194:4–8.

137. Scarpino S, Cancellario D'Alena F, et al. Papillary carcinoma of the thyroid: evidence for a role for hepatocyte growth factor (HGF) in promoting tumour angiogenesis. J Pathol. 2003;199:243–50.

138. Wiseman SM, Masoudi H, Niblock P. Anaplastic thyroid carcinoma: expression profile of targets for therapy offers new insights for disease treatment. Ann Surg Oncol. 2007;14:719–29.

139. Lam AK, Lau KK, Gopalan V, et al. Quantitative analysis of the expression of TGF-alpha and EGFR in papillary thyroid carcinoma: clinicopathological relevance. Pathology. 2011;43:40–7.

140. Degl' Innocenti D, Alberti C, Castellano G, et al. Integrated ligand-receptor bioinformatic and in vitro functional analysis identifies active TGFA/EGFR signaling loop in papillary thyroid carcinomas. PLoS One. 2010;5:e12701.

141. Ulisse S, Delcros JG, Baldini E, et al. Expression of Aurora kinases in human thyroid carcinoma cell lines and tissues. Int J Cancer. 2006;119:275–82.

142. Keen N, Taylor S. Aurora-kinase inhibitors as anticancer agents. Nat Rev Cancer. 2004;4:927–36. Review.

143. Keen N, Taylor S. Mitotic drivers-inhibitors of the Aurora B kinase. Cancer Metastasis Rev. 2009;28:185–95.

144. Wunderlich A, Fischer M, Schlosshauer T, et al. Evaluation of Aurora kinase inhibition as a new therapeutic strategy in anaplastic and poorly differentiated follicular thyroid cancer. Cancer Sci. 2011;102:762–8.

145. Sherman SI, Wirth LJ, Droz JP, et al. Motesanib diphosphate in progressive differentiated thyroid cancer. N Engl J Med. 2008;359:31–42.

146. Kloos RT, Ringel MD, Knopp MV, et al. Phase II trial of sorafenib in metastatic thyroid cancer. J Clin Oncol. 2009;27:1675–84.

147. Leboulleux S, Bastholt L, Krause TM, et al. Vandetanib in locally advanced or metastatic differentiated thyroid cancer (papillary or follicular; DTC): a randomized double blind phase II trial. Ann Oncol. 2010;21 (suppl_8): viii315.

148. Bible KC, Suman VJ, Molina JR, et al. Efficacy of pazopanib in progressive, radioiodine-refractory, metastatic differentiated thyroid cancers: results of a phase 2 consortium study. Lancet Oncol. 2010;11:962–72.

149. Lucas AS, Cohen EE, Cohen RB, et al. Phase II study and tissue correlative studies of AZD6244 (ARRY-142886) in iodine-131 refractory papillary thyroid carcinoma (IRPTC) and papillary thyroid carcinoma (PTC) with follicular elements. J Clin Oncol, 2010;28 (8_suppl): 5536.

150. Sherman SI, Jarzab B, Cabanillas ME, et al. A phase II trial of the multitargeted kinase inhibitor E7080 in advanced radioiodine (RAI)-refractory differentiated thyroid cancer (DTC). J Clin Oncol, 2011;29 (15_suppl): 5503.

151. de Groot JW, Zonnenberg BA, van Ufford-Mannesse PQ, et al. A phase II trial of imatinib therapy for metastatic medullary thyroid carcinoma. J Clin Endocrinol Metab. 2007;92:3466–9.

152. Frank-Raue K, Fabel M, Delorme S, et al. Efficacy of imatinib mesylate in advanced medullary thyroid carcinoma. Eur J Endocrinol. 2007;157:215–20.

153. Schlumberger MJ, Elisei R, Bastholt L, et al. Phase II study of safety and efficacy of motesanib in patients with progressive or symptomatic, advanced or metastatic medullary thyroid cancer. J Clin Oncol. 2009;27:3794–801.

154. Lam ET, Ringel MD, Kloos RT, et al. Phase II clinical trial of sorafenib in metastatic medullary thyroid cancer. J Clin Oncol. 2010;28:2323–30.

155. Robinson BG, Paz-Ares L, Krebs A, et al. Vandetanib (100 mg) in patients with locally advanced or metastatic hereditary medullary thyroid cancer. J Clin Endocrinol Metab. 2010;95:2664–71.

156. Wells SA Jr, Robinson BG, Gagel RF et al. Vandetanib in Patients With Locally Advanced or Metastatic Medullary Thyroid Cancer: A Randomized, Double-Blind Phase III Trial.J Clin Oncol. 2012;30:134–41.

157. Wells SA, Jr, Gosnell JE, Gagel RF, et al. vandetanib for the treatment of patients with locally advanced or metastatic hereditary medullary thyroid cancer. J Clin Oncol. 2010;28:767–72.

158. De Souza JA, Busaidy N, Zimrin A, et al. Phase II trial of sunitinib in medullary thyroid cancer (MTC). J Clin Oncol, 2010; 28 (8_suppl): 5504.

159. Cohen EE, Rosen LS, Vokes EE, et al. Axitinib is an active treatment for all histologic subtypes of advanced thyroid cancer: results from a phase II study. J Clin Oncol. 2008;26:4708–13.

160. Gupta-Abramson V, Troxel AB, Nellore A, et al. Phase II trial of sorafenib in advanced thyroid cancer. J Clin Oncol. 2008;26:4714–9.

161. Pennell NA, Daniels GH, Haddad RI, et al. A phase II study of gefitinib in patients with advanced thyroid cancer. Thyroid. 2008;18:317–23.

162. Cohen EE, Needles BM, Cullen KJ, et al. Phase 2 study of sunitinib in refractory thyroid cancer. J Clin Oncol, 2008;26 (15_suppl): 6025.

163. Carr LL, Mankoff DA, Goulart BH, et al. Phase II study of daily sunitinib in FDG-PET-positive, iodine-refractory differentiated thyroid cancer and metastatic medullary carcinoma of the thyroid with functional imaging correlation. Clin Cancer Res. 2010;16:5260–8.

164. Nagaiah G, Fu P, Wasman JK, et al. Phase II trial of sorafenib (bay 43-9006) in patients with advanced anaplastic carcinoma of the thyroid (ATC). J Clin Oncol, 2009;27 (15_suppl): 6058.

165. Coxon A, Bready JV, Hughes P, et al. Motesanib diphosphate (AMG 706) inhibits the growth of

166. Kurzrock R, Sherman SI, Ball DW, et al. Activity of XL184 (Cabozantinib), an oral tyrosine kinase inhibitor, in patients with medullary thyroid cancer. J Clin Oncol. 2011;29:2660–6.

167. Capdevila J, Argiles G, Rodriguez-Frexinos V, et al. New approaches in the management of radioiodine-refractory thyroid cancer: the molecular targeted therapy era. Discov Med. 2010;9:153–62.

168. Ricarte-Filho JC, Ryder M, Chitale DA, et al. Mutational profile of advanced primary and metastatic radioactive iodine-refractory thyroid cancers reveals distinct pathogenetic roles for BRAF, PIK3CA, and AKT1. Cancer Res. 2009;69: 4885–93.

169. Brose MS, Troxel AB, Redlinger M, et al. Effect of BRAFV600E on response to sorafenib in advanced thyroid cancer patients. J Clin Oncol, 2009;27 (15_suppl): 6002.

170. Sala E, Mologni L, Truffa S, et al. BRAF silencing by short hairpin RNA or chemical blockade by PLX4032 leads to different responses in melanoma and thyroid carcinoma cells. Mol Cancer Res. 2008;6:751–9.

171. Flaherty K, Puzanov I, Sosman J, et al. Phase I study of PLX4032: proof of concept for V600E BRAF mutation as a therapeutic target in human cancer. J Clin Oncol, 2009;27 (15_suppl): 9000.

172. Schwartz GK, Robertson S, Shen A, et al. A phase I study of XL281, a selective oral RAF kinase inhibitor, in patients with advanced solid tumors. J Clin Oncol, 2009;27 (15_suppl): 3513.

173. Gramza AW, Patterson J, Peters J, et al. Activity of novel RET genotypes associated with medullary thyroid cancer. J Clin Oncol, 2010;28 (8_suppl): 5559.

174. Tuccinardi T, Manetti F, Schenone S, et al. Construction and validation of a RET TK catalytic domain by homology modeling. J Chem Inf Model. 2007;47:644–55.

175. Cabanillas ME, Waguespack SG, Bronstein Y, et al. Treatment with tyrosine kinase inhibitors for patients with differentiated thyroid cancer: the M. D. Anderson experience. J Clin Endocrinol Metab. 2010;95:2588–95.

176. Broutin S, Ameur N, Lacroix L, et al. Identification of soluble candidate biomarkers of therapeutic response to sunitinib in medullary thyroid carcinoma in preclinical models. Clin Cancer Res. 2011;17: 2044–54.

177. Bass MB, Sherman SI, Schlumberger MJ, et al. Biomarkers as predictors of response to treatment with motesanib in patients with progressive advanced thyroid cancer. J Clin Endocrinol Metab. 2010;95: 5018–27.

178. Akeno-Stuart N, Croyle M, Knauf JA, et al. The RET kinase inhibitor NVP-AST487 blocks growth and calcitonin gene expression through distinct mechanisms in medullary thyroid cancer cells. Cancer Res. 2007;67:6956–64.

179. Harvey RD, Kauh JS, Ramalingam SS, et al. Combination therapy with sunitinib and bortezomib in adult patients with radioiodine refractory thyroid cancer. J Clin Oncol. 2010;abs 5589.

180. Gramza AW, Wells SA, Balasubramaniam S, et al. Phase I/II trial of vandetanib and bortezomib in adults with locally advanced or metastatic medullary thyroid cancer: phase I results. J Clin Oncol. 2011:abs 5565.

181. Hong DS, Cabanillas ME, Wheler J, et al. Inhibition of the Ras/Raf/MEK/ERK and RET kinase pathways with the combination of the multikinase inhibitor sorafenib and the farnesyltransferase inhibitor tipifarnib in medullary and differentiated thyroid malignancies. J Clin Endocrinol Metab. 2011;96:997–1005.

182. Motzer RJ, Escudier B, Oudard S, et al. Phase 3 trial of everolimus for metastatic renal cell carcinoma: final results and analysis of prognostic factors. Phase 3 trial of everolimus for metastatic renal cell carcinoma: final results and analysis of prognostic factors. Cancer. 2010;116:4256–65.

183. Edgerly M, Fojo T. Is there room for improvement in adverse event reporting in the era of targeted therapies? J Natl Cancer Inst. 2008;100:240–2.

184. Hu-Lowe DD, Zou HY, Grazzini ML, et al. Nonclinical antiangiogenesis and antitumor activities of axitinib (AG-013736), an oral, potent, and selective inhibitor of vascular endothelial growth factor receptor tyrosine kinases 1, 2, 3. Clin Cancer Res. 2008;14:7272–83.

185. Soria JC, Deutsch E. Hemorrhage caused by antiangiogenic therapy within previously irradiated areas: expected consequence of tumor shrinkage or a warning for antiangiogenic agents combined to radiotherapy? Ann Oncol. 2011;22:1247–9.

186. Rixe O, Billemont B, Izzedine H. Hypertension as a predictive factor of Sunitinib activity. Ann Oncol. 2007;18:1117.

187. Ravaud A, Sire M. Arterial hypertension and clinical benefit of sunitinib, sorafenib and bevacizumab in first and second-line treatment of metastatic renal cell cancer. Ann Oncol. 2009;20:966–7.

188. Dahlberg SE, Sandler AB, Brahmer JR, et al. Clinical course of advanced non-small-cell lung cancer patients experiencing hypertension during treatment with bevacizumab in combination with carboplatin and paclitaxel on ECOG 4599. J Clin Oncol. 2010;28:949–54.

189. Österlund P, Soveri LM, Isoniemi H, et al. Hypertension and overall survival in metastatic colorectal cancer patients treated with bevacizumab-containing chemotherapy. Br J Cancer. 2011;104: 599–604.

190. Friberg G, Kasza K, Vokes EE, et al. Early hypertension (HTN) as a potential pharmacodynamic (PD) marker for survival in pancreatic cancer (PC) patients (pts) treated with bevacizumab (B) and gemcitabine (G). J Clin Oncol, 2005; 23 (16_suppl): 3020.

191. Bono P, Elfving H, Utriainen T, et al. Hypertension and clinical benefit of bevacizumab in the treatment

of advanced renal cell carcinoma. Ann Oncol. 2009;20:393–4.

192. Scartozzi M, Galizia E, Chiorrini S, et al. Arterial hypertension correlates with clinical outcome in colorectal cancer patients treated with first-line bevacizumab. Ann Oncol. 2009;20:227–30.

193. Rini BI, Schiller JH, Fruehauf JP, et al. Diastolic blood pressure as a biomarker of axitinib efficacy in solid tumors. Clin Cancer Res. 2011;17:3841–9.

194. Sipos JA, Wang D, Wei L, et al. VEGF polymorphisms predict adverse events in patients taking sorafenib for refractory thyroid cancer. International Thyroid Congress 2010, abs 0C-089.

195. D'Amato RJ, Loughnan MS, Flynn E, et al. Thalidomide is an inhibitor of angiogenesis. Proc Natl Acad Sci U S A. 1994;91:4082–5.

196. Ain KB, Lee C, Williams KD. Phase II trial of thalidomide for therapy of radioiodine-unresponsive and rapidly progressive thyroid carcinomas. Thyroid. 2007;17(7):663–70.

197. Ain KB, Lee C, Holbrook KM, et al. Phase II study of lenalidomide in distantly metastatic, rapidly progressive, and radioiodine-unresponsive thyroid carcinomas: preliminary results. J Clin Oncol, 2008; 26 (15_suppl): 6027.

198. Mooney CJ, Nagaiah G, Fu P, et al. A phase II trial of fosbretabulin in advanced anaplastic thyroid carcinoma and correlation of baseline serum-soluble intracellular adhesion molecule-1 with outcome. Thyroid. 2009;19:233–40.

199. Sosa JA, Elisei R, Jarzab B, et al. A randomized phase II/III trial of a tumor vascular disrupting agent fosbretabulin tromethamine (CA4P) with carboplatin (C) and paclitaxel (P) in anaplastic thyroid cancer (ATC): final survival analysis for the FACT trial. J Clin Oncol, 2011;29 (15_suppl): 5502.

200. Woyach JA, Kloos RT, Ringel MD, et al. Lack of therapeutic effect of the histone deacetylase inhibitor vorinostat in patients with metastatic radioiodine-refractory thyroid carcinoma. J Clin Endocrinol Metab. 2009;94:164–70.

201. Kiazano M, Kitazono M, Chuman Y, Aikou T, Fojo T. Construction of gene therapy vectors targeting thyroid cells: enhancement of activity and specificity with histone deacetylase inhibitors and agents modulating the cyclic adenosine 3′,5′-monophosphate pathway and demonstration of activity in follicular and anaplastic thyroid carcinoma cells. J Clin Endocrinol Metab. 2001;86:834–40.

202. Sherman EJ, Fury MG, Tuttle RM, et al. Phase II study of depsipeptide (DEP) in radioiodine (RAI)-refractory metastatic nonmedullary thyroid carcinoma. J Clin Oncol, 2009;27 (15_suppl): 6059.

203. Catalano MG, Pugliese M, Poli R, et al. Effects of the histone deacetylase inhibitor valproic acid on the sensitivity of anaplastic thyroid cancer cell lines to imatinib. Oncol Rep. 2009;21:515–21.

204. Catalano MG, Fortunati N, Pugliese M, et al. Valproic acid induces apoptosis and cell cycle arrest in poorly differentiated thyroid cancer cells. J Clin Endocrinol Metab. 2005;90:1383–9.

205. Braiteh F, Soriano AO, Garcia-Manero G, et al. Phase I study of epigenetic modulation with 5-aza-cytidine and valproic acid in patients with advanced cancers. Clin Cancer Res. 2008;14:6296–301.

206. Short SC, Suovuori A, Cook G, et al. A phase II study using retinoids as redifferentiation agents to increase iodine uptake in metastatic thyroid cancer. Clin Oncol (R Coll Radiol). 2004;16:569–74.

207. Coelho SM, Corbo R, Buescu A, et al. Retinoic acid in patients with radioiodine non-responsive thyroid carcinoma. J Endocrinol Invest. 2004;27:334–9.

208. Simon D, Köhrle J, Schmutzler C, et al. Redifferentiation therapy of differentiated thyroid carcinoma with retinoic acid: basics and first clinical results. Exp Clin Endocrinol Diabetes. 1996;104 Suppl 4:13–5.

209. Tepmongkol S, Keelawat S, Honsawek S, et al. Rosiglitazone effect on radioiodine uptake in thyroid carcinoma patients with high thyroglobulin but negative total body scan: a correlation with the expression of peroxisome proliferator-activated receptor-gamma. Thyroid. 2008;18:697–704.

210. Koong SS, Reynolds JC, Movius EG, et al. Lithium as a potential adjuvant to 131I therapy of metastatic, well differentiated thyroid carcinoma. J Clin Endocrinol Metab. 1999;84:912–6.

211. Mitsiades CS, Kotoula V, Poulaki V, et al. Epidermal growth factor receptor as a therapeutic target in human thyroid carcinoma: mutational and functional analysis. J Clin Endocrinol Metab. 2006;91:3662–6.

212. Marsee DK, Venkateswaran A, Tao H, et al. Inhibition of heat shock protein 90, a novel RET/PTC1-associated protein, increases radioiodide accumulation in thyroid cells. J Biol Chem. 2004;279:43990–7.

213. Elisei R, Vivaldi A, Ciampi R, et al. Treatment with drugs able to reduce iodine efflux significantly increases the intracellular retention time in thyroid cancer cells stably transfected with sodium iodide symporter complementary deoxyribonucleic acid. J Clin Endocrinol Metab. 2006;91:2389–95.

214. Braga-Basaria M, Hardy E, Gottfried R. 17-Allylamino-17-demethoxygeldanamycin activity against thyroid cancer cell lines correlates with heat shock protein 90 levels. J Clin Endocrinol Metab. 2004;89:2982–8.

Targeted Therapies for Non-small-Cell Lung Cancer

4

Giulio Metro and Lucio Crinò

Introduction

Lung cancer is among the most commonly diagnosed cancers worldwide, representing the first cause of cancer-related death in both the USA and Europe [1, 2]. However, although it has been recently registered a slight decline in its incidence in western countries, the incidence of lung cancer in developing regions is still rising. Non-small-cell lung cancer (NSCLC) accounts for approximately 80% of all lung cancers, being often diagnosed at an advanced stage when treatment options are limited. Unfortunately, chemotherapy and radiation therapy used for the management of advanced disease have significant therapeutic and safety limitations. These limitations often result into poor clinical outcome, which is best exemplified by the dismal median survival of 8–11 months commonly reported for advanced NSCLC patients treated with standard platinum-based first-line chemotherapy [3]. For this reason, biological treatment approaches that demonstrate efficacy in targeting specifically cancer cells have become a priority. In recent years, with rapid advances in the molecular and biological understanding of the process of carcinogenesis, angiogenesis, and cell growth regulation, several new strategies have emerged for the medical treatment of NSCLC patients [4]. Particularly, agents targeting the epidermal growth factor receptor (EGFR) or the vascular endothelial growth factor (VEGF) have significantly improved clinical outcome when used alone or in combination with chemotherapy for the treatment of advanced NSCLC patients selected or not for certain biological characteristics [5–12]. Nevertheless, although these agents offer new hopes for patients with NSCLC, definitive cure is not achievable in case of advanced disease, and survival outcome is still disappointing, thus highlighting the urgent need for further therapeutic improvement.

In this chapter, we review the targeted therapies currently available for the treatment of patients with advanced NSCLC, also discussing the most appealing biological agents under clinical development.

Chemotherapy Overview

Since the publication of the meta-analysis of 1995, platinum-based chemotherapy has been regarded as the standard of care of patients with advanced NSCLC [13]. In the 1990s, several trials evaluated the role of new cytotoxics, such as taxanes, gemcitabine, and vinorelbine, in combination with platinum. These studies demonstrated that the combination of a new drug with a platinum

G. Metro, M.D. • L. Crinò, M.D. (✉)
Santa Maria della Misericordia Hospital,
Medical Oncology, Azienda Ospedaliera di Perugia,
via Dottori, 1, 06156, Perugia, Italy
e-mail: lcrino@unipg.it

M. Bologna (ed.), *Biotargets of Cancer in Current Clinical Practice*, Current Clinical Pathology,
DOI 10.1007/978-1-61779-615-9_4, © Springer Science+Business Media, LLC 2012

derivative produces better results compared with single-agent chemotherapy, an older two-drug combination, or an older three-drug regimen, at least in terms of response rate [14–21]. For these reasons, the combination of cisplatin or carboplatin with a new cytotoxic became the standard of care for the treatment of advanced NSCLC patients. Subsequently, several phase III trials compared among them these new platinum-based doublets to determine the best regimen of all [22–24]. These trials demonstrated a substantial equivalence of the new regimens, with a median survival of 8–9 months, with differences only in terms of costs and toxicity profile. Such discouraging results led to the design of new trials incorporating novel cytotoxics such as pemetrexed, a potent inhibitor of thymidylate synthase. Importantly, pemetrexed has been shown to be beneficial specifically for advanced NSCLC patients with non-squamous histology where, in combination with cisplatin, yielded a significantly greater overall survival (OS) compared with a reference regimen of cisplatin–gemcitabine (11.8 months vs. 10.4 months, respectively, HR=0.81, 95% CI 0.70–0.94, $P=0.005$) [25]. This result, in turn, allowed for the first time in clinical practice for chemotherapy treatment diversification according to tumor histotype. However, at the present time, targeted therapies seem to be the only way through which the clinical outcome of advanced NSCLC can be improved further.

Targeted Therapies: Existing Treatments

Anti-epidermal Growth Factor Receptor Agents

Ever since its identification, the epidermal growth factor receptor (EGFR) has emerged as a protein playing a major role in the development and growth of several human malignancies, including lung cancer [26]. Therefore, given its important contribution to multiple tumorigenic processes of lung cancer such as cancer cell proliferation, angiogenesis, and metastasization, EGFR was undoubtedly regarded as a target for the development of anticancer therapies [27]. More in detail, the EGFR family includes four distinct receptors: EGFR/HER1/erbB-1, HER2/erbB-2, HER3/erbB-3, and HER4/erbB-4 (Fig. 4.1). Upon ligand binding,

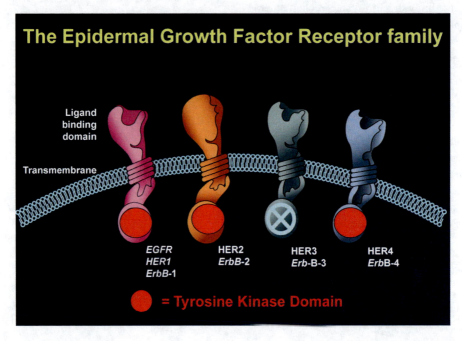

Fig. 4.1 The four distinct receptors of the EGFR family. Interestingly, while no ligand has been identified for the HER2 orphan receptor, no kinase activity has been documented for HER3

EGFR undergoes homo- or heterodimerization with other receptors of the same family, particularly HER2, with subsequent phosphorylation and activation of the intracellular tyrosine kinase (TK) domain, recruitment of second messengers, and intensification of the anti-apoptotic signaling, mainly via the PI3K/Akt and Ras/Raf/MAPK pathways [28]. Interestingly, no ligand has been identified for the HER2 orphan receptor, which allows HER2 to be actively involved in EGFR-mediated signaling through formation of heterodimers.

The main strategies aimed at inhibiting the EGFR pathway include small molecules interfering with the TK activity of the intracellular domain such as EGFR-TK inhibitors (TKIs), or agents directed against the extracellular domain of the receptor such as anti-EGFR monoclonal antibodies.

Reversible EGFR-Tyrosine Kinase Inhibitors

Gefitinib and erlotinib are selective and reversible EGFR-TKIs that act by blocking the phosphorylation of the EGFR-TK domain through competition with adenosine triphosphate (ATP) for binding at the active site of the receptor itself [29]. Two phase III studies comparing erlotinib or gefitinib to placebo in pretreated NSCLC showed a survival improvement for individuals receiving the EGFR-TKI [30, 31] which, in the case of gefitinib, was statistically significant only for patients with certain clinical or biological characteristics such as never-smoking history, Asian ethnicity, and increased EGFR gene copy number as assessed by fluorescence in situ hybridization (FISH) [31, 32]. However, only one study, namely, the BR.21 trial, showed that erlotinib improves OS in a statistically significant manner for the whole population (6.7 months vs. 4.7 months, respectively, HR=0.70, 95% CI 0.58–0.85, $P<0.001$). Therefore, based on these data, erlotinib and not gefitinib was granted approval by regulatory agencies (the FDA in 2004 and the European Medicines Agency in 2005) for the treatment of chemotherapy-resistant advanced NSCLC patients.

Importantly, ever since their identification in 2004, somatic activating kinase mutations in the EGFR gene have emerged as the most important predictor of response to either gefitinib or erlotinib (Fig. 4.2) [33–35], with several retrospective and prospective studies showing that advanced NSCLC patients harboring an activating EGFR mutation may experience responses in up to 90% of cases [4]. More recently, prospective studies demonstrated that gefitinib or erlotinib are associated with a significant improvement in terms of overall response rate (ORR) and progression-free survival (PFS) in EGFR-mutated untreated advanced NSCLC patients compared with platinum-based chemotherapy, clearly supporting the up-front use of a reversible EGFR-TKI in the so biologically selected group of patients (Table 4.1) [5–9]. Importantly, four of these studies tested gefitinib [5–8], and all but one study (EURTAC) were conducted in Asiatic patients [5–9, 36]. Based on these data, gefitinib was granted marketing authorization by European Medicines Agency for the treatment of advanced NSCLC patients with sensitizing mutations of the EGFR gene across all lines of therapy. However, even though no data have been officially presented yet, Roche has recently announced that the EURTAC study was closed early after that a planned interim analysis showed a statistically significant prolongation of PFS for erlotinib compared with platinum-based chemotherapy [36]. Therefore, it is likely that, similar to gefitinib, erlotinib will soon be approved for the treatment of EGFR-mutated advanced NSCLC patients.

Importantly, although EGFR mutations appear more frequently in patients with certain clinical features (female sex, never-smoking history, Asian ethnicity, adenocarcinoma histology) [37], it would be faulty to rule out the possibility of an EGFR mutation solely on the basis of clinical characteristics [7–9, 38]. However, it cannot be entirely ignored that never-smoking history and adenocarcinoma histology are the major enrichment factors for molecular screening. Therefore, in order to render EGFR mutational analysis cost-effective, it seems reasonable to prioritize EGFR mutation testing to non-squamous tumors, limiting testing of squamous tumors only to patients who refer a never-smoking history [39].

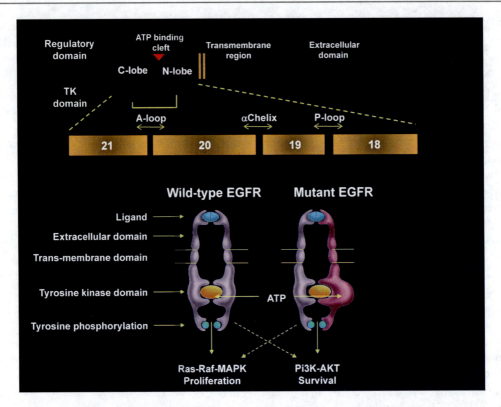

Fig. 4.2 Somatic activating mutations of the EGFR gene involve exons 18–21 which encode for the ATP-binding site within the intracellular tyrosine kinase domain of the receptor. EGFR mutation results into constitutive activation of the signaling pathway downstream EGFR, with preferential involvement of the PI3K/Akt pathway

Table 4.1 Randomized studies establishing a role for a reversible EGFR-TKI in the treatment of EGFR-mutated advanced NSCLC patients

Study	EGFR-TKI	No. of EGFR mutation-positive pts	ORR (EGFR-TKI vs. chemotherapy)	PFS (EGFR-TKI vs. chemotherapy)
IPASS [5]	Gefitinib	261	71.2% vs. 47.3%	HR = 0.48, 95% CI, 0.36–0.64, $P < 0.001$
First-SIGNAL [6]	Gefitinib	42	84.6% vs. 37.5%	8.5 vs. 6.7 months HR = 0.61, 95% CI, 0.30–1.22, $P < 0.0849$
WJTOG3405 [7]	Gefitinib	177	62.1% vs. 32.2%	9.2 vs. 6.3 months HR = 0.48, 95% CI, 0.33–0.71, $P < 0.0001$
NEJGSG002 [8]	Gefitinib	228	73.7% vs. 30.7%	10.4 vs. 5.5 months HR = 0.36, 95% CI, 0.25–0.51, $P < 0.001$
OPTIMAL [9]	Erlotinib	150	82.9% vs. 25%	13.1 vs. 4.6 months HR = 0.16, 95% CI, 0.10–0.26, $P < 0.001$
EURTAC [36]	Erlotinib	130	NA	NA

EGFR-TKI epidermal growth factor receptor tyrosine kinase inhibitor, *NA* not available, *ORR* overall response rate, *PFS* progression-free survival, *pts* patients

Specific EGFR-activating mutations are either short, in-frame nucleotide deletions, in-frame duplications/insertions, or single-nucleotide substitutions clustered around the ATP-binding pocket [40]. To date, in-frame deletions in exon 19 (del19) and exon 21 substitution (L858R)

are the best characterized mutations, together representing 85–90% of all EGFR mutations in NSCLC [40]. Interestingly, clinical data seem to indicate that patients harboring the del19 mutation are more susceptible to the activity of reversible EGFR-TKIs compared to those carrying the L858R mutation [38, 41]. However, the molecular mechanisms underlying this apparent discrepancy in drug sensitivity between del19 and L858R mutations have yet to be elucidated.

An interesting area of research has been the one searching for the best way to integrate reversible EGFR-TKIs with chemotherapy. The concomitant approach has been clearly shown to be unsuccessful since four large phase III trials failed to demonstrate an improvement in survival when a reversible EGFR-TKI was administered concomitantly with platinum-based first-line chemotherapy [42–45]. The INTACT 1 & 2, TRIBUTE, and TALENT trials randomly assigned more than 4,000 chemonaïve advanced NSCLC patients to standard chemotherapy (cisplatin plus gemcitabine or carboplatin plus paclitaxel) vs. the same combination plus gefitinib (INTACT 1 & 2) or erlotinib (TALENT and TRIBUTE). However, although no differences in survival were observed between the two arms of treatment, some benefit was noted at the end of chemotherapy, particularly for never smokers, suggesting that a sequential approach could be more effective than a concomitant strategy [46]. For this reason, reversible EGFR-TKIs have been subsequently tested in a sequential or intercalated-with-chemotherapy approach (during chemotherapy but in the rest periods), based on the preclinical evidence that the administration of the biological agent after chemotherapy would enhance the cytostatic effects deriving from the blockade of the EGFR pathway [47]. Consistently with this hypothesis, three recent phase III studies strongly supported the use of gefitinib or erlotinib as maintenance treatment when administered sequentially after chemotherapy [48–50]. The West Japan Thoracic Oncology Group randomly assigned 604 chemonaïve advanced NSCLCs to platinum-based chemotherapy up to 6 cycles vs. 3 cycles of chemotherapy followed by maintenance gefitinib until progression [48]. Although the primary end point of survival was not reached, median PFS was significantly prolonged in the gefitinib arm (4.6 vs. 4.3 months, HR = 0.68, 95% CI 0.57–0.80, $P < 0.001$), with a modest but statistically significant survival improvement in the adenocarcinoma population (15.4 vs. 14.3 months, HR = 0.65). Another study enrolling again Asian patients only, the FASTACT trial, randomized advanced NSCLCs to either erlotinib intercalated with platinum-based chemotherapy and then given sequentially until progression or platinum-based chemotherapy alone for a maximum of 6 cycles [49]. This trial, besides showing again a significant prolongation of PFS in favor of the EGFR-TKI arm (29.4 vs. 23.4 weeks, HR = 0.47, 95% CI 0.33–0.68, $P = 0.0002$), also suggested that this benefit was largely due to the sequential administration of erlotinib rather than to the intercalated one since the separation of the PFS curves started approximately after 6 months of treatment start, namely at a the time when chemotherapy was stopped in both arms. More recently, the SATURN study definitively established a role for maintenance erlotinib in the treatment of advanced NSCLC patients [50]. In the SATURN trial, a total of 889 patients with no evidence of disease progression after 4 cycles of platinum-based first-line chemotherapy were randomized to either erlotinib 150 mg/d or placebo until progression or unacceptable toxicity. The study met its primary end point by showing a significantly longer PFS in favor of maintenance erlotinib (12.3 vs. 11.1 weeks, HR = 0.71, 95% CI 0.62–0.82, $P < 0.0001$). Importantly, a significant improvement in PFS was also seen for EGFR wild-type tumors (HR = 0.78, 95% CI 0.63–0.96, $P = 0.0185$), although, as expected, EGFR mutation-positive patients were those who experienced the greatest PFS benefit of all (HR = 0.10, 95% CI 0.04–0.25, $P < 0.0001$). Median OS was also significantly increased in the whole population (12 vs. 11 months, HR = 0.81, 95% CI 0.70–0.95, $P = 0.0088$), and it was not reached for the subgroup of EGFR mutation-positive patients. Notably, a striking 2.3-month difference in OS was seen for patients who had stable disease after first-line chemotherapy (HR = 0.72, 95% CI 0.59–0.79, $P = 0.0019$), while there was only a

0.5-month OS improvement in patients who had experienced a previous complete or partial response to chemotherapy (HR=0.94, 95% CI 0.74–1.20, P=0.618). This finding is consistent with the fact that patients with advanced NSCLC whose tumors remain largely unchanged after initial chemotherapy (stable disease) are those who progress faster, are more resistant to further lines of chemotherapy, and have a poorer prognosis compared to patients with a complete or partial response to initial chemotherapy [51]. Therefore, this implies that the "stable disease" group would be the one that probably benefits the most from a maintenance treatment as this patient population may not be able and fit enough to receive further lines of treatment once the disease has progressed. Based on the results of the SATURN trial, erlotinib has gained approval in the USA for maintenance treatment of advanced NSCLC patients after 4 cycles of standard platinum-based first-line chemotherapy and in Europe for patients with stable disease after 4 cycles of platinum-based first-line chemotherapy.

Monoclonal Antibodies Against EGFR: Cetuximab

Cetuximab is the most widely tested anti-EGFR antibody in NSCLC, namely, a human-murine chimeric anti-EGFR IgG monoclonal antibody that binds to the extracellular domain of EGFR. Consistent with the preclinical observation that cetuximab may potentiate the antitumor effects of chemotherapy [52, 53], randomized trials of chemotherapy with or without cetuximab have challenged the paradigm of the platinum doublets as the gold standard of advanced NSCLC treatment. In fact, to date, two large phase III randomized trials have suggested a potential benefit for the combination of platinum-based chemotherapy with cetuximab (to which we will refer as cetuximab-based therapy) over the same chemotherapy regimen alone [10, 54]. The FLEX trial was a large phase III study randomly assigning EGFR-expressing patients to cisplatin-vinorelbine or the same regimen plus cetuximab. A total of 1,688 patients were screened, of which 1,442 (85%) were EGFR positive by immunohistochemistry, and 1,125 were enrolled into the trial. In this

study, the addition of cetuximab to chemotherapy led to a significant improvement in response rate (36% vs. 29%, P=0.012) with a significant survival benefit (11.3 vs. 10.1 months, P=0.044), even though the benefit in survival was marginal (HR=0.87) [10]. These results have been confirmed in another phase III study named BMS099 randomly assigning 676 chemonaïve advanced NSCLC patients to carboplatin plus a taxane (paclitaxel or docetaxel) vs. the same chemotherapy regimen plus cetuximab [54]. Importantly, patients were enrolled into the study regardless of EGFR expression in tumor tissue. Although the primary end point of PFS was not met (4.4 vs. 4.2 months, P=0.23), response rate (25% vs. 17%, P=0.007) and survival (9.6 vs. 8.3 months) favored the cetuximab arm with a reduction in the risk of death comparable to that of the FLEX trial (HR=0.89) which, however, was not statistically significant (P=0.16). More recently, a meta-analysis of 2,018 patients from four randomized trials (1,003 patients treated with cetuximab plus chemotherapy and 1,015 patients treated with chemotherapy alone), which included among others also the FLEX and BMS099 studies, showed that cetuximab-based therapy is associated with a significant improvement in objective response rate (odds ratio=1.463, 95% CI 1.201–1.783, P<0.001) and reduction in the risk of progression (HR=0.89, 95% CI 0.814–0.993, P=0.036) and death (HR=0.87, 95% CI 0.795–0.969, P=0.010) compared to chemotherapy alone, which was present irrespective of the histological subtype of the tumor or the type of platinum doublet employed [55]; however, given the marginal benefit favoring cetuximab-based therapy, it is evident that there is a consistent proportion of patients not benefiting at all from cetuximab treatment. Against this background, the identification of clinical or biological markers that could predict sensitivity to cetuximab would be of great value for treatment tailoring. In the cetuximab arms of both the FLEX and BMS 099 trials, the patients who developed an early rash (the main side effect of cetuximab) were those who seemed to benefit the most from cetuximab-based therapy, particularly in terms of OS [54, 56]. More in detail, in a prespecified analysis of the FLEX trial, median OS with cetuximab-based therapy was 15 months for the 290 patients who developed an acne-like rash of any grade within the first 3 weeks (and were still alive after the first cycle) compared to 8.8 months for the 228 patients without an acne-like rash ($P < 0.0001$, HR = 0.63) [56]. However, although these data suggest the existence of a mechanism linking the anticancer activity of cetuximab in patients with advanced NSCLC and the early incidence of an acne-like rash, it is still not clear what this mechanism might be. Therefore, additional studies are needed to determine the clinical relevance of this observation.

As for tissue biomarkers, the presence of activating EGFR mutations, a critical factor for response to EGFR-TKIs, does not seem to be relevant for cetuximab sensitivity [57–59]. In addition, in contrast to metastatic colorectal cancer where the presence of wild-type KRAS oncogene is required for the therapeutic efficacy of cetuximab [60], in NSCLC the benefit from cetuximab seems to be unrelated to the mutational status of the KRAS oncogene [58, 59]. On the other hand, increased EGFR gene copy number as detected by FISH might be associated with increased sensitivity to cetuximab, as suggested by the Southwest Oncology Group (SWOG) randomized phase II trial (S0342) comparing chemotherapy (carboplatin–paclitaxel) plus cetuximab vs. sequential treatment (the same chemotherapy followed by cetuximab) in untreated advanced NSCLC patients [61]. In this study, in which 106 patients were assigned to concurrent treatment and 117 to the sequential approach, no difference in response rate, PFS and OS was observed. However, EGFR FISH-positive patients treated with cetuximab experienced a significantly longer PFS and OS compared to the EGFR FISH-negative ones (PFS: 6 vs. 3 months, respectively, $P = 0.0008$; OS: 15 vs. 7 months, respectively, $P = 0.04$) [62]. Nevertheless, the value of FISH analysis in predicting the benefit to cetuximab treatment still needs prospective validation, which is currently matter of investigation of the randomized phase III SWOG 0819 study [63]. For this reason, at the present time, no fully reliable

Table 4.2 Clinical and/or biological markers investigated as potential predictors of improved OS on cetuximab-based therapy

Clinical and biological marker	Predictivity for improved OS
First-cycle rash	++
Increased EGFR gene copy number	+/–
EGFR mutation	–
Wild-type KRAS	–

tissue biomarker exists in clinical practice for selecting NSCLC patients candidate to cetuximab-based therapy (Table 4.2).

Antiangiogenic Agents

Angiogenesis, namely, the development of new vessels from parent blood vessels, is an essential stage for the growth and survival of most solid tumors, including lung cancer [64]. A dominant process regulating angiogenesis is the interaction between the vascular endothelial growth factor proteins (VEGFs), particularly VEGF-A (or VEGF), and their receptors (VEGFRs). More in detail, VEGFRs are specifically expressed on the surface of endothelial cells and, like VEGFs, are regulated by hypoxia [65]. Three different forms of VEGFRs have been identified: VEGFR-1 (Flt-1) has the highest binding affinity for VEGF but generates relatively little kinase activity; VEGFR-2 (KDR or Flk-1) is the isotype mostly associated with endothelial cell proliferation and chemotaxis; VEGFR-3 (Flt-4) seems to regulate lymphangiogenesis [66]. Because of its pivotal role in cancer, disruption of cellular signaling of the VEGF/VEGFR pathway represents an attractive therapeutic target. There are two main ways through which the VEGFRs activity can be blocked, either by monoclonal antibodies against VEGF or VEGFRs or by molecules that inhibit the VEGFRs tyrosine kinase activity.

Monoclonal Antibodies Against VEGF: Bevacizumab

The recombinant humanized monoclonal antibody against VEGF named bevacizumab was the first angiogenesis inhibitor to demonstrate efficacy in solid tumors [67]. In NSCLC, a randomized phase II trial of chemonaïve patients treated with standard platinum-based chemotherapy plus placebo or bevacizumab (at either 7.5 mg/kg or 15 mg/kg) demonstrated a higher ORR and longer PFS and OS in favor of the higher dose of bevacizumab compared with the placebo arm [68]. Importantly, patients with squamous cell histology as well as those with tumor cavitation and disease location close to major blood vessels were found to be at higher risk for fatal tumor-related bleeding events. Based on these findings, the Eastern Cooperative Oncology Group (ECOG) conducted a large phase III trial (E4599) comparing a standard platinum-based doublet consisting of carboplatin–paclitaxel with the same regimen plus bevacizumab at the dose of 15 mg/kg in 878 untreated advanced NSCLC patients (Table 4.3) [11]. To reduce the risk of side effects, the study excluded patients with squamous histology, gross hemoptysis, or brain metastases. Importantly, in this trial, the addition of bevacizumab to standard chemotherapy resulted into superiority of all clinical variables vs. chemotherapy alone, including OS ($P=0.003$, HR$=0.79$). Therefore, the E4599 trial was a cornerstone study in the treatment of advanced NSCLC because for the first time by combining a biological agent to chemotherapy, median survival exceeded 1 year (12.3 vs. 10.3 months in favor of bevacizumab plus chemotherapy). More recently, another large phase III trial conducted in Europe (AVAiL) randomly assigned untreated NSCLC patients to cisplatin–gemcitabine or the same regimen plus two different doses of bevacizumab (7.5 and 15 mg/kg) (Table 4.3) [12, 69]. Again, the AVAiL study excluded patients with squamous histology, gross hemoptysis, brain metastases as well as tumor invading major blood vessels, and patients with uncontrolled hypertension. Although the primary end point of the study was reached in that a significant improvement in PFS was shown for patients receiving bevacizumab, no benefit in survival was observed for the bevacizumab arms. More in detail, PFS was 6.1 months in the cisplatin–gemcitabine arm vs. 6.7 and 6.5 months in the bevacizumab 7.5 mg/kg ($P=0.0003$) and

15 mg/kg arms ($P=0.045$) [12]. On the other hand, median survival was 13.1 vs. 13.6 (HR$=0.93$) and 13.4 months (HR$=1.03$) for the chemotherapy alone, bevacizumab 7.5 mg/kg, and bevacizumab 15 mg/kg arms, respectively [69]. Although a confounding effect of second- and third-line therapies could explain the lack of survival benefit in favor of bevacizumab in the AVAiL trial, it is not possible to exclude that cisplatin–gemcitabine might not the best regimen with which bevacizumab should be combined. At the present time, current data suggest that carboplatin–paclitaxel is the preferable regimen to be used in combination with bevacizumab at the dose of 15 mg/kg. In addition, the use of bevacizumab in combination with a paclitaxel-containing regimen is supported by the preclinical evidence of synergism of this combination based on the fact that paclitaxel induces a mobilization spike in bone marrow-derived circulating endothelial progenitor cells which is prevented by the co-administration of an antiangiogenic agent [70]. Accordingly, a single-arm, multicenter, international trial evaluating the safety and efficacy of bevacizumab in combination with a range of chemotherapy regimens in over 2,000 patients (SAiL) showed that bevacizumab in combination with a taxane can yield a median PFS and OS as high as 8.3 and 15.5 months, respectively [71]. However, the results of the SAiL study were important in that they confirmed in a "real-life" population that bevacizumab plus chemotherapy is associated with a well-established and manageable safety profile (Fig. 4.3). At the moment, bevacizumab is the only antiangiogenic agent available for the treatment of non-squamous NSCLC based on improved survival shown in randomized trials in combination with platinum-based chemotherapy [11, 72], and either European guidelines or US NCI guidelines recommend the inclusion of bevacizumab in first-line chemotherapy regimens in selected patients with stage IV nonsquamous NSCLC [73, 74].

However, there are several pending issues about the use of bevacizumab in advanced NSCLC not only limited to the optimal dosage to employ or to which chemotherapy regimen should be used in combination. Other unresolved

4 Targeted Therapies for Non-small-Cell Lung Cancer

Table 4.3 Phase III trials with bevacizumab plus chemotherapy in the first-line treatment of advanced NSCLC

Trial	Regimen	No. pts	ORR (%)	ORR p value	PFS (months)	PFS p value	OS (months)	OS p value
E4599 [11]	CP + B 15 mg/kg	434	35		6.2		12.3	
	vs			<0.001[a]		<0.001[a]		0.0003[a]
	CP	444	15		4.5		10.3	
AVAiL [12, 69]	CG + B 7.5 mg/kg	345	34	<0.0001[a,b]	6.7	0.003[a,b]	13.6	0.420[b]
	CG + B 15 mg/kg	351	30	0.0023[a,b]	6.5	0.03[a,b]	13.4	0.761[b]
	CG + placebo	347	20		6.1		13.1	

B bevacizumab, *CG* cisplatin plus gemcitabine, *CP* carboplatin plus paclitaxel, *ORR* overall response rate, *OS* overall survival, *PFS* progression-free survival, *pts* patients

[a] Statistically significant

[b] Compared to the placebo arm

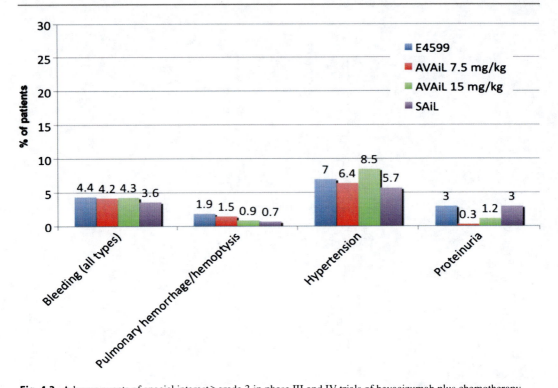

Fig. 4.3 Adverse events of special interest ≥ grade 3 in phase III and IV trials of bevacizumab plus chemotherapy

issues include the duration of bevacizumab treatment and patient selection according to criteria other than histology. With regard to the first issue, current evidence suggests that bevacizumab should be administered until disease progression as it was in the E4599 and AVAiL trials. Interestingly, such a conduct is also supported by the preclinical evidence that early withdrawal of anti-VEGF therapy results into rapid vessel regrowth, thus corroborating the fact that bevacizumab should be given at least until disease progression in clinical practice [75]. On the other hand, current clinical research is focusing on trying to identify clinical and/or biological markers of bevacizumab efficacy. Although the development of hypertension during treatment with bevacizumab plus chemotherapy might be associated with improved clinical outcome [76], to date, no biological marker useful for selecting patients candidate to bevacizumab treatment has been identified. Finally, ongoing clinical trials are investigating prospectively the efficacy and safety of bevacizumab in patients previously excluded from large phase III trials, particularly individuals with brain metastases and squamous cell histology [4].

Targeted Therapies Under Clinical Development

Targeting Anaplastic Lymphoma Kinase in Lung Cancer: Crizotinib

Chromosomal rearrangements involving the tyrosine kinase ALK occur in a variety of human malignancies including NSCLC [77]. First discovered in 2007 [78], the echinoderm microtubule-associated protein-like 4 (EML4)-ALK fusion oncogene derives from an inversion on the short arm of chromosome 2 that joins exons 1–13 of EML4 to exons 20–29 of ALK. This fusion oncogene results into ligand-independent dimerization of ALK, leading to "oncogene addiction" through constitutive activation of kinase activity (reviewed in [77]). The preclinical evidence showing that small molecules inhibiting ALK could effectively block the growth of NSCLC cell lines harboring the EML4-ALK translocation via downregulation of the Ras/Mek/Erk and PI3K/Akt signaling pathways [79] as well as induce tumor regression in EML4-ALK-positive transgenic mice [80], prompted the rapid validation of ALK as a therapeutic target in ALK-rearranged NSCLC patients. Notably, in NSCLC patients, the EML4-ALK fusion oncogene is usually associated with peculiar clinical and/or pathological characteristics such as young age of tumor onset, never- or light-smoking history, and adenocarcinoma histology, particularly of the signet ring cell type [77]. Therefore, while in the overall population the frequency of this genetic alteration is generally low (approximately 3%), it can be detected with higher frequency in patients selected on the basis of the above mentioned characteristics, being present in 35–45% of adenocarcinoma patients with a never- or light-smoking history without an EGFR mutation [81, 82].

Crizotinib (PF02341066), a small molecule TKI targeting both ALK and the MET receptor (the latter being encoded by the MET proto-oncogene), is the first ALK-targeted therapy that has been tested for the treatment of patients with advanced NSCLC selected on the basis of the positivity for the EML4-ALK fusion oncogene [83, 84]. A phase I study investigating crizotinib in 113 EML4-ALK-positive patients (as assessed by FISH analysis) reported an ORR of 56% among the 105 evaluable patients with a median PFS of 9.2 months for the whole study population [83, 84]. These outstanding results, which came without relevant drug-related toxicity, were even more remarkable considering that 93% of patients had received one or more lines of therapy and 30% had received more than 3 prior lines. Notably, response was independent of the number of prior treatments, gender, age, and Eastern Cooperative Oncology Group performance status. On this basis, an ongoing phase III study (PROFILE 1007) is comparing standard second-line chemotherapy vs. crizotinib in EML4-ALK-positive advanced NSCLC pretreated with one line of platinum-based therapy [85] (Table 4.4). Another trial (PROFILE 1005) is a single-arm phase II study whose eligible patients include those who received standard chemotherapy on PROFILE 1007 and discontinued treatment due to disease progression, thus serving as a mechanism by which PROFILE 1007 patients can cross over into the crizotinib arm (Table 4.4) [86]. Finally, a study is comparing crizotinib vs. standard first-line chemotherapy in EML4-ALK-positive patients with adenocarcinoma histology (Table 4.4) [87]. Importantly, recent sequencing of the ALK-TK domain has revealed the presence of two de novo mutations each of which confers resistance to treatment with crizotinib, thus opening a new scenario for the clinical development of agents with the potential of overcoming such mechanisms of resistance [88].

Overcoming Resistance to Reversible EGFR-TKIs

Unfortunately, approximately 20–30% of all EGFR-mutated patients do not respond to a reversible EGFR-TKI [5–9, 38]. Moreover, virtually all EGFR-mutated patients who initially benefit from gefitinib or erlotinib eventually develop progressive disease, usually after a median 14 months since treatment initiation [89]. Against this background, the identification of the molecular mechanisms that underlie either primary or acquired resistance to reversible EGFR-TKIs is of crucial importance to prevent, delay, or overcome resistance to treatment. To date, a few mechanisms of resistance to reversible EGFR-TKIs have been identified. Preclinically, primary resistance has been associated with in-frame insertion mutations in exon 20 [90]. Consistent with these data, most patients with tumors harboring exon 20 insertions have been shown to be resistant to gefitinib [91]. As for acquired resistance, in approximately 50% of patients resistance this can be attributed to the occurrence of a secondary T790M missense mutation in exon 20 of the EGFR kinase domain [92–94]. However, recent evidence suggests that the T790M mutation be involved also in primary resistance, becoming evident during exposure to reversible EGFR-TKIs as a result of evolutionary selection of clones of tumor cells

Table 4.4 Ongoing studies evaluating crizotinib for the treatment of EML4-ALK-positive advanced NSCLC patients

Clinical trial gov identifier	Phase (planned accrual)	Patient selection	Prior treatment	Study design	Primary end point	Status
NCT00932893 (PROFILE 1007) [85]	III (318 pts)	EML4-ALK positivity[a]	No more than 1 line of therapy which must have been platinum-based	2nd line chemotherapy[b] vs. crizotinib	PFS	Ongoing
NCT00932451 (PROFILE 1005) [86]	II (400 pts)	EML4-ALK positivity[a]	≥2 lines of therapy[c]	Crizotinib monotherapy	ORR	Ongoing
NCT0_154140 (PROFILE 1014) [87]	III (334 pts)	EML4-ALK positivity[a] Adenocarcinoma histology	None	Cisplatin or carboplatin[d]/ pemetrexed vs. crizotinib	PFS	Ongoing

ORR overall response rate, *PFS* progression-free survival, *pts* patients

[a] As assessed by fluorescence in situ hybridization (test provided by a central laboratory)

[b] Pemetrexed or docetaxel

[c] May have received pemetrexed or docetaxel from previous phase III trial (PROFILE 1007) and discontinued treatment due to response evaluation criteria in solid tumors (RECIST)-defined progression

[d] Investigator's choice

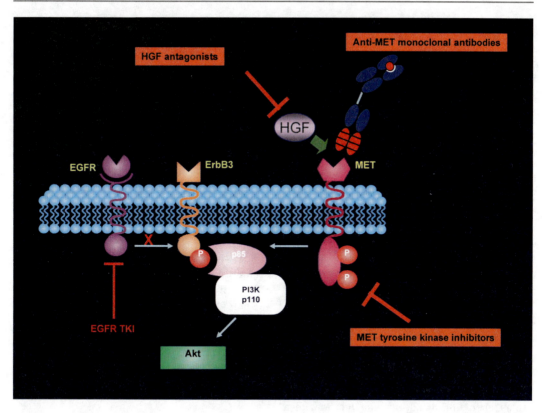

Fig. 4.4 The MET receptor signals through the HER3-mediated activation of the PI3K/Akt pathway and can therefore bypass EGFR. Here are also shown the therapeutic strategies under investigation in order to inhibit the signaling network derived from the interaction between the MET receptor and its ligand, namely, HGF

with a preexisting T790M mutation [95]. More recently, two other less common secondary mutations have been identified as "de novo" alterations in patients with acquired resistance to reversible EGFR-TKIs, namely, the D761Y (exon 19) and T854A (exon 21) mutations [94, 96]. In addition, another mechanism of acquired resistance to EGFR-TKIs has been described by Engelman et al. [97]. They isolated gefitinib-resistant clones from HCC827 lung cancer cells harboring EGFR-activating mutations and found that resistant cells maintained HER3- and Akt-mediated signaling activation in presence of gefitinib owing to focal amplification of the MET proto-oncogene (Fig. 4.4). Importantly, inhibition of MET signaling in these cells was able to restore sensitivity to gefitinib or erlotinib, indicating that the concomitant use of an EGFR-TKI with a MET inhibitor could potentially revert resistance to gefitinib or erlotinib. In addition, studies on NSCLC specimens obtained from human material found that MET amplification occurs in about 20% of EGFR-mutated patients with acquired resistance to EGFR-TKIs [97, 98]. In contrast, the same phenomenon occurs in 3–7.2% NSCLCs not treated with TKIs, thus confirming that also MET could be a relevant therapeutic target for some individuals with primary resistance to EGFR-TKIs [98, 99]. Occasionally, resistant tumors with MET amplification may have a concurrent secondary T790M mutation [98, 100].

Irreversible EGFR-TKIs: The Emerging Role of Afatinib

Currently, no approved therapy exists for advanced NSCLC patients who fail chemotherapy and progress after benefiting from a reversible EGFR-TKI [101]. Although some patients might keep deriving benefit from continued EGFR inhibition with gefitinib or erlotinib [102], the clinical value of such a conduct remains questionable [103].

Irreversible inhibition of the EGFR-TK domain has the theoretical potential to overcome resistance to gefitinib or erlotinib by forming a permanent covalent attachment to the intracellular domain of EGFR (reviewed in [104]). In fact, upon irreversible inhibition, EGFR functioning can resume only through the synthesis of a new receptor protein. On this basis, several irreversible EGFR-TKIs are under development for clinical use in the treatment of advanced NSCLC, the majority of which target simultaneously multiple receptors of the EGFR family. Among them, the dual EGFR/HER2 inhibitor afatinib (BIBW 2992) seems to be one of the most appealing drugs, based on the preclinical activity shown not only in NSCLC cell lines harboring the gefitinib- or erlotinib-resistant T790M mutation but also on the effectiveness demonstrated in xenograft models with the EGFR L858R/T790M double-mutant tumors, including a murine lung tumor with a "de novo" EGFR L858R/T790M-driven lung cancer [105]. Notably, afatinib was also found to be active in NSCLC cell lines expressing the secondary resistance mutation T854A [96]. Collectively, these preclinical data strongly suggest that afatinib may overcome acquired resistance to reversible EGFR-TKIs. Consistent with this preclinical evidence, afatinib has been recently shown to improve significantly ORR, PFS, and quality of life compared with placebo in a phase III trial (LUX-Lung 1) of biologically unselected patients with advanced adenocarcinoma of the lung who had progressed after ≤2 lines of chemotherapy (including one platinum-based regimen) and ≥12 weeks of treatment with gefitinib or erlotinib [106, 107]. Of note, by restricting the analysis only to the patients who harbored clinical features highly associated with sensitivity to reversible EGFR-TKIs (duration of prior treatment with gefitinib or erlotinib ≥48 weeks and complete or partial response on prior gefitinib or erlotinib), a striking 3.4-month difference in PFS in favor of afatinib was seen over placebo (4.4 months vs. 1.0 month, respectively,

HR=0.28), which is in line with the hypothesis that afatinib may overcome clinically acquired resistance to EGFR-TKIs.

Intriguingly, afatinib-mediated irreversible blockade of EGFR could not only overcome but also prevent/delay the onset of acquired resistance in EGFR-mutated NSCLC patients since preclinical evidence suggests that acquired resistance develops at a lower frequency with irreversible EGFR-TKIs than with reversible agents [108]. To this regard, afatinib showed greater potency than gefitinib or erlotinib in reducing survival of NSCLC cell lines harboring wild-type EGFR and the activating L858R mutation [105]. Consistently, a phase II trial (LUX-Lung 2) of afatinib given as first-line treatment of patients with EGFR-mutated advanced NSCLC showed median PFS and OS of 14 and 24 months [109], respectively, which are among the best outcome results when compared with similar studies employing reversible EGFR-TKIs (Table 4.5) [110–120], thus suggesting that afatinib provides a very prolonged inhibition of the EGFR target.

MET Inhibitors

MET inhibitors represent another class of drugs under active clinical development for the treatment of NSCLC, particularly for patients with acquired resistance to EGFR-TKIs. There are several ways to inhibit the MET signaling pathway, including anti-MET antibodies, inactivation of the MET ligand, namely, the hepatocyte growth factor (HGF), or inhibition of MET tyrosine kinase activity (Fig. 4.4) (reviewed in [121]). Importantly, because MET amplification and T790M mutation often occur in the same patient, probably the best strategy is to combine an EGFR-TKI with an MET inhibitor. Accordingly, a recent randomized phase II study of pretreated, EGFR-TKI-naïve advanced NSCLC patients showed that the combination of ARQ-197, a MET-TKI, with erlotinib can prolong significantly PFS over erlotinib plus placebo, thus emerging as a novel mechanism with the potential of preventing/delaying the onset of resistance to treatment with a reversible EGFR-TKI [122]. Similarly, another randomized phase II study of advanced NSCLC patients showed

4 Targeted Therapies for Non-small-Cell Lung Cancer

Table 4.5 Prospective single-arm studies evaluating an EGFR-TKI for the treatment of EGFR-mutated advanced NSCLC (modified from Cappuzzo)

Reference	#	Line	Drug	PFS (months)	OS (months)
LUX-Lung 2 [109]	129	I/II	Afatinib	14.0	24.0
Rosell [38]	217	I/II	Erlotinib	14	27
Asahina [110]	16	I	Gefitinib	8.9	Not reached
Inoue [111]	30	I	Gefitinib	6.5	17.8
Inoue [112]	16	I	Gefitinib	9.7	Not reported
Sequist [113]	34	I	Gefitinib	9.2	17.5
Yang [114]	55	I	Gefitinib	8	24
Sugio [115]	20	I/II	Gefitinib	7.1	20
Sunaga [116]	21	I/II	Gefitinib	12.9	Not reached
Sutani [117]	38	I/II	Gefitinib	9.4	15.4
Yoshida [118]	27	I/II	Gefitinib	7.7	Not reached
Han [119]	17	I/II+	Gefitinib	21.7	30.5
Tamura [120]	28	I/II/III	Gefitinib	11.5	Not reached

OS overall survival, *PFS* progression-free survival

that the addition of MET-mAb, an anti-MET monoclonal antibody, to erlotinib can improve PFS and OS compared to erlotinib plus placebo only in patients with high immunohistochemical expression of the MET receptor [123]. Such a finding, which was the result of a prespecified analysis, reinforces the importance of patient selection for a given targeted therapy to show clinical efficacy.

Antiangiogenic Therapy Beyond Bevacizumab: Multitargeted Kinase Inhibitors

Several multitargeted kinase inhibitors are being or have been evaluated for the treatment of advanced NSCLC almost inevitably with disappointing results in terms of efficacy. Vandetanib is a multitargeted inhibitor of VEGFR-2 and -3, EGFR, and RET kinases. This drug was developed based on the assumption that dual EGFR/ VEGFRs inhibition would prove more beneficial than blocking a single pathway [124]. In phase I and multiple randomized phase II studies, vandetanib was established as a promising novel targeted agent for the treatment of patients with advanced NSCLC, also supporting its potential role when administered in combination with

chemotherapy [125]. Recently, the results of three phase III studies investigating vandetanib in advanced NSCLC have been published [126–128]. The ZODIAC and ZEAL trials investigated whether the addition of vandetanib to single-agent chemotherapy would improve the efficacy of docetaxel or pemetrexed, respectively, in pretreated patients [126, 127]. Importantly, both trials showed that the addition of vandetanib to chemotherapy provides only a modest improvement in ORR and PFS compared with chemotherapy, although PFS prolongation reached statistical significance only in the ZODIAC study [126]. The third phase III study (ZEST) compared vandetanib with erlotinib in pretreated advanced NSCLCs [128]. This study did not meet the primary end point of demonstrating a statistically significant prolongation of PFS for the vandetanib arm. However, vandetanib and erlotinib showed equivalent efficacy in terms of PFS and survival in a preplanned noninferiority analysis. Nevertheless, taken together, although these data show that vandetanib may potentiate the efficacy of chemotherapy, it is not clear which subgroup of NSCLC patients may benefit the most from vandetanib treatment. Therefore, future studies should better address the issue of patient selection possibly searching for biomarkers of efficacy.

Sorafenib is a small molecule inhibiting several members of the receptor tyrosine kinase (RTK) family, particularly aiming at VEGFR-2, raf-kinases, PDGF-β, and c-KIT. Sorafenib was tested as monotherapy in chemonaïve advanced NSCLC patients where it showed an activity of 12% with a disease control rate of 36% [129]. In another phase II trial of previously treated NSCLCs, sorafenib demonstrated a more limited activity [130]. However, although no responses were observed, 59% of patients achieved disease stabilization [130]. Unfortunately, a recent phase III study (ESCAPE) testing carboplatin–paclitaxel with or without sorafenib as first-line treatment of advanced NSCLC suffered from early closure after the independent Data Monitoring Committee concluded that the study would not meet its primary end point of improved OS for the sorafenib arm [131]. The reason for this failure is likely to ascribe to the greater mortality registered in the sorafenib arm which apparently could not be explained by an increase in sorafenib-related adverse events.

To conclude, neoangiogenesis remains a potential relevant target in the treatment of advanced NSCLC, but the inconclusive results of multitargeted TKIs, the lack of biomarker selection, and the consistent benefit only in the bevacizumab prospective trials represent a strong limitation and a relevant concern in translating antiangiogenic therapy in the general clinical practice of advanced NSCLC.

Non-small-Cell Lung Cancer in Never Smokers

About 20% of lung cancer cases worldwide are not attributable to tobacco smoking as they arise in never smokers (<100 cigarettes in a lifetime), where lung cancer often shows peculiar clinicopathological features (Fig. 4.5) (reviewed in [132]).

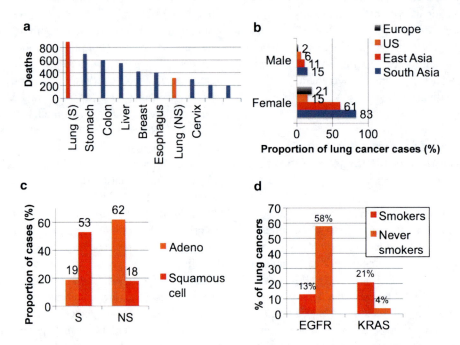

Fig. 4.5 (**a**) Epidemiologic data show that lung cancer arising in never smokers is among the top ten causes of cancer-related deaths in both sexes worldwide. (**b**) Lung cancer in never smokers occurs more frequently in women than men, regardless of geography. However, the proportion of female lung cancer cases is particularly high in East and South Asia. (**c**) Lung cancer in never smokers originates predominantly in distal airways, the most common histology being adenocarcinoma. (**d**) Lung cancer in never smokers has a different pattern of molecular alterations compared with lung cancer arising in smokers. For instance, EGFR mutations are more frequently found in adenocarcinomas arising in never smokers, whereas KRAS mutations are detected more often in lung cancer arising in smokers

Ever since never-smoking status was found to be the strongest clinical predictor of treatment sensitivity in early clinical studies of reversible EGFR-TKIs [30, 31], it became evident that lung cancer arising in never smokers may represent a distinct disease entity to whose pathogenesis contribute multiple factors other than smoking, including environmental, hormonal, viral, and genetic ones. More in detail, with regard to genetic factors, it is now clear that the likelihood of a tumor to harbor a somatic mutation in exons 18–21 of the EGFR gene is inversely proportional to smoking exposure [133] and that, besides activating EGFR mutations, several other TK mutations are detected in lung cancer from never smokers at higher frequencies compared with lung cancer in smokers, such as EML4-ALK fusions and HER2 insertions [134, 135]. This, in turn, may render this disease largely susceptible of being treated successfully with targeted therapies aimed at the oncogenic mutant kinase responsible for a given disease process. On the whole, these data strongly suggest that lung cancer arising in never smokers is a disease distinct from the more common tobacco-associated forms of lung cancer. However, further efforts are needed in order to fully recognize the diverse molecular alterations underlying this condition before the armamentarium of targeted therapies aimed at this disease entity can be implemented.

Conclusions and Future Perspectives

NSCLC is a heterogeneous tumor whose growth depends on the dysregulation of multiple signaling pathways. The introduction in the clinic of several biological therapies, each one targeting specific key cancer molecular profiles, represents a major step forward in the treatment of this disease. Also, it is now clear that not all targeted therapies are the same, which is best exemplified by the fact that their use in combination with standard chemotherapy has not always led to an improvement in clinical outcome. On the other hand, in the next future, it can be anticipated that tumor heterogeneity could be best targeted through simultaneous biological blockade of multiple dysregulated pathways. However, above all, the identification of patients who will benefit from such treatment used either alone or in combination regimens would allow physicians to deliver effective treatments to sensitive patients while preventing others from suffering the side effects of inactive drugs. In addition, biomarkers of response to certain biological agents may differ according to the type of malignancy. For instance, in colorectal cancer, the presence of wild-type KRAS was found to be a strong predictor of sensitivity to cetuximab [60]. In contrast, wild-type KRAS does not appear to have the same predictive value in NSCLC [58, 59]. For this reason, ongoing trials of targeted therapies are being often designed in an attempt to elucidate what biomarkers could best predict sensitivity to treatment. To this regard, the lesson learned from reversible EGFR-TKIs may represent a proof of concept. In fact, after the accumulation of clinical data showing that the presence of somatic activating EGFR mutations in the tumor were able to select a population with high likelihood of benefiting from such agents, phase III trials have been conducted in order to validate successfully this biomarker in a prospective manner [5–9, 36]. If rationally designed, future trials in NSCLC will keep contributing to a better understanding of the role of targeted therapies with regard to optimal dose, schedule, combination strategies, and above all, patient selection.

References

1. Jemal A, Siegel R, Xu J, Ward E. Cancer statistics, 2010. CA Cancer J Clin. 2010;60:277–300.
2. Ferlay J, Parkin DM, Steliarova-Foucher E. Estimates of cancer incidence and mortality in Europe in 2008. Eur J Cancer. 2010;46:765–81.
3. Ramalingam S, Belani C. Systemic chemotherapy for advanced non-small cell lung cancer: recent advances and future directions. Oncologist. 2008;13 Suppl 1:5–13.
4. Metro G, Cappuzzo F. New targeted therapies for non-small-cell lung cancer. Therapy. 2009;6:335–50.
5. Mok TS, Wu YL, Thongprasert S, et al. Gefitinib or carboplatin-paclitaxel in pulmonary adenocarcinoma. N Engl J Med. 2009;361:947–57.
6. Lee JS, Park K, Kim SW, et al. A randomized phase III study of gefitinib (IRESSA™) versus standard

chemotherapy (gemcitabine plus cisplatin) as a first-line treatment for never-smokers with advanced or metastatic adenocarcinoma of the lung. J Thor Oncol. 2009;4(suppl):4 (abstract).

7. Mitsudomi T, Morita S, Yatabe Y, et al. Gefitinib versus cisplatin plus docetaxel in patients with non-small-cell lung cancer harbouring mutations of the epidermal growth factor receptor (WJTOG3405): an open label, randomised phase 3 trial. Lancet Oncol. 2010;11:121–8.

8. Maemondo M, Inoue A, Kobayashi K, et al. Gefitinib or chemotherapy for non-small-cell lung cancer with mutated EGFR. N Engl J Med. 2010;362:2380–8.

9. Zhou C, Wu YL, Chen G, et al. Efficacy results from the randomised phase III OPTIMAL (CTONG 0802) study comparing first-line erlotinib versus carboplatin plus gemcitabine, in chinese advanced non-small-cell lung cancer patients with EGFR activating mutations. Ann Oncol. 2010;21 Suppl 8:13 (abstract).

10. Pirker R, Pereira JR, Szczesna A, et al. Cetuximab plus chemotherapy in patients with advanced non-small-cell lung cancer (FLEX): an open-label randomised phase III trial. Lancet. 2009;373:1525–31.

11. Sandler A, Gray R, Perry MC, et al. Paclitaxel-carboplatin alone or with bevacizumab for non-small-cell lung cancer. N Engl J Med. 2006;355: 2542–50.

12. Reck M, von Pawel J, Zatloukal P, et al. Phase III trial of cisplatin plus gemcitabine with either placebo or bevacizumab as first-line therapy for nonsquamous non-small-cell lung cancer: AVAiL. J Clin Oncol. 2009;27:1227–34.

13. Chemotherapy in non-small cell lung cancer: a meta-analysis using updated data on individual patients from 52 randomised clinical trials. Non-small Cell Lung Cancer Collaborative Group. BMJ. 1995;311: 899–909

14. Cardenal F, Lopez-Cabrerizo M, Anton A, et al. Randomized phase III study of gemcitabine-cisplatin versus etoposide-cisplatin in the treatment of locally advanced or metastatic non-small-cell lung cancer. J Clin Oncol. 1999;17:12–8.

15. Crino L, Scagliotti GV, Ricci S, et al. Gemcitabine and cisplatin versus mitomycin, ifosfamide, and cisplatin in advanced non-small-cell lung cancer: a randomized phase III study of the Italian Lung Cancer Project. J Clin Oncol. 1999;17:3522–30.

16. Sandler A, Nemunaitis J, Dehnam C, et al. Phase III study of gemcitabine plus cisplatin versus cisplatin alone in patients with locally advanced or metastatic non–small-cell lung cancer. J Clin Oncol. 2000;18: 122–30.

17. Giaccone G, Splinter TA, Debruyne C, et al. Randomized study of paclitaxel-cisplatin versus cisplatin-teniposide in patients with advanced non-small-cell lung cancer. The European Organization for Research and Treatment of Cancer Lung Cancer Cooperative Group. J Clin Oncol. 1998;16.2133–41.

18. Wozniak AJ, Crowley JJ, Balcerzak SP, et al. Randomized trial comparing cisplatin with cisplatin plus vinorelbine in the treatment of advanced non-

small-cell lung cancer: a Southwest Oncology Group study. J Clin Oncol. 1998;16:2459–65.

19. Bonomi P, Kim K, Fairclough D, et al. Comparison of survival and quality of life in advanced non–small-cell lung cancer patients treated with two dose levels of paclitaxel combined with cisplatin versus etoposide with cisplatin: results of an Eastern Cooperative Oncology Group trial. J Clin Oncol. 2000;18:623–31.

20. Le Chevalier T, Brisgand D, Douillard JY, et al. Randomized study of vinorelbine and cisplatin versus vindesine and cisplatin versus vinorelbine alone in advanced non-small-cell lung cancer: results of a European multicenter trial including 612 patients. J Clin Oncol. 1994;12:360–7.

21. Danson S, Middleton MR, O'Byrne KJ, et al. Phase III trial of gemcitabine and carboplatin versus mitomycin, ifosfamide, and cisplatin or mitomycin, vinblastine, and cisplatin in patients with advanced nonsmall cell lung carcinoma. Cancer. 2003;98: 542–53.

22. Schiller JH, Harrington D, Belani CP, et al. Comparison of four chemotherapy regimens for advanced non-small-cell lung cancer. N Engl J Med. 2002;346:92–8.

23. Scagliotti GV, De Marinis F, Rinaldi M, et al. Phase III randomized trial comparing three platinum-based doublets in advanced non-small cell lung cancer. J Clin Oncol. 2002;20:4285–92.

24. Smit EF, van Meerbeeck JP, Lianes P, et al. Three-arm randomized study of two cisplatin-based regimens and paclitaxel plus gemcitabine in advanced non-small-cell lung cancer: a phase III trial of the European Organization for Research and Treatment of Cancer Lung Cancer Group—EORTC 0897. J Clin Oncol. 2003;21:3909–17.

25. Scagliotti GV, Parikh P, von Pawel J, et al. Phase III study comparing cisplatin plus gemcitabine with cisplatin plus pemetrexed in chemotherapy-naive patients with advanced-stage non-small-cell lung cancer. J Clin Oncol. 2008;26:3543–51.

26. Huang SM, Harari PM. Epidermal growth factor receptor inhibition in cancer therapy: biology, rationale and preliminary clinical results. Invest New Drugs. 1999;17:259–69.

27. Metro G, Finocchiaro G, Toschi L, et al. Epidermal growth factor receptor (EGFR) targeted therapies in non-small cell lung cancer (NSCLC). Rev Recent Clin Trials. 2006;1:1–13.

28. Mendelsohn J, Baselga J. Epidermal growth factor receptor targeting in cancer. Semin Oncol. 2006;33: 369–85.

29. Sharma SV, Bell DW, Settleman J, Haber DA. Epidermal growth factor receptor mutations in lung cancer. Nat Rev Cancer. 2007;7:169–81.

30. Shepherd FA, Rodrigues Pereira J, Ciuleanu T, et al. Erlotinib in previously treated non-small-cell lung cancer. N Engl J Med. 2005;353:123–32.

31. Thatcher N, Chang A, Parikh P, et al. Gefitinib plus best supportive care in previously treated patients with refractory advanced non-small-cell lung cancer: results from a randomised, placebo-controlled,

multicentre study (Iressa Survival Evaluation in Lung Cancer). Lancet. 2005;366:1527–37.

32. Hirsch FR, Varella-Garcia M, Bunn Jr PA, et al. Molecular predictors of outcome with gefitinib in a phase III placebo-controlled study in advanced non-small-cell lung cancer. J Clin Oncol. 2006;24:5034–42.

33. Paez JG, Jänne PA, Lee JC, et al. EGFR mutations in lung cancer: correlation with clinical response to gefitinib therapy. Science. 2004;304:1497–500.

34. Lynch TJ, Bell DW, Sordella R, et al. Activating mutations in the epidermal growth factor receptor underlying responsiveness of non-small-cell lung cancer to gefitinib. N Engl J Med. 2004;350:2129–39.

35. Pao W, Miller V, Zakowski M, et al. EGF receptor gene mutations are common in lung cancers from "never smokers" and are associated with sensitivity of tumors to gefitinib and erlotinib. Proc Natl Acad Sci U S A. 2004;101:13306–11.

36. Roche-Media releases : http://www.roche.com/media/media_releases/med-cor-2011-01-28.htm Access Date April 1st, 2011

37. Mitsudomi T, Kosaka T, Yatabe Y. Biological and clinical implications of EGFR mutations in lung cancer. Int J Clin Oncol. 2006;11:190–8.

38. Rosell R, Moran T, Queralt C, et al. Screening for epidermal growth factor receptor mutations in lung cancer. N Engl J Med. 2009;361:958–67.

39. Gridelli C, De Marinis F, Di Maio M, et al. Gefitinib as first-line treatment for patients with advanced non-small-cell lung cancer with activating epidermal growth factor receptor mutation: implications for clinical practice and open issues. Lung Cancer. 2011;72(1): 3–8.

40. Murray S, Dahabreh IJ, Linardou H, et al. Somatic mutations of the tyrosine kinase domain of epidermal growth factor receptor and tyrosine kinase inhibitor response to TKIs in non-small cell lung cancer: an analytical database. J Thorac Oncol. 2008;3:832–9.

41. Jackman DM, Yeap BY, Sequist LV, et al. Exon 19 deletion mutations of epidermal growth factor receptor are associated with prolonged survival in non-small cell lung cancer patients treated with gefitinib or erlotinib. Clin Cancer Res. 2006;12:3908–14.

42. Giaccone G, Herbst RS, Manegold C, et al. Gefitinib in combination with gemcitabine and cisplatin in advanced non-small-cell lung cancer: a phase III trial-INTACT 1. J Clin Oncol. 2004;22:777–84.

43. Herbst RS, Giaccone G, Schiller JH, et al. Gefitinib in combination with paclitaxel and carboplatin in advanced non-small-cell lung cancer: a phase III trial-INTACT 2. J Clin Oncol. 2004;22:22785–794.

44. Herbst RS, Prager D, Hermann R, et al. TRIBUTE — A phase III trial of erlotinib hydrochloride (OSI-774) combined with carboplatin and paclitaxel chemotherapy in advanced non-small-cell lung cancer. J Clin Oncol. 2005;23:5892–9.

45. Gatzemeier U, Pluzanska A, Szczesna A, et al. Phase III study of erlotinib in combination with cisplatin and gemcitabine in advanced non-small cell lung cancer: the tarceva lung cancer investigation trial. J Clin Oncol. 2007;25:1545–52.

46. Eberhard DA, Johnson BE, Amler LC, et al. Mutations in the epidermal growth factor receptor and in KRAS are predictive and prognostic indicators in patients with non-small-cell lung cancer treated with chemotherapy alone and in combination with erlotinib. J Clin Oncol. 2005;23:5900–9.

47. Gandara D, Narayan S, Lara Jr PN, et al. Integration of novel therapeutics into combined modality therapy of locally advanced non-small cell lung cancer. Clin Cancer Res. 2005;11 Suppl 13:5057–62.

48. Takeda K, Hida T, Sato T, et al. Randomized phase III trial of platinum-doublet chemotherapy followed by gefitinib compared with continued platinum-doublet chemotherapy in Japanese patients with advanced non-small-cell lung cancer: results of a west Japan thoracic oncology group trial (WJTOG0203). J Clin Oncol. 2010;28:753–60.

49. Mok TS, Wu YL, Yu CJ, et al. Randomized, placebo-controlled, phase II study of sequential erlotinib and chemotherapy as first-line treatment for advanced non-small-cell lung cancer. J Clin Oncol. 2009;27:5080–7.

50. Cappuzzo F, Ciuleanu T, Stelmakh L, et al. Erlotinib as maintenance treatment in advanced non-small-cell lung cancer: a multicentre, randomised, placebo-controlled phase 3 study. Lancet Oncol. 2010;11:521–9.

51. Lara Jr PN, Redman MW, Kelly K, et al. Disease control rate at 8 weeks predicts clinical benefit in advanced non-small-cell lung cancer: results from Southwest Oncology Group randomized trials. J Clin Oncol. 2008;26:463–7.

52. Steiner P, Joynes C, Bassi R, et al. Tumor growth inhibition with cetuximab and chemotherapy in non-small cell lung cancer xenografts expressing wild-type and mutated epidermal growth factor receptor. Clin Cancer Res. 2007;13:1540–51.

53. Raben D, Helfrich B, Chan DC, et al. The effects of cetuximab alone and in combination with radiation and/or chemotherapy in lung cancer. Clin Cancer Res. 2005;11(2 Pt 1):795–805.

54. Lynch TJ, Patel T, Dreisbach L, et al. Cetuximab and first-line taxane/carboplatin chemotherapy in advanced non-small-cell lung cancer: results of the randomized multicenter phase III trial BMS099. J Clin Oncol. 2010;28:911–7.

55. Thatcher N, Lynch TJ, Butts C, et al. Cetuximab plus platinum-based chemotherapy as 1st line treatment in patients with non-small-cell lung cancer (NSCLC): a meta-analysis of randomized phase II/III trials. J Thorac Oncol. 2009;4:S297 (abstract).

56. Gatzemeier U, von Pawel J, Vynnychenko I, et al. First-cycle rash and survival in patients with advanced non-small-cell lung cancer receiving cetuximab in combination with first-line chemotherapy: a subgroup analysis of data from the FLEX phase 3 study. Lancet Oncol. 2011;12:30–7.

57. Mukohara T, Engelman JA, Hanna NH, et al. Differential effects of gefitinib and cetuximab on non-small-cell lung cancers bearing epidermal growth factor receptor mutations. J Natl Cancer Inst. 2005;97:1185–94.

58. Khambata-Ford A, Harbison CT, Hart LL, et al. K-Ras mutations (MT) and EGFR-related markers as potential predictors of cetuximab benefit in 1st line advanced NSCLC: results from the BMS099 study. J Thorac Oncol. 2008;3:S304 (abstract).

59. Gatzemeier U, Paz-Ares L, Rodrigues Pereira J, et al. Molecular and clinical biomarkers of cetuximab efficacy: data from the phase III FLEX study in non-small-cell lung cancer (NSCLC). J Thorac Oncol. 2009;4:S324 (abstract).

60. Jiang Y, Mackley H, Cheng H, Ajani JA. Use of K-Ras as a predictive biomarker for selecting anti-EGF receptor/pathway treatment. Biomark Med. 2010;4:535–41.

61. Herbst RS, Chansky K, Kelly K, et al. A phase II randomized selection trial evaluating concurrent chemotherapy plus cetuximab or chemotherapy followed by cetuximab in patients with advanced non-small cell lung cancer (NSCLC): final report of SWOG 0342. J Clin Oncol. 2007;25:7545 (abstract).

62. Hirsch FR, Herbst RS, Olsen C, et al. Increased EGFR gene copy number detected by fluorescent in situ hybridization predicts outcome in non-small-cell lung cancer patients treated with cetuximab and chemotherapy. J Clin Oncol. 2008;26:3351–7.

63. Carboplatin and paclitaxel with or without bevacizumab and/or cetuximab in treating patients with stage IV or recurrent non-small cell lung cancer. Available at: http://clinicaltrials.gov/ct2/results?term=NCT00946712 [Date accessed April 1st, 2011]

64. Carmeliet P, Jain RK. Angiogenesis in cancer and other disease. Nature. 2000;407:249–57.

65. Ferrara N. Molecular and biological properties of vascular endothelial growth factor. J Mol Med. 1999;77:527–43.

66. Kukk E, Lymboussaki A, Taira S, et al. VEGF-C receptor binding and pattern of expression with VEGFR-3 suggests a role in lymphatic vascular development. Development. 1996;122:3829–37.

67. Presta LG, Chen H, O'Connor SJ, et al. Humanization of an anti-vascular endothelial growth factor monoclonal antibody for the therapy of solid tumors and other disorders. Cancer Res. 1997;57:4593–9.

68. Johnson DH, Fehrenbacher L, Novotny WF, et al. Randomized phase II trial comparing bevacizumab plus carboplatin and paclitaxel with carboplatin and paclitaxel alone in previously untreated locally advanced or metastatic non-small-cell lung cancer. J Clin Oncol. 2004;22:2184–91.

69. Reck M, von Pawel J, Zatloukal P, et al. Overall survival with cisplatin-gemcitabine and bevacizumab or placebo as first-line therapy for nonsquamous non-small-cell lung cancer: results from a randomised phase III trial (AVAiL). Ann Oncol. 2010;21:1804–9.

70. Shaked Y, Henke E, Roodhart JM, et al. Rapid chemotherapy-induced acute endothelial progenitor cell mobilization. implications for antiangiogenic drugs as chemosensitizing agents. Cancer Cell. 2008; 14:263–73.

71. Crinò L, Dansin E, Garrido P, et al. Safety and efficacy of first-line bevacizumab-based therapy in advanced non-squamous non-small-cell lung cancer (SAiL, MO19390): a phase 4 study. Lancet Oncol. 2010;11:733–40.

72. Soria J, Mauguen A, Reck M, et al. Meta-analysis of randomized phase II/III trials adding bevacizumab to platin-based chemotherapy as 1st-line treatment in patients with advanced non-small cell lung cancer (NSCLC). Ann Oncol. 2010;21 Suppl 8:437 (abstract).

73. D'Addario G, Früh M, Reck M, et al. Metastatic non-small-cell lung cancer: ESMO Clinical Practice Guidelines for diagnosis, treatment and follow-up. Ann Oncol. 2010;21 Suppl 5:116–9.

74. National Cancer Institute. Stage IV non-small cell lung cancer http://www.cancer.gov/cancertopics/pdq/treatment/non-small-cell-lung/healthprofessional/page11. [Date accessed April 1st, 2011]

75. Mancuso MR, Davis R, Norberg SM, et al. Rapid vascular regrowth in tumors after reversal of VEGF inhibition. J Clin Invest. 2006;116:2610–21.

76. Dahlberg SE, Sandler AB, Brahmer JR, et al. Clinical course of advanced non-small-cell lung cancer patients experiencing hypertension during treatment with bevacizumab in combination with carboplatin and paclitaxel on ECOG 4599. J Clin Oncol. 2010;28:949–54.

77. Shaw AT, Solomon B. Targeting anaplastic lymphoma kinase in lung cancer. Clin Cancer Res. 2011. DOI: 10.1158/1078-0432.CCR-10-1591

78. Soda M, Choi YL, Enomoto M, et al. Identification of the transforming EML4-ALK fusion gene in non-small-cell lung cancer. Nature. 2007;448:561–6.

79. Koivunen JP, Mermel C, Zejnullahu K, et al. EML4-ALK fusion gene and efficacy of an ALK kinase inhibitor in lung cancer. Clin Cancer Res. 2008;14:4275–83.

80. Soda M, Takada S, Takeuchi K, et al. A mouse model for EML4-ALK-positive lung cancer. Proc Natl Acad Sci U S A. 2008;105:19893–7.

81. Shaw AT, Yeap BY, Mino-Kenudson M, et al. Clinical features and outcome of patients with non-small-cell lung cancer who harbor EML4-ALK. J Clin Oncol. 2009;27:4247–53.

82. Camidge DR, Kono SA, Flacco A, et al. Optimizing the detection of lung cancer patients harboring anaplastic lymphoma kinase (ALK) gene rearrangements potentially suitable for ALK inhibitor treatment. Clin Cancer Res. 2010;16:5581–90.

83. Kwak EL, Bang YJ, Camidge DR, et al. Anaplastic lymphoma kinase inhibition in non-small-cell lung cancer. N Engl J Med. 2010;363:1693–703.

84. Camidge DR, Bang YJ, Iafrate AJ, et al. Clinical activity of crizotinib (PF-02341066), in ALK-positive patients with advanced non-small cell lung cancer. Ann Oncol. 2010;21 Suppl 8:366 (abstract).

85. An investigational drug, PF-02341066 is being studied versus standard of care in patients with advanced non-small cell lung cancer with a specific gene pro-

file involving the anaplastic lymphoma kinase (ALK) gene. Available at: http://clinicaltrials.gov/ct2/results? term=NCT00932893. [Date accessed April 1st, 2011].

86. An investigational drug, PF-02341066 is being studied in patients with advanced non-small cell lung cancer with a specific gene profile involving the anaplastic lymphoma kinase (ALK) gene. Available at: http://clinicaltrials.gov/ct2/results? term=NCT00932451. [Date accessed April 1st, 2011].

87. A clinical trial testing the efficacy of crizotinib versus standard chemotherapy pemetrexed plus cisplatin or carboplatin in patients with ALK positive non squamous cancer of the lung. Available at: http://clinicaltrials.gov/ct2/results?term=NCT01154140. [Date accessed April 1st, 2011].

88. Choi YL, Soda M, Yamashita Y, et al. EML4-ALK mutations in lung cancer that confer resistance to ALK inhibitors. N Engl J Med. 2010;363:1734–9.

89. Paz-Ares L, Soulières D, Melezínek I, et al. Clinical outcomes in non-small-cell lung cancer patients with EGFR mutations: pooled analysis. J Cell Mol Med. 2010;14:51–69.

90. Greulich H, Chen TH, Feng W, et al. Oncogenic transformation by inhibitor-sensitive and -resistant EGFR mutants. PloS Med. 2005;2:e313.

91. Wu JY, Wu SG, Yang CH, et al. Lung cancer with epidermal growth factor receptor exon 20 mutations is associated with poor gefitinib treatment response. Clin Cancer Res. 2008;14:4877–82.

92. Kobayashi S, Boggon TJ, Dayaram T, et al. EGFR mutation and resistance of non-small-cell lung cancer to gefitinib. N Engl J Med. 2005;352:786–92.

93. Pao W, Miller VA, Politi KA, et al. Acquired resistance of lung adenocarcinomas to gefitinib or erlotinib is associated with a second mutation in the EGFR kinase domain. PloS Med. 2005;2:e73.

94. Balak MN, Gong Y, Riely GJ, et al. Novel D761Y and common secondary T790M mutations in epidermal growth factor receptor-mutant lung adenocarcinomas with acquired resistance to kinase inhibitors. Clin Cancer Res. 2006;12:6494–501.

95. Maheswaran S, Sequist LV, Nagrath S, et al. Detection of mutations in EGFR in circulating lung-cancer cells. N Engl J Med. 2008;359:366–77.

96. Bean J, Riely GJ, Balak M, et al. Acquired resistance to epidermal growth factor receptor kinase inhibitors associated with a novel T854A mutation in a patient with EGFR-mutant lung adenocarcinoma. Clin Cancer Res. 2008;14:7519–25.

97. Engelman JA, Zejnullahu K, Mitsudomi T, et al. MET amplification leads to gefitinib resistance in lung cancer by activating ERBB3 signaling. Science. 2007;316:1039–43.

98. Bean J, Brennan C, Shih JY, et al. MET amplification occurs with or without T790M mutations in EGFR mutant lung tumors with acquired resistance to gefitinib or erlotinib. Proc Natl Acad Sci U S A. 2007;104:20932–7.

99. Cappuzzo F, Jänne PA, Skokan M, et al. MET increased gene copy number and primary resistance to gefitinib therapy in non-small-cell lung cancer patients. Ann Oncol. 2009;20:298–304.

100. Oxnard GR, Arcila ME, Sima C, et al. Acquired resistance to EGFR tyrosine kinase inhibitors in EGFR mutant lung cancer: distinct natural history of patients with tumors harboring the T790M mutation. Clin Cancer Res. 2011;17:1616–22.

101. Jackman D, Pao W, Riely GJ, et al. Clinical definition of acquired resistance to epidermal growth factor receptor tyrosine kinase inhibitors in non-small-cell lung cancer. J Clin Oncol. 2010;28:357–60.

102. Riely GJ, Kris MG, Zhao B, et al. Prospective assessment of discontinuation and reinitiation of erlotinib or gefitinib in patients with acquired resistance to erlotinib or gefitinib followed by the addition of everolimus. Clin Cancer Res. 2007;13:5150–5.

103. Costa DB, Nguyen KS, Cho BC, et al. Effects of erlotinib in EGFR mutated non-small cell lung cancers with resistance to gefitinib. Clin Cancer Res. 2008;14:7060–7.

104. Belani CP. The role of irreversible EGFR inhibitors in the treatment of non-small cell lung cancer: overcoming resistance to reversible EGFR inhibitors. Cancer Invest. 2010;28:413–23.

105. Li D, Ambrogio L, Shimamura T, et al. BIBW2992, an irreversible EGFR/HER2 inhibitor highly effective in preclinical lung cancer models. Oncogene. 2008;27:4702–11.

106. Miller VA, Hirsh V, Cadranei J, et al. Phase IIB/III double-blind randomized trial of afatinib (BIBW 2992, an irreversible inhibitor of EGFR/HER1 and HER2)+best supportive care (BSC) versus placebo in patients with NSCLC failing 1–2 lines of chemotherapy and erlotinib or gefitinib (LUX-LUNG 1). Ann Oncol. 2010;21(Suppl 8):LBA1(abstract)

107. Miller VA, Hirsh V, Cadranei J, et al. Subgroup analysis of LUX-Lung 1 : a randomized phase III trial of afatinib (BIBW 2992)+best supportive care (BSC) versus placebo+BSC in patients with NSCLC failing 1–2 lines of chemotherapy and erlotinib or gefitinib. Presented at 2010 Chicago multidisciplinary symposium in thoracic oncology. Chicago, IL, USA, 9–11 December 2010.

108. Kwak EL, Sordella R, Bell DW, et al. Irreversible inhibitors of the EGF receptor may circumvent acquired resistance to gefitinib. Proc Natl Acad Sci U S A. 2005;102:7665–70.

109. Yang CH, Shih JY, Su WC, et al. A phase II of afatinib (BIBW 2992) in patients with adenocarcinoma of the lung and activating EGFR mutations. Ann Oncol. 2010;21 Suppl 8:367 (abstract).

110. Asahina H, Yamazaki K, Kinoshita I, et al. A phase II trial of gefitinib as first-line therapy for advanced non-small cell lung cancer with epidermal growth factor receptor mutations. Br J Cancer. 2006;95: 998–1004.

111. Inoue A, Kobayashi K, Usui K, et al. First-line gefitinib for patients with advanced non-small-cell lung cancer harboring epidermal growth factor receptor

111. mutations without indication for chemotherapy. J Clin Oncol. 2009;27:1394–400.
112. Inoue A, Suzuki T, Fukuhara T, et al. Prospective phase II study of gefitinib for chemotherapy-naive patients with advanced non-small-cell lung cancer with epidermal growth factor receptor gene mutations. J Clin Oncol. 2006;24:3340–6.
113. Sequist LV, Martins RG, Spigel D, et al. First-line gefitinib in patients with advanced non-small-cell lung cancer harboring somatic EGFR mutations. J Clin Oncol. 2008;26:2442–9.
114. Yang CH, Yu CJ, Shih JY, et al. Specific EGFR mutations predict treatment outcome of stage IIIB/IV patients with chemotherapy-naive non-small-cell lung cancer receiving first-line gefitinib monotherapy. J Clin Oncol. 2008;26:2745–53.
115. Sugio K, Uramoto H, Onitsuka T, et al. Prospective phase II study of gefitinib in non-small cell lung cancer with epidermal growth factor receptor gene mutations. Lung Cancer. 2009;64:314–8.
116. Sunaga N, Tomizawa Y, Yanagitani N, et al. Phase II prospective study of the efficacy of gefitinib for the treatment of stage III/IV non-small cell lung cancer with EGFR mutations, irrespective of previous chemotherapy. Lung Cancer. 2007;56:383–9.
117. Sutani A, Nagai Y, Udagawa K, et al. Gefitinib for non-small-cell lung cancer patients with epidermal growth factor receptor gene mutations screened by peptide nucleic acid-locked nucleic acid PCR clamp. Br J Cancer. 2006;95:1483–9.
118. Yoshida K, Yatabe Y, Park J, et al. Prospective validation for prediction of gefitinib sensitivity by epidermal growth factor receptor gene mutation in patients with non-small cell lung cancer. J Thorac Oncol. 2007;2:22–8.
119. Han SW, Kim TY, Hwang PG, et al. Predictive and prognostic impact of epidermal growth factor receptor mutation in non small-cell lung cancer patients treated with gefitinib. J Clin Oncol. 2005;23:2493–501.
120. Tamura K, Okamoto I, Kashii T, et al. Multicentre prospective phase II trial of gefitinib for advanced non-small cell lung cancer with epidermal growth factor receptor mutations: results of the West Japan Thoracic Oncology Group trial (WJTOG0403). Br J Cancer. 2008;98:907–14.
121. Toschi L, Jänne PA. Single-agent and combination therapeutic strategies to inhibit hepatocyte growth factor/MET signaling in cancer. Clin Cancer Res. 2008;14:5941–6.
122. Spigel D, Ervin T, Ramlau R, et al. Randomized multicenter double-blind placebo-controlled phase II study evaluating metmab, an antibody to met receptor, in combination with erlotinib, in patients with advanced non-small-cell lung cancer. Ann Oncol. 2010;21(Suppl 8):LBA15(abstract).
123. Sequist LV, Akerley WL, Brugger W, et al. Final results from ARQ 197–209: a global randomized placebo-controlled phase II clinical trial of erlotinib plus ARQ 197 versus erlotinib plus placebo in previously treated EGFR-inhibitor naïve patients with advanced non-small cell lung cancer. Ann Oncol. 2010;21 Suppl 8:363 (abstract).
124. Bianco R, Rosa R, Damiano V, et al. Vascular endothelial growth factor receptor-1 contributes to resistance to anti-epidermal growth factor receptor drugs in human cancer cells. Clin Cancer Res. 2008;14:5069–80.
125. Natale RB. Dual targeting of the vascular endothelial growth factor receptor and epidermal growth factor receptor pathways with vandetinib (ZD6474) in patients with advanced or metastatic non-small cell lung cancer. J Thorac Oncol. 2008;3(6 Suppl 2):128–30.
126. Herbst RS, Sun Y, Eberhardt WE, et al. Vandetanib plus docetaxel versus docetaxel as second-line treatment for patients with advanced non-small-cell lung cancer (ZODIAC): a double-blind, randomised, phase 3 trial. Lancet Oncol. 2010;11:619–26.
127. de Boer RH, Arrieta O, Yang CH, et al. Vandetanib plus pemetrexed for the second-line treatment of advanced non-small-cell lung cancer: a randomized, double-blind phase III trial. J Clin Oncol. 2011;29:1067–74.
128. Natale RB, Thongprasert S, Greco FA, et al. Phase III trial of vandetanib compared with erlotinib in patients with previously treated advanced non-small-cell lung cancer. J Clin Oncol. 2011;29:1059–66.
129. Dy GK, Hillman SL, Rowland Jr KM, et al. A front-line window of opportunity phase 2 study of sorafenib in patients with advanced nonsmall cell lung cancer: North Central Cancer Treatment Group Study N0326. Cancer. 2010;116:5686–93.
130. Blumenschein Jr GR, Gatzemeier U, Fossella F, et al. Phase II, multicenter, uncontrolled trial of single-agent sorafenib in patients with relapsed or refractory, advanced non-small-cell lung cancer. J Clin Oncol. 2009;27:4274–80.
131. Scagliotti G, Novello S, von Pawel J, et al. Phase III study of carboplatin and paclitaxel alone or with sorafenib in advanced non-small-cell lung cancer. J Clin Oncol. 2010;28:1835–42.
132. Sun S, Schiller JH, Gazdar AF. Lung cancer in never smokers—a different disease. Nat Rev Cancer. 2007;7:778–90.
133. Pham D, Kris MG, Riely GJ, et al. Use of cigarette-smoking history to estimate the likelihood of mutations in epidermal growth factor receptor gene exons 19 and 21 in lung adenocarcinomas. J Clin Oncol. 2006;24:1700–4.
134. Cappuzzo F, Bemis L, Varella-Garcia M. HER2 mutation and response to trastuzumab therapy in non-small-cell lung cancer. N Engl J Med. 2006;354:2619–21.
135. Sun Y, Ren Y, Fang Z, et al. Lung adenocarcinoma from East Asian never-smokers is a disease largely defined by targetable oncogenic mutant kinases. J Clin Oncol. 2010;28:4616–20.

Non-Hodgkin's Lymphomas

5

Roberta Zappasodi and Massimo Di Nicola

Epidemiology, Pathogenesis, and Classification

Non-Hodgkin's lymphomas (NHLs) are a group of malignancies that arise from mature T or B lymphocytes in the lymphoid tissue, which includes the lymph nodes, spleen, and other organs of the immune system. NHL is the fifth most common cancer in the USA, with an increasing incidence in the past three decades [1]. In the Western world, about 45 new cases of lymphoma are diagnosed per 100,000 people per year [2], with an even higher incidence in elderly people. The age-adjusted incidence of NHL rose by more than 79% from 1975 to 2005, representing an average annual percentage increase of about 2.6%, one of the highest registered. The reasons for this increase are not certain, and there are probably multiple causes, including human immunodeficiency virus (HIV) infection or acquired immune deficiency syndrome (AIDS) and the massive introduction of herbicides and pesticides containing organochlorine, organophosphate, and phenoxy acid, all compounds that are linked to lymphoma. Exposure to certain

R. Zappasodi, Ph.D. • M. Di Nicola, M.D. (✉)
"C. Gandini" Bone Marrow Transplantation Unit,
Department of Medical Oncology,
Fondazione IRCCS Istituto Nazionale dei Tumori,
Via Venezian, 1, Milan 20133, Italy
e-mail: massimo.dinicola@istitutotumori.mi.it

viruses and bacteria, such as Epstein–Barr virus (EBV) and *Helicobacter pylori*, is associated with NHL. Furthermore, inherited syndromes, such as Sjögren and Klinefelter syndromes, can predispose individuals to the later development of NHL. The concept of predisposition genes is under study to determine if they play a role in the sporadic occurrence of NHL in otherwise healthy individuals.

About 85% of NHL is of B-cell origin, the rest are T-cell or natural killer (NK) cell malignancies. Exciting progress has been made in the past 20 years to elucidate the cellular origin of human B-cell lymphomas and the identification of key transforming events, in particular the role of chromosomal translocations in lymphoma pathogenesis. B-cell development in the bone marrow (BM) takes place in distinct differentiation steps that are defined by a specific structure of the B-cell receptor (BCR). BCR development occurs via an "error-prone" process involving double-strand DNA breaks and the combinatorial rearrangement of the V, D, and J gene segments in the heavy (H) immunoglobulin (Ig) chain locus and the V and J gene segments in the light (L) Ig chain loci [3] (Fig. 5.1).

Mature (naïve) B cells carry a BCR composed of two identical heavy chains and two identical light-chain Ig polypeptides that are covalently linked by disulfide bridges [4]. Antigen recognition by naïve B cells, in conjunction with signals from T cells, favors their recruitment into secondary

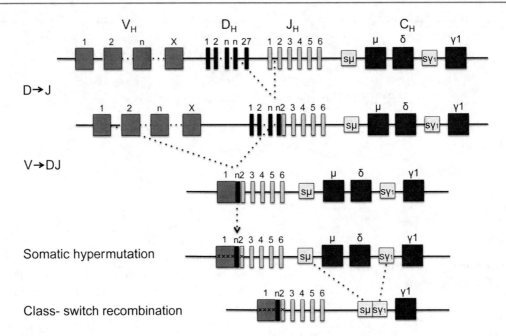

Fig. 5.1 Molecular processes that remodel immunoglobulin genes. Immunoglobulins (Igs) are expressed exclusively by B cells, after rearrangement of variable (V) regions, which interact with antigen, and constant (C) regions, which mediate their effector functions. (A) "V(D) J recombination" happen in the V regions of both heavy- (H) and light-chain (not shown) genes. About 50 functional VH gene segments, 27 DH segments, and 6 JH segments are available in the germline, allowing the generation of a diverse repertoire of VH gene rearrangements. The diversity is further increased by the addition or removal of nucleotides at the joining sites of the gene segments. The process of somatic hypermutation is activated when B cells reach the germinal center (GC, shown in more details in Fig. 5.2) and leads to the introduction of point mutations, deletions, or duplications in the rearranged V region of Ig genes ("X" in the figure). Class switching leads to the replacement of the IgM (Cμ) and IgD (Cδ) C-region gene segments with the IgG (Cγ1) ones by recombination at the switch regions (Sμ and Sγ1) and gives rise to an Ig with different effector functions but the same antigen-binding domain

lymphoid follicles where they undergo the germinal-center (GC) reaction. Thanks to the expression and activity of activation-induced cytidine deaminase (AID) enzyme, these cells undergo somatic hypermutation of VH genes, which create a population of B cells with increased (or decreased) affinity for a particular antigen, and class-switch recombination at the IgH locus, which changes the IgH class from IgM to IgG, IgA, or IgE. These processes typically happen in the dark zone of the GC, where B cells, stimulated by the surrounding antigen-specific T cells and antigen-bearing follicular dendritic cells (DCs), start to rapidly divide, becoming centroblasts. Even though centroblasts block the DNA damage response evoked by AID-dependent mutations and DNA breaks, they are usually prone to cell death due to their unique regulatory network. These cells periodically enter the light zone of the GC, where, as non-dividing centrocytes, they start to assay their capability to recognize the antigens that are presented by follicular DCs. The concomitant CD40 co-stimulation by T helper cells favors the transition of centrocytes to proliferating centroblast until B cells with high BCR-antigenic epitope affinity are positively selected [5] (Fig. 5.2). As a result, the most suitable B-cell clone(s), able to specifically clear pathogens and protect the host tissues, are preferentially expanded [6]. These genetic modifications are essential for a normal immune response, but they are also a source of DNA damage that can predispose to lymphomas.

A huge amount of tightly controlled transcription factors are involved in the B-cell activation/differentiation process in the GC. A key regulator of GC reaction is BCL-6 that represses many

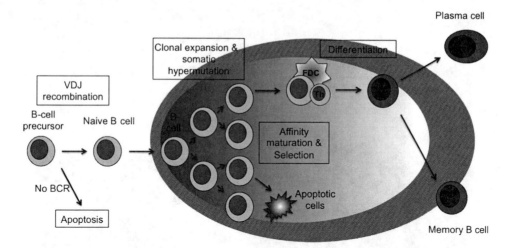

Fig. 5.2 B-cell development. Naïve antigen-activated B cells that receive "helper" signals are driven into B-cell follicles in secondary lymphoid organs, such as lymph nodes, where they establish germinal centers (GC). Proliferating GC B cells displaced the naive IgM+IgD+ B cells to the outside of the follicle, where they form a mantle zone (*dotted*). Within GC, a *dark zone*, with proliferating GC B cells (*dark gray*), and a *light zone*, containing resting GC B cells (*light gray*), can be distinguished (*left* and *right sides*, respectively). Proliferating GC B cells undergo somatic hypermutation in Ig V regions, and when they acquire an increased affinity for the antigen, they are positively selected through the interaction with CD4+ T cells (Th) and follicular dendritic cells (FDC) in the *light zone*. A fraction of these GC B cells undergo class-switch recombination and, finally, differentiate into memory B cells or plasma cells and leave the GC microenvironment

genes responsible for cell death, response to DNA damage, and plasma cell differentiation [7]. To differentiate into plasma cells, indeed, GC B lymphocytes need to upregulate interferon regulatory factor 4 (IRF4), a transcription factor that increases the expression of the BCL6 repressor Blimp-1, thus promoting terminal differentiation [8, 9].

B-cell malignancies can arise at each of these steps during B-cell differentiation. Therefore, the structure of BCR, the expression patterns of differentiation markers, and the specific tissue localization of a neoplastic clone serve to define the origin and the subtype of human B-cell lymphomas [10–12] (Fig. 5.3). In addition, carrying the same BCR on the surface, B-cell NHLs are distinguished by the unique antigenic determinants of BCR hypervariable regions, termed idiotype (Id), which represent one among few tumor-specific antigens identified until now.

According to these features, the World Health Organization (WHO) classification has identified 12 subtypes of B-cell NHL [13], which are listed in Table 5.1. Follicular lymphoma (FL) and diffuse large B-cell lymphoma (DLBCL) are the two most prevalent NHL subtypes and together account for about 50% of cases. Reciprocal chromosomal translocations involving one of the Ig loci and a proto-oncogene constitute the hallmark, and thus a diagnostic marker, of many types of B-cell lymphoma [14, 15] (Table 5.1). Indeed, translocations involve cyclin D1 in mantle cell lymphoma (MCL), B-cell lymphoma 2 (BCL-2) in FL, BCL-6 in DLBCL, c-myc in Burkitt's lymphoma, and PAX5 in lymphoplasmacytoid lymphoma. Mutations in tumor-suppressor genes (such as TP53 and the gene encoding IκBα), genomic amplifications (such as REL), and translocations not involving Ig loci (API2–MALT1) have also been implicated in the pathogenesis of B-cell lymphomas (Table 5.1). Such genetic alterations can result (1) as mistakes occurring during Ig V(D)J gene segment recombination in early B-cell development in the BM [16], (2) as by-products of the somatic hypermutation process [17], and (3) during class-switch recombination in the GC. The last two processes are typical features of B-cell development and occur exclusively in the GC [18], partly explaining why B cells are more

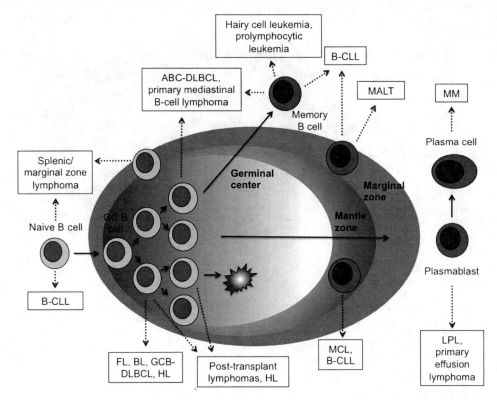

Fig. 5.3 Cellular origins of human B-cell lymphomas. Human B-cell lymphomas are assigned to their proposed normal B-cell counterpart. Most lymphomas are derived from germinal-center (GC) B cells or from B cells that have passed through the GC, indicating its role in the pathogenesis of B-cell lymphoma. *FL* follicular lymphoma, *BL* Burkitt's lymphoma, *DLBCL* diffuse large B-cell lymphoma, *GCB* germinal-center B-cell-like, *ABC* activated B-cell-like, *CLL* chronic lymphocytic leukemia, *MCL* mantle cell lymphoma, *MZL* marginal zone lymphoma, *LPL* lymphoplasmacytoid lymphoma, *MM* multiple myeloma, *MALT* mucosa-associated lymphoid tissue lymphoma, *HL* Hodgkin's lymphoma

prone to undergo malignant transformation than T cells and why most B-cell lymphomas derive from GC B cells or their descendants (Fig. 5.3). While carrying the differentiation program of the normal B-cell counterpart, lymphoma cells gradually lose its physiologic regulation. As an example, normal centroblasts lack the antiapoptotic activities of BCL2 and the proliferation stimuli of nuclear factor-kB (NF-kB) and c-myc signaling pathways and hence are poised to die [19, 20]. Malignant centroblasts avoid cell death by acquiring activating translocations of BCL2 or c-myc or by constitutively activating NF-kB. The survival and/or proliferation advantages provided by the constitutive expression of an oncogene and the deletion/inactivation of a tumor-suppressor gene represent the driving force for the uncontrolled expansion of a B-cell clone.

Clinically, NHLs are classified according to the Cotswolds modification of the Ann Arbor staging system into four stages based on anatomic sites of involvement and the presence of disease above or below the diaphragm (Fig. 5.4). For each stage, lymphomas are further divided into two subsets according to the presence (A) or not (B) of systemic symptoms (night sweats, weight loss of >10%, or fevers) (Fig. 5.4).

Commonly, NHLs are further characterized as either "aggressive" or "indolent" (http://www.nih.gov/), even though the WHO lymphoma classification [13] does not include this terminology. Rapidly progressing high-grade or aggressive NHLs account for about 60% of cases in the USA, with DLBCL being the most common subtype. Slow-growing indolent NHLs encompass the low-grade and some categories of intermediate-grade

Table 5.1 B-cell lymphoma classification

Lymphoma	Frequency among lymphomas (%)	Proposed cellular origin	Chromosome translocation (frequency)	Tumor-suppressor gene mutation (frequency)	Viruses (frequency)	Other alterations (frequency)
B-CLL	7	CD5+ small B cells memory, naive, or marginal-zone B cells	–	ATM (30), TP53 (15)	–	Deletion on 13q14 (60)
MCL	5	CD5+ mantle-zone B cells	CCND1–IgH (95)	ATM (40)	–	Deletion on 13q14 (50–70)
FL	20	GC B cells	BCL2–IgH (90)	–	–	–
MALT	7	Marginal-zone B cells	API2–MALT1 (30), BCL10–IgH (5), MALT1–IgH (15–20), FOXP1–IgH (10)	CD95 (5–80)	Indirect role of *Helicobacter pylori* in gastric MALT lymphomas	–
MZL	2	Marginal-zone or monocytoid B cells	–	–	–	–
Splenic MZL	1	Subset of small IgD+ naive B cells that have partially differentiated into marginal-zone B cells	–	–	–	Deletion on 7q22-36 (40)
BL	2	GC B cells	MYC–IgH or MYC–IgL (100)	TP53 (40), RB (20–80)	EBV (endemic, 95; sporadic, 30)	–
DLBCL	30–40	Post-GC B cells	BCL6–various (35) BCL2–IgH (15–30) MYC–IgH or MYC–IgL (15)	CD95 (10–20), ATM (15), TP53 (25)	–	Aberrant hypermutation of multiple proto-oncogenes (50)
Primary mediastinal B-cell lymphoma	2	Thymic B cells	–	SOCS1 (40)	–	Aberrant hypermutation of multiple proto-oncogenes (40)
Posttransplant lymphoma	<1	GC B cells	–	–	EBV (90)	–
Primary effusion lymphoma	<0.5	(Post) GC B cells	–	–	HHV8 (95), EBV (70)	–
LPL; Waldenström macroglobulinemia	1	(Post) GC B cells	PAX5–IgH (50)	–	–	–

B-CLL B-cell chronic lymphocytic leukemia, *MCL* mantle cell lymphoma, *FL* follicular lymphoma, *MALT* mucosa-associated lymphatic tissue lymphoma, *MZL* marginal zone lymphoma, *BL* Burkitt's lymphoma, *DLBCL* diffuse large B-cell lymphoma, *LPL* lymphoplasmacytic lymphoma, *GC* germinal center

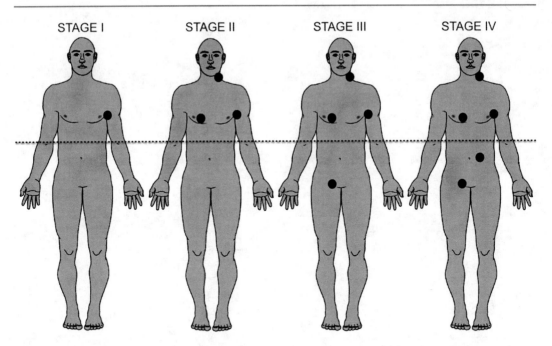

Fig. 5.4 Ann Arbor staging system. Schematic examples of stage I–IV disease are shown. Stage I: single lymph node or single extralymphatic site; stage II: two or more tumor sites in the same side with respect to the diaphragm or contiguous extralymphatic site; stage III: involvement of both sites of the diaphragm or spleen, or contiguous extralymphatic sites or both; stage IV: diffuse or disseminated involvement of one or more extralymphatic sites and/or lymph nodes. *Dotted line* indicated the diaphragm; *black-filled circles* represent involved tumor sites

subtypes, with FL being the most frequent. Both intermediate/aggressive and indolent diseases are diagnosed at stage III or IV in more than 50 and 80 % of cases, respectively. In contrast with other types of cancer, stage IV NHL may be still highly curable, depending on the patient's specific subtype of disease. Since the subtype and stage of NHL and whether it is the indolent or aggressive form determines appropriate treatment, an accurate diagnosis is required to optimize the management of NHL patients.

DLBCL

DLBCL is a cancer of large B cells that most commonly grows in a diffuse pattern completely subverting the normal lymphoid architecture. Besides this common feature, it represents a clinically, biologically, and pathologically heterogeneous entity, in which multiple morphologic variants have been recognized according to the WHO Classification of Tumors of Hematopoietic and Lymphoid Tissues [13]. Remarkable progress has been made during the past decade in understanding the biological heterogeneity of DLBCL. Very recently, gene expression profile (GEP) has allowed to recognize three molecular subtypes of histologically indistinguishable DLBCL with different clinical behaviors and prognosis: the activated B-cell-like (ABC) subtype, the germinal-center B-cell-like (GCB) subtype, and primary mediastinal B-cell lymphoma (PMBL) [21, 22]. The extended differences in gene expression and genetic abnormalities among these subtypes suggest that they arise from distinct B-cell precursors and progress differently toward malignant transformation. Increasing evidences indicate that the most probable precursors of GCB, ABC, and PMBL lymphoma subtypes are represented by germinal cell blasts, plasmablasts, and thymic B cells, respectively. The malignant clone in GCB lymphomas is blocked in the GC reaction as it continues to undergo somatic hypermutation even though it has often switched IgH classes [23]. These tumors are characterized by quite specific genetic lesions, including the t(14;18) translocation deletion of the tumor suppressor PTEN, amplification of the microRNA cluster miR-17-92 (which downregulates PTEN55), and p53 mutations [21, 24].

Constitutive activation of the NF-kB pathway, in ABC lymphomas, inducing the expression of the transcription factor IRF4, leads to their characteristic plasma-cell expression program [25]. However, the malignant clone acquires genetic lesions that, interfering with Blimp-1 transcription factor, block full differentiation into plasma cells [24]. Accordingly, these lymphomas still contain high amounts of AID and have not yet undergone class-switch recombination, even though their IgH genes are heavily mutated [23]. Molecular explanations of the constitutive activation of NF-kB in ABC lymphomas include the presence of activating mutations in the oncogene CARDD11 (in approximately 10% of patients) and a chronic active form of BCR that triggers NF-kB pathway through the canonical signaling cascade (see paragraph 2) [26, 27]. A selective trait of ABC lymphomas is the presence of aggregated and immobilized BCR on the tumor cell surface, which does not happen in GCB and PMBL cells. About 20% of ABC lymphomas indeed carry mutations in the BCR subunits CD79A or CD79B that increase BCR expression and reduce activation of its negative feedback [26]. Mutant CD79 proteins are rare or absent in GCB and other lymphoma subtypes, whereas they are positively selected in the ABC subtype as a tumor driving force [26]. Additional genetic alterations typically associated with ABC lymphomas include the amplification of BCL2 locus, which leads to BCL2 overexpression, the deletion of INK4A–ARF and p14ARF loci, which encodes, respectively, an inhibitor of senescence and of p53 activation [24]. Antiapoptotic protein overexpression and loss of tumor suppressors are responsible for the limited activity of chemotherapy and the poor prognosis of ABC lymphomas [24].

PMBL, the least common DLBCL subtypes, usually manifests in young adults (median age, 30–35 years), especially women, as a mediastinal mass in a thymic remnant. PMBL patients had a relatively favorable clinical outcome, with a 5-year survival rate of 64% compared with 46% for other DLBCL patients. GEP analysis is crucial for the diagnosis of PMBL, since its clinical features alone cannot reliably distinguish this tumor from the other subtypes [22]. PMBL genetic signature shares some similarities with that of Hodgkin's lymphoma (HL), which can also arise from a thymic B cell. In particular, both malignancies show the amplification of a region on chromosome 9p24, encoding JAK2, a tyrosine kinase that phosphorylates and activates the transcription factor STAT6, and the deletion of SOCS1, a suppressor of JAK signaling [24]. The immunosuppressor genes PDL1 (also called CD274) and PDL2 (also called CD273), SMARCA2, a putative chromatin regulator, and JMJD2C, a histone demethylase family member, being located in the 9p24 region, may result amplified, thus contributing to the malignant phenotype [22]. Very recently, it has been demonstrated that JAK2 and JMJD2C cooperate in PMBL and HL to reduce heterochromatin foci at oncogene loci, such as that of c-myc, thus promoting their transcription [28]. In contrast to HL, however, PMBL typically expresses genes of mature B cells [22].

Due to the difficulties to introduce GEP technology in the clinical practice, immunohistochemical algorithms, based on GCET1, CD10, BCL-6, MUM-1, and FOXP1 expression, have been proposed and validated for classification of DLBCL into GCB and ABC subtypes [29]. Besides providing a diagnostic tool, the molecular classification of DLBCL might be exploited for its prognostic value, since it has been shown that GCB, ABC, and PMBL differ in clinical presentation, responsiveness to chemotherapy, and targeted therapy, with GCB phenotype being associated with the most favorable survival [30].

Additional key prognostic factors of DLBCL have been found in the composition of the tumor microenvironment [30], as defined by two main genetic signatures. The expression of genes indicating extracellular matrix deposition (fibronectin, osteonectin, various collage and laminin isoforms as well as genes that encode modifiers of collagen synthesis) and infiltration of the tumors by cells of the myeloid/monocytic lineage, identified as stromal-1 signature, is commonly associated with an improved overall survival, (OS) probably due to its association with an antilymphoma reaction of the innate immunity. Conversely, stromal-2 signature, which encodes well-known markers of endothelial cells (von Willebrand factor, CD31, EGFL7, MMRN2, GRP116, and SPARCL1) and key regulators of angiogenensis (vascular endothelial growth factor receptor, GRB10, integrin alpha 9, TEK, the receptor tyrosin kinase of angiopoietin, ROBO4, and ERG), indicating the presence of a more advanced-stage hypervascularized lymphoma, is associated with an inferior prognosis [30].

Clearly, clinical trials for the assessment of novel therapeutic strategies for the treatment of DLBCL should consider GEP in order to highlight distinct clinical outcome for these three disease entities. Increasing the appreciation of the molecular basis for DLBCL subtypes will improve the understanding of the oncogenic mechanisms that cause these diseases toward the development of rational and disease-specific treatments. Because oncogenic pathways appear to be differentially activated in these subtypes of DLBCL, future advances in therapy should target these differences. For example, the possibility to distinguish DLBCL with a stromal-2 signature may allow to better select patients for an antiangiogenic therapy. In addition, the evidence that even in DLBCL survival is influenced by a particular composition of the tumor microenvironment may lead to the development of more effective combination therapy targeting both oncogenic pathways in the malignant clone and protumorigenic interactions with non-malignant cells.

FL

FL represents not only the most common indolent NHL but also the second most frequent subtype of lymphoma worldwide, accounting for approximately 20% of malignant lymphomas in adults, and 40% of all lymphomas diagnosed in the USA and in Western Europe [31]. FL is derived from GC B cells and maintains the GEP of this stage of differentiation [32]. Morphologically, the disease is composed of a mixture of centrocytes and centroblasts and is graded from 1 to 3, depending on the proportion of large cells per high-power field. Grades 1 and 2 are indolent disease. The rare subtype grade 3B is more aggressive and should be discriminated from lower-grade cases. FL cells express a surface Ig (more frequently IgM+/−IgD > IgG > IgA), B-cell-associated antigens (CD19, CD20, CD22, CD79A, and CD79B), and 60% express CD10. The hallmark of FL is the chromosomal translocation t(14;18), present in 70–95% of the cases, which results in the constitutive expression of the antiapoptotic protein BCL2, and thus allows to distinguish reactive from neoplastic follicles [33, 34]. As other indolent lymphomas, FL is characterized by extreme and often unpredictable clinical variability, with a continuous pattern of relapse that sometimes leads to a rapid unexpected clinical worsening, and remains incurable with the available therapies [35]. As an example, 15–60% of FLs undergo transformation into the more aggressive histologic malignancy DLBCLs, following molecular mechanisms that are not entirely known and in a largely unpredictable way [36–38]. Transformed lymphomas are usually quite aggressive and poorly responsive to chemotherapy [39], with a median survival from transformation of about 18 months [40, 41]. Thus, the accurate biomolecular characterization of tumor features associated with progression or response after therapy is essential to identify predictive and prognostic biomarkers and molecular targets for new drug development, thereby enabling the improvement of the clinical management for FL patients.

Multiple lines of evidence indicate the participation of immune cells also in the biology and pathogenesis of FL [42–44]. An important example is the demonstration that removing bacteria or viruses, such as *Helicobacter pylori* and hepatitis C virus and EBV, from the lymphoma microenvironment may efficiently arrest tumor growth [45–47]. Tumor-infiltrating immune cells, including T lymphocytes, macrophages, and DCs, can provide contact-dependent or independent signals for lymphoma cell survival [48, 49]. FL cell growth strictly depends on stromal cells and, in particular, upon CD40 stimulation by follicular DC to avoid apoptosis [50, 51]. The same interactions may directly or indirectly favor the establishment of immunosuppressive tumor microenvironment. FL cells can attract or locally convert FOXP3+ regulatory T cells (Tregs) [52], which in turn may suppress antitumor immunity by impairing T-cell activation [53–55] and by inducing the development of M2 regulatory macrophages, thus amplifying the mechanisms of tumor immune evasion [56–58]. Noteworthy, the gene and immunohistochemical signatures of non-tumor cells in the neoplastic tissue currently represent the best predictor for FL patient survival [32, 43, 58, 59]. In particular, two immunological signatures within the tumor tissue have been found to perfectly discriminate between favorable and poor prognosis, with the former being predicted by immune response-1 signature, which reflects the expression of T-cell genes, and the latter by immune response-2 signature, which includes genes preferentially expressed by macrophages and DCs [32].

These results suggest that interactions between the tumor and the microenvironment are established early in the course of the disease and may determine its long-term outcomes.

Therefore, the concomitant study of the intrinsic tumor features, the functional composition of the non-malignant microenvironment, and constitutive patient-related properties may be very useful to improve the management of indolent NHL patients and develop alternative therapies aimed at interfering with the prosurvival interaction between tumor and inflammatory cells.

Standard Therapeutic Approaches

Among NHL malignancies, treatment regimens often overlap. However, the accurate diagnosis of lymphoma histology and subgroup is mandatory to address patients to the most suitable treatment. The choice of the most adequate therapeutic intervention also depends upon patients' risk, which is assessed on the basis of the five independently prognostic factors (age, high-level serum LDH, stage, performance status, and extranodal site of disease) included in the International Prognostic Index (IPI).

Since the introduction of monoclonal antibodies (mAbs) for the treatment of lymphoma, the standard of choice as first-line therapy has been their combination with chemotherapy, namely, chemoimmunotherapy [60]. The most widely used mAb is rituximab, a chimeric unconjugated Ab against the CD20 antigen licensed by the Food and Drug Administration (FDA) and the European Agency for the Evaluation of Medicinal Products to treat DLBCL as well as relapsed or refractory, low-grade CD20+ B-cell NHL as a single agent; non-progressing (including stable disease), low-grade, CD20+ B-cell NHL, as a single agent, after first-line cyclophosphamide, vincristine, and prednisone (CVP) chemotherapy; previously untreated indolent, CD20+ B cell NHL in combination with CVP chemotherapy [61]. Multiple randomized clinical trials have demonstrated a significant survival benefit with the addition of rituximab to first-line chemotherapy in patients with FL and DLBCL [62–68].

The aggressiveness of the disease requires therapy to be started in a timely way once the diagnosis has been made. Rituximab plus cyclophosphamide, doxorubicin, vincristine, and prednisone (R-CHOP), eventually followed by involved-field radiation therapy in cases achieving a partial response, represents the standard induction regimens for stage I–II aggressive lymphoma patients [69] (Fig. 5.5). Stage II–IV patients are treated with the same regimens for repeated cycles as maintenance therapy [69] or may be addressed to clinical trials as frontline option (Fig. 5.5). Interestingly, rituximab-containing regimens have shown to improve survival for DLBCL patients regardless of age [70], and R-CHOP is currently considered the standard of choice for the treatment of aggressive lymphoma even in elderly patients [71]. However, young patients with intermediate risk according to IPI score are usually treated with more intense combination chemoimmunotherapy. On the basis of previous findings about the clinical benefit

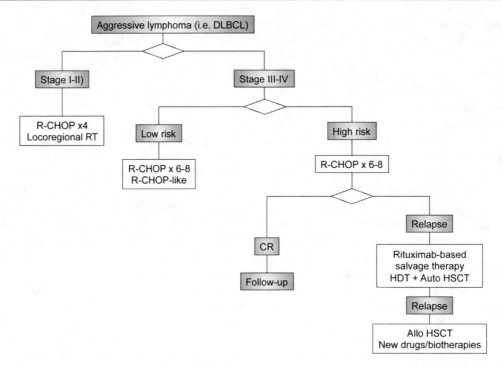

Fig. 5.5 Therapeutic algorithm for the treatment of aggressive NHL. *R-CHOP* rituximab plus cyclophosphamide, doxorubicin, vincristine, and prednisone; *RT* radiotherapy; *HDT* high-dose therapy; *Auto HSCT* autologous hematopoietic stem cell transplantation; *Allo HSCT* allogeneic hematopoietic stem cell transplantation; *CR* complete remission

associated with the administration of chemotherapy at 14-day instead of 21-day interval [72, 73], two large phase III studies are now comparing the clinical benefit of co-administering rituximab under this more intense schedule in newly diagnosed patients with DLBCL.

In case of refractory or relapsed disease, patients can be treated with different second-line regimens in combination with rituximab on the basis of the possibility for the patients to proceed to high-dose therapy (HDT) and autologous hematopoietic stem cell transplantation (HSCT) [69], which represents the standard of choice for patients that respond to salvage therapy (Fig. 5.5). Relapsed diseases following second-line therapies alone or plus HSCT are usually treated in clinical trials, with palliative RT or the supportive care on the basis of the patients [69] (Fig. 5.5).

FL and indolent B-cell lymphomas present relevant therapeutic challenges, with no current regimen offering curative treatment. Due to the indolent course of low-grade lymphomas, a major clinical question is how to identify the patients that may benefit from early therapy [74]. The institution of therapy for indolent NHL currently depends on patients' prognostic/risk factors, measured according to the modified IPI score (FLIPI) to take into account hemoglobin and β2-microglobulin serum levels, as well as the number and size of the involved sites and BM involvement [75–77]. Using these parameters, three risk groups have been identified, with 91, 69, and 51% progression free survival (PFS) and 99, 96, and 84% survival rate at 3 years for patients at low, intermediate, and high risk, respectively. Although FLIPI score helps to risk-stratify patients, there is a need for robust biomarkers of disease outcome.

At present, asymptomatic patients are usually managed following the so-called watch and wait approach until clear indications for treatment initiation [78] (Fig. 5.6). Indeed, no survival advantage has been demonstrated when patients in these conditions have been immediately treated [79]. However, when newly diagnosed indolent

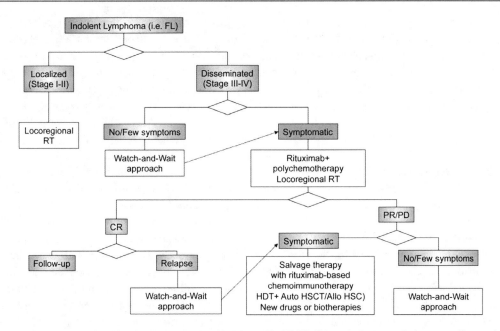

Fig. 5.6 Therapeutic algorithm for the treatment of indolent NHL. *RT* radiotherapy, *HDT* high-dose therapy, *Auto HSCT* autologous hematopoietic stem cell transplantation, *Allo HSCT* allogeneic hematopoietic stem cell transplantation, *CR* complete remission

NHL is limited (stage I or II), immediate involved-field radiation therapy (IFRT) is usually recommended since it has the potential to eradicate the disease [80, 81] (Fig. 5.6).

Once treatment is indicated, also for indolent NHL patients, the standard of care is represented by combination chemotherapy (CVP, CHOP) and rituximab [60]. Rituximab has also been evaluated as first-line monotherapy treatment of low-grade NHL, showing encouraging results [82–85]. More aggressive frontline therapies are usually considered for patients with a rapidly progressing disease, which represents an indicator of poor prognosis [86]. Randomized clinical trials have demonstrated that 2-year maintenance with rituximab after immunochemotherapy increases the PFS of the first-line or first-relapse FL patients [87, 88].

Treatment at relapse is defined according to patients' performance status, previous therapy, and duration of response and includes again expectant management, or rituximab as single agent [89, 90] or in combination with chemotherapy. Autologous HSCT has achieved encouraging results in young patients with chemosensitive disease [91–94]. However, it is applicable in only a minority of patients, due to extensive prior therapy and frequent marrow involvement (Fig. 5.6). By contrast, allogeneic HSCT is increasingly used as salvage therapy for relapsed or refractory indolent lymphomas, due to the lower risk of relapse, and the long-term (PFS) observed after allogeneic compared to autologous HSCT [95] (Fig. 5.6). Donor lymphocyte infusion (DLI) has demonstrated a significant therapeutic activity in case of relapse after allogeneic HSCT, thus pointing to the efficacy of a graft-versus-lymphoma (GVL) effect in indolent lymphomas [96–99].

An excellent therapeutic alternative for any lines of treatment of indolent NHL is the enrolment of the patients in randomized clinical trials due to the slow-progressing nature of the disease and the possibility to keep it in check.

In summary, the introduction of rituximab in polychemotherapy approaches has vastly improved the survival of NHL patients and has revolutionized the treatment of all B-cell NHL subtypes. However, given the difficulties in the management of relapse/resistance to rituximab, it seems that treatment of NHL has now reached a new plateau and there remains ample room for improving remission duration and the clinical outcome of relapsed patients. Novel agents under investigation for specifically targeting lymphoma cells may provide opportunities to spur the clinical efficacy of chemoimmunotherapy toward the cure of relapsed or refractory NHL.

Novel Antilymphoma Therapies

Cytotoxic Drugs

Bendamustine is certainly one among the most interesting new cytotoxic drugs for the treatment of lymphomas. It is a bifunctional alkylating agent, developed more than 40 years ago, that has been recently reevaluated for the treatment of hematologic diseases. After the demonstration of its ability to achieve the highest overall response rate (ORR) observed for a single agent in patients with rituximab-refractory, indolent or transformed lymphomas [100], it was evaluated in a multicenter open-label phase III study for the treatment of previously untreated indolent lymphoma patients where in addition to rituximab provided a superior PFS and complete response rate compared to R-CHOP with significantly fewer toxicity [101]. These findings led to the approval of bendamustine for the treatment of relapsed indolent NHL after rituximab therapy. Conversely, its role for the treatment of aggressive lymphomas has not yet been established.

Pralatrexate is a new antifolate compound that targets tumor cells with enhanced selectivity compared to methotrexate, thanks to its ability to enter cells expressing reduced folate carrier type 1 (RFC-1), which is expressed only in malignant and fetal tissue [102]. Like other antifolates, it reversibly inhibits the enzyme dihydrofolate reductase, which is required for the nucleoside thymidine and purine base synthesis, thus interfering with DNA and RNA synthesis. It represents the first and only drug approved for the treatment of relapsed or refractory peripheral T-cell lymphoma (PTCL) (http://ir.allos.com/phoenix.zhtml?c=125475&p=irolnewsArticle&ID=1335492&highlight).

However, in relapsed/refractory B-cell lymphoma it achieved only the disease stabilization in some patients [103]. Differences in RFC-1 expression between neoplastic T and B lymphocytes could represent one potential explanation of the different activity of pralatrexate in malignancies originating from these cells. The dose-limiting toxicity for pralatrexate is mucositis, which could be abrogated with folic acid and vitamin B12 supplementation. Pralatrexate is now being evaluated in a phase I/II trial in combination with gemcitabine for the treatment of non-Hodgkin's lymphoma.

Pixantrone, an antitumor antibiotic family member, is an analog of mitoxantrone and acts as a topoisomerase II inhibitor and intercalating agent. It was developed to reduce anthracycline-related cardiotoxicity while retaining antitumor efficacy. Besides demonstrating promising clinical activity with reduced toxicity in heavily pretreated NHL (http://www.prnewswire.com/cgi-bin/stories.pl?ACCT=104&STORY=/www/story/07-11-2007/0004623260), it showed increased clinical efficacy compared to other chemotherapeutic drugs used as third-line therapy in a phase III randomized trial with relapsed aggressive NHL patients [104]. Pixantrone is now being tested in earlier indications.

Among new chemotherapeutic regimens for NHL, it is worth mentioning the combination of gemcitabine and oxaliplatin, which demonstrated a significant clinical efficacy and a good safety profile in relapsed DLBCL that are not suitable candidates for HSCT [28].

Signal Transduction Inhibitor Therapy for Lymphoma

Main Signal Transduction Pathways in B-Cell NHL

The signaling pathways commonly deregulated in B-cell lymphomas are as follows: (a) the B-cell receptor/spleen tyrosine kinase (BCR/Syk) pathway, (b) the NF-kB pathway, (c) the phosphatidylinositol 3-kinase/mammalian target of rapamycin (PI3K/mTOR) pathway, (d) the protein kinase C-beta (PKC-β) pathway, and (e) the MAP kinase/Ras pathway (Fig. 5.7).

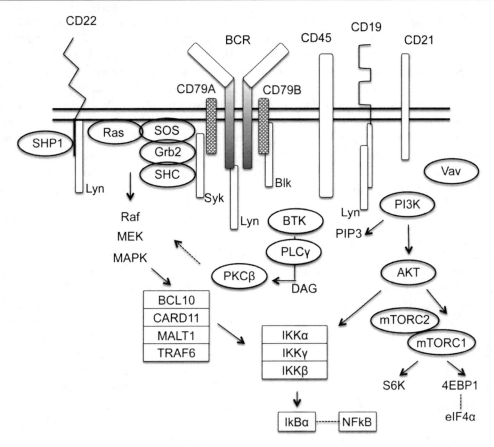

Fig. 5.7 BCR signaling pathways. The B-cell antigen receptor (BCR) includes an antigen-binding portion, represented by a membrane immunoglobulin (Ig) molecule, and Igα/Igβ subunits (CD79A/CD79B) that form heterodimers and associate to the BCR heavy Ig chains. Antigen binding leads to the aggregation of multiple molecules of BCR and adaptor proteins, including co-stimulator and co-inhibitor receptors. This rapidly initiates the transduction of intracellular signals through the activation of Src family kinases Lyn, phosphorylation of Igα/Igβ intracellular tails, and activation of SYK and BTK tyrosine kinases. As a result, the signaling cascades regulated by PLCγ, PI3K, and Vav are stimulated leading to deep changes in cell metabolism, gene expression, and cytoskeletal organization. BCR activation can concurrently induce signals of survival, tolerance (anergy) or apoptosis, proliferation, and differentiation, with the final cellular response being determined by the maturation status of the cell, the nature of the antigen, the magnitude and duration of the stimulation, and the activation of other co-receptors, such as CD40, CD22, CD19, CD45, PIR-B, Fcγ RIIB1, and BAFF-R. Negative feedback loops, including those mediated by SHIP and SHIP1 activation following stimulation of co-inhibitor receptors, such as CD22, FcgRIIB1, and PIR-B, regulate the magnitude and duration of BCR signaling, leading to the ultimate internalization of BCR

The primary BCR dependency of B-cell lymphoma survival has been confirmed in recent studies reporting that blocking its driven signals is sufficient to inhibit B-cell lymphoma growth both in vitro and in vivo [105, 106]. Under physiologic conditions, BCR engagement leads to activation of the SRC family kinase (SFK) that phosphorylates tyrosines in immunoreceptor tyrosine-based activation motifs (ITAMs) of the BCR subunits CD79A and CD79B. Phosphorylated CD79 acts as a docking site for SYK kinase that, becoming activated, initiates the signaling cascade leading to extracellular signal-regulated kinase 1 and 2 (ERK 1/2) and mitogen-activated protein kinase (MAPK) activation. BCR ITAMs also provide a negative regulation for BCR activation. Their phosphorylation promotes the recruitment of CD22 to BCR complex via the tyrosine kinase Lyn and activation of the SH2-domain-containing protein tyrosine phosphatase 1 (SHP1) that dephosphorylates BCR, switching off the signal. Phosphatidylinositol 3-kinase (PI3K) is concurrently recruited to B-cell co-receptor CD19, where it promotes the activation of mTOR and the generation of the membrane lipid phosphatidylinositol 3,4,5-triphopshate (PIP3). PIP3 complexes with Bruton's tyrosine kinase (BTK) and phospholipase Cγ (PLCγ), thus favoring IP3 release for PKCβ activation and diacylglycerol (DAG) signaling for the induction of Ras/Raf pathway that controls multiple cellular processes, including cell proliferation, differentiation, and transformation. These events are crucial for the phosphorylation and plasma membrane translocation of CARDD11 that is required for IKK-mediated phosphorylation of IkBα and the activation of the antiapoptotic NF-kB signaling cascade.

In lymphoma cells, constitutive BCR signaling can be promoted either by the specific ligand or by activating mutations in ITAMs or CARDD11 [26], and overexpression of one of its component, such as SYK, or directly BCR [106]. Furthermore, signal mediators, such as Ras and Raf, that control proliferation and survival via their downstream targets MEK and ERK are frequently mutated in B-cell malignancies [107].

As such, there are now extensive efforts to target key molecules in these signaling cascades for therapeutic benefit.

In addition to BCR, B-cell-activating factor receptor (BAFF-R) can provide survival signals in most mature B-cell lymphoproliferative disorders. Mainly via the alternative route, BAFF-R triggering leads to NF-kB activation and upregulation of antiapoptotic BCL-2 members such as BCL-xL or BCL-2, promoting survival [108].

Recently, the existence of autocrine/paracrine mechanisms responsible for the constitutive activation of Notch signaling has been identified as a novel mechanism underlying B-CLL cell apoptosis resistance. Interestingly, Notch-signaling stimulation by Jagged1, one of its ligand, is accompanied by increased NF-kB activity and expression of the antiapoptotic molecules c-IAP2 and XIAP [109].

The PI3K/AKT/mTOR axis is constitutively activated in the majority of B-cell lymphomas [110]. The mTOR kinase is an essential mediator of growth signals that originate from PI3K and AKT stimulation and are counterbalanced via the AMP-activated protein kinase system. It represents a critical pathway in the signaling of normal and malignant cell processes of growth and proliferation. Downstream targets of mTOR, p70 S6 kinase, and 4E binding protein 1 (4EBP1) are important regulators of protein synthesis and cell-cycle progression.

The mTOR kinase, a key member of the pathway, exists in two different complexes referred to as mTORC1 and mTORC2, with the former containing Raptor (regulatory-associated protein of mTOR) and mLST8 (mammalian lethal with Sec13 protein 8), and the latter Rictor (rapamycin-insensitive companion of mTOR) and mSIN1 (mammalian stress-activated protein kinase interacting protein), besides the common catalytic subunit mTOR [111]. mTORC1 positively controls cell growth and proliferation and is characterized by rapamycin sensitivity, whereas mTORC2 is the rapamycin-insensitive part of the pathway and regulates AKT activation [111]. Unraveling the relative importance of mTORC1 and mTORC2 in cancer cells is not only interesting but has relevance for drug development using mTOR-targeted agents.

PKC-β is another pivotal enzyme in the B-cell signaling pathway. In lymphocytes, PKC-β I and PKC-β II are the major isoforms of this enzyme, and they are commonly overexpressed in NHL. Interestingly, different studies have demonstrated that PKC-β protein or mRNA overexpression represents an adverse prognostic factor for Immunochemotherapy-treated DLBCL patients within low and high IPI risk groups and in all molecular entities [112]. These studies have provided the rationale to develop inhibitors of the PKC-β pathway.

The growing appraisal of the intracellular machinery and signaling cascades that are active in lymphoma has allowed dissecting and revealing multiple potential targets for therapy. Several novel agents are currently under clinical evaluation, with most having demonstrated clinically relevant activity in malignant lymphoma as monotherapy [27].

Inhibitors of BCR Signaling Pathway

The inhibition of the SRC family kinases SYK and BTK has been long regarded as a mean to block active BCR signaling in B-cell malignancies. Fostamatinib disodium (R788) is the oral prodrug of R406 that acts as an ATP competitor to inhibit SYK. In preclinical studies, R406 blocked proliferation and induced apoptosis of DLBCL cell lines with tonic BCR signaling, showing a particular activity in cell lines that expressed high levels of cell-surface immunoglobulin [113]. However, R406 has shown in vitro antitumor activity even against SYK-independent DLBCL, suggesting that its effects may result from the concurrent inhibition of additional kinases [26]. In a phase I/II trial, it has induced 22, 10, 55, and 11% ORR, with long-lasting remissions, in refractory or relapsed patients with, respectively, DLBCL, FL, CLL/SLL, and MCL [114].

As an alternative strategy, PCI-32765, a potent oral inhibitor of the SYK-downstream-kinase BTK, is showing clinical activity against B-cell NHL in early-phase trials [115]. Importantly, in all treated patients, the full occupancy of BTK active site in PBMC was demonstrated within few hours after drug administration [115].

Targeting PKCβ, the common downstream target of SYK and BTK, has been also exploited to inhibit BCR signaling in B-cell lymphomas. Enzastaurin is an oral serine/threonine kinase inhibitor that targets PKCβ and PI3K/AKT pathways, leading to apoptosis, reduction of tumor cell proliferation, and suppression of tumor-induced angiogenesis in several preclinical models of B-cell malignancies [116, 117]. Phase II studies with single-agent enzastaurin showed limited clinical responses in patients with aggressive lymphomas, but a significant increase in the time to progression (TTP) [118, 119]. In indolent lymphoma, it is currently showing a higher therapeutic activity, achieving an ORR of 25% in FL patients [120]. The ability of this oral agent to induce disease stabilization and its excellent tolerability has led to a large phase III study of enzastaurin versus placebo in patients with high-risk DLBCL that achieve remission after induction therapy. Information from this trial will likely be crucial for the approval of this agent for the treatment of aggressive NHL.

PI3K/AKT/mTOR Pathway Inhibitors

Four different isoforms exist for PI3K subunit p110, with p101δ being predominant in hematologic cells and overexpressed in B-cell malignancies, where it is often constitutively activated or stimulated by microenvironmental signals. P101δ has thus been considered a selective target for antilymphoma therapy. CAL-101 is an orally bioavailable potent and highly selective inhibitor of this PI3K isoform. It blocks proliferation and induces apoptosis in different B-cell malignancies, including FL, MCL, and CLL [121]. CAL-101 is demonstrating substantial single-agent activity in relapsed or refractory hematologic diseases, including NHL and CLL [122–124]. In preclinical models, enhanced antitumor effects have been observed combining CA-101 with existing chemoimmunotherapeutic agents [125]. Initial results from ongoing early-phase clinical trials in patients with indolent NHL or CLL have shown that CA-101 can be successfully combined with bendamustine or rituximab. No unexpected adverse events have been reported, while clinical responses were achieved in all patients enrolled, supporting further clinical evaluation of these regimens [126].

Perifosine (1,1-dimethyl-4 [(octadecyloxy) hydroxyphosphinyl]oxy]-piperidinium inner salt, Keryx Biopharmaceutical) is a new synthetic, orally available, anticancer agent within the alkylphospholipid class that blocks AKT activation. Inhibiting AKT, perifosine has shown to directly induce cell death in in vitro and in vivo in preclinical experiments; however, additional evidences indicate that perifosine may also act by inhibiting the MAPK and JNK pathways [127]. Perifosine is currently under clinical evaluation for the treatment of several solid tumors and, more recently, also multiple myeloma and Waldenström macroglobulinemia. This experience will be important for potential future investigation in lymphoma.

Additional strategies to interfere with oncogenic activation of PI3K signaling include the direct inhibition of mTOR. Currently, 4 mTOR inhibitors are being tested in the clinic: the orally available rapamycin (also called sirolimus), everolimus (RAD001), the intravenous temsirolimus (CC-779), and deforolimus. Rapamycin was the first among these agents to be used clinically and is thus considered the parent drug of mTOR inhibitors. It is a macrolide antibiotic and was approved as an oral immunosuppressant to prevent acute transplant rejection in 1999 [111]. The other agents within this class are rapamycin analogs and thus called rapalogs. By targeting mTORC1, they primarily block cell proliferation and induce G1 cell-cycle arrest as a result of the reduced activation of cyclin D1 by mTORC1 [110]. Since cyclin D1 overexpression is the hallmark of MCL, mTORC1 inhibitors were first tested in this type of lymphoma. Two initial phase II studies with single-agent temsirolimus in heavily pretreated patients with advanced MCL showed a substantial induction of clinical response with manageable toxicity of myelosuppression [128, 129]. A subsequent randomized phase III study found a significant increase of both ORR and PFS in patients treated with temsirolimus compared to those receiving the investigators' choice of therapy [130] and led to its approval, in 2010, for the treatment of relapsed or refractory MCL. Recent results from initial clinical evaluation of temsirolimus in relapsed NHL different from MCL have revealed significant activity, with the highest ORR and the longest PFS being reported for FL patients [131].

Preclinical studies showing the ability of everolimus to impair the growth of aggressive lymphoma cell lines and sensitize these cells to several cytotoxic agents [132] set the rationale for the clinical evaluation of everolimus in lymphoma patients. Phase II studies demonstrated the safety and the substantial antitumor effects of single-agent everolimus in both indolent [133] and aggressive NHL [134], thus providing the rationale for inhibiting mTOR pathway to treat these diseases. Larger studies are undergoing to assess the activity of temsirolimus and everolimus monotherapy in DLBCL patients as consolidation after induction therapy, and in combination with chemoimmunotherapy for untreated MCL patients. In addition, other more potent compounds

interfering with the mTOR pathway have been developed, some of which are still reached the clinical evaluation (the PI3K inhibitor GDC-0941 (NCT00876122), such as the pan-PI3K/mTOR inhibitor GDC-0980 (NCT00854126), SF1126 (NCT00907205), and XL765 (NCT00485719).

An increased activity of mTORC2, followed by the phosphorylation of its target AKT, has been frequently observed upon treatment with rapamycin or rapalogs, suggesting that blocking mTORC1 may favor the activation of mTORC2, thus leading to tumor resistance. Importantly, the combination of rapalogs and pan-inhibitors of histone deacetylase (HDAC) (see section "Epigenetic Drugs"), which can reduce AKT activation by enhancing protein phosphatase 1 activity and directly targeting mTORC2, has revealed synergistic antitumor effects in lymphoma preclinical models, providing the proof of concept for concurrently targeting mTORC1 and mTORC2 to overcome the onset of potential resistances [110]. These findings highlight the value of pathway-targeted combination therapy to achieve maximal blockade of signaling pathways for cancer treatment.

Ras Inhibitors

Ras inhibitors have only recently started to be evaluated as potential antilymphoma treatment. Since prenylation (farnesylation) is required for the Ras protein to function and activate its downstream targets Raf, MEK1/2, ERK 1/2, and MAPK, the use of farnesyltransferase inhibitors has been exploited to interfere with this pathway for therapeutic purpose. The oral farnesyltransferase inhibitor tipifarnib has shown some clinical activity with manageable toxicities, when tested as single agent for the treatment of relapsed aggressive B-cell lymphomas (DLBCL and MCL) in phase II trials, thus providing the rationale for its further clinical evaluation in combination with conventional chemoimmunotherapy to increase and stabilize clinical responses [135].

Sorafenib (BAY 43-9006) is another agent that can interfere with Ras pathway. However, although developed as a Raf-1 inhibitor, it has subsequently shown a wider spectrum of activity against multiple other kinases, including FLT3, platelet-derived growth factor receptor, vascular endothelial growth factor receptor 1 (VEGFR1), and VEGFR2 [136]. Sorafenib has been approved for the treatment of advanced renal cell carcinoma and hepatocellular carcinoma. Recently, its antitumor activity has started to be evaluated in preclinical lymphoma and multiple myeloma models. Initial results provide the proof of concept for combining sorafenib with MEK1/2 inhibitors (e.g., PD184352, AZD6244, TAK-733) to potentiate its antilymphoma activity [73].

Proteasome Inhibitors

Proteasome inhibitors interfere with the ubiquitin–proteasome pathway, which, targeting proteins for degradation in eukaryotic cells, is essential for protein turnover and cellular homeostasis [88]. Interestingly, malignant cells have generally more proteasomes compared to normal cells. Since many proteins involved in the regulation of the cell cycle, apoptosis, and in the activation of transcription factors are substrates for ubiquitination and proteasome-mediated degradation, interference with this pathway is considered a promising strategy for anticancer therapy. One of the most widely recognized mechanisms of antitumor activity of proteasome inhibitors is their ability to repress NF-kB signal transduction cascade, by reducing the proteasome-mediated degradation of its super-repressor, IkB [137]. The stabilization of IkB, which binds to NF-kB and prevents its nuclear translocation, is likely to be an effective strategy for the treatment of tumors showing a positive stimulation of NF-kB signaling pathway, such as the ABC subtype of DLBCL [25] and multiple myeloma [138]. The most extended study of proteasome inhibitors has been indeed conducted in multiple myeloma, with the first-in-class inhibitor, bortezomib, being now approved for the treatment of patients with relapsed or refractory disease after at least one prior regimen. Additional investigation is now directed toward the evaluation of its combination with several agents commonly used for the treatment of multiple myeloma, such as melphalan, doxorubicin, dexamethasone, thalidomide, and prednisone, in previously untreated patients affected by multiple myeloma. More recently, bortezomib started to be tested also for the treatment of relapsed B-cell NHL, achieving significant activity against MCL patients [139, 140], who can now see this agent among their therapeutic option. Bortezomib monotherapy showed to induce a substantial response rates also in relapsed or refractory indolent NHL patients in phase II studies [141]; however, time to response was found to be longer in these patients compared to those with MCL [142].

The ability of bortezomib to interfere with several pathways that are commonly associated with resistance to therapy, such as NF-kB, cyclin, p53, and Bcl-2 protein regulation [88], has led to the study of its combination with cytotoxic agents, thus widening the possibility of clinically effective synergistic activity with conventional therapy. Interestingly, in a small study, bortezomib combined with chemotherapy resulted in significantly improved ORR (83% vs. 13%; $p < 0.001$) and median OS (10.8 months vs. 3.4 months; $p = 0.003$) in ABC compared with GCB DLBCL, providing the rationale for a differential therapeutic approach in genetically distinct DLBCL subtypes [88, 143]. If confirmed in larger studies, the combination of a CHOP-like chemotherapy with bortezomib would represent the first differential therapy for the two major biological subtypes of DLBCL.

Despite robust antitumor activity in the clinic, bortezomib therapy is hindered by a treatment-emergent peripheral neuropathy. With the validation of the proteasome as target for cancer therapy, several new proteasome inhibitors have been thus developed with the aim to reduce toxicity and potential resistance associated with bortezomib treatment.

Within the class of peptide boronic acid analogs, which reversibly inhibit the proteasome, MLN9708 (Millennium Pharmaceuticals, Inc.) [144] and CEP-18770 (Cephalon) [145] have recently entered phase I trials for the treatment of lymphomas.

Among the peptides epoxyketone derivatives, which irreversibly block proteasome activities, carfilzomib (PR-171) and PR-047 have demonstrated significant cytotoxic activity against several hematologic and solid malignancies in a preclinical setting, showing enhanced potency compared with bortezomib and synergistic antitumor effects in combination with dexamethasone [146], and other novel selective inhibitors [147] without significant increase of toxicity. Carfilzomib is also currently achieving successful response rates within the clinical setting, being the second-generation proteasome inhibitor in the more advanced phase of clinical development for the treatment of multiple myeloma [148].Several natural compounds have also revealed potent activity as proteasome inhibitors. NPI-0052 is a small β-lactone compound derived from fermentation of *Salinispora tropica*, a gram-positive actinomycete that acts, as carfilzomib and PR-047, as an irreversible proteasome inhibitor. In preclinical studies, it has shown similar single-agent activity against multiple myeloma, HL, NHL, and leukemia compared with carfilzomib, including the ability to partially overcome bortezomib resistance in vitro [149]. It has also provided substantial synergistic effects with lenalidomide, HDAC inhibitors (HDACi), agents triggering TRAIL receptor, pan-BCL-2 inhibitors, and also bortezomib in lymphomas, leukemia, and multiple myeloma. Phase I trials with NPI-0052 in hematologic malignancies and solid tumors are underway.

Results from these studies will provide decisive information, whereby their different pharmacologic characteristics, compared to bortezomib, can really translate into distinct efficacy and/or safety profiles.

As an alternative strategy to increase specificity and reduce side effects associated with ubiquitous proteasome inhibitors, the selective targeting of immunoproteasome has been also investigated. Indeed, the predominant expression of immunoproteasome in hematologic cells may allow a wider therapeutic window to direct the inhibitory activity toward malignant cells of hematologic origin, sparing normal tissue. IPSI-00, the most potent immunoproteasome-specific inhibitor developed so far, has shown enhanced cytotoxic effects on tumor cells from a hematologic origin and the ability to overcome resistance to conventional and novel drugs, including bortezomib [150]. These findings have provided the rationale for the translation of immunoproteasome-specific inhibitors to the clinical evaluation.

Epigenetic Drugs

Heritable changes in gene expression that are not codified by DNA sequence are defined as epigenetics. The most common mechanisms of epigenetic regulation include the methylation of CpG islands within the DNA and the acetylation of lysine residues in the N-terminal histone tails. Usually, methylated DNA or deacetylated histones are associated with a condensed chromatin structure that results in the repression of gene transcription. DNA methyltransferase/demethylase and histone acetyltransferase (HAT)/HDACs enzymes coordinately act to shut down or activate the expression of specific genes' tails [151]. It is now widely accepted that changes in the patterns of epigenetic regulation, altering the expression of tumor-suppressor genes and oncogenes, may contribute to neoplastic transformation genes [151]. In contrast to genetic mutations, epigenetic changes may be pharmacologically reverted through the inhibition of the enzymes responsible for the altered epigenetic pattern.

HDAC family members are categorized within four main classes, with class I including the nuclear HDACs 1, 2, and 3 and the nuclear/cytoplasmic HDAC 8; class II, the nuclear/cytoplasmic 4, 5, 7, and 9 and HDACs 6 and 10, which are preferentially located into the cytoplasm; class III, sirtuins 1–7 (SIRT), which are homologous to the yeast-repressing protein Sir2; and class IV, the nuclear/cytoplasmic HDAC 11 as the only member. Besides controlling the transcription status of many genes through histone deacetylation [152], HDACs can also regulate the function of several non-histone proteins (Fig. 5.8). Indeed, lysine acetylation/deacetylation represent an additional level of control for the function of several proteins that, having a crucial role in the cellular homeostasis, need to be tightly regulated, suchasp53,E2F,c-myc,NF-kB,hypoxia-inducible factor-1α (HIF-1α), and STAT3 transcription factors, as well as α-tubulin and heat shock protein (HSP) 90 [153] (Fig. 5.8).The altered activity of HDACs may thus contribute by several fronts to malignant transformation. Hematologic neoplasms have been found to be particularly associated with the aberrant recruitment of HDACs to gene promoters, with acute promyelocytic

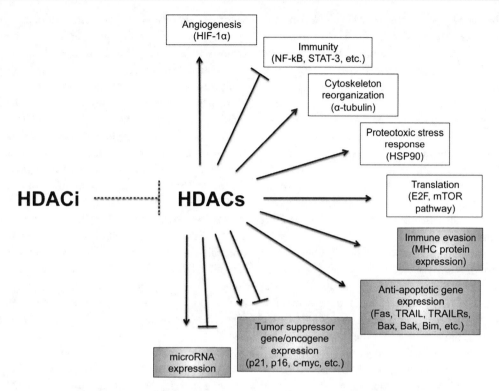

Fig. 5.8 Function of HDACs and effects of HDACi. Main cellular pathways affected by histone deacetylase enzymes (HDACs) (*gray boxes*, transcriptional effects; *white boxes*, posttranslational effects). *Arrows* and *perpendicular lines* indicate, respectively, positive and negative effects. HDAC inhibitors (HDACi) act by reverting HDAC activity on each pathway (*dotted perpendicular line*)

leukemia representing the first example of the causative role of HDACs in cancer. BCL-6 and c-myc are some examples of transcription factors that cooperate with HDACs in order to repress target genes [19, 154]. These proteins are often found aberrantly expressed in B-cell lymphomas and can contribute to the neoplastic process by transcriptionally silencing of tumor-suppressor genes. Therefore, HDACs are considered a promising target for anticancer therapy and in particular for the treatment of hematologic malignancies.

Several structurally distinct classes of HDACi have been developed, including hydroxamic acids, cyclic peptides, electrophilic ketones, short-chain fatty acids, and benzamides. In general, transformed cells are more sensitive to HDACi compared to normal cells. Importantly, these inhibitors can also kill non-proliferating tumor cells, while sparing normal cells, providing a significant advantage over conventional anticancer agents that selectively target proliferating tumor cells [155]. Common effects of HDAC inhibition include cell-cycle arrest in G1 and/or G2 phase, with the resulting block of cell growth [156], the induction of apoptosis via the extrinsic (death receptor) and intrinsic (mitochondrial) pathways [157], the inhibition of tumor angiogenesis, via the downregulation of proangiogenic factors [158], and metastatization, through the upregulation of metastatic suppressor genes and downregulation of prometastatic factors [159], and a positive immunomodulation resulting from the induction of major histocompatibility complex (MHC) class I and II protein expression [21] and alteration of cytokine secretion [22] (Fig. 5.8).

Hydroxamic acid derivatives represent the most widely studied category of HDACi. Compounds within this class that have reached the clinical development include vorinostat (SAHA, Zolinza®), panobinostat (LBH589), belinostat (PXD-101), givinostat (ITF2357), PCI

24781, and R306465 (JNJ-16241199). Vorinostat, a hydroxamate pan-inhibitor of class I and II HDACs, was the first HDACi to be approved by the FDA in October 2006 for the treatment of refractory cutaneous T-cell lymphoma (CTCL). Phase I and II studies have indicated an acceptable safety profile and preliminary activity of vorinostat as monotherapy in patients with relapsed or refractory aggressive and indolent B-cell NHL [160, 161]. Panobinostat potently inhibits class I, II, and IV HDACs. As single agent, it has shown antitumor activity in patients with several hematologic malignancies [162]. It is currently being studied in combination with novel agents, including AKT inhibitors and everolimus for the treatment of relapsed B-cell NHL [27]. Belinostat is another hydroxamate-based HDACi, whose clinical development is more advanced for the treatment of PTCL and CTCL compared to B-cell malignancies. However, results collected so far from a phase I study with escalating doses of belinostat in patients with B-NHL indicate a good safety profile and a certain clinical activity [163].

The natural cyclic peptide romidepsin (depsipeptide, Istodax®) is the second HDACi approved by the FDA (November 2009) for the treatment of CTCL patients after at least one prior systemic therapy. Although it can inhibit both class I and II HDACs, at low nanomolar levels, it exhibits a preferential activity against class I HDACs and is therefore considered a class-selective inhibitor in contrast to vorinostat [164]. The drug approval was based on two single-arm, multicenter, open-label trials that demonstrated a consistent ORR (34 and 35%), a remarkable long response duration and manageable side effects [165]. A combination of romidepsin and bortezomib is currently being investigated in a phase II study in patients with refractory multiple myeloma.

HDACi belonging to the benzamide class in clinical development include mocetinostat (MGCD0103) and etinostat. Mocetinostat is an oral, class I-selective HDACi that has demonstrated single-agent activity in refractory or relapsed NHL in phase II trials [166, 167].

The structurally simplest class of HDACi is represented by short-chain fatty acids, including valproic acid (VPA), butyric acid, and phenylbutyrate. Despite low inhibitory potency, these compounds have reached the clinical evaluation for the treatment of hematologic malignancies. VPA, a widely known antiepileptic drug, has been shown to preferentially inhibit class I HDACs leading to differentiation of transformed cells [168]. Due to the long-lasting clinical experiences with VPA and its well-characterized manageable side effects, this compound is currently investigated as an antileukemic agent in different trials.

Efforts have been made for the identification of valid surrogate biomarkers for the activity of HDACi, as well as potential predictors for their clinical efficacy. The acetylation of target proteins in PBMC or tumor tissues before and after treatment was not found to reproducibly correlate with the clinical activity of these agents [169]. The measurement of HDAC enzyme activity seems to be a more sensitive method for the assessment of the pharmacodynamic effects of HDACi; however, the correlation between HDAC enzyme activity and clinical effects of HDACi still needs to be determined [170]. Interestingly, the presence of high levels of activated STAT1, STAT3, and STAT5 in lymphoma cell lines that poorly respond to vorinostat treatment in vitro, and in pretreatment tumor biopsies from CTCL patients that did not respond to vorinostat indicated that STAT signaling pathway may represent a predictive biomarker for vorinostat response and/or may be involved in vorinostat resistance. Jak inhibitors, which can block this pathway, have shown to sensitize vorinostat-resistant cancer cell lines to HDACi, thus suggesting that the combination of HDACi and Jak inhibitors may represent a promising therapeutic strategy to overcome resistance [171]. SB1518 is an orally bioavailable inhibitor of JAK2 and the JAK2 mutant JAK2V617F that has shown antilymphoma activity in a phase I study [172]. Given the crucial role of Jak2 pathway in the PMBL subtype of DLBCL, as well as HL, combination regimens with HDACi and Jak2 have been proposed as a potential effective strategy for the treatment of these diseases [28].

Future preclinical and clinical studies will be crucial to elucidate whether and in which combination HDACi may be successfully exploited for the treatment of B-cell lymphomas.

In contrast to HDACs that posttranslationally modify cellular proteins, DNA methyltransferases (DNMT)1, DNMT3A, and DNMT3B catalyze the transfer of methyl groups to cytosine moieties within CpG dinucleotides of DNA. This results in the reduction of the binding of specific transcription factors and favors the recruitment of methyl-binding proteins and their preferential partners HDACs and histone metyl transferase, thus leading to gene silencing.

Due to their ability of silencing the expression of growth inhibitory and/or cell death promoting proteins, DNMTs are thought to play a key role in carcinogenesis. Overexpression of DNMT1/3A/3B is indeed a common feature of cancer, and it is frequently associated with increased tumor malignancy [173]. Therefore, the inhibition of these enzymes has also been exploited as a potential therapeutic anticancer strategy.

The nucleoside analog DNMT inhibitors (DNMTi), 5-azacytidine (azacitidine; Pharmion Corporation) and 5-aza-2'-deoxycytidine (decitabine; MGI Pharma), are approved for the treatment of myelodysplastic syndrome [174].

The simultaneous targeting of two epigenetic pathways is now being investigated with the aim to provide synergic antitumor effects and longer-lasting responses. Initial clinical trials of 5-azacytidine in combination with belinostat or VPA in patients with advanced myeloid malignancies, leukemia, and myelodysplastic syndromes show promising [108, 175]. Further studies with epigenetic agents in combination regimens will allow understanding whether they can be successfully exploited even for the treatment of B-cell lymphomas.

Agents Targeting the Apoptotic Pathway

The intrinsic apoptosis pathway is controlled at the mitochondrial level by Bcl-2 proteins. Bcl-2 family members are defined by the presence of at least one of the Bcl-2 homology domains (BH1-BH4). They may have either pro- (Bax, Bak, and the 3 (BH3)-only proteins) or antiapoptotic

functions (BCL-2, BCL-B, BCL-Xl, A1, and Mcl-1) depending on the domains expressed. When apoptosis pathway is triggered, BH3-only proteins bind Bcl-2 antiapoptotic proteins, thus allowing the release of Bax and Bak, which in turn induce the outflow of cytochrome c from the mitochondria into the cytoplasm where it activates the caspase cascade that leads to apoptosis. The upregulation of antiapoptotic Bcl-2 proteins is associated with tumorigenesis and resistance to chemotherapy. Bcl-2 is overexpressed in the majority of FL due to the translocation t(14;18) that lead to the juxtaposition of Bcl-2 gene next to the IgH promoter regions and in about 40% of DLBCL. Therefore, it represents a rationale target for the treatment of these diseases. The first construct targeting Bcl-2 that entered the clinical development was the specific antisense-nucleotide oblimersen. It is now being studied for the treatment of indolent lymphomas, where it has shown more convincing activity with respect to that achieved in aggressive lymphomas [176].

Successively, a major interest has been directed toward the development of small specific inhibitors of Bcl-2 proteins. The most widely exploited strategy in this setting has pointed to the generation of agents that, resembling BH3-only proteins, could bind to BCL-2, BCL-X_L, and BCL-W, thus displacing the proapoptotic BCL-2 proteins. For this reason, they are commonly called BH3 mimetics. ABT-263 is an orally available small-molecule BH3 mimetic that primarily inhibits BCL-X_L. In a phase I/II study in patients with previously treated lymphoid malignancies, it has demonstrated activity primarily against CLL, with dose-dependent acute thrombocytopenia being the major toxicity [177]. Combination with other agents may be required to increase the therapeutic efficacy of ABT-263 in other lymphomas. Obatoclax, a novel BH3 mimetic, has shown to sensitize rituximab-resistant B-cell lymphomas to treatment with bortezomib [178]. Promising results are being achieved from the initial clinical evaluation of the combination of obatoclax and bortezomib for the treatment of relapsed MCL [179].

Another potential therapeutic target within the apoptotic pathway is survivin, a bifunctional inhibitor of apoptosis that is overexpressed in most human neoplasm, but absent in normal tissues [180]. YM155 is a small inhibitor of survivin that has demonstrated to improve the antitumor effects of rituximab in DLBCL and to achieve significant responses in NHL patients in a phase I/II study [109].

The extrinsic or death receptor-dependent apoptosis pathway also offers novel strategies of intervention for the treatment of lymphoma. Death receptors, including Fas (CD95/Apo1), TNF receptor 1 (p55), TRAMP (WSL-1/Apo3/DR3/LARD), TRAIL-R1 (DR4), and TRAIL-R2 (DR5/Apo2/KILLER), belong to the tumor necrosis factor receptor (TNFR) superfamily, which trigger apoptosis upon ligand binding. Upon activation, the intracellular domain of death receptors interacts with Fas- and TNFR-associated death domain (FADD and TRADD) for the activation of caspase 8, which, in turn, triggers the caspase signaling cascade and the intrinsic apoptosis via the cleavage and activation of the BH3-only protein Bid. TRAIL-R1 and TRAIL-R2 agonist Abs as well as recombinant TRAIL are currently being investigated in early-phase clinical trials for the treatment of lymphoma [181–184]. To enhance the therapeutic efficacy of targeting TRAIL-Rs, cell-based vehiculation of the full-length membrane-bound TRAIL has been also evaluated in preclinical studies, showing a potent antitumor activity involving both direct and antiangiogenic mechanisms [185].

Signals from the tumor suppressor p53 are also crucial for the decision between life and death. P53 is physiologically inhibited by the human homolog of murine double-minute protein 2 (mdm2), which is often upregulated in B-cell lymphomas. Nutlin-3 is a small-molecule antagonist of mdm2 that has shown preclinical activity against MCL [186]. This compound, together with other mdm2 antagonists, which are under development, is expected to represent novel options for the treatment of lymphomas carrying wild-type p53.

Immunotherapy

MAb Therapy

With the advent of mAb technology [187, 188], more than ten cell-surface molecules have been

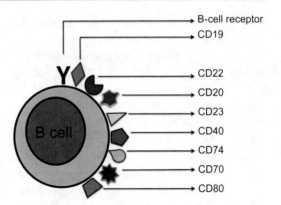

Fig. 5.9 B-cell antigen targets. B-cell-surface-associated antigens that have been exploited as immunotherapeutic targets for the treatment of B-cell malignancies

identified on B cells, with different expression levels at various stages of their development. Most of these antigens are found also on the malignant B-cell counterpart and have been thus exploited as molecular targets for mAb therapy (Fig. 5.9).

To date, CD20 has been the most commonly targeted antigen by mAb therapy for B-cell malignancies, because of its advantageous characteristics of being expressed at high levels on the surface of most malignant B cells, where it is tightly bound, with little modulation and no secretion or rapidly shedding in circulation. Furthermore, CD20 expression is absent on the early B-cell precursors allowing repopulation of the B-cell compartment after treatment [189]. In addition, CD20 seems to have an important role in the physiology of B-cell activation and cell-cycle regulation [190]. Thus, apart from its binding to normal B cells, CD20 represents an ideal target for B-cell lymphoma. The chimeric human–mouse IgG1 kappa anti-CD20 mAb rituximab was the first mAb to be approved by the FDA in 1997 for treatment of relapsed or refractory CD20+ indolent B-cell NHL [61]. On binding to CD20, rituximab induces Ab-dependent cell cytotoxicity (ADCC), Complement-dependent cytotoxicity CDC, and apoptosis of neoplastic B cells by promoting calcium influx and caspase activation [191, 192] and sensitizes malignant B cells to chemotherapy [193]. Rituximab has been the most valuable addition to the treatment for B-cell NHL since 20 years and is now considered the cornerstone of therapy in both indolent and aggressive B-cell lymphomas. Nevertheless, 30–50% of the patients do not respond to rituximab in first-line or more advanced treatment settings, respectively [89], and approximately 60% of initial responders no longer benefit from retreatment [194]. The success of rituximab, but also its recognized limitations, has stimulated investigational efforts to develop newer-generation anti-CD20 mAbs, as well as mAbs targeting different surface antigens expressed on malignant B cells (Fig. 5.9 and Table 5.2). Several approaches are under evaluation, including humanization of the molecule, to decrease its infusion reactions and immunogenicity, improved side-effect profile and enhancement of binding affinity. Modification of the Fc portion is also being performed to optimize effector functions, particularly ADCC. Second-generation anti-CD20 mAbs include ofatumumab, veltuzumab, and ocrelizumab that are humanized or fully human IgG1, with an unmodified Fc region (Table 5.2).

Ofatumumab (HuMax-CD20) is a fully human IgG1 Ab that binds to an extracellular CD20 epitope distinct from that recognized by rituximab, resulting in a stronger CDC but less apoptosis induction [195]. It has provided encouraging results in recent phase I/II studies in refractory/relapsed CLL and FL [112, 196] that led to its accelerated FDA approval for the treatment of refractory/relapsed CLL. Clinical investigation to confirm the clinical benefit of ofatumumab in rituximab-refractory CLL as well as other B-NHLs is underway.

Veltuzumab (hA20) is a recombinant humanized monoclonal IgG1 with identical variable complementarity-determining regions (CDRs) compared with rituximab, except from a single amino acid change, which does not alter CD20 binding avidity, but significantly reduced mAb off rates and enhanced CDC [197]. Veltuzumab has proven active and safe at lower doses than rituximab in phase I/II studies in patients with recurrent B-cell lymphomas [198, 199].

Ocrelizumab is a humanized version of the murine 2H7 Ab with enhanced ADCC in vitro [200]. After reaching phase III clinical trials for the treatment of autoimmune diseases, its development has been suspended due to the occurrence of lethal opportunistic infections. However, its clinical evaluation in patients with hematologic malignancies is still ongoing [113].

Given the finding that FcγRIII amino acid 158 polymorphism (valine/phenylalanine) can impair rituximab-mediated ADCC [201, 202], third-generation mAbs have been developed with an Fc region designed to improve therapeutic performance by adapting their effector functions. Three such engineered anti-CD20 Abs—AME-133v [203], PRO131921 (rhuMAb v114) (NCT00452127), and have entered clinical trials, GA-101 with GA101 having reached the most advanced phases [204]—of clinical development. All of them have demonstrated an increased capability to mediate ADCC as compared with rituximab, and GA-101 has also shown to better induce direct apoptosis in malignant B cells.

Novel anti-CD20 mAbs have demonstrated the same favorable toxicity profiles as rituximab. In general, pharmacodynamic parameters do not correlate with response, and no clear dose–effect relationships have been detected. They are associated with significant efficacy, although response rates in rituximab-refractory patients are modest. Therefore, mAb therapies for B-cell NHL targeting neoplastic B-cell targets distinct from CD20 are developing exponentially in number, with the aim of identifying more active and specific treatments. CD22, CD23, CD40, CD80, CD70, and CD74 are among the most widely exploited biotargets for novel antilymphoma passive immunotherapy (Fig. 5.9). However, being involved in the normal B-cell functions, these antigens are not tumor specific. Nevertheless, the humanized anti-CD22 monoclonal IgG epratuzumab [205], the primate-human chimeric anti-CD23 and anti-CD80 monoclonal IgG1 lumiliximab (IDEC-152) [206], and galiximab [207] have shown promising clinical results and a good safety profile in phase I/II trials for relapsed/refractory NHL (Table 5.2). Moreover, the combinations of epratuzumab or galiximab with rituximab demonstrated significant clinical activity with limited toxicity [208, 209], with the latter showing even better outcomes than either agent alone [210]. Epratuzumab or lumiliximab with chemoimmunotherapy or standard chemotherapy proved feasible and safe approaches for NHL patients, which compared also favorably with historical

Table 5.2 Novel mAbs in clinical development for B-cell malignancies

Study	Agent	Type	Description	Target	Status	Dose	Patients	Results ORR (%)	CR (%)
Hagenbeek et al. ASH 2005, abstract 5760 [288]	Ofatumumab (HuMax-CD20)	mAb	Human	CD20	Phase I/II	300–1,000 mg/m^2/week (×4)	Relapsed/refractory FL ($n=38$)	63	
Hagenbeek et al. ASH 2009, abstract 935 [289]	Ofatumumab (HuMax-CD20)	mAb	Human	CD20	Phase I/II	300 mg (dose 1), 500 or 1,000 mg (dose 2–8)/m^2/week (×8)	Rituximab refractory FL ($n=116$)	10	1
Coiffier et al. (2008) [112]	Ofatumumab (HuMax-CD20)	mAb	Human	CD20	Phase I/II	100–2,000 mg/m^2/week (×4)	Relapsed/refractory CLL ($n=33$)	44	
Coiffier et al. ASH 2010, abstract 3955 [290]	Ofatumumab (HuMax-CD20)	mAb	Human	CD20	Phase II	300 mg (dose 1), 1,000 mg (dose 1–8)/m^2/week (×8)	Relapsed/refractory DLBCL ($n=81$)	11	4
Kipps et al. ASCO 2009, abstract 7043 [291]	Ofatumumab (HuMax-CD20)	mAb	Human	CD20	Phase III	300 mg (dose 1), 2,000 mg (dose 2–12)/m^2/week (×8) and /months (×4)	Refractory CLL (interim analysis $n=138$)	58	
Morschhauser et al. 2009 [292]	Veltuzumab (hA20)	mAb	Humanized	CD20	Phase I/II	80–750 mg/m^2/week (×4)	Relapsed/refractory B-cell NHL ($n=82$)	40	21
Salles et al. ASH 2010, abstract 286 [293]	GA101	mAb	Humanized	CD20	Phase II	1,600 mg (d1 and d8); 800 mg (d22, q21) (×8)	Relapsed/refractory indolent NHL ($n=22$)	55	9
Cartron et al. ASH 2010, abstract 2878 [294]	GA101	mAb	Humanized	CD20	Phase II	1,600 mg (d1 and d8); 800 mg (d22, q21) (×9)	Relapsed/refractory aggressive NHL ($n=19$)	32	
Leonard et al. (2003) [205]	Epratuzumab	mAb	Humanized mLL2	CD22	Phase I/II	120–1,000 mg/m^2/week (×4)	Relapsed/refractory FL ($n=55$)	18	6
Leonard et al. (2004) [295]	Epratuzumab	mAb	Humanized mLL2	CD22	Phase I/II	120–1,000 mg/m^2/week (×4)	Relapsed/refractory aggressive lymphomas ($n=56$)	10	5
Leonard et al. (2008) [296]	Epratuzumab	mAb	Humanized mLL2	CD22	Phase II	360 mg/m^2/week (×4)	Relapsed/refractory FL ($n=41$)	54	24
	Rituximab	mAb	Mouse-chimeric	CD20		375 mg/m^2/2 weeks (×4)			
Grant et al. ASH 2010, abstract 427 [297]	Epratuzumab	mAb	Humanized mLL2	CD22	Phase II	360 mg/m^2/week (×4) and /2 months (×4)	Untreated FL ($n=60$)	84	33
	Rituximab	mAb	Mouse-chimeric	CD20		375 mg/m^2/2 weeks (×4) and /2 months (×4)			

5 Non-Hodgkin's Lymphomas

Reference	Agent	Type	Origin	Target	Phase	Dose	Population		
Micallef et al. ASCO 2009, abstract 8508 [211]	Epratuzumab	mAb	Humanized mLL2	CD22	Phase II	360 mg/m²/week (×4)	Untreated DLBCL	95	72
	Rituximab	mAb	Mouse-chimeric	CD20		375 mg/m²/2 weeks (×4)			
	CHOP								
Fayad et al. ASH 2006, abstract 2711 [230]	Inotuzumab ozogamicin (CMC-544)	ADC (calicheamicin conjugated)	Humanized	CD22	Phase I	1.8 mg/m², every 28 days	Relapsed/refractory FL or DLBCL (n=34)	53	24
Tobiani et al. ASH 2008, abstract 1565 [298]	Inotuzumab ozogamicin (CMC-544)	ADC (calicheamicin conjugated)	Humanized	CD22	Phase I	1.8 mg/m², every 28 days	Relapsed/refractory FL (n=13)	85	54
Fayad et al. ASH 2008, abstract 266 [231]	Inotuzumab ozogamicin (CMC-544)	ADC (calicheamicin conjugated)	Humanized	CD22	Phase I/II	1.8 mg/m² on day 2, every 28 days	Relapsed/refractory FL or DLBCL (n=30)	80	43
	Rituximab	mAb	Mouse-chimeric	CD20					
Goy et al. ASH 2010, abstract 430 [299]	Inotuzumab ozogamicin (CMC-544)	ADC	Humanized	CD22	Phase II	1.8 mg/m² on day 2, every 28 days	Rituximab relapsed/refractory indolent NHL (n=43)	53	19
Byrd et al. (2010) [300]	Lumiliximab	mAb	Primate-chimeric	CD23	Phase I/II	375 mg/m² (n=3) or 500 mg/m² (n=28)	Relapsed/refractory CLL (n=31)	65	52
	FCR								
Advani et al. (2009) [301]	Dacetuzumab (SGN-40)	mAb, mild agonist	Humanized	CD40	Phase I	2–8 mg/kg/week (×6)	Relapsed/refractory B-cell NHL (n=50)	12	2
Kivekas et al. (2002) [302]	Galiximab	mAb	Primate-chimeric	CD80	Phase I/II	500 mg/m²/week (×4)	Relapsed/refractory FL (n=38)	11	5
Friedberg et al. ASH 2008, abstract 1004 [210]	Galiximab	mAb	Primate-chimeric	CD80	Phase II	500 mg/m²/week (×4)	Relapsed/refractory FL (n=64)	64	17
	Rituximab	mAb	Mouse-chimeric	CD20		375 mg/m²/2 week (×4)			
Czuczman et al. ASH 2008, abstract 1003 [209]	Galiximab	mAb	Primate-chimeric	CD80	Phase II	500 mg/m²/week (×4) and /2 months (×4)	Untreated FL (n=61)	70	38
	Rituximab	mAb	Mouse-chimeric	CD20		375 mg/m²/2 weeks (×4)			
Brence-Bruckler et al. ASH 2010, abstract 428 [303]	Galiximab	mAb	Primate-chimeric	CD80	Phase II	500 mg/m²/week (×4)	Relapsed/refractory FL (n=337)	51	20
	Rituximab	mAb	Mouse-chimeric	CD20		375 mg/m²/2 weeks (×4)			

Mos, months; wk, week.

controls receiving the same treatment without these novel agents [211, 212]. Such encouraging results have prompted the initiation of randomized phase III trials to evaluate the clinical benefit of combining rituximab with galiximab and polychemotherapy with lumiliximab.

Due to the crucial role of CD40 engagement on the surface of lymphoma B cells for their proliferation and survival [213, 214], CD40 has been largely studied as a potential biotarget for these diseases. HCD122 (formerly CHIR-12.12) and dacetuzumab (SGN-40) are, respectively, a fully human and a humanized anti-CD40 monoclonal IgG1 that, blocking CD40/CD40L-mediated signaling, induce proapoptotic signals and provide ADCC, resulting in clearance of malignant B cells [215, 216]. Clinical evaluation of the tolerability of HCD122 is underway in phase I trials for NHL or HL, multiple myeloma, and relapsed CLL. Dacetuzumab has already reached phase II clinical trials that indicate some effects as monotherapy in patients with heavily pretreated DLBCL [217] (Table 5.2). Ongoing studies are exploring its activity in combination with conventional therapies in multiple myeloma, DLBCL, and low-grade NHL.

MAbs targeting CD70 and CD74 are the last ones entering preclinical and initial clinical development for the treatment of B-cell malignancies [218]. CD70 has the advantage of being expressed prevalently on neoplastic B cells and rarely on normal B or T lymphocytes [219]. CD70 targeting on lymphoma cells with the specific fully human MDX-1411 mAb has resulted in potent ADCC induction [220]. CD74 is a type-II transmembrane chaperone molecule, expressed on normal and malignant B cells, monocytes and histiocytes. It mediates several prosurvival signals and favors tumor immune escape by impairing the binding of antigenic peptides to HLA-DR [221, 222]. The anti-CD74 mAb milatuzumab (hLL1, IMMU-115) has shown to cause very modest ADCC or CDC, but in the presence of an appropriate cross-linking agent, it can inhibit cell proliferation and promote apoptosis in vitro, resulting in significant prolongation of survival in lymphoma mouse models [223, 224].

All these results have been seen with great enthusiasm, even though, as yet, none have demonstrated significant efficacy over that seen with rituximab. Retrospective analysis of failures and successes of mAb therapy has resulted in the reemphasis of three major caveats of this approach: (1) identity of the target antigens, (2) the limited understanding of the mechanisms of action of the mAbs, and (3) resistance induction [225–227]. Tumor specificity, essential biologic activity, the absence of mutation in the target epitope, and minimal shedding or extracellular secretion are the most important properties that an ideal mAb target should have. However, B-cell-surface proteins identified to date do not concomitantly display all of these features. Therefore, novel Ab-based immunotherapeutics continue to be under evaluation to improve the current therapies for B-cell malignancies.

The strategy to conjugate mAbs with toxin(s) (immunotoxin(s)) has been developed to more efficiently target rapidly modulating antigens and induce tumor cell death. However, this approach has been limited by the induction of immune responses to the mAb and the toxin as well as non-specific toxicity [228]. This has led to the generation of agents with an improved safety profile. The calicheamicin-conjugated anti-CD22 mAb inotuzumab ozogamicin (CMC-544) is such an example [229] that, having demonstrated significant single-agent activity in relapsed FL and DLBCL [230], is now under clinical investigation in combination with rituximab [231] (Table 5.2).

In contrast to unmodified mAb and drug/toxin mAb conjugates, tumor-specific mAbs complexed to a radioisotope (131I, 90Y) do not need to bind to each tumor cell or penetrate homogeneously into the neoplastic tissue to exert their effects. The ionizing energy emitted from therapeutic isotopes can kill cells several cell diameters away (cross fire effect), thus resulting in a more efficient tumor targeting. Two radiolabeled mAbs directed against CD20 have been tested for the treatment of relapsed/refractory NHL after first-line chemotherapy: 131I-tositumomab (Bexxar) and 90Y-ibritumomab tiuxetan (Zevalin) [78, 232]. Both have provided high response rate in large cohorts of patients with relapsed/refractory FL [233–236]. 90Y-ibritumomab showed also greater efficacy than rituximab as single agent in a randomized trial [237]. For the majority of patients, however, the response duration is relatively short, and at present, it is difficult to predict the best candidates for this treatment.

Therefore, the need for more cost-effective immunotherapeutics has led to the development of novel scaffold strategies, many of which are based on the use of mAb fragments or single-domain Abs. The aim is to increase target multi-specificity, an increased ability to recruit effector cells, and to bind cryptic epitopes.

Small-modular immunopharmaceuticals (SMIPs) are single-chain polypeptides with a target-binding domain attached to an effector domain through a flexible hinge domain, the latter designed to govern the engagement of receptors on immune cells for enhanced ADCC activity [238]. TRU-015 and TRU-016 are recently developed anti-CD20 and anti-CD37 SMIPs that have demonstrated more potent ADCC than rituximab in CLL and NHL. Ongoing research is investigating the potential clinical use of these SMIPs in B-cell lymphomas [239, 240].

Bispecific T-cell engager (BiTE) Abs, which consist of two single-chain Abs, one specific for CD3, a subunit of T-cell receptor complex, and the other for a tumor-associated antigen (TAA), currently represent the most promising novel immunotherapeutics [241]. Blinatumomab (MT103/MEDI538; bscCD3xCD19) is the first BiTE Ab tested clinically in patients with relapsed NHL that has provided excellent antitumor activity in patients with FL, MCL, and CLL in a recent phase I clinical trial [242]. Ongoing phase II studies will clarify the role of this compound for the treatment of B-cell malignancies.

Active Immunotherapy

Multiple observations that, in cancer patients, the presence of Ab and/or T-cell responses against the autologous malignancy is associated with a significant improved survival [243] have led to the development of strategies able to actively generate such immunity. In contrast to passive immunotherapy, therapeutic anticancer vaccines have the potential to stimulate an endogenous tumor-specific immune response and the generation of an immunological memory, which, in turn, may favor the long-term control of the disease.

Indolent B-cell NHLs have long been regarded as particularly immune responsive based on reports of spontaneous regressions [38] and high response rates to mAbs [89, 244]. In addition, multiple evidences supporting the association between the prognosis of indolent lymphomas and the presence of different subsets of tumor-infiltrating non-malignant immune cells further indicate that the immune system plays a major role in the control of these diseases. Therefore, active immunotherapy has been considered a valid option to be exploited for the treatment of indolent NHL patients.

A therapeutic cancer vaccine usually comprises (1) a unique/tumor-specific (products of mutated genes, altered cell surface glycolipids and glycoproteins or viral antigens) or a shared self-antigen/TAA (proteins exogenously expressed in tumors but found in normal tissues), eventually loaded into professional APCs (i.e., DCs), (2) a carrier, and (3) an adjuvant (Fig. 5.10). Given the low immunogenicity of most TAA (in particular self-antigens) and the immunosuppressive network established by tumor cells, antigen delivering strategies and immunostimulatory agents included in the vaccine formulation are crucial to allow shaping the proper adaptive antitumor immune response for the induction of a tumor-specific immunological memory and long-lasting clinical benefit. Some of the most largely exploited adjuvants and carrier proteins in active immunotherapy include Freund's adjuvant, keyhole limpet hemocyanin (KLH) [245], bacilli Calmette–Guerin (BCG), syntax adjuvant formulation-1 (SAF-1) [246], granulocyte/monocyte colony-stimulating factor (GM-CSF) [247], and toll-like receptor (TLR) ligands (imiquimod for TLR-7/8, CpG for TLR-9) [248].

Id represents a unique TAA for mature B-cell malignancies including B-cell lymphomas and has been, therefore, the most widely exploited antigen in vaccination against these diseases. Originally generated by hybridoma technology, Id protein can now be produced by recombinant technology, cloning Ig genes into stable cell lines,

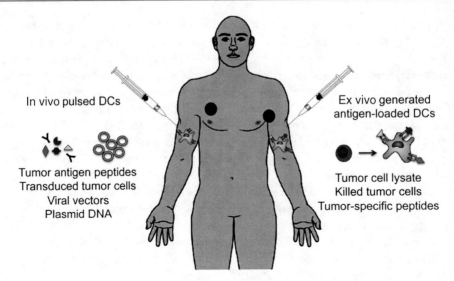

Fig. 5.10 Active immunotherapeutic strategies. *Left*: injection of the immunogenic agents (tumor antigen peptides, tumor cells transduced to express the antigen, viral vector or plasmid DNA encoding for the tumor antigen) for a random in vivo target of DCs. *Right*: injection of ex vivo-generated tumor antigen-loaded (derived from tumor cell lysate, killed tumor cells, or recombinant technology) DCs

for its use as a vaccine. The first demonstration in mice of the ability of Id protein to generate a protective tumor-specific immune response came from a pioneering study by Lynch et al. in multiple myeloma models [249]. Initial preclinical studies were thus performed immunizing with the soluble Id proteins alone [250, 251]. Successively, it was demonstrated that the KLH conjugation could significantly improve the immunogenicity of tumor-Id in the 38C13 lymphoma model [114]. Interestingly, the antitumor effect of Id-KLH was associated with the induction of a specific humoral response and was preferentially achieved in animals with low tumor burden [114]. Using the same lymphoma model, a further improvement was achieved when low doses of GM-CSF were co-administered with the vaccine [252]. Indeed, GM-CSF showed to enhance the protective antitumor immunity elicited by Id-KLH in a way that was strictly dependent upon the specific activation of a T-cell adaptive response [252]. Collectively, results achieved in preclinical studies with Id vaccines allowed to predict that Id conjugated to a carrier protein, namely, KLH, and co-administered with GM-CSF into patients with limited disease could represent the best strategy to induce a clinically relevant tumor-specific immunity.

Phase I/II studies in FL patients in complete clinical remission or with residual disease after chemotherapy demonstrated the ability of vaccination with Id-KLH to induce a specific adaptive immunity, eventually associated with a therapeutic effect [253–257]. Interestingly, the study by Inoges et al. [257] showed that the clinical responses achieved by vaccination in patients in clinical remission after induction therapy were significantly longer compared to the previous ones achieved in the same patients after frontline standard therapy. In particular, all patients showing an Id-specific immunity after vaccination experienced the most longer-lasting second complete remission, indicating, for the first time in human, that vaccine-induced Id-specific immune activation and clinical efficacy were most likely associated [257] (Table 5.3). The critical role of immune responses in vaccinated patients highlighted a major concern considering the drastic B-cell depletion caused by rituximab, which was becoming the standard of care for B-cell lymphoma. Two clinical trials thus evaluated the immunogenicity and the clinical efficacy of the

Table 5.3 Main features and interpretation of clinical trials assessing the clinical benefit of Id vaccines for FL

	University of Navarra, Spain	Genitope	Favrille	NCI/Biovest
Vaccine	Generic	MyVax	FavId	BiovaxID
Patients	FL, first relapse	FL, untreated	FL, untreated or relapsed	FL, untreated
Source of tumor	Excisional biopsy	FNA/core biopsy	FNA/core biopsy	Excisional biopsy
Idiotype production	Heterohybridoma technology	Recombinant DNA technology	Recombinant DNA technology	Heterohybridoma technology
Induction therapy	Six cycles of CHOP or CNOP	CVP (8 cycles every 3 weeks)	Rituximab (weekly ×4)	PACE/R-CHOP (6–8 cycles every 4 weeks)
Type of comparison (experimental/control)	Same patients: second compared with first CR	2/1 randomization	1/1 randomization	2/1 randomization
Patient status before vaccination	Second CR	First CR or PR	First CR, PR, or SD	First CR or CRu
Vaccination	Id-KLH+GM-CFSE (sc, 23–30 months of active vaccination)	Id-KLH+GM-CFSE or KLH+GM-CSF (sc, 7 doses)	Id-KLH+GM-CFSE or placebo+GM-CSF (sc, until PD)	Id-KLH+GM-CFSE or KLH+GM-CSF (sc, 5 doses)
Number of patients (actual/expected)	25/25	Vaccine: 192/240; control: 95/120	Vaccine: 174 instead of 171; control: 175 instead of 171	Vaccine: 76/250; control: 41/125
Primary end point	Second CR > first CR and 13 months	PFS ($p<0.01$)	TTP ($p<0.01$)	DFS ($p<0.01$)
Results	20 of 20 immune responders achieved both end points; 5 of 5 immune non-responders did not	Median PFS, 19.1 (experimental) vs. 23.3 (control) months ($p=0.297$)	Median TTP, 9 (experimental) vs. 12.6 (control) months ($p=0.019$)	Median DFS, 44.2 (experimental) vs. 30.6 (control) months ($p=0.045$)
Potential caveats	Small proof-of-principle study	More patients than expected (at least one-quarter) relapsed or progressed within 9 months from randomization	Too few CR induction before vaccination; severe B cell depletion by rituximab in most vaccinated patients	Missed target ITT and statistically significant
Refs	Inoges et al. [257]	Levy et al. [261]	Freedman et al. [260]	Schuster et al. [262]

CHOP cyclophosphamide, doxorubicin, vincristine, and prednisone; CNOP cyclophosphamide, mitoxantrone, vincristine, and prednisone; R Rituximab; CRu complete response unconfirmed; CVP cyclophosphamide, vincristine, and prednisone; DFS disease-free survival; GM-CSF granulocyte-macrophage colony-stimulating factor; ITT intent to treat; KLH keyhole limpet hemocyanin; n.s not significant; PACE prednisone, doxorubicin, cyclophosphamide, and etoposide; PFS progression-free survival; CR complete response; PR partial response; SD stable disease; TTP time to progression

Id-KLH+GM-CSF vaccine following induction therapy with rituximab, showing that antitumor T-cell responses were not affected after rituximab therapy [258, 259]. Remarkably, the study by Koc et al. demonstrated an improved TTP for patients receiving vaccination after rituximab compared to the historical controls treated with rituximab alone, suggesting a potential clinical benefit provided by active immunotherapy after rituximab induction therapy.

Therefore, three large-scale randomized phase III clinical trials were initiated with the aim of demonstrating a clear-cut survival improvement in vaccinated patients. These studies used either hybridoma-derived Id (BiovaxID, Biovest International Inc., Worcester, MA) or recombinant Id (MyVax, Genitope Corporation, Fremont, CA; FavId, Favrille, San Diego, CA) in grade 1–3 FL patients experiencing at least disease stabilization (Favrille study [260]), partial (Genitope study) [261], or complete (Biovest study) [262] remission after standard course of rituximab, CVP or prednisone, doxorubicin, cyclophosphamide, and etoposide (PACE), respectively (Table 5.3). Only the Biovest study showed an amelioration of the clinical outcome in patients receiving the anti-Id vaccination, as they experienced a prolongation of chemotherapy-induced remission compared to those in the control arm [262]. However, the targeted level of statistical significance for this end point was missed, as was the expected intention to treat. Therefore, the clinical benefit of Id vaccination still remains to be formally demonstrated. These studies, however, did not prove that the negative results were due to the failure of the vaccine rather than to defects in study design. The prevaccine treatment modality has been recognized as one of the major flaws of these studies: rituximab-treated patients started vaccination with severely depleted numbers of circulating B cells, CVP did not always produce durable response, and PACE regimen proved inappropriate in the rituximab era, thus explaining the very limited patient enrolment and randomization. In addition, given the heterogeneous (1) natural history of indolent NHL, (2) influence of these tumors on host defenses, (3) responsiveness of these patients to the Id antigen, and (4) the antitumor effects of an immune response induced by Id vaccines coupled with the possible emergence of target antigen mutation or downregulation over the course of the disease, the use of standard phase III randomized trials does not seem the most appropriate to assess the clinical benefit of patient-specific Id vaccines [263]. As suggested by Inoges et al. [257], the study of Id vaccination in lymphoma patients in first relapse and/or progression after chemotherapy would allow the possibility to compare the length of the clinical responses obtained with the subsequent treatments (standard chemotherapy vs. vaccination protocol). In this regard, a longer duration of the vaccine-induced second clinical response compared to the first in a substantial proportion of patients has been proposed as the major end point for regulatory approval without facing the specific complications of a randomization [263]. Randomization to either idiotypic vaccination or maintenance rituximab after chemotherapy has been also suggested with the non-inferiority of Id vaccines compared to rituximab as a second independent main clinical end point, possibly allowing regulatory approval [263].

As an additional option to target DC in vivo and to immunize cancer patients, viral vectors and plasmid DNA encoding TAAs have been exploited (Fig. 5.10). This strategy requires in vivo transfection and antigen production. The optimized gene sequence is delivered intradermally, subcutaneously (gene gun device), or to the muscle (intramuscular injection and electroporation), which allows, respectively, the in vivo transfection of professional APC (epidermal keratinocytes and Langerhans DCs) or myocytes and secondary cross-presentation of tumor antigens by recruited DCs. The advantages of DNA-based vaccines over other immunization strategies include the possibility of incorporating multiple epitope-encoding DNA regions to target several antigens in a single vaccine formulation, the low cost, and the easy procedure required for their generation. Initial clinical trials in lymphoma with Id-encoding DNA have demonstrated the safety and immunological efficacy of this strategy, with no relevant levels of integration into host cellular DNA, or the development of antinuclear auto-Abs [264, 265]. However, one note of caution is the possibility that vaccine antigen uptake and presentation may take place in the improper DC subset without the adequate stimuli, thus resulting in tolerance or an unwanted type of immunity rather than in the priming of an antitumor adaptive immune response [266].

As opposite to in vivo targeting of DCs, when generated ex vivo, they are properly matured starting from CD34+ hematopoietic progenitors or, more commonly, from peripheral blood (PB)-derived monocytes [266] (Fig. 5.10). Following incubation with a cocktail of maturation cytokines [267], they are loaded with tumor antigens as to recapitulate ex vivo the early phase of DC activation. Timmermann et al. reported an ORR of 36% in relapsed FL patients with residual diseases after vaccination with DC loaded with Id or Id-KLH [268]. More recently, a pilot study, in which heavily pretreated indolent NHL patients with measurable disease were treated with killed whole autologous tumor-cell DC vaccines, demonstrated a strict correlation between a multifaceted immune activation and the induction of clinical responses (33%) [269, 270]. Responder patients showed, indeed, both T- and B-cell antitumor immunity, the activation of NK cells and the downregulation of circulating and tumor-infiltrating Tregs [269, 270]. Whole tumor-cell-based vaccines might potentially induce autoimmunity but have the advantage of widening the spectrum of target TAAs, reducing the risk of the emergence of immune escape variants. Importantly, in this study, no autoimmune reactions were observed, indicating the feasibility of vaccinating indolent NHL patients using tumor-loaded DCs [269].

Clinical efficacy of DC-based vaccines in lymphoma patients seems to be superior compared to that achieved by Id-specific vaccines. However, variables associated with employing DC vaccines are numerous and require precise consideration for their therapeutic efficacy. They include the source or DC lineage to use, the antigen-engulfing strategy, the DC maturation and/or activation levels to achieve ex vivo, and the route of vaccine administration.

A novel autologous tumor-derived proteoliposomal vaccine formulation achieved very promising results in a phase I trial with a small number of patients with previously untreated or treated stage III or IV FL grade 1 or 2 [271]. Vaccine was generated using cell membrane proteins extracted from lymph node biopsies that were incorporated into liposomes with interleukin(IL)-2 as an adjuvant, following a very easy and rapid procedure compared to the labor-intensive method for the generation of Id- or DC-based approaches. The treatment was well tolerated without any signs of autoimmune reaction. It achieved one complete remission and one stabilization of the disease that were associated with a significant induction of tumor-specific T-cell responses [271]. These results support the development of more advanced clinical trials, in particular in the setting of low tumor burden, to test the efficacy and clinical benefit of this vaccine formulation over conventional standard management of FL patients.

Alternatively, given the growing appreciation that some conventional treatments possess the immune stimulatory property of inducing immunogenic tumor cell death [272], then they, in association with DC-activating agents, may be exploited to target TAAs to DCs in vivo. Recently, the proof of principle that this strategy, namely, in situ vaccination, can be feasible, safe, and potentially clinically efficacious has been provided in a pilot study in which low-grade NHL patients were treated with low-dose radiotherapy with intratumor injection of a TLR9 agonist [273]. If confirmed, and supported by a clear biologic mechanisms in a wider series of patients, then these promising results may not only provide important information on underlying tumor immunity but, interestingly, may have the potential to pave the way for a future novel straightforward, non-customized active immunotherapy approach. Such an option will be widely applicable without the need of following clinical grade procedures for the production of the vaccine.

Collectively, results achieved in clinical trials have shown that it is possible to boost cellular immune responses against autologous B-cell tumor in the majority of vaccinated patients. However, the frequent unfavorable clinical outcome suggests that such antitumor immunity is often hampered in vivo and cannot achieve therapeutic effects. In addition, according to the initial observation in mouse models, vaccination has demonstrated to most likely provide a therapeutic advantage when tumor size is limited. Immune tolerance mechanisms activated by neoplastic cells to avoid immune-mediated tumor control and eventually clearance thus represent major obstacles to the biological and clinical efficacy of anticancer immunotherapy. Most of these mechanisms are becoming clear, thus allowing the design of novel immunotherapeutic strategies in which vaccination may be combined with approaches able to revert tolerance and/or enhance immune activation [274]. Finally, since rituximab has become the standard of care for the treatment of B-cell NHL, in the future, large-scale studies should test the therapeutic advantage of antitumor vaccination after rituximab induction therapy.

Immunomodulatory Drugs

The immunomodulatory (IMiD) class of antineoplastic agents includes thalidomide and its derivatives lenalidomide, pomalidomide, and actimid. These compounds have initially been studied for the treatment of multiple myeloma and myelodysplastic syndrome achieving significant results. Compared to the parent compound, thalidomide analogs have equal or greater antitumor activity and less neurotoxicity. Although the precise mechanism of action of these agents is still unclear, they have demonstrated multiple effects not only on tumor cells but also on the tumor microenvironment. They directly impair tumor cell proliferation by inhibiting NF-kB, MAPK, STAT3, and AKT pathways and increasing the expression of the tumor suppressor p21 for the block of cell-cycle G1 phase [118, 275]. In addition, they favor the induction of apoptosis stimulating the intrinsic pathway. Effects on the tumor microenvironment include the downregulation of crucial cytokines for the survival and growth of hematologic malignancies (TNF-α, IL-6, IL-8, VEGF), the stimulation of T/NK cells effector functions, and the inhibition of Tregs [275–277].

Lenalidomide as monotherapy has demonstrated clinical activity against relapsed or refractory aggressive and indolent NHL, achieving an ORR of, respectively, 35 and 23%, with the most remarkable responses being observed in MCL patients [278, 279]. The single-agent activity in a relapsed setting has led to new trials with lenalidomide in combination with other agents. Based upon the findings that lenalidomide-mediated activation of NK cells may improve rituximab-induced ADCC, the combination of these two agents has started to be evaluated in clinical trials in patients with relapsed indolent lymphomas following rituximab therapy [280] or with previously untreated disease [281]. Initial results are promising; however, longer follow-up in a wider series of patients is required to clearly understand the clinical improvements of this combination and to bring forward its development to phase III studies. Lenalidomide is also currently being investigated in combination with R-CHOP21 in patients with newly diagnosed aggressive B-cell lymphomas and as maintenance therapy for patients with DLBCL [282].

Conclusions and Perspectives

A variety of novel targeted agents are demonstrating promising activity in NHL. Their study has rationally proceeded from basic laboratory research to preclinical test, followed, in case of successful results, by clinical evaluation. This intense process has rapidly led to the availability of several novel agents that are currently being investigated in NHL, including at least 3 proteasome inhibitors, at least 3 mTOR inhibitors, 6 PI3K inhibitors, at least 15 HDACi, and a number of new-generation anti-CD20 mAbs and mAbs with different specificities. Novel anti-CD20 mAbs offer the potential for enhancing the activity of rituximab, while agents directed against different targets the possibility for novel more active combinations. Signal transduction inhibitors represent an emerging invaluable therapeutic option for lymphomas. Several agents designed for interfering with crucial pathways of B-cell NHL, such as those mediated by PI3K, BCR, and PKC, are being evaluated in clinical trials. However, the clinical benefit of new compounds, used alone and in combination regimens, still needs to be validated in randomized comparative trials with rituximab alone and/or in rituximab-refractory patients. A clear understanding of the off-target effects and the toxicity profile of these agents together with the identification of biomarkers and predictors for response will be critical to identify optimal drug combinations and the most efficacious treatment schedule for being evaluated in more advanced clinical trials. Indeed, we are now only starting to appreciate the tip of the iceberg of the complex regulatory signaling network that targeted agents provide, besides the inhibition of the specific biotarget.

The list of anticancer agents that can favor immune activation against tumor is incredibly growing. Novel and conventional therapies have shown the capability to render malignant cells more immunogenic and, thus, susceptible to a specific immune attack, or to, respectively, stimulate and inhibit effector and regulatory immune cells directly or as bystander effects induced in the tumor microenvironment [272]. Recently, the proof of principle that passive immunotherapy with rituximab may also elicit a tumor-specific T-cell immunity has been provided, demonstrating the "vaccinal properties" of a mAb therapy [283]. These findings open new possibilities for the design of rational chemoimmunotherapy combination strategies for maximal cytotoxic and antitumor immune effects.

Another relevant property of certain anticancer agents for the design of rational combination regimens is their ability of targeting molecules per se non-oncogenic but crucial for the maintenance of oncogenic pathways in cancer cells. It is becoming clearer and clearer that cancer cells, due to their genomic instability, exceed telomeres shortening, altered protein content caused by overexpression of oncogenes and prosurvival factors, and adaptation to hypoxic conditions, are more dependent on stress response pathways for their survival compared to normal cells. Thus therapeutic agents interfering with these functions should display a sufficiently large therapeutic window for killing malignant while sparing normal cells and are now considered attractive agents to be used in combination regimens for improving the treatment of cancer. As an example, cancer cells counteract proteotoxic stress by overexpressing HSPs that promote the proper folding or the proteolytic degradation of the client

proteins. HSP90 has been found to chaperone several proteins involved in the pathogenesis of lymphoma, including AKT, NF-kB complexes, anaplastic lymphoma kinase (ALK), and BCL-6 [284, 285]. Its targeting has been thus seen as an attractive way to concurrently affect multiple oncogenic pathways in lymphoma cells, and a logical strategy to be combined with conventional (gemcitabine, cytarabine, or cisplatin) as well as novel anticancer agents (HDACi, proteasome inhibitors, etc.) [134, 286, 287].

The clinical study of the new available agents presents also substantial challenge. Indeed, given that many of the new molecules are rather cytostatic than cytotoxic, the absence of response in heavily pretreated patients in phase I and II trials may not necessarily means lack of efficacy. Therefore, it will be important to redefine the major goal of early clinical evaluation with such drugs to test their potential benefit in combination with established regimens in more advanced studies.

Finally, on the basis of the positive experience achieved with the molecular studies of DLBCL, one can speculate that, in the future, GEP will lead to a better definition of lymphoma subtypes and to the use of risk analysis to individualized treatment. Indeed, molecular profiling may allow to identify the most relevant signaling pathways within a tumor and to determine the most suitable nodes to be inhibited using a specific and more effective treatment. In addition, it is likely that the possibility of monitoring the activity of the targeted pathway before and during therapy will provide novel predictor markers of response.

With these continuing advances, we can most likely envisage the possibility of a significant improvement for the management of lymphoma patients.

References

1. Jemal A, Siegel R, Xu J, Ward E. Cancer statistics, 2010. CA Cancer J Clin. 2010;60(5):277–300.
2. Fisher SG, Fisher RI. The epidemiology of non-Hodgkin's lymphoma. Oncogene. 2004;23(38):6524–34.
3. Brack C, Hirama M, Lenhard-Schuller R, Tonegawa S. A complete immunoglobulin gene is created by somatic recombination. Cell. 1978;15(1):1–14.

4. Rajewsky K. Clonal selection and learning in the antibody system. Nature. 1996;381(6585):751–8.
5. Batista FD, Harwood NE. The who, how and where of antigen presentation to B cells. Nat Rev Immunol. 2009;9(1):15–27.
6. LeBien TW, Tedder TF. B lymphocytes: how they develop and function. Blood. 2008;112(5):1570–80.
7. Shaffer AL, Yu X, He Y, Boldrick J, Chan EP, Staudt LM. BCL-6 represses genes that function in lymphocyte differentiation, inflammation, and cell cycle control. Immunity. 2000;13(2):199–212.
8. Klein U, Casola S, Cattoretti G, et al. Transcription factor IRF4 controls plasma cell differentiation and class-switch recombination. Nat Immunol. 2006;7(7): 773–82.
9. Shaffer AL, Lin KI, Kuo TC, et al. Blimp-1 orchestrates plasma cell differentiation by extinguishing the mature B cell gene expression program. Immunity. 2002;17(1):51–62.
10. Epstein FH, Küppers R, Klein U, Hansmann M-L, Rajewsky K. Cellular origin of human B-cell lymphomas. N Engl J Med. 1999;341:1520–9.
11. Shaffer AL, Rosenwald A, Staudt LM. Lymphoid malignancies: the dark side of B-cell differentiation. Nat Rev Immunol. 2002;2(12):920–32.
12. Küppers R. Mechanisms of B-cell lymphoma pathogenesis. Nat Rev Cancer. 2005;5:251–62.
13. The JES. WHO classification of lymphomas: implications for clinical practice and translational research. Hematology (Am Soc Hematol Educ Program). 2008;2009:523–31.
14. Küppers R, Dalla-Favera R. Mechanisms of chromosomal translocations in B cell lymphomas. Oncogene. 2001;20:5580–94.
15. Willis TG, Dyer MJ. The role of immunoglobulin translocations in the pathogenesis of B-cell malignancies. Blood. 2000;96(3):808–22.
16. Jäger U, Böcskör S, Le T, et al. Follicular lymphomas' BCL-2/IgH junctions contain templated nucleotide insertions: novel insights into the mechanism of t(14;18) translocation. Blood. 2000;95:3520–9.
17. Bross L, Fukita Y, McBlane F, Démolliére C, Rajewsky K, Jacobs H. DNA double-strand breaks in immunoglobulin genes undergoing somatic hypermutation. Immunity. 2000;13(5):589–97.
18. Esser C, Radbruch A. Immunoglobulin class switching: molecular and cellular analysis. Annu Rev Immunol. 1990;8(1):717–35.
19. Pasqualucci L, Bereschenko O, Niu H, et al. Molecular pathogenesis of non-Hodgkin's lymphoma: the role of Bcl-6. Leuk Lymphoma. 2003;44 Suppl 3:S5–12.
20. Klein U, Tu Y, Stolovitzky GA, et al. Transcriptional analysis of the B cell germinal center reaction. Proc Natl Acad Sci USA. 2003;100(5):2639–44.
21. Magner WJ, Kazim AL, Stewart C, et al. Activation of MHC class I, II, and CD40 gene expression by histone deacetylase inhibitors. J Immunol. 2000; 165(12):7017–24.
22. Lemoine M, Younes A. Histone deacetylase inhibitors in the treatment of lymphoma. Discov Med. 2010;10(54):462–70.
23. Lenz G, Nagel I, Siebert R, et al. Aberrant immunoglobulin class switch recombination and switch translocations in activated B cell-like diffuse large B cell lymphoma. J Exp Med. 2007;204(3):633–43.
24. Lenz G, Wright GW, Emre NC, et al. Molecular subtypes of diffuse large B-cell lymphoma arise by distinct genetic pathways. Proc Natl Acad Sci USA. 2008;105(36):13520–5.
25. Davis RE, Brown KD, Siebenlist U, Staudt LM. Constitutive nuclear factor kappaB activity is required for survival of activated B cell-like diffuse large B cell lymphoma cells. J Exp Med. 2001;194(12): 1861–74.
26. Davis RE, Ngo VN, Lenz G, et al. Chronic active B-cell-receptor signalling in diffuse large B-cell lymphoma. Nature. 2010;463(7277):88–92.
27. Reeder CB, Ansell SM. Novel therapeutic agents for B-cell lymphoma: developing rational combinations. Blood. 2011;117(5):1453–62.
28. Rui L, Emre NC, Kruhlak MJ, et al. Cooperative epigenetic modulation by cancer amplicon genes. Cancer cell. 2010;18(6):590–605.
29. Choi WW, Weisenburger DD, Greiner TC, et al. A new immunostain algorithm classifies diffuse large B-cell lymphoma into molecular subtypes with high accuracy. Clin Cancer Res. 2009;15(17):5494–502.
30. Lenz G, Wright G, Dave SS, et al. Stromal gene signatures in large-B-cell lymphomas. N Engl J Med. 2008;359(22):2313–23.
31. Armitage JO, Weisenburger DD. New approach to classifying non-Hodgkin's lymphomas: clinical features of the major histologic subtypes. Non-Hodgkin's Lymphoma Classification Project. J Clin Oncol. 1998;16(8):2780–95.
32. Dave SS, Wright G, Tan B, et al. Prediction of survival in follicular lymphoma based on molecular features of tumor-infiltrating immune cells. N Engl J Med. 2004;351(21):2159–69.
33. Ngan B-Y, Chen-Levy Z, Weiss LM, Warnke RA, Cleary ML. Expression in non-Hodgkin's lymphoma of the bcl-2 protein associated with the t(14;18) chromosomal translocation. N Engl J Med. 1988; 318(25):1638–44.
34. Pezzella F, Tse AG, Cordell JL, Pulford KA, Gatter KC, Mason DY. Expression of the bcl-2 oncogene protein is not specific for the 14;18 chromosomal translocation. Am J Pathol. 1990;137(2):225–32.
35. Hiddemann W, Buske C, Dreyling M, et al. Treatment strategies in follicular lymphomas: current status and future perspectives. J Clin Oncol. 2005;23(26): 6394–9.
36. Rosenberg SA. Follicular lymphoma revisited. J Clin Oncol. 2008;26(4):515–6.
37. Lossos IS. Higher-grade transformation of follicular lymphoma – a continuous enigma. Leukemia. 2005; 19(8):1331–3.

38. Horning SJ, Rosenberg SA. The natural history of initially untreated low-grade non-Hodgkin's lymphomas. N Engl J Med. 1984;311(23):1471–5.
39. O'Brien ME, Easterbrook P, Powell J, et al. The natural history of low grade non-Hodgkin's lymphoma and the impact of a no initial treatment policy on survival. Q J Med. 1991;80(292):651–60.
40. Rohatiner AZ, Lister TA. The clinical course of follicular lymphoma. Best Pract Res Clin Haematol. 2005;18(1):1–10.
41. Montoto S, Davies AJ, Matthews J, et al. Risk and clinical implications of transformation of follicular lymphoma to diffuse large B-cell lymphoma. J Clin Oncol. 2007;25(17):2426–33.
42. Herreros B, Sanchez-Aguilera A, Piris MA. Lymphoma microenvironment: culprit or innocent? Leukemia. 2008;22(1):49–58.
43. Glas AM, Knoops L, Delahaye L, et al. Gene-expression and immunohistochemical study of specific T-cell subsets and accessory cell types in the transformation and prognosis of follicular lymphoma. J Clin Oncol. 2007;25(4):390–8.
44. Alvaro T, Lejeune M, Salvado MT, et al. Immunohistochemical patterns of reactive microenvironment are associated with clinicobiologic behavior in follicular lymphoma patients. J Clin Oncol. 2006; 24(34):5350–7.
45. Wotherspoon AC, Doglioni C, Diss TC, et al. Regression of primary low-grade B-cell gastric lymphoma of mucosa-associated lymphoid tissue type after eradication of Helicobacter pylori. Lancet. 1993;342(8871):575–7.
46. Hermine O, Lefrere F, Bronowicki JP, et al. Regression of splenic lymphoma with villous lymphocytes after treatment of hepatitis C virus infection. N Engl J Med. 2002;347(2):89–94.
47. Sagaert X, De Wolf-Peeters C, Noels H, Baens M. The pathogenesis of MALT lymphomas: where do we stand? Leukemia. 2007;21(3):389–96.
48. Dave SS. Follicular lymphoma and the microenvironment. Blood. 2008;111(9):4427–8.
49. de Jong D. Molecular pathogenesis of follicular lymphoma: a cross talk of genetic and immunologic factors. J Clin Oncol. 2005;23(26):6358–63.
50. Eray M, Postila V, Eeva J, et al. Follicular lymphoma cell lines, an in vitro model for antigenic selection and cytokine-mediated growth regulation of germinal centre B cells. Scand J Immunol. 2003;57(6): 545–55.
51. Goval JJ, Thielen C, Bourguignon C, et al. The prevention of spontaneous apoptosis of follicular lymphoma B cells by a follicular dendritic cell line: involvement of caspase-3, caspase-8 and c-FLIP. Haematologica. 2008;93(8):1169–77.
52. Farinha P, Al-Tourah A, Gill K, Klasa R, Connors JM, Gascoyne RD. The architectural pattern of FOXP3-positive T cells in follicular lymphoma is an independent predictor of survival and histologic transformation. Blood. 2010;115:289–95.
53. Yang Z-Z, Novak AJ, Stenson MJ, Witzig TE, Ansell SM. Intratumoral CD4+CD25+ regulatory T-cell-mediated suppression of infiltrating CD4+ T cells in B-cell non-Hodgkin lymphoma. Blood. 2006;107(9): 3639–46.
54. Yang ZZ, Novak AJ, Ziesmer SC, Witzig TE, Ansell SM. CD70+ non-Hodgkin lymphoma B cells induce Foxp3 expression and regulatory function in intratumoral CD4+CD25- T cells. Blood. 2007;110(7): 2537–44.
55. Ai WZ, Hou JZ, Zeiser R, Czerwinski D, Negrin RS, Levy R. Follicular lymphoma B cells induce the conversion of conventional CD4+ T cells to T-regulatory cells. Int J Cancer. 2009;124(1):239–44.
56. Tiemessen MM, Jagger AL, Evans HG, van Herwijnen MJC, John S, Taams LS. CD4+CD25+Foxp3+ regulatory T cells induce alternative activation of human monocytes/macrophages. Proc Natl Acad Sci USA. 2007;104(49):19446–51.
57. Alvaro T, Lejeune M, Camacho FI, et al. The presence of STAT1-positive tumor-associated macrophages and their relation to outcome in patients with follicular lymphoma. Haematologica. 2006;91: 1605–12.
58. Farinha P, Masoudi H, Skinnider BF, et al. Analysis of multiple biomarkers shows that lymphoma-associated macrophage (LAM) content is an independent predictor of survival in follicular lymphoma (FL). Blood. 2005;106(6):2169–74.
59. Lee AM, Clear AJ, Calaminici M, et al. Number of CD4+ cells and location of forkhead box protein P3-positive cells in diagnostic follicular lymphoma tissue microarrays correlates with outcome. J Clin Oncol. 2006;24(31):5052–9.
60. Keating MJ, O'Brien S, Albitar M, et al. Early results of a chemoimmunotherapy regimen of fludarabine, cyclophosphamide, and rituximab as initial therapy for chronic lymphocytic leukemia. J Clin Oncol. 2005;23(18):4079–88.
61. Leget GA, Czuczman MS. Use of rituximab, the new FDA-approved antibody. Curr Opin Oncol. 1998; 10(6):548–51.
62. Marcus R, Imrie K, Belch A, et al. CVP chemotherapy plus rituximab compared with CVP as first-line treatment for advanced follicular lymphoma. Blood. 2005;105(4):1417–23.
63. Hiddemann W, Kneba M, Dreyling M, et al. Frontline therapy with rituximab added to the combination of cyclophosphamide, doxorubicin, vincristine, and prednisone (CHOP) significantly improves the outcome for patients with advanced-stage follicular lymphoma compared with therapy with CHOP alone: results of a prospective randomized study of the German Low-Grade Lymphoma Study Group. Blood. 2005;106(12):3725–32.
64. Herold M, Haas A, Srock S, et al. Rituximab added to first-line mitoxantrone, chlorambucil, and prednisolone chemotherapy followed by interferon maintenance prolongs survival in patients with advanced follicular

lymphoma: an East German Study Group Hematology and Oncology Study. J Clin Oncol. 2007;25(15): 1986–92.

65. Schulz H, Bohlius JF, Trelle S, et al. Immunochemotherapy with rituximab and overall survival in patients with indolent or mantle cell lymphoma: a systematic review and meta-analysis. J Natl Cancer Inst. 2007;99(9):706–14.

66. Tan D, Horning SJ. Follicular lymphoma: clinical features and treatment. Hematol Oncol Clin North Am. 2008;22(5):863–82.

67. Vose JM, Link BK, Grossbard ML, et al. Phase II study of rituximab in combination with chop chemotherapy in patients with previously untreated, aggressive non-Hodgkin's lymphoma. J Clin Oncol. 2001;19(2):389–97.

68. Press OW, Leonard JP, Coiffier B, Levy R, Timmerman J. Immunotherapy of non-Hodgkin's lymphomas. Hematology Am Soc Hematol Educ Program. 2001(1);221–40.

69. Zelenetz AD, Abramson JS, Advani RH, et al. NCCN Clinical Practice Guidelines in Oncology: non-Hodgkin's lymphomas. J Natl Compr Canc Netw. 2010;8(3):288–334.

70. Pfreundschuh M, Trumper L, Osterborg A, et al. CHOP-like chemotherapy plus rituximab versus CHOP-like chemotherapy alone in young patients with good-prognosis diffuse large-B-cell lymphoma: a randomised controlled trial by the MabThera International Trial (MInT) Group. Lancet Oncol. 2006;7(5):379–91.

71. Habermann TM, Weller EA, Morrison VA, et al. Rituximab-CHOP versus CHOP alone or with maintenance rituximab in older patients with diffuse large B-cell lymphoma. J Clin Oncol. 2006;24(19):3121–7.

72. Pfreundschuh M, Trumper L, Kloess M, et al. Two-weekly or 3-weekly CHOP chemotherapy with or without etoposide for the treatment of elderly patients with aggressive lymphomas: results of the NHL-B2 trial of the DSHNHL. Blood. 2004;104(3):634–41.

73. Pfreundschuh M, Schubert J, Ziepert M, et al. Six versus eight cycles of bi-weekly CHOP-14 with or without rituximab in elderly patients with aggressive CD20+ B-cell lymphomas: a randomised controlled trial (RICOVER-60). Lancet Oncol. 2008;9(2): 105–16.

74. Gribben JG, How I. treat indolent lymphoma. Blood. 2007;109(11):4617–26.

75. Solal-Celigny P, Roy P, Colombat P, et al. Follicular lymphoma international prognostic index. Blood. 2004;104(5):1258–65.

76. Buske C, Hoster E, Dreyling M, Hasford J, Unterhalt M, Hiddemann W. The Follicular Lymphoma International Prognostic Index (FLIPI) separates high-risk from intermediate- or low-risk patients with advanced-stage follicular lymphoma treated front-line with rituximab and the combination of cyclophosphamide, doxorubicin, vincristine, and prednisone (R-CHOP) with respect to treatment outcome. Blood. 2006;108(5):1504–8.

77. Federico M, Bellei M, Marcheselli L, et al. Follicular lymphoma international prognostic index 2: a new prognostic index for follicular lymphoma developed by the international follicular lymphoma prognostic factor project. J Clin Oncol. 2009;27(27):4555–62.

78. Vitolo U, Ferreri AsJM, Montoto S. Follicular lymphomas. Crit Rev Oncol Hematol. 2008;66(3): 248–61.

79. Hoppe RT, Kushlan P, Kaplan HS, Rosenberg SA, Brown BW. The treatment of advanced stage favorable histology non-Hodgkin's lymphoma: a preliminary report of a randomized trial comparing single agent chemotherapy, combination chemotherapy, and whole body irradiation. Blood. 1981; 58(3):592–8.

80. Vaughan Hudson B, Vaughan Hudson G, MacLennan KA, Anderson L, Linch DC. Clinical stage 1 non-Hodgkin's lymphoma: long-term follow-up of patients treated by the British National Lymphoma Investigation with radiotherapy alone as initial therapy. Br J Cancer. 1994;69(6):1088–93.

81. Wilder RB, Jones D, Tucker SL, et al. Long-term results with radiotherapy for Stage I-II follicular lymphomas. Int J Radiat Oncol Biol Phys. 2001;51(5): 1219–27.

82. Colombat P, Salles G, Brousse N, et al. Rituximab (anti-CD20 monoclonal antibody) as single first-line therapy for patients with follicular lymphoma with a low tumor burden: clinical and molecular evaluation. Blood. 2001;97(1):101–6.

83. Hainsworth JD, Burris 3rd HA, Morrissey LH, et al. Rituximab monoclonal antibody as initial systemic therapy for patients with low-grade non-Hodgkin lymphoma. Blood. 2000;95(10):3052–6.

84. Hainsworth JD. Monoclonal antibody therapy in lymphoid malignancies. Oncologist. 2000;5(5): 376–84.

85. Solal-Celigny P. Rituximab as first-line monotherapy in low-grade follicular lymphoma with a low tumor burden. Anticancer Drugs. 2001;12 Suppl 2:S11–4.

86. Brice P, Bastion Y, Lepage E, et al. Comparison in low-tumor-burden follicular lymphomas between an initial no-treatment policy, prednimustine, or interferon alfa: a randomized study from the Groupe d'Etude des Lymphomes Folliculaires. Groupe d'Etude des Lymphomes de l'Adulte. J Clin Oncol. 1997;15(3):1110–7.

87. van Oers MH, Klasa R, Marcus RE, et al. Rituximab maintenance improves clinical outcome of relapsed/resistant follicular non-Hodgkin lymphoma in patients both with and without rituximab during induction: results of a prospective randomized phase 3 intergroup trial. Blood. 2006;108(10):3295–301.

88. Salles G, Seymour JF, Offner F, et al. Rituximab maintenance for 2 years in patients with high tumour burden follicular lymphoma responding to rituximab plus chemotherapy (PRIMA): a phase 3, randomised controlled trial. Lancet. 2011;377(9759):42 51.

89. McLaughlin P, Grillo-Lopez AJ, Link BK, et al. Rituximab chimeric anti-CD20 monoclonal antibody

therapy for relapsed indolent lymphoma: half of patients respond to a four-dose treatment program. J Clin Oncol. 1998;16(8):2825–33.

90. McLaughlin P, Hagemeister FB, Grillo-Lopez AJ. Rituximab in indolent lymphoma: the single-agent pivotal trial. Semin Oncol. 1999;26(5 Suppl 14): 79–87.

91. Freedman AS, Ritz J, Neuberg D, et al. Autologous bone marrow transplantation in 69 patients with a history of low-grade B-cell non-Hodgkin's lymphoma. Blood. 1991;77(11):2524–9.

92. Freedman AS, Neuberg D, Mauch P, et al. Long-term follow-up of autologous bone marrow transplantation in patients with relapsed follicular lymphoma. Blood. 1999;94(10):3325–33.

93. Apostolidis J, Gupta RK, Grenzelias D, et al. High-dose therapy with autologous bone marrow support as consolidation of remission in follicular lymphoma: long-term clinical and molecular follow-up. J Clin Oncol. 2000;18(3):527–36.

94. Rohatiner AZ, Nadler L, Davies AJ, et al. Myeloablative therapy with autologous bone marrow transplantation for follicular lymphoma at the time of second or subsequent remission: long-term follow-up. J Clin Oncol. 2007;25(18):2554–9.

95. Toze CL, Barnett MJ, Connors JM, et al. Long-term disease-free survival of patients with advanced follicular lymphoma after allogeneic bone marrow transplantation. Br J Haematol. 2004;127(3):311–21.

96. Gribben JG, Zahrieh D, Stephans K, et al. Autologous and allogeneic stem cell transplantations for poor-risk chronic lymphocytic leukemia. Blood. 2005; 106(13):4389–96.

97. Morris E, Thomson K, Craddock C, et al. Outcomes after alemtuzumab-containing reduced-intensity allogeneic transplantation regimen for relapsed and refractory non-Hodgkin lymphoma. Blood. 2004; 104(13):3865–71.

98. Rezvani AR, Storer B, Maris M, et al. Nonmyeloablative allogeneic hematopoietic cell transplantation in relapsed, refractory, and transformed indolent non-Hodgkin's lymphoma. J Clin Oncol. 2008;26(2):211–7.

99. Khouri IF, McLaughlin P, Saliba RM, et al. Eight-year experience with allogeneic stem cell transplantation for relapsed follicular lymphoma after nonmyeloablative conditioning with fludarabine, cyclophosphamide, and rituximab. Blood. 2008; 111(12):5530–6.

100. Friedberg JW, Cohen P, Chen L, et al. Bendamustine in patients with rituximab-refractory indolent and transformed non-Hodgkin's lymphoma: results from a phase II multicenter, single-agent study. J Clin Oncol. 2008;26(2):204–10.

101. Czuczman MS, Rummel MJ. Clinical Roundtable Monograph: recent advances in NHL. Highlights from the 51st ASH Annual Meeting and Exposition, December 5–8, 2009, New Orleans, Louisiana. Clin Adv Hematol Oncol. 2010;8(2):A1–11.

102. Sirotnak FM, DeGraw JI, Colwell WT, Piper JR. A new analogue of 10-deazaaminopterin with markedly enhanced curative effects against human tumor xenografts in mice. Cancer Chemother Pharmacol. 1998;42(4):313–8.

103. O'Connor OA, Hamlin PA, Portlock C, et al. Pralatrexate, a novel class of antifol with high affinity for the reduced folate carrier-type 1, produces marked complete and durable remissions in a diversity of chemotherapy refractory cases of T-cell lymphoma. Br J Haematol. 2007;139(3):425–8.

104. Engert A, Herbrecht R, Santoro A, Zinzani PL, Gorbatchevsky I. EXTEND PIX301: a phase III randomized trial of pixantrone versus other chemotherapeutic agents as third-line monotherapy in patients with relapsed, aggressive non-Hodgkin's lymphoma. Clin Lymphoma Myeloma. 2006;7(2): 152–4.

105. Gururajan M, Dasu T, Shahidain S, et al. Spleen tyrosine kinase (Syk), a novel target of curcumin, is required for B lymphoma growth. J Immunol. 2007;178(1):111–21.

106. Gururajan M, Jennings CD, Bondada S. Cutting edge: constitutive B cell receptor signaling is critical for basal growth of B lymphoma. J Immunol. 2006;176(10):5715–9.

107. Platanias LC. Map kinase signaling pathways and hematologic malignancies. Blood. 2003;101(12): 4667–79.

108. Soriano AO, Yang H, Faderl S, et al. Safety and clinical activity of the combination of 5-azacytidine, valproic acid, and all-trans retinoic acid in acute myeloid leukemia and myelodysplastic syndrome. Blood. 2007;110(7):2302–8.

109. Tolcher AW, Mita A, Lewis LD, et al. Phase I and pharmacokinetic study of YM155, a small-molecule inhibitor of survivin. J Clin Oncol. 2008;26(32): 5198–203.

110. Gupta M, Ansell SM, Novak AJ, Kumar S, Kaufmann SH, Witzig TE. Inhibition of histone deacetylase overcomes rapamycin-mediated resistance in diffuse large B-cell lymphoma by inhibiting Akt signaling through mTORC2. Blood. 2009;114(14):2926–35.

111. Bjornsti MA, Houghton PJ. The TOR pathway: a target for cancer therapy. Nat Rev Cancer. 2004;4(5): 335–48.

112. Coiffier B, Lepretre S, Pedersen LM, et al. Safety and efficacy of ofatumumab, a fully human monoclonal anti-CD20 antibody, in patients with relapsed or refractory B-cell chronic lymphocytic leukemia: a phase 1–2 study. Blood. 2008;111(3):1094–100.

113. Kausar F, Mustafa K, Sweis G, et al. Ocrelizumab: a step forward in the evolution of B-cell therapy. Expert Opin Biol Ther. 2009;9(7):889–95.

114. Kaminski MS, Kitamura K, Maloney DG, Levy R. Idiotype vaccination against murine B cell lymphoma. Inhibition of tumor immunity by free idiotype protein. J Immunol. 1987;138(4):1289–96.

115. Advani R, Sharman JP, Smith SM, et al. Effect of Btk inhibitor PCI-32765 monotherapy on responses in patients with relapsed aggressive NHL: Evidence of antitumor activity from a phase I study. J Clin Oncol. 2010;28:15s(suppl; abstr 8012).

116. Nowakowski GS, Maurer MJ, Habermann TM, et al. Statin use and prognosis in patients with diffuse large B-cell lymphoma and follicular lymphoma in the rituximab era. J Clin Oncol. 2010;28(3):412–7.

117. Kwak LW, Campbell M, Levy R. Idiotype vaccination post-bone marrow transplantation for B-cell lymphoma: initial studies in a murine model. Cancer Detect Prev. 1991;15(4):323–5.

118. Anderson KC. Lenalidomide and thalidomide: mechanisms of action–similarities and differences. Semin Hematol. 2005;42(4 Suppl 4):S3–8.

119. Morschhauser F, Seymour JF, Kluin-Nelemans HC, et al. A phase II study of enzastaurin, a protein kinase C beta inhibitor, in patients with relapsed or refractory mantle cell lymphoma. Ann Oncol. 2008;19(2):247–53.

120. Schwartzberg L, Hermann RC, Flinn IW, et al. Enzastaurin in patients with follicular lymphoma: Results of a phase II study. J Clin Oncol. 2010;28:15s, (suppl; abstr 8040).

121. Lannutti BJ, Meadows SA, Herman SE, et al. CAL-101, a p110delta selective phosphatidylinositol-3-kinase inhibitor for the treatment of B-cell malignancies, inhibits PI3K signaling and cellular viability. Blood. 2011;117(2):591–4.

122. Furman et al. ASCO 2010, abstract 3032.

123. Kahl et al. ASH annual meeting 2010, abstract 1777.

124. Furman et al. ASH annual meeting 2010, abstract 55.

125. Hoellenriegel et al. ASH annual meeting 2010, abstract 48.

126. Flinn et al. ASH annual meeting 2010, abstract 2832.

127. Hideshima T, Catley L, Yasui H, et al. Perifosine, an oral bioactive novel alkylphospholipid, inhibits Akt and induces in vitro and in vivo cytotoxicity in human multiple myeloma cells. Blood. 2006;107(10):4053–62.

128. Witzig TE, Geyer SM, Ghobrial I, et al. Phase II trial of single-agent temsirolimus (CCI-779) for relapsed mantle cell lymphoma. J Clin Oncol. 2005;23(23):5347–56.

129. Ansell SM, Inwards DJ, Rowland Jr KM, et al. Low-dose, single-agent temsirolimus for relapsed mantle cell lymphoma: a phase 2 trial in the North Central Cancer Treatment Group. Cancer. 2008;113(3):508–14.

130. Hess G, Herbrecht R, Romaguera J, et al. Phase III study to evaluate temsirolimus compared with investigator's choice therapy for the treatment of relapsed or refractory mantle cell lymphoma. J Clin Oncol. 2009;27(23):3822–9.

131. Smith SM, van Besien K, Karrison T, et al. Temsirolimus has activity in non-mantle cell non-Hodgkin's lymphoma subtypes: The University of Chicago phase II consortium. J Clin Oncol. 2010;28(31):4740–6.

132. Haritunians T, Mori A, O'Kelly J, Luong QT, Giles FJ, Koeffler HP. Antiproliferative activity of RAD001 (everolimus) as a single agent and combined with other agents in mantle cell lymphoma. Leukemia. 2007;21(2):333–9.

133. Zent CS, LaPlant BR, Johnston PB, et al. The treatment of recurrent/refractory chronic lymphocytic leukemia/small lymphocytic lymphoma (CLL) with everolimus results in clinical responses and mobilization of CLL cells into the circulation. Cancer. 2010;116(9):2201–7.

134. Best OG, Singh N, Forsyth C, Mulligan SP. The novel Hsp-90 inhibitor SNX7081 is significantly more potent than 17-AAG against primary CLL cells and a range of haematological cell lines, irrespective of lesions in the TP53 pathway. Br J Haematol. 2010;151(2):185–8.

135. Widmann T, Sester U, Gartner BC, et al. Levels of CMV specific CD4 T cells are dynamic and correlate with CMV viremia after allogeneic stem cell transplantation. PLoS One. 2008;3(11):e3634.

136. Held G, Schubert J, Pfreundschuh M. [Treatment of hematological malignancies with monoclonal antibodies]. Internist (Berl). 2008;49(8):929–30, 932–4, 936–7.

137. Orlowski RZ, Baldwin Jr AS. NF-kappaB as a therapeutic target in cancer. Trends Mol Med. 2002;8(8):385–9.

138. Chauhan D, Uchiyama H, Akbarali Y, et al. Multiple myeloma cell adhesion-induced interleukin-6 expression in bone marrow stromal cells involves activation of NF-kappa B. Blood. 1996;87(3):1104–12.

139. Goy A, Younes A, McLaughlin P, et al. Phase II study of proteasome inhibitor bortezomib in relapsed or refractory B-cell non-Hodgkin's lymphoma. J Clin Oncol. 2005;23(4):667–75.

140. Goy A, Bernstein SH, Kahl BS, et al. Bortezomib in patients with relapsed or refractory mantle cell lymphoma: updated time-to-event analyses of the multicenter phase 2 PINNACLE study. Ann Oncol. 2009;20(3):520–5.

141. Di Bella N, Taetle R, Kolibaba K, et al. Results of a phase 2 study of bortezomib in patients with relapsed or refractory indolent lymphoma. Blood. 2010;115(3):475–80.

142. O'Connor OA, Portlock C, Moskowitz C, et al. Time to treatment response in patients with follicular lymphoma treated with bortezomib is longer compared with other histologic subtypes. Clin Cancer Res. 2010;16(2):719–26.

143. Dunleavy K, Pittaluga S, Czuczman MS, et al. Differential efficacy of bortezomib plus chemotherapy within molecular subtypes of diffuse large B-cell lymphoma. Blood. 2009;113(24):6069–76.

144. Kupperman et al. ASCO 2009, abstract 5636.

145. Piva R, Ruggeri B, Williams M, et al. CEP-18770: a novel, orally active proteasome inhibitor with a tumor-selective pharmacologic profile competitive with bortezomib. Blood. 2008;111(5):2765–75.

146. Kuhn DJ, Chen Q, Voorhees PM, et al. Potent activity of carfilzomib, a novel, irreversible inhibitor of the ubiquitin-proteasome pathway, against preclinical models of multiple myeloma. Blood. 2007;110(9):3281–90.

147. Paoluzzi L, Gonen M, Gardner JR, et al. Targeting Bcl-2 family members with the BH3 mimetic AT-101

markedly enhances the therapeutic effects of chemotherapeutic agents in in vitro and in vivo models of B-cell lymphoma. Blood. 2008;111(11):5350–8.

148. O'Connor OA, Stewart AK, Vallone M, et al. A phase 1 dose escalation study of the safety and pharmacokinetics of the novel proteasome inhibitor carfilzomib (PR-171) in patients with hematologic malignancies. Clin Cancer Res. 2009;15(22):7085–91.

149. Chauhan D, Catley L, Li G, et al. A novel orally active proteasome inhibitor induces apoptosis in multiple myeloma cells with mechanisms distinct from Bortezomib. Cancer cell. 2005;8(5):407–19.

150. Kuhn DJ, Hunsucker SA, Chen Q, Voorhees PM, Orlowski M, Orlowski RZ. Targeted inhibition of the immunoproteasome is a potent strategy against models of multiple myeloma that overcomes resistance to conventional drugs and nonspecific proteasome inhibitors. Blood. 2009;113(19):4667–76.

151. Jones PA, Baylin SB. The epigenomics of cancer. Cell. 2007;128(4):683–92.

152. Pandolfi PP. Histone deacetylases and transcriptional therapy with their inhibitors. Cancer Chemother Pharmacol. 2001;48 Suppl 1:S17–9.

153. Glozak MA, Sengupta N, Zhang X, Seto E. Acetylation and deacetylation of non-histone proteins. Gene. 2005;363:15–23.

154. Kurland JF, Tansey WP. Myc-mediated transcriptional repression by recruitment of histone deacetylase. Cancer Res. 2008;68(10):3624–9.

155. Burgess A, Ruefli A, Beamish H, et al. Histone deacetylase inhibitors specifically kill nonproliferating tumour cells. Oncogene. 2004;23(40):6693–701.

156. Bolden JE, Peart MJ, Johnstone RW. Anticancer activities of histone deacetylase inhibitors. Nat Rev Drug Discov. 2006;5(9):769–84.

157. Ma X, Ezzeldin HH, Diasio RB. Histone deacetylase inhibitors: current status and overview of recent clinical trials. Drugs. 2009;69(14):1911–34.

158. Deroanne CF, Bonjean K, Servotte S, et al. Histone deacetylases inhibitors as anti-angiogenic agents altering vascular endothelial growth factor signaling. Oncogene. 2002;21(3):427–36.

159. Liu LT, Chang HC, Chiang LC, Hung WC. Histone deacetylase inhibitor up-regulates RECK to inhibit MMP-2 activation and cancer cell invasion. Cancer Res. 2003;63(12):3069–72.

160. Kirschbaum et al. ASCO 2007, abstracts 18515.

161. Kirschbaum et al. ASH annual meeting 2008, abstract 1564.

162. Ottmann et al. ASH annual meeting 2008, abstract 958.

163. Zain et al. ASCO 2009, abstract 8580.

164. Furumai R, Matsuyama A, Kobashi N, et al. FK228 (depsipeptide) as a natural prodrug that inhibits class I histone deacetylases. Cancer Res. 2002;62(17): 4916–21.

165. Piekarz RL, Frye R, Turner M, et al. Phase II multi-institutional trial of the histone deacetylase inhibitor romidepsin as monotherapy for patients with cutaneous T-cell lymphoma. J Clin Oncol. 2009;27(32): 5410–7.

166. Crump et al. ASCO 2008, abstract 8528.

167. Younes et al. ASH annual meeting 2007, abstract 2571.

168. Gottlicher M, Minucci S, Zhu P, et al. Valproic acid defines a novel class of HDAC inhibitors inducing differentiation of transformed cells. EMBO J. 2001;20(24):6969–78.

169. Chung EJ, Lee MJ, Lee S, Trepel JB. Assays for pharmacodynamic analysis of histone deacetylase inhibitors. Expert Opin Drug Metab Toxicol. 2006; 2(2):213–30.

170. Bonfils C, Kalita A, Dubay M, et al. Evaluation of the pharmacodynamic effects of MGCD0103 from pre-clinical models to human using a novel HDAC enzyme assay. Clin Cancer Res. 2008;14(11):3441–9.

171. Fantin VR, Loboda A, Paweletz CP, et al. Constitutive activation of signal transducers and activators of transcription predicts vorinostat resistance in cutaneous T-cell lymphoma. Cancer Res. 2008;68(10): 3785–94.

172. Younes et al. ASH annual meeting 2010, abstract 2830.

173. Ganesan A, Nolan L, Crabb SJ, Packham G. Epigenetic therapy: histone acetylation, DNA methylation and anti-cancer drug discovery. Curr Cancer Drug Targets. 2009;9(8):963–81.

174. Garcia-Manero G. Demethylating agents in myeloid malignancies. Curr Opin Oncol. 2008;20(6):705–10.

175. Odenike et al. ASCO 2008, abstract 7057.

176. Pro B, Leber B, Smith M, et al. Phase II multicenter study of oblimersen sodium, a Bcl-2 antisense oligonucleotide, in combination with rituximab in patients with recurrent B-cell non-Hodgkin lymphoma. Br J Haematol. 2008;143(3):355–60.

177. Wilson et al. ASCO 2009, abstract 8574.

178. Hernandez-Ilizaliturr et al. ASH annual meeting 2009, abstract 114:288.

179. Goy et al. ASH annual meeting 2008, abstract 2569.

180. Andersen MH, Svane IM, Becker JC, Straten PT. The universal character of the tumor-associated antigen survivin. Clin Cancer Res. 2007;13(20):5991–4.

181. Oldenhuis et al. ASCO 2008, abstract 3540.

182. Younes et al. ASH annual meeting 2009, abstract 1708.

183. Ling et al. ASCO 2006, abstract 3047.

184. Yee et al. ASCO 2007, abstract 8078.

185. Lavazza C, Carlo-Stella C, Giacomini A, et al. Human CD34+ cells engineered to express membrane-bound tumor necrosis factor-related apoptosis-inducing ligand target both tumor cells and tumor vasculature. Blood. 2010;115:2231–40.

186. Tabe Y, Sebasigari D, Jin L, et al. MDM2 antagonist nutlin-3 displays antiproliferative and proapoptotic activity in mantle cell lymphoma. Clin Cancer Res. 2009;15(3):933–42.

187. Kohler G, Milstein C. Continuous cultures of fused cells secreting antibody of predefined specificity. Nature. 1975;256(5517):495–7.

188. Stashenko P, Nadler LM, Hardy R, Schlossman SF. Characterization of a human B lymphocyte-specific antigen. J Immunol. 1980;125(4):1678–85.

189. Cragg MS, Walshe CA, Ivanov AO, Glennie MJ. The biology of CD20 and its potential as a target for mAb therapy. Curr Dir Autoimmun. 2005;8:140–74.

190. Jazirehi AR, Bonavida B. Cellular and molecular signal transduction pathways modulated by rituximab (rituxan, anti-CD20 mAb) in non-Hodgkin's lymphoma: implications in chemosensitization and therapeutic intervention. Oncogene. 2005;24(13):2121–43.

191. Golay J, Zaffaroni L, Vaccari T, et al. Biologic response of B lymphoma cells to anti-CD20 monoclonal antibody rituximab in vitro: CD55 and CD59 regulate complement-mediated cell lysis. Blood. 2000;95(12):3900–8.

192. Pedersen IM, Buhl AM, Klausen P, Geisler CH, Jurlander J. The chimeric anti-CD20 antibody rituximab induces apoptosis in B-cell chronic lymphocytic leukemia cells through a p38 mitogen activated protein-kinase-dependent mechanism. Blood. 2002;99(4):1314–9.

193. Alas S, Emmanouilides C, Bonavida B. Inhibition of interleukin 10 by rituximab results in down-regulation of bcl-2 and sensitization of B-cell non-Hodgkin's lymphoma to apoptosis. Clin Cancer Res. 2001;7(3):709–23.

194. Davis TA, Grillo-Lopez AJ, White CA, et al. Rituximab anti-CD20 monoclonal antibody therapy in non-Hodgkin's lymphoma: safety and efficacy of re-treatment. J Clin Oncol. 2000;18(17):3135–43.

195. Teeling JL, French RR, Cragg MS, et al. Characterization of new human CD20 monoclonal antibodies with potent cytolytic activity against non-Hodgkin lymphomas. Blood. 2004;104(6):1793–800.

196. Hagenbeek A, Gadeberg O, Johnson P, et al. First clinical use of ofatumumab, a novel fully human anti-CD20 monoclonal antibody in relapsed or refractory follicular lymphoma: results of a phase 1/2 trial. Blood. 2008;111(12):5486–95.

197. Goldenberg DM, Rossi EA, Stein R, et al. Properties and structure-function relationships of veltuzumab (hA20), a humanized anti-CD20 monoclonal antibody. Blood. 2009;113(5):1062–70.

198. Morschhauser F, Leonard JP, Fayad L, et al. Humanized anti-CD20 antibody, veltuzumab, in refractory/recurrent non-Hodgkin's lymphoma: phase I/II results. J Clin Oncol. 2009;27(20):3346–53.

199. Milani C, Castillo J. Veltuzumab, an anti-CD20 mAb for the treatment of non-Hodgkin's lymphoma, chronic lymphocytic leukemia and immune thrombocytopenic purpura. Curr Opin Mol Ther. 2009;11(2):200–7.

200. Vugmeyster Y, Beyer J, Howell K, et al. Depletion of B cells by a humanized anti-CD20 antibody PRO70769 in Macaca fascicularis. J Immunother. 2005;28(3):212–9.

201. Cartron G, Dacheux L, Salles G, et al. Therapeutic activity of humanized anti-CD20 monoclonal antibody and polymorphism in IgG Fc receptor FcgammaRIIIa gene. Blood. 2002;99(3):754–8.

202. Weng WK, Levy R. Two immunoglobulin G fragment C receptor polymorphisms independently predict response to rituximab in patients with follicular lymphoma. J Clin Oncol. 2003;21(21):3940–7.

203. Bowles JA, Wang SY, Link BK, et al. Anti-CD20 monoclonal antibody with enhanced affinity for CD16 activates NK cells at lower concentrations and more effectively than rituximab. Blood. 2006;108(8):2648–54.

204. Salles GA. ASH annual meeting 2009, abstract 1704.

205. Leonard JP, Coleman M, Ketas JC, et al. Phase I/II trial of epratuzumab (humanized anti-CD22 antibody) in indolent non-Hodgkin's lymphoma. J Clin Oncol. 2003;21(16):3051–9.

206. Pathan NI, Chu P, Hariharan K, Cheney C, Molina A, Byrd J. Mediation of apoptosis by and antitumor activity of lumiliximab in chronic lymphocytic leukemia cells and CD23+ lymphoma cell lines. Blood. 2008;111(3):1594–602.

207. Czuczman MS, Thall A, Witzig TE, et al. Phase I/II study of galiximab, an anti-CD80 antibody, for relapsed or refractory follicular lymphoma. J Clin Oncol. 2005;23(19):4390–8.

208. Leonard JP, Coleman M, Ketas J, et al. Combination antibody therapy with epratuzumab and rituximab in relapsed or refractory non-Hodgkin's lymphoma. J Clin Oncol. 2005;23(22):5044–51.

209. Czuczman M. ASH annual meeting 2008, abstract 1003.

210. Friedberg et al. ASH annual meeting 2008, abstract 1004.

211. Micallef et al. ASCO 2009, abstract 8508.

212. Byrd et al. ASH annual meeting 2006, abstract 32.

213. Grdisa M. Influence of CD40 ligation on survival and apoptosis of B-CLL cells in vitro. Leuk Res. 2003;27(10):951–6.

214. Kater AP, Evers LM, Remmerswaal EB, et al. CD40 stimulation of B-cell chronic lymphocytic leukaemia cells enhances the anti-apoptotic profile, but also Bid expression and cells remain susceptible to autologous cytotoxic T-lymphocyte attack. Br J Haematol. 2004;127(4):404–15.

215. Luqman M, Klabunde S, Lin K, et al. The antileukemia activity of a human anti-CD40 antagonist antibody, HCD122, on human chronic lymphocytic leukemia cells. Blood. 2008;112(3):711–20.

216. Law CL, Gordon KA, Collier J, et al. Preclinical antilymphoma activity of a humanized anti-CD40 monoclonal antibody, SGN-40. Cancer Res. 2005;65(18):8331–8.

217. Advani et al. ASH annual meeting 2008, abstract 1000.

218. Kaufman et al. ASCO 2009, abstract 8593.

219. Hintzen RQ, Lens SM, Beckmann MP, Goodwin RG, Lynch D, van Lier RA. Characterization of the human CD27 ligand, a novel member of the TNF gene family. J Immunol. 1994;152(4):1762–73.

220. Israel BF, Gulley M, Elmore S, Ferrini S, Feng WH, Kenney SC. Anti-CD70 antibodies: a potential treatment for EBV+ CD70-expressing lymphomas. Mol Cancer Ther. 2005;4(12):2037–44.

221. Starlets D, Gore Y, Binsky I, et al. Cell-surface CD74 initiates a signaling cascade leading to cell proliferation and survival. Blood. 2006;107(12):4807–16.

222. Roche PA, Cresswell P. Invariant chain association with HLA-DR molecules inhibits immunogenic peptide binding. Nature. 1990;345(6276):615–8.

223. Stein R, Mattes MJ, Cardillo TM, et al. CD74: a new candidate target for the immunotherapy of B-cell neoplasms. Clin Cancer Res. 2007;13(18 Pt 2):5556s–63.

224. Stein R, Qu Z, Cardillo TM, et al. Antiproliferative activity of a humanized anti-CD74 monoclonal antibody, hLL1, on B-cell malignancies. Blood. 2004; 104(12):3705–11.

225. Davis TA, Czerwinski DK, Levy R. Therapy of B-cell lymphoma with anti-CD20 antibodies can result in the loss of CD20 antigen expression. Clin Cancer Res. 1999;5(3):611–5.

226. Cartron G, Watier H, Golay J, Solal-Celigny P. From the bench to the bedside: ways to improve rituximab efficacy. Blood. 2004;104(9):2635–42.

227. Zhou X, Hu W, Qin X. The role of complement in the mechanism of action of rituximab for B-cell lymphoma: implications for therapy. Oncologist. 2008;13(9):954–66.

228. Messmann RA, Vitetta ES, Headlee D, et al. A phase I study of combination therapy with immunotoxins IgG-HD37-deglycosylated ricin A chain (dgA) and IgG-RFB4-dgA (Combotox) in patients with refractory CD19(+), CD22(+) B cell lymphoma. Clin Cancer Res. 2000;6(4):1302–13.

229. DiJoseph JF, Armellino DC, Boghaert ER, et al. Antibody-targeted chemotherapy with CMC-544: a CD22-targeted immunoconjugate of calicheamicin for the treatment of B-lymphoid malignancies. Blood. 2004;103(5):1807–14.

230. Fayad L, Patel H, Verhoef G, et al. Clinical Activity of the Immunoconjugate CMC-544 in B-Cell Malignancies: Preliminary Report of the Expanded Maximum Tolerated Dose (MTD) Cohort of a Phase 1 Study. (ASH Annual Meeting Abstracts). Blood. 2006;108(11): abstract 2711.

231. Fayad et al. ASH annual meeting 2008, abstract 266.

232. Emmanouilides C. Radioimmunotherapy for Waldenstrom's macroglobulinemia. Semin Oncol. 2003;30(2):258–61.

233. Fisher RI, Kaminski MS, Wahl RL, et al. Tositumomab and iodine-131 tositumomab produces durable complete remissions in a subset of heavily pretreated patients with low-grade and transformed non-Hodgkin's lymphomas. J Clin Oncol. 2005;23(30):7565–73.

234. Kaminski MS, Radford JA, Gregory SA, et al. Re-treatment with I-131 tositumomab in patients with non-Hodgkin's lymphoma who had previously responded to I-131 tositumomab. J Clin Oncol. 2005;23(31):7985–93.

235. Witzig TE, Flinn IW, Gordon LI, et al. Treatment with ibritumomab tiuxetan radioimmunotherapy in patients with rituximab-refractory follicular non-Hodgkin's lymphoma. J Clin Oncol. 2002;20(15):3262–9.

236. Witzig TE, White CA, Gordon LI, et al. Safety of yttrium-90 ibritumomab tiuxetan radioimmunotherapy for relapsed low-grade, follicular, or transformed non-Hodgkin's lymphoma. J Clin Oncol. 2003;21(7): 1263–70.

237. Witzig TE, Gordon LI, Cabanillas F, et al. Randomized controlled trial of yttrium-90-labeled ibritumomab tiuxetan radioimmunotherapy versus rituximab immunotherapy for patients with relapsed or refractory low-grade, follicular, or transformed B-cell non-Hodgkin's lymphoma. J Clin Oncol. 2002;20(10):2453–63.

238. Gill DS, Damle NK. Biopharmaceutical drug discovery using novel protein scaffolds. Curr Opin Biotechnol. 2006;17(6):653–8.

239. Hayden-Ledbetter MS, Cerveny CG, Espling E, et al. CD20-directed small modular immunopharmaceutical, TRU-015, depletes normal and malignant B cells. Clin Cancer Res. 2009;15(8):2739–46.

240. Burge DJ, Bookbinder SA, Kivitz AJ, Fleischmann RM, Shu C, Bannink J. Pharmacokinetic and pharmacodynamic properties of TRU-015, a CD20-directed small modular immunopharmaceutical protein therapeutic, in patients with rheumatoid arthritis: a Phase I, open-label, dose-escalation clinical study. Clin Ther. 2008;30(10):1806–16.

241. Brischwein K, Parr L, Pflanz S, et al. Strictly target cell-dependent activation of T cells by bispecific single-chain antibody constructs of the BiTE class. J Immunother. 2007;30(8):798–807.

242. Bargou R, Leo E, Zugmaier G, et al. Tumor regression in cancer patients by very low doses of a T cell-engaging antibody. Science. 2008;321(5891): 974–7.

243. Koos D, Josephs SF, Alexandrescu DT, et al. Tumor vaccines in 2010: need for integration. Cellular Immunol. 2010;263:138–47.

244. Forstpointner R, Unterhalt M, Dreyling M, et al. Maintenance therapy with rituximab leads to a significant prolongation of response duration after salvage therapy with a combination of rituximab, fludarabine, cyclophosphamide, and mitoxantrone (R-FCM) in patients with recurring and refractory follicular and mantle cell lymphomas: results of a prospective randomized study of the German Low Grade Lymphoma Study Group (GLSG). Blood. 2006;108(13):4003–8.

245. Harris JR, Markl J. Keyhole limpet hemocyanin: molecular structure of a potent marine immunoactivator. A review. Eur Urol. 2000;37 Suppl 3:24–33.

246. Hsu FJ, Caspar CB, Czerwinski D, et al. Tumor-specific idiotype vaccines in the treatment of patients with B-cell lymphoma – long-term results of a clinical trial. Blood. 1997;89(9):3129–35.

247. Li J, Song W, Czerwinski DK, et al. Lymphoma immunotherapy with CpG oligodeoxynucleotides requires TLR9 either in the host or in the tumor itself. J Immunol. 2007;179(4):2493–500.

248. Datta SK, Cho HJ, Takabayashi K, Horner AA, Raz E. Antigen-immunostimulatory oligonucleotide conjugates: mechanisms and applications. Immunol Rev. 2004;199:217–26.

249. Lynch RG, Graff RJ, Sirisinha S, Simms ES, Eisen HN. Myeloma proteins as tumor-specific transplantation antigens. Proc Natl Acad Sci USA. 1972; 69(6):1540–4.

250. Freedman PM, Autry JR, Tokuda S, Williams Jr RC. Tumor immunity induced by preimmunization with BALB/c mouse myeloma protein. J Natl Cancer Inst. 1976;56(4):735–40.

251. Stevenson GT, Elliott EV, Stevenson FK. Idiotypic determinants on the surface immunoglobulin of neoplastic lymphocytes: a therapeutic target. Fed Proc. 1977;36(9):2268–71.

252. Kwak LW, Young HA, Pennington RW, Weeks SD. Vaccination with syngeneic, lymphoma-derived immunoglobulin idiotype combined with granulocyte/macrophage colony-stimulating factor primes mice for a protective T-cell response. Proc Natl Acad Sci USA. 1996;93(20):10972–7.

253. Kwak LW, Campbell MJ, Czerwinski DK, Hart S, Miller RA, Levy R. Induction of immune responses in patients with B-cell lymphoma against the surface-immunoglobulin idiotype expressed by their tumors. N Engl J Med. 1992;327(17):1209–15.

254. Bendandi M, Gocke CD, Kobrin CB, et al. Complete molecular remissions induced by patient-specific vaccination plus granulocyte-monocyte colony-stimulating factor against lymphoma. Nat Med. 1999;5(10):1171–7.

255. Redfern CH, Guthrie TH, Bessudo A, et al. Phase II trial of idiotype vaccination in previously treated patients with indolent non-Hodgkin's lymphoma resulting in durable clinical responses. J Clin Oncol. 2006;24(19):3107–12.

256. Yanez R, Barrios Y, Ruiz E, Cabrera R, Diaz-Espada F. Anti-idiotypic Immunotherapy in follicular lymphoma patients: results of a long follow-up study. J Immunother. 2008;31(3):310–2.

257. Inoges S, Rodriguez-Calvillo M, Zabalegui N, et al. Clinical benefit associated with idiotypic vaccination in patients with follicular lymphoma. J Natl Cancer Inst. 2006;98(18):1292–301.

258. Neelapu SS, Kwak LW, Kobrin CB, et al. Vaccine-induced tumor-specific immunity despite severe B-cell depletion in mantle cell lymphoma. Nat Med. 2005;11(9):986–91.

259. Koc et al. ASH annual meeting 2005, abstract 772.

260. Freedman A, Neelapu SS, Nichols C, et al. Placebo-controlled phase III trial of patient-specific immunotherapy with mitumprotimut-T and granulocyte-macrophage colony-stimulating factor after rituximab in patients with follicular lymphoma. J Clin Oncol. 2009;27(18):3036–43.

261. Levy et al. ASCO 2008, abstract LB-204.

262. Schuster et al. ASCO 2009, abstract 2;27 Suppl:18s.

263. Bendandi M. Idiotype vaccines for lymphoma: proof-of-principles and clinical trial failures. Nat Rev Cancer. 2009;9(9):675–81.

264. Timmerman JM, Singh G, Hermanson G, et al. Immunogenicity of a plasmid DNA vaccine encoding chimeric idiotype in patients with B-cell lymphoma. Cancer Res. 2002;62(20):5845–52.

265. Hawkins RE, Zhu D, Ovecka M, et al. Idiotypic vaccination against human B-cell lymphoma. Rescue of variable region gene sequences from biopsy material for assembly as single-chain Fv personal vaccines. Blood. 1994;83(11):3279–88.

266. Palucka AK, Ueno H, Fay JW, Banchereau J. Taming cancer by inducing immunity via dendritic cells. Immunol Rev. 2007;220:129–50.

267. Sallusto F, Lanzavecchia A. Efficient presentation of soluble antigen by cultured human dendritic cells is maintained by granulocyte/macrophage colony-stimulating factor plus interleukin 4 and downregulated by tumor necrosis factor alpha. J Exp Med. 1994;179(4):1109–18.

268. Timmerman JM. Idiotype-pulsed dendritic cell vaccination for B-cell lymphoma: clinical and immune responses in 35 patients. Blood. 2002;99(5):1517–26.

269. Di Nicola M, Zappasodi R, Carlo-Stella C, et al. Vaccination with autologous tumor-loaded dendritic cells induces clinical and immunologic responses in indolent B-cell lymphoma patients with relapsed and measurable disease: a pilot study. Blood. 2009; 113(1):18–27.

270. Zappasodi R, Pupa SM, Ghedini GC, et al. Improved clinical outcome in indolent B-cell lymphoma patients vaccinated with autologous tumor cells experiencing immunogenic death. Cancer Res. 2010;70(22):9062–72.

271. Neelapu SS, Gause BL, Harvey L, et al. A novel proteoliposomal vaccine induces antitumor immunity against follicular lymphoma. Blood. 2007;109(12): 5160–3.

272. Zitvogel L, Apetoh L, Ghiringhelli FO, Kroemer G. Immunological aspects of cancer chemotherapy. Nat Rev Immunol. 2008;8(1):59–73.

273. Brody JD, Ai WZ, Czerwinski DK, et al. In situ vaccination with a TLR9 agonist induces systemic lymphoma regression: a phase I/II study. J Clin Oncol. 2010;28:4324–32.

274. Neelapu SS, Kwak LW. Cancer vaccines: up, down, … up again? Blood. 2009;113(1):1–2.

275. Vallet S, Palumbo A, Raje N, Boccadoro M, Anderson KC. Thalidomide and lenalidomide: mechanism-based potential drug combinations. Leuk Lymphoma. 2008;49(7):1238–45.

276. Zhu D, Corral LG, Fleming YW, Stein B. Immunomodulatory drugs Revlimid (lenalidomide) and CC-4047 induce apoptosis of both hematological and solid tumor cells through NK cell activation. Cancer Immunol Immunother. 2008;57(12):1849–59.

277. Chang DH, Liu N, Klimek V, et al. Enhancement of ligand-dependent activation of human natural killer T cells by lenalidomide: therapeutic implications. Blood. 2006;108(2):618–21.

278. Wiernik PH, Lossos IS, Tuscano JM, et al. Lenalidomide monotherapy in relapsed or refractory aggressive non-Hodgkin's lymphoma. J Clin Oncol. 2008;26(30):4952–7.

279. Witzig TE, Wiernik PH, Moore T, et al. Lenalidomide oral monotherapy produces durable responses in relapsed or refractory indolent non-Hodgkin's lymphoma. J Clin Oncol. 2009;27(32):5404–9.

280. Dutia et al. ASH annual meeting 2009, abstract 1679.

281. Fowler et al. ASH annual meeting 2009, abstract 1714.
282. Nowakowski et al. ASH annual meeting 2009, abstract 1669.
283. Hilchey SP, Hyrien O, Mosmann TR, et al. Rituximab immunotherapy results in the induction of a lymphoma idiotype-specific T-cell response in patients with follicular lymphoma: support for a "vaccinal effect" of rituximab. Blood. 2009;113(16): 3809–12.
284. Cerchietti LC, Lopes EC, Yang SN, et al. A purine scaffold Hsp90 inhibitor destabilizes BCL-6 and has specific antitumor activity in BCL-6-dependent B cell lymphomas. Nat Med. 2009;15(12):1369–76.
285. Whitesell L, Lindquist SL. HSP90 and the chaperoning of cancer. Nat Rev Cancer. 2005;5(10):761–72.
286. Younes et al. ASH annual meeting 2009, abstract 3744.
287. Rao et al. ASH annual meeting 2010, abstract 2856.
288. Hagenbeek A, Plesner T, Johnson P, et al. HuMax-CD20, a novel fully human anti-CD20 monoclonal antibody: results of a phase I/II trial in relapsed or refractory follicular non-Hodgkins's lymphoma. (ASH annual meeting abstracts). Blood. 2005;106(11):abstract 5760.
289. Hagenbeek A, Fayad L, Delwail V, et al. Evaluation of ofatumumab, a novel human CD20 monoclonal antibody, as single agent therapy in rituximab-refractory follicular lymphoma. (ASH annual meeting abstracts). Blood. 2009;114(22):abstract 935.
290. Coiffer B, Bosly A, Wu KL, et al. Ofatumumab monotherapy for treatment of patients with relapsed/progressive diffuse large B-cell lymphoma: results from a multicenter phase II study. Blood. 2010;116(21):abstract 3955.
291. Kipps T, Osterborg A, Mayer J, et al. Clinical improvement with a novel CD20 mAb, ofatumumab, in fludarabine-refractory chronic lymphocytic leukemia (CLL) also refractory to alemtuzumab or with bulky lymphadenopathy. J Clin Oncol. 2009;27:15s (suppl; abstract 7043).
292. Morschhauser F, Leonard JP, Fayad L, et al. Humanized anti-CD20 antibody, veltuzumab, in refractory/recurrent non-Hodgkin's lymphoma: phase I/II results. J Clin Oncol. 2009;27(20):3346–53.
293. Salles GA, Morschhauser F, Thieblemont C, et al. Promising efficacy with the new anti-CD20 antibody GA101 in heavily pre-treated NHL patients—updated results with encouraging progression free survival (PFS) data from a phase II study in patients with relapsed/refractory indolent NHL (iNHL). (ASH annual meeting abstracts). Blood. 2010; 116(21):abstract 2868.
294. Cartron G, Thieblemont C, Solal-Celigny P, et al. Promising efficacy with the new anti-CD20 antibody GA101 in heavily pre-treated NHL patients—first results from a phase II study in patients with relapsed/refractory DLBCL and MCL. (ASH annual meeting abstracts). Blood. 2010;116(21):abstract 2878.
295. Leonard JP, Coleman M, Ketas JC, et al. Epratuzumab, a humanized anti-CD22 antibody, in aggressive non-Hodgkin's lymphoma: phase I/II clinical trial results. Clin Cancer Res. 2004;10:5327–34.
296. Leonard JP, Schuster SJ, Emmanouilides C, et al. Durable complete responses from therapy with combined epratuxumab and rituximab: final results from an international multicenter, phase 2 study in recurrent, indolent, non-Hodgkin lymphoma. Cancer. 2008:113(10):2714–23.
297. Grant B, Leonard JP, Jeffrey L, et al. Combination biologic therapy as initial treatment for follicular lymphoma: initial results from CALGB 50701—a phase II trial of extended induction epratuzumab (anti-CD22) and rituximab (anti-CD20). (ASH annual meeting abstracts). Blood. 2010;116(21): abstract 427.
298. Tobanai K, Ogura M, Hatake K, et al. Phase I and pharmacokinetic study of inotuzumab ozogamicin (CMC- 544) as a single agent in Japanese patients with follicular lymphoma pretreated with rituximab. (ASH annual meeting abstracts). Blood. 2008; 118(11):abstract 1565.
299. Goy A, Leach J, Ehmann WC, et al., Inotuzumab ozogamicin (CMC-544) in patients with indolent B-cell NHL that is refractory to rituximab alone, rituximab and chemotherapy, or radioimmunotherapy: preliminary safety and efficacy from a phase 2 trial. (ASH annual meeting abstracts). Blood. 2010;116(21):abstract 430.
300. Byrd J, Kipps TJ, Flinn IW, et al. Phase 1/2 study of lumiliximab combined with fludarabine, cyclophosphamide, and rituximab in patients with relapsed or refractory chronic lymphocytic leukemia. Blood. 2010;115(3):489–95.
301. Advani R, Forero-Torres A, Furman RR, et al. Phase I study of the humanized anti-CD40 monoclonal antibody dacetuzumab in refractory or recurrent non-Hodgkin's lymphoma. J Clin Oncol. 2009;27(32): 4371–77.
302. Kivekas I, Hulkkonen J, Hurme M, Vilpo L, Vilpo J. CD80 antigen expression as a predictor of ex vivo chemosensitivity in chronic lymphocytic leukemia. Leuk Res. 2002;26(5):443–6.
303. Bence-Bruckler I, Macdonald D, Stiff PJ, et al. A phase 2, double-blind, placebo-controlled trial of rituximab + galiximab vs rituximab + placebo in advanced follicular non-Hodgkin's lymphoma (NHL). (ASH annual meeting abstracts). Blood. 2010;116(21):abstract 428.

Leukemias

6

Lia Ginaldi and Massimo De Martinis

Abbreviations

ABC	Antibody binding capacity
ADCC	Antibody-dependent cellular cytotoxicity
ALL	Acute lymphoid leukemia
AML	Acute myeloid leukemia
APL	Acute promyelocytic leukemia
Ara-C	Cytarabine
ATO	Arsenic trioxide
ATRA	All-trans-retinoic acid
BAALC	Brain cells and acute leukemia, cytoplasmic
B-CLL	B-cell chronic lymphocytic leukemia
BCP-ALL	B-cell precursor acute lymphoblastic leukemia
BCR	B-cell receptor
cAMP	Cyclic adenosine monophosphate
CDC	Complement-dependent cytotoxicity
CDK	Cyclin-dependent kinase
CLL	Chronic lymphocytic leukemia
CML	Chronic myeloid leukemia
CN	Cytogenetically normal
CR	Complete remission
ET	Essential thrombocythemia
EVI1	Ecotropic viral integration site 1
FCR	Fludarabine, cyclophosphamide, rituximab
FISH	Fluorescent in situ hybridization
FLT3	FMS-like tyrosine kinase 3
GO	Gemtuzumab ozogamicin
HCL	Hairy cell leukemia
HDACs	Histone deacetylases
HIF-1α	Hypoxia-inducible transcription factor-1 α
HMOX-1	Heme oxygenase
HSC	Hematopoietic stem cells
IL	Interleukin
IFN-α	Interferon alfa
IgVH	Immunoglobulin heavy-chain variable gene
IKZF1	IKAROS family zinc finger 1
ITDs	Internal tandem duplications
ITIMs	Immune tyrosine-based inhibitory motifs
LSC	Leukemic stem cell
MCL	Mantle cell lymphoma
MDS	Myelodysplastic syndrome
MESF	Molecules of equivalent soluble fluorophore
MMPs	Matrix metalloproteinases
MN1	Meningioma 1
MoAb	Monoclonal antibody
MPD	Myeloproliferative disorder
MPN	Myeloproliferative neoplasm
NFκB	Nuclear factor kappa B
NPM1	Nucleophosmin 1
NRP-1	Neuropilin-1
NR	Nonresponder
NRR	Negative regulatory region

L. Ginaldi, M.D. (✉) • M. De Martinis, M.D.
Department of Internal Medicine and Public Health,
University of L'Aquila, Coppito, L'Aquila 67100, Italy
e-mail: lia.ginaldi@cc.univaq.it;
massimo.demartinis@cc.univaq.it

M. Bologna (ed.), *Biotargets of Cancer in Current Clinical Practice*, Current Clinical Pathology,
DOI 10.1007/978-1-61779-615-9_6, © Springer Science+Business Media, LLC 2012

PCD	Programmed cell death
PCR	Polymerase chain reaction
Ph-chromosome	Philadelphia chromosome
PI3K	Phosphoinositide 3-kinase
PLL	Prolymphocytic leukemia
PMF	Primary myelofibrosis
PML-RARα	Promyelocytic leukemia–retinoic acid receptor-α
PR	Partial remission
PTD	Partial tandem duplications
PV	Polycythemia vera
R	Responder
RARG	Retinoic acid receptor-γ
RoS	Reactive oxygen species
siRNA	Short-interfering RNA
SLVL	Splenic lymphoma with villous lymphocytes
SMIPs	Small-molecule immunopharmaceuticals
T-ALL	T-lineage ALL
TCRAD	T-cell receptor α–δ
TCRB	T-cell receptor β
TH	T helper
TKIs	Tyrosine kinase inhibitors
TNF-α	Tumor necrosis factor-alpha
T-PLL	T-prolymphocytic leukemia
VDR	Vitamin D receptor
VEGF	Vascular endothelial growth factor
WT1	Wilms tumor 1
XiaP	X-linked inhibitor of apoptosis

Introduction

Leukemias are a heterogeneous group of hematologic malignancies derived from stem cells or blasts in the hemopoietic bone marrow and characterized by uncontrolled neoplastic proliferation and suppression of normal hemopoiesis. Depending on the cell line from which the leukemic clone evolves, leukemias can be divided into myeloid or lymphoid. Within these two subsets, we can further differentiate acute and chronic leukemias, based on the disease course. Each of these broad subsets includes several pathological entities that differ in clinical and biological characteristics, as well as with regard to prognosis and

response to therapy. The outcome of the majority of these diseases has changed profoundly in recent years, thanks to huge advances in basic and clinical research. The identification of important biological markers allowed the differentiation of patients with different prognostic features, suggesting innovative and successful therapeutic approaches and the planning of targeted therapies.

The pathways that regulate proliferation, differentiation, apoptosis, and cell invasiveness are the basis of neoplastic transformation and are the target of this new therapeutic approach. Some of these innovative drugs are now commonly used in the treatment of leukemia.

Paradigmatic example is the understanding of molecular pathophysiology of the BCR–ABL rearrangement in Philadelphia chromosome (Ph)-positive chronic myeloid leukemia (CML) which led to the extraordinarily rapid development of multiple selective BCR–ABL tyrosine kinase inhibitors (TKIs). Imatinib mesylate, the first BCR–ABL-targeted drug, proved superior to the old standard of therapy of interferon and hydroxyurea. However, as many as 20% of newly diagnosed patients do not respond, and an equivalent number fail, due to the development of imatinib-resistant mutations. There are now three new TKIs available that inhibit BCR–ABL (nilotinib, dasatinib, and bosutinib) and provide further treatment options in patients who fail imatinib treatment as well as in newly diagnosed CML patients in the chronic phase of their disease. These new compounds improved 10-year survival of CML patients from the historic experience of approximately 20% to an estimated rate of 85% [1, 2].

An improved survival has also been obtained in chronic lymphocytic leukemia (CLL), by using chemoimmunotherapy involving the combination of fludarabine, cyclophosphamide, and rituximab (FCR), an anti-CD20 monoclonal antibody (MoAb) [3, 4]. Furthermore, several other MoAbs against different myeloid and lymphoid cell lineage antigens have been synthesized and introduced in clinical trials as biodrugs for chronic as well as acute leukemias.

In acute lymphoid leukemia (ALL), modern intensive chemotherapy regimens now result in cure rates of 90% in children and 40% in adults [5]. Similarly, high-dose cytarabine-based regimens in acute myeloid leukemia (AML) now result in cure rates of 60–80% [6]. Combining chemotherapy with targeted therapies involving TKIs has increased the estimated 5-year survival rates in Ph-positive ALL subsets from less than 10% to approximately 50% [7]. Anti-CD20 MoAb combined with short-term, dose-intensive chemotherapy increased survival rates in the subset of CD20-positive B-lineage ALL and in Burkitt ALL, ranging in this latter from less than 20% to approximately 70% [8].

Several molecular aberrations with important prognostic implications have recently been identified in patients with AML exhibiting "normal" diploid karyotype: these discoveries enabled the planning of a more rationally targeted therapy, including the use of allogeneic stem-cell transplantation in first remissions for higher-risk patients as well as avoidance of transplantation in better-risk individuals, such as those with NPM1 mutations. Moreover, a large number of AML patients with FLT3 gene mutations could benefit from the targeted therapy with FLT3 inhibitors [9]. Therapeutic strategies that use all-trans-retinoic acid and arsenic trioxide (ATO), either alone or in combination with chemotherapy, are now associated with cure rates of 80% in acute promyelocytic leukemia (PML) [8].

The introduction of hypomethylating agents in the therapy of myelodysplastic syndromes (MDS) and the discovery of the important role of the JAK2-mutated signaling pathways in myeloproliferative disorders (MPD) with the consequent development of JAK2 inhibitors resulted in improved survival when compared with supportive care alone and/or traditional chemotherapy. Subsets of low-risk MDS with 5q deletion and red-cell transfusion dependency had dramatic benefit from therapy with the immunomodulant agent lenalidomide [10], and several JAK2 inhibitors are now showing promise in the treatment of myelofibrosis [11].

With the increasing pathogenetic discoveries and the consequent production of many new drugs, leukemia landscape is changing rapidly. Some of the most important biotargets of leukemia and their clinical implications will be addressed in this chapter with attention paid to the emerging molecular features, to provide an updated overview of the current knowledge in this rapidly developing field.

Monoclonal Antibody Therapy

MoAb treatments of leukemia have improved outcomes and reduced toxicity compared to more conventional chemotherapy regimens. The reduced toxicity results from the more targeted killing of neoplastic cells and a relative lack of toxicity to nonneoplastic cells. Several potential MoAb effector mechanisms have been highlighted (Fig. 6.1), including complement-mediated cytotoxicity, antibody-dependent cellular cytotoxicity, inhibition of cell growth, induction of apoptosis, and sensitization to chemotherapy or radiation. Because of this latter mechanism, best results are obtained when MoAbs are used in combination with chemotherapy.

Resistance to the MoAb therapy may be due to increased MoAb metabolism, reduced tumor penetration, impaired MoAb binding, loss or downregulation of the antigen, resistance of leukemic cells to MoAb effector mechanisms [12, 13], and impaired immune effector cell recruitment or function [14]. In fact, one of the possible causes of MoAb target therapy failure could be a low antigen expression on leukemic cells, either typical of the leukemia phenotype or due to therapy-induced receptor downregulation. The synthesis of engineered antibodies with high avidity for the antigen may be useful in these cases. For example, leukemic cells from CLL patients exhibit CD20 expression intensity lower than normal peripheral blood lymphocytes, and this is an important parameter of immunophenotypic diagnosis (Fig. 6.2). Receptor expression intensity could also differentiate CLL from other B-cell neoplastic diseases (Fig. 6.3). Another B-cell antigen, CD19, is expressed with different intensity on normal and leukemic cells (Figs. 6.4 and 6.5) [15]. Similarly, CD52 antigen is expressed on most normal and neoplastic lymphoid cells with different intensity (Figs. 6.6 and 6.7) [16].

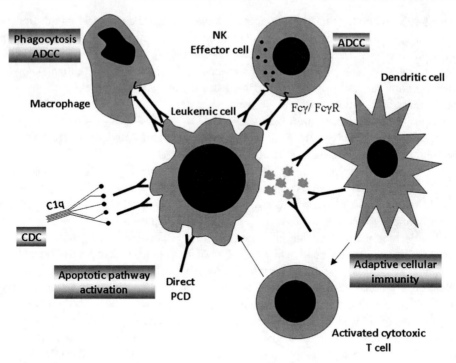

Fig. 6.1 Potential MoAb effector mechanisms in leukemia therapy. MoAbs kill their target by multiple mechanisms. The Fc arm of the immunoglobulin recruits and activates Fc-R-expressing immune effector cells, including macrophages and NK cells, which in turn eliminate the target cell by release of cytotoxic mediators in antibody-dependent cell cytotoxicity (ADCC) (NK cells and macrophages) or direct phagocytosis (macrophages). Another antileukemic effect could be mediated by complement-dependent cytotoxicity (CDC): complement fixation occurs when C1q, the globular head of C1, binds the Fc portion of two IgG molecules, which triggers a series of enzymatic reactions in cascade that generate pores in the cell membrane (membrane attack complex) leading ultimately to cell lysis. Apoptosis or programmed cell death (PCD) is induced by direct and indirect mechanisms. Adaptive cellular immunity is potentially enhanced by promoting the uptake of tumor antigens by dendritic cells and cross-presentation to T cells, which differentiate into cytotoxic T cells that evoke an antitumor cellular immune response, inducing a sort of vaccination effect

The reshaped humanized IgG1 anti-CD52 MoAb (campath-IH) has been used in the treatment of hemopoietic and nonhemopoietic diseases for its ability to induce lymphocyte depletion both in vitro and in vivo. Good activity has been shown in patients with chronic T- and B-cell leukemias, in particular T-prolymphocytic leukemia (T-PLL). However, the response to treatment is not uniform, and this variability may depend on differences in the level of antigen expression on the leukemic cells (Fig. 6.8). Although other factors may play a role in the response to MoAb therapy, the quantitative estimation of the target antigen expression may drive the selection of those patients with a higher probability of responding to target therapy.

Several MoAbs have been utilized in clinical practice for targeted therapy of leukemia, while others are in a preclinical phase of study (Table 6.1).

CD20 is a B-cell activation and growth regulator receptor, which represents an excellent target for MoAb therapy: it is expressed at all stages of B-cell maturation but not on precursor B cells or other cells, and it is not shed or internalized after binding with antibody. The effectiveness of rituximab correlates with the level of CD20 expression. Not all B-cell leukemias express high levels of CD20. For example, CLL characteristically expresses CD20 at low levels. Rituximab depletes both normal and neoplastic CD20+ B cells. Patients tolerate the decrease in B cells

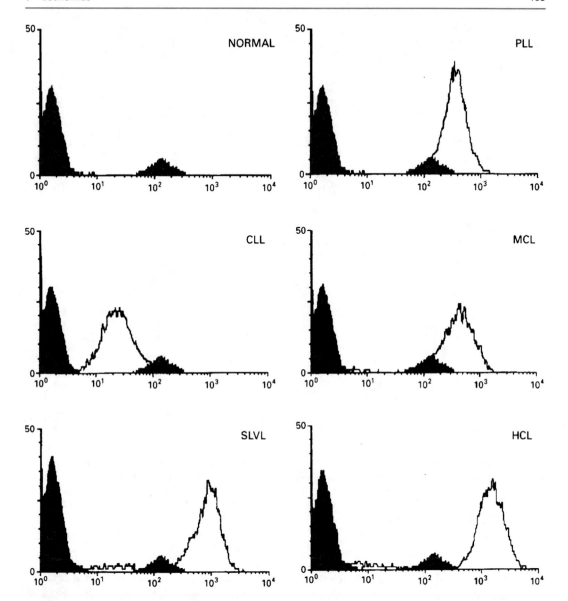

Fig. 6.2 Different CD20 expression patterns in B-cell leukemias. Overlays of single-parameter histograms showing different CD20 expression patterns in B-cell leukemias compared with normal (full histogram). CLL has lower CD20 density compared to prolymphocytic leukemia (PLL), mantle cell lymphoma (MCL), splenic lymphoma with villous lymphocytes (SLVL), and hairy cell leukemia (HCL). (Reproduced from [15]. With permission from BMJ Publishing Group Ltd)

better than a decrease in other leukocytes: immunoglobulin stores can be replenished relatively easily from donor immunoglobulin whereas antibody therapies to other targets such as CD33 or CD52 cause decreased granulocytes and increased infection risk that is not so easily rectified. Rituximab toxicities include non-infection-associated side effects due to immune reactions to the product or to lysis of the neoplastic B cells. The more severe immune reactions have been labeled a "cytokine release syndrome" [17].

Ofatumumab is a second-generation, fully humanized, anti-CD20 MoAb with enhanced Fc effector function based on an IgG1-kappa immunoglobulin framework [18]. It theoretically improves complement activation and access by

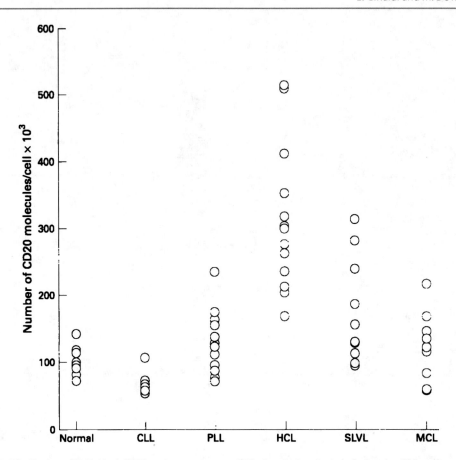

Fig. 6.3 Distribution of individual CD20 antigen concentration among B-cell leukemias. Antigen molecules/cell, detected by quantitative flow cytometry and expressed as antibody binding capacity (ABC) values, for CD20 in normal peripheral blood lymphocytes and B-cell leukemias. *CLL* chronic lymphocytic leukemia, *PLL* prolymphocytic leukemia, *HCL* hairy cell leukemia, *SLVL* splenic lymphoma with villous lymphocytes, *MCL* mantle cell lymphoma. (Reproduced from [15]. With permission from BMJ Publishing Group Ltd)

effector cells to kill the target by ADCC [19]. Alemtuzumab is a humanized MoAb against CD52, an antigen expressed on lymphocytes (T and B), monocytes, and subpopulations of granulocytes. The function of CD52 is unknown, but it is expressed at high levels on CLL and not expressed on most marrow stem cells. Alemtuzumab has been approved as a single agent for treatment of CLL [20, 21]. CD33 is a cell surface glycoprotein commonly expressed on myeloid cells including myeloid leukemia cells. CD33, involved in sialic acid-dependent cell interactions and adhesion of myeloid cells at certain stages of their differentiation, contains immune tyrosine-based inhibitory motifs (ITIMs), thus serving as an inhibitory receptor. Engagement of CD33 by MoAb induces apoptosis and inhibits proliferation in normal myeloid cells and leukemia cells from patients with AML and CML [17].

Gemtuzumab ozogamicin (GO) is a calicheamicin-conjugated anti-CD33 MoAb approved for therapy of relapsed AML. This humanized IgG4 MoAb induced remissions in 31% of patients with tolerable side effects [22]. Another MoAb directed to CD33, lintuzumab, has been developed. It is a humanized MoAb whose activity depends solely on its inherent properties of mediating direct effects through binding to CD33 and activating effector cells through its Fc domain. Lintuzumab has demonstrated its ability to decrease the production of

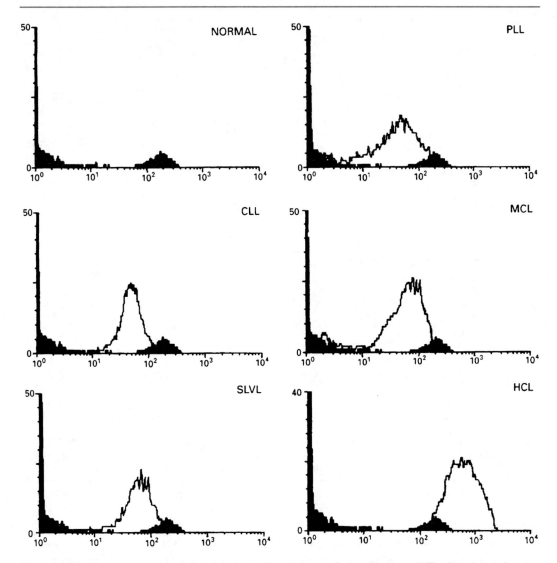

Fig. 6.4 CD19 expression in normal and leukemic B cells. Overlays of single-parameter histograms showing the difference in CD19 expression between normal peripheral blood B cells (displayed in *black*) and B-cell leukemias. CD19 is lower than in normal B lymphocytes in all B-lineage leukemias except HCL. *CLL* chronic lymphocytic leukemia, *PLL* prolymphocytic leukemia, *HCL* hairy cell leukemia, *SLVL* splenic lymphoma with villous lymphocytes, *MCL* mantle cell lymphoma. (Reproduced from [15]. With permission from BMJ Publishing Group Ltd)

proinflammatory cytokines by AML cells and mediate ADCC and phagocytosis of AML cells. Lintuzumab has been used in studies of the treatment of AML converting patients with minimal residual disease into molecular remission [23].

Leukemic stem cells (LSCs), different from normal hematopoietic stem cells (HSC), are a small subpopulation within the leukemic bulk, with the peculiar property of propagating the leukemic growth. Targeting this LSC population of cells holds the promise of higher cure rates by elimination of the total population of leukemia, not just the more prevalent non-stem cell fraction. Thus, it is important to determine the antigenic targets on this population for treatment with MoAbs with or without other therapy. Candidate

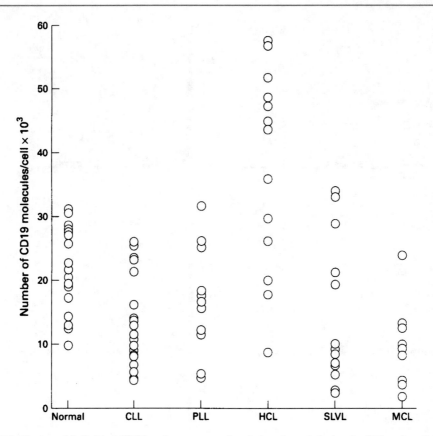

Fig. 6.5 Distribution of individual CD19 antigen concentration among B-cell leukemias. Individual ABC values for CD19 in normal peripheral blood B cells and B-lineage leukemias, showing the extremely expression variability among the different disease entities. *CLL* chronic lymphocytic leukemia, *PLL* prolymphocytic leukemia, *HCL* hairy cell leukemia, *SLVL* splenic lymphoma with villous lymphocytes, *MCL* mantle cell lymphoma. (Reproduced from [15]. With permission from BMJ Publishing Group Ltd)

antigens include the cell adhesion family receptor CD44, the leukemic stem cell-associated antigen CD123, and CD33 [24].

CD44 is a receptor for hyaluronic acid and can also interact with other ligands, such as osteopontin, collagens, and matrix metalloproteinases (MMPs). While not uniquely expressed on AML stem/progenitor cells, it nevertheless is present on AML cells and may be a good target for therapy.

The mechanisms underlying this effect may include interference with transport to stem cell-supportive niches and alteration of AML-LSC fate, thus identifying CD44 as a key regulator of AML LSCs [25]. The CD123 antigen is functionally the interleukin-3 receptor. This receptor is found on pluripotent progenitor cells, induces tyrosine phosphorylation within the cell, and promotes proliferation and differentiation within the hematopoietic cell lines. CD123 is expressed on LSC but not normal HSC and thus may be a suitable target for antibody-mediated therapy. A MoAb is available that targets this antigen. Other methods of targeting CD123 include the use of antibody fragments coupled to toxins, such as diphtheria or pseudomonas exotoxins. These compounds have promising activities in preclinical studies [26].

Rituximab (CD20 MoAb) and epratuzumab (CD22 MoAb) in combination with chemotherapy for newly diagnosed BCR–ABL-negative B-lineage ALL are giving promising results. Aside from CD20 and CD22, ALL cells do express antigens that are targetable by MoAbs

6 Leukemias

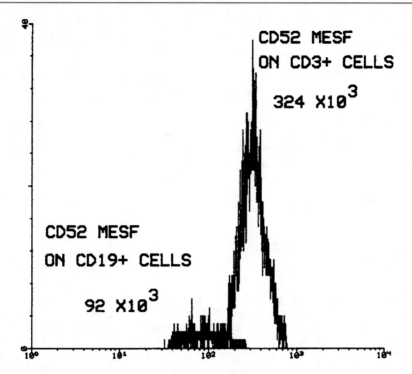

Fig. 6.6 CD52 expression on normal peripheral B and T lymphocytes. Overlay of fluorescein-conjugated (FITC)-campath-1H histograms, gated on CD3+T lymphocytes and CD19+B lymphocytes from a normal control, showing the difference in CD52 density between T and B cells. The strong CD52+cells are CD3+T lymphocytes while the weak CD52+cells are CD19+B lymphocytes. (Reprinted from [16]. With permission from Elsevier)

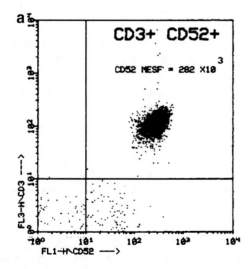 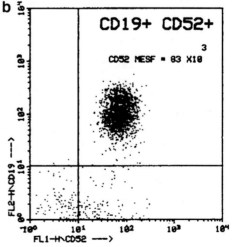

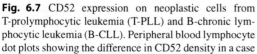

Fig. 6.7 CD52 expression on neoplastic cells from T-prolymphocytic leukemia (T-PLL) and B-chronic lymphocytic leukemia (B-CLL). Peripheral blood lymphocyte dot plots showing the difference in CD52 density in a case of (**a**) T-PLL and in a (**b**) B-CLL patient. In T-PLL cells, there is a significantly higher expression of CD52 compared to B-CLL cells. (Reprinted from [16]. With permission from Elsevier)

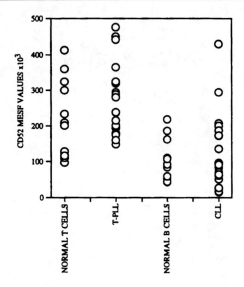 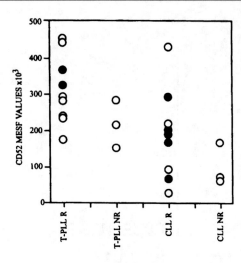

Fig. 6.8 CD52 expression on normal and leukemic lymphoid cells and correlation with response to therapy in patients treated with anti-CD52 MoAb. Distribution of individual values of CD52 MESF in T and B lymphocytes from normal controls, T-PLL and CLL cases, (**a**) and distribution of individual CD52 MESF values in leukemic cells from T-PLL and CLL patients who underwent campath treatment (**b**). Patients are divided into responders (R), including complete remissions (CR) and partial remissions (PR), and nonresponders (NR). Solid symbols are patients with partial remission. The intensity of the expression of CD52 is significantly higher in T-CLL, such as T-PLL, compared with B-CLL. Moreover, the differences in CD52 expression are somewhat higher in campath responder patients than in nonresponders. (Reprinted from [16]. With permission from Elsevier)

including CD52, and CD19, and even the myeloid antigen CD33 in some cases. Thus, existing monoclonal antibodies may be effective for ALL [17].

Chronic Myeloid Leukemia

According to the 2008 WHO classification system for myeloid neoplasms [27], CML can be considered as a classic BCR–ABL-positive myeloproliferative neoplasm (MPN), together with other classic MPN, such as JAK2 V617F-positive polycythemia vera (PV), essential thrombocythemia (ET), and primary myelofibrosis (PMF).

CML is a clonal disorder caused by the malignant transformation of a pluripotent stem cell. It is characterized by a genetic abnormality, the Philadelphia chromosome, identified as the balanced translocation t(9;22) (q34;q11), which is present in more than 90% of adult CML patients, as well as in 15–30% of adult ALL and 2% of AML. This translocation fuses the genes encoding BCR and ABL and results in expression of the constitutively active protein tyrosine kinase BCR–ABL. Different molecular weight isoforms are generated, based on different breakpoints and mRNA splicing. Most chronic myelogenous leukemia patients have a fusion protein of 210 kDa, while approximately 30% of Ph+ALL cases and few chronic myelogenous leukemias are associated with 190 kDa BCR–ABL1 protein [28]. CML is a progressive neoplasm typically comprising three clinically recognized phases: the majority of patients are diagnosed during the indolent chronic phase, which is followed by an accelerated phase and a terminal blastic phase. As patients progress through the different phases, cytogenetic abnormalities may be detected in addition to the Ph-chromosome (clonal evolution). Mutations and deletions in specific genes may also occur (e.g., p53, p16/INK4a, and RB). There are increasing evidences that Src family kinases are involved in chronic myelogenous leukemia progression through induction of cytokine

Table 6.1 Monoclonal antibodies (MoAb) as therapeutic agents in leukemia

MoAb	Target antigen	Description	Therapeutic indication	Properties
Rituximab	CD20	Chimeric	CLL, phase III trial ALL	FcγR binding with complement activation, caspase activation (CDC, apoptosis)
Ofatumumab	CD20	Fully human	Refractory CLL	Slow off-rate, enhanced FcγR binding, complement dependent cytotoxicity (CDC)
Obinutuzumab GA101	CD20	Humanized, glycoengineered (afucosylated Fc)	Phase III trial refractory CLL	Enhanced FcγR IIIa, increased ADCC, direct PCD, lacking ability to translocate CD20 into membrane rafts or activate C'
Ocrelizumab PRO131921	CD20	Humanized with modified Fc	Phase I/II trials in refractory CLL	Enhanced FcγR IIIa binding and ADCC ability
Epratuzumab	CD22	Humanized	Phase III trial BCR–ABL-negative B-ALL	ADCC
Lumiliximab	CD23	Chimeric	Phase I/II trial CLL	Immunomodulator
Lintuzumab	CD33	Humanized	Phase III trial AML	Decreased inflammatory cytokine production by AML, Fc-mediated effector cell activation, ADCC, phagocytosis
Gemtuzumab/ozogamicin GO	CD33	Humanized, calicheamicin-conjugated	AML	Internalization, hydrolytical cleavage, calicheamicin DNA binding and breaking
H90	CD44	Chimeric	Preclinical studies in AML	Interference with stem cell-supportive niche signals, abrogation of LSC homing
Alemtuzumab campath	CD52	Humanized	CLL	CDC, ADCC, PCD
7G3	CD123	Humanized	Preclinical studies in AML	IL-3 receptor targeting and neutralization, LSC homing inhibition
Apolizumab	HLA-DRB	Humanized	Preclinical studies in CLL	Fc-mediated effector functions
Bevacizumab	VEGF	Humanized	Phase II trials in AML	Neutralization of angiogenesis

C' complement, *CDC* complement-dependent cytotoxicity, *ADCC* antibody-dependent cellular cytotoxicity, *PCD* programmed cell death, *LSC* leukemic stem cell

independence and apoptotic protection [29]. The identification of the crucial role of BCR–ABL1 has allowed the development of imatinib mesylate, the first therapy to target this pathogenetic transcript, which acts by competitively binding the inactive form of BCR–ABL1, preventing a switch to the active form and partially blocking the enzyme ATP binding site. This action also prevents BCR–ABL1 autophosphorylation, activation, and signal transduction. Imatinib, which inhibits the tyrosine kinase activity of BCR–ABL, was introduced as a first-line treatment for CML almost 10 years ago and radically improved the outcome of patients with CML. Imatinib has been the standard therapy for CML due to its remarkable activity and mild toxicity. It now constitutes the first-line therapy for the majority of CML patients diagnosed in chronic phase and the minority diagnosed in advanced phase. Today, most patients have the expectation of a favorable outcome when treated with standard-dose imatinib. Patients treated with imatinib showed a cumulative complete cytogenetic response rate of approximately 89%, an estimated survival rate of 85% and freedom from progression rate of 92%, with an event-free survival of 81. CML patients who consistently tested negative for BCR–ABL by reverse transcription PCR for at least 2 years may safely stop imatinib, provided they are subjected to intense monitoring to detect disease recurrence. It is estimated that 10% of patients with CML may be eligible for a trial of imatinib discontinuation [30].

Clinical trials in which CML patients in chronic phase were randomly assigned to receive imatinib or interferon alfa (IFN-α) plus cytarabine (Ara-C) established imatinib as the standard therapy [31]. However, in this trial, 17% of patients never achieved a complete cytogenetic response, and approximately 15% of responders eventually lost it; moreover, nearly 5% were intolerant to imatinib. Thus, at least one-third of all patients did not have an acceptable outcome. Therefore, a significant proportion of patients do not achieve the optimal desirable outcome [32]. Effective salvage therapy followed the recognition of some of the most common mechanisms of resistance.

Some patients develop imatinib resistance, and some events (loss of response, progression to advanced phase) still occur, even in low rate, also in patients who previously demonstrated complete response. It has been shown that continuous and adequate imatinib dosing is essential to the achievement of therapeutic goals [33]. Nonadherence can lead to unnecessary diagnostic testing, changes in dose or regimen, misleading results, and inconsistent response rates (suboptimal responses or failure) [34]. Therefore, second-generation TKIs, namely dasatinib, nilotinib, and bosutinib, have been recently developed [29].

Clinical trials assessing the newer TKIs (dasatinib, nilotinib, and bosutinib) as first-line therapies in newly diagnosed chronic phase CML are ongoing. Despite the responses observed with imatinib, a proportion of patients develop resistance to imatinib or cannot tolerate its side effects. This led to the development of newer TKIs of BCR–ABL, including dasatinib, nilotinib, and bosutinib, that were initially tested in clinical studies of patients with prior imatinib therapy [35].

Dasatinib and nilotinib, the two most extensively studied second-generation TKIs, have been approved for use as second-line therapy in CML patients with imatinib resistance or intolerance. Both agents show significant clinical efficacy and a favorable toxicity profile. With dasatinib, a complete cytogenetic remission occurs in 51% of patients, with a 24-month progression-free survival of 81% [36]. Nilotinib induced remission in 44%, with a 24-month progression-free survival of 64% [37]. Bosutinib, the other second-generation TKI under development, appears to have also significant clinical activity, with a remission rate of 50% [38]. The excellent results obtained with imatinib when used as initial therapy, and the availability of effective salvage therapy, therefore redefined the CML treatment algorithm [39]. IFN-α was for many years the standard therapy for CML because it induced cytogenetic remissions in a significant number of patients. With imatinib and other TKIs, it is possible to achieve complete cytogenetic remission [polymerase chain reaction (PCR)-undetectable

BCR–ABL transcript] in many more patients. Another attractive approach could be the combination of TKIs with IFN-α [32].

Chronic Lymphocytic Leukemia

CLL is the most common mature B-cell neoplasm. It is a clonal disorder resulting in the accumulation of B lymphocytes coexpressing CD5, CD19, and CD23 [3]. The goal of therapy in CLL is now to achieve complete remission, eradicate minimal residual disease, and improve survival [4]. The molecular profile of CLL provides insight into disease pathogenesis and provides useful information on time to progression, need for therapy, and overall survival. A molecular profile can be built from assessment of a large number of biomarkers that have been identified [mutational status of the immunoglobulin heavy-chain variable gene (IgVH)], use of IgVH, and expression of 70-kDa zeta-associated protein (ZAP70) and CD38. One or more chromosome abnormalities can be found in more than 80% of CLL patients by using fluorescent in situ hybridization (FISH), including del13q, del11q, trisomy 12, del17p, and del6q [40, 41]. Fifty percent of CLL patients have undergone somatic hypermutation in IgVH, and these patients have a more indolent clinical course and longer survival than those without somatic hypermutation. Analysis of variable region sequences demonstrates that CLL cells use a biased repertoire of V genes with overrepresentation of certain Ig gene segments. Patients with CLL cells that use IGHV3-21 have relatively aggressive disease [4]. Surrogate markers of IgVH mutational status, such as expression of ZAP70 and CD38, have been assessed, and both have prognostic significance. However, there is not an absolute relationship between ZAP70 expression and IgVH mutational status, with discrepancies occurring in up to 25% of patients [40]. Discordant cases may have other biologic features with poor prognostic implications such as del17p, del11q, or use of IGHV3-21 [4, 8].

Currently, the most effective treatment for CLL consists of a combination of FCR. Although this approach has encouraging results, patients with CLL eventually relapse and require additional therapies. Patients with unmutated immunoglobulin heavy-chain (IgVH) genes as well as del(17p13.1) and del(11q22.3) are more likely to become refractory to conventional therapies. These CLL cases might benefit from novel agents. Many of the current therapeutic regimens for CLL are myelotoxic, immunosuppressive, and associated with infectious complications. Targeted therapies can often minimize these complications [42]. Emerging therapies ranging from new monoclonal antibodies to small molecules that interfere with vital pathways in signal transduction and cell cycle regulation are currently being developed, including the immunomodulator lenalidomide; monoclonal antibodies, such as lumiliximab, GA-101, and small-molecule immunopharmaceuticals (SMIPs); BCL-2 inhibitors, such as oblimersen, obatoclax, and ABT-263; and protein kinase inhibitors, such as flavopiridol, spleen TKIs, and phosphatidylinositol 3-kinase inhibitors [4].

CD20 is a B-cell activation and growth regulator receptor expressed at all stages of B-cell maturation but not on precursor B cells or other cells. Rituximab, the first anti-CD20 MoAb, is extensively employed in the clinical practice as single agent or in combination with conventional chemotherapeutical drugs [43]. Recent data suggest that the main antileukemic effect of rituximab is mediated through the induction of apoptosis, whereas complement-mediated cytotoxicity could be a minor component for clearance of tumor cells and even be detrimental to therapeutic efficacy. Rituximab induces caspase activation in CLL patients which correlates with tumor cell depletion [44]. Apoptosis could be directly mediated by anti-CD20 MoAb or indirectly through FcγR-expressing effector cells or could be mediated through sensitizing tumor cells to chemotherapy-induced cell death [14].

Several new anti-CD20 MoAbs have been generated to enhance therapeutic function in rituximab-refractory patients and/or enhance activity over rituximab in newly diagnosed patients. Their structures have been engineered to provide theoretical advantages over rituximab and are currently undergoing clinical investigation.

A newly approved agent, ofatumumab, is a fully human anti-CD20 MoAb that differs from rituximab by binding to a different CD20 epitope and directing more potent complement-dependent cytotoxicity, even against cells expressing lower levels of CD20 [18]. Ofatumumab has been utilized in patients refractory to fludarabine and alemtuzumab (anti-CD52, campath) in various clinical trials. Lenalidomide is an immunomodulatory drug currently approved for the treatment of multiple myeloma as well as 5q-deletion MDS. It exerts antiangiogenic properties, tumor necrosis factor-alpha (TNF-α) inhibition, modulation of T- and NK cell-mediated immunologic responses, and induction of apoptosis [45]. Furthermore, lenalidomide upregulates the expression of costimulatory CD80 and CD150 on CLL cells, leading, respectively, to T- and normal B-cell activation, which correlates with the cytokine release syndrome observed during treatment and enhanced immunoglobulin production [46]. The MoAb lumiliximab is directed against CD23, a surface glycoprotein commonly expressed on the surface of CLL cells but rarely found on other cells. It strongly induces apoptosis in CD23+ CLL cells [47] and shows a favorable safety profile in relapsed/refractory CLL. Lumiliximab also enhances the effects of fludarabine and rituximab, providing rationale for their combined use. GA-101 (obinutuzumab), a third-generation MoAb with higher affinity binding to CD20 type II epitope, shows an enhanced ability to induce ADCC compared to other anti-CD20 MoAbs, such as rituximab. Alemtuzumab (anti-CD52) is now approved for use in previously untreated CLL, having been approved initially for fludarabine-refractory patients. SMIPs are peptides designed to contain the variable region from a specific antibody and a constant region encoding IgG1 domains. TRU-016 is engineered to contain a variable region from anti-CD37 antibodies. CD37 is a glycoprotein strongly expressed on the surface of normal B cells as well as B-CLL. It mediates signal transduction for cell growth and development. The expression of CD37 is particularly strong on CLL cells

compared to CD20 [48]. TRU-016 has shown significant antitumor activity by NK-mediated antibody-dependent cellular cytotoxicity against human B-cell neoplasms. BCL-2 inhibitors are modulators of the BCL-2 pathway. The majority of CLLs overexpress the antiapoptotic BCL-2 family members BCL-2, BCL-XL, and MCL-1. These proteins sequester the proapoptotic proteins BAX and BAK, thereby preventing apoptosis. Oblimersen is a single-stranded DNA oligonucleotide that can bind to the first six codons of BCL-2, thereby inhibiting its transcription and impairing tumor cell viability [3]. Obatoclax is a small molecule mimicking the BH3 peptidic domain that acts as a pan-inhibitor of BCL-2 family proteins, resulting in apoptosis. Other BCL-2 inhibitors, such as ABT-263 and AT-101, induce apoptosis in CLL cells by binding to antiapoptotic BCL-2 family proteins BCL-XL, BCL-2, and BCL-W but not MCL-1 or A1, and BCL-2, BCL-XL, and MCL-1, respectively, with synergistic effects with cyclophosphamide and rituximab [49]. Flavopiridol is a pan-inhibitor of cyclin-dependent kinases, including CDK9, and can induce apoptosis in primary human CLL cells [50]. SNS-032 is another small-molecule inhibitor of CDK2, CDK7, and CDK9 currently being studied in a multicenter phase I trial in relapsed/refractory CLL and multiple myeloma [51, 52]. Preclinical studies demonstrate potent induction of apoptosis in CLL cells irrespective of prior drug exposure, IgVH gene mutational status, or the presence of high-risk cytogenetic abnormalities. The B-cell receptor (BCR) signals are transduced by the nonreceptor spleen tyrosine kinase (Syk). Activation of Syk leads to the activation of phosphatidylinositol 3-kinases (PI3K) and AKT and the phosphorylation of multiple signaling proteins including RAS, PLC-gamma, and MAP kinases, resulting in cell survival. Syk is expressed mainly in hematopoietic cells, and its expression is upregulated in CLL, making it a potential target for CLL treatment [53, 54]. Fostamatinib disodium is the first clinically available oral Syk TKI. Class I PI3Ks are a family of intracellular signaling proteins that are essential components of migratory, proliferative, survival, and differentiation pathways in many cell types, including those of hematopoietic origin. Upon PI3K activation, the p110 catalytic subunit generates the lipid second messenger phosphatidylinositol-trisphosphate, which acts as a binding site for recruitment and activation of numerous intracellular signaling enzymes. Sustained activation of the PI3K pathway can occur following BCR stimulation and has a pivotal role in the survival of CLL. CAL-101 is an oral small-molecule inhibitor of PI3K. Mammalian target of rapamycin (mTOR) is a kinase involved in cellular growth and proliferation that transduces signals from the PI3/AKT pathway, which is commonly activated in hematologic malignancies [55]. CLL cells exposed to the mTOR inhibitor rapamycin have reduced expression of cyclin D3, cyclin E, and cyclin A. Inhibition of this pathway is currently the focus of numerous research efforts. Rapamycin, also known as sirolimus, acts as an immunosuppressive agent as well as a growth inhibitory agent [56]. Everolimus is a more readily bioavailable derivative of sirolimus [57]. Dasatinib is a TKI approved by the FDA for the management of all phases of CML and adults with Ph+ALL with resistance or intolerance to prior therapy. In addition to inhibition of BCR–ABL, dasatinib has inhibitory activity on Src family kinases, including LYN, which is often unregulated and constitutively activated in CLL cells [58]. Dasatinib can induce apoptosis in CLL cells in vitro. Dasatinib can also sensitize CLL cells to other chemotherapy agents by inhibiting the antiapoptotic program induced by CD40 stimulation. Heat shock protein 90 (Hsp90) is a chaperone protein involved in the proper folding, assembly, transport, and function of important mediators of cell signaling and cell cycle control, such as tyrosine kinase–associated protein of 70 kDa (ZAP-70). The Hsp90 inhibitor BIIB021 is currently being evaluated in a phase I trial in relapsed/refractory CLL. The histone deacetylase inhibitor valproic acid was recently shown to induce apoptosis by modulating antiapoptotic and proapoptotic genes. Furthermore, valproic acid also appears to increase the chemosensitivity of CLL cells to fludarabine, flavopiridol, bortezomib, thalidomide, and lenalidomide. SDF-1/CXCR4 axis plays a central role in CLL cell trafficking and survival; CXCR4 antagonists impair migration of CLL cells to the microenvironment and result in increased susceptibility to chemotherapeutic agents [59]. Plerixafor, a CXCR4 antagonist, has been experimented in combination with rituximab in patients with relapsed CLL [3].

Acute Myeloid Leukemia

AML is a very heterogeneous clonal disorder characterized by the accumulation of somatically acquired genetic alterations in hematopoietic progenitor cells that alter normal mechanisms of self-renewal, proliferation, and differentiation. Nonrandom chromosome abnormalities occur in 50–60% of patients. In some instances, such as the acute promyelocytic subtype, cytogenetic corroboration is essential confirmation of that subtype, which is now regarded and treated as a separate entity [60, 61].

In recent years, gene mutations and deregulated expression of genes and noncoding RNAs (microRNAs) have been identified, unraveling the enormous molecular genetic heterogeneity within distinct cytogenetically defined subsets of AML, in particular the large group of cytogenetically normal (CN) AML [62–64].

An increasing number of cases of AML can be categorized on the basis of their underlying genetic defects. From a clinical perspective, specific chromosome abnormalities and molecular genetic changes are among the most important prognostic markers and therefore may be used for stratification of patients with AML to risk adapted therapeutic strategies. Novel therapies are being developed that target some of the identified genetic defects to optimize the treatment of distinct subtypes of AML. Although many promising biotargets have been identified, to date, only diagnosis of NPM1, CEBPA, and FLT3 mutations has entered clinical practice and affects diagnosis, risk assessment, and also guidance of therapy. Nucleophosmin 1 (NPM1) is a nuclear-cytoplasmic shuttling phosphoprotein with pleiotropic functions. NPM1 gene mutations, resulting in its delocalization into the cytoplasm, are found in approximately one-third of adult cases of AML, making it the most frequent mutation known in this disease to date [65]. NPM1 mutations have been associated with achievement of complete remission and favorable outcome [60]. CEBPA is a key leucine zipper containing transcription factor regulating differentiation of several cell types, including myeloid precursors. CEBPA biallelic mutations in AML have been identified, affecting the N-terminal region (truncated CEBPA isoform with dominant-negative properties) and the C-terminal basic region-leucine zipper domain (decreased DNA-binding or dimerization activity) [66]. The end result of such mutations is often a null phenotype. CEBPA mutations are predominantly found in CN-AML and in cases with 9q deletion [60]. Among CN-AML, CEBPA mutations have consistently been associated with a relatively favorable outcome [67]. In both cases, therapeutic recommendation is standard induction chemotherapy followed by three to four cycles of high-dose cytarabine [6, 9].

Activating mutations in the FMS-like tyrosine kinase 3 (FLT3), a tyrosine kinase receptor, important in the development of myeloid and lymphoid lineages, occur in 25–30% AML. FLT3 mutations result in internal tandem duplications (ITDs) in the juxtamembrane domain or mutations of the activating loop of the kinase. FLT3-ITD provides proliferative advantage and antiapoptotic signals and predicts shorter complete remission duration [68]. Several TKIs with FLT3 inhibitory activity have been introduced in clinical trials with best results in combination with chemotherapy. Prognosis of CN-AML with FLT3-ITD is significantly inferior compared with CN-AML without this mutation when treated with current standard chemotherapy [69], and allogeneic hemopoietic stem-cell transplantation is an attractive option for these patients. Given the poor results after standard chemotherapy in FLT3-ITD AML, new modalities need to be evaluated. FLT3 inhibitors in combination with chemotherapy as a frontline approach to patients with AML with activating FLT3 mutations are underway.

KIT, another member of the class III receptor tyrosine kinase family, and its ligand, stem-cell factor, have a key role in differentiation and activation of hemopoietic progenitors. KIT mutations have been associated with inferior outcome [70]. Activating mutations of the c-KIT receptor result in drug resistance and cytokine-independent proliferation through activation of STAT3 signaling [62]. IDH1 (cytosolic) and IDH2 (mitochondrial) are enzymes catalyzing oxidative decarboxylation of isocitrate to α-ketoglutarate. They are involved in cellular defense against oxidative damage. Both IDH1 and IDH2 mutants cause loss of the physiologic enzyme function and create a novel ability of the enzymes to convert α-ketoglutarate into 2-hydroxyglutarate, a putative oncogenic metabolite [71]. This mutation predicts worse outcome for patients without FLT3-ITD [72–74]. Wilms tumor 1 (WT1) transcription factor is implicated in regulation of apoptosis of hemopoietic progenitors. Its mutations are found in 10–13% of CN-AML and are associated with inferior outcome. Increased expression of WT1 has been used as a surrogate marker for minimal residual disease in AML. RUNX1 is deregulated in AML by chromosomal translocations and by mutations clustering in the Runt domain of the gene. RUNX1 mutations have been associated with undifferentiated (M0) morphology and with specific chromosome aberrations, such as trisomy 21 and trisomy 13. Mutations of this transcription factor gene are associated with lower complete remission rate and with inferior survival [68]. MLL is a binding protein that regulates gene expression through epigenetic mechanisms. Partial tandem duplications (PTD) of MLL oncogene are found in 5–11% of patients with CN-AML and frequently in those with AML with trisomy 11 [9, 67, 72]. MLL-PTD have been shown to contribute to leukemogenesis through DNA hypermethylation and epigenetic silencing of tumor suppressor genes, pointing to a potential role of DNA methyltransferase and/or histone deacetylase inhibitors in the treatment of this AML subset. MLL-PTD have been associated with inferior CR duration and relapse-free survival [67].

Low expression of the brain cells and acute leukemia, cytoplasmic (BAALC) gene product, the human member of a novel mammalian neuroectoderm gene lineage implicated in hematopoiesis and acute leukemia, is associated with favorable outcome in CN-AML [75]. The MN1 (meningioma 1) gene was first identified as a fusion partner of the TEL gene in reciprocal translocations. Recent studies have shown that MN1 overexpression is associated with poor response to induction chemotherapy and higher relapse rate and worse overall survival [76, 77]. ERG amplification with consecutive gene overexpression was observed in AML with complex aberrant karyotypes and has an adverse prognostic significance in CN-AML [67]. Deregulated expression of EVI1 (ecotropic viral integration site 1) is found in virtually all AML, with inv(3) (q21q26.2/t)(3,3)(q21; q26.2) leading to rearrangement of the EVI1 and RPN1 genes. High EVI1 expression predicts poor outcome. Aberrant expression of multiple microRNAs has recently been reported in AML [61]. MicroRNAs are naturally occurring noncoding RNAs that are cleaved from hairpin precursors and hybridize to imprecisely complementary mRNA of protein-coding genes, thereby leading to downregulation of the encoded proteins by RNA degradation or translation inhibition [78]. Deregulation of microRNAs and in turn of their target genes has been found to contribute to malignant transformation [79].

Immunophenotyping using multiparameter flow cytometry is used to determine lineage involvement of a newly diagnosed acute leukemia [80]. Quantification of expression patterns of several surface and cytoplasmic antigens is necessary for lineage assignment and to detect aberrant immunophenotypes allowing for measurement of minimal residual disease. AMLs with minimal differentiation frequently express early hematopoiesis-associated antigens (e.g., CD34, CD38, and HLA-DR) and lack most markers of myeloid and monocytic maturation; megakaryoblasts from acute megakaryoblastic leukemia typically express one or more of the platelet glycoproteins CD41 and/or CD61, and less commonly CD42. Some AMLs with recurrent genetic abnormalities are associated with characteristic immunophenotypic features. For example, AMLs with t(8;21) frequently express the lymphoid markers CD19 or, to a lesser extent, CD7; they may also express CD56; AMLs with inv(16) frequently express the T lineage-associated marker CD2 and AMLs with NPM1 mutation typically have high CD33 but absent or low CD34 expression [6]. Some of these antigens are becoming therapeutic targets. GO is a calicheamicin-conjugated anti-CD33 humanized MoAb approved for therapy of relapsed AML [81]. GO induced remissions in 31% of patients with tolerable side effects. Lintuzumab is another anti-CD33 MoAb [82, 83] whose activity depends on its properties of activating effector cells through its Fc domain. Lintuzumab decreases the production of proinflammatory cytokines by AML cells and mediates ADCC and phagocytosis of AML cells [23]. Lintuzumab has been used in the treatment of AML converting patients with minimal residual disease into molecular remission [17]. CD44 functions as a key regulator of AML LSCs. It is a receptor for hyaluronic acid and can also interact with other ligands, such as osteopontin, collagens, and MMPs and may be a good target for therapy [25].

The interleukin-3 receptor CD123 on pluripotent progenitor cells induces tyrosine phosphorylation and promotes proliferation and differentiation [26]. Anti-CD123 fragments coupled to toxins, such as diphtheria or pseudomonas exotoxins, have promising activities in preclinical studies [84].

D-cyclins regulate cell cycle progression and proliferation by acting in a complex with cyclin-dependent kinases (CDKs) to promote the phosphorylation of the retinoblastoma protein and initiate cellular transition from G1 to the S phase. Overexpression of D-cyclins occurs in many tumors and leads to increased cell proliferation and chemoresistance [85]. In contrast, inhibition of the expression of D-cyclins decreases cellular proliferation and induces apoptosis [86]. D-cyclins, universally dysregulated in multiple myeloma, are also overexpressed in a subset of patients with AML and are associated with poor outcome. Compounds with inhibitory activity are glucocorticoids [87], cyproheptadine [88], kinetin riboside [89], and the novel compound S14161, which inhibits D-cyclin transactivation via inhibition of phosphoinositide 3-kinase (PI3K) activity. This latter displayed preclinical activity in myeloma and leukemia cells in vitro and in vivo [85].

Acute Lymphoblastic Leukemia

Acute lymphoblastic leukemia (ALL) is a neoplasm of lymphoid progenitors that may be of B- or T-lymphoid lineage (B-ALL or T-ALL) and is the most common malignancy of childhood [90]. The outcome of ALL therapy has improved dramatically in recent decades, with cure rates exceeding 80% [91]. However, up to one-quarter of patients relapse, which carries a poor prognosis [92]. Current treatment regimens use intensive combination chemotherapy with little scope for significant intensification due to excessive short- and long-term side effects. Consequently, further improvements in the outcome of ALL therapy require the development of new, targeted, and less toxic therapies [7].

Because of the highly specific treatments available for unique ALL subtypes, it is essential to differentiate Philadelphia (Ph) chromosome positive from Ph-negative ALL, and mature ALL from B- or T-cell precursor ALL. Age and white blood cell count are important risk factors. Older adults are regarded as a prognostically unfavorable group. Regarding immunophenotype, in B-cell precursor ALL, a CD10-negative pro-B phenotype has high risk, especially when associated with t(4;11). Ph-negative common ALL (CD10+) is standard risk. The pre-B subtype expressing cytoplasmic heavy chains has a bad outlook when harboring MLL rearrangements. CD20 antigen is expressed in nearly half of BCP-ALL and may be prognostically adverse [5]. In T-cell precursor ALL, the prognosis is worse for CD1a-negative, CD3-negative cases compared to the CD1a-positive cortical/thymic phenotype [90].

ALL is characterized by recurring genetic alterations, including aneuploidy and structural rearrangements that commonly result in the expression of chimeric fusion genes, for example, BCR–ABL1 and MLL rearrangements, or

dysregulate genes by juxtaposition to antigen receptor gene loci [93]. Several of these, such as MLL rearrangement and low hypodiploidy, are associated with a high risk of relapse. A substantial minority of patients lack a known, recurring gross chromosomal alteration. Consequently, there has been intensive effort in recent years to use high-resolution genomic profiling to identify novel genetic alterations that contribute to leukemogenesis, influence treatment responsiveness, and ultimately may be translated to the clinic as new prognostic tools and therapeutic targets.

In B-lineage ALL, there are recurring genetic alterations in genes encoding regulators of lymphoid development (e.g., PAX5, IKZF1, and EBF1), transcription factors (ETV6, ERG), lymphoid signaling molecules (BTLA, CD200, BLNK, VPREB1), regulators of cell cycle and tumor suppressors (CDKN2A/CDKN2B, ATM, RB1, PTEN), and less commonly regulators of drug responsiveness (e.g., the glucocorticoid receptor NR3C1) [94, 95]. Genetic alterations targeting lymphoid development are key determinants of both the pathogenesis of B-ALL and responsiveness to therapy [96]. Different alterations targeting lymphoid development exhibit markedly variable associations with treatment outcome. PAX5 is the most common target of genetic alteration in B-ALL [97]. Deletion or sequence mutation of the early lymphoid transcription factor gene IKZF1 (encoding IKAROS) is associated with very poor outcome. IKAROS family zinc finger 1 (IKZF1) mutations are prevalent in blast phase CML or BCR–ABL+ALL, suggesting a pathogenetic contribution to leukemia transformation [98]. Mutation of IKZF1 is associated with an up to threefold increased risk of treatment failure in ALL [96, 99]. Consequently, there has been considerable interest in testing for IKZF1 alterations at the time of diagnosis to assist with risk stratification. Expression of the constitutively active tyrosine kinase BCR–ABL1 is a hallmark of CML and a subset of ALL (Ph+ALL). Prior to the advent of TKIs, Ph+ALL was associated with very poor outcome [64]. Targeted therapy with TKIs for Ph+ALL and with anti-CD20 MoAb added to hyperfractionated cyclophosphamide, vincristine, adriamycin, dexamethasone plus methotrexate, high-dose cytarabine regimen for Ph + B-ALL, improved patient survival; clinical trials combining chemotherapy plus rituximab (anti-CD20) and epratuzumab (anti-CD22) are in progress [5]. IKZF1 alterations are present in more than 80% of Ph + ALL cases in both adults and children and at the progression of CML to lymphoid blast crisis but are uncommon in other subtypes of ALL [100]. These findings suggest that IKZF1 alteration is a key determinant of the lineage and progression of Ph-positive leukemia. Approximately one-third of these Ph-like ALL have rearrangements of CRLF2, which encodes the cytokine receptor-like factor two that forms a heterodimer with interleukin-7 receptor alpha for the cytokine thymic stromal lymphopoietin. Up to 60% of patients with CRLF2 rearrangements have concomitant activating mutations in the kinase or pseudokinase domains of JAK1 and JAK2 [101]. Several selective JAK1/2 inhibitors are being investigated for the treatment of myeloproliferative diseases [102]. JAK inhibitors show activity as single agents or combined with chemotherapy in patients with these alterations.

The vast majority of cases of ALL appear to originate from putative developmental lesions in normal B-cell precursor clones during early phases of ontogeny and express D19 coreceptor. CD19 is a B-lineage restricted molecule that functions as a key regulator of transmembrane signals. Recently, a CD19-specific recombinant human protein (CD-L) has been tested as antileukemic agent in B-ALL. CD19-L, as well as anti-CD19 MoAb, induces apoptosis of normal and malignant B cells, suggesting that CD19 participates in regulation of immune responses and prevention of autoimmunity by mediating negative selection of hyperactive or autoreactive B-cell clones via apoptosis [103].

Genomic profiling has been successfully used to identify new sequence alterations in T-ALL, including deletions dysregulating LMO2 [104], amplification of MYB [105], amplification associated with the NUP214-ABL1 rearrangement [106], and deletion and sequence mutation of PTEN109 [107] and WT1 [108]. However, few associations between individual genetic alterations and outcome in T-ALL have been identified [101].

The less common T-lineage ALL (T-ALL) has an inferior outcome compared to B-ALL [109]. It represents about 15% of pediatric and 25% of adult ALLs. It is an aggressive hematologic tumor resulting from the malignant transformation of immature T-cell progenitors. The outcome of T-ALL patients has improved remarkably over the last two decades as a result of the introduction of intensified chemotherapy protocols. However, these treatments are associated with significant toxicity, and the treatment of patients presenting with primary resistant disease or those relapsing after a transient response remains challenging.

The most common genetic alteration in T-ALL is the presence of deletions in the CDKN2A tumor suppressor locus containing the P16/INK4A and the P14/ARF tumor suppressor genes, which control cell cycle progression and p53-mediated apoptosis, respectively. In addition, over 50% of T-ALLs harbor activating mutations in the NOTCH signaling pathway [110, 111]. T-ALL-associated chromosomal translocations typically result in the juxtaposition of a selective group of oncogenic transcription factors next to strong regulatory elements located in the vicinity of the T-cell receptor β (TCRB) gene in chromosome 7q34 or the T-cell receptor α–δ (TCRAD) locus in chromosome 14q11 [112].

Aberrant NOTCH signaling is a central player in T-ALL, and the NOTCH pathway represents an important potential therapeutic target. The NOTCH1 receptor is a transmembrane protein that functions as a ligand-activated transcription factor [110], directly transducing information from extracellular signals into changes in gene expression in the nucleus. It is composed of an N-terminal extracellular subunit (NEC) and a C-terminal transmembrane and intracellular subunit (NTM). In addition, it contains a negative regulatory region (NRR) which prevents the spontaneous activation of the receptor in the absence of ligand. Under physiologic conditions, the ligand–receptor interaction induces a conformational change in the NRR regulatory region and triggers a first cleavage of the surface domain by metalloproteases followed by a second proteolytic cleavage catalyzed by the γ-secretase complex in the transmembrane region of the receptor [113]. Thus, the γ-secretase complex releases the intracellular domain of NOTCH1 (ICN1) into the cytosol and allows its translocation into the nucleus, where it recruits members of the mastermind (MAML) family of coactivators and p300, and, through these interactions, activates gene expression. Finally, the polyubiquitination and proteasomal degradation of the activated receptor takes place in the nucleus [110]. In the lymphoid system, NOTCH signals provided by the thymic microenvironment are essential for the specification of α/β T-cell progenitors [114]. During this process, several important factors are transcriptionally controlled by NOTCH, including the pre-T-cell receptor α, the IL7 receptor α [115], and MYC [116]. NOTCH1 signaling is also critically required to sustain cell metabolism via activation of the PI3K–AKT cascade. Activating mutations in NOTCH1 typically result in the disruption of molecular locks responsible for preventing the spontaneous activation of the receptor at the membrane or mediating the termination of NOTCH1 signaling in the nucleus. Various genes and pathways are controlled by NOTCH1 in T-cell transformation [117]. In addition to its direct effect on anabolic genes and facilitating cell growth via upregulation of MYC [116], NOTCH1 facilitates the activation of the PI3K–AKT–mTOR signaling pathway, a critical regulator of cell growth and metabolism. Oncogenic NOTCH1 signaling also promotes G1/S cell cycle progression [118] through transcriptional upregulation of CCND3, CDK4, and CDK6 [119]. Moreover, inhibition of NOTCH signaling in T-ALL is associated with upregulation of the cyclin-dependent kinase inhibitors CDKN2D and CDKN1B [118]. Finally, NOTCH1 signaling can also regulate the survival of T-ALL cells by increasing expression of IkB kinase and consequently upregulating NFκB activity [120].

The critical role of this interaction is demonstrated by the antileukemic effects of NFκB inhibition in T-ALL and the strict requirement of NFκB signaling for NOTCH-induced transformation [121]. The most exciting opportunity derived from the identification of NOTCH1 mutations in T-ALL is the possibility of developing anti-NOTCH1-targeted therapies. The γ-secretase complex, responsible for the proteolytic processing

and activation of NOTCH signaling, can be inhibited with small-molecule inhibitors (GSIs), which block the activity of NOTCH receptors and reduce proliferation by inducing G1 cell cycle arrest [112]. Because of their gastrointestinal toxicity, intermittent dosing schemes as well as combined chemotherapy or other molecularly targeted drugs have been experimented, such as combination therapies of GSIs with CDK inhibitors, drugs targeting NFκB signaling, or small-molecule inhibitors of CK21 and the PI3K–AKT–mTOR pathway [118, 122]. Glucocorticoid treatment seems to have a direct protective effect against GSI-induced intestinal toxicity. The use of synthetic peptides blocking the NOTCH transcriptional complex directly in the cell nucleus is under investigation. It has recently shown that SAHM1, a cell-permeable peptide targeting NOTCH, has specific antileukemic effects both in human T-ALL cell lines and in a mouse model of NOTCH1-induced T-ALL [123]. Finally, given that NOTCH proteins are surface molecules, specific antibodies could provide selective blocking of NOTCH1 while preserving the activity of the other NOTCH family members [112, 124].

The PI3K/AKT/mTOR pattern of signal transduction has a critical function in proliferation, cell cycle progression, apoptosis, and metabolism. AKT kinase is activated in response to PI3K directly and is the most important effector of PI3K. It is capable of integrating signals from outside and inside the cell, such as signals related to the state energy, in the presence of nutrients and growth factors. T-ALL is characterized by the constitutive activation of the PI3K/AKT/mTOR axis, and many compounds that target the PI3K/AKT/mTOR have been developing [85].

Acute Promyelocytic Leukemia

Acute promyelocytic leukemia (APL) is a rare disease in which biotargeted therapies have a central role in clinical practice. APL had a bad prognosis, particularly because of fatal coagulation disorders, before the introduction of anthracyclines, which allowed the cure of some APL

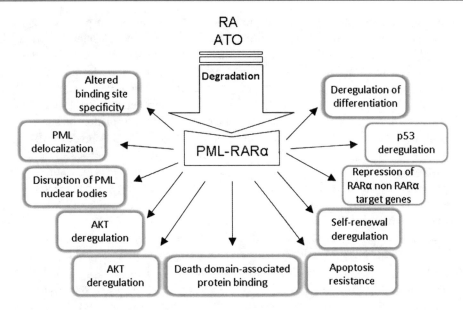

Fig. 6.9 PML-RARα as a gain-of-function fusion protein. PML-RARα functions as a multifaceted protein that deregulates differentiation and self-renewal of myeloid progenitors and confers resistance to apoptosis. It represses RARα and non-RARα target genes and disrupts PML nuclear bodies. This results in immortal proliferation and inhibition of terminal differentiation. Mechanistically, therapy-induced transcriptional activation (or derepression) is responsible for APL cell differentiation, and PML-RARα degradation by RA or ATO results in APL eradication. Arsenic trioxide targets PML through oxidation-triggered disulfide bond formation and direct binding. This results in PML and PML-RARα sumoylation, ubiquitylation, and proteasome-mediated degradation

patients. The subsequent introduction of all-trans-retinoic acid (ATRA) and the pure form of ATO improved the response of these patients leading to a dramatic change in the prognosis of this disease [125]. The simultaneous administration of ATRA and anthracycline-based chemotherapy is currently considered the standard induction treatment for newly diagnosed patients [126]. Various clinical regimens combining RA, ATO, and anthracyclines now definitively cure up to 90% of APL patients. This combination results in extremely high antileukemic efficacy, leading to complete remission rates of 90–95%. In several recent clinical trials, more than 90% of patients are disease-free and off-treatment after 5 years [127]. In particular, treatment regimens combining RA and ATO, including some without any DNA-damaging chemotherapy, have cured most patients [128, 129].

The specific PML-retinoic acid receptor-α (RARα) oncogene fusion and/or the t(15;17) translocation, detected by PCR, FISH, and conventional karyotyping, respectively, are the hallmarks of this leukemia. Additional alterations, for example, NRAS mutation, FMS-related tyrosine kinase 3 (FLT3) activation, and MYC overexpression, increase disease penetrance or favor its progression but do not have the same central role as PML-RARα in the hierarchy of genetic alterations [8, 127].

PML-RARα gene fusion initiates leukemogenesis by blocking the normal myeloid differentiation program and increasing self-renewal of APL progenitor cells (Fig. 6.9). RA and ATO cure this leukemia, by targeting PML-RARα gene fusion for degradation, triggering rapid APL cell differentiation into granulocytes. The combination of RA with anthracyclines cures 70% of patients. Moreover, ATO triggers apoptosis and partial maturation of human APL cells, but together with cytokines or cyclic AMP (cAMP), it also promotes terminal differentiation. Both RA and ATO can trigger differentiation. RARα is an RA-responsive transcription factor, and PML is the organizer of nuclear subdomains that are linked to posttranslational modifications and the control of stem-cell self-renewal. The PML-RARα fusion protein retains all the functional domains of RARα. PML-RARα transforms hematopoietic progenitors through the transcriptional repression of RARα target genes in a dominant-negative manner, resulting in enhanced recruitment of corepressors and histone deacetylases (HDACs) onto RARα target genes, enforcing DNA methylation. As RARα signaling regulates myeloid differentiation, its inhibition could explain the block in differentiation that is observed in APL cells. Pharmacological doses of RA convert PML-RARα into a transcriptional activator, thus enhancing expression of crucial RARα targets and restoring the normal differentiation [130].

Transcriptional repression of RARα target genes is not the only molecular mechanism initiating APL leukemogenesis. For example, PML-RARα activates the expression of cyclin-dependent kinase inhibitor 1A (CDKN1A encoding p21), which could allow HSC to tolerate DNA damage, indirectly contributing to transformation. PML-RARα also induces massive histone modifications or DNA methylation [131].

Heterotetramers of PML-RARα linked to RXRα bind several DNA target sequences that are not efficiently recognized by the normal RXRα–RARα heterodimers, thus contributing to widespread transcriptional deregulation. These de novo binding sites include sites that are recognized by other nuclear receptors controlling myeloid differentiation or stem-cell self-renewal, such as retinoic acid receptor-γ (RARG), vitamin D receptor (VDR), and thyroid hormone receptors. These non-RARα binding sites constitute a considerable proportion of the recently determined natural targets of PML-RARα in human APL cells, exemplifying a dramatic gain of function of the oncogenic fusion. As for many other transcription factors, PML-RARα sumoylation induces transcriptional repression. PML-RARα may also function by interfering with poorly defined PML-controlled pathways implicated in apoptosis resistance and have been recently linked to defective p53 activation [8].

PML-RARα modulates several key pathways that cooperate to enforce leukemic transformation.

PML-RARα degradation pathway involves proteases, activated by RA-induced differentiation, that cleave the PML moiety of PML-RARα [132, 133]. The second degradation pathway directly couples RA-induced transcriptional activation to proteasome-mediated RARα degradation. A third pathway involves formation of autophagic vesicles. In contrast, ATO degrades PML-RARα by targeting its PML moiety and accordingly also degrades the normal PML protein. ATO induces the formation of reactive oxygen species (RoS), which trigger the formation of PML intermolecular disulfide cross-links that induce multimerization, targeting nuclear bodies, and allow PML sumoylation in trans by ubiquitin-conjugating enzyme nine. In mouse models, RoS inducers (such as paraquat and α-tocopheryl succinate) have resulted in disease regression and/or dramatic prolongation of survival [134]. This observation sheds new light on the basis for the efficacy of anthracyclines in APL. Similar to ATO, anthracyclines induce massive RoS production.

Rare variant translocations, all involving RARα, account for 1–2% of patients with APL. The most common results in a PLZF-RARα fusion protein that is associated with RA-resistant APL. Resistance was proposed to result from an additional corepressor binding site in PLZF, which precludes RA-dependent target gene activation and thus differentiation [8]. High-dose RA treatment results in PLZF-RARα degradation, by the same mechanism as RARα and PML-RARα.

Clinical and basic research have allowed most patients with APL to be definitively cured, even with some treated without DNA-damaging agents. Greatly simplified clinical protocols associating frontline RA and ATO should lead not only to extremely high levels of cure but also to a higher quality of life and fewer days spent as an inpatient [135].

JAK2 + Myeloproliferative Neoplasms

The classical Philadelphia chromosome-negative myeloproliferative neoplasms (Ph-negative MPNs) include PV, ET, and PMF [136] Ph-negative MPNs are chronic myeloid neoplasms which are thought to arise from a

6 Leukemias

Table 6.2 JAK tyrosine inhibitors tested in myeloproliferative neoplasms (MPN)

Compound	Mainly inhibited transcription factor	Stage of development
Ruxolitinib (INCB018424)	JAK1, JAK2	Phase III
TG101348	JAK2, JAK2 V617F	Phase II
Lestaurtinib (CEP-701)	JAK2 V617F, FLT3, RET, TRKA	Phase II
XL019	JAK2	Phase I/II (halted for neurological toxicity)
SB1518	JAK2, JAK2 V617F	Phase I
CYT387	JAK1, JAK2	Phase I/II
AZD1480	JAK1, JAK2	Phase I/II
Tasocitinib (CP-690550)	JAK1, JAK2, JAK3	Phase II/III

primitive HSC which has undergone malignant transformation. Several MPN-associated mutations, not mutually exclusive, are currently known. They mainly originate at the progenitor cell level, but they do not necessarily represent the primary clonogenic event. Clinical manifestations include variable degrees of erythrocytosis, thrombocytosis, and leukocytosis, or cytopenias, extramedullary hematopoiesis (e.g., splenomegaly), increased risk for thrombosis, and transformation to AML. Patients with PV and ET are usually treated with cytoreductive agents (e.g., hydroxyurea, anagrelide, busulfan, and pipobroman) which can effectively control elevated blood cell counts and decrease the risk of thrombosis but may also be associated with an increased risk of transformation to AML [137, 138]. Apart from hydroxyurea, there are few drugs available for treating these patients without incurring in significant late side effects. For patients with MF, therapy is usually palliative and directed to alleviation of symptoms caused by splenomegaly and/or cytopenias. Recently, great advances were made in the understanding of the pathogenesis of these disorders with the discovery of an activating mutation of the JAK2 tyrosine kinase (TK) (JAK2 V617F) in patients with Ph-negative MPNs [139, 140]. The JAK2 V617F mutation leads to constitutive signaling through the JAK2 TK, leading to increased cellular proliferation and resistance to apoptosis in hematopoietic cells. More importantly, the discovery of JAK2 V617F led to the development of JAK2 inhibitors for therapy of patients with Ph-negative MPNs, following the same rationale used to target BCR–ABL1 in CML with imatinib.

Preclinical studies have confirmed activity of these compounds, with induction of apoptosis in both in vitro and in vivo models [141, 142], and several JAK inhibitors were entering clinical trials for patients with MF and later PV/ET, with differences in potency and kinase specificity (Table 6.2).

Most TKIs in current clinical development are small molecules that act by competing with adenosine triphosphate (ATP) for the ATP-binding catalytic site in the TK domain since ATP is the source of phosphate groups utilized by TK for phosphorylating protein targets [143]. The V617F mutation locates outside the TK domain of JAK2, and current JAK2 inhibitors target both wild-type and mutated JAK2 indiscriminately. This could explain why these drugs are active in patients with both wild-type and mutated JAK2 [11]. Therapy with JAK2 inhibitors may induce rapid and marked reductions in spleen size and can lead to remarkable improvements in constitutional symptoms and overall quality of life. Because JAKs are involved in the pathogenesis of inflammatory and immune-mediated disorders, JAK inhibitors are also being tested in clinical trials in patients with rheumatoid arthritis and psoriasis, as well as for the treatment of other autoimmune diseases and for the prevention of allograft rejection. In these pathologies, the main effect is the inhibition of T helper 1 (TH1) and TH17 inflammatory pathways [144]. Preliminary results indicate that these agents hold great promise for the treatment of JAK-driven disorders [145–147].

Myelodysplastic Syndromes

MDS, commonly considered preleukemic diseases, are characterized by clonal hematopoiesis, aberrant differentiation, peripheral cytopenias, and risk of progression to AML. The spectrum of genetic abnormalities in MDS implicates a wide range of molecular mechanisms in the pathogenesis of these disorders, including activation of tyrosine kinase signaling, genomic instability, impaired differentiation, altered ribosome function, and changes in the bone marrow microenvironment [148]. Table 6.3 shows the more frequent genetic abnormalities in MDS [10].

The term "epigenetic" refers to the heritable component of cellular phenotypes that are not mediated by changes to the genomic DNA sequence. The most relevant molecular mediators of the epigenetic state in MDS are gene expression patterns maintained by methylation of cytosine residues in DNA and covalent

Table 6.3 Genetic, epigenetic, and microenvironmental abnormalities in myelodysplastic syndromes

Chromosomal abnormalities	Pathogenetic mechanisms	Clinical features
Chromosome 5q deletions	Haploinsufficiency for RPS14, RPS14, miRNAs	Better prognosis, high lenalidomide response rate erythroid phenotype
Chromosome 7 and 7q deletions	Mutations in EZH2	Poor prognosis
Trisomy 8	Unknown	Intermediate risk, marker of progression in AML and responsiveness to immunosuppressors
Chromosome Y and 20q deletions	Unrelated to disease pathogenesis	Marker of clonal hematopoiesis
Chromosome 3q26 abnormalities	Altered expression of EVII	Poor prognosis
Chromosome 17 abnormalities	TP53 disruption	Intermediate risk when isolated
Isodicentric chromosome Xq13	Unknown	Intermediate risk when isolated presence of ring sideroblasts
T(6;9)(p23;q34) translocation	Generation of the DEK-NUP214 fusion gene	Intermediate risk when isolated
Gene mutations		
TET2	α-Ketoglutarate-dependent dioxygenase gene	Frequently present in low-risk MDS cases
ASXL1	Additional sex comb-like 1 gene encoding a member of the polycomb family of chromatin-binding proteins	Uncertain prognostic significance
RUNX1	Member of the transcriptional core-binding factor gene family (CBFA2 or AML1); DNA binding domain disruption	High risk of progression to AML; frequently found in secondary MDS
IDH1, IDH2	Isocitrate dehydrogenase genes encoding nicotinamide adenine dinucleotide phosphate-dependent enzymes; altered catalytic function	High risk of progression to AML; associated with advanced disease
FLT3, KIT, PDGFR, MPL	Constitutive tyrosine kinase activation	Rare in MDS, more frequent in MPN; more advanced disease and progression to AML, except for MPL
JAK2	Constitutive tyrosine kinase activation	Uncertain prognostic significance

(continued)

6 Leukemias

Table 6.3 (continued)

Chromosomal abnormalities	Pathogenetic mechanisms	Clinical features
CBL	TK-associated ubiquitin ligase functioning as negative regulator; STAT5 phosphorylation and growth factor hypersensitivity	Poor prognosis
NRAS, KRAS	GPTase activity loss and constitutive activation of serine/threonine kinase	Frequent; poor prognosis and progression to AML
TP53	Tumor suppressor gene	More frequent in secondary MDS; poor prognosis; resistance to therapy
Epigenetics		
DNA cytosine residue methylation	Hypermethylation target genes: CDKN2A/B, CTNNA1, CDH1, etc. silencing of promoters of tumor suppressor gene expression	Uncertain prognostic significance; rationale for the use of demethylating agents
Histone covalent modification	Enzymatic histone modification and altered interaction with DNA and other chromatin-binding proteins	Uncertain prognostic significance; rationale for the use of histone-modifying enzymes
Bone marrow microenvironment signals		
VEGF	Hypoxia-induced increase and neoangiogenesis	Uncertain prognostic significance
Proinflammatory cytokines	Immune system activation, cell–cell and cell–stroma interactions	Uncertain prognostic significance

modification of histones. DNA methyltransferases convert cytosine bases into 5-methylcytosines. Abnormal DNA methylation can alter gene interaction with DNA-binding proteins, such as transcription factors and histone-modifying enzymes. Typically, methylation of promoters leads to silencing of neighboring genes and represents a mechanism for loss of tumor suppressor gene expression. In MDS and AML, several genes have been described as targets of DNA hypermethylation. These include the cell cycle regulators CDKN2A (p14 and p16) and CDKN2B (p15), CTNNA1, E-cadherin (CDH1), and many others [149, 150]. These observations provide a rationale for the use of demethylating agents in MDS. The nucleoside analog azacitidine and its 2′-deoxy counterpart decitabine are inhibitors of DNMTs and have been approved for the treatment of MDS in the USA. Both medications have good response rates in MDS with 30–73% of patients experiencing a 50% or better decrease in transfusion dependence [151]. Inhibition of histone-modifying enzymes represents another potential epigenetic target for MDS therapy. Abnormalities of the bone marrow microenvironment are well documented in MDS and other myeloid malignancies. Levels of vascular endothelial growth factor (VEGF) and several inflammatory cytokines are elevated in the bone marrow of patients with MDS [152]. These changes are thought to be the result of the complex interplay between the abnormal hematopoietic cells and the adaptive immune response they instigate: activation of the innate immune system and autocrine or cell contact-mediated interactions with the stroma. Such alterations to the microenvironment can negatively impact normal hematopoiesis, providing a potential explanation for why cytopenias can occur even when MDS cells occupy only a fraction of the bone marrow [10].

Patients are divided into low- and high-risk categories. Without therapy, prognosis of patients with high-risk MDS is poor, and treatments should be directed to improve survival. Prognosis of patients with low-risk MDS is more heterogeneous, and therapies are usually directed to minimize transfusion needs and potentially to alter the natural course of the disease. Treatment options for patients with high-risk MDS include hypomethylating agents (azacitidine and decitabine), intensive chemotherapy, and allogeneic stem-cell transplantation. The use of the hypomethylating agents has transformed the approach to these patients, in particular older individuals, for whom intensive chemotherapy and bone marrow transplantation are not indicated. In low-risk MDS, treatment strategies are used sequentially: observation in patients with low risk and no transfusion dependency, growth factors, and lenalidomide for patients with alteration of chromosome 5 and anemia. The use of hypomethylating agents is less understood in this group of patients. Bone marrow transplantation is usually reserved for patients with low-risk MDS closer to the time of transformation [148, 153].

Leukemic Microenvironment and Leukemic Stem Cell

Acute myelogenous leukemia is propagated by a subpopulation of LSCs. Unresponsiveness to initial treatment and/or relapses are often the consequence of LSC resistance to current therapies. Like normal HSCs, LSCs reside in a mostly quiescent state [8] which renders them substantially more resistant to standard chemotherapy than bulk leukemia populations. Both intrinsic and extrinsic components influence LSC survival. Among intrinsic factors, there are regulators of cell cycle and prosurvival pathways, such as nuclear factor kappa B (NFκB) and AKT. The extrinsic components are generated by the bone marrow microenvironment and include chemokine receptors (CXCR4), adhesion molecules (VLA-4 and CD44), and hypoxia-related proteins. New targeted strategies exploit potentially unique properties of the LSCs and their microenvironment. The specific LSC phenotype allows

primitive leukemia cells to be distinguished from normal stem and progenitor cells [154].

The NFκB and AKT pathways are constitutively activated in AML stem cells [155], representing central targets in LSC-specific therapies [156]. For example, the inhibition of AKT by using phosphatidylinositol-3 kinase (PI3K) inhibitors has been shown to augment LSC-targeted therapies. In addition to its role as survival signal via modulation of the proapoptotic factor BAD, the activity of the PI3K pathway has also recently been implicated in antioxidant defenses. Treatment with PI3K inhibitors effectively blocks induction of heme oxygenase (HMOX-1), acting to increase oxidative stress in AML cells through the inhibition of cellular antioxidant mechanisms. Interestingly, oxidative stress may reduce self-renewal, leading to either differentiation or death of primitive AML cells. Bcl-XL and Bcl-2 antiapoptotic proteins, highly expressed in leukemic progenitor cells, could be targeted by specific modulators, such as ABT-263, which is undergoing phase I and II clinical trials as single agent or in combination with MoAbs in CLL and ALL. ATO, widely utilized in APL therapy, is a strong inhibitor of the NFκB pathway and also induces high levels of oxidative stress. Multiple agents that inhibit PI3K pathway components are in development, and derivatives of the mTOR inhibitor are also available (e.g., temsirolimus). In addition, there is strong interest in targeting the Wnt/beta-catenin pathway with several types of agents currently under investigation [157, 158]. Activation of the principal self-renewal pathways through Wnt/beta-catenin and NOTCH signaling can be caused by microenvironmental stimuli and is amenable to therapeutic interventions [159]. Microenvironment plays a pivotal role in survival and drug resistance of LSCs [160], and this finding has generated novel approaches targeting the microenvironmental niche. This latter supports LSC survival through production of cytokines, chemokines, and intracellular signals initiated by cellular adhesion. Recent data indicate that, in parallel with leukemogenic events in the hematopoietic system, the niche is converted into an environment with dominant signals that favor cell proliferation and growth [161, 162]. The interaction between

CXCL12 (stromal cell-derived factor-1 alpha) and its receptor CXCR4 on leukemic progenitor cells contributes to their homing to the bone marrow microenvironment. CXCR4 levels are significantly elevated and associated with poor outcome in patients with AML. Administration of anti-CXCR4 antibody to mice engrafted with primary AML cells resulted in a dramatic decrease in the levels of human AML cells in the BM, blood, and spleen. Integrins are also required for LSC attachment to the bone marrow microenvironment, and interaction between very late antigen-4 on leukemic cells and fibronectin in the niche is crucial for the persistence of minimal residual disease in AML. CD44 adhesion molecule is another key regulator of AML LSCs homing to microenvironmental niches [25, 163]. Disruption of migratory and adhesion signals represents the strategy of blocking LSC homing to a BM niche and/or sensitizing leukemic cells to chemotherapy or kinase inhibitors. Targeting CXCR4 with small-molecule pharmacologic inhibitors has been shown to be efficacious in preclinical models of CLL, ALL, and AML [164]. Leukemic cells are able to proliferate even under hypoxic conditions [165]. In bone marrow specimens from ALL patients, there is overexpression of the key hypoxia mediator hypoxia-inducible transcription factor-1 α (HIF-1α). Several strategies specifically targeting HIF-1α are being explored, including antisense oligonucleotide against HIF-1α and small-molecule HIF-1α inhibitors [166]. Hypoxia is the major stimulus for angiogenesis through upregulation of VEGF. Increased angiogenesis is observed in MDS, AML, and ALL. Targeting angiogenesis is the most clinically advanced approach for influencing leukemia microenvironment. The anti-VEGF MoAb bevacizumab is the first antiangiogenic agent that has been validated in cancer therapy. Bevacizumab, combined with cytarabine and mitoxantrone, has been demonstrated to improve the overall response rate of 48% in a phase II study in AML patients [167–169]. Other types of antiangiogenic agents, such as TKIs (sunitinib and sorafenib) and anticytokine drugs (thalidomide and lenalidomide), have now entered clinical practice [170]. Although these agents may affect endothelial bone marrow niches, they may, in turn, enforce expansion of hypoxic niches and possibly promote chemoresistance. Structural chromosomal changes have been found in bone marrow stromal cells from patients with MDS and AML, suggesting an aberrant microenvironment in leukemia [171]. The transmembrane neuropilin-1 (NRP-1) receptor, a glycoprotein initially identified on neurons and endothelial cells, offers a potential drug delivery approach for therapies against AML and ALL, due to its role in angiogenesis and progression of hematologic malignancies in bone marrow microenvironment [165]. NRP-1 is highly expressed in diverse tumors [171] where it correlates with cell growth, vascularization, and invasiveness. Its expression can be stimulated in response to tissue injury or hypoxic conditions [172]. NRP-1 expression is increased in the bone marrow of ALL and AML patients compared with normal bone marrow and high levels of NRP-1 correlates with disease severity and progression. Since angiogenesis is an important requirement for the development and progression of human hematologic malignancies [173], NRP-1 can be, therefore, considered as a potential target in leukemia therapies, suggesting the potential for ligand-directed drug delivery [174].

TP53 and Apoptosis

The p53 protein is a transcription factor that controls cellular responses to stress by inducing cell cycle arrest, apoptosis, and cellular senescence. Impairment of p53 function (Fig. 6.10) occurs in the majority of tumors as a result of mutations in TP53 gene itself or abrogation of signaling pathways regulating p53 protein. Direct inactivation of p53 protein can also occur as a result of the binding of virus proteins. For example, preclinical studies suggest that p53 may be an excellent candidate tumor antigen [175]. The tumor-specific, high expression levels of TP53 and its frequent mutation in human cancers suggest that p53 may be perceived by the immune system as a target antigen. This has led to a number of active clinical trials using immunization with large peptides derived from p53 [176]. The MDM2 ubiquitin ligase regulates p53 by targeting it for

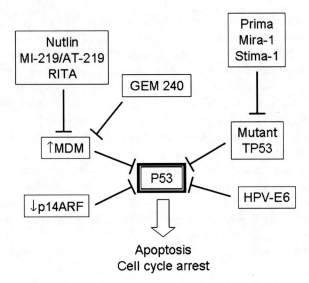

Fig. 6.10 Possible inactivation mechanisms of p53 responses in hematologic malignancies and main therapeutical approaches targeting dysfunctional p53 pathways currently in development. Normally, p53 functions as a transcription factor which upregulates key genes involved in cell cycle arrest and apoptosis. p53 dysregulation may be achieved in different ways: (1) p14ARF promoter methylation downregulating p14ARF expression, (2) MDM2 gene amplification, (3) TP53 missense and nonsense mutations, (4) p53 protein degradation by human papillomavirus E6 (HPV-E6). Agents targeting the p53 pathway currently in development for leukemias include MDM2 antagonists (nutlin, MI-219/AT-219, RITA), reactivators of mutant p53 (PRIMA, MIRA-1, STIMA-1), and antisense MDM2 oligonucleotides (GEM240)

ubiquitin-dependent proteasomal degradation [177]. MDM2 gene amplification is frequently found in cancer with consequent downregulation of p53 activity [178]. Similarly, methylation at the CDKN2A locus can epigenetically silence the expression of the p14ARF protein blocking the ability of activated oncogenes to stabilize the p53 response [179]. In hematologic malignancies such as acute and chronic lymphoid leukemias, the induction of p53 function using nutlin-3, a small-molecule inhibitor of MDM2, can induce apoptosis in malignant cells [180], whereas normal cells tolerate MDM2 inhibition with low-grade toxic effects in normal tissues. Another MDM2 inhibitor from the nutlin series, rG7112, is being tested in phase I trials. The small-molecule reactivation of p53 and induction of tumor cell apoptosis (RITA) [181] seems to act differently to the nutlins by binding directly to p53 and blocking its ability to interact with MDM2 but not its ability to activate p53-dependent apoptosis. The induction of apoptosis by nutlin-3 is specific to wild-type TP53 and synergistically enhances the cytotoxicity of doxorubicin and cytarabine in AML blasts but not in normal hematopoietic progenitor cells with minimal side effects. Treatment with nutlin-3 also resulted in TP53-dependent upregulation of NOTCH1 in CLL [182]; the combination with γ-secretase inhibitors, which block the activation of NOTCH receptors, enhanced its cytotoxic effects, suggesting therapeutic potential for this drug combination. Another study reported that combining treatment of nutlin-3 with inhibition of XiaP (X-linked inhibitor of apoptosis, which is highly expressed in AML and protects malignant cells from apoptosis) produced synergistic apoptogenic activities in blast cells isolated from AML patients [183]. A novel potential role for nutlin and p53-activating drugs is in protecting normal tissues from the side effects of chemotherapy, through the cell cycle arrest functions of p53 in normal tissues (cyclotherapy). In this approach, nutlin would protect normal tissues from the effects of conventional cytotoxic agents resulting in improvement of their therapeutic window, fewer toxic effects, and possibility of increasing the doses of the active agents [175].

Conclusion and Perspectives

New advances in understanding the biology of leukemias and the development of modern therapies are occurring at a rapid pace. The increasingly detailed understanding of the pathophysiology and molecular pathogenesis of leukemia has led to the identification of important biotargets against which highly effective and selective new compounds have been synthesized [184].

The new lines of research are directed to the identification of agents that interfere in a selective manner against specific molecular targets to increase the selectivity and reduce systemic side effects. This kind of approach to disease configurates an excellent example of modern translational and personalized medicine [185]. Genomics and proteomics have increased our understanding of the mechanisms of leukemogenesis, resistance to therapy, and relapses [37], with results derived from clinical trials using new biotargeted drugs, moving observations from the bedside to the bench and vice versa. The use of functional genomic approaches, such as siRNA screens, may identify novel targets and pathways in many leukemias. Lessons learnt from first-generation targeted agents have aided the design and evaluation of second-generation compounds. Better understanding of the mechanism of action of a drug may also help in defining potential mechanisms of resistance. Profiling of human leukemia-derived cell lines with combinatorial libraries might yield ligand peptide sequences that bind to specific internalizing receptors on cell surfaces and may potentially lead to the discovery of new or unrecognized therapeutic targets. Such targeting motifs could also serve as vehicles for the preferential delivery of cytotoxic agents to leukemic cells [17, 184].

New preclinical strategies are being used to evaluate novel agents, such as inhibitors of phosphatidylinositol 3-kinase for T acute lymphoblastic leukemias (T-ALL) characterized by the constitutive activation of this kinase, and to identify promising combinations of targeted drugs [186–188]. These strategies should include the identification of molecular changes that are essential for the survival and proliferation of leukemic cells, for example, by using multiparametric flow cytometry to detect cell-specific surface markers characteristic of distinct bone marrow populations [189–191], together with annexin V staining to detect apoptotic cells [192, 193]. The identification of specific cell surface markers on putative LSC, and their separation from other tumor cells by flow cytometry, might enable research into their biological properties, including their sensitivity to drugs [60, 194].

However, only about 5% of identified compounds targeting specific molecules or pathways essential for the survival and proliferation of leukemic cells demonstrate sufficient clinical efficacy in phase III trials, recapitulating disease complexity and molecular heterogeneity [195]. The most effective treatment to inhibit the survival of leukemic blasts depends on the mechanism of activation in each different type of leukemia [166]. The clinical development of drugs directed against biological targets should be aimed not only to inhibit the signaling pathway but inhibition should also lead to a clinical response in the patient [196, 197]. Better knowledge of oncogenic signaling mechanisms and the mechanisms of action of their inhibitors is probably the most effective way to obtain such goal.

References

1. Saglio G, Kim DW, Issaragrisil S, et al. Nilotinib versus imatinib for newly diagnosed chronic myeloid leukaemia. N Engl J Med. 2010;362:2251–9.
2. DeVita VT, Canellos GP. New therapies and standard of care in oncology. Nat Rev Clin Oncol. 2011; 8:67–8.
3. Abou-Nassar K, Brown RJ. Novel agents for the treatment of chronic lymphocytic leukaemia. Clin Adv Hematol Oncol. 2010;8:1–10.
4. Gribben JG, O'Brien S. Update on therapy of chronic lymphocytic leukaemia. J Clin Oncol. 2011;29: 544–50.
5. Bassan R, Hoelzer D. Modern therapy of acute lymphoblastic leukaemia. J Clin Oncol. 2011;29: 532–43.

6. Dohner H, Estey EH, Amadori S, et al. Diagnosis and management of acute myeloid leukaemia in adults: recommendations from an international expert panel, on behalf of the European LeukaemiaNet. Blood. 2010;15:396–400.
7. Mullighan CG. New strategies in acute lymphoblastic leukaemia: translating advances in genomics into clinical practice. Clin Cancer Res. 2010;17: 396–400.
8. de Thè H, Chen Z. Acute promyelocytic leukaemia: novel insights into the mechanisms of cure. Nat Rev Cancer. 2010;10:775–83.
9. Burnett A, Wetzler M, Löwenberg B. Therapeutic advances in acute myeloid leukemia. J Clin Oncol. 2011;29:487–94.
10. Bejar R, Levine R, Ebert BL. Unraveling the molecular pathophysiology of myelodysplastic syndromes. J Clin Oncol. 2011;29:504–15.
11. Santos FP, Verstovsek S. JAK2 inhibitors: what's the true therapeutic potential? Blood Rev. 2011;25:53–63.
12. Czuczman MS, Olejniczak S, Gowda A, et al. Acquirement of rituximab resistance in lymphoma cell lines is associated with both global CD20 gene and protein down-regulation regulated at the pretranscriptional and posttranscriptional levels. Clin Cancer Res. 2008;14:1561–70.
13. Hiraga J, Tomita A, Sugimoto T, et al. Downregulation of CD20 expression in B-cell lymphoma cells after treatment with rituximab-containing combination chemotherapies: its prevalence and clinical significance. Blood. 2009;113:4885–93.
14. Alduaij W, Illidge TM. The future of anti-CD20 monoclonal antibodies: are we making progress? Blood. 2011;117:2993–3001.
15. Ginaldi L, De Martinis M, Matutes E, et al. Levels of expression of CD19 and CD20 in chronic B cell leukaemias. J Clin Pathol. 1998;51:364–9.
16. Ginaldi L, De Martinis M, Matutes E, et al. Levels of expression of CD52 in normal and leukemic B and T cells: correlation with in vivo therapeutic responses to Campath-1H. Leuk Res. 1998;22:185–91.
17. Ball ED, Broome HE. Monoclonal antibodies in the treatment of hematologic malignancy. Best Pract Res Clin Haematol. 2010;23:403–16.
18. Wierda WG, Kipps TJ, Mayer J, et al. Ofatumumab as single-agent CD20 immunotherapy in fludarabine-refractory chronic lymphocytic leukaemia. J Clin Oncol. 2010;28:1749–55.
19. Richards JO, Karki S, Lazar GA, et al. Optimization of antibody binding to FcgammaRIIa enhances macrophage phagocytosis of tumor cells. Mol Cancer Ther. 2008;7:2517–27.
20. Hillmen P, Skotnicki AB, Robak T, et al. Alemtuzumab compared with chlorambucil as firstline therapy for chronic lymphocytic leukaemia. J Clin Oncol. 2007;25:5616–23.
21. Keating MJ, Flinn I, Jain V, et al. Therapeutic role of alemtuzumab (Campath-1H) in patients who have failed fludarabine: results of a large international study. Blood. 2002;99:3554–61.
22. Ball ED, Medeiros BC, Balaian L, et al. A phase I/II trial of 5-azacytidine prior to gemtuzumab ozogamicin (GO) for patients with relapsed acute myeloid leukaemia with correlative biomarker studies. Blood. 2009;114 (Abstract 2049).
23. Sutherland MK, Yu C, Lewis TS, et al. Anti-leukemic activity of lintuzumab (SGN-33) in preclinical models of acute myeloid leukaemia. MAbs. 2009;1: 481–90.
24. Krause DS, Van Etten RA. Right on target: eradicating leukemic stem cells. Trends Mol Med. 2007;13:470–81.
25. Jin L, Hope KJ, Zhai Q, et al. Targeting of CD44 eradicates human acute myeloid leukemic stem cells. Nat Med. 2006;12:1167–74.
26. Du X, Ho M, Pastan I. New immunotoxins targeting CD123, a stem cell antigen on acute myeloid leukaemia cells. J Immunother. 2007;30:607–13.
27. Vardiman JW, Thiele J, Arber DA, et al. The 2008 revision of the World Health Organization (WHO) classification of myeloid neoplasms and acute leukaemia: rationale and important changes. Blood. 2009;114:937–51.
28. le Coutre P, Schwarz M, Kim TD. New developments in tyrosine kinase inhibitor therapy for newly diagnosed chronic myeloid leukaemia. Clin Cancer Res. 2010;16:1771–80.
29. Breccia M, Efficace F, Alimena G. Imatinib treatment in chronic myelogenous leukaemia: what have we learned so far? Cancer Lett. 2011;300:115–21.
30. Mahon FX, Réa D, Guilhot J. Discontinuation of imatinib in patient with chronic myeloid leukaemia who have maintained complete molecular remission for at least 2 years: the prospective, multicentre stop imatinib (STIM) trial. Lancet Oncol. 2010;11: 1029–35.
31. O'Brien SG, Guilhot F, Larson RA, et al. Imatinib compared with interferon and low-dose cytarabine for newly diagnosed chronic-phase chronic myeloid leukaemia. N Engl J Med. 2003;348:994–1004.
32. Cortes J, Hochhaus A, Hughes T, Kantarjian H. Front-line and salvage therapies with tyrosine kinase inhibitors and other treatments in chronic myeloid leukaemia. J Clin Oncol. 2011;29:524–31.
33. Druker BJ, Guilhot F, O'Brien SG. Five-year followup of patients receiving imatinib for chronic myeloid leukaemia. N Engl J Med. 2006;355:2408–17.
34. Ibrahim AR, Eliasson L, Apperley JF, Milojkovic D, et al. Poor adherence is the main reason for loss of CCyR and imatinib failure for chronic myeloid leukaemia patients on long-term therapy. Blood. 2011; 117:3733–6.
35. Wei G, Rafiyath S, Liu D. First-line treatment for chronic myeloid leukaemia: dasatinib, nilotinib, or imatinib. J Hematol Oncol. 2010;3:47.
36. Hochhaus A, Baccarani M, Deininger M, et al. Dasatinib induces durable cytogenetic responses in patients with chronic myelogenous leukaemia in chronic phase with resistance or intolerance to imatinib. Leukemia. 2008;22:1200–6.

37. Kantarjian H, Giles F, Bhalla K, et al. Update on imatinib-resistant chronic myeloid leukaemia patients in chronic phase (CML-CP) on nilotinib therapy at 24 months: clinical response, safety, and long-term outcomes. Blood. 2009;114 (Abstract 1129).
38. Cortes J, Kantarjian H, Brummendorf TH, et al. Safety and efficacy of bosutinib (SKI-606) in patients with chronic phase chronic myeloid leukaemia following resistance or intolerance to imatinib. J Clin Oncol. 2010;28:487s (Abstract 6502).
39. Deininger M. Curing CML with imatiib-a dream come true? Nat Rev Clin Oncol. 2001;8:127–8.
40. Bosch F, Muntanola A, Gine E, et al. Clinical implications of ZAP-70 expression in chronic lymphocytic leukaemia. Cytometry B Clin Cytom. 2006; 70:214–7.
41. Del Principe MI, Del Poeta G, Buccisano F, et al. Clinical significance of ZAP-70 protein expression in B-cell chronic lymphocytic leukaemia. Blood. 2006;108:853–61.
42. Knauf WU, Lissichkov T, Aldaoud A, et al. Phase III randomized study of bendamustine compared with chlorambucil in previously untreated patients with chronic lymphocytic leukaemia. J Clin Oncol. 2009; 27:4378–84.
43. Lim SH, Beers SA, French RR, et al. Anti-CD20 monoclonal antibodies: historical and future perspectives. Haematologica. 2010;95:135–43.
44. de Haij S, Jansen JH, Boross P, et al. In vivo cytotoxicity of type I CD20 antibodies critically depends on Fc receptor ITAM signaling. Cancer Res. 2010;70: 3209–17.
45. Chang DH, Liu N, Klimek V, et al. Enhancement of ligand-dependent activation of human natural killer T cells by lenalidomide: therapeutic implications. Blood. 2006;108:618–21.
46. Aue G, Njuguna N, Tian X, et al. Lenalidomide-induced upregulation of CD80 on tumor cells correlates with T-cell activation, the rapid onset of a cytokine release syndrome and leukemic cell clearance in chronic lymphocytic leukaemia. Haematologica. 2009;94:1266–73.
47. Pathan NI, Chu P, Hariharan K, Cheny C, Molina A, Byrd J. Mediation of apoptosis by and antitumor activity of lumiliximab in chronic lymphocytic leukaemia cells and CD23 lymphoma cell lines. Blood. 2008;111:1594–602.
48. Zhao X, Lapalombella R, Joshi T, et al. Targeting CD37-positive lymphoid malignancies with a novel engineered small modular immunopharmaceutical. Blood. 2007;110:2569–77.
49. Paoluzzi L, Gonen M, Gardner JR, et al. Targeting Bcl-2 family members with the BH3 mimetic AT-101 markedly enhances the therapeutic effects of chemotherapeutic agents in in vitro and in vivo models of B-cell lymphoma. Blood. 2008;111:5350–8.
50. Lin TS, Ruppert AS, Johnson AJ, et al. Phase II study of flavopiridol in relapsed chronic lymphocytic leukaemia demonstrating high response rates in

genetically high-risk disease. J Clin Oncol. 2009; 27:6012–8.
51. Wierda WG, Chen R, Plunkett W, et al. A phase 1 trial of SNS-032, a potent and specific CDK 2, 7 and 9 inhibitor, in chronic lymphocytic leukaemia and multiple myeloma. Blood (ASH Annual Meeting Abstracts). 2008;112 (Abstract 3178).
52. Flynn JM, Johnson AJ, Andritsos L, et al. The cyclin dependent kinase inhibitor SCH 727965 demonstrates promising pre-clinical and early clinical activity in chronic lymphocytic leukaemia. Blood (ASH Annual Meeting Abstracts). 2009;114 (Abstract 886).
53. Gobessi S, Laurenti L, Longo PG, et al. Inhibition of constitutive and BCR-induced Syk activation down-regulates Mcl-1 and induces apoptosis in chronic lymphocytic leukaemia B cells. Leukemia. 2009;23: 686–97.
54. Friedberg JW, Sharman J, Sweetenham J, et al. Inhibition of Syk with fostamatinib disodium has significant clinical activity in non Hodgkin's lymphoma and chronic lymphocytic leukemia. Blood. 2010;115:2578–85.
55. Shaw RJ, Cantley LC. Ras, PI(3)K and mTOR signaling controls tumour cell growth. Nature. 2006; 441:424–30.
56. Aleskog A, Norberg M, Nygren P, et al. Rapamycin shows anticancer activity in primary chronic lymphocytic leukemia cells in vitro, as single agent and in drug combination. Leuk Lymphoma. 2008;49:2333–43.
57. Decker T, Sandherr M, Goetze K, et al. A pilot trial of the mTOR (mammalian target of rapamycin) inhibitor RAD001 in patients with advanced B-CLL. Ann Hematol. 2009;88:221–7.
58. Contri A, Brunati AM, Trentin L, et al. Chronic lymphocytic leukemia B cells contain anomalous Lyn tyrosine kinase, a putative contribution to defective apoptosis. J Clin Invest. 2005;115:369–78.
59. Stamatopoulos B, Meuleman N, De Bruyn C, et al. The histone deacetylase inhibitor suberoylanilide hydroxamic acid (SAHA) downregulates the CXCR4 chemokine receptor and impairs migration of chronic lymphocytic leukemia cells. Haematologica. 2009; 95:S83.
60. Marcucci G, Haferlach T, Dohner H. Molecular genetics of adult acute myeloid leukemia: prognostic and therapeutic implications. J Clin Oncol. 2011; 29:475–86.
61. Mrozek K, Radmacher MD, Bloomfield CD, et al. Molecular signatures in acute myeloid leukemia. Curr Opin Hematol. 2009;16:64–9.
62. Garzon R, Garofalo M, Martelli MP, et al. Distinctive microRNA signature of acute myeloid leukemia bearing cytoplasmic mutated nucleophos- min. Proc Natl Acad Sci U S A. 2008;105:3945–50.
63. Debernardi S, Skoulakis S, Molloy G, et al. MicroRNA miR-181a correlates with morphological sub-class of acute myeloid leukemia and the expression of its target genes in global genome-wide analysis. Leukemia. 2007;21:912–6.

64. Pui CH, Carroll WL, Meshinchi S, Arceci RJ. Biology, risk stratification, and therapy of pediatric acute leukemias. J Clin Oncol. 2011;29:551–65.

65. Damm F, Heuser M, Morgan M, et al. Single nucleotide polymorphism in the mutational hotspot of WT1 predicts a favorable outcome in cytogenetically normal acute myeloid leukemia. J Clin Oncol. 2010;28:578–85.

66. Ho PA, Alonzo TA, Gerbing RB, et al. Prevalence and prognostic implications of CEBPA mutations in pediatric acute myeloid leukemia (AML): a report from the Children's Oncology Group. Blood. 2009; 113:6558–66.

67. Mrozek K, Marcucci G, Paschka P, et al. Clinical relevance of mutations and gene-expression changes in adult acute myeloid leukemia with normal cytogenetics: are we ready for a prognostically prioritized molecular classification? Blood. 2007;109:431–48.

68. Gaidzik VI, Schlenk RF, Moschny S, et al. Prognostic impact of WT1 mutations in cytogenetically normal acute myeloid leukemia: a study of the German-Austrian AML Study Group. Blood. 2009;113: 4505–11.

69. Mead AJ, Linch DC, Hills RK, et al. FLT3 tyrosine kinase domain mutations are biologically distinct from and have a significantly more favorable prognosis than FLT3 internal tandem duplications in patients with acute myeloid leukemia. Blood. 2007; 110:1262–70.

70. Paschka P. Core binding factor acute myeloid leukemia. Semin Oncol. 2008;35:410–7.

71. Ward PS, Patel J, Wise DR, et al. The common feature of leukemia-associated IDH1 and IDH2 mutations is a neomorphic enzyme activity converting alpha-ketoglutarate to 2-hydroxyglutarate. Cancer Cell. 2010;17:225–34.

72. Marcucci G, Maharry K, Wu YZ, et al. IDH1 and IDH2 gene mutations identify novel molecular subsets within de novo cytogenetically normal acute myeloid leukemia: a Cancer and Leukemia Group B study. J Clin Oncol. 2010;28:2348–55.

73. Paschka P, Schlenk RF, Gaidzik VI, et al. IDH1 and IDH2 mutations are frequent genetic alterations in acute myeloid leukemia (AML) and confer adverse prognosis in cytogenetically normal AML with NPM1 mutation without FLT3-ITD. J Clin Oncol. 2010;28:3636–43.

74. Boissel N, Nibourel O, Renneville A, et al. Prognostic impact of isocitrate dehydrogenase enzyme isoforms 1 (IDH1) and 2 (IDH2) mutations in acute myeloid leukemia: a study by the Acute Leukemia French Association (ALFA) group. J Clin Oncol. 2010;28: 3717–23.

75. Becker H, Marcucci G, Maharry K, et al. Favorable prognostic impact of NPM1 mutations in older patients with cytogenetically normal de novo acute myeloid leukemia and associated gene- and microRNA-expression signatures: a Cancer and Leukemia Group B study. J Clin Oncol. 2010;28: 596–604.

76. Heuser M, Argiropoulos B, Kuchenbauer F, et al. MN1 over expression induces acute myeloid leukemia in mice and predicts ATRA resistance in patients with AML. Blood. 2007;110:1639–47.

77. Langer C, Marcucci G, Holland KB, et al. Prognostic importance of MN1 transcript levels, and biologic insights from MN1-associated gene and microRNA expression signatures in cytogenetically normal acute myeloid leukemia: a Cancer and Leukemia Group B study. J Clin Oncol. 2009;27:3198–204.

78. Bartel DP. MicroRNAs: target recognition and regulatory functions. Cell. 2009;136:215–33.

79. Calin GA, Croce CM. MicroRNA signatures in human cancers. Nat Rev Cancer. 2006;6:857–66.

80. Haferlach C, Mecucci C, Schnittger S, et al. AML with mutated NPM1 carrying a normal or aberrant karyotype show overlapping biologic, pathologic, immunophenotypic, and prognostic features. Blood. 2009;114:3024–32.

81. Lowenberg B, Beck J, Graux C, et al. Gemtuzumab ozogamicin as postremission treatment in AML at 60 years of age or more: results of a multicenter phase 3 study. Blood. 2010;115:2586–91.

82. Ball ED, Balaian L. Cytotoxic activity of gemtuzumab ozogamicin (Mylotarg) in acute myeloid leukemia correlates with the expression of protein kinase Syk. Leukemia. 2006;20:2093–101.

83. Migkou M, Dimopoulos MA, Gavriatopoulou M, et al. Applications of monoclonal antibodies for the treatment of hematological malignancies. Expert Opin Biol Ther. 2009;9:207–20.

84. Jin L, Lee EM, Ramshaw HS, et al. MAb-mediated targeting of CD123, IL-3 receptor alpha chain, eliminates human acute myeloid leukemic stem cells. Cell Stem Cell. 2009;5:31–42.

85. Mao X, Cao B, Wood TE, et al. A small-molecule inhibitor of D-cyclin transactivation displays preclinical efficacy in myeloma and leukemia via phosphoinositide 3-kinase pathway. Blood. 2011;117: 1986–97.

86. Baughn LB, Di Liberto M, Wu K, et al. A novel orally active small molecule potently induces G1 arrest in primary myeloma cells and prevents tumor growth by specific inhibition of cyclin dependent kinase 4/6. Cancer Res. 2006;66:7661–7.

87. Mao X, Zhu X, Hurren R, et al. Dexamethasone increases ubiquitin transcription through an SP-1 dependent mechanism in multiple myeloma cells. Leuk Res. 2008;32:1480–2.

88. Mao X, Liang SB, Hurren R, et al. Cyproheptadine displays preclinical activity in myeloma and leukemia. Blood. 2008;112:760–9.

89. Tiedemann RE, Mao X, Shi CX, et al. Identification of kinetin riboside as a repressor of CCND1 and CCND2 with preclinical antimyeloma activity. J Clin Invest. 2008;118:1750–64.

90. Pui CH, Robison LL, Look AT. Acute lymphoblastic leukaemia. Lancet. 2008;371:1030–43.

91. Pui CH, Pei D, Sandlund JT, et al. Long-term results of St Jude Total Therapy Studies 11, 12, 13A, 13B,

and 14 for childhood acute lymphoblastic leukemia. Leukemia. 2009;24:371–82.

92. Nguyen K, Devidas M, Cheng SC, et al. Factors influencing survival after relapse from acute lymphoblastic leukemia: a Children's Oncology Group study. Leukemia. 2008;22:2142–50.

93. Harrison CJ. Cytogenetics of paediatric and adolescent acute lymphoblastic leukaemia. Br J Haematol. 2009;144:147–56.

94. Mullighan CG, Downing JR. Genome-wide profiling of genetic alterations in acute lymphoblastic leukemia: recent insights and future directions. Leukemia. 2009;23:1209–18.

95. Beroukhim R, Mermel CH, Porter D, et al. The landscape of somatic copy-number alteration across human cancers. Nature. 2010;463:899–905.

96. Kuiper RP, Waanders E, Van Der Velden VH, et al. IKZF1 deletions predict relapse in uniformly treated pediatric precursor B-ALL. Leukemia. 2010;24: 1258–64.

97. Nebral K, Denk D, Attarbaschi A, et al. Incidence and diversity of PAX5 fusion genes in childhood acute lymphoblastic leukemia. Leukemia. 2009;23: 134–43.

98. Mullighan CG, Miller CB, Radtke I, et al. BCR-ABL1 lymphoblastic leukaemia is characterized by the deletion of Ikaros. Nature. 2008;453:110–4.

99. Virely C, Moulin S, Cobaleda C, et al. Haploinsufficiency of the IKZF1 (IKAROS) tumor suppressor gene cooperates with BCR-ABL in a transgenic model of acute lymphoblastic leukemia. Leukemia. 2010;24:1200–4.

100. Schwab CJ, Jones LR, Morrison H, et al. Evaluation of multiplex ligation-dependent probe amplification as a method for the detection of copy number abnormalities in B-cell precursor acute lymphoblastic leukemia. Genes Chromosomes Cancer. 2010;49: 1104–13.

101. Mullighan CG. New strategies in acute lymphoblastic leukemia: translating advances in genomics into clinical practice. Clin Cancer Res. 2001;17: 396–400.

102. Harvey RC, Mulligan CG, Chen IM, et al. Rearrangement of CRLF2 is associated with mutation of JAK kinases, alteration of IKZF1, Hispanic/Latino ethnicity, and a poor outcome in pediatric B-progenitor acute lymphoblastic leukemia. Blood. 2010;115:5312–21.

103. Uckun FM, Sun L, Qazi S, et al. Recombinant human CD19-ligand protein as a potent anti-leukaemic agent. Br J Haematol. 2001;153:15–23.

104. Van Vlierberghe P, van Grotel M, Beverloo HB, et al. The cryptic chromosomal deletion del(11) (p12p13) as a new activation mechanism of LMO2 in pediatric T-cell acute lymphoblastic leukemia. Blood. 2006;108:3520–9.

105. Lahortiga I, De Keersmaecker K, Van Vlierberghe P, et al. Duplication of the MYB oncogene in T cell acute lymphoblastic leukemia. Nat Genet. 2007; 39:593–5.

106. Graux C, Cools J, Melotte C, et al. Fusion of NUP214 to ABL1 on amplified episomes in T-cell acute lymphoblastic leukemia. Nat Genet. 2004;36: 1084–9.

107. Palomero T, Sulis ML, Cortina M, et al. Mutational loss of PTEN induces resistance to NOTCH1 inhibition in T-cell leukemia. Nat Med. 2007;13:1203–10.

108. Tosello V, Mansour ML, Barnes K, et al. WT1 mutations in T-ALL. Blood. 2009;114:1038–45.

109. Aifantis I, Raetz E, Buonamici S. Molecular pathogenesis of T-cell leukaemia and lymphoma. Nat Rev Immunol. 2008;8:380–90.

110. Aster JC, Pear WS, Blacklow SC. Notch signaling in leukemia. Annu Rev Pathol. 2008;3:587–613.

111. Ferrando AA. The role of NOTCH1 signaling in T-ALL. Hematol Am Soc Hematol Educ Program. 2009:353–61.

112. Paganin M, Adolfo Ferrando A. Molecular pathogenesis and targeted therapies for NOTCH1-induced T-cell acute lymphoblastic. Blood Rev. 2011;25: 83–90.

113. van Tetering G, van Diest P, Verlaan I, et al. Metalloprotease ADAM10 is required for Notch1 site 2 cleavage. J Biol Chem. 2009;284:31018–27.

114. Hozumi K, Mailhos C, Negishi N, et al. Delta-like 4 is indispensable in thymic environment specific for T cell development. J Exp Med. 2008;205:2507–13.

115. Gonzalez-Garcia S, Garcia-Peydro M, Martin-Gayo E, et al. CSL-MAML-dependent Notch1 signaling controls T lineage specific IL-7R{alpha} gene expression in early human thymopoiesis and leukemia. J Exp Med. 2009;206:779–91.

116. Weng AP, Millholland JM, Yashiro-Ohtani Y, et al. c- Myc is an important direct target of Notch1 in T-cell acute lymphoblastic leukemia/lymphoma. Genes Dev. 2006;20:2096–109.

117. Margolin AA, Palomero T, Sumazin P, et al. ChIP-on-chip significance analysis reveals large-scale binding and regulation by human transcription factor oncogenes. Proc Natl Acad Sci U S A. 2009;106: 244–9.

118. Rao SS, O'Neil J, Liberator CD, et al. Inhibition of NOTCH signaling by gamma secretase inhibitor engages the RB pathway and elicits cell cycle exit in T-cell acute lymphoblastic leukemia cells. Cancer Res. 2009;69:3060–8.

119. Joshi I, Minter LM, Telfer J, et al. Notch signaling mediates G1/S cell-cycle progression in T cells via cyclin D3 and its dependent kinases. Blood. 2009; 113:1689–98.

120. Song LL, Peng Y, Yun J, et al. Notch-1 associates with IKK alpha and regulates IKK activity in cervical cancer cells. Oncogene. 2008;27:5833–44.

121. Vilimas T, Mascarenhas J, Palomero T, et al. Targeting the NF-kappaB signaling pathway in Notch1-induced T-cell leukemia. Nat Med. 2007; 13:70–7.

122. Cullion K, Draheim KM, Hermance N, et al. Targeting the Notch1 and mTOR pathways in a mouse T-ALL model. Blood. 2009;113:6172–81.

123. Moellering RE, Cornejo M, Davis TN, et al. Direct inhibition of the NOTCH transcription factor complex. Nature. 2009;462:182–8.
124. Wu Y, Cain-Hom C, Choy L, et al. Therapeutic antibody targeting of individual Notch receptors. Nature. 2010;464:1052–7.
125. Sanz MA, Lo-Coco F. Arsenic trioxide: its use in the treatment of acute promyelocytic leukemia. Am J Cancer. 2006;5:183–91.
126. Sanz MA, Grimwade D, Tallman MS, et al. Management of acute promyelocytic leukemia: recommendations from an expert panel on behalf of the European leukemia net. Blood. 2009;113:1875–91.
127. Sanz MA, Lo-Coco F. Modern approaches to treating acute promyelocytic leukemia. J Clin Oncol. 2011;29:495–503.
128. de la Serna J, Montesinos P, Vellenga E, et al. Causes and prognostic factors of remission induction failure in patients with acute promyelocytic leukemia treated with all-trans retinoic acid and idarubicin. Blood. 2008;111:3395–402.
129. Sanz MA, Montesinos P, Rayon C, et al. Risk-adapted treatment of acute promyelocytic leukemia based on all-trans retinoic acid and anthracycline with addition of cytarabine in consolidation therapy for high-risk patients: further improvements in treatment outcome. Blood. 2010;115:5137–46.
130. Licht JD. Reconstructing a disease: what essential features of the retinoic acid receptor fusion on coproteins generate acute promyelocytic leukemia? Cancer Cell. 2006;9:73–4.
131. Martens JH, Brinkman AB, Simmer F, et al. PML-RARalpha/RXR alters the epigenetic landscape in acute promyelocytic leukemia. Cancer Cell. 2010;17:173–85.
132. Curing KSC. Curing APL: differentiation or destruction? Cancer Cell. 2009;15:7–8.
133. Licht JD. Acute promyelocytic leukemia weapons of mass differentiation. N Engl J Med. 2009;360:928–30.
134. Jeanne M, Lallemand-Breitenbach V, Ferhi O, et al. PML/RARA oxidation and arsenic binding initiate the antileukemia response of As2O3. Cancer Cell. 2010;18:88–98.
135. Tallman MS, Altman JK. How I treat acute promyelocytic leukemia. Blood. 2009;114:5126–35.
136. Tefferi A, Vainchenker W. Myeloproliferative neoplasms: molecular pathophysiology, essential clinical understanding, and treatment strategies. J Clin Oncol. 2011;29:573–82.
137. Tefferi A. Novel mutations and their functional and clinical relevance in myeloproliferative neoplasms: JAK2, MPL, TET2, ASXL1, CBL, IDH and IKZF1. Leukemia. 2010;24:1128–38.
138. Voskaridou E, Christoulas D, Bilalis A, et al. The effect of prolonged administration of hydroxyu.rea on morbidity and mortality in adult patients with sickle cell syndromes: results of a 17-year, single center trial (LaSHS). Blood. 2010;115:2354–63.

139. Baxter EJ, Scott LM, Campbell PJ, et al. Acquired mutation of the tyrosine kinase JAK2 in human myeloproliferative disorders. Lancet. 2005;365:1054–61.
140. Abdel-Wahab O, Manshouri T, Patel J, et al. Genetic analysis of transforming events that convert chronic myeloproliferative neoplasms to leukemias. Cancer Res. 2010;70:447–52.
141. Quintas-Cardama A, Kantarjian HM, Manshouri T, et al. Lenalidomide plus prednisone results in durable clinical, histopathologic, and molecular responses in patients with myelofibrosis. J Clin Oncol. 2009;27:4760–6.
142. Tefferi A, Lasho TL, Mesa RA, et al. Lenalidomide therapy in del(5)(q31)-associated myelofibrosis: cytogenetic and JAK2V617F molecular remissions. Leukemia. 2007;21:1827–8.
143. Mishchenko E, Tefferi A. Treatment options for hydroxyurea-refractory disease complications in myeloproliferative neoplasms: JAK2 inhibitors, radiotherapy, splenectomy and transjugular intra hepatic portosystemic shunt. Eur J Haematol. 2010;85:192–9.
144. Agrawal M, Garg RJ, Cortes J, et al. Experimental therapeutics for patients with myeloproliferative neoplasias. Cancer. 2011;15(117):662–76.
145. Quintás-Cardama A, Kantarjian H, Cortes J, Verstovsek S. Janus kinase inhibitors for the treatment of myeloproliferative neoplasias and beyond. Nat Rev Drug Discov. 2011;10:127–40.
146. Jones AV, Kreil S, Zoi K, et al. Widespread occurrence of the JAK2V617F mutation in chronic myeloproliferative disorders. Blood. 2005;106:2162–8.
147. Santos FP, Kantarjian HM, Jain N, et al. Phase 2 study of CEP-701, an orally available JAK2 inhibitor, in patients with primary or post-polycythemia vera/essential thrombocythemia myelofibrosis. Blood. 2010;115:1131–6.
148. Giralt S, Horowitz M, Weisdorf D, Cutler C. Review of stem-cell transplantation for myelodysplastic syndromes in older patients in the context of the decision memo for allogeneic hematopoietic stem cell transplantation for myelodysplastic syndrome emanating from the centers for medicare and medicaid services. J Clin Oncol. 2011;29:566–72.
149. Shen L, Kantarjian H, Guo Y, et al. DNA methylation predicts survival and response to therapy in patients with myelodysplastic syndromes. J Clin Oncol. 2010;28:605–13.
150. Jiang Y, Dunbar A, Gondek LP, et al. Aberrant DNA methylation is a dominant mechanism in MDS progression to AML. Blood. 2009;113:1315–25.
151. Fenaux P, Mufti GJ, Hellstrom-Lindberg E, et al. Efficacy of azacitidine compared with that of conventional care regimens in the treatment of higher-risk myelodysplastic syndromes: a randomised, open-label, phase III study. Lancet Oncol. 2009;10:223–32.
152. Tsimberidou AM, Estey E, Wen S, et al. The prognostic significance of cytokine levels in newly

diagnosed acute myeloid leukemia and high-risk myelodysplastic syndromes. Cancer. 2008;113: 1605–13.

153. Garcia-Manero G, Pierre Fenaux P. Hypomethylating agents and other novel strategies in myelodysplastic syndromes. J Clin Oncol. 2011;29:516–23.

154. van Rhenen A, van Dogen GA, Kelder A, et al. The novel AML stem cell associated antigen CLL-1 aids in discrimination between normal and leukemic stem cell. Blood. 2007;110:2659–66.

155. Guzman ML, Swiderski CF, Howard DS, et al. Preferential induction of apoptosis for primary human leukemic stem cells. Proc Natl Acad Sci U S A. 2002;99:16220–5.

156. Hassane DC, Guzman ML, Corbett C, et al. Discovery of agents that eradicate leukemia stem cells using an in silico screen of public gene expression data. Blood. 2008;111:5654–62.

157. MacDonald BT, Tamai K, He X. Wnt/betacatenin signaling: components, mechanisms, and diseases. Dev Cell. 2009;17:9–26.

158. Chen B, Dodge ME, Tang W, et al. Small molecule-mediated disruption of Wnt-dependent signaling in tissue regeneration and cancer. Nat Chem Biol. 2009;5:100–7.

159. Wang Y, Krivtsov AV, Sinha AU, et al. The Wnt/beta-catenin pathway is required for the development of leukemia stem cells in AML. Science. 2010;327:1650–3.

160. Meads MB, Gatenby RA, Dalton WS. Environment-mediated drug resistance: a major contributor to minimal residual disease. Nat Rev Cancer. 2009;9:665–74.

161. Naveiras O, Daley GQ. Stem cells and their niche: a matter of fate. Cell Mol Life Sci. 2006;63:760–6.

162. Colmone A, Amorim M, Pontier AL, et al. Leukemic cells create bone marrow niches that disrupt the behavior of normal hematopoietic progenitor cells. Science. 2008;322:1861–5.

163. Ishikawa F, Yoshida S, Saito Y, et al. Chemotherapy-resistant human AML stem cells home to and engraft within the bone-marrow endosteal region. Nat Biotechnol. 2009;25:1315–21.

164. Zeng Z, Shi YX, Samudio IJ, et al. Targeting the leukemia microenvironment by CXCR4 inhibition overcomes resistance to kinase inhibitors and chemotherapy in AML. Blood. 2009;113:6215–24.

165. Karjalainen K, Jaalouk DE, Bueso-Ramos CE, et al. Targeting neuropilin-1 in human leukemia and lymphoma. Blood. 2011;117:920–7.

166. Konopleva MY, Jordan CT. Leukemia stem cells and microenvironment: biology and therapeutic targeting. J Clin Oncol. 2011;29:591–9.

167. Wang Y, Liu Y, Malek SN, et al. Targeting HIF1α eliminates cancer stem cells in hematological malignancies. Cell Stem Cell. 2011;8:399–411.

168. Karp JE, Gojo I, Pili R, et al. Targeting vascular endothelial growth factor for relapsed and refractory adult acute myelogenous leukemias: therapy with sequential 1-beta-d arabinofuranosylcytosine, mitoxantrone, and bevacizumab. Clin Cancer Res. 2004;10:3577–85.

169. Lam BS, Adams GB. Blocking HIF1α activity eliminates hematological cancer stem cells. Cell Stem Cell. 2011;8:354–6.

170. Vignoli A, Marchetti M, Russo L, et al. LMWH bemiparin and ULMWH RO-14 reduce the endothelial angiogenic features elicited by leukemia, lung cancer, or breast cancer cells. Cancer Invest. 2011;29: 153–61.

171. Blau O, Hofmann WK, Baldus CD, et al. Chromosomal aberrations in bone marrow mesenchymal stromal cells from patients with myelodysplastic syndrome and acute myeloblastic leukaemia. Exp Hematol. 2007;35:221–9.

172. Bielenberg DR, Pettaway CA, Takashima S, Klagsbrun M. Neuropilin in neoplasms: expression, regulation, and function. Exp Cell Res. 2006;312: 584–93.

173. Pan Q, Chanthery Y, Liang WC, et al. Blocking neuropilin-1 function has an additive effect with anti-VEGF to inhibit tumor growth. Cancer Cell. 2007;11: 53–67.

174. Vales A, Kondo R, Aichberger KJ. Myeloid leukemias express a broad spectrum of VEGF receptors including neuropilin-1 (NRP-1) and NRP-2. Leuk Lymphoma. 2007;48(10):1997–2007.

175. Cheok CF, Verma CS, Baselga J, Lane DP. Translating p53 into the clinic. Nat Rev Clin Oncol. 2011;8: 25–37.

176. Hoffmann TK, Donnenberg AD, Finkelstein SD, et al. Frequencies of tetramer T cells specific for the wild type sequence p53264–272 peptide in the circulation of patients with head and neck cancer. Cancer Res. 2002;62:3521–9.

177. Allende VN, Saville MK. Targeting the ubiquitin proteasome system to activate wildtype p53 for cancer therapy. Semin Cancer Biol. 2010;20:29–39.

178. Marine JC, Lozano G. Mdm2 mediated ubiquitylation: p53 and beyond. Cell Death Differ. 2010;17: 93–102.

179. Dickens MP, Fitzgerald R, Fischer PM. Small molecule inhibitors of MDM2 as new anticancer therapeutics. Semin Cancer Biol. 2010;20:10–8.

180. Secchiero P, di Iasio MG, Gonelli A, Zauli G. The MDM2 inhibitor Nutlins as an innovative therapeutic tool for the treatment of haematological malignancies. Curr Pharm Des. 2008;14:2100–10.

181. Grinkevich VV, Nikulenkov F, Shi Y, et al. Ablation of key oncogenic pathways by RITA reactivated p53 is required for efficient apoptosis. Cancer Cell. 2009;15:441–53.

182. Carter BZ, Mak DH, Schober WD, et al. Simultaneous activation of p53 and inhibition of XIAP enhance the activation of apoptosis signaling pathways in AML. Blood. 2010;115:306–14.

183. Secchiero P, Melloni E, di Iasio MG, et al. Nutlin 3 up regulates the expression of Notch1 in both

184. Ocana A, Pandiella A, Siu LL, Tannock IF. Preclinical development of molecular-targeted agents for cancer. Nat Rev Clin Oncol. 2011;8:200–9.

185. Sawyers CL. Translational research: are we on the right track? 2008 American Society for Clinical Investigation Presidential Address. J Clin Invest. 2008;118:3798–801.

186. Chiarini F, Grimaldi C, Ricci F, et al. Activity of the novel dual phosphatidylinositol 3-kinase/mammalian target of rapamycin inhibitor NVP-BEZ235 against T-cell acute lymphoblastic leukemia. Cancer Res. 2010;70:8097–107.

187. Smith MA. Update on developmental therapeutics for acute lymphoblastic leukemia. Curr Hematol Malig Rep. 2009;4:175–82.

188. Fullmer A, O'Brien S, Kantarjian H, Jabbour E. Novel therapies for relapsed acute lymphoblastic leukemia. Curr Hematol Malig Rep. 2009;4:148–56.

189. Real PJ, Ferrando AA. NOTCH inhibition and glucocorticoid therapy in T-cell acute lymphoblastic leukemia. Leukemia. 2009;23:1374–7.

190. Babusikova O, Stevulova L, Fajtova M. Immunophenotyping parameters as prognostic factors in T-acute leukemia patients. Neoplasma. 2009;56:508–13.

191. Ginaldi L, Farahat N, Matutes E, et al. Differential expression of T cell antigens in normal peripheral blood lymphocytes: a quantitative analysis by flow cytometry. J Clin Pathol. 1996;49:539–44.

192. Ginaldi L, Matutes E, Farahat N, et al. Differential expression of CD3 and CD7 in T-cell malignancies. Br J Haematol. 1996;93:921–7.

193. Baskic D, Ilic N, Popovic S, Djurdjevic P, et al. In vitro induction of apoptotic cell death in chronic lymphocytic leukemia by two natural products: preliminary study. J BUON. 2010;15:732–9.

194. Sarma SN, Kim YJ, Song M, Ryu JC. Induction of apoptosis in human leukemia cells through the production of reactive oxygen species and activation of HMOX1 and Noxa by benzene, toluene, and o-xylene. Toxicology. 2011;280:109–17.

195. Zhao WL. Targeted therapy in T-cell malignancies: dysregulation of the cellular signaling pathways. Leukemia. 2010;24:13–21.

196. Walsby E, Lazenby M, Pepper C, Burnett AK. The cyclin-dependent kinase inhibitor SNS-032 has single agent activity in AML cells and is highly synergistic with cytarabine. Leukemia. 2011;25: 411–9.

197. Taghdisi SM, Abnous K, Mosaffa F, Behravan J. Targeted delivery of daunorubicin to T-cell acute lymphoblastic leukemia by aptamer. J Drug Target. 2010;18:277–81.

Breast Cancer

7

Nadia Rucci, Luca Ventura, and Anna Teti

Structure and Regulation of Normal Breast

Anatomy of Mammary Gland

The mammary gland is a specialized accessory gland of the skin. According to the histological features, it can be classified as an exocrine, tubular-alveolar gland organized in 15–20 lobes defined by connective tissue septa. Each lobe has a cone shape, with its apex close to the nipple and the base facing the deep fascia (Fig. 7.1a), and is in turn composed of several groups of lobules containing alveoli, the smallest secretory units of the mammary gland (Fig. 7.1b). At variance with the other composed glands, human breast lacks an external connective capsule and does not have a principal excretory duct branching into progressively smaller and smaller ductules. Indeed, each lobe is drained by a duct, called lactiferous duct, and all these ducts converge in the nipple, below the areola, where they expand to form the lactiferous sinus (Fig. 7.1a). The portion of the gland opposite to the nipple includes the most actively growing terminal ductal structures, named terminal end buds (TEBs) (Fig. 7.1c).

The number of ductules is closely related to the functional state of the breast, varying from 8 to 200, and reaching the maximum number (over 400) during pregnancy. The glandular structure, which represents the parenchymal compartment, is surrounded by a loose specialized stroma, differing from the interlobar stroma because of a higher vascularization and cellularity. Another peculiarity of the mammary gland is the presence of adipose tissue between the lobes, which increases with age.

The branching ductal system of the mammary gland, except for the terminal part of the lactiferous duct, is lined by a continuous inner layer of luminal epithelial cells and an outer layer of myoepithelial cells resting on the basal lamina (Fig. 7.1c). Both cell types originate from the ectoderm, then epithelial cells differentiate in a tissue-specific manner, while the other type acquires a contractile myoepithelial phenotype [1]. Major ducts are usually lined by a single or pseudostratified layer of cuboidal or low columnar epithelial cells, the latter well joined by junctional complexes. In contrast, TEBs are lined by a multilayered epithelium composed of large cuboidal cells having a high rate of proliferation (Fig. 7.1c). On the basal surface of the end beneath the basal lamina are the so-called cap cells, which lack of differentiated features, thus representing a multipotent stem cell population, capable of differentiating into both ductal and myoepithelial cell types [2].

N. Rucci, Ph.D. • A. Teti, Ph.D. (✉)
Department of Experimental Medicine,
University of L'Aquila, Via Vetoio, Coppito 2,
L'Aquila 67100, Italy
e-mail: teti@univaq.it

L. Ventura, M.D.
Department of Pathology, San Salvatore Hospital,
L'Aquila, Italy

M. Bologna (ed.), *Biotargets of Cancer in Current Clinical Practice*, Current Clinical Pathology,
DOI 10.1007/978-1-61779-615-9_7, © Springer Science+Business Media, LLC 2012

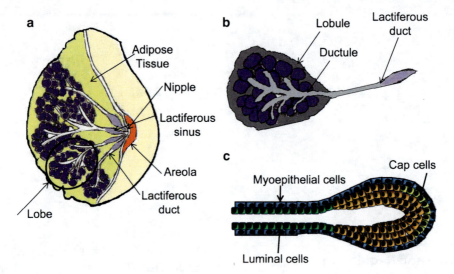

Fig. 7.1 The human mammary gland. (**a**) Schematic representation of the whole mammary gland, showing the lobes, the adipose tissue surrounding them and the branching of ducts which, once leaved the lobe, reach the nipple where they enlarge to form the lactiferous sinus. (**b**) Schematic representation of one breast lobe, showing the presence of the lobules and ductules branching into the lobe. (**c**) Cartoon showing the terminal end bud (TEB), which is composed of an outer layer of myoepithelial cells and an inner multilayer of epithelial cells. Cap cells are the putative terminal end bud stem cells

Luminal cells are cuboidal polarized cells anchored to myoepithelial cells and to the basal lamina. They have an apical and a basolateral domain expressing sialomucin and adhesion molecules, respectively. Moreover, these cells express oestrogen and progesterone receptors (ER, PR). The cytoplasm of the luminal cells presents with electron-dense secretory granules stained with ruthenium red, indicating an acidic mucopolysaccharide content [3].

Myoepithelial cells are flat-shaped cells located between the secretory cells and the basal lamina to which they are anchored. They are contractile cells enveloping the secretory cells, thus facilitating milk ejection. This contraction, as described in more detail below, is induced by oxytocin stimulation. Several markers have been identified for these cells, although none of them are exclusively expressed by myoepithelial cells. Among them are the oxytocin receptors, S-100 protein, glial fibrillary acidic protein (GFAP), vimentin, nerve growth factor (NGF) receptor, smooth muscle myosin heavy chain (SMM-HC) and a p53 homologue, named p63, which seems to be the most specific since it stains nuclei of myoepithelial cells without reacting with myofibroblasts or secretory cells [4, 5].

Several reports showed a role for myoepithelial cells in tumourigenesis since loss of their function could allow progression of epithelial cancer [6–8]. Indeed, it has been demonstrated that some proteins expressed by these cells, including connexin 43, cytokeratin 5 and smooth muscle actin and TIMP-1 could have an antitumourigenic activity [8–12].

Physiology and Regulation of Mammary Gland

Except for the pregnancy period, breast is an inactive gland with a lesser developed parenchymatous tissue surrounded by adipose and connective tissue. At birth, the mammary gland is not completely formed but begins to develop during the early pubertal period when the primitive ductal structures enlarge and branch. The number of ductules increases with age, reaching the maximum in pregnant women, whereas they regress with the onset of menopause.

With the onset of the ovulatory menstrual cycle, the branching of ductal system acquires a more complex structure, while lobular structures form at the end of the terminal ducts to produce the so-called terminal ductal lobular units [TDLUs, also named TEBs (Fig. 7.1c)]. Two principal hormones contribute to the development of the mammary gland: oestradiol and progesterone. Indeed, whereas the former stimulates ductal elongation and progesterone receptor expression, progesterone induces lobulo-alveolar development.

During pregnancy, the high levels of oestrogen and progesterone trigger mammary gland hyperplasia, thus inducing a further branching and enlargement of the ductal tree, together with proliferation of the alveoli, at the expense of the adipose tissue that is reduced. This massive enlargement of the breast continues throughout pregnancy, together with the hypertrophy of parenchyma cells and the distension of alveoli and ducts, reaching its maximal effect during lactation [13].

After the delivery, prolactin secreted by the pituitary gland stimulates milk production, which is continuous, while milk emission is episodic, with the principal stimulus of milk ejection being mechanic, due to baby suckling. Indeed, between one feeding and another, the major part of the milk is stored in the alveolar and ductal lumen; baby sucking stimulates the release of prolactin by the anterior lobe of the pituitary gland, while the posterior lobe releases oxytocin. The latter, in turn, induces the contraction of the myoepithelial cells surrounding the alveoli, thus favouring milk ejection [13].

All the components of the milk are produced by alveolar cells. Different secretory processes are synchronized in the mammary epithelial cells to secrete all the components of the milk. The protein components of milk, such as casein, together with lactose, are released by a mechanism of merocrine secretion. Indeed, these secretory vesicles represent the source of most of the constituents of the aqueous phase of milk including citrate, nucleotides, calcium, phosphate and probably monovalent ions and glucose. These latter two components are also transferred outside by a direct transport across the apical membrane of the mammary alveolar cell. Finally, lipids, organized in droplets, are secreted by an apocrine mechanism [13].

Pathogenesis of Breast Cancer

Breast cancer represents the second most common cause of cancer-related mortality in women, with an estimate of at least one million of women diagnosed per year worldwide [14]. Nevertheless, an earlier detection of this disease, together with the assessment of a more efficacious adjuvant therapy, led to a 24% reduction of breast cancer mortality, especially for young patients with oestrogen receptor-positive breast cancer [15, 16].

As for the other types of cancers, despite the many efforts, the mechanisms underlying tumour onset have not been completely elucidated and are still debated. A classic theory, known as sporadic clonal evolution model, hypothesizes that any breast epithelial cell could be subjected to random mutations. These mutated cells escape the mechanisms of DNA repair and/or apoptosis and acquire an advantage in terms of ability to proliferate, thus perpetuating the harboured mutations to their progeny in a clonal way [17].

Although this theory has never been disproved and could be valid for several types of cancer, over the last years, a new theory has more and more emerged, which identifies tumour stem cells as the principal players of carcinogenesis, recurrence and resistance to therapy [18].

Normal breast stem cells, like any other normal stem cell, are tissue-resident cells, located within a specialized niche in the basal epithelial compartment, characterized by self-renewal activity and multi-lineage differentiation at the same time and with the ability to recapitulate the breast tubule-lobular architecture of the mammary gland [19]. It has been estimated that 1 breast stem cell for 2,000 epithelial cells is present [19, 20], carrying a phenotype characterized by high levels of CD44 receptor and of aldehyde dehydrogenase 1 (ALDH1) and low levels of CD24, with no expression of oestrogen or progesterone receptors [21, 22]. How regulation of this stem pool is accomplished has not been completely understood. Indeed, it has been recently demonstrated that mouse mammary stem

Table 7.1 Summary of the mechanisms involved in breast cancer tumourigenesis

Hormone treatment
Oestrogen and progesterone alone or in combination
Epigenetic mechanisms
Histone acetylation/deacetylation
DNA methylation
MicroRNAs (miRNAs)
Genetic predisposition
BRCA1 and BRCA2 germ line mutations

cells are highly responsive to steroid hormone signalling, despite lacking the ER and PR, and that ovariectomy markedly diminished their number and growth [23]. A parallel work also showed a crucial role of progesterone on adult mammary stem cell pool expansion, by an indirect mechanism, that is the stimulation by progesterone of ductal epithelial cells to release the cytokine RANKL (receptor activator of NF-kappaB ligand), which in turn elicits expansion of stem cell population [24].

As far as the involvement of mammary stem cells in carcinogenesis is concerned, these cells could be a good candidate for the accumulation of genetic and epigenetic modifications, leading to the development of a tumour stem cell. The latter, by asymmetric division, maintains a tumour stem cell pool and triggers the onset of tumour growth, leading to the different breast cancer subtypes [18].

Mechanisms Involved in Breast Cancer Tumourigenesis

As defined by Anderson [25], breast tumourigenesis is the result of a benign to malignant progression due to the accumulation of multiple genetic changes that allows the evolution from normal breast epithelium through benign proliferative lesions to atypical proliferative lesions and then to in situ carcinoma and invasive tumours. This progression is due to a common fault caused not only by genetic changes but also by epigenetic factors and hormonal treatments as summarized in Table 7.1 and described in more detail below.

Hormones and Breast Cancer

It has been well established that the ovarian hormones progesterone and oestrogens are linked to breast cancer. Indeed, use of oestrogens as oral contraceptive or for therapy (i.e. hormonal replacement therapy), early menarche, late menopause, nulliparity and late first full-term pregnancy are all the principal hallmarks of increased breast cancer risk [25–27]. In support of this evidence, it is known that treatment with antioestrogens reduces the incidence of breast cancer in high-risk women [28].

As far as the progesterone is concerned, there is less evidence about its involvement in breast tumourigenesis. While progestins included in combined oral contraceptives can prevent ovarian and endometrial cancer [29], it has been reported that a combination of oestrogen and progestins in post-menopausal women subjected to hormone replacement therapy slightly, but significantly, increases the risk of breast cancer over time when compared with oestrogen alone [30]. Indeed, data to this regard are not completely clear since it is also known that early pregnancy in rodents and humans or treatment of rodents with low doses of oestrogen plus progestins produces a mammary gland phenotype that is refractory to subsequent chemically induced carcinogenesis [31]. Other studies conducted in mice demonstrated that the synthetic progestin medroxyprogesterone acetate (MPA), when employed in combination with the carcinogen dimethylbenz[a] anthracene (DMBA), significantly accelerates the development and increases the incidence of breast tumours [32]. Conversely, it was found that combination treatment with different progestin antagonists and different antioestrogens has greater antitumour efficacy than single therapy. A positive effect of antiprogestins was also observed in post-menopausal patients with metastatic breast cancer [33]. Finally, two studies from Beral [34] and Rossouw [35] suggest that hormone replacement therapy with oestrogen plus progestin is associated with an increased risk of breast cancer.

Concerning the mechanisms of tumourigenesis induced by progesterone, two recent independent works call into question the RANKL, whose role in normal mammary gland development has

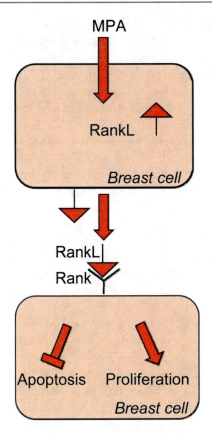

Fig. 7.2 Effect of progesterone on RANKL/RANK signalling. Medroxyprogesterone acetate (MPA) stimulates RANKL secretion in epithelial breast cells. RANKL interacts with its receptor RANK, thus triggering breast cell proliferation and protecting them from apoptosis

been clearly established [36]. Schramek and colleagues found that in vivo administration of MPA in female mice drives a massive secretion of RANKL by progesterone receptor (PR)-positive epithelial breast cells, which in turn interacts with its receptor RANK expressed by mammary epithelial cells triggering their proliferation as well as protecting them from apoptosis [37] (Fig. 7.2). Moreover, progesterone-induced RANKL/RANK pathways also provide a survival advantage to damaged mammary epithelium, which is a hallmark for the onset of mammary carcinogenesis [37, 38]. The parallel study from Gonzalez-Suarez et al. [39] showed an increased pre-neoplasia and breast tumour formation in mice overexpressing RANK, while treatment with RANK-Fc, which blocks the RANKL pathway, reduced tumourigenesis in MPA plus carcinogenic-treated mice as well as in a spontaneous mammary tumour model. Finally, Jones et al. demonstrated the ability of RANKL to stimulate human epithelial cancer cells and melanoma cells migration [40].

These findings acquire additional value if we consider the role of RANKL/RANK in the development of breast cancer bone metastases. Indeed, this cancer has a high prevalence to induce osteolytic bone metastases, which rely on the so-called "vicious circle", a phenomenon triggered by the interplay between osteoclasts, the bone cells devoted to resorb bone, and tumour cells. In this context, RANKL plays a prominent role since it is one of the most powerful inducers of osteoclastogenesis and bone resorption [41]. Indeed, in a mouse model of melanoma metastasis, in vivo neutralization of RANKL by its decoy receptor osteoprotegerin dramatically reduced bone lesions [40]. Consistently, it has been recently demonstrated that in the MDA-MB-231 human breast cancer cell line treatment with RANKL stimulated EMMPRIN expression, which in turn induced the MMP-9 and VEGF genes and increased the incidence of osteolytic lesions in vivo [42]. Finally, a recent work showed that tumour-infiltrating regulatory T cells stimulated mammary cancer metastasis through the RANKL/RANK signalling [43].

Epigenetic Factors and Breast Cancer

The term "epigenetic" identifies specific mechanisms able to change gene activity with no alteration of the primary DNA sequence. Several biological processes have an epigenetic regulation, including genome reprogramming during differentiation and development, genomic imprinting and X-chromosome inactivation. Two main epigenetic mechanisms regulating gene transcription have been characterized so far: chemical histone tail modifications and DNA methylation, both interacting with each other for the regulation of gene transcription.

Histone modifications include acetylation or deacetylation of lysine residues located in the N-terminal tail of histones which changes chromatin compactness, leading to active transcription or transcriptional repression, respectively [44].

DNA methylation consists of the addition of a methyl group to the 5-carbon of the cytosine ring within CpG (cytosine-p-guanine) dinucleotides, a reaction catalyzed by the DNA methyltransferase (DNMT). Over 60% of genes harbour CpG dinucleotides in their promoting region, and it has been shown that several genes normally unmethylated in the non-malignant tissue became aberrantly methylated in the tumour, most of them being tumour suppressing genes [45, 46].

Breast cancer is usually characterized by global DNA hypomethylation, together with a 50% reduction of 5-methylcysteine levels compared to normal tissue. Hypomethylation involves especially repetitive DNA sequences and pericentromeric satellite DNA [47] as well as specific genes including urokinase plasminogen activator, the breast cancer-specific protein 1/synuclein-y gene (SNCG) and the multidrug resistance 1 (MDR1) gene [48–50].

Another epigenetic mechanism regulating gene transcription is accomplished by microRNAs (miRNAs), recently identified as a class of small (20–30 nucleotides) non-coding RNAs that match the 3′ untranslated regions (3′UTR) of a target mRNA, leading to its degradation or inhibition of translation [51]. So far, several miRNAs have been implicated in tumourigenesis, that is, let-7 family mRNAs, whose depletion in breast, lung and colon cells causes enhanced tumourigenicity [44, 52], and miR-21, whose overexpression in breast cancer increased tumour invasion and metastasis [53, 54]. A recent genome-wide profiling study of miRNAs identified 15 differentially expressed miRNAs, most of them downregulated, that were able to distinguish between breast cancer and normal breast [53]. Other studies identified a cluster of miRNAs that correlate with the HER2/neu or oestrogen receptor (ER) status in breast tumours [55].

Genetic Mutations Predisposing to Breast Cancer

Mutations in the BRCA1 and BRCA2 genes account for the majority of hereditary breast cancers, with a risk of developing breast cancer ranging from 50% to 80% [56]. In 1990, genetic studies provided initial evidence that the risk of breast cancer in some families was linked to chromosome 17q21, which was characterized by autosomal dominant inheritance with incomplete penetrance [57]. Few years later, BRCA1 was identified as the breast cancer susceptibility gene together with BRCA2, the latter located on chromosome 13q12.3 [58, 59]. Of note, these two genes are not only associated with an increased risk of breast cancer but also with increased susceptibility to ovarian, pancreatic, prostatic and male breast cancers [60].

More than 200 different germ line mutations associated with cancer susceptibility have been identified so far, most of them generating loss of function due to a premature truncation of the protein. In contrast, somatic disease-causing mutations in either of these genes are extremely rare in sporadic breast cancers [61].

Both BRCA1 and BRCA2 are involved in the mechanisms of DNA repair. Indeed, several studies demonstrated the involvement of BRCA1 and BRCA2 in complexes that activate the repair of double-strand breaks (DSBs) and initiate homologous recombination, linking the maintenance of genomic integrity to tumour suppression. Recent evidence shows that BRCA1 contributes to the regulation of c-Abl activity, a tyrosine kinase that induces apoptosis under the effect of genotoxic agents [62]. BRCA1 has also been implicated in the transcriptional regulation of several genes activated in response to DNA damage and as coactivator for p53 [63, 64].

BRCA1-associated breast cancers are usually diagnosed in younger patients (premenopausal) and show characteristic histological features, being in most cases poorly differentiated infiltrating ductal carcinomas of high grade and ER, PR and HER2/neu negative (triple negative). Other typical features are the positivity for cytokeratins 5 and 6, the overexpression of cyclin E and p53, while p27 is downregulated [65]. BRCA2-associated breast cancers are also generally of high grade, although they share pathologic characteristics more similar to that of non-carriers [64]. Moreover, tumours from BRCA1 mutation carriers have been found to be frequently of the basal subtype, whereas BRCA2 tumours fall mainly within the luminal category [66].

As far as the prognosis of BRCA-associated breast cancer is concerned, this matter is complex and still debated. Since BRCA-related breast cancers occur earlier in life and usually cannot be treated with common hormone therapy due to the fact that they are mainly oestrogen receptor negative, many breast cancer patients with BRCA mutations have shorter survival. Indeed, a prospective study examining 5-year disease-free survival and overall survival show that BRCA1 mutation carriers had a worse (survival) prognosis compared to non-carriers [67], while the study from Rennert [68] showed that there is no significant difference in overall survival between BRCA1-BRCA2 mutant carriers and non-carriers. Moreover, a meta-analysis study performed by Lee and colleagues investigated the effect of BRCA1/2 mutation on short-term and long-term breast cancer survival, finding that short-term prognosis of BRCA1 mutation was significantly worse than non-carriers, while in BRCA2 mutation, it was similar to non-carrier patients [69]. Finally, the risk of contralateral breast cancer seems to be higher in the mutant carrier group relative to non-carrier patient [69], while the risk of metastasis is similar between the two groups [70].

Breast Cancer Diagnosis

The diagnostic approach to breast lesions has dramatically changed in the last 10 years. The use of frozen section examination for intraoperative diagnosis underwent a rapid decline following the adoption of preoperative diagnostic strategies, including the fine needle aspiration cytology and the needle core biopsy. These are simple procedures, applicable to outpatients in order to allow decisions prior to hospital admission and surgery. Moreover, the use of mammography and population-based screening programmes has led to an increase of non-palpable breast lesions, outnumbering biopsies for palpable masses. Nevertheless, in a large number of cases, differentiation between benign and malignant lesions is still based on histologic examination. Therefore, a close cooperation of the pathologists with surgeons, radiologists and oncologists is needed to avoid suboptimal patient management.

The role of histopathology in breast cancer diagnosis has remained unchanged in its importance over the years since it is essential to differentiate the pathological changes of benign disease towards neoplastic lesions. Cancer diagnosis is usually confirmed preoperatively and sometimes during the operation. After surgery, the pathologist is required to provide an evaluation of the features determining prognosis and the requirement of further treatments.

Diagnostic Procedures

According to the timing and the techniques employed, the procedures for breast cancer diagnosis may be distinguished in preoperative, intraoperative and operative (Table 7.2).

Preoperative Diagnostic Procedures

Fine Needle Aspiration Cytology (FNAC). FNAC is a fast, inexpensive and minimally invasive procedure that can confirm malignancy, although it cannot differentiate between in situ and invasive carcinoma [71]. It is usually performed free hand for palpable masses or under image guidance for non-palpable lesions. The accuracy of FNAC depends on adequate and representative sampling, suitable technical procedures and interpretation by an expert cytopathologist [72]. Following the triple approach (clinical, radiologic and cytologic), the accuracy rate for palpable lesions is 99% [72]. Dealing with non-palpable lesions, sensitivity decreases to 87%, with specificity virtually about 100% [73]. Standardized

Table 7.2 Description of the principal breast cancer diagnostic procedures

Preoperative diagnostic procedures
Fine needle aspiration cytology (FNAC)
Needle core biopsy (NCB)
Intraoperative diagnostic procedures
Frozen section examination
Operative diagnostic procedures
Open biopsy (incisional or excisional)
Quadrantectomy
Mastectomy (radical, simple, subcutaneous)
Sentinel lymph node dissection (SLND)
Axillary lymph node dissection

reporting is required in order to assure a clear interpretation by clinicians and correlation with following biopsies.

According to the current reporting system [74], the following five diagnostic categories are classified: C1: unsatisfactory; C2: benign; C3: atypia, probably benign; C4: suspicious of malignancy and C5: malignant.

Needle core biopsy (NCB). NCB has been introduced and rapidly developed more recently, almost totally replacing FNAC. It can be performed under local anaesthesia in the outpatient setting. A stereotactic approach is preferable for non-palpable lesions, especially in areas harbouring microcalcifications [75].

By simultaneously evaluating cellular features and tissue architecture, NCB allows to differentiate invasive from in situ carcinoma and easily identify the majority of benign lesions [71, 75]. Moreover, grade assessment of malignant lesions is easier on biopsy material, which also allows to perform ancillary testing [71, 76, 77].

Standardized reporting systems include the following five categories [78]: B1: normal tissue/inadequate sample, B2: benign lesion, B3: lesion of uncertain malignant potential, B4: lesion suspicious of malignancy and B5: malignant lesion.

FNAC and NCB are widely used, achieving high rates of sensitivity and specificity [71]. The utility of both procedures is limited mainly by sampling errors. Despite image-guided sampling, the results of both methods are sometimes inconclusive, resulting in repeat of the procedures or in open biopsy [75].

Intraoperative Diagnostic Procedures

Frozen section examination. Frozen section assessment may be useful in lesions exceeding 1 cm in largest diameter, representing a highly accurate method [73]. In smaller or ill-defined nodules, this procedure should be avoided since the right area is often difficult to be identified, the tissue for definitive examination may be exhausted and the architecture of the residual tissue distorted [75]. Moreover, other information, such as tumour size and margins status, is difficult to provide intraoperatively. The use of frozen sections should be limited to cases in which a

preoperative diagnosis could not be yielded and/or if the intraoperative diagnosis can modify the therapeutic approach.

Operative Diagnostic Procedures

Each specimen collected should be submitted fresh and untouched, immediately after the operation, to allow optimal processing by the pathology team [75, 79]. Because most of the breast surgical specimens lack natural landmarks, they need to be oriented according to markers (wires) placed by the surgeon. In addition, given the already mentioned importance of pathological-radiological correlation, evaluation of the radiographs represents an integral part of specimen examination, providing information about disease locations and the sectioning strategy.

Open biopsy. This could include the incisional biopsy (partial removal of the lesion) that is occasionally performed to give tissue for intraoperative consultation and the excisional biopsy, where the whole nodule with variable portions of surrounding normal tissue is removed and the specimen to be processed is oriented in order to evaluate the margins status [79]. This procedure is applied when facing clinically benign lesions, but it is also performed in a two-step surgical approach or in elderly patients.

Quadrantectomy. The removal of an artificially subdivided portion (quadrant) of mammary gland with overlying skin represents the standard operation for breast cancer, usually associated with sentinel lymph node dissection (see further). Although the amount of tissue may vary, the documentation of five fundamental tumour margins (superior, inferior, lateral, medial, deep) together with a skin sample is always needed [73, 75, 79, 80].

Mastectomy. Surgical specimens from radical (removal of breast with overlying skin and axillary lymph nodes), simple (without nodes) and subcutaneous (without overlying skin) mastectomy became more and more infrequent in these recent years of conservative surgery. Sampling strategy is similar to that mentioned for quadrantectomies, with the adjunction of nipple/areola region.

Sentinel lymph node dissection (SLND). SLN biopsy has become an invaluable alternative to total lymph node dissection in order to determine nodal spread of the cancer [81, 82]. It is well known that sentinel nodes have a higher chance of containing metastases than do other lymph nodes. Despite controversies about optimal evaluation methods, the lack of standardized protocols and persisting uncertainties about the clinical implications of isolated tumour cells and micrometastases, the removal of sentinel lymph node and its thorough examination represent the standard method for predicting the status of non-sentinel lymph nodes [81, 83].

The gross specimen should be dissected carefully to check any node present, as not infrequently more than one node is removed. Multilevel assessment is mandatory; thus, each single node is serially sectioned at 2-mm interval and entirely processed for histology. The preparation of stained and unstained sections (for additional immunohistochemistry) at intervals of 50–100 μm until exhaustion of the block allows to examine the sentinel node status with sufficient reliability. Immunohistochemistry is not mandatory [83], but it is reported able to reveal occult metastases in nodes appearing negative on routine stains [82]. Intraoperative examination is usually limited to nodes grossly suspicious for malignancy [79] but might be routinely done by frozen sections or imprint cytology, with advantages and disadvantages in both methods [84–86].

Axillary (non-sentinel) lymph node dissection. Total axillary dissection should be performed only after a nodal FNAB or NCB or SLND positive for carcinoma. After careful gross dissection of nodes from the fat, each palpable node is submitted to histology, and at least two sections at different levels are obtained. This represents an effective compromise to the removal and complete staging of the disease.

Ancillary Studies

Along with classic prognostic factors (histological type, grade, size, margin status, lymphovascular invasion), additional features of prognostic and/or predictive significance may be important in determining the risk of recurrence and choosing

appropriate treatment [79, 87, 88]. Some of these factors are routinely determined in histopathology laboratories by molecular morphology (immunohistochemistry and fluorescence in situ hybridization) methods, whereas other markers are variably used (see further).

Classification of Breast Carcinoma

From a classical point of view, two main distinctions are made between intraductal and invasive forms and between ductal and lobular histologic types. Carcinoma in situ is a neoplastic epithelial proliferation within breast ducts and always limited by the basement membrane of the ducts. Along with other forms of intraepithelial proliferative lesions, it represents a precursor of invasive carcinoma and may occur in coexistence with it (Fig. 7.3). Invasive carcinoma shows a range of histological subtypes, but the majority of cases are classified as invasive ductal carcinoma, not otherwise specified. The second most frequent form is invasive lobular carcinoma (Fig. 7.3).

Although recent studies on gene expression profiling have been able to identify different subtypes of tumours with different prognostic implications [89], histological typing remains the golden standard for the classification of breast carcinomas, providing useful prognostic information. A comprehensive classification of epithelial malignant lesions, based on the histological classification published by the World Health Organization [74], is provided in Table 7.3.

Histopathology of Breast Carcinoma

Below is a brief description of the most frequent histopathological features of breast cancer cases [73, 75, 79].

Intraductal Proliferative Lesions. They are traditionally classified in different categories, including both "benign" entities as well as ductal carcinoma in situ (DCIS). DCIS may show a variety of microscopic growth patterns and three different cytological grades. All these entities often coexist together or with invasive ductal

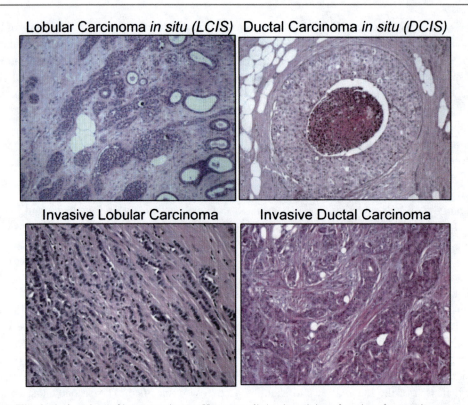

Fig. 7.3 Histological sections of breast carcinoma. Haematoxylin/eosin staining of sections from various types of carcinomas. Original magnification ×100

Table 7.3 Histological classification of the principal breast epithelial malignant lesions

Intraductal proliferative lesions
Ductal hyperplasia
Flat epithelial atypia
Columnar cell hyperplasia
Atypical ductal hyperplasia (ADH)
Ductal carcinoma in situ (DCIS)
Lobular intraepithelial neoplasia
Lobular carcinoma in situ (LCIS)
Atypical lobular hyperplasia
Intraductal papillary neoplasia
Intraductal papilloma
Atypical papilloma
Intraductal/intracystic papillary carcinoma
Microinvasive carcinoma
Infiltrating epithelial tumours
Invasive ductal carcinoma (IDC), not otherwise specified (NOS)
Invasive lobular carcinoma
Tubular carcinoma
Invasive cribriform carcinoma
Adenoid cystic carcinoma
Secretory carcinoma
Apocrine carcinoma
Invasive micropapillary carcinoma
Invasive papillary carcinoma
Mucinous carcinoma
Medullary carcinoma
Neuroendocrine tumours
Metaplastic carcinoma
Lymphoepithelioma-like carcinoma
Squamous carcinoma
Lipid-rich carcinoma
Oncocytic carcinoma
Acinic cell carcinoma
Glycogen-rich clear cell carcinoma
Sebaceous carcinoma
Inflammatory carcinoma
Carcinoma with osteoclastic giant cells
Carcinoma with choriocarcinomatous features
Melanotic carcinoma
Basal-like carcinoma

carcinoma. A recently introduced classification of intraductal proliferations considers all these lesions as true neoplastic processes, naming them ductal intraepithelial neoplasia (DIN). Translational scheme between old and new classification systems are available [75].

Lobular Intraepithelial Neoplasia (LIN). This is a solid and often occlusive proliferation of small and loosely cohesive epithelial cells within TDLUs, with (lobular carcinoma in situ, LCIS) or without (atypical lobular hyperplasia) expansion of the lobules. LIN is often an incidental finding and may progress to invasive carcinoma.

Intraductal Papillary Neoplasia. These are ductal proliferations, with peculiar morphology and clinical behaviour. Papillomas are made of fibro-vascular stalks covered by myoepithelial cells and non-atypical epithelial cells. They may be solitary (central, located in a larger duct) or multifocal (peripheral, involving TDLUs). They may show secondary alterations (haemorrhagic necrosis, squamous metaplasia, sclerosis) and often result in bloody nipple discharge. When epithelial cells display intraepithelial proliferative lesions, the lesion is designed as atypical papilloma. Whether or not atypical, a papilloma always behaves in a benign fashion.

Intraductal/intracystic (non-invasive) papillary carcinoma has the same architecture of benign lesions but lacks myoepithelial layer. It has an excellent outcome, but it may be very difficult to distinguish true infiltration from epithelial elements entrapped or displaced within the stroma.

Microinvasive Carcinoma. It describes a focus of invasive carcinoma usually <1 mm in diameter within CIS and is associated with a very low risk of metastasis.

Infiltrating Epithelial Tumours. A great number of invasive breast cancers (see Table 7.3) are *invasive ductal carcinoma* (Fig. 7.3), not otherwise specified (IDC, NOS). Special histological types of invasive carcinoma have distinct clinico-pathological features and different outcomes. To be considered of special type, at least 90% of the

tumour should have the characteristic morphology of that particular type. Mixed carcinomas contain more than 50% of characteristic morphology and have intermediate outcomes. When characteristic morphology is less than 50%, the tumour is classified as NOS.

Invasive lobular carcinoma (ILC) is the second most common histotype after IDC, NOS, and is characterized by scattered non-cohesive cells, often arranged in single rows or concentrically around benign epithelial structures (targetoid growth) (Fig. 7.3). Intracytoplasmic mucin-containing vacuoles or lumina are also present, to complete the classic morphologic triad of this type. Nuclear atypia is almost always mild, except in the pleomorphic variant of ILC.

Tubular carcinoma (unusual) is composed of tubules lined by a single layer of cells with mild nuclear atypia and desmoplastic stroma. The prognosis is excellent.

Invasive cribriform carcinoma (rare) is often mixed with the tubular variant, with similar cells arranged in cribriform structures. This type has a good prognosis.

Adenoid cystic carcinoma (rare) is histologically identical to that of salivary gland origin. It is characteristically ER and PR negative and has an excellent prognosis.

Secretory carcinoma (rare) is characterized by a multicystic growth of cells with abundant intra- and extracellullar eosinophilic secretions. The prognosis is very good.

Apocrine carcinoma (unusual) harbours cells with abundant granular eosinophilic cytoplasm with large vesicular nuclei and prominent nucleoli. They express androgen receptor and gross cystic disease fluid protein 15 but lack ER and PR.

Invasive micropapillary carcinoma (rare) is composed of small solid clusters of malignant cells lying within clear stromal spaces. Despite the high occurrence rate of nodal metastases, the prognosis is not necessarily poor.

Invasive papillary carcinoma represents the association of an invasive component with an intraductal/intracystic papillary carcinoma, associated with a very good prognosis.

Mucinous carcinoma (unusual) is a well-circumscribed nodule made of small tumour cell nests floating within mucin pools. The prognosis is good.

Medullary carcinoma (unusual) is a well-circumscribed lesion with high-grade tumour cells arranged in a syncytial pattern of growth with a marked lymphocytic infiltrate. The prognosis is excellent.

Neuroendocrine carcinoma (unusual) has the characteristic organoid growth pattern with cellular features (and clinical behaviour) depending on the differentiation grade, with nuclei made of finely granular chromatin.

Metaplastic carcinoma is a rare, heterogeneous group of lesions containing variable amounts of neoplastic epithelial and/or mesenchymal elements.

All the other types mentioned in Table 7.3 are extremely rare findings.

Basal-Like Breast Carcinoma (BLBC). This is a recently emerged subgroup of tumours identified by gene expression profiling [89, 90] but displaying a characteristic morphology and immunophenotype [90]. From the morphological point of view, the vast majority of basal-like carcinoma is represented by poorly differentiated carcinomas [87, 90]. Despite the absence of an international consensus about the immunohistochemical requirements to diagnose such tumours, basal-like breast carcinoma usually expresses basal cytokeratins and lacks hormone receptors and HER2/neu (triple-negative tumour) [75, 90]. There is a marked parallelism between triple-negative breast carcinomas (see further) and basal-like breast carcinomas, but these are not equivalent terms [90]. These features allow us to

make the diagnosis at the pathology level [90]. Recent studies suggest that BLBCs originate from mammary stem cells and are associated with the worst clinical outcome [75, 90, 91].

Additional Prognostic and Predictive Markers

The most important goal in patients affected by cancer is to determine their outcome, a very difficult task in which some value is provided by TNM staging system [92]. Multiple elements related to prognosis and prediction were identified and still continue to be taken into account. Beside "classical" factors, such as histological type, grade and vascular invasion, additional prognostic and predictive markers may be investigated in biopsies or surgical tissues and using ancillary techniques. Some of these factors are recommended in daily practice, and the results must be cited in the final report.

Oestrogen and Progesterone Receptors

Hormone receptor expression represents the first additional marker introduced in breast cancer diagnosis [93]. The expression of ER and PR by tumours has a weak prognostic significance but represents an excellent predictive factor, correlating with low histologic grade and responsiveness to hormonal treatment [79, 87]. ER and PR are nowadays routinely evaluated with immunohistochemistry on paraffin sections (Fig. 7.4a). The actual percentage of ER-positive neoplastic cells (stained nuclei) is included in the pathology report, to identify patients likely to benefit for adjuvant hormonal therapy.

Tumour Proliferation Rate

It is usually measured by immunohistochemical detection of Ki-67 (MIB-1 monoclonal antibody). The percentage of positive nuclei of the neoplastic cells correlates with prognosis and tumours with a high proliferation rate have a worse prognosis. When combined with other routinely used proliferative indicators, such as mitotic index, MIB-1 index may be of help in identifying patients sensitive to adjuvant treatments [88, 94].

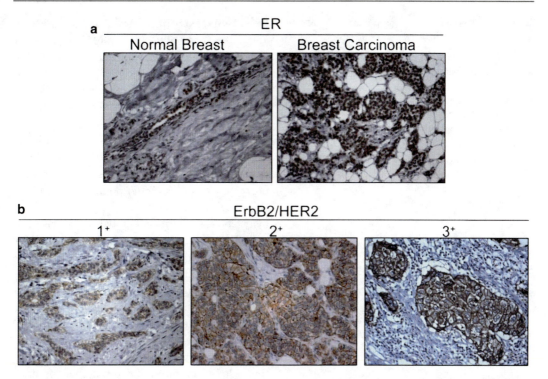

Fig. 7.4 Immunohistochemical analysis. (**a**) Histological sections from normal breast and breast carcinoma samples were evaluated for ER (oestrogen receptor) protein expression by immunohistochemistry analysis. (**b**) Histological sections from breast carcinomas immunostained for ErbB2/HER2 and scored according to the levels of cell membrane expression of ErbB2/HER2 (1⁺=low positivity, 2⁺=medium positivity, 3⁺=high positivity). Original magnification ×100

Human Epidermal Growth Factor Receptor 2/neu Status

HER2/neu (c-erbB2) is a membrane tyrosine kinase and a proto-oncogene that encodes the production of HER2, a cell surface protein important in cell regulation. When activated, it provides the cell with potent proliferative and antiapoptosis signals [95]. Abnormalities of such gene (amplification with resultant protein overexpression) occur especially in poorly differentiated, ER and PR negative, highly proliferating breast carcinomas [96]. Using paraffin-embedded sections, gene amplification can be detected by fluorescence in situ hybridization (FISH), but protein overexpression is cheaply investigated by IHC (Fig. 7.4b). HER2 status represents an adverse prognostic factor and an eligibility criterion for immunotherapy with trastuzumab, which significantly reduces mortality [95, 96] (see further).

Other prognostic factors, such as DNA ploidy and p53 protein overexpression correlate with shorter survivals, but there is little evidence to support their routine use at present time.

Breast Cancer Therapy

Several improvements of the therapeutic strategies allowed recently to increase patient's quality of life as well as life expectancy. Another issue that is more and more emerging is the possibility of a combination versus single chemotherapy. Recent randomized phase III studies showed that a combination of chemotherapeutic agents increased the response rate and improved the time to tumour progression [97]. In this section, we show the main therapies employed and their specific application according to tumour phenotype (Table 7.4).

Table 7.4 Classification of the principal therapeutic approaches employed in breast cancer therapy

Antioestrogen therapy
Selective oestrogen receptor modulators (SERMs): Tamoxifen, raloxifen
Aromatase inhibitors: First generation: aminoglutethimide Second generation: fadrozole, anastrozole, letrozole Third generation: exemestane
Selective oestrogen receptor downregulators (SERD): Fulvestrant
Chemotherapy
Anthracyclines: Doxorubicin
Taxanes: Paclitaxel, docetaxel
Epothilones
Targeted therapy
Epidermal growth factor receptor (EGFR) family inhibitors: Trastuzumab, gefitinib, erlotinib, pertuzumab
Dual EGFR and HER2 inhibitors: Lapatinib
Inhibitors of Ras pathway: Tipifarnib
Anti-VEGF drugs: Bevacizumab

Antioestrogen Therapy

This therapy lasts over the years since it is still one of the most successful for patients with ER-positive metastatic breast cancer with no compromised visceral tissues [98]. Indeed, it has been clearly demonstrated that adjuvant endocrine therapy has contributed to the reduction of breast cancer mortality.

It has been estimated that ER-positive breast cancer constitutes about 60% of breast cancers arising in premenopausal women and 80% of those diagnosed after menopause [99, 100]. However, not all ER-positive tumours are sensitive to endocrine regulation, and the degree of sensitivity is variable in terms of grade of tumour shrinkage and duration of effect, the latter issue strictly related to the occurring of the resistance towards this therapy, an event that is very frequent [101].

As described below in more detail, the two most commonly used approaches in hormone therapy are oestrogen antagonists and oestrogen deprivation.

Selective Oestrogen Receptor Modulators

Tamoxifen is one of the first SERMs employed in the clinical practice. This drug acts as a competitive inhibitor, by binding to ER. When oestrogen binds to its receptor, ER acquires changed shape, thus gaining the ability to interact with coactivators of transcription (Fig. 7.5a). Tamoxifen binds to ER, but this binding fails to allow a conformational change, so that ER is no longer able to interact with nuclear coactivators, with the resulting repression of ER transcriptional activity [102] (Fig. 7.5b). The overall effect on the cell is cytostatic since hormonal growth signal has been turned off. Breast cancer cells treated with tamoxifen stop growing at the point between the G1 and the S phases of the cell cycle.

Tamoxifen proved to be mainly effective in the adjuvant therapy, thus significantly reducing the risk of recurrence and death in patients with ER-positive breast cancer [103, 104]. However, as for other therapies, one of the pitfalls of tamoxifen administration is the occurrence of drug resistance, frequently seen during long-term therapy. Moreover, it has been described that tamoxifen could acquire an agonistic effect, so that tumour cells could proliferate in response to both oestrogen and tamoxifen [105, 106].

Raloxifen is a second generation SERM approved by US Food and Drug Administration (FDA) for prevention and treatment of osteoporosis, which proved to be effective like tamoxifen on ER-positive breast carcinomas, with a lesser toxicity in terms of endometrial cancer and thromboembolic events [107]. Other SERMs showed no further therapeutic advantages if compared to tamoxifen or raloxifen.

Selective Oestrogen Receptor Downregulators

Among this class, there is fulvestrant (ICI 182,780/Faslodex), an antioestrogen with no agonist activity which, at variance with tamoxifen, binds to ER and blocks its signalling by promoting ER degradation [108]. This leads to a dramatic reduction of ER cellular levels and is also associated with a significant reduction of PR. Fulvestrant is indicated for the treatment of hormone receptor-positive metastatic breast

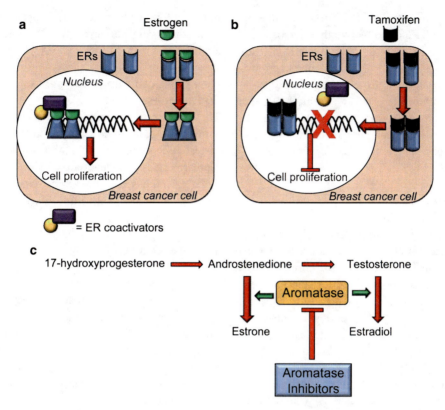

Fig. 7.5 Antioestrogen therapy. (**a**) Schematic representation of the mechanism of action of oestrogen, which interacts with its cytoplasm receptor, thus inducing a conformational change. After dimerization, the ER/oestrogen complex translocates to the nucleus where it interacts with coactivators of transcription, thus triggering specific target gene transcription, which in turn promotes cell proliferation. (**b**) Tamoxifen binds to ER, but this binding fails to allow a conformational change, so that ER is no longer able to interact with nuclear coactivators, with the resulting repression of ER transcriptional activity. (**c**) Schematic representation of the effect of aromatase inhibitors on oestrogen synthesis

cancer in postmenopausal women with disease progression following antioestrogen therapy.

Aromatase Inhibitors

This is another therapeutic approach able to block oestrogen synthesis by inhibiting the aromatization of androgens and their conversion to oestrogens in peripheral tissues. Aromatase is an enzyme of the cytochrome P-450 family that catalyzes the conversion of androstenedione and testosterone to estrone and estradiol (Fig. 7.5c). The gene that encodes this enzyme is expressed in several human tissues and cells such as ovarian granulosa cells, placental syncytiotrophoblast, adipocytes, skin fibroblasts and brain. In reproductive-age women, the ovary is the most important site of oestrogen biosynthesis, and this takes place in a cyclic fashion. On the other hand, in postmenopausal women, oestrogen formation takes place in extraglandular tissues such as the adipose tissue and the skin.

It seems that aromatase inhibitors are more effective than tamoxifen as adjuvant therapy of ER-positive breast cancer patients, with longer disease-free survival and without the risk of endometrial hyperplasia, cancer and thromboembolic events. By contrast, while tamoxifen can have oestrogen-like effects on bone, aromatase inhibitors could induce bone loss [109].

The third-generation aromatase inhibitors include anastrozole and letrozole, which are nonsteroidal aromatase inhibitors, and exemestane, a steroid similar to androstenedione that binds and irreversibly inhibits aromatase (Table 7.4). These compounds showed greater efficacy against advanced breast cancer if compared to tamoxifen [101]. Indeed, exemestane resulted to be more effective than tamoxifen in terms of objective response rate, while letrozole is significantly better in terms of time to progression and quality-adjusted time without symptoms, with no differences in toxicity [110–112]. Comparison among the three aromatase inhibitors shows no differences in terms of overall survival and progression-free survival [101].

Chemotherapy

A substantial body of evidence has shown that breast cancer is among the most chemosensitive solid tumours. However, as for hormone-based therapy, intrinsic or acquired resistance to these treatments is still a common feature that limits the benefits and should encourage the identification of novel therapeutic strategies.

Anthracyclines

These are the most employed cytotoxic drugs for the treatment of breast cancer, with particular regard to adjuvant therapy, although it has also been hypothesized to have a potential leukaemogenic effect, together with cardiac dysfunction, especially in the metastatic setting and heart failure [113, 114]. However, data to this regard are still conflicting. Indeed, Zambetti and colleagues [115] showed that along 10 years of follow-up, the use of doxorubicin at a dose commonly applied in regimen of adjuvant chemotherapy did not lead to cardiac complications that counterbalance the benefit of treatment in patients with operable breast cancer. Similar results were observed by Ganz [116].

Taxanes

This is a group of cytotoxic drugs interacting with microtubules of mitotic spindles, thus blocking mitosis. Among them, the most employed in metastatic setting are paclitaxel and docetaxel [97, 117]. Taxanes represent a valid alternative for anthracyclines, as demonstrated by recent trials showing an efficacy of these compounds slightly higher than those of anthracyclines in the metastatic setting [118], with no cardiotoxicity. Moreover, a recent study indicated that docetaxel

plus cyclophosphamide was more effective than adriamycin plus cyclophosphamide in the adjuvant treatment of breast cancer [119].

New Chemotherapeutic Agents: Epothilones

These new drugs share a similar mechanism of action with taxanes, having the advantage of a lower susceptibility to tumour resistance, thus representing a useful alternative for breast cancer patients who have acquired a resistance to other currently available treatments [120, 121].

Targeted Therapy

This term was coined to identify a therapy able to target a specific molecular pathway involved in the growth and progression of cancer, thus inhibiting crucial processes such as cell proliferation, migration and invasion and angiogenesis. Below is enclosed a brief description of the most important targeted therapies employed in breast cancer treatment.

Epidermal Growth Factor Receptor Family Inhibitors

EGFR is a receptor tyrosine kinase belonging to a wide family including four homologous receptors: EGFR, also known as ErbB1 or HER1; ErbB2 (HER2/*neu*); ErbB3 (HER3); and ErbB4 (HER4) which are the most commonly studied proto-oncogenes in the recent years. Figure 7.6a shows the main pathways triggered by the four receptors, whose ligands are structurally related polypeptides grouped in the epidermal growth factor (EGF) family. The proto-oncogenic role relies on an abnormal activation of these receptors due to gain of function somatic mutations, gene amplification or protein overexpression. Indeed, HER1 and HER2 are frequently overexpressed in many tumours, among them breast cancer, where they promote breast cancer cell proliferation and invasiveness; therefore, their expression is correlated with a poor outcome [122–124]. It has been estimated that HER2/neu amplification could increase the number of receptors on the tumour cell surface from 20,000 to

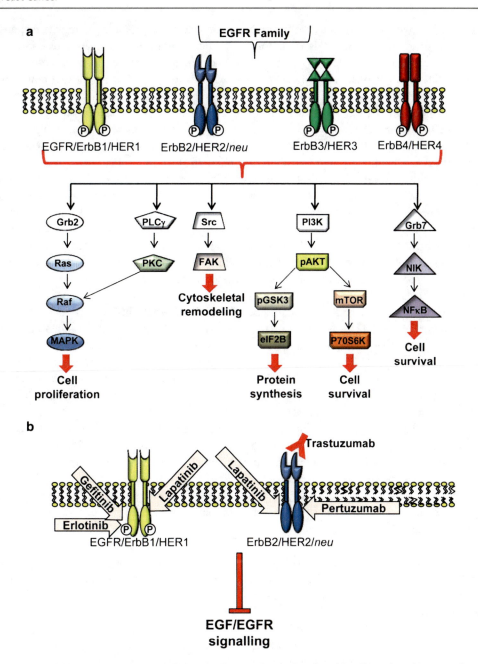

Fig. 7.6 The EGFR pathway. (**a**) EGFR family includes four main tyrosine kinase receptors, named EGFR *alias* ErbB1 (HER1), ErbB2 (HER2/neu), ErbB3 (HER3) and ErbB4 (HER4), which under physiological conditions interact with their specific ligands and autophosphorylate, thus triggering several molecular pathways and leading to downstream effects, including cell cytoskeletal remodelling, cell proliferation and survival. (**b**) Principal drugs targeting EGFR receptors

2 million, thus promoting their proliferation and survival [123] and resulting in a more aggressive breast cancer and a reduced disease-free survival [125]. Therefore, blocking EGFR signalling represents a good target for a therapeutic strategy (Fig. 7.6b).

In clinical practice, HER2/neu overexpression identifies the candidate patients for treatment with EGFR family inhibitor, such as trastuzumab (Fig. 7.4b). Trastuzumab (Herceptin) is a milestone in the HER2-targeted therapy. This is a recombinant humanized monoclonal antibody able to bind the extracellular domain of HER2 with a consequent block of HER2 signalling [126]. Starting in 1998, when it was approved by FDA, several clinical trials have been performed, showing that trastuzumab significantly improved disease-free and overall survival in metastatic breast cancer patients [127–129]. Since 2006, trastuzumab has been approved in a combination therapy together with adjuvant chemotherapy for the treatment of HER2/*neu*-positive, node-positive breast cancer patients. This combination therapy significantly improved response and progression rates, with an increase of quality of life and a reduction of 33% mortality and 50% recurrence [130]. However, one pitfall of trastuzumab is that over one-third of patients could acquire resistance to this therapy.

Trastuzumab-DM1 is a recently synthesized molecule consisting of an antibody, trastuzumab, linked to maytansine, also known as DM1, which is an antimicrotubule drug. This "combination drug" has the advantage that trastuzumab targets DM1 specifically into tumour cells. Two phase III studies are ongoing on HER2-positive metastatic breast cancer patients, testing the activity of this compound versus lapatinib plus capecitabine therapy or versus docetaxel plus trastuzumab [97].

Gefitinib (ZD1839) and erlotinib (OSI-774) are two recent selective EGFR inhibitors belonging to the anilinoquinazoline family and able to reversibly bind EGF receptor, thus preventing its autophosphorylation [131, 132]. Phase I and II studies have been performed with gefitinib, alone or in combination with chemotherapy which, however, showed the lack of improvement of disease-free survival and overall response rate [97]. In contrast, preliminary results of two phase II trials comparing anastrozole or tamoxifen with or without gefitinib showed that patients experienced a prolonged progression-free survival with hormone therapy plus gefitinib [133].

As far as erlotinib is concerned, a recent study showed that this drug, in combination with capecitabine and docetaxel in patients with meta-static breast cancer, gave a complete response in 2 patients, while 12 had a partial response [134]. Other preclinical studies are still in progress.

Pertuzumab (2C4) belongs to a new class of drugs that blocks EGFR dimerization by binding the dimerization domain of HER2; moreover, this binding site does not overlap with the domain recognized by trastuzumab, thus allowing a combination therapy with these two antibodies. Indeed, preclinical studies demonstrated a synergistic effect between these two compounds on breast cancer cell survival [135], and a clinical benefit of this combination therapy has been reported in patients overexpressing HER2, although a cardiac toxicity, asymptomatic in most cases, has been also found [136].

Dual EGFR and HER2 Inhibitors

These compounds are able to target both EGFR and HER2 receptors, thus resulting in a more efficient inhibition of breast cancer cell growth. Among them, there is lapatinib (GW572016), the most advanced dual EGFR/HER2 inhibitor in breast cancer. Although there is not significant benefit as monotherapy, a preclinical study showed a synergistic effect of lapatinib with trastuzumab [137], while preliminary data indicate that this combination therapy significantly improved progression-free survival [138]. Moreover, a preclinical study showed that lapatinib is able to restore sensitivity in tamoxifen-resistant breast cancer cells [139], while combination therapy with letrozole in postmenopausal women with HER2-positive, hormone-sensitive metastatic breast cancer improved progression-free survival [140].

Inhibitors of Ras Pathway

Ras protein is involved in cell growth-stimulating signalling, and its constitutive activation, due to point mutations, could be found in 5% of breast cancer patients. One of the most advanced Ras pathways inhibitor is tipifarnib (R115777). Combination therapy with tipifarnib plus doxorubicin and cyclophosphamide gave encouraging results since 7 out of 21 treated patients had a pathological complete response [141]. Other interesting results were also observed in metastatic breast cancer patients treated with tipifarnib plus fulvestrant [142].

Antiangiogenic Drugs

This therapeutic strategy could also be considered a targeted therapy, mostly directed against the vascular endothelial growth factor (VEGF), which plays a key role in the neovasculature accomplished during tumourigenesis as well as during tumour metastasis.

Bevacizumab is a monoclonal antibody able to neutralize all the six isoforms of VEGF (i.e. VEGF-A, B, C, D, placental growth factor-1 and placental growth factor-2). Clinical trials showed that this compound can be employed in combination with chemotherapy without toxic effects. A phase III study of bevacizumab as first-line treatment for patients with metastatic breast cancer showed a significant increase of the progression-free survival parameters in patients treated with this compound plus paclitaxel versus single treatment with paclitaxel [143]. Currently, bevacizumab is in clinical trial as neoadjuvant treatment.

Conclusions

Breast cancer represents the second most common cause of cancer-related mortality in women, with an estimate of at least one million women diagnosed per year worldwide [14]. As for the other types of cancer, the mechanisms underlying tumour onset have not been completely elucidated. What is clearly known is that progression towards a malignant condition is a complex phenomenon due to a common fault caused not only by genetic (i.e. accumulation of somatic mutations) but also by epigenetic and environmental factors. Moreover, among the other types of tumours, breast cancer is a quite heterogeneous disease, with several subtypes characterized by distinct morphological features and clinical behaviours.

Nevertheless, since 1990, overall breast cancer mortality has decreased, especially for young patients with ER-positive breast cancers [15, 16]. This is at least in part due to an earlier diagnosis of the disease, through the use of more efficacious diagnostic techniques, together with the implementation of population-based screening programmes, which allow to identify non-palpable breast lesions. Moreover, the close cooperation of the pathologists with surgeons, radiologists and oncologists is always desirable to avoid suboptimal patient management.

Another issue crucial to increase patient's quality of life as well as their life expectancy is the advance in terms of therapeutic strategies, such as the combination therapy. Indeed, several randomized phase III studies have compared single-agent chemotherapy versus combination chemotherapy, and one of the most recent studies showed that a combination of chemotherapeutic agents improved the response rate and increased the time to tumour progression. Moreover, a therapeutic strategy more and more adopted over the years is the so-called targeted therapy, that is, a therapy able to target a specific molecular pathway involved in the growth and progression of cancer, thus inhibiting crucial processes such as cell proliferation, migration, invasion and angiogenesis.

Finally, it should be pointed out that improvements of the diagnostic and therapeutic strategies rely mainly on basic and preclinical research, which needs to be encouraged since the knowledge of the molecular mechanisms underlying tumour onset and progression are the starting point to the identification of more selective tumour markers as well as alternative therapies that could be more efficacious and could counteract the occurrence of the resistance towards a canonical therapy.

References

1. Rønnov-Jessen L, Petersen OW, Bissell MJ. Cellular changes involved in conversion of normal to malignant breast: importance of the stromal reaction. Physiol Rev. 1996;76:69–125.
2. Daniel CW, Silberstein GB. Postnatal development of the rodent mammary gland. In: Neville MC, Daniel CW, editors. The mammary gland. New York: Plenum Press; 1987. p. 3–36.
3. Eusebi V, Pich A, Macchiorlatti E, Bussolati G. Morpho-functional differentiation in lobular carcinoma of the breast. Histopathology. 1977;1:301–14.

4. Foschini MP, Scarpellini F, Grown AM, Eusebi V. Differential expression of myoepithelial markers in salivary, sweat and mammary glands. Int J Surg Pathol. 2000;8:29–37.

5. Barbareschi M, Pecciarini L, Cangi MG, Macrì E, Rizzo A, Viale G, Doglioni C. p63, a p53 homologue, is a selective nuclear marker of myoepithelial cells of the human breast. Am J Surg Pathol. 2001;25:1054–60.

6. Radice GL, Ferreira-Cornwell MC, Robinson SD, Rayburn H, Chodosh LA, Takeichi M, Hynes RO. Precocious mammary gland development in P-cadherin-deficient mice. J Cell Biol. 1997;139:1025–32.

7. Sternlicht MD, Kedeshian P, Shao ZM, Safarians S, Barsky SH. The human myoepithelial cell is a natural tumor suppressor. Clin Cancer Res. 1997;3:1949–58.

8. Slade MJ, Coope RC, Gomm JJ, Coombes RC. The human mammary gland basement membrane is integral to the polarity of luminal epithelial cells. Exp Cell Res. 1999;247:267–78.

9. Zajchowski DA, Band V, Trask DK, Kling D, Connolly JL, Sager R. Suppression of tumor-forming ability and related traits in MCF-7 human breast cancer cells by fusion with immortal mammary epithelial cells. Proc Natl Acad Sci U S A. 1990;87:314–8.

10. Sager R, Anisowicz A, Neveu M, Liang P, Sotiropoulou G. Identification by differential display of alpha 6 integrin as a candidate of tumor suppressor gene. FASEB J. 1993;7:964–70.

11. Hirschi KK, Xu CE, Tsukamoto T, Sager R. Gap junction genes Cx26 and Cx43 individually suppress the cancer phenotype of human mammary carcinoma cells and restore differentiation potential. Cell Growth Diff. 1996;7:861–70.

12. Gomm JJ, Browne PJ, Coope RC, Bansal GS, Yiangou C, Johnston CL, Mason R, Coombes RC. A paracrine role for myoepithelial cell-derived FGF2 in the normal human breast. Exp Cell Res. 1997;234:165–73.

13. Alberts B, Bray D, Lewis J, Raff M, Roberts K, Watson JD. Specialized tissues, stem cells and tissue renewal. Molecular biology of the cell. 4th ed. New York: Garland Science; 2002.

14. Garcia S, Dalès JP, Charafe-Jauffret E, Carpentier-Meunier S, Andrac-Meyer L, Jacquemier J, Andonian C, Lavaut MN, Allasia C, Bonnier P, Charpin C. Poor prognosis in breast carcinomas correlates with increased expression of targetable CD146 and c-met and with proteomic basal-like phenotype. Hum Pathol. 2007;38:830–41.

15. Berry DA, Cronin KA, Plevritis SK, Fryback DG, Clarke L, Zelen M, Mandelblatt JS, Yakovlev AY, Habbema JD, Feuer EJ. Cancer intervention and surveillance modeling network (CISNET) collaborators. N Engl J Med. 2005;353:1784–92.

16. Jatoi I, Chen BE, Anderson WF, Rosenberg PS. Breast cancer mortality trends in the United States

according to estrogen receptor status and age at diagnosis. J Clin Oncol. 2007;25:1683–90.

17. Steeg PS. Tumor metastasis: mechanistic insights and clinical challenges. Nat Med. 2006;12:895–904.

18. Wicha MS, Liu S, Dontu G. Cancer stem cells: an old idea-a paradigm shift. Cancer Res. 2006;66:1883–90.

19. Villadsen R, Fridriksdottir AJ, Rønnov-Jessen L, Gudjonsson T, Rank F, LaBarge MA, Bissell MJ, Petersen OW. Evidence for a stem cell hierarchy in the adult human breast. J Cell Biol. 2007;177:87–101.

20. Gudjonsson T, Villadsen R, Nielsen HL, Rønnov-Jessen L, Bissell MJ, Petersen OW. Isolation, immortalization, and characterization of a human breast epithelial cell line with stem cell properties. Genes Dev. 2002;16:693–706.

21. Ginestier C, Hur MH, Charafe-Jauffret E, Monville F, Dutcher J, Brown M, Jacquemier J, Viens P, Kleer CG, Liu S, Schott A, Hayes D, Birnbaum D, Wicha MS, Dontu G. ALDH1 is a marker of normal and malignant human mammary stem cells and a predictor of poor clinical outcome. Cell Stem Cell. 2007;1:555–67.

22. Dontu G, El-Ashry D, Wicha MS. Breast cancer, stem/progenitor cells and the estrogen receptor. Trends Endocrinol Metab. 2004;15:193–7.

23. Asselin-Labat ML, Vaillant F, Sheridan JM, Pal B, Wu D, Simpson ER, Yasuda H, Smyth GK, Martin TJ, Lindeman GJ, Visvader JE. Control of mammary stem cell function by steroid hormone signalling. Nature. 2010;465:798–802.

24. Joshi PA, Jackson HW, Beristain AG, Di Grappa MA, Mote PA, Clarke CL, Stingl J, Waterhouse PD, Khokha R. Progesterone induces adult mammary stem cell expansion. Nature. 2010;465:803–7.

25. Anderson E. The role of oestrogen and progesterone receptors in human mammary development and tumorigenesis. Breast Cancer Res. 2002;4:197–201.

26. Laron Z, Pauli R, Pertezelan A. Clinical evidence on the role of estrogens in the development of the breasts. Proc R Soc Edinburgh B1. 1989;95:13–22.

27. Key TJA, Pike MC. The role of oestrogens and progestagens in the epidemiology and prevention of breast cancer. Eur J Cancer Clin Oncol. 1984;24:29–43.

28. Fisher B, Costantino JP, Wickerham DL, Redmond CK, Kavanah M, Cronin W, Vogel V, Robidoux A, Dimitrov N, Atkins J, Daly M, Wieand S, Tan-Chiu E, Ford L, Wolmark N. Tamoxifen for prevention of breast cancer: report of the National Surgical Adjuvant Breast and Bowel project P-1 study. J Natl Cancer Inst. 1998;90:1371–88.

29. Pike MC, Spicer DV. Hormonal contraception and chemoprevention of female cancers. Endocr Relat Cancer. 2000;7:73–83.

30. Ross RK, Paganini-Hill A, Wan PC, Pike MC. Effect of hormone replacement therapy on breast cancer

31. Medina D, Sivaraman L, Hilsenbeck SG, Conneely O, Ginger M, Rosen J, O'Malley BW. Mechanisms of hormonal prevention of breast cancer. Ann N Y Acad Sci. 2001;952:23–35.

32. Aldaz CM, Liao QY, LaBate M, Johnston DA. Medroxyprogesterone acetate accelerates the development and increases the incidence of mouse mammary tumors induced by dimethylbenzanthracene. Carcinogenesis. 1996;17:2069–72.

33. Klijn JG, Setyono-Han B, Foekens JA. Progesterone antagonists and progesterone receptor modulators in the treatment of breast cancer. Steroids. 2000;65:825–30.

34. Beral V. Breast cancer and hormone-replacement therapy in the Million Women Study. Lancet. 2003;362:419–27.

35. Rossouw J, Anderson GL, Prentice RL, LaCroix AZ, Kooperberg C, Stefanick ML, Jackson RD, Beresford SA, Howard BV, Johnson KC, Kotchen JM, Ockene J. Risks and benefits of estrogen plus progestin in healthy postmenopausal women: principal results from the Women's Health Initiative randomized controlled trial. JAMA. 2002;288:321–33.

36. Fata JE, Kong YY, Li J, Sasaki T, Irie-Sasaki J, Moorehead RA, Elliott R, Scully S, Voura EB, Lacey DL, Boyle WJ, Khokha R, Penninger JM. The osteoclast differentiation factor osteoprotegerin-ligand is essential for mammary gland development. Cell. 2000;103:41–50.

37. Schramek D, Leibbrandt A, Sigl V, Kenner L, Pospisilik JA, Lee HJ, Hanada R, Joshi PA, Aliprantis A, Glimcher L, Pasparakis M, Khokha R, Ormandy CJ, Widschwendter M, Schett G, Penninger JM. Osteoclast differentiation factor RANKL controls development of progestin-driven mammary cancer. Nature. 2010;468:98–102.

38. Hanahan D, Weinberg RA. The hallmarks of cancer. Cell. 2000;100:57–70.

39. Gonzalez-Suarez E, Jacob AP, Jones J, Miller R, Roudier-Meyer MP, Erwert R, Pinkas J, Branstetter D, Dougall W. RANK ligand mediates progestin-induced mammary epithelial proliferation and carcinogenesis. Nature. 2010;468:103–7.

40. Jones DH, Nakashima T, Sanchez OH, Kozieradzki I, Komarova SV, Sarosi I, Morony S, Rubin E, Sarao R, Hojilla CV, Komnenovic V, Kong YY, Schreiber M, Dixon SJ, Sims SM, Khokha R, Wada T, Penninger JM. Regulation of cancer cell migration and bone metastasis by RANKL. Nature. 2006;440:692–6.

41. Boyle WJ, Simonet WS, Lacey DL. Osteoclast differentiation and activation. Nature. 2003;423:337–42.

42. Rucci N, Millimaggi D, Mari M, Del Fattore A, Bologna M, Teti A, Angelucci A, Dolo V. Receptor activator of NF-kappaB ligand enhances breast cancer-induced osteolytic lesions through upregulation of the extracellular matrix metalloproteinase inducer/CD147. Cancer Res. 2010;70:6150–60.

43. Tan W, Tan W, Zhang W, Strasner A, Grivennikov S, Cheng JQ, Hoffman RM, Karin M. Tumour-infiltrating regulatory T cells stimulate mammary cancer metastasis through RANKL-RANK signalling. Nature. 2011;470:548–53.

44. Veeck J, Esteller M. Breast cancer epigenetics: from DNA methylation to microRNAs. J Mammary Gland Biol Neoplasia. 2010;15:5–17.

45. Merlo A, Herman JG, Mao L, Lee DJ, Gabrielson E, Burger PC, Baylin SB, Sidransky D. 5'CpG island methylation is associated with transcriptional silencing of the tumor suppressor p16/CDKN2/MTS1 in human cancer. Nat Med. 1995;1:686–92.

46. Esteller M, Silva JM, Dominguez G, Bonilla F, Matiaz-Guiu X, Lerma E, Bussaglia E, Prat J, Harkes IC, Repasky EA, Gabrielson E, Schutte M, Baylin SB, Herman JG. Promoter hypermethylation and BRCA1 inactivation in sporadic breast and ovarian tumors. J Natl Cancer Inst. 2000;92:564–9.

47. Alves G, Tatro A, Fanning T. Differential methylation of human LINE-1 retrotransposons in malignant cells. Gene. 1996;176:39–44.

48. Guo Y, Pakneshan P, Gladu J, Slack A, Szyf M, Rabbani SA. Regulation of DNA methylation in human breast cancer. Effect on the urokinase-type plasminogen activator gene production and tumor invasion. J Biol Chem. 2002;277:41571–9.

49. Gupta A, Godvin AK, Vanderveer L, Lu A, Liu J. Hypomethylation of the synuclein gamma gene CpG island promotes its aberrant expression in breast carcinoma and ovarian carcinoma. Cancer Res. 2003;63:644–73.

50. Sharma G, Mirza S, Parshad R, Srivastava A, Datta Gupta S, Pandya P, Ralhan R. CpG hypomethylation of MDR1 gene in tumor and serum of invasive ductal breast carcinoma patients. Clin Biochem. 2010;43:373–9.

51. He L, Hannon GJ. MicroRNAs: small RNAs with a big role in gene regulation. Nat Rev Genet. 2004;5:522–31.

52. Yu F, Yao H, Zhu P, Zhang X, Pan Q, Gong C, Huang Y, Hu X, Su F, Lieberman J, Song E. Let-7 regulates self renewal and tumorigenicity of breast cancer cells. Cell. 2007;131:1109–23.

53. Iorio MV, Ferracin M, Liu CG, Veronese A, Spizzo R, Sabbioni S, Magri E, Pedriali M, Fabbri M, Campiglio M, Ménard S, Palazzo JP, Rosenberg A, Musiani P, Volinia S, Nenci I, Calin GA, Querzoli P, Negrini M, Croce CM. MicroRNA gene expression deregulation in human breast cancer. Cancer Res. 2005;65:7065–70.

54. Zhu S, Wu H, Wu F, Nie D, Sheng S, Mo YY. Micro RNA-21 targets tumor suppressor genes in invasion and metastasis. Cell Res. 2008;18:350–9.

55. Mattie MD, Benz CC, Bowers J, Sensinger K, Wong L, Scott GK, Fedele V, Ginzinger D, Getts R, Haqq C. Optimized high-throughput microRNA expression profiling provides novel biomarker assessment of clinical prostate and breast cancer biopsies. Mol Cancer. 2006;5:24.

56. Antoniou A, Pharoa PD, Narod S, Risch HA, Eyfjord JE, Hopper JL, Loman N, Olsson H, Johannsson O, Borg A, Pasini B, Radice P, Manoukian S, Eccles DM, Tang N, Olah E, Anton-Culver H, Warner E, Lubinski J, Gronwald J, Gorski B, Tulinius H, Thorlacius S, Eerola H, Nevanlinna H, Syrjäkoski K, Kallioniemi OP, Thompson D, Evans C, Peto J, Lalloo F, Evans DG, Easton DF. Average risks of breast and ovarian cancer associated with BRCA1 or BRCA2 mutations detected in case Series unselected for family history: a combined analysis of 22 studies. Am J Hum Genet. 2003;72:1117–30.

57. Hall JM, Lee MK, Newman B, Morrow JE, Anderson LA, Huey B, King MC. Linkage of early-onset familial breast cancer to chromosome 17q21. Science. 1990;250:1684–9.

58. Miki Y, Swensen J, Shattuck-Eidens D, Futreal PA, Harshman K, Tavtigian S, Liu Q, Cochran C, Bennett LM, Ding W, et al. A strong candidate for the breast and ovarian cancer susceptibility gene BRCA1. Science. 1994;266:66–71.

59. Wooster R, Neuhausen SL, Mangion J, Quirk Y, Ford D, Collins N, Nguyen K, Seal S, Tran T, Averill D, et al. Localization of a breast cancer susceptibility gene, BRCA2, to chromosome 13q12-13. Science. 1994;265:2088–90.

60. Rahman N, Stratton MR. The genetics of breast cancer susceptibility. Annu Rev Genet. 1998;32:95–121.

61. Yoshida K, Miki Y. Role of BRCA1 and BRCA2 as regulators of DNA repair, transcription, and cell cycle in response to DNA damage. Cancer Sci. 2004;95:866–71.

62. Foray N, Marot D, Randrianarison V, Venezia ND, Picard D, Perricaudet M, Favaudon V, Jeggo P. Constitutive association of BRCA1 and c-Abl and its ATM-dependent disruption after irradiation. Mol Cell Biol. 2002;22:4020–32.

63. MacLachlan TK, Takimoto R, El-Deiry WS. BRCA1 directs a selective p53-dependent transcriptional response towards growth arrest and DNA repair targets. Mol Cell Biol. 2002;22:4280–92.

64. Zhang H, Somasundaram K, Peng Y, Tian H, Bi D, Weber BL, El-Deiry WS. BRCA1 physically associates with p53 and stimulates its transcriptional activity. Oncogene. 1998;16:1713–21.

65. Atchley DP, Albarracin CT, Lopez A, Valero V, Amos CI, Gonzales-Angulo AM, Hortobagyi GN, Arun BK. Clinical and pathologic characteristics of patients with BRCA-positive and BRCA-negative breast cancer. J Clin Oncol. 2008;26:4282–8.

66. Bordeleau L, Panchal S, Goodwin P. Prognosis of BRCA-associated breast cancer: a summary of evidence. Breast Cancer Res Treat. 2010;119:13–24.

67. Moller P, Evans DG, Reis MM, Gregory H, Andersen E, Maehle L, Lalloo G, Howell A, Apold J, Clark N, Lucassen A, Steel CM. Surveillance for familial breast cancer: differences in outcome according to BRCA mutation status. Int J Cancer. 2007;121.1017–20.

68. Rennert G, Bisland-Naggan S, Barnett-Grinness O, Bar-Joseph N, Zhang S, Rennert HS, Narod SA. Clinical outcomes of breast cancer in carriers of BRCA1 and BRCA2 mutations. N Engl J Med. 2007;357:115–23.

69. Lee EH, Park SK, Park B, Kim SW, Lee MH, Ahn SH, Son BH, Yoo KY, Kang D, KHOBRA Research Group, Korean Breast Cancer Society. Effect of BRCA1/2 mutation on short-term and long-term breast cancer survival: a systematic review and meta-analysis. Breast Cancer Res Treat. 2010;122:11–25.

70. Brekelmans CT, Tilanus-Linthorst MM, Seynaeve C, vd Ouweland A, Menke-Pluymers MB, Bartels CC, Kriege M, van Geel AN, Burger CW, Eggermont AM, Meijers-Heijboer H, Klijn JG. Tumour characteristics, survival and prognostic factors of hereditary breast cancer from BRCA2-, BRCA1- and non-BRCA1/2 families as compared to sporadic breast cancer cases. Eur J Cancer. 2007;43:867–76.

71. Tse GM, Tan PH. Diagnosing breast lesions by fine needle aspiration cytology or core biopsy: which is better? Breast Cancer Res Treat. 2010;123:1–8.

72. Sloane JP, Trott PA, Lakhani SR. Biopsy pathology of the breast. 2nd ed. London: Oxford University Press; 2001.

73. Rosai J. Surgical pathology. St. Louis: Mosby; 2004.

74. Tavassoli FA, Devilee P. World Health Organization classification of tumours. Pathology and genetics of tumours of the breast and female genital organs. Lyon: IARC Press; 2003.

75. Tavassoli FA, Eusebi V. Tumors of the mammary gland AFIP. Atlas of tumor pathology, fourth series, fascicle 10. Washington, DC: Armed Forces Institute of Pathology; 2009.

76. Kwok TC, Rakha EA, Lee AHS, Grainge M, Green AR, Ellis IO, Powe DG. Histological grading of breast cancer on needle core biopsy: the role of immunohistochemical assessment of proliferation. Histopathology. 2010;57:212–9.

77. Purdie C, Jordan LB, McCullough JB, Edwards SL, Cunningham J, Walsh M, Grant E, Pratt N, Thompson AL. HER2 assessment on core biopsy specimens using monoclonal antibody CB11 accurately determines HER2 status in breast carcinoma. Histopathology. 2010;56:702–7.

78. Ellis IO, Humphreys S, Michell M, et al. Best practice no. 179. Guidelines for breast needle core biopsy handling and reporting in breast screening assessment. J Clin Pathol. 2004;57:897–902.

79. Humphrey PA, Dehner LP, Pfeifer JD, editors. The Washington manual of surgical pathology. Philadelphia: Lippincott Williams & Wilkins; 2008.

80. Hodi Z, Ellis IO, Elston CW, Pinder SE, Donovan G, Macmillan RD, Lee AHS. Comparison of margin assessment by radial and shave sections in wide local excision specimens for invasive carcinoma of the breast. Histopathology. 2010;56:573–80.

81. Viale G, Mastropasqua MG, Maiorano E, Mazzarol G. Pathologic examination of the axillary sentinel lymph nodes in patients with early-stage breast

carcinoma: current and resolving controversies on the basis of the European Institute of Oncology experience. Virchows Arch. 2006;448:241–7.

82. Treseler P. Pathologic examination of the sentinel lymph node: what is the best method? Breast J. 2006;12:S143–151.

83. Cserni G. Histopathologic examination of the sentinel lymph nodes. Breast J. 2006;12:S152–156.

84. Creager AJ, Geisinger KR. Intraoperative evaluation of sentinel lymph nodes for breast carcinoma: current methodologies. Adv Anat Pathol. 2002;9:233–43.

85. Francz M, Egervari K, Szollosi Z. Intraoperative evaluation of sentinel lymph nodes in breast cancer: comparison of frozen sections, imprint cytology and immunocytochemistry. Cytopathology. 2011;22:36–42.

86. Upender S, Mohan H, Handa U, Attri AK. Intraoperative evaluation of sentinel lymph nodes in breast carcinoma by imprint cytology, frozen section and rapid immunohistochemistry. Diagn Cytopathol. 2009;37:871–5.

87. Fernandes RCM, Bevilacqua JLB, Soares IC, Siqueira SAC, Pires L, Hegg R, Carvalho FM. Coordinated expression of ER, PR, and HER2 define different prognostic subtypes among poorly differentiated breast carcinomas. Histopathology. 2009;55:346–52.

88. Spyratos F, Ferrero Poüs M, Trassard M, Hacène K, Phillips E, Tubiana-Hulin M, Le Doussal V. Correlation between MIB-1 and other proliferation markers: clinical implications of the MIB-1 cutoff value. Cancer. 2002;94:2151–9.

89. Perou CM, Sørlie T, Eisen MB, van de Rijn M, Jeffrey SS, Rees CA, Pollack JR, Ross DT, Johnsen H, Akslen LA, Fluge O, Pergamenschikov A, Williams C, Zhu SX, Lønning PE, Børresen-Dale AL, Brown PO, Botstein D. Molecular portraits of human breast tumours. Nature. 2000;406:747–52.

90. Haupt B, Ro JY, Schwartz MR. Basal-like breast carcinoma. A phenotypically distinct entity. Arch Pathol Lab Med. 2010;134:130–3.

91. Lerma E, Barnadas A, Prat J. Triple negative breast carcinomas: similarities and differences with basal like carcinomas. Appl Immunohistochem Mol Morphol. 2009;17:483–94.

92. Edge SB, Byrd DR, Compton CC, Fritz AG, Green FL, Trotti A. AJCC Cancer staging handbook. New York: Springer; 2010. p. 419–60.

93. Santeusanio G, Mauriello A, Ventura L, Liberati F, Colantoni A, Lasorella R, Spagnoli LG. Immunohistochemical analysis of estrogen receptors in breast carcinomas using monoclonal antibodies that recognize different domains of the receptor molecule. Appl Immunohistochem Mol Morphol. 2000;8:275–84.

94. Elston CW, Ellis IO. Pathologic prognostic factors in breast cancer. I. The value of histological grade in breast cancer: experience from a large study with long-term follow-up. Histopathology. 1991;19:403–10.

95. Gutierrez C, Schiff R. HER2. Biology, detection, and clinical implications. Arch Pathol Lab Med. 2011;135:55–62.

96. Barros FFT, Powe DG, Ellis IO, Green AR. Understanding the HER family in breast cancer: interaction with ligands, dimerization and treatments. Histopathology. 2010;56:560–72.

97. Alvarez RH. Present and future evolution of advanced breast cancer therapy. Breast Cancer Res. 2010;12:S1.

98. Howell A, Dowsett M. Endocrinology and hormone therapy in breast cancer: aromatase inhibitors versus antiestrogens. Breast Cancer Res. 2004;6:269–74.

99. Heldring N, Pike A, Andersson S, Matthews J, Cheng G, Hartman J, Tujague M, Ström A, Treuter E, Warner M, Gustafsson JA. Estrogen receptors: how do they signal and what are their targets. Physiol Rev. 2007;87:905–31.

100. Jensen EV, Jacobson HJ, Walf AA, Frye CA. Estrogen action: a historic perspective on the implications of considering alternative approaches. Physiol Behav. 2010;99:151–62.

101. Riemsma R, Forbes CA, Kessels A, Lykopoulos K, Amonkar MM, Rea DW, Kleijnen J. Systemic review of aromatase inhibitors in the first-line treatment for hormone sensitive advanced or metastatic breast cancer. Breast Cancer Res Treat. 2010;123:9–24.

102. Osborne CK. Tamoxifen in the treatment of breast cancer. N Engl J Med. 1998;339:1609–18.

103. Early Breast Cancer Trialists'Collaborative Group (EBCTCG). Effects of chemotherapy and hormonal therapy for early breast cancer on recurrence and 15-year survival: an overview of the randomized trial. Lancet. 2005;365:1687–717.

104. Orlando L, Schiavone P, Fedele P, Calvani N, Nacci A, Rizzo P, Marino A, D'Amico M, Sponziello F, Mazzoni E, Cinefra M, Fazio N, Maiello E, Silvestris N, Colucci G, Cinieri S. Molecularly targeted endocrine therapies for breast cancer. Cancer Treat Rev. 2010;36S3:S67–71.

105. Fisher B, Dignan J, Bryant J, Wolmark N. Five versus more than five years of tamoxifen for lymph node-negative breast cancer: updated findings from the national Surgical Adjuvant Breast and Bowel Project B-14 randomized trial. J Natl Cancer Inst. 2001;93:684–90.

106. Riggs I, Hartman IC. Selective estrogen-receptor modulators: mechanism of action and application to clinical practice. N Engl J Med. 2003;348:618–29.

107. Vogel VG, Costantino JP, Wickerham DL, Cronin WM, Cecchini RS, Atkins JN, Bevers TB, Fehrenbacher L, Pason ER, Wade JL, Robidoux W, Ford LG, Jordan VC, Wolmark N. National Surgical Adjuvant Breast and Bowel project. Update of the National adjuvant breast and bowel project: study of tamoxifen and raloxifen (STAR) P-2 trial: preventing breast cancer. Cancer Prev Res. 2010;3:696–706.

108. Kansra S, Yamagat S, Sneade L, Foster L, Ben-Jonathan N. Differential effects of estrogen receptor

108. antagonists on pituitary lactotroph proliferation and prolactin release. Mol Cell Endocrinol. 2005;239: 27–36.

109. Mazziotti G, Canalis E, Giustina A. Drug induced osteoporosis: mechanisms and clinical implications. Am J Med. 2010;123:877–84.

110. Mouridsen H, Sun Y, Gershanovich M, Perez-Carrion R, Becquart D, Chaudri-Ross HA, Lang R. Superiority of letrozole to tamoxifen in the first-line treatment of advanced breast cancer: evidence from metastatic subgroups and a test of functional ability. Oncologist. 2004;9:489–96.

111. Mouridsen HT. Letrozole in advanced breast cancer: the PO25 trial. Breast Cancer Res Treat. 2007;105 Suppl 1:19–29.

112. Irish W, Sherril B, Cole B, Gard C, Glendenning GA, Mourdsen H. Quality-adjusted survival in a crossover trial of letrozole versus tamoxifen in postmenopausal women with advanced breast cancer. Ann Oncol. 2005;16:1458–62.

113. Von I, Off DD, Layard MW, Basa P, Davis Jr HL, Von Hoff AL, Rozencweig M, Muggia FM. Risk factors for doxorubicin-induced congestive heart failure. Ann Intern Med. 1979;91:710–7.

114. Jones LW, Haykowsky MJ, Swartz JJ, Douglas PS, Mackey JR. Early breast cancer therapy and cardiovascular injury. J Am Coll Card. 2007;50: 1435–41.

115. Zambetti M, Moliterni A, Materazzo C, Stefanelli M, Cipriani S, Valagussa P, Bonadonna G, Gianni L. Long-term cardiac sequelae in operable breast cancer patients given adjuvant chemotherapy with or without doxorubicin and breast irradiation. J Clin Oncol. 2001;19:37–43.

116. Ganz PA, Hussey MA, Moinpour CM, Unger JM, Hutchins LF, Dakhil SR, Giguere JK, Goodwin JW, Martino S, Albain KS. Late cardiac effects of adjuvant chemotherapy in breast cancer survivors treated on Southwest Oncology Group protocol s8897. J Clin Oncol. 2008;26:1223–30.

117. Esteva FJ, Valero V, Pusztai L, Boehnke-Michaud L, Buzdar AU, Hortobagyi GN. Chemotherapy of metastatic breast cancer: what to expect in 2001 and beyond. Oncologist. 2001;6:133–46.

118. Sledge GW, Neuberg D, Bernardo P, Ingle JN, Martino S, Rowinsky EK, Wood WC. Phase III trial of doxorubicin, paclitaxel, and the combination of doxorubicin and paclitaxel as front-line chemotherapy for metastatic breast cancer: an intergroup trial (E1193). J Clin Oncol. 2003;21:588–92.

119. Jones S, Holmes FA, O'Shaughnessy J, Blum JL, Vukelja SJ, McIntyre KJ, Pippen JE, Bordelon JH, Kirby RL, Sandbach J, Hyman WJ, Richards DA, Mennel RG, Boehm KA, Meyer WG, Asmar L, Mackey D, Riedel S, Muss H, Savin MA. Docetaxel with cyclophosphamide is associated with an overall survival benefit compared with doxorubicin and cyclophosphamide: 7-year follow-up of US Oncology Research Trial 9735. J Clin Oncol. 2009; 27:1177–83.

120. Wartmann M, Altmann KH. The biology and medicinal chemistry of epothilones. Curr Med Chem Anticancer Agents. 2002;2:123–48.

121. Lee FY, Borzilleri R, Fairchild CR, Kim SH, Long BH, Reventos-Suarez C, Vite GD, Rose WC, Kramer RA. BMS-247550: a novel epothilone analog with a mode of action similar to paclitaxel but possessing superior antitumor efficacy. Clin Cancer Res. 2001;7:1429–37.

122. Slamon DJ, Clark GM, Wong SG, Levin WJ, Ulrich A, McGuire WL. Human breast cancer: correlation of relapse and survival with amplification of the HER-2/neu oncogene. Science. 1987;235:177–82.

123. Yarden Y, Sliwkowski MX. Untangling the ErbB signalling network. Nat Rev Mol Cell Biol. 2001;2:127–37.

124. Angelucci A. Targeting ERBB receptors to inhibit metastasis: old hopes and new certainties. Curr Cancer Drug Targets. 2009;9:1–18.

125. Ariga R, Zariff A, Korasick J, Reddy V, Siziopikou K, Gattuso P. Correlation of HER2/neu gene amplification with other prognostic and predictive factors in female breast carcinoma. Breast J. 2005;11: 278–80.

126. Baselga J, Norton L, Albanell J, Kim YM, Mendelshon J. Recombinant humanized anti-HER2 antibody (Herceptin) enhances the antitumor activity of paclitaxel and doxorubicin against Her2/neu over-expressing human breast cancer xenografts. Cancer Res. 1998;58:2825–31.

127. Piccart-Gebhart MJ, Procter M, Leyland-Jones B, Goldhirsch A, Untch M, Smith I, Gianni L, Baselga J, Bell R, Jackisch C, Cameron D, Dowsett M, Barrios CH, Steger G, Huang CS, Andersson M, Inbar M, Lichinitser M, Lang I, Nitz U, Iwata H, Thomssen C, Lohrisch C, Suter TM, Ruschoff J, Suto T, Greatorex V, Ward C, Straehle C, McFadden E, et al. Trastuzumab after adjuvant chemotherapy in HER2-positive breast cancer. N Engl J Med. 2005; 353:1659–72.

128. Buzdar AU, Ibrahim NK, Francis D, Booser DJ, Thomas ES, Theriault RL, Pusztai L, Green MC, Arun BK, Giordano SH, Cristofanilli M, Frye DK, Smith TL, Hunt KK, Singletary SE, Sahin AA, Ewer MS, Buchholz TA, Berry D, Hortobagy GN. Significant higher pathologic complete remission rate after neoadjuvant therapy with trastuzumab, paclitaxel, and epirubicin chemotherapy: results of randomized trial in human epidermal growth factor receptor 2-positive operable breast cancer. J Clin Oncol. 2005;23:3676–85.

129. Romond EH, Perez FA, Bryant J, Suman VJ, Geyer Jr CE, Davidson NF, Tan-Chiu E, Martino S, Paik S, Kaufman PA, Swain SM, Pisansky TM, Fehrenbacher L, Kutteh LA, Vogel VG, Visscher DW, Yothers G, Jenkins RB, Brown AM, Dakhil SR, Mamounas EP, Lingle WL, Klein PM, Ingle JN, Wolmark N. Trastuzumab plus adjuvant chemotherapy for operable HER2-positive breast cancer. N Engl J Med. 2005;353:1673–84.

130. Smith I, Procter M, Gelber RD, Guillaume S, Feyerlislova A, Dowsett M, Goldhirsch A, Untch M, Mariani G, Baselga J, Kaufmann M, Cameron D, Bell R, Bergh J, Coleman R, Wardley A, Harbeck N, Lopez RI, Mallmann P, Gelmon K, Wilcken N, Wist E. 2-year follow-up of trastuzumab after adjuvant chemotherapy in HER2-positive breast cancer: a randomized controlled trial. Lancet. 2007;369: 29–36.

131. Pollack VA, Savage DM, Baker DA, Tsaparikos KE, Sloan DE, Meyer JD, Barbacci EG, Pustilnik LR, Smolarek TA, Davis JA, Vaidya MP, Arnold LD, Doty JL, Iwara KK, Morin MJ. Inhibition of epidermal growth factor receptor-associated tyrosine phosphorylation in human carcinomas with CP-358,774: dynamics of receptor inhibition in situ and anti tumor effects in athimic mice. J Pharmacol Exp Ther. 1999;291:739–48.

132. Baselga J. Targeting the epidermal growth factor receptor: a clinical reality. J Clin Oncol. 2001;19: 41S–4S.

133. Cristofanelli M, Schiff R, Valero V, Iacona R, Yu J, Speake G, Smith I, Osborne CK. Exploratory subset analysis according to prior endocrine treatment of two randomized phase II trials comparing gefitinib (G) with placebo (P) in combination with tamoxifen (T) or anastrozole (A) in hormone receptor positive (HR+) metastatic breast cancer (MBC). In: 2009 ASCO Annual Meeting. J Clin Oncol 2009;27(Suppl 15):Abstract 1014

134. Twelves C, Trigo JM, Jones R, De Rosa F, Rakhit A, Fettner S, Wright T, Baselga J. Erlotinib in combination with capecitabine and docetaxel in patients with metastatic breast cancer: a dose-escalation study. Eur J Cancer. 2008;44:419–26.

135. Nahta R, Hung MC, Esteva FJ. The HER-2-targeting antibodies trastuzumab and pertuzumab synergistically inhibit the survival of breast cancer cells. Cancer Res. 2004;64:2343–6.

136. Portera CC, Walshe JM, Rosing DR, Denduluri N, Berman AW, Vatas U, Velarde M, Chow CK, Steinberg SM, Nguyen D, Yang SX, Swain SM. Cardiac toxicity and efficacy of trastuzumab combined with pertuzumab in patients with [corrected] human epidermal growth factor receptor 2-positive metastatic breast cancer. Clin Cancer Res. 2008; 14:2710–6.

137. Konecny GE, Pegran MD, Venkatesan N, Finn R, Yang G, Rahmeh M, Untch M, Rusnak DW, Spehar G, Mullin RJ, Keith BR, Gilmer TM, Berger M, Podratz KC, Slamon DJ. Activity of the dual kinase inhibitor lapatinib (GW572016) against HER-2-overexpressing and trastuzumab-treated breast cancer cells. Cancer Res. 2006;66:1630–9.

138. O'Shaughnessy J, Blackwell K, Burstein H, Storniolo AM, Sledge G, Baselga J, Koehler M, Laabs S, Florance A, Roychowdhury DF. A randomized study of lapatinib alone or in combination with trastuzumab in heavily pretreated HER2+ metastatic breast cancer progression on trastuzumab therapy. In: 2008 ASCO Annual Meeting. J Clin Oncol. 2008;26: Abstract 1015.

139. Chu QS, Cianfrocca ME, Goldstein LJ, Gale M, Murray N, Loftiss J, Arya N, Koch KM, Pandite L, Fleming RA, Paul E, Rowinsky EK. A phase I and pharmacokinetic study of lapatinib in combination with letrozole in patients with advanced cancer. Clin Cancer Res. 2008;14:4484–90.

140. Johnston S, Pippen Jr JE, Pivot X, Lichinitser M, Sadeghi S, Dieras V, Gomez H, Romieu G, Manikhas A, Kennedy J, Press MF, Maltzman J, Florance A, O'Rourke L, Olive C, Stein S, Pegram M. Lapatinib combined with letrozole versus letrozole and placebo as first-line therapy for postmenopausal hormone receptor-positive metastatic breast cancer. J Clin Oncol. 2009;27:5538–46.

141. Sparano JA, Moulder S, Kazi A, Vahdat L, Li T, Pellegrino C, Munster P, Malafa M, Lee D, Hoschander S, Hopkins U, Hershman D, Wright JJ, Sebti SM. Targeted inhibition of farnesyltransferase in locally advanced breast cancer: a phase I and II trial of tipifarnib plus dose-dense doxorubicin and cyclophosphamide. J Clin Oncol. 2006;24:3013–8.

142. Li T, Christos PJ, Sparano JA, Hershman DL, Hoschander S, O'Brien K, Wright JJ, Vahdat LT. Phase II trial of the farnesyltransferase inhibitor tipifarnib plus fulvestrant in hormone receptor-positive metastatic breast cancer: New York Cancer Consortium Trial P6205. Ann Oncol. 2009;20:642–7.

143. Miller K, Wang M, Gralow J, Dickler M, Cobleigh M, Perez EA, Shenkier T, Cella D, Davidson NE. Paclitaxel plus bevacizumab versus paclitaxel alone for metastatic breast cancer. N Engl J Med. 2007; 357:2666–76.

Oesophago-Gastric Cancer

8

Alex M. Reece-Smith, Simon L. Parsons, and Sue A. Watson

Introduction

Gastric cancer currently represents the second most common cause of cancer-associated death in the world [1], and as such is one of the leading causes of mortality globally. Oesophageal cancer also presents an important global health issue as the sixth most common cause of cancer-associated death globally; however, it has risen to great prominence over recent decades due to the alarming rise in incidence of certain forms of the disease [2]. In the USA, there has been sixfold increase in incidence in adenocarcinoma of the oesophagus and gastro-oesophageal junction (GOJ) over recent decades [3], this being, in part, due to the ageing populations in these countries as well as the increasing incidence of obesity which results in increased gastro-oesophageal reflux [4].

A.M. Reece-Smith, M.B.B.S., M.R.C.S.
Division of Pre-Clinical Oncology PRECOS Ltd,
School of Clinical Sciences, University of Nottingham,
Queen's Medical Centre, D Floor, West Block,
Nottingham, NG7 2UH, UK

S.L. Parsons, D.M., F.R.C.S.
Oesophago-gastric surgery, Nottingham University
Hospitals NHS Trust,
Nottingham, Nottinghamshire, UK

S.A. Watson, Ph.D. (✉)
Division of Pre-Clinical Oncology,
School of Clinical Sciences, University of Nottingham,
Queen's Medical Centre, D Floor, West Block,
Nottingham, NG7 2UH, UK
e-mail: sue.watson@nottingham.ac.uk

The incidence of these diseases vary across the globe in response to genetic variation as well as variations in exposure to carcinogens particularly in the form of tobacco and dietary factors including alcohol and obesity as mentioned above.

Biologically, the cancers of the gastro-oesophageal region fall broadly into one of six categories, namely, cancers of the distal stomach, the proximal stomach, the gastro-oesophageal junction, oesophageal adenocarcinomas (excluding Barrett's carcinomas), Barrett's carcinomas and oesophageal squamous cell carcinomas.

Aetiology

Distal gastric cancers are primarily related to *Helicobacter pylori* infection [5], and subsequent to the discovery and treatment of this pathogen, there has been a reduction in the incidence of this form of cancer. Conversely, *H. pylori* infection has a protective effect against oesophageal adenocarcinoma according to meta-analysis of a number of studies [6]. However, eradication therapy had not been shown to be contributing to the rise in incidence of cancer or gastro-oesophageal reflux disease (GORD) [7].

Genetic predisposition is likely to play a role in carcinogenesis in individuals as well as differential population risks around the globe. The incidence of alcohol dehydrogenase and aldehyde dehydrogenase polymorphisms shows heterogeneity across continents and appears to confer higher risk of squamous oesophageal cancers in

Asian populations [8], and twin studies report a genetic predisposition to GORD [9, 10]. Alcohol is a well-established contributing factor to the development of oesophageal squamous cell carcinoma, particularly when taken in excess, and tobacco smoke is similarly associated. However, whilst these risk factors are known to contribute to GORD, the link to oesophageal adenocarcinoma is only confirmed in smoking but not alcohol [11].

The Spectrum of Pathology in the Stomach and Oesophagus

The differentiation between Barrett's carcinoma and other adenocarcinoma of the oesophagus continues to develop. Indeed, the definition of Barrett's continues to be a matter of debate with some recent definitions excluding the previous requirement for histological confirmation of intestinal metaplasia that is pathognomonic of the condition [12]. Whilst, in part, this is a response to the practicalities of histologically assessing an area of field change, it is also symptomatic of an awareness that the many lower oesophageal cancers occur in patients with no history of Barrett's and also that the presence of glandular mucosa above the GOJ appears to confer to a similar cancer risk as those who develop metaplasia in the lower oesophagus [13].

The differentiation between lower oesophageal adenocarcinomas and GOJ carcinomas was initially a clinical observation regarding the poorer survival noted in patients with GOJ tumours, and even amongst tumours at the GOJ, there are clear cut clinical differences dependent on the precise relationship to the junction, leading to the adoption of the Siewert classification system [14]. Defining the biological properties that give rise to these differences continues to be an area of investigation and as yet not sufficiently defined to have led divergence from the established standards of care for these tumours. However, genetic characteristics are being documented that may lead to better understanding of the disease in these different areas. For example, COX-2 expression has been noted to be increased in lower oesophageal cancers but not in GOJ cancers [15, 16], and whilst this has not led

to successful therapeutic strategies, it does point to biological differences between sites that are important to consider in the successful design of clinical trials. However, other genetic changes appear to be consistent between cancers of the lower oesophagus and the GOJ, with one study finding a similar pattern of gain and loss of gene function across the 2 areas and thereby distinguished them from gastric cancers that displayed a different pattern. These changes included upregulation of EGFR and CDK6 genes in oesophageal and GOJ cancers [17].

This chapter is divided into sections that will explore the biology of individual clinically relevant biotargets and then review current clinical evidence regarding therapies developed that take advantage of these targets. Where possible, it will seek to differentiate between the anatomical subtypes of cancer in order to determine the utility of the biotarget in precise situations; however, this is not always possible due to the limited evidence which has often combined the groups, for example, to increase recruitment in clinical trials. In these situations, only the evidence available can be reported even though further definition will develop in time.

Epidermal Growth Factor Receptor

EGFR is the cell surface receptor for the epidermal growth factor family of ligands which cause dimerisation of the receptor and resulting autophosphorylation of the intracellular tyrosine kinase. Activation of the tyrosine kinase initiates a number of signalling pathways including the RAS/RAF/MEK/ERK and PI3K and JAK/STAT pathways (Fig. 8.1) [18–22]. The receptor itself is a glycoprotein with a molecular weight of 170 kDa and is transcribed from a gene on chromosome 7p12 [23].

Pathways activated by EGFR have been implicated in cell growth, survival, proliferation and differentiation and may become dysregulated during the development of a variety of cancers. This makes it an attractive target for therapy, and a variety of methods of targeting this class of receptor have developed over recent years and successfully transferred into clinical practice.

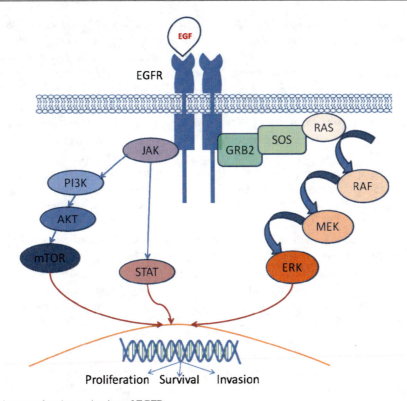

Fig. 8.1 Pathways related to activation of EGFR

A great deal is known of the interactions of these pathways with EGF signalling, and this has demonstrable clinical utility as seen in the use of cetuximab (an EGFR inhibitor) in colorectal metastases which is used only in patients with wild-type RAS, which has been shown to be of greater importance than the EGFR phenotype of the tumour [24].

In total, there are 4 subclasses of protein named EGFR, EGFR2, EGFR3 and EGFR4, although the alternative nomenclature human epidermal receptor (HER) and the gene symbol ErbB remain in use, particularly in regard to EGFR2 (HER2, ErbB2). EGFR 3 and 4 have only been assessed to a minor degree in oesophageal cancer, although an understanding of the role of these molecules in breast cancer is beginning to emerge. They have been reported as markers of good prognosis or to have a role in regulating response to existing targeted agents, and as such no interest has yet to be shown in these molecules as potential targets for treatment [25]. However, a single study has suggested that EGFR 3 may be associated with diffuse-type gastric cancer and also worse overall survival, leaving the possibility that the storey may be different in subtypes of gastro-oesophageal cancer [26].

EGFR2 (HER2)-targeted agents have an established role in the treatment of breast cancer, and the introduction of trastuzumab and related targeted agents for the treatment of oesophago-gastric cancers will be discussed in the light of positive phase III trials in a separate section (HER2) with this section, concentrating exclusively on EGFR.

EGFR inhibitors have also been shown to be effective agents in the treatment of EGFR mutant non-small-cell lung cancer. At present, no phase III trial information is published regarding the use of these same agents in oesophago-gastric cancer, but the results of phase II trials are encouraging and are discussed below.

Even though EGFR inhibitors such as gefitinib, erlotinib and trastuzumab have been shown to be effective agents, their use has required targeting in a variety of ways. Current clinical practice targets trastuzumab treatment essentially to those who express the HER2 protein on immunohistochemistry [27]. However, in lung cancer, the tyrosine kinase inhibitors have been shown to primarily benefit those with mutations of EGFR gene but to have minimal effects in those who simply express the protein and a debated effect in those over-expressing the gene [28–31], and in colon cancer, mutations in the downstream KRAS gene have been shown to negate the effects of cetuximab on expressed EGFR protein [24]. These differences emphasise the need for preselection of well-defined targets at a genetic or molecular level and well-designed clinical trials with adequate analysis of those patients that respond to the treatment and those that do not. This is particularly the case in oesophago-gastric cancer (E-GC) where a variety of sub-classifications exist. Many studies have initially assessed a mixture of oesophageal, gastric and junctional tumours and have included adenocarcinomas, Barrett's carcinomas and squamous carcinomas without adequately reporting the outcomes in the subgroups. In reviewing the literature below, an attempt has been made to precisely define the findings in these individual biological categories and also to report on the geographical origin of the patients involved in order to remain mindful of the genetic differences that may exist particularly between Caucasian populations and those from East Asian countries.

EGFR in Oesophageal SCC

Between studies that have assessed EGFR protein expression, there has been significant variation in the methodology to determine the degree of expression. Some studies report the presence of any degree of staining on immunohistochemistry (IHC), and others have performed semi-quantitative assessment by grading the intensity of staining, often using methods similar to those used clinically in HER2 staining, which define those cases with moderate to intense staining for the receptor to be positive. There is also significant heterogeneity noted within individual

tumours and as such a further method of scoring computes a composite score from the percentage area stained and staining intensity. Three Japanese studies [32–34] of between 62 and 217 patients and one Thai study of 55 patients [35] have determined the expression of EGFR protein by IHC in oesophageal SCC and have reported it in between 34% (in the smallest Japanese series) and 80% (in the Thai series), with all reports from groups who removed patients considered to have low-intensity staining, although each used slightly different methods to determine which patients were excluded. Similarly, a Chinese study of 62 patients found 75.8% of cases to be positive for EGFR mRNA in SCC [36]. One group reported that a higher proportion of the EGFR-positive group achieved complete pathological response to chemoradiotherapy than those with EGFR-negative tumours [34]; however, other studies report no difference in survival in patients expressing EGFR [32, 33]. One study went on to perform fluorescent in situ hybridisation (FISH) analysis of those expressing EGFR and found that 28% of the 53 cases assessed over-expressed EGFR (13% of the total population) [33]. The Thai study found gene amplification in 15% of cases, but this included analysis of EGFR IHC-negative patients of whom 7% were FISH positive [35]. In a study that analysed a small number of lymph nodes involved with metastatic disease, it was found that, in some cases, only 50% of nodes possessed the same over-expression seen in the primary tumour suggesting that amplification may be an early process in carcinogenesis that is not integral to the metastatic process [33]. A final Japanese study reported EGFR gene amplification by slot-blot analysis of 107 SCC cases and detected amplification in 12%, all of which had stage 3 or 4 disease, but multivariate analysis confirmed EGFR amplification to be an independent determinant of poor survival [37].

Within Europe, two studies have been conducted of EGFR expression in SCC, each analysing approximately 100 patients from France and Holland [38, 39]. EGFR expression was reported in between 40% and 68.2% of cases with both using concordant methods of scoring EGFR positivity when there was moderate or intense staining. The French study also reported that a diffuse rather than mosaic pattern of staining correlated with poor survival. A further German study reviewed a similar number of patients and reported 98.8% positivity. However, this study did not perform semi-quantitative analysis of the immunostaining and so may represent an over-estimate of the biologically significant expression [40], and a further small Irish study using semi-quantitative scoring consistent with other European sites also provides a consistent result of 64.3% [41].

Overall, it appears difficult to distinguish a difference between European and East Asian SCC populations based on EGFR protein expression using current evidence. FISH analysis of gene amplification has only been assessed in Japanese patients but has consistently been reported as 12% or 13% in both studies [33, 37]. From the evidence available, conclusive prognostic use for EGFR staining has been demonstrated, with only one study reporting a poor survival in patients with high EGFR expression. This has been important to determine in order to make a valid assessment of phase II trial evidence for the novel agents that target EGFR. In trials recruiting EGFR-positive patients with SCC, we could at present assume that these patients have a survival expectation that is little different to the EGFR-negative population prior to intervention.

EGFR in Oesophageal and GOJ Adenocarcinoma

Studies examining the incidence of EGFR protein expression in oesophageal and GOJ cancer have been more consistent although still included some variability in the reporting of immunostaining. The evidence comes exclusively from primarily Caucasian populations in the USA and Europe but has often included oesophageal and GOJ tumours together which has made it difficult to determine if these areas are biologically different in terms of the EGF contribution to carcinogenesis. Three such studies used similar semi-quantitative scoring systems that excluded weakly staining patients to find positivity for EGFR in 24–55% of patients [17, 42, 43].

A study that restricted itself to oesophageal adenocarcinomas reported positivity in 39% of 38 cases; however, this included patients with weak or focal staining [44]. Two studies limited to Barrett's carcinomas found EGFR amplification in 8% of cases [45, 46].

Only one study has reported mutation rates in oesophageal adenocarcinoma, which were present in 11.7% of cases [47].

With regard to prognostic information, none of the studies demonstrated a significant survival difference on multivariate analysis; however, two studies demonstrated a trend towards worse survival in EGFR-positive patients that may have reached significance with a larger sample size or longer follow-up [42, 44].

EGFR in Gastric Cancer

In gastric cancer, the evidence is more robust, particularly due to two large East Asian studies of more than 400 patients each and using consistent semi-quantitative scoring methods. One study only found positive staining in 2.1% of cases and only 10.4% even when weakly stained cases were included [48]. The other study found positivity in 27.4% of cases [49]. Both studies undertook FISH analysis and found this to be positive in 1.6% and 5.5% of cases. Smaller Asian studies have also found protein expression in 7.3% of early gastric cancers and 30% of advanced gastric cancers [50, 51], whilst EGFR mutations have been detected in 5.1% of cases in the only small series available [52].

In European studies, EGFR expression has been scored again using variations on semi-quantitative methods that measure intensity and area stained, and this makes direct comparison difficult. Two studies report the proportion of positive cases to be between 14.8% and 33% [53, 54]. However, the scoring system used by the second group used a lower threshold for positivity in terms of area and intensity and so may represent fairly consistent populations. One of these studies reported EGFR expression to be associated with worse prognosis, particularly when combined with VEGF expression as well [53]. Similar poor survival was noted in a Mexican study that reported EGFR moderate/intense positivity in 28% of cases [55].

Summary of EGFR in Gastro-Oesophageal Cancer

SCCs appear to demonstrate EGFR positivity in a higher proportion of cases than adenocarcinomas of the oesophagus, and proportions may be consistent between East Asian and European populations. Although, a high degree of heterogeneity exists between results in SCC, it may be that greater than 50% of cases express EGFR. In adenocarcinomas of the oesophagus and GOJ, there is EGFR expression in approximately 40% of cases in Caucasian populations, whilst EGFR expression is low in gastric cancer. Present evidence might suggest a trend to higher positivity in Caucasian populations in gastric cancer, in whom approximately 20% of cases appear positive compared to 10% or less in East Asian populations.

There is some evidence to suggest that EGFR positivity may increase with advancing disease and that survival may be slightly worse in patients with EGFR-positive cancers.

In NSCLC, the efficacy of EGFR TKIs is largely restricted to those cancers that have activating mutations of the EGFR gene rather than simply those that express the EGFR protein. Whilst this does mean that it is a dramatically limited population of patients that benefit from this treatment, the precise targeting of the treatment allows for other individuals to avoid the side effects of unsuccessful therapy. In oesophageal cancer, the incidence of mutations in the EGFR gene is similarly low, but clinical trials so far have not identified the need to limit EGFR inhibitor treatment to patients carrying mutations.

EGFR Inhibitors

The EGFR inhibitors in current clinical use are either receptor tyrosine kinase inhibitors or monoclonal antibodies against the extracellular domain of the receptor. These antibodies competitively inhibit the receptor ligands by binding to the receptor and on binding can induce dimerisation of the receptor and its subsequent down-regulation, whilst the tyrosine kinase inhibitors (including erlotinib and gefitinib) are small molecules that primarily act by competing for ATP binding sites on the intracellular tyrosine kinase [18].

EGFR Inhibitors in Oesophageal and GOJ Cancer

Gefitinib is currently approved for use in other cancer types including as a first-line agent in non-small-cell lung cancer, and two European phase II trials have reported on the safety of this drug. In one trial, 27 patients were recruited with advanced oesophageal or GOJ adenocarcinoma more than 2 months since completing any first-line treatments. These patients were assessed for response to gefitinib radiologically after 1 month of treatment, and response rate was found to be 11%, with a total of 37% achieving disease control and a median progression-free survival of 1.9 months across the study population [56]. Results similar to this were also reported in a preliminary report of a US phase II trial [57].

The other European trial of gefitinib as a second-line treatment of advanced oesophageal or GOJ cancer included patients with either adenocarcinoma or SCC. This study recruited 36 patients of which only 1 (2.8%) patient achieved a partial response, with another 10 (27.8%) maintaining stable disease on reassessment at 8 weeks. This study found k-ras mutations in 2 of the non-responder patients, but no EGFR mutations in the cohort. However, they did find high EGFR expression in 37.5% of those tested, and this was more prevalent in SCCs with disease control rate reported to be 66.7% in patients with high EGFR expression, although this failed to convert into statistically superior survival outcomes [58].

An American study examining Erlotinib in a phase II setting initially recruited 43 GOJ cancer patients and 25 gastric cancer patients, with outcomes reported separately. All had advanced adenocarcinoma, but none had been treated for metastatic disease previously. There were 4 responses (9%) in the GOJ arm including one complete response. In total, 10 patients had stable disease or a response to treatment (23.8%). Eighty-six percent of 42 patients tested for EGFR expression were positive, but again no EGFR mutations were detected, and there was no correlation between EGFR expression and response to erlotinib. Median survival in the GOJ and gastric arms were 6.7 and 3.5 months, respectively [59], but without details of the EGFR expression status of the patients included, it is impossible to determine if these differences are due to the higher proportion of GOJ cancers expected to express EGFR.

Cetuximab in combination with cisplatin and 5-FU has been trialled against chemotherapy alone and achieved a 19% response rate and 75% control rate with a trend to benefit with the addition of cetuximab which did not reach significance in any survival outcomes [60].

EGFR Inhibitors in Gastric Cancer

A US phase II trial of Erlotinib reported above also recruited 25 gastric cancer patients. This arm of the study closed early due to there being only one patient with a stable disease response [59]. However, other studies have observed more promising levels of response.

A Korean phase II trial of cetuximab in combination with FOLFOX treatment treated 40 patients with advanced gastric cancer and found EGFR expression in 12 (30%), and these patients had longer time to progression outcomes. This group also measured serum concentrations of the ligands EGF and TGF-alpha and reported that 100% of patients with EGFR protein expression who had low serum EGF/TGF-alpha responded to treatment. A total of eight patients in this responder group had follow-up blood tests of which seven showed a rise in EGF levels at the time of disease progression. No patients had EGFR amplifications [51].

An Italian Phase II trial of cetuximab in combination with FOLFIRI in advanced gastric cancer included 38 patients known to be EGFR positive. The study design included four patients who had tumours involving the GOJ. They reported a response rate of 44.1% and disease control in 91.2%. They found no correlation between the degree of IHC positivity for EGFR or in the proportion of the tumour examined that stained positive. Complete response was seen in 11.8%. Median time to progression was 8 months and predicted median survival 16 months [61]. Whilst this may not provide conclusive evidence of a benefit from the addition of the targeted therapy, these results are favourable compared to a number of trials using similar regimes without cetuximab [62–65].

The same group have more recently reported similar findings from a further phase II study combining cetuximab with a different combination chemotherapy including docetaxel and cisplatin, although this trial returned a slightly lower stable disease rate possibly due to the absence of a fluoypyrimidine in the combination [66].

Panitumumab is a similar humanised IgG2 monoclonal antibody that has been optimised for entry into phase III studies and is likely to target the same disease as treated by cetuximab [67].

Results appear to suggest that patients with high EGFR protein expression are more likely to respond to EGFR inhibitor therapy and the additional quantification of EGF levels may also allow further identification of patients most likely to respond to these targeted agents. As discussed above, the expression of EGFR appears to be more frequent in cancers of the oesophagus or GOJ, and so phase III trials in progress have justifiably chosen to assess the benefits of gefitinib and cetuximab primarily in oesophageal and junctional cancer and initial results may appear in 2012. The subgroup analysis of any such trial may yet reveal important understanding of the mechanism of efficacy of these drugs in gastro-oesophageal cancer. The impact of mutations of the EGFR gene and genes downstream such as KRAS have yet to be determined, and similarly, the effects of gene amplifications, found in smaller portions of the population, are not yet understood. However, it appears that response may primarily be related to protein expression in a similarly way that HER2 inhibitors are used in breast cancer, and if this proves to be the case, this form of treatment will mark a huge step forward in the treatment of these cancers due to the relatively common expression of these markers particularly in squamous oesophageal cancer.

Human Epidermal Growth Factor Receptor 2

As discussed previously, HER2 belongs to the EGFR family of receptors. However, the terminology 'receptor' is a little misleading because at present no physiological ligands or binding sites for a ligand has been identified [20, 68]. However, the molecule is integral in heterodimerisation of other members of the EGFR family and so might perhaps have been more appropriately termed a co-receptor (Fig. 8.2). Structurally, it is similar to the other members of the EGFR family consisting of an extracellular glycoprotein, a small transmembrane section and an intracellular tyrosine kinase. The molecular weight of the HER2 receptor is 185 kDa, with the gene being located on chromosome 17 q21 [69].

The receptor was initially identified in breast cancer as a marker of poor prognosis, [70] and trastuzumab was subsequently developed as a successful therapy targeted to inhibit the receptor by preventing its binding to other members of the EGFR family in metastatic breast cancer and in the adjuvant setting [71]. HER2 inhibitors constrain the same pathways discussed in the previous section regarding EGFR, which promote cell growth, survival, proliferation and differentiation, and of which a developing understanding will allow greater definition of the mechanisms of resistance to these therapies [72]. Indeed, whilst no mutations of the HER2 gene have been identified as an absolute indication or contraindication to therapy, as in lung cancer, for example, there may yet prove to be downstream mutations that will aid in the refining of the treatment group [73].

Subsequently, research focused on determining other targets for this therapeutic approach and O-GCs have proven to be a prosperous area. Below, the evidence will be discussed that has sought to determine the role of HER2 in this group of cancers, to determine if the assumptions made in breast cancer with regard to prognosis and treatment remain true in E-GC. Once again, the evidence will be assessed to determine if generalisations can be made across the anatomical regions of the gastro-oesophageal tract as well as across geographical and racially different populations.

The identification of the target is arguably as important as the development of the therapy, and whilst a great deal of work has been done in breast cancer to refine and validate methods of detecting patients suitable for therapy, the evidence will show that whilst many similarities

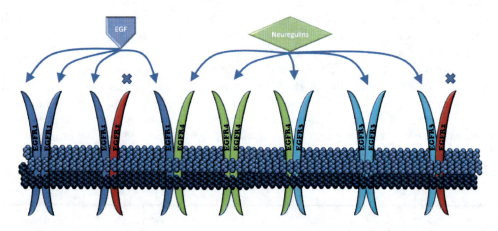

Fig. 8.2 Dimerisation of EGF family receptors in response to the EGF ligand as well as the neuregulin ligands

exist in the utilisation of HER2-targeted therapies in O-GC, there are differences in the detailed application that shall be reviewed.

Identification of HER2 Status

Whilst the incidence of HER2 staining varies across the different areas of the stomach and oesophagus, it currently appears that the accurate determination of HER2 status can be achieved in a manner similar to that used in breast cancer, whereby intensity of IHC staining is scored on a scale of 0 to 3+ (Table 8.1).

Consensus has been reached with regard to scoring of HER2 staining in E-GC and essentially the system of HercepTest, as used in breast cancer, with FISH correlation of indeterminate cases has been adopted for E-GC. In this system, samples that score 3+ on IHC are considered positive, and those that stain 2+ are only positive provided gene amplification is demonstrated. The only modification required for E-GC being that samples with incomplete basolateral membranous staining should also be considered positive should they stain with sufficient intensity because the receptors are frequently lacking on the luminal surface of cells [74]. This system appears to be clinically validated to some degree in gastric cancer with the publication of the ToGA trial, discussed below, which used this scoring system and provides initial evidence that clinical outcomes following treatment with an HER2 inhibitor may correspond to this scoring system and a high concordance has been demonstrated between HER2 expression and gene amplification using this

system [75–77]. However, the evidence is not conclusive as yet, and hopefully further progress will continue to finely tune the distinction between those who will benefit from treatment and those who will not. Other scoring systems in the past have placed greater emphasis on the proportion of the tumour that expresses HER2, and this is a notable omission of the current consensus guidance. This is of particular importance in gastric cancer in which heterogeneity of the HER2 status has been reported in 4.8% of cases, a figure far higher than in breast cancer where there is heterogeneity in 1.4% of cases [74] (Fig. 8.3).

For clinical utility, this heterogeneity can never be fully assessed histologically to determine patient treatment due to the difficulty in sampling the whole disease, but questions persist regarding the efficacy of treatment in patients with less than 10% of the disease over-expressing HER2 even though some concordance has been shown in the clinical features of patient groups when either a 5% or 10% cut-off point has been used [78]. Developments to determine HER2 status through novel imaging techniques remain largely preclinical or in preliminary phase assessment but may provide the extra detail required in the future to determine whether a patient, who may have disease at multiple sites, has a sufficient burden of disease with HER2 over-expression to warrant treatment [79, 80]. In the mean time, tumour heterogeneity poses a difficult problem in these tumour types. Advanced cases do not warrant resection, and so the diagnosis and treatment is guided by biopsy material which is primarily derived endoscopically with no way of

Table 8.1 Consensus IHC scoring for HER2

IHC score	Staining classification
0	Staining in less than 10% of cell membranes
1+	Faint staining in more than 10% of cell membranes or incomplete membrane staining
2+	Weak to moderate complete or basolateral membrane staining in more than 10% of cells
3+	Moderate to intense complete or basolateral membrane staining in more than 10% of cells

A score of 3+ is regarded as positive. 2+ is equivocal, and gene amplification analysis may be important in determining clinical benefit from HER2-targeted therapies in these patients [Adapted from Hofmann M, Stoss O, Shi D, et al. Assessment of a HER2 scoring system for gastric cancer: results from a validation study. *Histopathology.* Jun 2008;52(7):797–805. With permission from John Wiley & Sons, Inc.]

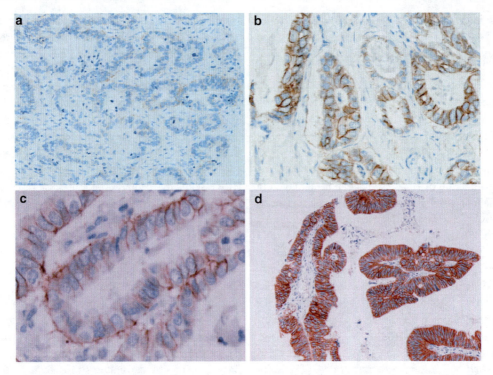

Fig. 8.3 HER2 staining by immunohistochemistry in E-GC cancer. (**a**) IHC 1+. (**b**) IHC 2+. (**c**) Example of basolateral staining in IHC 2+. (**d**) IHC 3+ [Kindly provided by Dr S. Madhusudan, Academic Department of Clinical Oncology, University of Nottingham]

targeting towards areas of positivity. Consensus guidance on HER2 scoring has removed the necessity for 10% staining in biopsy material, but as yet no study has determined how many false-negatives will occur with different biopsy regimens [74]. The heterogeneity in these advanced cases may also occur between the primary and secondary sites, and as such patients will continue to have HER2 primary lesions treated when the main secondary disease burden may be HER2 negative and others undertreated because the HER2-positive disease is only found at secondary sites [77, 81, 82].

Unfortunately, many studies previously have not used standardised scoring techniques, and this does cloud the interpretation of many previous results. It is also difficult to account for differences in tissue handling and the variability seen between commercially available assays which have been demonstrated in the past to be unacceptably high [83], as well as individual variation in scoring by pathologists who historically may or may not have accounted for variable intensity of staining in surrounding normal tissue [84].

As we have seen, there is some variation in the techniques used to identify patients for HER2-targeted treatments. This has been highlighted by a study that compared different thicknesses of section that FISH was performed on and found considerable higher detection was possible in thicker sections [85]. With time, there has been a degree of standardisation, but developments continue to occur. The role of gene amplification in determining the patient population continues to be researched, and until a simple, cheap and reliable method of testing is developed, treatment will be rationed in some quarters to those with IHC 3+ staining [86] who have proven clinical benefit with treatment. Whilst FISH has been used successfully in breast cancer to determine which IHC2+ patients are most likely to benefit, an alternative technology, CISH (chromogenic in situ hybridisation), has been developed that has advantages over FISH in terms of ease of use and longevity of staining for future reference whilst maintaining accurate identification of amplification [87]. This is due to lesser need for specialised fluorescent microscopy and practitioners skilled in its interpretation and does not suffer from fading of the fluorescent signal with time. These benefits importantly lead to cost savings that may yet have an impact on the adoption of amplification screening for equivocal cases, and CISH has already been shown to have a high concordance with FISH results [88, 89].

It is a more common occurrence for HER2 protein expression to be unrelated to gene amplification in GEC than in breast cancer, highlighting the importance for further research to continue to define the therapeutic implications of the possible combinations of HER2 expression [74], especially as amplification appears to be more homogenous in cancer samples than the protein expression [87].

HER2 Expression in Gastric Cancer

The high prevalence of gastric cancer in East Asian countries again ensures that there is a large amount of evidence available regarding the incidence of HER2 expression in this population. Protein expression has been determined to occur in between 8% and 18.6% of cases [26, 88, 90–95], and the correlation of HER2 with intestinal type histology, as opposed to diffuse type, is an almost universal finding throughout the studies [26, 88, 91, 93–95]. However, most studies have not used consensus scoring to determine clinical benefit, and as such the proportion expected to benefit from HER2-receptor-targeted therapy will be lower. One study reported 3+ IHC scores in 6% of patients [88], and gene amplification has been reported in 7.1–7.8% of cases [93, 96], and these figures are a more likely estimate of the proportion of East Asian gastric cancer patients likely to benefit from drugs such as trastuzumab. HER2 expression has often been shown to be present in higher stage disease [26, 90, 92, 93] and at times has correlated with survival on

multivariate analysis [26, 88, 90, 91]. As in breast cancer, only a small proportion of those patients with IHC2+ staining will be demonstrated to have gene amplification, with studies reporting this in 11.1–20% of patients [88, 93].

It seems likely that HER2 expression is similar in European populations with the literature reporting 3+ or similar staining in between 3.4% and 13% of cases [75, 76, 78, 97]. Gene amplification has been reported in 8.2% and 16% of cases [75, 76, 98]. The only study that has found a worse survival in European HER2 gastric cancers appears anomalous due to the exceptionally high incidence of HER2 staining (91%) [99]. However, there is other heterogeneity in survival. The largest European study combined datasets from the UK and Germany, but subgroup analysis found that the German HER2 group tended towards worse survival, whilst the British group tended towards improved prognosis and so overall the results cancelled each other out [78].

These figures, of course, represent the populations that the trials have sampled. Predominantly, these are populations with localised or locally advanced disease in patients that have undergone resection with curative intent. Whilst many have not excluded patients undergoing palliative resection, these studies are inevitably biassed towards earlier stage disease and, since they have demonstrated that HER2 positive disease correlates with increased disease stage, the assumption would be that HER2-positive rates are higher in advanced disease. The ToGA trial, discussed later, treated patients with HER2-positive advanced disease, and an analysis of those screened in recruitment for the trial has been reported as an abstract. This found that in approximately 3,000 advanced gastric cancers from around the globe, 20.9% were either IHC 3+ or FISH positive.

In summary, the expression of HER2 seems comparable between Europe and East Asia, but in spite of a large number of trials, it remains uncertain as to whether HER2-positive gastric cancers represent a subgroup with worse prognosis. The implication of this is that any therapy trialled to target HER2 must expect survival figures which improve upon current expectations using present standard of care treatment.

HER2 in Oesophageal Adenocarcinoma

Few studies have reported results specifically in oesophageal adenocarcinoma but have rather included these cases in mixed analyses with either GOJ or SCCs. However, one study has reported gene amplification in 15% of cases [77], and others report protein expression in 15.3–23% of cases [100, 101], although both have not specifically identified those who might benefit from HER2 inhibitor therapy according to consensus scoring and so the clinically relevant group is presumed to be closer to the lower end of these figures.

Various studies have focused on Barrett's carcinomas specifically, although all are set in primarily Caucasian populations. These have found some degree of IHC staining in 9.8–26% of cases [85, 102, 103], and gene amplification has been reported in 10.5–19% of cases [85, 104]. Two of these studies have reported worse survival in HER2-positive patients [102, 104].

Overall, it is difficult to determine if the Barrett's carcinoma subgroup of oesophageal adenocarcinomas has a different pattern of HER2 expression, with approximately 15% of these cases having clinically relevant expression levels.

HER2 in Oesophageal SCC

There is a great deal of heterogeneity in reported incidence of HER2 expression in SCC with very low incidence reported in a number of studies. Even though an early study found some degree of protein expression present in 26% of cases [101], three other European studies have since reported expression or amplification in between 2.8% and 5% when scoring using, what has been determined to be, more clinically relevant systems [38, 77, 100]. A subsequent Swedish study found 13% of SCC cases to intensely stain for HER2 but less than a third of IHC 3+ cases in this mixed study of adeno- and squamous carcinoma were found to have corresponding gene amplification [105].

East Asian populations have returned more mixed results with one study finding 13.6% of patients to be IHC 2/3+ and clinically relevant gene amplification in a total of 9% [106], but other studies reported 2+/3+ staining in 7.7–9% of cases [35, 107] which is an overestimate of the treatable population as demonstrated by one of the studies that found no cases of 3+ staining and only 2% gene amplification due to infrequent amplification in IHC2+ disease [35], whilst a single South American study found cases to be IHC 3+ 6% of the time [108].

When patients with locally advanced disease were biopsied prior to chemoradiotherapy, it was found that within those who proved to be resistant to oncological treatment, there was a high proportion of HER2-positive cases (71.4%) [109]. However, this study reports a total of 55.9% IHC 2/3+ staining, and no survival difference was noted due to HER2 status even though the treatment resistant group overall had lower survival than the sensitive group. Although this is an unexpectedly high incidence of HER2 staining, the relationship to resistance to therapy is mirrored by another study that found high HER2 mRNA expression correlated with resistance to chemoradiotherapy in a study group containing more than 60% SCCs [110].

Whilst there may be few cases of SCC that express HER2 to a sufficient degree to warrant targeted treatment, it may be that these patients do still benefit from such therapy. The expense of screening for HER2 in SCCs for so few cases may be prohibitive at times, but if this group of patients proves to be resistant to conventional therapy, then the cost to benefit ratio is improved.

HER2 Expression in GOJ Cancers

In an analysis of patients with advanced disease screened during recruitment to the ToGA trial, the incidence of HER2 expression was considerably higher in GOJ tumours than the gastric cancers that were assessed, with IHC- or FISH-positive results in 33.2% of cases [111]. As mentioned previously, the high rates reported partly reflect the advanced stage of the disease in this patient group, but other trials that have included GOJ tumours in mixed populations of gastro-oesophageal cancers have also reported high expression of HER2 at 23–28% [81, 98, 101, 112].

The high expression of HER2 in GOJ cancers appears to be the primary reason for regional variations in HER2 expression with countries that have a higher proportion of GOJ cancers, compared to gastric or oesophageal cancers, having the highest frequency of HER2-positive expression [113].

HER2 Inhibitors in Gastric and Junctional Cancers

The advent of a successful phase III trial of trastuzumab in advanced gastric and GOJ cancers has demonstrated that targeted therapies may have a role in the treatment of O-GC, but at present, it remains the only targeted drug to come into mainstream usage. The results of the ToGA trial [114] that has prompted this will be discussed in detail below, but the future role for other drugs still in development as well as the expanding role of trastuzumab will also be reviewed.

The ToGA trial randomised 584 patients with either advanced gastric (approx. 80%) or GOJ (approx. 20%) cancer from centres across Europe, Asia, Central and South America to Cisplatin and 5-Fluorouracil either with or without trastuzumab. All patients were either FISH positive or IHC3+ in either arm of the study with no option for crossover. Both arms were demographically comparable, and HER2 status was determined in line with consensus guidance. Median follow-up was approximately 18 months with the study powered to detect an increase in overall survival of 3 months. The primary outcome was reached with median survival in the treatment arm of 13.8 months compared to 11.1 months in the control arm ($p = 0.0046$). Overall response rate was 47% with a further 32% maintaining stable disease and 12% suffering progressive disease. Interestingly, those patients included due to FISH positivity that did not have IHC 3+ protein expression appeared to gain less benefit from the treatment. Previously, it has been shown that

mRNA levels correlated strongly with gene amplification [115], and as such there may be post-transcriptional regulation that is of great importance in determining protein expression. In patients with IHC2+/FISH+ disease, the confidence interval of the hazard ratio was 0.51–1.11 showing evidence of a possible benefit in this group, although further research will be required in the future to determine the optimal treatment regimes in equivocal cases. Overall, no difference was noted in adverse effects, although the treatment arm particularly had higher frequencies of diarrhoea, stomatitis and fatigue. Cardiac events were rare with a total of 5% of the trastuzumab group suffering >10% decrease in LVEF (left ventricular ejection fraction) to a value <50%, compared to 1% in the control arm. Only approximately 20% of cases were GOJ tumours, and, as such, the hazard ratio for this subgroup does not demonstrate benefit as unequivocally as the gastric tumours with a confidence interval of 0.42–1.08, but with this strong suggestion of benefit in the biologically different GOJ tumours, it must be hoped that oesophageal squamous and adenocarcinomas that similarly express HER2 could also prove to be usefully targeted by trastuzumab.

Currently, no evidence exists for the use of trastuzumab in an adjuvant or neoadjuvant setting in the treatment of early stage disease.

There are several phase II trials in progress for lapatinib (HER2/EGFRi) and also a phase III trial (LOGIC) which will again target patients with advanced disease anywhere in the gastro-oesophageal tract for treatment provided they are shown to be HER2 positive. Although the drug is a dual inhibitor, it appears in preclinical testing that the drug is primarily active in HER2-positive cells [116, 117].

HER2 Inhibitors in Oesophageal Cancers

A phase II trial of cisplatin and paclitaxel in combination with radiation and trastuzumab selected only HER2 2+- and 3+-positive patients with distal oesophageal adenocarcinoma for treatment.

The study only consisted of 19 patients, but more than 70% of these had coeliac, portal, cervical or retroperitoneal lymphadenopathy. As such, the group was weighted towards patients who had advanced disease that might become resectable following down-staging therapy. In HER2 3+ patients, there was a 57% complete response rate, and in the HER2 2+ group, five patients were included who were FISH negative, one of which had a complete response to chemoradiotherapy. Six patients underwent surgical exploration following what was assessed to be complete response, but two of these were found to have metastatic disease, which presumably remained either because it fell outside the radiation field or because it did not respond to the various chemotherapies as well as the primary disease. However, the residual disease in all cases was not assessed further for biomarkers of response. Median survival for the whole group was 24 months, but the cohort was not powered to demonstrate differences between subgroups [118].

No reported trials have yet included squamous cell cancers within their cohorts; however, evidence is building that there is clinically relevant expression of targets to a greater or lesser extent throughout the gastro-oesophageal tract and that response to trastuzumab can be predicted using standardised scoring systems similar to that reported in breast cancer. Research continues to define the precise role for trastuzumab, and, following the same path as breast cancer before it, the development of second generation inhibitors and dual inhibitors will hopefully add to this progress.

VEGF

The ability of cancers to facilitate neoangiogenesis has long been understood to be vital in the progression of tumours beyond a given size [119] and has subsequently been termed a 'hallmark of cancer' [120]. As such, it provides an enticing biotarget that could be taken advantage of in all solid tumour types, and indeed, clinical efficacy of inhibitors have been subsequently demonstrated in a wide variety of tumour types including lung, colon and breast amongst others.

Table 8.2 Dimerisation occurs during binding between members of the VEGF family and the receptors shown were indicated by an 'X'

	Growth factor				
Receptor	VEGF-A	VEGF-B	VEGF-C	VEGF-D	PIGF
VEGFR1	X	X			X
VEGFR2	X		X		
VEGFR3			X	X	
NP1 and 2	X				

Based on data from Refs. [123, 130–134]

However, the gains in terms of overall survival have often been limited, and with the toxicity that has been attributed to these agents, their utility in clinical practice remains a topic of debate. This section will seek to briefly outline the role of this growth factor in carcinogenesis in oesophagogastric cancer and will then explore the developing role of its inhibition in the treatment of this disease. Whilst these agents have not yet demonstrated the efficacy required to put them into wide spread clinical use, there has been some encouraging initial trial data, with the results of a number of phase III trials pending. Should ongoing clinical trials successfully identify biomarkers of response and non-response to these agents, they may yet have an important role to play in personalised therapy.

There are a number of VEGF subclasses including VEGF-A, VEGF-B, VEGF-C and VEGF-D, as well as other members of the PDGF superfamily such as PIGF (placental growth factor), and these are functionally and structurally related [121–123]. VEGF-E and VEGF-F have also been identified encoded in orf virus or as a component of snake venom [124]. These subclasses also may individually exist in a number of different isoforms [125, 126]. The growth factors themselves consist of glycoproteins of approximately 45 kDa molecular weight, dependent upon the specific isoform, and these interact with the receptors VEGFR-1, VEGFR-2 and VEGFR-3. VEGF-A may also act as a ligand for the neuropilins NP-1 and NP-2 which behave as co-receptors to enhance the binding of VEGFR [127–129]. The specificity of the individual growth factors with the ligands is detailed on Table 8.2.

The receptors are primarily expressed on vascular endothelium, with the exception of

VEGFR-3 which is found in lymphatic vessels following their development from a common embryological source [135], and they are also present on a number of haemopoietic cells. Activation of these receptors produces a variety of biological effects, through the initiation of cellular transduction pathways including Raf-MEK-MAP-kinases, PI3K-AKT and TSAb-Src pathways [136, 137].

These contribute towards angiogenesis through processes including alteration of vascular permeability and vasodilatation, and increasing endothelial cell proliferation and migration [138]. However, these are equally relevant in the development of side effects due to its inhibition. The molecule of primary importance in clinical practice is the VEGF-A class, which is generally referred to simply as VEGF, and this text will continue in this manner from here onwards. The interaction of prime importance that VEGF will perform is with the VEGFR-2 tyrosine kinase, and this will contribute to vasodilation as well as the proliferation and migration of vascular endothelial cells. The vasodilatory effects also create hyperpermeability of capillaries which in turn allows the extravasation of plasma proteins which can subsequently create extracellular matrix for the proliferating endothelial cells [139].

VEGF levels are found to be elevated in cancer patients due to release from a variety of sources including the tumour cells and surrounding stroma [140], although skeletal muscle and platelets represent the major reservoir of VEGF in the body [141]. The promotion of VEGF expression can occur in a wide variety of ways including the stimulation of cells via other cytokines, such as HGF or TGFβ, or due to the hypoxic tumour micro-environment [137, 142, 143]. The presence of increasing levels of VEGF in the serum has been correlated with worse survival and increasing stage of disease in gastric cancer [144–146] and has been shown to decrease following curative surgical intervention after a short-term rise in VEGF levels secondary to surgical trauma [147]. In oesophageal SCC, high VEGF was associated with increasing stage and decreased response to subsequent chemoradiotherapy and worse survival [148, 149]. Similarly, tissue sections from gastric cancer

have been found to have VEGF present when stained immunohistochemically, and these positive patients also had a worse overall survival and were more likely to have metastatic disease [150]. Also, receptors for VEGF are found in stromal vessels in between 42% and 87% of gastric cancer cases (dependent on the specific receptor stained for using IHC), and these cases also had poor survival [151].

The side effects of VEGF inhibitor therapies particularly related to the mode of action are thromboembolic events, hypertension, gastrointestinal bleeding and perforation and problems with wound healing. Although no evidence exists within the field of gastro-oesophageal surgery, the evidence from colorectal cancer trials provides a model for abdominal surgery that can be usefully extrapolated with due caution. It has been suggested that surgeons should aim to delay surgery by 6–8 weeks following the completion of bevacizumab therapy used in the neoadjuvant setting for colorectal cancer due to poor wound healing and liver regeneration demonstrated in in vivo models, although the more rapid elimination of tyrosine kinase inhibitors might allow surgery after just 1 week [152]. However, in the emergency surgical setting, following incidental or complications related to chemotherapy, the delayed wound healing remains an unavoidable issue with this type of therapy.

Two large studies have reported that complications in regard to wound healing were encountered in 1.7–5% of patients who received treatment at a variety of time points following surgery, and this was significantly increased in the study that randomised to chemotherapy with or without bevacizumab [153, 154].

VEGF Inhibitors

Inhibition of vascular endothelial growth factor in order to suppress angiogenesis has been known to be an effective way of inhibiting tumour growth in vivo for some time [155], and this has led to the development of a variety of inhibitors including monoclonal antibodies and tyrosine kinase inhibitors. Specifically, bevacizumab (a monoclonal antibody to VEGF) and sorafenib and sunitinib (small molecule VEGF-R inhibitors also inhibiting PDGFR) have been carried forward into some degree of clinical usage in gastro-oesophageal cancer types, although a number of other related agents will surely follow, especially if biomarkers of response to these drugs can improve their efficacy by more accurately identifying patients who might benefit from them. The integral role of angiogenesis in tumour development provides some rational to the non-targeted use of these drugs, but with many clinical trials failing to show sufficient benefit improvements in the tailoring appears to be vital if they are to move in to widespread clinical usage. A variety of markers of response have indeed been demonstrated but clinical validation is yet to be completed and incorporated into successful phase III trials [156].

Sorafenib has been used in a single phase II trial in combination with docetaxel and cisplatin for 44 patients with advanced or metastatic gastric or GOJ adenocarcinomas. This study found that 41% of patients experienced a partial response to the combination and overall survival was 13.6 months, although 64% experienced grade 3 or 4 neutropaenia and there were also 3 cases of grade 3 or 4 thrombotic complications and 1 rectal perforation [157]. With regard to efficacy, these results may be demonstrating some benefit with this treatment especially considering that approximately 3 quarters of the participants had GOJ tumours that carry a worse prognosis compared to distal gastric cancers; however at present, the drug remains in phase II trials with different combination regimes in gastric and oesophageal cancer [158–160].

Two phase II trials of sunitinib have recently been reported. When used in the second-line setting in gastric cancer, only 2.6% of patients demonstrated a response, although 32% maintained stable disease, and overall survival was 6.8 months. The main toxicities reported were grade 3 or 4 thrombocytopenia or neutropenia, which both occurred in approximately a third of patients [161]. As such, it shows no advantage over existing treatments in this setting, but it is yet to be determined if the different mode of action means that it may be of use in a combination

therapy regime. Another study of 51 patients who had exhausted various treatment options reported an overall survival approaching 6 months at an international meeting. The cohort included GOJ cancers which may account for the lower survival in spite of the consistent 32% disease control rate [162].

At present, no evidence exists for the use of sunitinib or sorafenib in advanced oesophageal cancers besides the few GOJ cancer patients included in other trials, although recruitment of patients to phase II trials in an adjuvant setting is ongoing [163–165] and if they can demonstrate a reduced side effect profile and more rapid clearance, these may yet have advantages over bevacizumab.

Bevacizumab is a humanised murine IgG1 antibody that binds to VEFG-A receptor to inhibit its function. This drug has reached later stages in development in a number of cancer types leading to its approval for use in some of these, albeit not without controversy following the FDA approval for use in breast cancer and subsequent withdrawal of this indication for the drug. Most phase II evidence regarding bevacizumab was produced through the study of gastric and GOJ tumours, with oesophageal cancers almost completely excluded. The drug was assessed in combination with a variety of other conventional agents with response rates of between 42% and 67% and reporting survival of 11.1–16.8 months, although there were also perforation rates of 2–8% and thromboembolic events in 25.5–39% [166–168].

Phase III evidence continues to be collected by a number of trial groups, but the AVAGAST trial has reported initial findings with final publication including pre-planned analysis of samples collected during the trial still awaited. The trial randomised 774 patients to a cisplatin/capecitabine combination with or without bevacizumab and found a median survival of 12.1 months in the treatment arm compared to 10.1 months in the placebo group which was not statistically significant. Progression-free survival was significantly increased with bevacizumab from 29.5 to 38 months, and the incidence of perforation and thromboembolism was actually lower in the treatment group, although the overall incidence of grade 3–5 complications was 6.2% with treatment compared to 0.5% without; wound problems being particularly prevalent in the bevacizumab arm (2.3% versus 0.3%). Although this does not provide evidence to support the use of this drug in this setting at present, the sample analysis may yet help to determine some means of targeting the treatment to those more likely to benefit, and to this end, the authors report that they have noticed that East Asian patients appear to have gained less benefit compared to the European and American groups. With nearly 50% of patients recruited from East Asian countries, it will be important to determine the reason for this difference in order to design more effective future trials [169].

In summary, VEGF inhibitor therapy has not been as successful as other targeted therapies during its introduction into clinical practice due to the greater evidence of side effects and the lack of validated biomarkers that can be used to target the drugs towards those most likely to benefit, and it is the development of these that may well determine their ongoing use outside the clinical trial setting.

EpCAM

EpCAM is a 40-kDa protein derived from the GA733-2 gene which acts as a cell adhesion molecule [170]. As such, it is present on various tissues in both health and disease; however, variations in its exposure allow it to be utilised as a biotarget with limited toxicity to normal epithelium because the intact basement membrane of normal tissue prevents binding of targeted drugs such as monoclonal antibodies and if used in the setting of a malignant effusion, as with catumaxomab discussed below, the mesothelial lining of the peritoneum is protective because this does not express EpCAM. In contrast, EpCAM is expected to be accessible for binding in solid tumours with antibodies passing through the increasingly permeable tumour capillaries or in body fluids such as ascites or pleural effusions.

Expression of EpCAM has been reported in a high proportion of cases of E-GC, although the precise number has varied widely from 34.3% to 100% [171–173]. This may be due to variation in reporting of staining intensity on immunohistochemistry, but one study has reported that intense staining was found in 41% of cases of oesophageal SCC [174]. In malignant effusions, expression of EpCAM may fall in the upper end of this range being found in 66.2–100% of cases from a variety of cancers associated with ascites [175–177].

With regard to prognosis, there is conflicting evidence in SCC that EpCAM-positive patients carry a prognosis different to negative groups [174, 178].

Monoclonal Antibodies to EpCAM

Catumaxomab is a trifunctional monoclonal antibody with two antigen-binding sites and a functional Fc domain, which will bind to EpCAM on the epithelial tumour cells. In addition, it binds to T-cells via CD3 and also activates Fc gamma-receptor I-, IIa- and III-positive accessory cells via its functional Fc domain [179].

Other monoclonal antibodies to EpCAM have been trialled in the past but failed to show efficacy in the adjuvant treatment of colon cancer [180].

However, the use of tri-functional EpCAM-targeted agents delivered directly to the intraperitoneal space in disseminated intra-abdominal malignancy may improve efficacy by providing localised treatment of EpCAM-positive tumour cells in the peritoneal cavity as well as having increased efficacy due to tri-functional binding. Disseminated intra-abdominal malignancy may cause malignant ascites, and one goal of treatment in this setting is to palliate the ascites, aside from improving survival.

Catumaxomab has been studied in phase I/II trials in patients with peritoneal carcinomatosis secondary to GI malignancy (mainly gastric and colonic). There was evidence of efficacy in a matched pair, case control analysis [181], and the drug continues in randomised phase III multicentre trials to further define the optimal treatment strategy for the drug and is due to commence recruitment of patients with peritoneal carcinomatosis secondary to gastric cancer in the second half of 2011.

Currently, a single phase II/III study has been published which recruited 258 patients, half of which had ovarian cancer and half of which had other cancers. In the non-ovarian group, approximately 50% had ascites secondary to gastric cancer. Ovarian and non-ovarian groups were analysed separately due to the different prognosis and treatment options in ovarian cancer.

Patients were randomised 2 to 1 to paracentesis with or without catumaxomab intraperitoneal infusion, and puncture-free survival in the non-ovarian patients was 37 days in the treatment arm compared to 14 in the control group; however, this was most marked in the gastric cancer patients in whom the puncture-free survival increased from 15 to 118 days and overall survival was also significantly increased from 44 to 71 days with treatment [179].

Phase II studies in operable gastric cancer have completed recruitment though publication is pending following a sufficient follow-up period [182].

In summary, catumaxomab is a monoclonal antibody to EpCAM, which is over-expressed on the majority of gastric cancers including oesophageal cancer. Although no evidence exists in oesophageal cancer at present, early results in advanced gastric cancer are encouraging though further studies are required, and at present the indications are limited to the specific disease setting of malignant ascites.

References

1. Parkin DM, Bray F, Ferlay J, Pisani P. Global cancer statistics, 2002. CA Cancer J Clin. 2005;55(2):74–108.
2. Devesa SS, Blot WJ, Fraumeni Jr JF. Changing patterns in the incidence of esophageal and gastric carcinoma in the United States. Cancer. 1998;83(10):2049–53.
3. Pohl H, Welch HG. The role of overdiagnosis and reclassification in the marked increase of esophageal adenocarcinoma incidence. J Natl Cancer Inst. 2005;97(2):142–6.
4. Jeon J, Luebeck EG, Moolgavkar SH. Age effects and temporal trends in adenocarcinoma of the esophagus and gastric cardia (United States). Cancer Causes Control. 2006;17(7):971–81.

5. Romano M, Ricci V, Zarrilli R. Mechanisms of disease: Helicobacter pylori-related gastric carcinogenesis–implications for chemoprevention. Nat Clin Pract Gastroenterol Hepatol. 2006;3(11):622–32.
6. Islami F, Kamangar F. Helicobacter pylori and esophageal cancer risk: a meta-analysis. Cancer Prev Res (Phila). 2008;1(5):329–38.
7. Malfertheiner P, Megraud F, O'Morain C, et al. Current concepts in the management of Helicobacter pylori infection: the Maastricht III Consensus Report. Gut. 2007;56(6):772–81.
8. Lao-Sirieix P, Caldas C, Fitzgerald RC. Genetic predisposition to gastro-oesophageal cancer. Curr Opin Genet Dev. 2010;20(3):210–7.
9. Cameron AJ, Lagergren J, Henriksson C, Nyren O, Locke 3rd GR, Pedersen NL. Gastroesophageal reflux disease in monozygotic and dizygotic twins. Gastroenterology. 2002;122(1):55–9.
10. Mohammed I, Cherkas LF, Riley SA, Spector TD, Trudgill NJ. Genetic influences in gastro-oesophageal reflux disease: a twin study. Gut. 2003;52(8):1085–9.
11. Wu AH, Wan P, Bernstein L. A multiethnic population-based study of smoking, alcohol and body size and risk of adenocarcinomas of the stomach and esophagus (United States). Cancer Causes Control. 2001;12(8):721–32.
12. Playford RJ. New British Society of Gastroenterology (BSG) guidelines for the diagnosis and management of Barrett's oesophagus. Gut. 2006;55(4):442.
13. Kelty CJ, Gough MD, Van Wyk Q, Stephenson TJ, Ackroyd R. Barrett's oesophagus: intestinal metaplasia is not essential for cancer risk. Scand J Gastroenterol. 2007;42(11):1271–4.
14. Siewert JR, Stein HJ. Classification of adenocarcinoma of the oesophagogastric junction. Br J Surg. 1998;85(11):1457–9.
15. Buskens CJ, Van Rees BP, Sivula A, et al. Prognostic significance of elevated cyclooxygenase 2 expression in patients with adenocarcinoma of the esophagus. Gastroenterology. 2002;122(7):1800–7.
16. Buskens CJ, Sivula A, van Rees BP, et al. Comparison of cyclooxygenase 2 expression in adenocarcinomas of the gastric cardia and distal oesophagus. Gut. 2003;52(12):1678–83.
17. Isinger-Ekstrand A, Johansson J, Ohlsson M, et al. Genetic profiles of gastroesophageal cancer: combined analysis using expression array and tiling array–comparative genomic hybridization. Cancer Genet Cytogenet. 2010;200(2):120–6.
18. Mendelsohn J, Baselga J. Status of epidermal growth factor receptor antagonists in the biology and treatment of cancer. J Clin Oncol. 2003;21(14):2787–99.
19. Shaw RJ, Cantley LC. Ras, PI(3)K and mTOR signalling controls tumour cell growth. Nature. 2006;441(7092):424–30.
20. Yarden Y, Sliwkowski MX. Untangling the ErbB signalling network. Nat Rev Mol Cell Biol. 2001;2(2):127–37.
21. Hackel PO, Zwick E, Prenzel N, Ullrich A. Epidermal growth factor receptors: critical mediators of

multiple receptor pathways. Curr Opin Cell Biol. 1999;11(2):184–9.

22. Oda K, Matsuoka Y, Funahashi A, Kitano H. A comprehensive pathway map of epidermal growth factor receptor signaling. Mol Syst Biol. 2005;1:2005.0010.

23. Wang Y, Minoshima S, Shimizu N. Precise mapping of the EGF receptor gene on the human chromosome 7p12 using an improved fish technique. Jpn J Hum Genet. 1993;38(4):399–406.

24. Rizzo S, Bronte G, Fanale D, et al. Prognostic vs predictive molecular biomarkers in colorectal cancer: is KRAS and BRAF wild type status required for anti-EGFR therapy? Cancer Treat Rev. 2010;36 Suppl 3:S56–61.

25. Koutras AK, Fountzilas G, Kalogeras KT, Starakis I, Iconomou G, Kalofonos HP. The upgraded role of HER3 and HER4 receptors in breast cancer. Crit Rev Oncol Hematol. 2010;74(2):73–8.

26. Zhang XL, Yang YS, Xu DP, et al. Comparative study on overexpression of HER2/neu and HER3 in gastric cancer. World J Surg. 2009;33(10):2112–8.

27. Hanna W. Testing for HER2 status. Oncology. 2001;61 Suppl 2:22–30.

28. Cappuzzo F, Ciuleanu T, Stelmakh L, et al. Erlotinib as maintenance treatment in advanced non-small-cell lung cancer: a multicentre, randomised, placebo-controlled phase 3 study. Lancet Oncol. 2010;11(6):521–9.

29. Sholl LM, Xiao Y, Joshi V, et al. EGFR mutation is a better predictor of response to tyrosine kinase inhibitors in non-small cell lung carcinoma than FISH, CISH, and immunohistochemistry. Am J Clin Pathol. 2010;133(6):922–34.

30. Cappuzzo F, Hirsch FR, Rossi E, et al. Epidermal growth factor receptor gene and protein and gefitinib sensitivity in non-small-cell lung cancer. J Natl Cancer Inst. 2005;97(9):643–55.

31. Hirsch FR, Varella-Garcia M, McCoy J, et al. Increased epidermal growth factor receptor gene copy number detected by fluorescence in situ hybridization associates with increased sensitivity to gefitinib in patients with bronchioloalveolar carcinoma subtypes: a Southwest Oncology Group Study. J Clin Oncol. 2005;23(28):6838–45.

32. Itakura Y, Sasano H, Shiga C, et al. Epidermal growth factor receptor overexpression in esophageal carcinoma. An immunohistochemical study correlated with clinicopathologic findings and DNA amplification. Cancer. 1994;74(3):795–804.

33. Hanawa M, Suzuki S, Dobashi Y, et al. EGFR protein overexpression and gene amplification in squamous cell carcinomas of the esophagus. Int J Cancer. 2006;118(5):1173–80.

34. Gotoh M, Takiuchi H, Kawabe S, et al. Epidermal growth factor receptor is a possible predictor of sensitivity to chemoradiotherapy in the primary lesion of esophageal squamous cell carcinoma. Jpn J Clin Oncol. 2007;37(9):652–7.

35. Sunpaweravong P, Sunpaweravong S, Puttawibul P, et al. Epidermal growth factor receptor and cyclin D1 are independently amplified and overexpressed in esophageal squamous cell carcinoma. J Cancer Res Clin Oncol. 2005;131(2):111–9.

36. Zhang G, Zhang Q, Yin L, et al. Expression of nucleostemin, epidermal growth factor and epidermal growth factor receptor in human esophageal squamous cell carcinoma tissues. J Cancer Res Clin Oncol. 2010;136(4):587–94.

37. Kitagawa Y, Ueda M, Ando N, Ozawa S, Shimizu N, Kitajima M. Further evidence for prognostic significance of epidermal growth factor receptor gene amplification in patients with esophageal squamous cell carcinoma. Clin Cancer Res. 1996;2(5):909–14.

38. Gibault L, Metges JP, Conan-Charlet V, et al. Diffuse EGFR staining is associated with reduced overall survival in locally advanced oesophageal squamous cell cancer. Br J Cancer. 2005;93(1):107–15.

39. Boone J, van Hillegersberg R, Offerhaus GJ, van Diest PJ, Borel Rinkes IH, Ten Kate FJ. Targets for molecular therapy in esophageal squamous cell carcinoma: an immunohistochemical analysis. Dis Esophagus. 2009;22(6):496–504.

40. Sarbia M, Ott N, Puhringer-Oppermann F, Brucher BL. The predictive value of molecular markers (p53, EGFR, ATM, CHK2) in multimodally treated squamous cell carcinoma of the oesophagus. Br J Cancer. 2007;97(10):1404–8.

41. Hickey K, Grehan D, Reid IM, O'Briain S, Walsh TN, Hennessy TP. Expression of epidermal growth factor receptor and proliferating cell nuclear antigen predicts response of esophageal squamous cell carcinoma to chemoradiotherapy. Cancer. 1994;74(6):1693–8.

42. Wang KL, Wu TT, Choi IS, et al. Expression of epidermal growth factor receptor in esophageal and esophagogastric junction adenocarcinomas: association with poor outcome. Cancer. 2007;109(4):658–67.

43. Langer R, Von Rahden BH, Nahrig J, et al. Prognostic significance of expression patterns of c-erbB-2, p53, p16INK4A, p27KIP1, cyclin D1 and epidermal growth factor receptor in oesophageal adenocarcinoma: a tissue microarray study. J Clin Pathol. 2006;59(6):631–4.

44. Wilkinson NW, Black JD, Roukhadze E, et al. Epidermal growth factor receptor expression correlates with histologic grade in resected esophageal adenocarcinoma. J Gastrointest Surg. 2004;8(4):448–53.

45. van Dekken H, Hop WC, Tilanus HW, et al. Immunohistochemical evaluation of a panel of tumor cell markers during malignant progression in Barrett esophagus. Am J Clin Pathol. 2008;130(5):745–53.

46. Miller CT, Moy JR, Lin L, et al. Gene amplification in esophageal adenocarcinomas and Barrett's with high-grade dysplasia. Clin Cancer Res. 2003;9(13):4819–25.

47. Kwak EL, Jankowski J, Thayer SP, et al. Epidermal growth factor receptor kinase domain mutations in esophageal and pancreatic adenocarcinomas. Clin Cancer Res. 2006;12(14 Pt 1):4283–7.

48. Takehana T, Kunitomo K, Suzuki S, et al. Expression of epidermal growth factor receptor in gastric carcinomas. Clin Gastroenterol Hepatol. 2003;1(6): 438–45.

49. Kim MA, Lee HS, Lee HE, Jeon YK, Yang HK, Kim WH. EGFR in gastric carcinomas: prognostic significance of protein overexpression and high gene copy number. Histopathology. 2008;52(6):738–46.

50. Lee SA, Choi SR, Jang JS, et al. Expression of VEGF, EGFR, and IL-6 in gastric adenomas and adenocarcinomas by endoscopic submucosal dissection. Dig Dis Sci. 2010;55(7):1955–63.

51. Han SW, Oh DY, Im SA, et al. Phase II study and biomarker analysis of cetuximab combined with modified FOLFOX6 in advanced gastric cancer. Br J Cancer. 2009;100(2):298–304.

52. Mimori K, Nagahara H, Sudo T, et al. The epidermal growth factor receptor gene sequence is highly conserved in primary gastric cancers. J Surg Oncol. 2006;93(1):44–6.

53. Lieto E, Ferraraccio F, Orditura M, et al. Expression of vascular endothelial growth factor (VEGF) and epidermal growth factor receptor (EGFR) is an independent prognostic indicator of worse outcome in gastric cancer patients. Ann Surg Oncol. 2008; 15(1):69–79.

54. Bamias A, Karina M, Papakostas P, et al. A randomized phase III study of adjuvant platinum/docetaxel chemotherapy with or without radiation therapy in patients with gastric cancer. Cancer Chemother Pharmacol. 2010;65(6):1009–21.

55. Gamboa-Dominguez A, Dominguez-Fonseca C, Quintanilla-Martinez L, et al. Epidermal growth factor receptor expression correlates with poor survival in gastric adenocarcinoma from Mexican patients: a multivariate analysis using a standardized immunohistochemical detection system. Mod Pathol. 2004; 17(5):579–87.

56. Ferry DR, Anderson M, Beddard K, et al. A phase II study of gefitinib monotherapy in advanced esophageal adenocarcinoma: evidence of gene expression, cellular, and clinical response. Clin Cancer Res. 2007;13(19):5869–75.

57. Adelstein DJ, Rybicki LA, Carroll MA, Rice TW, Mekhail T. Phase II trial of gefitinib for recurrent or metastatic esophageal or gastroesophageal junction (GOJ) cancer. J Clin Oncol. 2005;23((16S)):4054.

58. Janmaat ML, Gallegos-Ruiz MI, Rodriguez JA, et al. Predictive factors for outcome in a phase II study of gefitinib in second-line treatment of advanced esophageal cancer patients. J Clin Oncol. 2006;24(10): 1612–9.

59. Dragovich T, McCoy S, Fenoglio-Preiser CM, et al. Phase II trial of erlotinib in gastroesophageal junction and gastric adenocarcinomas: SWOG 0127. J Clin Oncol. 2006;24(30):4922–7.

60. Lorenzen S, Schuster T, Porschen R, et al. Cetuximab plus cisplatin-5-fluorouracil versus cisplatin-5-fluorouracil alone in first-line metastatic squamous cell carcinoma of the esophagus: a randomized phase II study of the Arbeitsgemeinschaft Internistische Onkologie. Ann Oncol. 2009;20(10):1667–73.

61. Pinto C, Di Fabio F, Siena S, et al. Phase II study of cetuximab in combination with FOLFIRI in patients with untreated advanced gastric or gastroesophageal junction adenocarcinoma (FOLCETUX study). Ann Oncol. 2007;18(3):510–7.

62. Kim BG, Oh SY, Kwon HC, et al. A phase II study of irinotecan with biweekly, low dose leucovorin and bolus and continuous infusion 5-fluorouracil (modified FOLFIRI) as first line therapy for patients with recurrent or metastatic gastric cancer. Am J Clin Oncol. 2010;33(3):246–50.

63. Kim JA, Lee J, Han B, et al. Docetaxel/cisplatin followed by FOLFIRI versus the reverse sequence in metastatic gastric cancer. Cancer Chemother Pharmacol. 2011;68(1):177–84.

64. Kim SH, Lee GW, Go SI, et al. A phase II study of irinotecan, continuous 5-fluorouracil, and leucovorin (FOLFIRI) combination chemotherapy for patients with recurrent or metastatic gastric cancer previously treated with a fluoropyrimidine-based regimen. Am J Clin Oncol. 2010;33(6):572–6.

65. Li Q, Chen J, Zhao X, et al. A pilot study of irinotecan combined with 5-fluorouracil and leucovorin for the treatment of Chinese patients with locally advanced and metastatic gastric cancer. Tumori. 2009;95(4):432–7.

66. Pinto C, Di Fabio F, Barone C, et al. Phase II study of cetuximab in combination with cisplatin and docetaxel in patients with untreated advanced gastric or gastro-oesophageal junction adenocarcinoma (DOCETUX study). Br J Cancer. 2009;101(8): 1261–8.

67. Okines AF, Ashley SE, Cunningham D, et al. Epirubicin, oxaliplatin, and capecitabine with or without panitumumab for advanced esophagogastric cancer: dose-finding study for the prospective multicenter, randomized, phase II/III REAL-3 trial. J Clin Oncol. 2010;28(25):3945–50.

68. Barros FF, Powe DG, Ellis IO, Green AR. Understanding the HER family in breast cancer: interaction with ligands, dimerization and treatments. Histopathology. 2010;56(5):560–72.

69. Coussens L, Yang-Feng TL, Liao YC, et al. Tyrosine kinase receptor with extensive homology to EGF receptor shares chromosomal location with neu oncogene. Science. 1985;230(4730):1132–9.

70. Gusterson BA, Gelber RD, Goldhirsch A, et al. Prognostic importance of c-erbB-2 expression in breast cancer. International (Ludwig) Breast Cancer Study Group. J Clin Oncol. 1992;10(7):1049–56.

71. Piccart-Gebhart MJ, Procter M, Leyland-Jones B, et al. trastuzumab after adjuvant chemotherapy in HER2-positive breast cancer. N Engl J Med. 2005;353(16):1659–72.

72. Nahta R, Yu D, Hung MC, Hortobagyi GN, Esteva FJ. Mechanisms of disease: understanding resistance to HER2-targeted therapy in human breast cancer. Nat Clin Pract Oncol. 2006;3(5):269–80.

73. Dave B, Migliaccio I, Gutierrez MC, et al. Loss of phosphatase and tensin homolog or phosphoinositol-3 kinase activation and response to trastuzumab or lapatinib in human epidermal growth factor receptor 2-overexpressing locally advanced breast cancers. J Clin Oncol. 2011;29(2):166–73.

74. Hofmann M, Stoss O, Shi D, et al. Assessment of a HER2 scoring system for gastric cancer: results from a validation study. Histopathology. 2008;52(7):797–805.

75. Marx AH, Tharun L, Muth J, et al. HER-2 amplification is highly homogenous in gastric cancer. Hum Pathol. 2009;40(6):769–77.

76. Barros-Silva JD, Leitao D, Afonso L, et al. Association of ERBB2 gene status with histopathological parameters and disease-specific survival in gastric carcinoma patients. Br J Cancer. 2009;100(3): 487–93.

77. Reichelt U, Duesedau P, Tsourlakis M, et al. Frequent homogeneous HER-2 amplification in primary and metastatic adenocarcinoma of the esophagus. Mod Pathol. 2007;20(1):120–9.

78. Grabsch H, Sivakumar S, Gray S, Gabbert HE, Muller W. HER2 expression in gastric cancer: Rare, heterogeneous and of no prognostic value—conclusions from 924 cases of two independent series. Cell Oncol. 2010;32(1–2):57–65.

79. Reddy S, Shaller CC, Doss M, et al. Evaluation of the anti-HER2 C6.5 diabody as a PET radiotracer to monitor HER2 status and predict response to trastuzumab treatment. Clin Cancer Res. 21 Dec 2010. doi: 10.1158/1078-0432.CCR-10-1654

80. Dijkers EC. Oude Munnink TH, Kosterink JG, et al. Biodistribution of 89Zr-trastuzumab and PET imaging of HER2-positive lesions in patients with metastatic breast cancer. Clin Pharmacol Ther. 2010; 87(5):586–92.

81. Yu GZ, Chen Y, Wang JJ. Overexpression of Grb2/HER2 signaling in Chinese gastric cancer: their relationship with clinicopathological parameters and prognostic significance. J Cancer Res Clin Oncol. 2009;135(10):1331–9.

82. Kim JH, Kim MA, Lee HS, Kim WH. Comparative analysis of protein expressions in primary and metastatic gastric carcinomas. Hum Pathol. 2009;40(3): 314–22.

83. Press MF, Hung G, Godolphin W, Slamon DJ. Sensitivity of HER-2/neu antibodies in archival tissue samples: potential source of error in immunohistochemical studies of oncogene expression. Cancer Res. 1994;54(10):2771–7.

84. Jacobs TW, Gown AM, Yaziji H, Barnes MJ, Schnitt SJ. Specificity of HercepTest in determining HER-2/neu status of breast cancers using the United States Food and Drug Administration-approved scoring system. J Clin Oncol. 1999;17(7):1983–7.

85. Rauser S, Weis R, Braselmann H, et al. Significance of HER2 low-level copy gain in Barrett's cancer: implications for fluorescence in situ hybridization testing in tissues. Clin Cancer Res. 2007;13(17): 5115–23.

86. Holden J, Garrett Z, Stevens A. NICE guidance on trastuzumab for the treatment of HER2-positive metastatic gastric cancer. Lancet Oncol. 2011;12(1): 16–7.

87. Yan B, Yau EX. Bte Omar SS, et al. A study of HER2 gene amplification and protein expression in gastric cancer. J Clin Pathol. 2010;63(9):839–42.

88. Park DI, Yun JW, Park JH, et al. HER-2/neu amplification is an independent prognostic factor in gastric cancer. Dig Dis Sci. 2006;51(8):1371–9.

89. Bartlett JM, Campbell FM, Ibrahim M, et al. A UK NEQAS ISH multicenter ring study using the Ventana HER2 dual-color ISH assay. Am J Clin Pathol. 2011;135(1):157–62.

90. Yonemura Y, Ninomiya I, Yamaguchi A, et al. Evaluation of immunoreactivity for erbB-2 protein as a marker of poor short term prognosis in gastric cancer. Cancer Res. 1991;51(3):1034–8.

91. Uchino S, Tsuda H, Maruyama K, et al. Overexpression of c-erbB-2 protein in gastric cancer. Its correlation with long-term survival of patients. Cancer. 1993;72(11):3179–84.

92. Mizutani T, Onda M, Tokunaga A, Yamanaka N, Sugisaki Y. Relationship of C-erbB-2 protein expression and gene amplification to invasion and metastasis in human gastric cancer. Cancer. 1993;72(7): 2083–8.

93. Takehana T, Kunitomo K, Kono K, et al. Status of c-erbB-2 in gastric adenocarcinoma: a comparative study of immunohistochemistry, fluorescence in situ hybridization and enzyme-linked immuno-sorbent assay. Int J Cancer. 2002;98(6):833–7.

94. Ishikawa T, Kobayashi M, Mai M, Suzuki T, Ooi A. Amplification of the c-erbB-2 (HER-2/neu) gene in gastric cancer cells. Detection by fluorescence in situ hybridization. Am J Pathol. 1997;151(3):761–8.

95. Nakajima M, Sawada H, Yamada Y, et al. The prognostic significance of amplification and overexpression of c-met and c-crb B-2 in human gastric carcinomas. Cancer. 1999;85(9):1894–902.

96. Park JB, Rhim JS, Park SC, Kimm SW, Kraus MH. Amplification, overexpression, and rearrangement of the erbB-2 protooncogene in primary human stomach carcinomas. Cancer Res. 1989;49(23): 6605–9.

97. Hilton DA, West KP. c-erbB-2 oncogene product expression and prognosis in gastric carcinoma. J Clin Pathol. 1992;45(5):454–6.

98. Tanner M, Hollmen M, Junttila TT, et al. Amplification of HER-2 in gastric carcinoma: association with Topoisomerase IIalpha gene amplification, intestinal type, poor prognosis and sensitivity to trastuzumab. Ann Oncol. 2005;16(2): 273–8.

99. Allgayer H, Babic R, Gruetzner KU, Tarabichi A, Schildberg FW, Heiss MM. c-erbB-2 is of independent prognostic relevance in gastric cancer and is associated with the expression of tumor-associated protease systems. J Clin Oncol. 2000;18(11): 2201–9.

100. Schoppmann SF, Jesch B, Friedrich J, et al. Expression of Her-2 in carcinomas of the esophagus. Am J Surg Pathol. 2010;34(12):1868–73.

101. Hardwick RH, Barham CP, Ozua P, et al. Immunohistochemical detection of p53 and c-erbB-2 in oesophageal carcinoma; no correlation with prognosis. Eur J Surg Oncol. 1997;23(1):30–5.

102. Flejou JF, Paraf F, Muzeau F, et al. Expression of c-erbB-2 oncogene product in Barrett's adenocarcinoma: pathological and prognostic correlations. J Clin Pathol. 1994;47(1):23–6.

103. Hardwick RH, Shepherd NA, Moorghen M, Newcomb PV, Alderson D. c-erbB-2 overexpression in the dysplasia/carcinoma sequence of Barrett's oesophagus. J Clin Pathol. 1995;48(2):129–32.

104. Brien TP, Odze RD, Sheehan CE, McKenna BJ, Ross JS. HER-2/neu gene amplification by FISH predicts poor survival in Barrett's esophagus-associated adenocarcinoma. Hum Pathol. 2000; 31(1):35–9.

105. Dreilich M, Wanders A, Brattstrom D, et al. HER-2 overexpression (3+) in patients with squamous cell esophageal carcinoma correlates with poorer survival. Dis Esophagus. 2006;19(4):224–31.

106. Mimura K, Kono K, Hanawa M, et al. Frequencies of HER-2/neu expression and gene amplification in patients with oesophageal squamous cell carcinoma. Br J Cancer. 2005;92(7):1253–60.

107. Wei Q, Chen L, Sheng L, Nordgren H, Wester K, Carlsson J. EGFR, HER2 and HER3 expression in esophageal primary tumours and corresponding metastases. Int J Oncol. 2007;31(3):493–9.

108. Sato-Kuwabara Y, Neves JI, Fregnani JH, Sallum RA, Soares FA. Evaluation of gene amplification and protein expression of HER-2/neu in esophageal squamous cell carcinoma using Fluorescence in situ Hybridization (FISH) and immunohistochemistry. BMC Cancer. 2009;9:6.

109. Akamatsu M, Matsumoto T, Oka K, et al. c-erbB-2 oncoprotein expression related to chemoradioresistance in esophageal squamous cell carcinoma. Int J Radiat Oncol Biol Phys. 2003;57(5):1323–7.

110. Miyazono F, Metzger R, Warnecke-Eberz U, et al. Quantitative c-erbB-2 but not c-erbB-1 mRNA expression is a promising marker to predict minor histopathologic response to neoadjuvant radiochemotherapy in oesophageal cancer. Br J Cancer. 2004;91(4):666–72.

111. Bang Y, Chung H, Xu J, et al. Pathological features of advanced gastric cancer (GC): Relationship to human epidermal growth factor receptor 2 (HER2) positivity in the global screening programme of the ToGA trial. 2009 ASCO Annu Meet. 27:15s. J Clin Oncol 2009:(suppl; abstr 4556).

112. Polkowski W, van Sandick JW, Offerhaus GJ, et al. Prognostic value of Lauren classification and c-erbB-2 oncogene overexpression in adenocarcinoma of the esophagus and gastroesophageal junction. Ann Surg Oncol. 1999;6(3):290–7.

113. Kang Y, Bang Y, Lordick S, et al. Incidence of gastric and gastro-esophageal cancer in the ToGA trial: Correlation with HER2 positivity. ASCO Gastrointest Cancers Symp. 2008. [Epub ahead of print] http://www.asco.org/ascov2/Meetings/Abstracts?&vmview=abst_detail_view&confID=53&abstractID=10587. Accessed 10 Feb 2012.

114. Bang YJ, Van Cutsem E, Feyereislova A, et al. trastuzumab in combination with chemotherapy versus chemotherapy alone for treatment of HER2-positive advanced gastric or gastro-oesophageal junction cancer (ToGA): a phase 3, open-label, randomised controlled trial. Lancet. 2010;376(9742): 687–97.

115. Tubbs RR, Pettay JD, Roche PC, Stoler MH, Jenkins RB, Grogan TM. Discrepancies in clinical laboratory testing of eligibility for trastuzumab therapy: apparent immunohistochemical false-positives do not get the message. J Clin Oncol. 2001;19(10):2714–21.

116. Konecny GE, Pegram MD, Venkatesan N, et al. Activity of the dual kinase inhibitor lapatinib (GW572016) against HER-2-overexpressing and trastuzumab-treated breast cancer cells. Cancer Res. 2006;66(3):1630–9.

117. Wainberg ZA, Anghel A, Desai AJ, et al. Lapatinib, a dual EGFR and HER2 kinase inhibitor, selectively inhibits HER2-amplified human gastric cancer cells and is synergistic with trastuzumab in vitro and in vivo. Clin Cancer Res. 2010;16(5):1509–19.

118. Safran H, Dipetrillo T, Akerman P, et al. Phase I/II study of trastuzumab, paclitaxel, cisplatin and radiation for locally advanced, HER2 overexpressing, esophageal adenocarcinoma. Int J Radiat Oncol Biol Phys. 2007;67(2):405–9.

119. Folkman J, Cole P, Zimmerman S. Tumor behavior in isolated perfused organs: in vitro growth and metastases of biopsy material in rabbit thyroid and canine intestinal segment. Ann Surg. 1966;164(3): 491–502.

120. Hanahan D, Weinberg RA. The hallmarks of cancer. Cell. 2000;100(1):57–70.

121. DiSalvo J, Bayne ML, Conn G, et al. Purification and characterization of a naturally occurring vascular endothelial growth factor.placenta growth factor heterodimer. J Biol Chem. 1995;270(13):7717–23.

122. Olofsson B, Pajusola K, Kaipainen A, et al. Vascular endothelial growth factor B, a novel growth factor for endothelial cells. Proc Natl Acad Sci U S A. 1996;93(6):2576–81.

123. Joukov V, Pajusola K, Kaipainen A, et al. A novel vascular endothelial growth factor, VEGF-C, is a ligand for the Flt4 (VEGFR-3) and KDR (VEGFR-2) receptor tyrosine kinases. EMBO J. 1996;15(7):1751.

124. Shibuya M. Vascular endothelial growth factor receptor-2: its unique signaling and specific ligand, VEGF-E. Cancer Sci. 2003;94(9):751–6.

125. Tischer E, Mitchell R, Hartman T, et al. The human gene for vascular endothelial growth factor. Multiple

125. protein forms are encoded through alternative exon splicing. J Biol Chem. 1991;266(18):11947–54.
126. Houck KA, Ferrara N, Winer J, Cachianes G, Li B, Leung DW. The vascular endothelial growth factor family: identification of a fourth molecular species and characterization of alternative splicing of RNA. Mol Endocrinol. 1991;5(12):1806–14.
127. Pellet-Many C, Frankel P, Jia H, Zachary I. Neuropilins: structure, function and role in disease. Biochem J. 2008;411(2):211–26.
128. Geretti E, Shimizu A, Klagsbrun M. Neuropilin structure governs VEGF and semaphorin binding and regulates angiogenesis. Angiogenesis. 2008;11(1):31–9.
129. Pan Q, Chathery Y, Wu Y, et al. Neuropilin-1 binds to VEGF121 and regulates endothelial cell migration and sprouting. J Biol Chem. 2007;282(33):24049–56.
130. Park JE, Chen HH, Winer J, Houck KA, Ferrara N. Placenta growth factor. Potentiation of vascular endothelial growth factor bioactivity, in vitro and in vivo, and high affinity binding to Flt-1 but not to Flk-1/KDR. J Biol Chem. 1994;269(41):25646–54.
131. Olofsson B, Korpelainen E, Pepper MS, et al. Vascular endothelial growth factor B (VEGF-B) binds to VEGF receptor-1 and regulates plasminogen activator activity in endothelial cells. Proc Natl Acad Sci U S A. 1998;95(20):11709–14.
132. Silvestre JS, Tamarat R, Ebrahimian TG, et al. Vascular endothelial growth factor-B promotes in vivo angiogenesis. Circ Res. 2003;93(2):114–23.
133. Cao Y, Chen H, Zhou L, et al. Heterodimers of placenta growth factor/vascular endothelial growth factor. Endothelial activity, tumor cell expression, and high affinity binding to Flk-1/KDR. J Biol Chem. 1996;271(6):3154–62.
134. Achen MG, Jeltsch M, Kukk E, et al. Vascular endothelial growth factor D (VEGF-D) is a ligand for the tyrosine kinases VEGF receptor 2 (Flk1) and VEGF receptor 3 (Flt4). Proc Natl Acad Sci U S A. 1998;95(2):548–53.
135. Kaipainen A, Korhonen J, Mustonen T, et al. Expression of the fms-like tyrosine kinase 4 gene becomes restricted to lymphatic endothelium during development. Proc Natl Acad Sci U S A. 1995; 92(8):3566–70.
136. Shibuya M, Claesson-Welsh L. Signal transduction by VEGF receptors in regulation of angiogenesis and lymphangiogenesis. Exp Cell Res. 2006;312(5): 549–60.
137. Kerbel RS. Tumor angiogenesis. N Engl J Med. 2008;358(19):2039–49.
138. Zeng H, Dvorak HF, Mukhopadhyay D. Vascular permeability factor (VPF)/vascular endothelial growth factor (VEGF) peceptor-1 down-modulates VPF/VEGF receptor-2-mediated endothelial cell proliferation, but not migration, through phosphatidylinositol 3-kinase-dependent pathways. J Biol Chem. 2001;276(29):26969–79.
139. Dvorak HF. Vascular permeability factor/vascular endothelial growth factor: a critical cytokine in tumor angiogenesis and a potential target for diagnosis and therapy. J Clin Oncol. 2002;20(21):4368–80.
140. Fukumura D, Xavier R, Sugiura T, et al. Tumor induction of VEGF promoter activity in stromal cells. Cell. 1998;94(6):715–25.
141. Kut C. Mac Gabhann F, Popel AS. Where is VEGF in the body? A meta-analysis of VEGF distribution in cancer. Br J Cancer. 2007;97(7):978–85.
142. Lee KH, Choi EY, Kim MK, et al. Hepatoma-derived growth factor regulates the bad-mediated apoptotic pathway and induction of vascular endothelial growth factor in stomach cancer cells. Oncol Res. 2010;19(2):67–76.
143. Breier G, Blum S, Peli J, et al. Transforming growth factor-beta and Ras regulate the VEGF/VEGF-receptor system during tumor angiogenesis. Int J Cancer. 2002;97(2):142–8.
144. Yoshikawa T, Tsuburaya A, Kobayashi O, et al. Plasma concentrations of VEGF and bFGF in patients with gastric carcinoma. Cancer Lett. 2000;153(1–2):7–12.
145. Hyodo I, Doi T, Endo H, et al. Clinical significance of plasma vascular endothelial growth factor in gastrointestinal cancer. Eur J Cancer. 1998; 34(13):2041–5.
146. Eroglu A, Demirci S, Ayyildiz A, et al. Serum concentrations of vascular endothelial growth factor and nitrite as an estimate of in vivo nitric oxide in patients with gastric cancer. Br J Cancer. 1999;80(10):1630–4.
147. Karayiannakis AJ, Syrigos KN, Polychronidis A, et al. Circulating VEGF levels in the serum of gastric cancer patients: correlation with pathological variables, patient survival, and tumor surgery. Ann Surg. 2002;236(1):37–42.
148. Shimada H, Takeda A, Nabeya Y, et al. Clinical significance of serum vascular endothelial growth factor in esophageal squamous cell carcinoma. Cancer. 2001;92(3):663–9.
149. Shih CH, Ozawa S, Ando N, Ueda M, Kitajima M. Vascular endothelial growth factor expression predicts outcome and lymph node metastasis in squamous cell carcinoma of the esophagus. Clin Cancer Res. 2000;6(3):1161–8.
150. Maeda K, Chung YS, Ogawa Y, et al. Prognostic value of vascular endothelial growth factor expression in gastric carcinoma. Cancer. 1996;77(5):858–63.
151. Hirashima Y, Yamada Y, Matsubara J, et al. Impact of vascular endothelial growth factor receptor 1, 2, and 3 expression on the outcome of patients with gastric cancer. Cancer Sci. 2008;100(2):310–5.
152. Bose D, Meric-Bernstam F, Hofstetter W, et al. Vascular endothelial growth factor targeted therapy in the perioperative setting: implications for patient care. Lancet Oncol. 2010;11(4):373–82.
153. Allegra CJ, Yothers G, O'Connell MJ, et al. Initial safety report of NSABP C-08: A randomized phase III study of modified FOLFOX6 with or without bevacizumab for the adjuvant treatment of patients with stage II or III colon cancer. J Clin Oncol. 2009;27(20):3385–90.
154. Van Cutsem E, Rivera F, Berry S, et al. Safety and efficacy of first-line bevacizumab with FOLFOX, XELOX, FOLFIRI and fluoropyrimidines in metastatic

colorectal cancer: the BEAT study. Ann Oncol. 2009;20(11):1842–7.

155. Kim KJ, Li B, Winer J, et al. Inhibition of vascular endothelial growth factor-induced angiogenesis suppresses tumour growth in vivo. Nature. 1993;362(6423):841–4.

156. Jain RK, Duda DG, Willett CG, et al. Biomarkers of response and resistance to antiangiogenic therapy. Nat Rev Clin Oncol. 2009;6(6):327–38.

157. Sun W, Powell M, O'Dwyer PJ, et al. Phase II study of sorafenib in combination with docetaxel and cisplatin in the treatment of metastatic or advanced gastric and gastroesophageal junction adenocarcinoma: ECOG 5203. J Clin Oncol. 2010;28(18):2947–51.

158. Ilson D, Shah MA, Kelsen DP, et al. Phase II trial of sorafenib in esophageal (E) and gastroesophageal junction (GOJ) cancer: response observed in adenocarcinoma. J Clin Oncol. 2010; 28 (suppl; abstr e14668)

159. Study of oxaliplatin and sorafenib combination to treat gastric cancer relapsed after a cisplatin based treatment http://clinicaltrials.gov/ct2/show/NCT01262482. Accessed 18 Apr 2011.

160. Sorafenib trial in advanced and/or recurrent gastric adenocarcinoma: treatment evaluation (STARGATE) http://clinicaltrial.gov/ct2/show/NCT01187212. Accessed 18 Apr 2011.

161. Bang YJ, Kang YK, Kang WK, et al. Phase II study of sunitinib as second-line treatment for advanced gastric cancer. Invest New Drugs. 12 May 2010. [Epub ahead of print].

162. Moehler MH, Hatmann JT, Lordick F, et al. An open-label, multicenter phase II trial of sunitinib for patients with chemorefractory metastatic gastric cancer. J Clin Oncol. 2010;28:(suppl; abstr e14503)

163. Horgan AM, Hornby J, Wong R, et al. Adjuvant sunitinib following trimodality therapy for locally advanced esophageal cancer (LAEC). ASCO. 2010:Abstract No. 105.

164. Sunitinib in treating patients with relapsed or refractory esophageal or gastroesophageal junction cancer http://clinicaltrials.gov/ct2/show/NCT00702884. Accessed 18 Apr 2011.

165. Sorafenib for patients with metastatic or recurrent esophageal and gastroesophageal junction cancer. http://clinicaltrials.gov/ct2/show/NCT00917462. Accessed 18 Apr 2011.

166. Shah MA, Ramanathan RK, Ilson DH, et al. Multicenter phase II study of irinotecan, cisplatin, and bevacizumab in patients with metastatic gastric or gastroesophageal junction adenocarcinoma. J Clin Oncol. 2006;24(33):5201–6.

167. Shah MA, Jhawer M, Ilson DH, et al. Phase II study of modified docetaxel, cisplatin, and fluorouracil with bevacizumab in patients with metastatic gastroesophageal adenocarcinoma. J Clin Oncol. 2011;29(7):868–74.

168. El-Rayes BF, Zalupski M, Bekai-Saab T, et al. A phase II study of bevacizumab, oxaliplatin, and docetaxel in locally advanced and metastatic gastric and gastroesophageal junction cancers. Ann Oncol. 2010;21(10):1999–2004.

169. Kang Y, Ohtsu A, Van Cutsem E, et al. AVAGAST: a randomized, double-blind, placebo-controlled, phase III study of first-line capecitabine and cisplatin plus bevacizumab or placebo in patients with advanced gastric cancer (AGC). JCO. 2010;28(Suppl 18): LBA4007

170. Heideman DA, Snijders PJ, Craanen ME, et al. Selective gene delivery toward gastric and esophageal adenocarcinoma cells via EpCAM-targeted adenoviral vectors. Cancer Gene Ther. 2001;8(5): 342–51.

171. Anders M, Sarbia M, Grotzinger C, et al. Expression of EpCam and villin in Barrett's esophagus and in gastric cardia. Dis Markers. 2008;24(6):287–92.

172. Joo M, Kim H, Kim MK, Yu HJ, Kim JP. Expression of Ep-CAM in intestinal metaplasia, gastric epithelial dysplasia and gastric adenocarcinoma. J Gastroenterol Hepatol. 2005;20(7):1039–45.

173. Wenqi D, Li W, Shanshan C, et al. EpCAM is overexpressed in gastric cancer and its downregulation suppresses proliferation of gastric cancer. J Cancer Res Clin Oncol. 2009;135(9):1277–85.

174. Stoecklein NH, Siegmund A, Scheunemann P, et al. Ep-CAM expression in squamous cell carcinoma of the esophagus: a potential therapeutic target and prognostic marker. BMC Cancer. 2006;6:165.

175. Passebosc-Faure K, Li G, Lambert C, et al. Evaluation of a panel of molecular markers for the diagnosis of malignant serous effusions. Clin Cancer Res. 2005;11(19 Pt 1):6862–7.

176. De Angelis M, Buley ID, Heryet A, Gray W. Immunocytochemical staining of serous effusions with the monoclonal antibody Ber-EP4. Cytopathology. 1992;3(2):111–7.

177. Diaz-Arias AA, Loy TS, Bickel JT, Chapman RK. Utility of BER-EP4 in the diagnosis of adenocarcinoma in effusions: an immunocytochemical study of 232 cases. Diagn Cytopathol. 1993;9(5):516–21.

178. Kimura H, Kato H, Faried A, et al. Prognostic significance of EpCAM expression in human esophageal cancer. Int J Oncol. 2007;30(1):171–9.

179. Heiss MM, Murawa P, Koralewski P, et al. The trifunctional antibody catumaxomab for the treatment of malignant ascites due to epithelial cancer: Results of a prospective randomized phase II/III trial. Int J Cancer. 2010;127(9):2209–21.

180. Fields AL, Keller A, Schwartzberg L, et al. Adjuvant therapy with the monoclonal antibody Edrecolomab plus fluorouracil-based therapy does not improve overall survival of patients with stage III colon cancer. J Clin Oncol. 2009;27(12):1941–7.

181. Strohlein MA, Lordick F, Ruttinger D, et al. Immunotherapy of peritoneal carcinomatosis with the antibody catumaxomab in colon, gastric, or pancreatic cancer: an open-label, multicenter, phase I/II trial. Onkologie. 2011;34(3):101–8.

182. clinicaltrials.gov. Phase II study with catumaxomab in patients with gastric cancer after neoadjuvant CTx and curative resection. ClinicalTrials.gov identifier: NCT00464893: http://clinicaltrials.gov/ct2/show/NCT00464893. Accessed 18 Apr 2011.

Colorectal Cancer

9

David N. Church, Rachel Susannah Midgley, and David J. Kerr

Epidemiology, Staging and Biology of CRC

Epidemiology

Colorectal cancer (CRC) is the third commonest cancer in the Western world, with an estimated 142,570 cases diagnosed in the USA in 2010 (SEER database). Worldwide, approximately 1.23 million new cases are diagnosed each year and 608,000 deaths from CRC occurred in 2008 [1]. The lifetime risk for CRC in the Western world is roughly 5–6%. Although familial cases—patients with two or more first- or second-degree relatives with CRC—comprise approximately 20% of disease, high-penetrance Mendelian conditions are responsible for a relatively small proportion (3–4%). Hereditary non-polyposis colorectal cancer (HNPCC), also known as Lynch syndrome,

D.N. Church, M.B.Ch.B., M.R.C.P., D.Phil.
University Department of Medical Oncology, Churchill Hospital, Oxford, Oxfordshire, UK

R.S. Midgley, M.B.Ch.B., F.R.C.P., Ph.D.
Department of Oncology, Churchill Hospital, Oxford, Oxfordshire, UK

D.J. Kerr, M.A., M.D., D.Sc., F.R.C.P., F.Med.Sci., C.B.E. (✉)
Nuffield Department of Clinical and Laboratory Sciences, University of Oxford, Oxford, Oxfordshire, OX3 7DQ, UK
e-mail: david.kerr@clinpharm.ox.ac.uk

results from germline mutation in mismatch repair proteins [2]. Defective DNA mismatch repair leads to accumulation of mutations with development of CRC typically in the 5th decade of life [2]. Carriers have a risk of 22–69% for CRC development before age 70 [3] and are also at significantly increased risk of tumours of the endometrium, ovary, stomach, uroepithelium, small bowel and bile duct [4]. In familial adenomatous polyposis (FAP), germline mutation of the *APC* tumour suppressor results in the development of hundreds to thousands of adenomatous polyps within the colorectum, with inevitable malignant change by the 4th to 5th decade of life [2]. Recent large-scale genome-wide association studies have begun to demonstrate the low-penetrance, common genetic variants that underlie many sporadic CRCs [5, 6].

Several dietary factors appear to modify the risk of CRC. An inverse association between folate intake and the incidence of colorectal adenomas and carcinomas has been shown in epidemiological studies [7], but trials of folate supplementation after CRC diagnosis demonstrated no reduction in risk of adenoma or carcinoma recurrence [8, 9]. Evidence also supports a role for calcium supplementation in the reduction of CRC incidence and adenoma recurrence [10–12]. Additional risk factors for CRC include smoking [13, 14] and high BMI [15], while physical exercise [16, 17] and aspirin use [18–20] reduce risk.

Table 9.1 AJCC/Dukes' staging systems for colorectal cancer and 5-year overall survival

AJCC/Dukes' stage	Anatomical extent of disease	5-Year overall survival
I/A	Confined to mucosa (T1) or muscularis propria (T2) No nodal involvement No distant metastases	93.2%
II/B	Tumour penetrates muscularis (T3) or invades adjacent organs or structures (T4) No nodal involvement No distant metastases	82.5%
III/C	Any tumour stage Nodal metastases No distant metastases	59.5%
IV/D	Any tumour stage Any nodal status Distant metastases	8.1%

Staging

The anatomical and histological progression of CRC is well understood. The classic model is the development of an adenomatous polyp, with malignant conversion leading to local invasion through submucosa, muscularis propria, and, eventually through the outer layers of the colon and into surrounding fat or adjacent structures. Invasion of lymphatic vessels facilitates spread to locally draining mesenteric lymph nodes and access to blood vessels enables spread to distant organs, most commonly the liver. The extent of local invasion, nodal and distant metastases remains the best prognosticators in CRC, as codified in the staging systems used clinically—the AJCC TNM [21] and the Dukes' systems. These are summarised in Table 9.1 together with the approximate 5-year survival associated with each stage. Further prognostication is provided by additional factors such as bowel obstruction or perforation at presentation, tumour vascular and lymphatic invasion, tumour grade and patient performance status [22]. However, even accounting for these, there remains substantial heterogeneity

in outcome within stage groups, indicating additional differences in tumour and patient biology not revealed by these indicators.

Biology

The adenoma–carcinoma sequence of CRC development described above is estimated to take place over 10–20 years. As a result of this stepwise progression, and the technical feasibility of obtaining pathological material from colonic biopsy and tumour resection, the molecular biology of CRC is better understood than that of many cancers. CRC can be divided into two principal pathological categories. The majority (65–70%) of cases are characterised by aneuploidy and chromosomal instability (CIN), while tumours from patients with HNPCC and approximately 15% of sporadic cancers [23, 24] demonstrate an alternative molecular phenotype of microsatellite instability (MSI), and typically retain diploid chromosome complement.

In a seminal paper published over two decades ago, Vogelstein et al. proposed a model of sequential mutations to account for adenoma–carcinoma progression in CIN CRC [25]. In this, inactivating mutations in tumour suppressor genes and activating mutations in oncogenes each confer a proliferative, survival or metastatic advantage to the tumour, enabling progression, invasion and ultimately metastasis. Early lesions were shown to lack APC, a tumour suppressor that encodes a negative regulator of Wnt signalling—a key developmental signalling pathway that promotes cell division [26]. Subsequent events include activating mutations in *KRAS*, a small GTPase downstream of many receptor tyrosine kinases (RTKs) including EGFR, which leads to constitutive activation of the MAPK pathway, resulting in further mitogenic effects, loss of chromosome 18q-containing *SMAD4*—a transcriptional regulator with tumour suppressive effects and loss of TP53, which results in resistance to apoptosis. Though this basic model has been validated by subsequent studies [27], it has also been substantially enriched by the demonstration that there are many more mutations and epigenetic changes

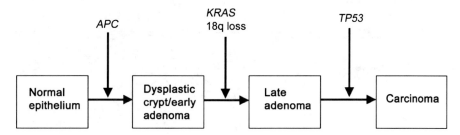

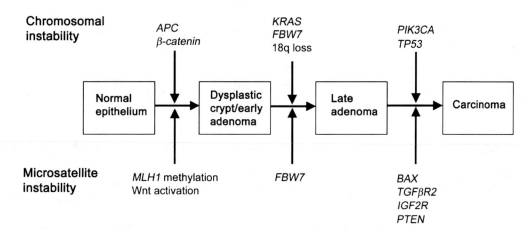

Fig. 9.1 Original and updated genetic models of adenoma–carcinoma sequence. (**a**) Model of carcinoma development proposed by Vogelstein and Kinzler. The first event is mutation of the tumour suppressor *APC*, resulting in constitutive activation of the Wnt pathway and the development of crypt dysplasia and early adenoma. Subsequent activation of the small GTPase KRAS by mutation at codons 12, 13 or 61 leads to activation of the MAPK pathway, while 18q deletion results in loss of SMAD4, a component of the transforming growth factor-β (TGFβ) pathway, leading to adenoma progression. Inactivating mutations in *TP53* result in progression to invasive carcinoma. (**b**) The refined model encompasses subsequent data since the pivotal work of Vogelstein and reflects the demonstration that CRC development can be broadly divided into two subclasses, depending on the underlying pattern of molecular aberrations—chromosomal instability (CIN) (*upper figure*) and microsatellite instability (MSI) (*lower figure*). CIN tumours largely develop according to the schematic proposed in (**a**), though further common mutations have been demonstrated, including inactivating mutations in the ubiquitin ligase *FBW7* and activating mutations in *PIK3CA*—encoding the catalytic subunit of PI3K. MSI tumours result from defective mismatch repair apparatus and are characterised by an alternative spectrum of mutations. Early lesions demonstrate Wnt pathway activation, while mutation in *BRAF* appears to substitute for *KRAS* mutation in promotion of adenoma progression. Inactivating mutations in tumour suppressors *TGFβR2*, *IGF2R* and *PTEN* characterise progression to carcinoma. It should be noted that both models are significant oversimplifications—recent work suggests CRC typically contains over ten driver mutations—and that many tumours demonstrate features of both

in CRC than previously realised [28]. A summary of the schematic proposed by Vogelstein et al. and an updated version are shown in Fig. 9.1.

MSI results from defective function of the DNA mismatch repair (MMR) proteins MLH1, MSH2, MSH6 and PMS1 MMR leading to slippage and duplication of repetitive microsatellite DNA elements during DNA replication. This results in mutation of genes that contain such repeats, including *TGFBR2* [29], *IGF2R* [30] and *BAX* [31], in addition to point mutations in other genes such as *BRAF* [32, 33]. Though this may result from germline mutation (HNPCC, discussed above), the commonest cause in sporadic carcinomas is the downregulation of *MLH1* by promoter methylation [34, 35]. Consequently, MSI tumours

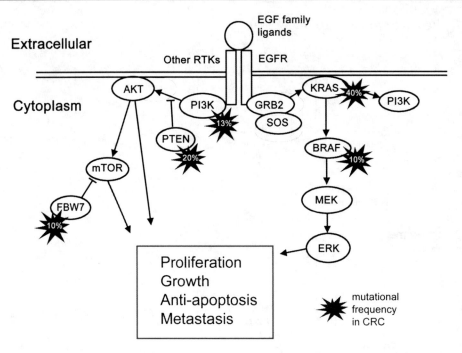

Fig. 9.2 Aberrant MAPK and PI3K pathway activation in colorectal cancer results from mutation. The MAPK and PI3K-AKT pathways are essential in cellular homeostasis, and their activation drives colorectal carcinoma (CRC) development via multiple mechanisms. Binding of extracellular ligand to RTKs including the epidermal growth factor receptor (EGFR) typically causes receptor dimerisation and autophosphorylation at tyrosine residues. These serve as docking moieties for adaptor proteins including GRB2 and the regulatory p85 subunit of PI3K (not shown). Though precise mechanisms vary, these typically act to recruit substrates to the plasma membrane where they are activated. In the case of the MAPK pathway, membrane localisation of the small GTPase KRAS by the GRB2-SOS complex causes it to exchange GDP for GTP, converting it from its inactive to active form. Activating *KRAS* mutations occur in 40% of CRC and abrogates the GTPase activity of KRAS, rendering it constitutively "switched on." BRAF is a serine–threonine kinase immediately downstream of KRAS and is mutated in 10% of CRC, particularly in MSI tumours. *BRAF* mutations substitute for *KRAS* mutation in activating the MAPK pathway, and the two events appear mutually exclusive. Downstream of BRAF, MEK and ERK activation leads to changes in transcriptional regulators such as Fos, Jun and EGR1 with net result of increased cellular proliferation, growth and migration. The PI3K pathway is also activated by RTKs via p85 recruitment, which causes the p110α subunit of PI3K to phosphorylate the membrane lipid phosphatidylinositol-4,5-bisphosphate (PIP2) at the 3′ position to generate phosphatidylinositol-3,4,5-trisphosphate (PIP3). By removal of the 3′ phosphate from PIP3, the tumour suppressor PTEN catalyses the reversal of this reaction. PIP3 recruits the serine–threonine kinase AKT to the plasma membrane, where it activated and proceeds to phosphorylate multiple substrates. Sequential phosphorylation events downstream of AKT include activation of mTOR, a key regulator of cell growth, activation of glycolytic pathways and inactivation of multiple anti-apoptotic proteins. The PI3K pathway is activated in the majority of CRC by multiple mechanisms, including activating mutations in *PIK3CA*, loss of PTEN and mutation in the ubiquitin ligase *FBW7*. Approximate mutational frequencies are indicated for pathway intermediates (PTEN is also silenced by promoter methylation). It should be noted that extensive crosstalks and feedbacks exist between the MAPK and PI3K (and additional) pathways, not shown for reasons of space

demonstrate a different mutational spectrum and histological features (proximal to splenic flexure, mucinous, poorly differentiated, lymphocytic invasion) to CIN tumours [36–38]. The potential utility of CIN and MSI status in tumours as prognostic and predictive markers is discussed below.

To summarise, recent data indicate that the simple model of CRC progression associated with predictable genetic changes requires embellishment. Though tumours are characterised by common themes of pathway activation, tumour suppressor loss and acquisition of metastatic ability, there exists a substantial variation between tumours in the actual genes mutated. A summary of the commonly deregulated pathways and mutations is shown in Fig. 9.2. The increased knowledge of the molecular biology of CRC has provided many new therapeutic targets, of which some have been successfully validated, as discussed below.

Current Standard of Care and Novel Biotargets

Multimodality Management of Colorectal Cancer

The management of CRC is multimodal and optimum therapy is determined by the tumour stage. Surgery to remove the primary tumour and draining lymph nodes is the only treatment required in stage I and low-risk stage II disease, and resection followed by adjuvant chemotherapy is generally recommended for high-risk stage II and all stage III tumours [39]. Although historically, patients with stage IV disease were managed with palliative chemotherapy alone, an expanding indication for surgery is the removal of hepatic metastases, which permits 5-year survival rates of 20–30% in appropriately staged patients [40,41]. Radiotherapy, though seldom used in management of colonic tumours, is an essential component of rectal tumour therapy either delivered as a short course prior to surgery or as a longer fractionation schedule combined with chemotherapy [42].

Chemotherapy in CRC

Metastatic CRC

The median survival of stage IV CRC with no treatment is less than 7.5 months [43]. Early clinical trials of chemotherapy in metastatic CRC (mCRC) demonstrated that 5-fluorouracil (FU), combined with leucovorin (LV), which improves fluorouracil (FU) response rate through modulation of thymidylate synthetase activity resulted in the extension of survival by a median of 3.7 months [44]. Irinotecan is an inhibitor of topoisomerase I, an enzyme required for the unwinding of DNA prior to replication or repair, and has activity in FU-refractory CRC. In a pivotal clinical

trial for first-line therapy of mCRC, the addition of irinotecan to FU (FOLFIRI) was shown to improve response rate (RR) (39% vs. 21%, $P<0.001$) and extend median overall survival (OS) (14.8 vs. 12.6 months, $P=0.04$) compared to FU alone [45]. Another agent with anti-tumour activity in FU-refractory CRC is oxaliplatin, a third-generation platinum that mediates cytotoxicity though addition of platinum adducts to DNA. Oxaliplatin improved RR (50.7% vs. 22.3%; $P=0.0001$), progression-free survival (PFS) (median, 9.0 vs. 6.2 months; $P=0.0003$) and OS (median, 16.2 vs. 14.7 months; $P=0.12$) when combined with FU (FOLFOX) in first-line therapy for advanced CRC compared to FU alone [46]. The clinical benefit of the addition of oxaliplatin and irinotecan to the therapeutic armamentarium is reflected in the improved overall survival of patients with stage IV CRC treated with all three drugs when compared with patients who were not able to receive such therapy [47]. Capecitabine (Xeloda™) is an oral fluoropyrimidine with at least equivalent efficacy to bolus FU in mCRC as monotherapy [48] or in combination with oxaliplatin (XELOX) [49]. It provides a convenient alternative to intravenous FU and has been widely adopted in clinical practice. Response rates and overall survival have been further improved, albeit modestly by the addition of targeted therapies to the above regimens in the last decade, as described below.

Adjuvant Therapy

The benefit of adjuvant chemotherapy in stage III disease was demonstrated in pivotal clinical trials, which showed that FU treatment reduced the absolute risk of disease relapse by approximately 15% [50]. The activity of irinotecan and oxaliplatin in the metastatic setting led to their evaluation in adjuvant therapy of stage II and III disease. Results were mixed; while the addition of oxaliplatin to FU-based therapy led to significant improvement in disease-free survival (DFS) and OS [51, 52], combination of irinotecan and FU failed to demonstrate superiority over FU alone in several large studies [53, 54]. Though the benefits of adjuvant therapy in stage II disease are smaller, the QUASAR trial demonstrated that FU-based therapy resulted in a 3.6% absolute benefit in survival compared to observation [55]. Subsequent data indicate that the addition of oxaliplatin to FU in stage II disease does not significantly improve this benefit, though the study was not powered for this analysis [51]. As in the metastatic setting, capecitabine can be substituted for FU monotherapy [56] and may be combined with oxaliplatin [57].

Novel Targets in CRC

Vascular Endothelial Growth Factor

Like other solid tumours, CRC is reliant on the development of new vasculature to maintain cellular viability and was therefore a logical target for antiangiogenic therapy. Bevacizumab (Avastin®), is a monoclonal antibody that targets vascular endothelial growth factor (VEGF)—an extracellular ligand that promotes angiogenesis and endothelial cell survival [58]. In a large phase III clinical trial, the addition of bevacizumab to FOLFIRI as first-line therapy of mCRC was associated with substantial improvement in PFS (10.6 vs. 6.2 months, $P<0.001$) and OS (20.3 vs. 15.6 months, $P<0.001$) [59]. Following these results, bevacizumab was widely adopted as part of first-line therapy for mCRC. Subsequent studies combining bevacizumab with FOLFOX or XELOX either as first-line therapy or following FOLFIRI also demonstrated improvements in PFS and OS [60, 61], though the OS improvements of 6–8 weeks were modest compared to the pivotal FOLFIRI trial. Unfortunately, despite efficacy in the metastatic setting, the addition of bevacizumab to FOLFOX for adjuvant therapy in the NSABP C-08 trial did not translate into improved 3-year DFS (77.4% vs.75.5% $P=$NS) [62]. Additionally, the AVANT study, though as yet unpublished, was discontinued early by the data monitoring committee due to lack of efficacy [63].

Epidermal Growth Factor Receptor

The epidermal growth factor receptor (EGFR) is a cell surface receptor tyrosine kinase expressed on epithelial cells, including CRC cells. Activation of EGFR by ligand binding induces a cascade of downstream phosphorylation events through the MAPK and PI3K pathways (Fig. 9.2). The resulting changes in gene transcription, protein localisation and protein activity act in concert to promote cell division, cell growth and cell survival [64]. Cetuximab and panitumumab are monoclonal antibodies that target the EGFR extracellular domain, and both have proven efficacy in advanced CRC. Several RCTs have demonstrated significant benefit from cetuximab or panitumumab treatment either as monotherapy [65, 66] or in combination with cytotoxics [67–69]. Notably, response to therapy in these studies was not correlated with EGFR expression [70]—highlighting the need for alternative biomarkers predictive of response. In light of the encouraging data in advanced disease, anti-EGFR therapy in the adjuvant setting was examined in a recently reported study. Disappointingly, the addition of cetuximab to FOLFOX chemotherapy showed a trend to inferiority to FOLFOX alone [71]. Thus, EGFR targeting cannot be recommended following resection of localised disease. The reasons for these discordant results are presently unclear, though they may reflect disparate biology of micro- and macrometastases.

Other Emerging Targets

PIK3CA, which encodes the catalytic subunit of PI3K, is activated by mutation in 13% of CRC [72]. This results in activation of the PI3K-AKT pathway and increased sensitivity to PI3K inhibition [73]. Several compounds targeting PI3K have been developed and are presently in early-phase clinical trials with promising results [74]. BRAF is a serine–threonine kinase downstream of KRAS and is mutated in approximately 10% of CRC [75, 76]. This mutation—a substitution

9 Colorectal Cancer

of glutamic acid for valine at residue 600 (V600E)—results in a constitutively active protein with downstream pathway activation. Recently, PLX4032, an inhibitor of mutated BRAF, has shown remarkable activity in metastatic melanoma [77]. An early trial of PLX4032 in BRAF V600E mutant pre-treated mCRC has demonstrated a more modest benefit (3.7 month PFS), though this remains a target worthy of further validation in the clinic [78]. Insulin-like growth factor receptor-1 (IGF1R) mediates signalling from insulin-like growth factors (IGF1 and IGF2). IGF1R is overexpressed in many solid tumours and is an emerging therapeutic target in breast and ovarian cancers [79]. Unfortunately, a phase II study of an anti-IGF1R monoclonal antibody in cetuximab-/panitumumab-refractory CRC demonstrated no anti-tumour activity [80]. Identification of additional therapeutic targets in CRC is the focus of intensive investigation.

Biomarkers in Clinical Practice

The generally accepted definition of a biomarker is a measurable variable that either varies categorically (present or absent) or continuously (low level to high level). Our definition in this chapter is broad—it may be a single biomarker with prognostic or predictive import or a multivariable prediction model (such as DNA microarray data). Broadly, biomarkers can be divided into three categories:

1. Prognostic biomarkers
   This is a biomarker, the level of which has implications for patient outcome independent of the treatment used.
2. Predictive biomarkers
   These comprise biomarkers' presence or absence or the relative level of which predicts response to therapy. If therapy is universally used, then a predictive biomarker will also have prognostic import.
3. Biomarkers correlating with treatment response
   This is a measurable substance, the levels of which correlate with response to therapy. The commonest example in CRC is the use of serum carcinoembryonic antigen (CEA) to monitor disease burden in response to palliative chemotherapy.

Though prognostic and predictive biomarkers have been the subject of many published papers, unfortunately, the majority of studies are small retrospective studies with poorly defined protocols for sample collection and analysis. These studies have a high risk of bias and false-positive results. In view of these difficulties, guidelines for assessing the level of evidence (LOE) for biomarkers have been published [81] as summarised below:

Categories that constitute levels of evidence determination for biomarker studies (from Simon et al. [81]):

A Prospective, controlled trial designed to address tumour marker. Specimens collected, processed and assayed in real time. Study powered to answer tumour marker question.
B Prospective trial not designed to address tumour marker, but incorporating tumour marker utility. Specimens collected, processed and archived prospectively using generic SOPs. Assayed after trial completion. Study powered to answer therapeutic question, but not marker question.
C Prospective observational registry, treatment and follow-up not dictated. Specimens collected, processed and archived prospectively using generic SOPs. Not prospectively powered.
D No prospective aspect to study. Specimens collected, processed and archived with no SOPs. Not prospectively powered.

Though it is preferable that it is subsequently confirmed, validation of a category A study is not required to obtain Level I evidence, while category B studies require validation to become LOE I and merit incorporation of results into clinical practice. Category B studies without validation and validated category C studies both fall into LOE II, while category C studies without validation merit LOE III. Category C studies are unlikely to change practice in the absence of strong supporting data. Category D studies are very likely to be due to the play of chance, are assigned LOE IV or V, and are hypothesis generating rather than practice changing.

Biomarkers in CRC: An Unmet Need

Despite accurate staging, CRC remains a heterogeneous disease, with 5-year survival varying from 72% to 83% in stage II disease and 44% to 83% in stage III disease [21]. Adjuvant chemotherapy reduces risk of relapse by 3–5% and 12–15% in stage II and III disease, respectively. However, most patients who receive treatment fail to benefit from therapy, while all are exposed to the toxicities and suffer the inconvenience of treatment. Stage II disease, in particular, provides an illustrative example of the need for improved predictors of outcome. Typically, patients with high-risk features (T4 tumour, vascular and lymphatic invasion, high tumour grade) are offered chemotherapy. Even with an optimistic estimation of therapeutic efficacy, 19 of every 20 such patients gain no benefit, as their disease was low risk and cured by surgery alone, or inherently chemotherapy resistant. The availability of accurate prognostic biomarkers would spare the former group chemotherapy, while predictive biomarkers would identify the latter group, enabling either omission of therapy or the use of an alternative regimen. Improved prognostic and predictive markers would also assist in individualising therapy for patients with stage III and IV disease.

A particularly important area is the identification of biomarkers that predict response to targeted therapies. These may be as simple as the presence of the target on or within the cell (e.g. overexpression of the HER2 receptor and benefit from trastuzumab in breast cancer) or the presence or absence of mutations—for instance, detectable aberrations downstream of the agent that interfere with therapeutic effect. The pressing need for these is underlined by the relatively modest clinical benefits associated with targeted therapies and their high cost compared to conventional cytotoxics.

Current and Emerging Biomarkers in CRC

Some biomarkers, such as the CEA tumour marker are long established in clinical practice, while others, such as *KRAS* mutation testing for prediction of response to anti-EGFR therapy, have entered use more recently. Yet other biomarkers remain unvalidated or demonstrate mixed results in studies. Here, we summarise the current status of established and emerging biomarkers, together with the LOE underlying their use. As previously discussed, distinction must be made between prognostic markers— which predict relapse or progression independent of future treatment effects and predictive markers—which predict response or resistance to a particular therapy [82, 83]. As several prognostic biomarkers also have predictive significance, the two are combined in the following section.

Tumour-Associated Proteins

CEA

CEA is a mucoprotein that is secreted by CRC cells and detectable within the serum. Although the specificity of CEA for CRC is high, its sensitivity is low, and therefore, CEA is not recommended by the American Society of Clinical Oncology (ASCO) or the European Group on Tumour Markers (EGTM) for screening of CRC [84]. However, measurement of CEA prior to resection of primary disease is recommended by ASCO and EGTM as it provides prognostic information independent of other variables [85, 86] and acts as baseline for subsequent assay [84, 87]. CEA levels prior to resection of liver metastases were also shown to be prognostic for risk of relapse in two large case series [88, 89], while a further study demonstrated that CEA of <30 ng/mL before resection of liver metastases was associated with median survival of 34.8 months, while patients with CEA>30 had median survival of 22 months [90].

Regular determination of CEA is also recommended in follow-up of patients following resection of CRC [84, 87] as a sensitive and cost-effective indicator of recurrence [91–94]. CEA provides no indication of the likelihood of tumour response to therapy and, therefore, has no value as a predictive marker.

Tumour DNA Repair and Chromosomal Instability

Mismatch Repair/Microsatellite Instability

MSI is defined as instability in at least two of five microsatellite markers within the tumour [95]. An association between MSI and favourable prognosis has been detected in several randomised clinical therapeutic trials (RCTs) [96–98] and confirmed in a meta-analysis comprising 7,642 patients, 1,277 of whom had MSI tumours. This demonstrated conclusively that patients with MSI tumours have better overall survival than those with microsatellite stable (MSS) tumours, with hazard ratio for death of 0.65 (95%; CI 0.59–0.71) [99]. Thus, defective MMR is a confirmed prognostic marker in CRC.

Incorporation of FU metabolites into DNA resulting in FU/G mispairs is one of the mechanisms by which the drug exerts its effects. These can be recognised and repaired by proficient MMR machinery [100, 101]. Of four prospective RCTs comparing adjuvant FU with no chemotherapy, two found that chemotherapy benefit was limited to patients with MSI-L or MSS tumours [102, 103], while two found no difference in outcome by tumour MSI status [96, 104]. Provocatively, both the meta-analysis referred to above and more recent meta-analyses have found no evidence of benefit from adjuvant FU chemotherapy in patients with MSI tumours, though small numbers and methodological heterogeneity limit firm conclusions [99, 105, 106]. However, patients with microsatellite unstable advanced CRC respond to FU chemotherapy [107, 108], and currently, the ability of microsatellite instability to predict FU efficacy is unclear. Further complication is created by the incorporation of oxaliplatin and irinotecan into treatment regimens, as preclinical and clinical data indicate that sensitivity to these agents is unaffected by perturbations in MMR apparatus [109–111]. Interestingly, a recent subgroup analysis of the CALGB 89803 adjuvant trial demonstrated improved outcome in patients with MSI-positive resected stage III CRC treated with FOLFIRI compared to patients with MSS tumours [112]. This difference was not seen in patients who received FU. These interesting results merit prospective investigation.

The Eastern Cooperative Oncology Group (ECOG) E5202 trial (ClinicalTrials.gov Identifier: NCT00217737) selects patients with resected stage II CRC according to MSI status and 18q loss of heterozygosity (LOH) (see below). Patients with MSI tumours without LOH are managed with observation alone. This trial has completed accrual and will provide valuable information of the safety of omission of chemotherapy in this patient group.

The 2006 ASCO panel on colorectal tumour markers concluded that although evidence suggested a favourable prognosis in MSI CRC compared to MSS, current data were insufficient to recommend the use of MSI status as a prognostic or predictive marker [84]. However, based upon the available current evidence, MSI is clearly a prognostic biomarker, though its potential role as a predictive biomarker requires clarification.

Chromosomal Instability

Chromosomal instability (CIN) is usually defined as loss and gain of chromosome complement, or structural changes in chromosomes, and is typically measured by flow cytometry. The 2006 ASCO tumour marker guidelines recommended that tumour aneuploidy could not be recommended for prognostication of CRC [84]. Subsequently, a meta-analysis of 10,126 patients in 63 studies has demonstrated unequivocally that CIN is a poor prognostic factor in CRC [113]. CIN was detected in 60% of CRC and was associated with HR for death of 1.45 (95%; CI of 1.35–1.55, $P < 0.001$). The effect was present in both stage II and III disease and independent of adjuvant FU therapy [113].

CIN results in tumour heterogeneity and rapid mutation which could predict for early selection of resistant clones in response to anti-neoplastic therapy [114]. CIN is associated with multidrug resistance in colorectal cell lines, and analysis of informative studies of adjuvant FU is consistent with reduced benefit from therapy in CIN-positive tumours [115]. However, prospective data linking CIN with decreased therapeutic efficacy are currently lacking.

Chromosome 18q Deletion

Deletions of the long arm of chromosome 18 are common in CRC [25] and have been associated with poor prognosis [116]. 18q loss can be detected either by loss of heterozygosity for polymorphic markers [97] or loss of DCC protein by IHC [117]. In addition to DCC, a netrin receptor involved in apoptosis, other candidate tumour suppressors on 18q include the transcription factor *SMAD4* and *SMAD22*. However, the above data are confounded by the association of 18q deletion as a marker of CIN, rather than an independent prognostic variable. 18q loss was used in ECOG E5202 to stratify patients into the poor-risk group who received adjuvant therapy—the results from this study should indicate whether prognosis in patients with stage II disease and retained 18q is sufficiently good to be spared chemotherapy.

Data on 18q loss as predictor of adjuvant chemotherapy benefit are conflicting; studies have suggested that compared with patients with 18q-positive tumours, outcomes are improved [118], no difference [96] or worse [98]. Thus, conclusions regarding the prognostic and predictive role of 18q loss are limited by confounding from CIN and the variable methodology used between studies. 18q loss is not currently recommended for either by the ASCO guidelines [84].

Tumour Apoptosis

P53

TP53 is the most commonly mutated tumour suppressor in human cancer (http://www-p53.iarc. fr/). The incidence of *TP53* mutations in CRC is approximately 40–50% [119], and it is thought to be a late event in adenoma to carcinoma transition [120]. Unfortunately, despite over 100 research papers involving over 18,000 patients

purporting to determine the prognostic effect of *TP53* mutation, no firm conclusions can be drawn from the systematic reviews of the literature [121, 122]. One systematic review showed that patients with abnormal TP53 measured either by immunohistochemistry or mutation were at increased risk of death with relative risk of 1.32 (95%; CI 1.23–1.42) and 1.31 (95%; CI 1.19–1.45), respectively [122]. This study also suggested that the risk associated with abnormal TP53 was greater in patients at lower risk of relapse. However, studies were heterogeneous, and TP53 status is not presently recommended in prognostication by most authorities [84]. The largest meta-analysis showed no effect of TP53 status on benefit from chemotherapy [122].

Tumour Proliferation

Ki67 Proliferative Index

A number of studies have assayed the role of CRC proliferative index in prognostication. Results are mixed; of ten studies using flow cytometry identified by the 2006 ASCO guidelines, five found that the percentage of cells in S phase was an independent prognostic factor, and five did not [84]. Thus, proliferative index in primary CRC cannot be recommended as prognostic at present.

Tumour Signalling Transduction

Like many other malignancies, activation of the MAPK and PI3K-AKT pathways due to mutation of multiple intermediates is near universal in CRC. Consequently, the prognostic and predictive import of these mutations has been the subject of intensive study.

EGFR

EGFR is the cell surface receptor for extracellular ligands from the neuregulin family [64] and is the target of the monoclonal antibodies cetuximab and panitumumab. EGFR is overexpressed in 40–80% of CRC, and overexpression generally appears to correlate with poor prognosis, though as studies are small and retrospective, the potential for publication bias is high [123–128]. Data linking an R497K polymorphism in EGFR—which results in decreased ligand binding and downstream pathway activation—to improved outcome require validation [129].

Interestingly, despite predictions, cetuximab efficacy does not correlate with levels of *EGFR* expression [66, 67, 130]. While increased *EGFR* copy number does correlate with response to EGFR targeting [131–134], its predictive ability is not sufficient to recommend its use as a biomarker at present [135]. Additionally, in contradistinction to non-small cell lung cancer, *EGFR* mutations do not predict anti-EGFR efficacy in CRC [136]. Recent retrospective data suggest that an *EGFR* A61G polymorphism may correlate with cetuximab efficacy in *KRAS* wild-type tumours, with increased response rate and overall survival in A/G heterozygote patients compared to homozygotes [137], though these data require confirmation.

EGFR overexpression cannot currently be recommended in prognostication and has no role in predicting cetuximab efficacy. The prognostic and predictive value of *EGFR* polymorphisms requires prospective validation.

KRAS

Point mutations in *KRAS* at codons 12, 13 and 61 occur in 30–40% of CRCs and are an early event in the adenoma–carcinoma sequence [75, 138]. These result in abrogation of KRAS GTPase activity with constitutive activation of the protein and downstream MAPK and PI3K-AKT pathways [139].

The role of *KRAS* mutations in CRC prognosis has been extensively investigated with mixed results. Though a large early study suggested that *KRAS* mutation is associated with poorer outcome, this finding was restricted to the G12V substitution and stage III disease only [138]. Although a subsequent study has also linked *KRAS* mutation with poor prognosis [140], several

large RCTs have found no correlation with survival [33, 121, 141, 142]. Thus, presently, there is no clear evidence that *KRAS* mutation is an independent prognostic factor in CRC, though emerging data suggest that it may predict for lung metastases at relapse [143].

KRAS mutations are predicted to cause constitutive activation of downstream pathways irrespective of RTK activation. Consequently, therapeutic approaches targeting RTKs may be futile in the presence of *KRAS* mutation. Conclusive demonstration that this is the case for the anti-EGFR monoclonal antibodies cetuximab and panitumumab in CRC has been provided by several RCTs [68, 69, 144–147]. In a recent systematic review, anti-EGFR therapy in patients with *KRAS* mutant tumours was shown to confer no significant benefit in progression-free or overall survival, in contrast to patients with *KRAS* wild-type tumours, in whom anti-EGFR treatment resulted in significant improvement in both parameters [148]. *KRAS* mutation is a highly specific negative biomarker of response to anti-EGFR therapy (specificity 93%), though its sensitivity is limited (47%), indicating the existence of additional resistance mechanisms [149]. Consequently, *KRAS* mutation testing is indicated for all patients being considered for anti-EGFR therapy [150]. Interestingly, a small number of patients with *KRAS*-mutated tumours respond to anti-EGFR therapies, possibly due to the particular codon or residues substituted [145, 151]. Though this does not affect current guidelines, further research is warranted. *KRAS* mutation does not predict response to cytotoxic therapy in the absence of anti-EGFR agents [152].

BRAF

BRAF is a serine–threonine kinase directly downstream of KRAS in the MAPK pathway. Mutations in *BRAF*, almost universally a valine to glutamic acid substitution at residue 600 (V600E), activate the MAPK pathway and are mutually exclusive with *KRAS* mutation [32, 76]. *BRAF* mutations are found in 5–10% of CRC overall, but at much higher frequency (40–60%)

in MSI tumours [75, 76, 140, 153, 154]. *BRAF* mutation appears to be associated with shorter survival in the context of advanced disease [76, 140, 154–157], though data on MSI tumours are conflicting [156]. Similar to *KRAS*, mutant *BRAF* is associated with lack of response to anti-EGFR therapy, indicating that it may be MAPK pathway activation that confers resistance [75, 158]. *BRAF* mutation (V600E) testing is likely to become commonplace in clinical practice over the coming years [135]. As discussed previously, although the remarkable results of targeting V600E mutant BRAF in melanoma have not been reproduced in early-phase studies of CRC, further research is ongoing.

NRAS

NRAS is a further member of the RAS family of oncogenes that also functions as a signal transducer downstream of EGFR. *NRAS* mutations have been detected in 2–5% of CRC [159, 160]. Emerging data indicate that *NRAS* mutation confers resistance to anti-EGFR therapy, though patient numbers are small [75].

PIK3CA

PIK3CA encodes the p100α catalytic subunit of PI3K [161]. Mutations typically occur at three hotspots (two in exon 9, one in exon 20) and render the protein constitutively active, resulting in activation of the PI3K-AKT pathway. *PIK3CA* mutations are found in 13–15% of CRC [72, 75, 162]. Data on the prognostic significance of *PIK3CA* mutation are limited, though a recent prospective study showed an association of mutation with poor prognosis in patients who had undergone curative resection. Interestingly, this effect was stronger in patients with *KRAS* wild-type tumours [162]. These interesting data require further analysis.

An emerging body of literature indicates that *PIK3CA* mutation in the context of wild-type *KRAS* and *BRAF* is predictive of lack of response to anti-EGFR therapy. However, data are not uniform and the relationship is not as strong as for *KRAS* or *BRAF* mutation [75, 163, 164]. Interestingly, in one study, only mutations in exon 20 predicted resistance to anti-EGFR therapy [75].

PTEN

PTEN is a lipid phosphatase and key negative regulator of the PI3K pathway. *PTEN* is mutated or epigenetically silenced in approximately 20% of CRC [155]. Data regarding the significance of PTEN as prognostic marker are conflicting [144, 155]. Though results are not universal, loss of PTEN by IHC appears to predict lack of benefit from anti-EGFR therapy [144, 164, 165]. Unfortunately, PTEN IHC is challenging, and standardisation of methodology is likely to be required for prospective studies in order to draw firm conclusions.

IGF2

IGF2 is an imprinted, paternally expressed growth factor which signals via IGF1R to activate the PI3K-AKT and MAPK pathways [166]. Regulation of *IGF2* expression is complex and involves an imprinting control region (ICR) and additional differentially methylated regions (DMRs) within the gene locus [167]. Loss of imprinting (LOI) of *IGF2* with biallelic expression is common in CRC and is detectable in the normal adjacent mucosa [168, 169]. A recent study has shown that *IGF2* DMR0 hypomethylation correlates with LOI and also demonstrated that DMR0 hypomethylation was associated with higher mortality in 1,033 patients in two prospective cohort studies [170]. These interesting results require validation in a prospective RCT.

Pharmacogenetics and Therapeutic Efficacy

The three principal cytotoxic drugs used in the management of CRC are all metabolised with differing efficiencies depending on germline

9 Colorectal Cancer

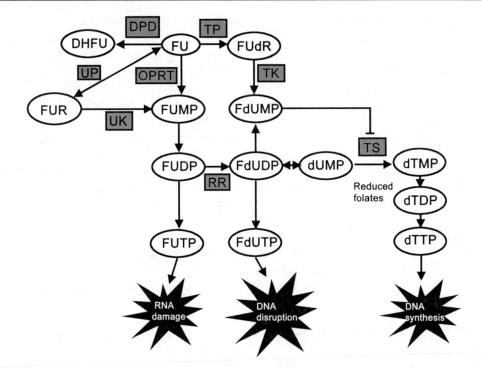

Fig. 9.3 5-Fluorouracil metabolism and variants. 5-Fluorouracil (FU) is converted into three principal active metabolites: fluorodeoxyuridine monophosphate (FdUMP), fluorodeoxyuridine triphosphate (FdUTP) and fluorouridine triphosphate (FUTP). Inhibition of thymidylate synthetase (TS) by FdUMP is an important mechanism of FU action and is enhanced by the presence of the reduced folate 5,10-methylenetetrahydrofolate. High intratumoral concentrations of TS are associated with poor prognosis and decreased benefit from FU. Incorporation of FdUTP into DNA also contributes to cytotoxicity, though may require an intact mismatch repair system to detect the modified base. Incorporation of FUTP into RNA disrupts normal processing and function and leads to toxicity through several mechanisms. The main mechanism of FU catabolism is by conversion to dihydrofluorouracil (DHFU) via the action of dihydropyrimidine dehydrogenase (DPD). Germline variants in the DPD activity are associated with FU toxicity. *dTMP* deoxythymidine monophosphate, *dTTP* deoxythymidine triphosphate, *dUMP* deoxyuridine monophosphate, *FdUDP* fluorodeoxyuridine diphosphate, *FUDP* fluorouridine diphosphate, *FUdR* fluorodeoxyuridine, *FUMP* fluorouridine monophosphate, *FUR* 5-fluorouridine, *OPRT* uridine monophosphate synthetase, *RR* ribonucleotide reductase, *TK* thymidine kinase, *TP* thymidine phosphorylase, *UK* uridine kinase, *UP* uridine phosphorylase

polymorphisms present in the population. As these result in varying exposure of patients to active drug, they may lead to differences in therapeutic efficacy and toxicity. As it has been in clinical practice for the longest duration, most of the available data pertain to FU, the metabolism of which is complex and summarised in Fig. 9.3. Most information on targeted therapies has focused on tumour resistance mechanisms, though emerging studies suggest that germline variants may also contribute to response.

Thymidylate Synthase

Thymidylate synthetase (TS) catalyses the formation of thymidylate, required for DNA replication and repair, and is thought to be the principal target for the main active metabolite of FU, fluorodeoxyuridine monophosphate (5-fdUMP). A systematic review and meta-analysis showed poorer overall survival patients with high tumour TS expression in both the adjuvant and metastatic settings. Interestingly, the prognostic effect of high TS was greatest in patients who did not receive chemotherapy [171]. TS expression is determined by germline polymorphisms—a variable tandem repeat in the promoter and a 6 base pair (6 bp) insertion and deletion polymorphism in the 3′ UTR. Approximately one quarter of the Caucasian population is homozygous for a double repeat (2R/2R) in the promoter, one quarter homozygous for a triple repeat (3R/3R) and half are heterozygous [172]. Although the 3R/3R repeat does not affect the level of TS mRNA, it is associated with significantly higher levels of TS protein [173]. The 6-bp deletion polymorphism in the 3′ UTR decreases mRNA stability and results in lower intratumoral TS expression [174]. Both preclinical and clinical evidence indicate that high TS correlates with decreased benefit from FU [171, 172, 175, 176].

Methyltetrahydrofolate Reductase

Methyltetrahydrofolate reductase (MTHFR) catalyses the irreversible conversion of 5-10-methylenetetrahydrofolate (5,10-mTHF) to 5-methyltetrahydrofolate (5-mTHF), thus reducing levels of the former, an essential cofactor in the conversion of deoxyuridine monophosphate to deoxythymidine monophosphate by TS. Two polymorphisms within *MTHFR* have been demonstrated to have functional significance: a C677T polymorphism associated with reduced enzymatic activity [177] and increased sensitivity to FU [178] and to a lesser degree an A1298C polymorphism. Though initial data suggested that *MTHFR* 677T polymorphism was associated increased sensitivity to FU [179, 180], other studies have detected no difference in outcome [181, 182]. Interestingly, a recent study suggests that favourable *MTHFR* polymorphisms predict response to FOLFOX in advanced CRC [183]. Both polymorphisms appear to predict capecitabine and FOLFOX toxicity [184, 185].

Thymidine Phosphorylase

Thymidine phosphorylase (TP) catalyses the conversion of FU to the active metabolite FUdR.

Data on its role as a biomarker are conflicting, however, as studies have suggested that high TP expression may either decrease [186] or not affect FU activation [187]. Further complication is afforded by the additional function of TP in promotion of angiogenesis—reflected in its alternative name, platelet-derived endothelial cell growth factor [188–191]. Though higher levels of TP in tumours have been associated with more extensive angiogenesis [192] and poorer outcome [191, 193, 194], firm conclusions cannot be drawn at present.

Dihydropyrimidine Dehydrogenase

Dihydropyrimidine dehydrogenase (DPD) is the principal enzyme in FU catabolism [195]. Levels of DPD in the population vary—3–5% of people are partially and 0.2% are completely DPD deficient. DPD deficiency results in the accumulation of active drug and is associated with FU toxicity [196]. However, the association of over 30 polymorphisms with DPD deficiency precludes screening for this prior to FU therapy [197]. Several studies have shown an inverse correlation between tumour DPD expression and survival following adjuvant FU treatment for CRC [198–200], while another study has shown that high FU clearance predicts poorer outcome in this context [201]. However, this requires confirmation.

Oxaliplatin Sensitivity

Reduced sensitivity to oxaliplatin has been linked to decreased tumour penetration, increased detoxification and increased removal of platinum DNA adducts by proficient repair mechanisms. Glutathione S-transferases are a family of enzymes that target drugs for excretion by conjugation with glutathione. GSTP1 targets platinum derivatives, including oxaliplatin for this process. Polymorphisms in GSTP1—I105V and A114V—result in decreased activity and have been associated with improved outcome and increased neuropathy after oxaliplatin treatment [202–205], though other studies have shown no correlation with either toxicity or outcome [206, 207]. Enhanced removal of platinum DNA adducts by nucleotide excision repair (NER) machinery would be predicted to result in decreased therapeutic efficacy. A recent systematic review of 17 published studies comprising 1,787 patients showed that polymorphisms in two NER genes, *ERCC1* C11615T and *ERCC2* T13181G, were predictive of substantial reduction in oxaliplatin effect (HR for survival 2.03 and 1.42, respectively) [208]. These interesting results require prospective validation.

Irinotecan Sensitivity

The active metabolite of irinotecan, SN38 is conjugated and detoxified by UDP-glucuronosyltransferase (UGT1A1). The *UGT1A1* promoter is polymorphic, with variation in the number of repeats of a TATA element, with increasing repeat number associated with decrease in enzyme activity—homozygosity for the 7-repeat allele, referred to as *UGT1A1*28*, is associated with significantly increased risk of toxicity from irinotecan, particularly at higher doses [205, 209, 210]. Though testing for the *UGT1A1*28* polymorphism was approved by the FDA in patients prior to irinotecan therapy, use has been patchy, possibly as a result of the decreased toxicity associated with lower irinotecan doses in combination regimens.

Determinants of Response/Toxicity to Targeted Therapies

Activation of antibody-dependent cell-mediated cytotoxicity (ADCC) contributes substantially to the therapeutic effect of trastuzumab and rituximab [211]. FcγR polymorphisms modify the killing function of effector immune cells and are associated with tumour response in patients treated with these agents. Although it appears clear that the predominant mechanisms of resistance to anti-EGFR monoclonal antibodies are tumour intrinsic, small studies have shown that FcγR polymorphisms

(*FCGR2A*-H131R and *FCGR3A*-V158F) are associated with cetuximab response [212, 213]. Although these interesting results suggest that ADCC contributes to cetuximab efficacy, they require prospective confirmation.

Emerging Platforms in Biomarker Analysis

Though yet to fully translate into advances in the clinic, high-throughput arrays and other emerging technologies provide hugely powerful platforms for analysis of tumours and facilitate a shift from hypothesis-driven research to unbiased interrogation of the whole genome, transcriptome and proteome (Fig. 9.4) [214–217]. With the rapidly decreasing cost and increasing capacity of next generation sequencing, it is likely in the not too distant future both mutational and expression analysis of tumours will be feasible on an individual patient basis [218]. The enormous amounts of data generated by these technologies pose significant logistical and statistical challenges to analysis and require careful experimental design for accurate biomarker identification and validation.

Gene-Expression Signatures

The first published gene signature in CRC was published in 2004 [219]. Based on analysis of 31 relapses in 71 patients, Wang et al. proposed a 23-gene prognostic signature as identifying patients likely to develop recurrent disease. However, validation of this set showed that this performed little better than chance (67% positive predictive value), and the same group demonstrated in a larger cohort that a reduced signature of seven genes performed better in an enlarged patient cohort [220]. Further small studies have also generated prognostic signatures in stage II and III CRC [221, 222]. Escherisch et al. analysed adenomas and stage II–IV CRC by microarray. They generated a 43-gene signature that was superior to TNM staging in prediction 36-month overall survival and validated this in an independent

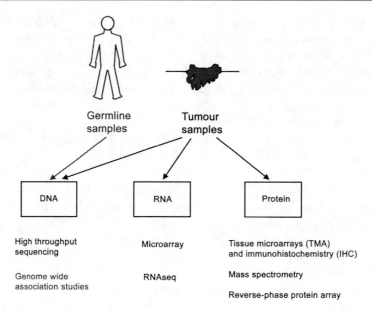

Fig. 9.4 High-throughput methodologies in colorectal cancer. Emerging platforms in the diagnosis and investigation of CRC include assays of change in genetic sequence, gene expression and protein expression. Most advanced in clinical development are gene-expression signatures (Onco*type* DX®, ColoPrint®), which use either RT-qPCR or microarray technology to assay the relative expression of hundreds to thousands of genes within tumour samples. By generation of prognostic and predictive signatures, these seek to enable individualised therapy by stratification of patients according to risk of relapse and likelihood of benefit from therapy. The rapid progress in sequencing technology is likely to permit the mutational analysis of tumours in the next few years, while RNAseq combines expression analysis with mutational detection of the transcriptome. Genome-wide association studies (GWAS) have been used to identify single nucleotide polymorphisms (SNPs) that confer increased risk of developing CRC and, more recently, to predict outcome. Proteomics provides several powerful platforms for tumour analysis, including high-throughput immunohistochemistry (IHC) via tissue microarrays (TMA) and mass-spectrometric approaches

cohort of 95 patients [223]. However, again, this awaits large-scale validation.

Recently, O'Connell et al. have published a recurrence score generated from 1,851 formalin-fixed, paraffin-embedded tumour samples from patients with stage II/III CRC enrolled in NSABP adjuvant trials C-01/C-02/C-04/C-06 and a cohort of untreated patients from the Cleveland Clinic. They performed reverse transcriptase quantitative PCR (RT-qPCR) for 761 candidate genes and found 48 genes significantly associated with recurrence and 66 predictive of FU benefit [224]. From these, they selected seven recurrence genes, six FU-benefit genes and five internal reference genes, and validated them in 1,436 patients with stage II CRC from the QUASAR trial. This 12-gene recurrence signature (commercially available as Onco*type* DX®) predicted recurrence risk ($P=0.004$) and retained significance ($P=0.008$) in multivariate analysis independent of MSI status, T-stage, tumour grade and lymphovascular invasion [225]. This recurrence score has also been shown to be prognostic in stage III disease [226]. Another group analysed fresh frozen tissue from 188 patients with stage I–IV CRC by microarray and generated an 18-gene signature (ColoPrint®). This was then validated in an independent dataset or 206 tumours. Classification of patients into low and high risk by the signature correlated with 5-year relapse-free survival of 87.6 and 67.2%, with hazard ratio of 2.5 (95% CI, 1.33–4.73; $P=0.005$), and the signature retained significance in multivariate analysis (HR=3.34; $P=0.017$) [227]. The PARSC trial seeks to compare the ColoPrint® signature with current prognostic factors in prediction of relapse in patients with resected stage II CRC and is currently recruiting [228]. However, practically speaking, the collection and storage of good quality fresh frozen tissue that is viable for this screening assessment is a huge challenge. A 33-gene signature has been generated from the NSABP C-07 trial using Illumina arrays and division of the study population into equally sized training and validation subsets. Classification of patients into low- and high-risk groups by the index predicated recurrence at 5 years (82.6% disease free vs. 64.3% disease free, $P<0.001$). Notably, the authors demonstrated that although the relative benefit from the addition of oxaliplatin to FU was similar in both risk categories, the absolute risk reduction from combination therapy was small enough in the low-risk group to be of questionable benefit [229]. These interesting results await further validation.

High-throughput platforms have substantial promise in the identification of patients likely to benefit from individual therapies, though this remains challenging due to the large sample sizes required in studies. In addition to the 6-gene FU benefit signature predictor referred to above, small studies have attempted to generate signatures predictive of therapeutic response. A small study generated a 14-gene signature predictive of FOLFIRI response in mCRC by microarray profiling of snap-frozen tissue [230]. Though this identified all responding patients, the study lacked an independent validation set, and, therefore, requires confirmation. Microarray analysis has also been used to predict response to cetuximab [231], and interestingly, the response signature overlaps significantly with the KRAS mutation signature [232].

Genome-Wide Association Studies

SNP array-based genome-wide association studies (GWAS) have proven a powerful platform for the discovery of CRC susceptibility loci [5, 6]. Functional SNPs in genes encoding kinases and cell cycle-associated proteins may be predicted to alter tumour phenotype and thus outcome. Though large numbers are required to gain suffi-

cient power to detect modifiers, one study in CRC has been reported in abstract form. In this, samples from 947 patients with stage II/III CRC were typed at 309,200 SNPs and analysed by Cox regression. Thirty-three SNPs were further analysed in three additional patient cohorts comprising 2,213 patients. In the final meta-analysis, one SNP met the significance level. This polymorphism, located near a gene that regulates cell motility and invasion conferred an HR for relapse of 1.46 (95%; CI 1.10–1.94) [233]. Based upon this analysis, it is unlikely that SNPs conferring HR>2.0 exist, though further studies may define lower risk loci.

Proteomics

Proteomics provides a powerful platform for the simultaneous analysis of multiple tumour-associated proteins. Mass spectrometry may be performed on serum or primary tumour tissue, and antibody-based approaches include IHC and reverse-phase protein array (RPPA). With the exception of IHC, methodologies are in a relatively early stage of development. Small studies using mass spectrometry have demonstrated characteristic tumour-associated and serum signatures [234, 235] that have promise in early CRC diagnosis. However, these require validation in large prospective studies. The advent of tissue microarrays (TMA) and automated image analysis enables high-throughput analysis of tumour protein expression [236]. These technologies have been utilised in CRC to demonstrate that intratumoral T-cell infiltration is associated with favourable prognosis, with superior prognostic value than TNM staging [237, 238]. The same group have recently published an additional retrospective study confirming these results [239], and this finding merits prospective confirmation. RPPA enables evaluation of pathway activation by quantification of phosphoproteins within tumours and has been utilised in CRC in small studies [240, 241].

While incorporation of proteomic analysis of tumours into routine clinical practice is unlikely to occur within the next few years, the technology has substantial promise to contribute to CRC detection and management in the future.

Conclusions

The duration for which validated biomarkers have been clinically utilised in CRC varies from greater than three decades in the case of CEA to less than 5 years for *KRAS* mutation testing. During this period, myriad other biomarkers have been postulated in small, retrospective studies, without confirmation in larger retrospective or prospective cohorts. This emphasises the requirement for evaluation of biomarkers in well-designed prospective clinical trials, where the potential for bias is minimised. Several approaches have been postulated to incorporate biomarker studies into clinical trial design in order to expedite biomarker validation and adoption into clinical practice [242]. A summary of the LOE supporting the use of selected established and emerging biomarkers is presented in Table 9.2. Currently, the evidence supports the use of only three of the many biomarkers discussed above in routine CRC clinical practice. A further two categories of biomarker are promising, but require additional validation before adoption into patient care (Table 9.3, Fig. 9.5).

Furthermore, the significance of individual CRC biomarkers has been reappraised and refined in light of increased understanding of tumour biology over recent years. For example, 18q deletion appears to be a surrogate for CIN rather than an independent prognostic factor, while the precise prognostic significance of *BRAF* V600E mutation requires clarification given its association with microsatellite instability. It is plausible that

Table 9.2 Levels of evidence supporting biomarker studies

Biomarker	Context	Valid biomarker	Level of evidence	Recommended by ASCO/ESMO guidelines
Serum carcinoembryonic antigen (CEA)	Prognosis	Yes	I	Yes
	Predictive	No	I	No
Microsatellite instability	Prognosis in stage II disease	Yes	I	ESMO only
	Predictive (FU benefit)	Unclear	NA	No
Chromosomal instability	Prognosis	Yes	I	No
	Predictive (FU benefit)	Unclear	NA	No
KRAS mutation	Prognostic	No	II	No
	Predictive (anti-EGFR therapy)	Yes	I	Yes
Gene-expression signatures	Prognostic (stage II)	Emerging	II	No
	Predictive (FU benefit)	Emerging	II	No

Table 9.3 Biomarkers supported by current clinical evidence and likely to be validated in the near future

Use supported by current evidence

Microsatellite instability in stage II CRC with T3 primary tumours. Patients with MSI^H tumours have excellent prognosis and are unlikely to benefit from adjuvant chemotherapy

KRAS mutation testing in patients considered for anti-EGFR therapy. Patients with *KRAS* mutant tumours do not benefit from cetuximab or panitumumab, and therapy should be reserved for patients with *KRAS* wild-type tumours

CEA testing prior to resection of primary tumour or liver metastases as an indicator of prognosis, and in follow-up following resection of the primary tumour in patients who would be considered for surgery should metastases develop

Likely to be validated in near future

Gene-expression signatures for prognostication in stage II disease (Onco*type* DX®, ColoPrint®)

BRAF, *NRAS* and *PIK3CA* mutation testing for prediction of benefit from anti-EGFR therapy

9 Colorectal Cancer

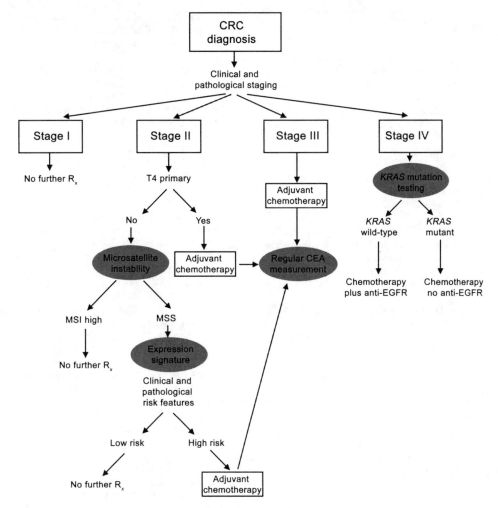

Fig. 9.5 Recommendations for biomarker-informed management of CRC. Evidence-based algorithm incorporating biomarkers for management of CRC. Patients with stage I disease have less than 10% chance of relapse and require no further therapy. Patients with stage II disease have variable prognosis; T4 stage of the primary tumour is the most significant pathological factor, and patients with T4 disease should be offered adjuvant chemotherapy if appropriate. Patients with MSI-high T3 tumours without nodal involvement have good prognosis, appear less likely to benefit from adjuvant chemotherapy and should be observed only (level I evidence). MSS T3 tumours should be stratified according to further pathological criteria—grade, vascular invasion—and are good candidates for gene-expression analysis of tumour to determine prognosis and inform therapy (level II evidence). All patients at significant risk of relapse (excluding stage I disease and low-risk stage II) require regular CEA measurement as part of follow-up, with the exception of patients who are not candidates for therapy at relapse (level I evidence). All patients with stage IV disease being considered for anti-EGFR therapy require *KRAS* mutation testing on tumours, with therapy not indicated if *KRAS* mutant (level I evidence)

additional markers will be discovered to co-segregate when analysed in toto.

Building on the bedrock outlined above, high-throughput technologies promise to enhance biomarker discovery and validation and have the potential to enable truly individualised therapies for patients with CRC. Perhaps the greatest challenge will be the integration of data from multiple analyses and platforms—germline and tumour genomic, proteomic, immunologic—to facilitate this. High-quality collaborations between basic scientists and clinicians and well-designed clinical trials are essential over the coming years if we are to achieve this aim.

References

1. Ferlay J, Shin HR, Bray F, Forman D, Mathers C, Parkin DM. Estimates of worldwide burden of cancer in 2008: GLOBOCAN 2008. Int J Cancer. 2010; 127(12):2893–917.
2. Lynch HT, de la Chapelle A. Hereditary colorectal cancer. N Engl J Med. 2003;348(10):919–32.
3. Barrow E, Alduaij W, Robinson L, et al. Colorectal cancer in HNPCC: cumulative lifetime incidence, survival and tumour distribution. A report of 121 families with proven mutations. Clin Genet. 2008;74(3):233–42.
4. Aarnio M, Sankila R, Pukkala E, et al. Cancer risk in mutation carriers of DNA-mismatch-repair genes. Int J Cancer. 1999;81(2):214–8.
5. Houlston RS, Cheadle J, Dobbins SE, et al. Meta-analysis of three genome-wide association studies identifies susceptibility loci for colorectal cancer at 1q41, 3q26.2, 12q13.13 and 20q13.33. Nat Genet. 2010;42(11):973–7.
6. Houlston RS, Webb E, Broderick P, et al. Meta-analysis of genome-wide association data identifies four new susceptibility loci for colorectal cancer. Nat Genet. 2008;40(12):1426–35.
7. Giovannucci E. Epidemiologic studies of folate and colorectal neoplasia: a review. J Nutr. 2002;132(8 Suppl):2350S–5.
8. Cole BF, Baron JA, Sandler RS, et al. Folic acid for the prevention of colorectal adenomas: a randomized clinical trial. JAMA. 2007;297(21):2351–9.
9. Logan RF, Grainge MJ, Shepherd VC, Armitage NC, Muir KR. Aspirin and folic acid for the prevention of recurrent colorectal adenomas. Gastroenterology. 2008;134(1):29–38.
10. Baron JA, Beach M, Mandel JS, et al. Calcium supplements for the prevention of colorectal adenomas. Calcium Polyp Prevention Study Group. N Engl J Med. 1999;340(2):101–7.
11. Grau MV, Baron JA, Sandler RS, et al. Prolonged effect of calcium supplementation on risk of colorectal adenomas in a randomized trial. J Natl Cancer Inst. 2007;99(2):129–36.
12. Cho E, Smith-Warner SA, Spiegelman D, et al. Dairy foods, calcium, and colorectal cancer: a pooled analysis of 10 cohort studies. J Natl Cancer Inst. 2004;96(13):1015–22.
13. Giovannucci E. An updated review of the epidemiological evidence that cigarette smoking increases risk of colorectal cancer. Cancer Epidemiol Biomarkers Prev. 2001;10(7):725–31.
14. Liang PS, Chen TY, Giovannucci E. Cigarette smoking and colorectal cancer incidence and mortality: systematic review and meta-analysis. Int J Cancer. 2009;124(10):2406–15.
15. Boutron-Ruault MC, Senesse P, Meance S, Belghiti C, Faivre J. Energy intake, body mass index, physical activity, and the colorectal adenoma-carcinoma sequence. Nutr Cancer. 2001;39(1):50–7.
16. Giovannucci E, Ascherio A, Rimm EB, Colditz GA, Stampfer MJ, Willett WC. Physical activity, obesity, and risk for colon cancer and adenoma in men. Ann Intern Med. 1995;122(5):327–34.
17. Wolin KY, Yan Y, Colditz GA, Lee IM. Physical activity and colon cancer prevention: a meta-analysis. Br J Cancer. 2009;100(4):611–6.
18. Flossmann E, Rothwell PM. Effect of aspirin on long-term risk of colorectal cancer: consistent evidence from randomised and observational studies. Lancet. 2007;369(9573):1603–13.
19. Din FV, Theodoratou E, Farrington SM, et al. Effect of aspirin and NSAIDs on risk and survival from colorectal cancer. Gut. 2010;59:1670–9.
20. Rothwell PM, Wilson M, Elwin CE, et al. Long-term effect of aspirin on colorectal cancer incidence and mortality: 20-year follow-up of five randomised trials. Lancet. 2010;376(9754):1741–50.
21. O'Connell JB, Maggard MA, Ko CY. Colon cancer survival rates with the new American Joint Committee on Cancer sixth edition staging. J Natl Cancer Inst. 2004;96(19):1420–5.
22. Compton CC, Fielding LP, Burgart LJ, et al. Prognostic factors in colorectal cancer. College of American Pathologists Consensus Statement 1999. Arch Pathol Lab Med. 2000;124(7):979–94.
23. Gonzalez-Garcia I, Moreno V, Navarro M, et al. Standardized approach for microsatellite instability detection in colorectal carcinomas. J Natl Cancer Inst. 2000;92(7):544–9.
24. Lothe RA, Peltomaki P, Meling GI, et al. Genomic instability in colorectal cancer: relationship to clinicopathological variables and family history. Cancer Res. 1993;53(24):5849–52.
25. Vogelstein B, Fearon ER, Hamilton SR, et al. Genetic alterations during colorectal-tumor development. N Engl J Med. 1988;319(9):525–32.
26. Taipale J, Beachy PA. The Hedgehog and Wnt signalling pathways in cancer. Nature. 2001;411(6835):349–54.
27. Markowitz SD, Bertagnolli MM. Molecular origins of cancer: molecular basis of colorectal cancer. N Engl J Med. 2009;361(25):2449–60.
28. Sjoblom T, Jones S, Wood LD, et al. The consensus coding sequences of human breast and colorectal cancers. Science. 2006;314(5797):268–74.
29. Parsons R, Myeroff LL, Liu B, et al. Microsatellite instability and mutations of the transforming growth factor beta type II receptor gene in colorectal cancer. Cancer Res. 1995;55(23):5548–50.
30. Souza RF, Appel R, Yin J, et al. Microsatellite instability in the insulin-like growth factor II receptor gene in gastrointestinal tumours. Nat Genet. 1996;14(3):255–7.
31. Rampino N, Yamamoto H, Ionov Y, et al. Somatic frameshift mutations in the BAX gene in colon cancers of the microsatellite mutator phenotype. Science. 1997;275(5302):967–9.
32. Rajagopalan H, Bardelli A, Lengauer C, Kinzler KW, Vogelstein B, Velculescu VE. Tumorigenesis:

RAF/RAS oncogenes and mismatch-repair status. Nature. 2002;418(6901):934.

33. Roth AD, Tejpar S, Delorenzi M, et al. Prognostic role of KRAS and BRAF in stage II and III resected colon cancer: results of the translational study on the PETACC-3, EORTC 40993, SAKK 60-00 trial. J Clin Oncol. 2010;28(3):466–74.

34. Potocnik U, Glavac D, Golouh R, Ravnik-Glavac M. Causes of microsatellite instability in colorectal tumors: implications for hereditary non-polyposis colorectal cancer screening. Cancer Genet Cytogenet. 2001;126(2):85–96.

35. Herman JG, Umar A, Polyak K, et al. Incidence and functional consequences of hMLH1 promoter hypermethylation in colorectal carcinoma. Proc Natl Acad Sci USA. 1998;95(12):6870–5.

36. Young J, Leggett B, Gustafson C, et al. Genomic instability occurs in colorectal carcinomas but not in adenomas. Hum Mutat. 1993;2(5):351–4.

37. Risio M, Reato G, di Celle PF, Fizzotti M, Rossini FP, Foa R. Microsatellite instability is associated with the histological features of the tumor in nonfamilial colorectal cancer. Cancer Res. 1996;56(23):5470–4.

38. Salahshor S, Kressner U, Fischer H, et al. Microsatellite instability in sporadic colorectal cancer is not an independent prognostic factor. Br J Cancer. 1999;81(2):190–3.

39. Labianca R, Nordlinger B, Beretta GD, Brouquet A, Cervantes A. Primary colon cancer: ESMO Clinical Practice Guidelines for diagnosis, adjuvant treatment and follow-up. Ann Oncol. 2010;21 Suppl 5:v70–7.

40. Goldberg RM, Fleming TR, Tangen CM, et al. Surgery for recurrent colon cancer: strategies for identifying resectable recurrence and success rates after resection. Eastern Cooperative Oncology Group, the North Central Cancer Treatment Group, and the Southwest Oncology Group. Ann Intern Med. 1998;129(1):27–35.

41. Fong Y, Cohen AM, Fortner JG, et al. Liver resection for colorectal metastases. J Clin Oncol. 1997;15(3):938–46.

42. Glimelius B, Pahlman L, Cervantes A. Rectal cancer: ESMO Clinical Practice Guidelines for diagnosis, treatment and follow-up. Ann Oncol. 2010;21 Suppl 5:v82–6.

43. Stangl R, Altendorf-Hofmann A, Charnley RM, Scheele J. Factors influencing the natural history of colorectal liver metastases. Lancet. 1994;343(8910):1405–10.

44. Simmonds PCC. Palliative chemotherapy for advanced colorectal cancer: systematic review and meta-analysis. Colorectal Cancer Collaborative Group. BMJ. 2000;321(7260):531–5.

45. Saltz LB, Cox JV, Blanke C, et al. Irinotecan plus fluorouracil and leucovorin for metastatic colorectal cancer. Irinotecan Study Group. N Engl J Med. 2000;343(13):905–14.

46. de Gramont A, Figer A, Seymour M, et al. Leucovorin and fluorouracil with or without oxaliplatin as first-line treatment in advanced colorectal cancer. J Clin Oncol. 2000;18(16):2938–47.

47. Grothey A, Sargent D, Goldberg RM, Schmoll HJ. Survival of patients with advanced colorectal cancer improves with the availability of fluorouracil-leucovorin, irinotecan, and oxaliplatin in the course of treatment. J Clin Oncol. 2004;22(7):1209–14.

48. Hoff PM, Ansari R, Batist G, et al. Comparison of oral capecitabine versus intravenous fluorouracil plus leucovorin as first-line treatment in 605 patients with metastatic colorectal cancer: results of a randomized phase III study. J Clin Oncol. 2001;19(8):2282–92.

49. Cassidy J, Clarke S, Diaz-Rubio E, et al. Randomized phase III study of capecitabine plus oxaliplatin compared with fluorouracil/folinic acid plus oxaliplatin as first-line therapy for metastatic colorectal cancer. J Clin Oncol. 2008;26(12):2006–12.

50. Efficacy of adjuvant fluorouracil and folinic acid in colon cancer. International Multicentre Pooled Analysis of Colon Cancer Trials (IMPACT) investigators. Lancet. 1995;345(8955):939–44.

51. Andre T, Boni C, Navarro M, et al. Improved overall survival with oxaliplatin, fluorouracil, and leucovorin as adjuvant treatment in stage II or III colon cancer in the MOSAIC trial. J Clin Oncol. 2009;27(19):3109–16.

52. Kuebler JP, Wieand HS, O'Connell MJ, et al. Oxaliplatin combined with weekly bolus fluorouracil and leucovorin as surgical adjuvant chemotherapy for stage II and III colon cancer: results from NSABP C-07. J Clin Oncol. 2007;25(16):2198–204.

53. Saltz LB, Niedzwiecki D, Hollis D, et al. Irinotecan fluorouracil plus leucovorin is not superior to fluorouracil plus leucovorin alone as adjuvant treatment for stage III colon cancer: results of CALGB 89803. J Clin Oncol. 2007;25(23):3456–61.

54. Van Cutsem E, Labianca R, Bodoky G, et al. Randomized phase III trial comparing biweekly infusional fluorouracil/leucovorin alone or with irinotecan in the adjuvant treatment of stage III colon cancer: PETACC-3. J Clin Oncol. 2009;27(19):3117–25.

55. Gray R, Barnwell J, McConkey C, Hills RK, Williams NS, Kerr DJ. Adjuvant chemotherapy versus observation in patients with colorectal cancer: a randomised study. Lancet. 2007;370(9604):2020–9.

56. Twelves C, Wong A, Nowacki MP, et al. Capecitabine as adjuvant treatment for stage III colon cancer. N Engl J Med. 2005;352(26):2696–704.

57. Rothenberg ML, Cox JV, Butts C, et al. Capecitabine plus oxaliplatin (XELOX) versus 5-fluorouracil/folinic acid plus oxaliplatin (FOLFOX-4) as second-line therapy in metastatic colorectal cancer: a randomized phase III noninferiority study. Ann Oncol. 2008;19(10):1720–6.

58. Ferrara N, Hillan KJ, Gerber HP, Novotny W. Discovery and development of bevacizumab, an anti-VEGF antibody for treating cancer. Nat Rev Drug Discov. 2004;3(5):391–400.

59. Hurwitz H, Fehrenbacher L, Novotny W, et al. Bevacizumab plus irinotecan, fluorouracil, and leucovorin for metastatic colorectal cancer. N Engl J Med. 2004;350(23):2335–42.

60. Saltz LB, Clarke S, Diaz-Rubio E, et al. Bevacizumab in combination with oxaliplatin-based chemotherapy as first-line therapy in metastatic colorectal cancer: a randomized phase III study. J Clin Oncol. 2008; 26(12):2013–9.

61. Giantonio BJ, Catalano PJ, Meropol NJ, et al. Bevacizumab in combination with oxaliplatin, fluorouracil, and leucovorin (FOLFOX4) for previously treated metastatic colorectal cancer: results from the Eastern Cooperative Oncology Group Study E3200. J Clin Oncol. 2007;25(12):1539–44.

62. Allegra CJ, Yothers G, O'Connell MJ, et al. Phase III trial assessing bevacizumab in stages II and III carcinoma of the colon: results of NSABP protocol C-08. J Clin Oncol. 2011;29(1):11–6.

63. Kerr DJ, Young AM. Targeted therapies: Bevacizumab – has it reached its final resting place? Nat Rev Clin Oncol. 2011;8(4):195–6.

64. Yarden Y, Sliwkowski MX. Untangling the ErbB signalling network. Nat Rev Mol Cell Biol. 2001; 2(2):127–37.

65. Jonker DJ, O'Callaghan CJ, Karapetis CS, et al. Cetuximab for the treatment of colorectal cancer. N Engl J Med. 2007;357:2040–8.

66. Van Cutsem E, Peeters M, Siena S, et al. Open-label phase III trial of panitumumab plus best supportive care compared with best supportive care alone in patients with chemotherapy-refractory metastatic colorectal cancer. J Clin Oncol. 2007;25(13):1658–64.

67. Cunningham D, Humblet Y, Siena S, et al. Cetuximab monotherapy and cetuximab plus irinotecan in irinotecan-refractory metastatic colorectal cancer. N Engl J Med. 2004;351(4):337–45.

68. Van Cutsem E, Kohne CH, Hitre E, et al. Cetuximab and chemotherapy as initial treatment for metastatic colorectal cancer. N Engl J Med. 2009;360(14): 1408–17.

69. Bokemeyer C, Bondarenko I, Makhson A, et al. Fluorouracil, leucovorin, and oxaliplatin with and without cetuximab in the first-line treatment of metastatic colorectal cancer. J Clin Oncol. 2009;27(5):663–71.

70. Chung KY, Shia J, Kemeny NE, et al. Cetuximab shows activity in colorectal cancer patients with tumors that do not express the epidermal growth factor receptor by immunohistochemistry. J Clin Oncol. 2005;23(9):1803–10.

71. Alberts SR, Sargent DJ, Smyrk TC, Shields AF, Chan E, Goldberg RM, Gill S, Kahlenberg MS, Thibodeau SN, Nair S. Adjuvant mFOLFOX6 with or without cetuxiumab (Cmab) in KRAS wild-type (WT) patients (pts) with resected stage III colon cancer (CC): Results from NCCTG Intergroup Phase III Trial N0147. J Clin Oncol. 2010;28(Suppl):18s. abstr CRA3507.

72. Samuels Y, Wang Z, Bardelli A, et al. High frequency of mutations of the PIK3CA gene in human cancers. Science. 2004;304(5670):554.

73. O'Brien C, Wallin JJ, Sampath D, et al. Predictive biomarkers of sensitivity to the phosphatidylinositol 3' kinase inhibitor GDC-0941 in breast cancer pre-clinical models. Clin Cancer Res. 2010;16(14): 3670–83.

74. Burris H, Roden J, Sharma S, Herbst RS, Tabernero J, Infante JR, Silva A, Demanse D, Hackl W, Baselga J. First-in-human phase I study of the oral PI3K inhibitor BEZ235 in patients (pts) with advanced solid tumors. J Clin Oncol. 2010;28(Suppl):15s. abstr 3005.

75. De Roock W, Claes B, Bernasconi D, et al. Effects of KRAS, BRAF, NRAS, and PIK3CA mutations on the efficacy of cetuximab plus chemotherapy in chemotherapy-refractory metastatic colorectal cancer: a retrospective consortium analysis. Lancet Oncol. 2010;11(8):753–62.

76. Farina-Sarasqueta A, van Lijnschoten G, Moerland E, et al. The BRAF V600E mutation is an independent prognostic factor for survival in stage II and stage III colon cancer patients. Ann Oncol. 2010; 21(12):2396–402.

77. Flaherty KT, Puzanov I, Kim KB, et al. Inhibition of mutated, activated BRAF in metastatic melanoma. N Engl J Med. 2010;363(9):809–19.

78. Kopetz S, Desai J, Chan E, Hecht JR, O'Dwyer PJ, Lee RJ, Nolop KB, Saltz L. PLX4032 in metastatic colorectal cancer patients with mutant BRAF tumors. J Clin Oncol. 2010;28(Suppl):15s. abstr 3534.

79. Chitnis MM, Yuen JS, Protheroe AS, Pollak M, Macaulay VM. The type 1 insulin-like growth factor receptor pathway. Clin Cancer Res. 2008;14(20): 6364–70.

80. Reidy DL, Vakiani E, Fakih MG, et al. Randomized, phase II study of the insulin-like growth factor-1 receptor inhibitor IMC-A12, with or without cetuximab, in patients with cetuximab- or panitumumab-refractory metastatic colorectal cancer. J Clin Oncol. 2010;28(27):4240–6.

81. Simon RM, Paik S, Hayes DF. Use of archived specimens in evaluation of prognostic and predictive biomarkers. J Natl Cancer Inst. 2009;101(21):1446–52.

82. Hayes DF, Bast RC, Desch CE, et al. Tumor marker utility grading system: a framework to evaluate clinical utility of tumor markers. J Natl Cancer Inst. 1996;88(20):1456–66.

83. McGuire WL, Clark GM. Prognostic factors and treatment decisions in axillary-node-negative breast cancer. N Engl J Med. 1992;326(26):1756–61.

84. Locker GY, Hamilton S, Harris J, et al. ASCO 2006 update of recommendations for the use of tumor markers in gastrointestinal cancer. J Clin Oncol. 2006;24(33):5313–27.

85. Park YJ, Park KJ, Park JG, Lee KU, Choe KJ, Kim JP. Prognostic factors in 2230 Korean colorectal

cancer patients: analysis of consecutively operated cases. World J Surg. 1999;23(7):721–6.

86. Park YJ, Youk EG, Choi HS, et al. Experience of 1446 rectal cancer patients in Korea and analysis of prognostic factors. Int J Colorectal Dis. 1999;14(2):101–6.

87. Duffy MJ, van Dalen A, Haglund C, et al. Clinical utility of biochemical markers in colorectal cancer: European Group on Tumour Markers (EGTM) guidelines. Eur J Cancer. 2003;39(6):718–27.

88. Fong Y, Fortner J, Sun RL, Brennan MF, Blumgart LHC. Clinical score for predicting recurrence after hepatic resection for metastatic colorectal cancer: analysis of 1001 consecutive cases. Ann Surg. 1999;230(3):309–18. discussion 318–21.

89. Nordlinger B, Guiguet M, Vaillant JC, et al. Surgical resection of colorectal carcinoma metastases to the liver. A prognostic scoring system to improve case selection, based on 1568 patients. Association Francaise de Chirurgie. Cancer. 1996;77(7):1254–62.

90. Bakalakos EA, Burak Jr WE, Young DC, Martin Jr EW. Is carcino-embryonic antigen useful in the follow-up management of patients with colorectal liver metastases? Am J Surg. 1999;177(1):2–6.

91. Graham RA, Wang S, Catalano PJ, Haller DGC. Postsurgical surveillance of colon cancer: preliminary cost analysis of physician examination, carcinoembryonic antigen testing, chest x-ray, and colonoscopy. Ann Surg. 1998;228(1):59–63.

92. Pietra N, Sarli L, Costi R, Ouchemi C, Grattarola M, Peracchia A. Role of follow-up in management of local recurrences of colorectal cancer: a prospective, randomized study. Dis Colon Rectum. 1998;41(9): 1127–33.

93. Arnaud JP, Koehl C, Adloff M. Carcinoembryonic antigen (CEA) in diagnosis and prognosis of colorectal carcinoma. Dis Colon Rectum. 1980;23(3):141–4.

94. Rosen M, Chan L, Beart Jr RW, Vukasin P, Anthone G. Follow-up of colorectal cancer: a meta-analysis. Dis Colon Rectum. 1998;41(9):1116–26.

95. Boland CR, Thibodeau SN, Hamilton SR, et al. A National Cancer Institute Workshop on Microsatellite Instability for cancer detection and familial predisposition: development of international criteria for the determination of microsatellite instability in colorectal cancer. Cancer Res. 1998;58(22):5248–57.

96. Barratt PL, Seymour MT, Stenning SP, et al. DNA markers predicting benefit from adjuvant fluorouracil in patients with colon cancer: a molecular study. Lancet. 2002;360(9343):1381–91.

97. Halling KC, French AJ, McDonnell SK, et al. Microsatellite instability and 8p allelic imbalance in stage B2 and C colorectal cancers. J Natl Cancer Inst. 1999;91(15):1295–303.

98. Watanabe T, Wu TT, Catalano PJ, et al. Molecular predictors of survival after adjuvant chemotherapy for colon cancer. N Engl J Med. 2001;344(16): 1196–206.

99. Popat S, Hubner R, Houlston RS. Systematic review of microsatellite instability and colorectal cancer prognosis. J Clin Oncol. 2005;23(3):609–18.

100. Carethers JM, Chauhan DP, Fink D, et al. Mismatch repair proficiency and in vitro response to 5-fluorouracil. Gastroenterology. 1999;117:123–31.

101. Fischer F, Baerenfaller K, Jiricny J. 5-Fluorouracil is efficiently removed from DNA by the base excision and mismatch repair systems. Gastroenterology. 2007;133(6):1858–68.

102. Ribic CM, Sargent DJ, Moore MJ, et al. Tumor microsatellite-instability status as a predictor of benefit from fluorouracil-based adjuvant chemotherapy for colon cancer. N Engl J Med. 2003;349:247–57.

103. Carethers JM, Smith EJ, Behling CA, et al. Use of 5-fluorouracil and survival in patients with microsatellite-unstable colorectal cancer. Gastroenterology. 2004;126:394–401.

104. Storojeva I, Boulay JL, Heinimann K, et al. Prognostic and predictive relevance of microsatellite instability in colorectal cancer. Oncol Rep. 2005; 14(1):241–9.

105. Guastadisegni C, Colafranceschi M, Ottini L, Dogliotti E. Microsatellite instability as a marker of prognosis and response to therapy: a meta-analysis of colorectal cancer survival data. Eur J Cancer. 2010;46(15):2788–98.

106. Des Guetz G, Schischmanoff O, Nicolas P, Perret GY, Morere JF, Uzzan B. Does microsatellite instability predict the efficacy of adjuvant chemotherapy in colorectal cancer? A systematic review with meta-analysis. Eur J Cancer. 2009;45(10):1890–6.

107. Liang JT, Huang KC, Lai HS, et al. High-frequency microsatellite instability predicts better chemosensitivity to high-dose 5-fluorouracil plus leucovorin chemotherapy for stage IV sporadic colorectal cancer after palliative bowel resection. Int J Cancer. 2002;101(6):519–25.

108. Kim GP, Colangelo LH, Wieand HS, et al. Prognostic and predictive roles of high-degree microsatellite instability in colon cancer: a National Cancer Institute-National Surgical Adjuvant Breast and Bowel Project Collaborative Study. J Clin Oncol. 2007;25(7):767–72.

109. Fink D, Zheng H, Nebel S, et al. In vitro and in vivo resistance to cisplatin in cells that have lost DNA mismatch repair. Cancer Res. 1997;57(10): 1841–5.

110. Vilar E, Scaltriti M, Balmana J, et al. Microsatellite instability due to hMLH1 deficiency is associated with increased cytotoxicity to irinotecan in human colorectal cancer cell lines. Br J Cancer. 2008;99(10):1607–12.

111. Fallik D, Borrini F, Boige V, et al. Microsatellite instability is a predictive factor of the tumor response to irinotecan in patients with advanced colorectal cancer. Cancer Res. 2003;63(18):5738–44.

112. Bertagnolli MM, Niedzwiecki D, Compton CC, et al. Microsatellite instability predicts improved response to adjuvant therapy with irinotecan, fluorouracil, and leucovorin in stage III colon cancer: Cancer and Leukemia Group B Protocol 89803. J Clin Oncol. 2009;27(11):1814–21.

113. Walther A, Houlston R, Tomlinson I. Association between chromosomal instability and prognosis in colorectal cancer: a meta-analysis. Gut. 2008; 57(7):941–50.
114. Gerlinger M, Swanton C. How Darwinian models inform therapeutic failure initiated by clonal heterogeneity in cancer medicine. Br J Cancer. 2010; 103(8):1139–43.
115. Lee AJ, Endesfelder D, Rowan AJ, et al. Chromosomal instability confers intrinsic multidrug resistance. Cancer Res. 2011;71(5):1858–70.
116. Popat S, Houlston RS. A systematic review and meta-analysis of the relationship between chromosome 18q genotype, DCC status and colorectal cancer prognosis. Eur J Cancer. 2005;41(14):2060–70.
117. Sun XF, Rutten S, Zhang H, Nordenskjold B. Expression of the deleted in colorectal cancer gene is related to prognosis in DNA diploid and low proliferative colorectal adenocarcinoma. J Clin Oncol. 1999;17(6):1745–50.
118. Martinez-Lopez E, Abad A, Font A, et al. Allelic loss on chromosome 18q as a prognostic marker in stage II colorectal cancer. Gastroenterology. 1998;114(6): 1180–7.
119. Iacopetta B. TP53 mutation in colorectal cancer. Hum Mutat. 2003;21(3):271–6.
120. Fearon ER, Vogelstein B. A genetic model for colorectal tumorigenesis. Cell. 1990;61(5):759–67.
121. Anwar S, Frayling IM, Scott NA, Carlson GL. Systematic review of genetic influences on the prognosis of colorectal cancer. Br J Surg. 2004;91(10):1275–91.
122. Munro AJ, Lain S, Lane DP. P53 abnormalities and outcomes in colorectal cancer: a systematic review. Br J Cancer. 2005;92(3):434–44.
123. Kountourakis P, Pavlakis K, Psyrri A, et al. Clinicopathologic significance of EGFR and Her-2/neu in colorectal adenocarcinomas. Cancer J. 2006;12(3):229–36.
124. Takahari D, Yamada Y, Okita NT, et al. Relationships of insulin-like growth factor-1 receptor and epidermal growth factor receptor expression to clinical outcomes in patients with colorectal cancer. Oncology. 2009;76(1):42–8.
125. Zlobec I, Vuong T, Hayashi S, et al. A simple and reproducible scoring system for EGFR in colorectal cancer: application to prognosis and prediction of response to preoperative brachytherapy. Br J Cancer. 2007;96(5):793–800.
126. Spano JP, Lagorce C, Atlan D, et al. Impact of EGFR expression on colorectal cancer patient prognosis and survival. Ann Oncol. 2005;16(1):102–8.
127. Goldstein NS, Armin M. Epidermal growth factor receptor immunohistochemical reactivity in patients with American Joint Committee on Cancer Stage IV colon adenocarcinoma: implications for a standardized scoring system. Cancer. 2001;92(5):1331–46.
128. Mayer A, Takimoto M, Fritz E, Schellander G, Kofler K, Ludwig H. The prognostic significance of proliferating cell nuclear antigen, epidermal growth factor receptor, and mdr gene expression in colorectal cancer. Cancer. 1993;71(8):2454–60.
129. Wang WS, Chen PM, Chiou TJ, et al. Epidermal growth factor receptor R497K polymorphism is a favorable prognostic factor for patients with colorectal carcinoma. Clin Cancer Res. 2007;13(12):3597–604.
130. Saltz LB, Meropol NJ, Loehrer Sr PJ, Needle MN, Kopit J, Mayer RJ. Phase II trial of cetuximab in patients with refractory colorectal cancer that expresses the epidermal growth factor receptor. J Clin Oncol. 2004;22:1201–8.
131. Sartore-Bianchi A, Moroni M, Veronese S, et al. Epidermal growth factor receptor gene copy number and clinical outcome of metastatic colorectal cancer treated with panitumumab. J Clin Oncol. 2007; 25(22):3238–45.
132. Cappuzzo F, Finocchiaro G, Rossi E, et al. EGFR FISH assay predicts for response to cetuximab in chemotherapy refractory colorectal cancer patients. Ann Oncol. 2008;19(4):717–23.
133. Moroni M, Veronese S, Benvenuti S, et al. Gene copy number for epidermal growth factor receptor (EGFR) and clinical response to antiEGFR treatment in colorectal cancer: a cohort study. Lancet Oncol. 2005;6(5):279–86.
134. Personeni N, Fieuws S, Piessevaux H, et al. Clinical usefulness of EGFR gene copy number as a predictive marker in colorectal cancer patients treated with cetuximab: a fluorescent in situ hybridization study. Clin Cancer Res. 2008;14(18):5869–76.
135. Bardelli A, Siena S. Molecular mechanisms of resistance to cetuximab and panitumumab in colorectal cancer. J Clin Oncol. 2010;28(7):1254–61.
136. Barber TD, Vogelstein B, Kinzler KW, Velculescu VE. Somatic mutations of EGFR in colorectal cancers and glioblastomas. N Engl J Med. 2004;351(27):2883.
137. Garm Spindler KL, Pallisgaard N, Rasmussen AA, et al. The importance of KRAS mutations and EGF61A>G polymorphism to the effect of cetuximab and irinotecan in metastatic colorectal cancer. Ann Oncol. 2009;20(5):879–84.
138. Andreyev HJ, Norman AR, Cunningham D, et al. Kirsten ras mutations in patients with colorectal cancer: the 'RASCAL II' study. Br J Cancer. 2001;85(5):692–6.
139. Downward J, Targeting RAS. signalling pathways in cancer therapy. Nat Rev Cancer. 2003;3(1):11–22.
140. Richman SD, Seymour MT, Chambers P, et al. KRAS and BRAF mutations in advanced colorectal cancer are associated with poor prognosis but do not preclude benefit from oxaliplatin or irinotecan: results from the MRC FOCUS trial. J Clin Oncol. 2009;27(35):5931–7.
141. Westra JL, Plukker JT, Buys CH, Hofstra RM. Genetic alterations in locally advanced stage II/III colon cancer: a search for prognostic markers. Clin Colorectal Cancer. 2004;4(4):252–9.

142. Ogino S, Meyerhardt JA, Irahara N, et al. KRAS mutation in stage III colon cancer and clinical outcome following intergroup trial CALGB 89803. Clin Cancer Res. 2009;15(23):7322–9.

143. Tie J, Lipton L, Desai J, et al. KRAS mutation is associated with lung metastasis in patients with curatively resected colorectal cancer. Clin Cancer Res. 2011;17(5):1122–30.

144. Loupakis F, Ruzzo A, Cremolini C, et al. KRAS codon 61, 146 and BRAF mutations predict resistance to cetuximab plus irinotecan in KRAS codon 12 and 13 wild-type metastatic colorectal cancer. Br J Cancer. 2009;101:715–21.

145. Karapetis CS, Khambata-Ford S, Jonker DJ, et al. K-ras mutations and benefit from cetuximab in advanced colorectal cancer. N Engl J Med. 2008;359(17):1757–65.

146. Amado RG, Wolf M, Peeters M, et al. Wild-type KRAS is required for panitumumab efficacy in patients with metastatic colorectal cancer. J Clin Oncol. 2008;26(10):1626–34.

147. Peeters M, Price TJ, Cervantes A, et al. Randomized phase III study of panitumumab with fluorouracil, leucovorin, and irinotecan (FOLFIRI) compared with FOLFIRI alone as second-line treatment in patients with metastatic colorectal cancer. J Clin Oncol. 2010;28(31):4706–13.

148. Dahabreh IJ, Terasawa T, Castaldi PJ, Trikalinos TA. Systematic review: anti-epidermal growth factor receptor treatment effect modification by KRAS mutations in advanced colorectal cancer. Ann Intern Med. 2011;154(1):37–49.

149. Linardou H, Dahabreh IJ, Kanaloupiti D, et al. Assessment of somatic k-RAS mutations as a mechanism associated with resistance to EGFR-targeted agents: a systematic review and meta-analysis of studies in advanced non-small-cell lung cancer and metastatic colorectal cancer. Lancet Oncol. 2008; 9(10):962–72.

150. Allegra CJ, Jessup JM, Somerfield MR, et al. American Society of Clinical Oncology provisional clinical opinion: testing for KRAS gene mutations in patients with metastatic colorectal carcinoma to predict response to anti-epidermal growth factor receptor monoclonal antibody therapy. J Clin Oncol. 2009;27(12):2091–6.

151. Benvenuti S, Sartore-Bianchi A, Di Nicolantonio F, et al. Oncogenic activation of the RAS/RAF signaling pathway impairs the response of metastatic colorectal cancers to anti-epidermal growth factor receptor antibody therapies. Cancer Res. 2007;67(6):2643–8.

152. Etienne-Grimaldi MC, Formento JL, Francoual M, et al. K-Ras mutations and treatment outcome in colorectal cancer patients receiving exclusive fluoropyrimidine therapy. Clin Cancer Res. 2008;14(15): 4830–5.

153. Palomaki GE, McClain MR, Melillo S, Hampel HL, Thibodeau SNC. EGAPP supplementary evidence review: DNA testing strategies aimed at reducing morbidity and mortality from Lynch syndrome. Genet Med. 2009;11(1):42–65.

154. Saridaki Z, Papadatos-Pastos D, Tzardi M, et al. BRAF mutations, microsatellite instability status and cyclin D1 expression predict metastatic colorectal patients' outcome. Br J Cancer. 2010;102(12): 1762–8.

155. Laurent-Puig P, Cayre A, Manceau G, et al. Analysis of PTEN, BRAF, and EGFR status in determining benefit from cetuximab therapy in wild-type KRAS metastatic colon cancer. J Clin Oncol. 2009;27: 5924–30.

156. Samowitz WS, Sweeney C, Herrick J, et al. Poor survival associated with the BRAF V600E mutation in microsatellite-stable colon cancers. Cancer Res. 2005;65(14):6063–9.

157. Tol J, Nagtegaal ID, Punt CJ. BRAF mutation in metastatic colorectal cancer. N Engl J Med. 2009;361(1):98–9.

158. Di Nicolantonio F, Martini M, Molinari F, et al. Wild-type BRAF is required for response to panitumumab or cetuximab in metastatic colorectal cancer. J Clin Oncol. 2008;26:5705–12.

159. Vaughn CP, Zobell SD, Furtado LV, Baker CL, Samowitz WS. Frequency of KRAS, BRAF, and NRAS mutations in colorectal cancer. Genes Chromosomes Cancer. 2011;50(5):307–12.

160. Irahara N, Baba Y, Nosho K, et al. NRAS mutations are rare in colorectal cancer. Diagn Mol Pathol. 2010;19(3):157–63.

161. Engelman JA, Luo J, Cantley LC. The evolution of phosphatidylinositol 3-kinases as regulators of growth and metabolism. Nat Rev Genet. 2006; 7(8):606–19.

162. Ogino S, Nosho K, Kirkner GJ, et al. PIK3CA mutation is associated with poor prognosis among patients with curatively resected colon cancer. J Clin Oncol. 2009;27(9):1477–84.

163. Sartore-Bianchi A, Martini M, Molinari F, et al. PIK3CA mutations in colorectal cancer are associated with clinical resistance to EGFR-targeted monoclonal antibodies. Cancer Res. 2009;69:1851–7.

164. Perrone F, Lampis A, Orsenigo M, et al. PI3KCA/PTEN deregulation contributes to impaired responses to cetuximab in metastatic colorectal cancer patients. Ann Oncol. 2009;20(1):84–90.

165. Frattini M, Saletti P, Romagnani E, et al. PTEN loss of expression predicts cetuximab efficacy in metastatic colorectal cancer patients. Br J Cancer. 2007;97(8):1139–45.

166. Foulstone E, Prince S, Zaccheo O, et al. Insulin-like growth factor ligands, receptors, and binding proteins in cancer. J Pathol. 2005;205(2):145–53.

167. Ito Y, Koessler T, Ibrahim AE, et al. Somatically acquired hypomethylation of IGF2 in breast and colorectal cancer. Hum Mol Genet. 2008;17(17): 2633–43.

168. Cui H, Cruz-Correa M, Giardiello FM, et al. Loss of IGF2 imprinting: a potential marker of colorectal cancer risk. Science. 2003;299(5613):1753–5.

169. Woodson K, Flood A, Green L, et al. Loss of insulin-like growth factor-II imprinting and the presence of screen-detected colorectal adenomas in women. J Natl Cancer Inst. 2004;96(5):407–10.

170. Baba Y, Nosho K, Shima K, et al. Hypomethylation of the IGF2 DMR in colorectal tumors, detected by bisulfite pyrosequencing, is associated with poor prognosis. Gastroenterology. 2010;139(6):1855–64.

171. Popat S, Matakidou A, Houlston RS. Thymidylate synthase expression and prognosis in colorectal cancer: a systematic review and meta-analysis. J Clin Oncol. 2004;22:529–36.

172. Marsh S, McKay JA, Cassidy J, McLeod HL. Polymorphism in the thymidylate synthase promoter enhancer region in colorectal cancer. Int J Oncol. 2001;19(2):383–6.

173. Kawakami K, Salonga D, Park JM, et al. Different lengths of a polymorphic repeat sequence in the thymidylate synthase gene affect translational efficiency but not its gene expression. Clin Cancer Res. 2001;7(12):4096–101.

174. Mandola MV, Stoehlmacher J, Zhang W, et al. A 6 bp polymorphism in the thymidylate synthase gene causes message instability and is associated with decreased intratumoral TS mRNA levels. Pharmacogenetics. 2004;14(5):319–27.

175. Suh KW, Kim JH, Kim YB, Kim J, Jeong S. Thymidylate synthase gene polymorphism as a prognostic factor for colon cancer. J Gastrointest Surg. 2005;9:336–42.

176. Pullarkat ST, Stoehlmacher J, Ghaderi V, et al. Thymidylate synthase gene polymorphism determines response and toxicity of 5-FU chemotherapy. Pharmacogenomics J. 2001;1(1):65–70.

177. Frosst P, Blom HJ, Milos R, et al. A candidate genetic risk factor for vascular disease: a common mutation in methylenetetrahydrofolate reductase. Nat Genet. 1995;10(1):111–3.

178. Sohn KJ, Croxford R, Yates Z, Lucock M, Kim YI. Effect of the methylenetetrahydrofolate reductase C677T polymorphism on chemosensitivity of colon and breast cancer cells to 5-fluorouracil and methotrexate. J Natl Cancer Inst. 2004;96(2):134–44.

179. Jakobsen A, Nielsen JN, Gyldenkerne N, Lindeberg J. Thymidylate synthase and methylenetetrahydrofolate reductase gene polymorphism in normal tissue as predictors of fluorouracil sensitivity. J Clin Oncol. 2005;23(7):1365–9.

180. Cohen V, Panet-Raymond V, Sabbaghian N, Morin I, Batist G, Rozen R. Methylenetetrahydrofolate reductase polymorphism in advanced colorectal cancer: a novel genomic predictor of clinical response to fluoropyrimidine-based chemotherapy. Clin Cancer Res. 2003;9(5):1611–5.

181. Afzal S, Jensen SA, Vainer B, et al. MTHFR polymorphisms and 5-FU-based adjuvant chemotherapy in colorectal cancer. Ann Oncol. 2009;20(10): 1660–6.

182. Etienne-Grimaldi MC, Francoual M, Formento JL, Milano G. Methylenetetrahydrofolate reductase (MTHFR) variants and fluorouracil-based treatments in colorectal cancer. Pharmacogenomics. 2007;8(11): 1561–6.

183. Etienne-Grimaldi MC, Milano G, Maindrault-Goebel F, et al. Methylenetetrahydrofolate reductase (MTHFR) gene polymorphisms and FOLFOX response in colorectal cancer patients. Br J Clin Pharmacol. 2010;69(1):58–66.

184. Sharma R, Hoskins JM, Rivory LP, et al. Thymidylate synthase and methylenetetrahydrofolate reductase gene polymorphisms and toxicity to capecitabine in advanced colorectal cancer patients. Clin Cancer Res. 2008;14(3):817–25.

185. Chua W, Goldstein D, Lee CK, et al. Molecular markers of response and toxicity to FOLFOX chemotherapy in metastatic colorectal cancer. Br J Cancer. 2009;101(6):998–1004.

186. Metzger R, Danenberg K, Leichman CG, et al. High basal level gene expression of thymidine phosphorylase (platelet-derived endothelial cell growth factor) in colorectal tumors is associated with nonresponse to 5-fluorouracil. Clin Cancer Res. 1998;4(10): 2371–6.

187. de Bruin M, van Capel T, Van der Born K, et al. Role of platelet-derived endothelial cell growth factor/thymidine phosphorylase in fluoropyrimidine sensitivity. Br J Cancer. 2003;88(6):957–64.

188. Usuki K, Saras J, Waltenberger J, et al. Platelet-derived endothelial cell growth factor has thymidine phosphorylase activity. Biochem Biophys Res Commun. 1992;184(3):1311–6.

189. Folkman J. What is the role of thymidine phosphorylase in tumor angiogenesis. J Natl Cancer Inst. 1996;88(16):1091–2.

190. Takebayashi Y, Yamada K, Maruyama I, Fujii R, Akiyama S, Aikou T. The expression of thymidine phosphorylase and thrombomodulin in human colorectal carcinomas. Cancer Lett. 1995;92(1):1–7.

191. Takebayashi Y, Akiyama S, Akiba S, et al. Clinicopathologic and prognostic significance of an angiogenic factor, thymidine phosphorylase, in human colorectal carcinoma. J Natl Cancer Inst. 1996;88(16):1110–7.

192. Matsuura T, Kuratate I, Teramachi K, Osaki M, Fukuda Y, Ito H. Thymidine phosphorylase expression is associated with both increase of intratumoral microvessels and decrease of apoptosis in human colorectal carcinomas. Cancer Res. 1999;59(19): 5037–40.

193. Tokunaga Y, Hosogi H, Hoppou T, Nakagami M, Tokuka A, Ohsumi K. Prognostic value of thymidine phosphorylase/platelet-derived endothelial cell growth factor in advanced colorectal cancer after surgery: evaluation with a new monoclonal antibody. Surgery. 2002;131(5):541–7.

194. van Halteren HK, Peters HM, van Krieken JH, et al. Tumor growth pattern and thymidine phosphorylase expression are related with the risk of hematogenous metastasis in patients with Astler Coller B1/B2 colorectal carcinoma. Cancer. 2001;91(9):1752–7.

195. Diasio RB, Harris BE. Clinical pharmacology of 5-fluorouracil. Clin Pharmacokinet. 1989;16(4):215–37.

196. van Kuilenburg AB, Haasjes J, Richel DJ, et al. Clinical implications of dihydropyrimidine dehydrogenase (DPD) deficiency in patients with severe 5-fluorouracil-associated toxicity: identification of new mutations in the DPD gene. Clin Cancer Res. 2000;6(12):4705–12.

197. van Kuilenburg AB. Dihydropyrimidine dehydrogenase and the efficacy and toxicity of 5-fluorouracil. Eur J Cancer. 2004;40(7):939–50.

198. Tsuji T, Sawai T, Takeshita H, et al. Tumor dihydropyrimidine dehydrogenase in stage II and III colorectal cancer: low level expression is a beneficial marker in oral-adjuvant chemotherapy, but is also a predictor for poor prognosis in patients treated with curative surgery alone. Cancer Lett. 2004;204(1):97–104.

199. Yamada H, Iinuma H, Watanabe T. Prognostic value of 5-fluorouracil metabolic enzyme genes in Dukes' stage B and C colorectal cancer patients treated with oral 5-fluorouracil-based adjuvant chemotherapy. Oncol Rep. 2008;19(3):729–35.

200. Soong R, Shah N, Salto-Tellez M, et al. Prognostic significance of thymidylate synthase, dihydropyrimidine dehydrogenase and thymidine phosphorylase protein expression in colorectal cancer patients treated with or without 5-fluorouracil-based chemotherapy. Ann Oncol. 2008;19(5):915–9.

201. Gusella M, Frigo AC, Bolzonella C, et al. Predictors of survival and toxicity in patients on adjuvant therapy with 5-fluorouracil for colorectal cancer. Br J Cancer. 2009;100(10):1549–57.

202. Stoehlmacher J, Park DJ, Zhang W, et al. Association between glutathione S-transferase P1, T1, and M1 genetic polymorphism and survival of patients with metastatic colorectal cancer. J Natl Cancer Inst. 2002;94(12):936–42.

203. Funke S, Timofeeva M, Risch A, et al. Genetic polymorphisms in GST genes and survival of colorectal cancer patients treated with chemotherapy. Pharmacogenomics. 2010;11(1):33–41.

204. Lecomte T, Landi B, Beaune P, Laurent-Puig P, Loriot MA. Glutathione S-transferase P1 polymorphism (Ile105Val) predicts cumulative neuropathy in patients receiving oxaliplatin-based chemotherapy. Clin Cancer Res. 2006;12(10):3050–6.

205. McLeod HL, Sargent DJ, Marsh S, et al. Pharmacogenetic predictors of adverse events and response to chemotherapy in metastatic colorectal cancer: results from North American Gastrointestinal Intergroup Trial N9741. J Clin Oncol. 2010;28(20):3227–33.

206. Kweekel DM, Gelderblom H, Antonini NF, et al. Glutathione-S-transferase pi (GSTP1) codon 105 polymorphism is not associated with oxaliplatin efficacy or toxicity in advanced colorectal cancer patients. Eur J Cancer. 2009;45(4):572–8.

207. Braun MS, Richman SD, Thompson L, et al. Association of molecular markers with toxicity outcomes in a randomized trial of chemotherapy for advanced colorectal cancer: the FOCUS trial. J Clin Oncol. 2009;27(33):5519–28.

208. Yin M, Yan J, Martinez-Balibrea E, et al. ERCC1 and ERCC2/XPD polymorphisms predict clinical outcomes of oxaliplatin-based chemotherapies in gastric and colorectal cancer: a systemic review and meta-analysis. Clin Cancer Res. 2011. doi:10.1158/1078-0432.

209. Ando Y, Saka H, Ando M, et al. Polymorphisms of UDP-glucuronosyltransferase gene and irinotecan toxicity: a pharmacogenetic analysis. Cancer Res. 2000;60(24):6921–6.

210. Hoskins JM, Goldberg RM, Qu P, Ibrahim JG, McLeod HL. UGT1A1*28 genotype and irinotecan-induced neutropenia: dose matters. J Natl Cancer Inst. 2007;99(17):1290–5.

211. Clynes RA, Towers TL, Presta LG, Ravetch JV. Inhibitory Fc receptors modulate in vivo cytotoxicity against tumor targets. Nat Med. 2000;6(4):443–6.

212. Zhang W, Gordon M, Schultheis AM, et al. FCGR2A and FCGR3A polymorphisms associated with clinical outcome of epidermal growth factor receptor expressing metastatic colorectal cancer patients treated with single-agent cetuximab. J Clin Oncol. 2007;25(24):3712–8.

213. Bibeau F, Lopez-Crapez E, Di Fiore F, et al. Impact of Fc{gamma}RIIa-Fc{gamma}RIIIa polymorphisms and KRAS mutations on the clinical outcome of patients with metastatic colorectal cancer treated with cetuximab plus irinotecan. J Clin Oncol. 2009;27(7):1122–9.

214. van't Veer LJ, Bernards R. Enabling personalized cancer medicine through analysis of gene-expression patterns. Nature. 2008;452(7187):564–70.

215. Feinberg AP. Phenotypic plasticity and the epigenetics of human disease. Nature. 2007;447(7143):433–40.

216. Brennan DJ, O'Connor DP, Rexhepaj E, Ponten F, Gallagher WM. Antibody-based proteomics: fast-tracking molecular diagnostics in oncology. Nat Rev Cancer. 2010;10(9):605–17.

217. Chin L, Gray JW. Translating insights from the cancer genome into clinical practice. Nature. 2008;452(7187):553–63.

218. Mardis ER. A decade's perspective on DNA sequencing technology. Nature. 2011;470(7333):198–203.

219. Wang Y, Jatkoe T, Zhang Y, et al. Gene expression profiles and molecular markers to predict recurrence of Dukes' B colon cancer. J Clin Oncol. 2004;22(9):1564–71.

220. Jiang Y, Casey G, Lavery IC, et al. Development of a clinically feasible molecular assay to predict recurrence of stage II colon cancer. J Mol Diagn. 2008;10(4):346–54.

221. Barrier A, Boelle PY, Roser F, et al. Stage II colon cancer prognosis prediction by tumor gene expression profiling. J Clin Oncol. 2006;24(29):4685–91.

222. Barrier A, Lemoine A, Boelle PY, et al. Colon cancer prognosis prediction by gene expression profiling. Oncogene. 2005;24(40):6155–64.

223. Eschrich S, Yang I, Bloom G, et al. Molecular staging for survival prediction of colorectal cancer patients. J Clin Oncol. 2005;23(15):3526–35.

224. O'Connell MJ, Lavery I, Yothers G, et al. Relationship between tumor gene expression and recurrence in four independent studies of patients with stage II/III colon cancer treated with surgery alone or surgery plus adjuvant fluorouracil plus leucovorin. J Clin Oncol. 2010;28(25):3937–44.

225. Kerr D, Gray R, Quirke P, Watson D, Yothers G, Lavery IC, Lee M, O'Connell MJ, Shak S, Wolmark N. A quantitative multigene RT-PCR assay for prediction of recurrence in stage II colon cancer: Selection of the genes in four large studies and results of the independent, prospectively designed QUASAR validation study. J Clin Oncol. 2009;27(Suppl):15s. abstr 4000.

226. O'Connell MJ, Lavery IC, Gray RG, Quirke P, Kerr DJ, Lopatin M, Yothers GA, Lee M, Langone K, Wolmark N. Comparison of molecular and pathologic features of stage II and stage III colon cancer in four large studies conducted for development of the 12-gene colon cancer recurrence score. Paper presented at: ASCO 2010 Gastrointestinal Cancers Symposium 2010, Chicago, IL.

227. Salazar R, Roepman P, Capella G, et al. Gene expression signature to improve prognosis prediction of stage II and III colorectal cancer. J Clin Oncol. 2011;29(1):17–24.

228. Salazar R, Marshall J, Stork-Sloots L, Simon I, Lutke Holzik M, Tabernero J, Van Der Hoeven JJ, Bibeau F, Rosenberg R. The PARSC trial, a prospective study for the assessment of recurrence risk in stage II colon cancer (CC) patients using ColoPrint. J Clin Oncol. 2010;28(Suppl):15s. abstr TPS199.

229. Pogue-Geile KL, Youthers GA, Gavin P, Fumagalli D, Kim C, Colangelo LH, Geyer CE, O'Connell MJ, Wolmark N, Paik S. Use of a prognostic (prog) gene index and nodal status to identify a subset of stage II and III colon cancer patients (pts) who may not need oxaliplatin (ox)-containing adjuvant chemotherapy. J Clin Oncol. 2010;28(Suppl):15s. abstr 3516.

230. Del Rio M, Molina F, Bascoul-Mollevi C, et al. Gene expression signature in advanced colorectal cancer patients select drugs and response for the use of leucovorin, fluorouracil, and irinotecan. J Clin Oncol. 2007;25(7):773–80.

231. Khambata-Ford S, Garrett CR, Meropol NJ, et al. Expression of epiregulin and amphiregulin and K-ras mutation status predict disease control in metastatic colorectal cancer patients treated with cetuximab. J Clin Oncol. 2007;25(22):3230–7.

232. de Reynies A, Boige V, Milano G, Faivre J, Laurent-Puig P. KRAS mutation signature in colorectal tumors significantly overlaps with the cetuximab response signature. J Clin Oncol. 2008;26(13):2228–30. author reply 2230–1.

233. Walther A, Domingo E, Mesher D, Johnstone E, Orntoft T, Sasieni P, Dunlop M, Tejpar S, Kerr DJ, Tomlinson I. Genome-wide association study for germline prognostic markers in colorectal cancer. J Clin Oncol. 2010;28(Suppl):15s. abstr 3514.

234. Gemoll T, Roblick UJ, Auer G, Jornvall H, Habermann JK. SELDI-TOF serum proteomics and colorectal cancer: a current overview. Arch Physiol Biochem. 2010;116(4–5):188–96.

235. Jimenez CR, Knol JC, Meijer GA, Fijneman RJ. Proteomics of colorectal cancer: overview of discovery studies and identification of commonly identified cancer-associated proteins and candidate CRC serum markers. J Proteomics. 2010;73(10):1873–95.

236. Camp RL, Chung GG, Rimm DL. Automated subcellular localization and quantification of protein expression in tissue microarrays. Nat Med. 2002;8(11):1323–7.

237. Pages F, Berger A, Camus M, et al. Effector memory T cells, early metastasis, and survival in colorectal cancer. N Engl J Med. 2005;353(25):2654–66.

238. Galon J, Costes A, Sanchez-Cabo F, et al. Type, density, and location of immune cells within human colorectal tumors predict clinical outcome. Science. 2006;313(5795):1960–4.

239. Mlecnik B, Tosolini M, Kirilovsky A, et al. Histopathologic-based prognostic factors of colorectal cancers are associated with the state of the local immune reaction. J Clin Oncol. 2011;29(6):610–8.

240. Gulmann C, Sheehan KM, Conroy RM, et al. Quantitative cell signalling analysis reveals downregulation of MAPK pathway activation in colorectal cancer. J Pathol. 2009;218(4):514–9.

241. Melle C, Bogumil R, Ernst G, Schimmel B, Bleul A, von Eggeling F. Detection and identification of heat shock protein 10 as a biomarker in colorectal cancer by protein profiling. Proteomics. 2006;6(8):2600–8.

242. Van Schaeybroeck S, Allen WL, Turkington RC, Johnston PG. Implementing prognostic and predictive biomarkers in CRC clinical trials. Nat Rev Clin Oncol. 2011;8(4):222–32.

Hepatocellular Carcinoma

10

Yasunori Minami and Masatoshi Kudo

Abbreviations

AFP	Alpha-fetoprotein
AFP-L3	Alpha-fetoprotein
Lens	Culinaris agglutinin 3
BCLC	Barcelona Clinic Liver Cancer
CTHA/CTAP	CT with hepatic arteriography and arterial portography
DCP	Des-gamma-carboxyprothrombin
Gd-DTPA	Gadolinium diethylenetriamine pentaacetic acid
Gd-EOB-DTPA	Gadolinium-ethoxybenzyl-diethylenetriamine pentaacetic acid
HBV	Hepatitis B virus
HCC	Hepatocellular carcinoma
HCV	Hepatitis C virus
MDCT	Multidetector row CT
MPR	Multiplanar reconstruction
NASH	Nonalcoholic steatohepatitis
PDGFR	Platelet-derived growth factor receptors
PIVKA-II	Prothrombin induced by vitamin K absence-II
SPIO	Superparamagnetic iron oxide
RCT	Randomized controlled trial

Y. Minami, M.D. • M. Kudo, M.D., Ph.D. (✉)
Department of Gastroenterology and Hepatology,
Kinki University School of Medicine,
377-2 Ohno-higashi, Osaka-Sayama,
Osaka 589-8511, Japan
e-mail: m-kudo@med.kindai.ac.jp

TACE	Transcatheter arterial chemoembolization
VEGFR	Vascular endothelial growth factor receptors

Hepatocellular carcinoma (HCC) is the sixth most common cancer in the world and the third most common cause of cancer mortality worldwide [1, 2]. Between 500,000 and 1 million new HCC cases are diagnosed each year worldwide, with an age-adjusted annual incidence of 14.9 per 100,000 in men and 5.5 per 100,000 in women [3, 4]. There are wide geographical variations in the incidence of the disease with the highest rates in the developing countries of Asia and Africa. However, the incidence of HCC is increasing in North America and Europe [5].

HCC Risk Factors

The most common risk factor for HCC is cirrhosis, which is present in 80–90% of HCC patients. It is hypothesized that cirrhotic hepatic necroinflammation from various etiologies leads to cirrhosis and HCC due to increased hepatocyte regeneration and hyperplasia predisposing to mutations and malignant transformation [6]. The interval from chronic liver disease to cirrhosis and HCC ranges from an average of two decades in hepatitis B virus (HBV) and hepatitis C virus (HCV) infection to 10–15 years for nonalcoholic steatohepatitis (NASH) and hereditary hemochromatosis [7, 8]. Established risk factors for HCC include chronic infection with HBV and/or HCV, old age, male sex, aflatoxin exposure, alcohol abuse, diabetes, NASH, hemochromatosis, and various host genetic factors.

HBV

Chronic hepatitis B contributes to more than 50% of HCC cases worldwide and 70–80% of HCC cases in the highly endemic regions of HBV [9]. Standard HBV vaccination programs are expected to decrease the prevalence of HCC among the vaccinated cohort. Immigration from HBV-endemic countries may also contribute to the increasing incidence of HCC. The incidence of HCC increases with age, reaching a peak among those aged 50–65 in HBV-endemic areas. However, in the last two decades in western countries, there has been a shift of incidence to patients aged 40–60 possibly because of an increase in HBV-infected individuals.

High viral loads (>10^4 copies/mL), genotype C, and mutations (especially in the Enh II/BCP/precore and pre-S regions) are independently associated with increased risks of HCC, indicating that these viral properties can be used for the prediction of HCC in HBV-infected individuals [10].

HCV

The risk of HCC in patients with chronic hepatitis C is greatest among patients who have established cirrhosis, where the incidence of HCC is between 2 and 8% per year [11]. However, although the incidence of HCV has also decreased since blood donor screening was started in 1990, the impact of the decrease in HCV will not become evident until after the year 2015. In the meantime, it is expected that the incidence of HCV-related HCC will continue to increase. An effective vaccine against HCV has yet to be developed because of the high mutation rate of the virus.

Age

Age-specific incidence rates are strongly affected by the etiology of the background liver disease. Advanced age is an independent risk factor for HCC, especially in areas where HCV infection is endemic [12].

Male Sex

Males are more likely to develop HCC than females. Male–female ratios are around 3:1 in high-risk countries and tend to be higher in patients with HBV than in those with HCV [12].

Aflatoxin

Aflatoxins are potent hepatocarcinogens produced by fungi and are contaminants of stored grains. When controlled for HBV infection, HCC incidence in Africa is correlated with the extent of aflatoxin exposure in diet. A consistent genetic mutation in codon 249 of the tumor suppressor p53 gene (GC to TA transversion) has been identified and positively correlated with aflatoxin exposure [12, 13].

Alcohol

Oral ingestion of alcohol produces a spectrum of liver impairments, from fat accumulation and acute necroinflammation to cirrhosis. HCC generally does not develop in the absence of cirrhosis, and heavy alcohol intake is the only obvious risk factor in some HCC patients without cirrhosis. The 5-year cumulative risk for HCC in alcoholic cirrhosis is 8% [13].

Obesity and Diabetes

The relative risk of HCC for obesity has been shown to increase to 4.52 for men and to 1.69 for women [14]. For diabetes, a Danish study showed that the risk of HCC was increased 4- and 2.1-fold in men and women, respectively.

NASH

At the time of diagnosis, advanced fibrosis is found in 30–40% of NASH patients, and 10–15% already have established cirrhosis [15, 16]. NASH patients share many of the systemic disorders that constitute insulin resistance syndrome: hyperlipidemia, hypertension, insulin resistance, obesity, iron accumulation in the liver, and hepatic steatosis. Hyperglyceridemia, diabetes, and normal aminotransferases are independent factors associated with HCC arising in NASH.

Hemochromatosis

The increased absorption of dietary iron and accumulation in tissue leads to heart failure and cirrhosis, primarily in C282Y homozygotes and C282Y/H63D compound heterozygotes [12]. The 5-year cumulative risk for HCC in hemochromatosis-associated cirrhosis is 21%, even greater than that for HCV cirrhosis in Europe and North America [13].

Surveillance

HCC surveillance can detect tumors early and increase the chance of a successful curative treatment. All patients at risk of developing HCC with potentially curative treatment available are recommended to undergo regular surveillance. High-risk populations (e.g., cirrhosis with HBV or HCV infection) with HCC have been clearly identified. At present, ultrasonography (US) and a serum AFP test at 6-month intervals are standard surveillance tools [11]. To improve the detection rate of early-stage HCC, the benefit of additional tests and a shorter surveillance interval should be confirmed by a randomized clinical trial [17]. The application of individualized prediction models to surveillance programs may improve the cost-effectiveness by focusing on high-risk groups. At least, cirrhotic patients with HBV and HCV should be recommended as candidates for surveillance [12].

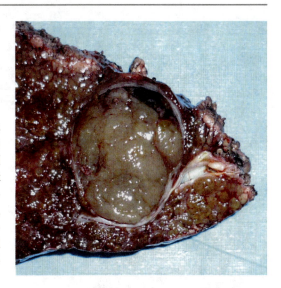

Fig. 10.1 Hepatocellular carcinoma, nodular type, in the context of a cirrhotic liver

Pathology

In terms of gross findings, the lesion may be a unifocal, multifocal or diffusely infiltrative soft tumor, and may be green in color, due to its bile content; extensive intrahepatic metastases are common; snake-like masses of tumor may involve the portal vein (35–80%), hepatic vein (20%), or inferior vena cava; and hemorrhages and necrotic areas are common. Microscopically, patterns are trabecular (most common) with 4+ cells surrounded by a layer of flattened endothelial cells, solid, pseudoglandular (acinar with proteinaceous material or bile in the lumina), and a fibrous capsule and septum [18–20] (Figs. 10.1 and 10.2).

The malignant transformation of hepatocytes to HCC is a multistep process associated with genetic mutations, allelic losses, epigenetic alterations, and perturbation of molecular cellular pathways [18–20]. The phenotypic expression of these changes can be manifested by precursor lesions, which accompany HCC spatially and temporally and are termed dysplastic nodules. These nodules show a distinct malignant transformation to HCC with a shift in vascular supply from the portal vein to the hepatic artery and an increase in size (Fig.10.3).

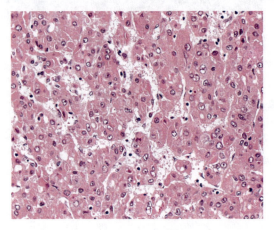

Fig. 10.2 Moderately differentiated hepatocellular carcinoma. Hepatocellular carcinoma composed of trabeculae with a thickness of three or more cell layers

Diagnosis

Diagnostic tests universally available to date are imaging modalities including contrast-enhanced US, CT, and MRI, and a tumor marker such as alpha-fetoprotein (AFP) [11, 12, 17].

The evaluation of intranodular hemodynamics is important for the diagnosis of HCC because the pathologic findings of HCC are closely related to the intranodular hemodynamics. HCC can be diagnosed radiologically, without the need for biopsy if typical imaging features are present [21–23]. In the arterial phase, HCC enhances more intensely than the surrounding liver because the liver tissue is mainly supplied by portal blood that does not contain contrast, whereas the HCC contains mostly arterial blood. In the delayed phase, the HCC enhances less than the surrounding liver. This is known as "washout," because HCC does not have a portal blood supply and the arterial blood flowing through the lesion no

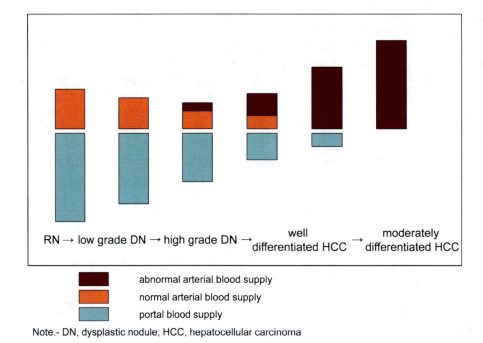

Fig. 10.3 Hepatocarcinogenesis. In the course of hepatocarcinogenesis, first, both arterial and portal supply decrease (due to a decrease in the portal tracts), then arterial supply returns to a level equivalent (due to newly formed abnormal arteries) to that in the surrounding liver, while portal supply continues to decrease, and finally portal supply vanishes, and only arterial blood (from newly formed abnormal arteries) supplies the lesion (moderately differentiated HCC)

10 Hepatocellular Carcinoma

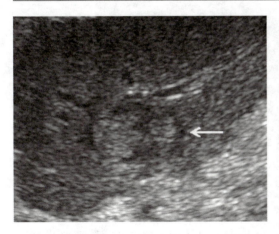

Fig. 10.4 B-mode US. The nodule demonstrated a halo image and mosaic pattern at the left lateral lobe of the liver on B-mode US

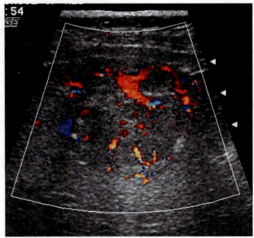

Fig. 10.5 Color Doppler imaging. Color Doppler image showed hypervascularity of the tumor

longer contains contrast, whereas the portal blood in the liver now contains contrast. The presence of arterial uptake followed by washout is highly specific for HCC.

Imaging

US

B-mode US is the most widely used modality for HCC screening and surveillance. Typical US findings of classical HCC are a mosaic pattern, septum formation, peripheral sonolucency (halo), lateral shadow produced by a fibrotic pseudocapsule, posterior echo enhancement, arterial hypervascularity with dilated intratumoral blood sinusoids, and perinodular daughter nodule formation [24] (Fig. 10.4). The halo sign corresponds to the thin fibrous capsule of the tumor [25, 26]. Correspondence between sonographic halo sign and histological capsule was reported to be 90.1%, and that between the presence of extracapsular invasion on US and on histology was 88.0%. Color Doppler imaging demonstrates arterial pulsating flows, such as basket pattern flow and "spot" pattern flow; these patterns represent a fine network of arterial vessels surrounding the tumor nodules [25, 26] (Fig. 10.5). Moreover, two breakthroughs in US, harmonic imaging and the development of second-generation contrast agents, have demonstrated the potential to dramatically broaden the scope of US diagnosis of hepatic tumors [27, 28]. Dynamic contrast harmonic US can depict tumor vascularity sensitively and accurately and is able to evaluate small hypervascular HCCs.

CT

With the advent of multidetector row CT (MDCT), high-resolution scanning of the entire upper abdomen during one breath-hold became feasible. The use of a thinner collimation leads to increased spatial resolution and reduced partial volume averaging. These volume data sets can be easily manipulated with three-dimensional imaging, potentially providing additional information to a conventional axial display. Thus, the image quality of MPR from thin axial slices may significantly improve. This may foster the routine use of coronal or sagittal reformats for CT evaluation of abdominal lesions.

The hallmark of HCC in a dynamic CT scan is the presence of arterial enhancement followed by washout of the tumor in the delayed phases [29] (Fig. 10.6). Furthermore, 3D CT angiography is a noninvasive volumetric imaging technique increasingly used for evaluation of vascular systems, and 3D CT angiography has important advantages over conventional angiography, such as reduced risk, diminished time, and better patient acceptance. With MDCT, 3D CT

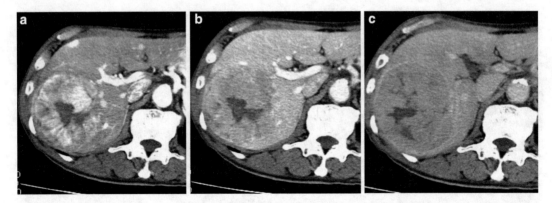

Fig. 10.6 Dynamic CT. (**a**) Axial CT scan obtained during hepatic arterial phase showed a huge hypervascular tumor in the right hepatic lobe. Unenhanced area at the center of the nodule indicated necrotic tissue. (**b**) CT during portal venous phase showed portal perfusion defect due to tumor. (**c**) The washout image was obtained during the equilibrium phase of dynamic CT

angiography crosses over vessel tortuosity and allows evaluation of vessel fragility [30, 31].

MRI

Some studies have indicated that the detectability of small nodules in the liver is significantly improved by MRI dynamic study using gadolinium diethylenetriamine pentaacetic acid (Gd-DTPA) in comparison with CT dynamic study [32, 33].

Superparamagnetic iron oxide (SPIO) particles are used as MR contrast media and are composed of iron oxide crystals coated with dextran or carboxydextran. These particles are sequestered by phagocytic Kupffer cells in the normal reticuloendothelial system, but are not retained in tumor tissue. Consequently, there are significant differences in T2/T2* relaxation between normal liver parenchyma and tumors, which result in increased lesion conspicuity and detectability. For focal hepatocellular lesions, it has been documented that SPIO-enhanced MR imaging exhibits a slightly better diagnostic performance than dynamic helical CT in the detection of hypervascular HCC [34, 35].

Gadolinium-ethoxybenzyl-diethylenetriamine pentaacetic acid (Gd-EOB-DTPA) is a new liver-specific contrast agent. Gd-EOB-DTPA-enhanced MR imaging enables improved detection of hepatic lesions over Gd-DTPA-enhanced MR imaging [36, 37]. A bolus injection of Gd-EOB-DTPA enables tumor vascularity to be evaluated in a manner similar to that with Gd-DTPA. Moreover, Gd-EOB-DTPA accumulates in normally functioning hepatocytes in the delayed phase (hepatobiliary phase). Thus, the liver parenchyma is enhanced, while HCCs appear as hypointense lesions, because they do not contain normally functioning hepatocytes (Fig. 10.7).

Hepatic Angiography

Hepatic angiography is an essential part of the workup performed prior to chemoembolization, and demonstrates homogeneously stained hypervascular HCCs with their feeding arteries [12] (Fig. 10.8). In addition, CT with hepatic arteriography and arterial portography (CTHA/CTAP) are often performed together and recognized as the most sensitive test for detecting individual liver lesions [38, 39]. CTHA is performed with the arterial catheter in the common hepatic artery. On CT images obtained with this technique, HCC tumors appear as uniformly enhancing hyperdense masses. CTAP is performed with the arterial catheter in the supermesenteric artery, producing a more consistent and homogeneous enhancement of the normal hepatic parenchyma. HCC tumors are exclusively shown as defects. These techniques are invasive; however, it has become possible to visualize the distribution of

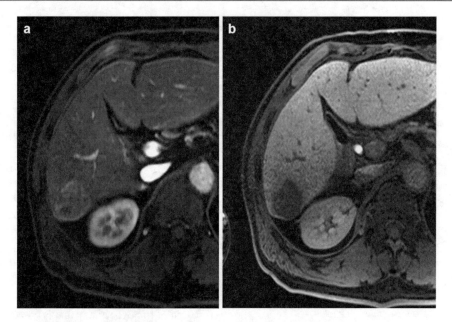

Fig. 10.7 Gd-EOB-DTPA-enhanced MRI. (**a**) Axial T1-weighted MR image showed that the lesion was hyperintense compared with the liver in the dynamic arterial phase. (**b**) HCCs show hypointensity in the hepatobiliary phase

the intrahepatic portal and arterial blood flow separately with extremely high contrast resolution.

Tumor Markers

AFP

AFP is a glycoprotein synthesized by the fetal yolk sac, fetal liver, testicular nonseminomatous germ cell cancers, and malignant hepatic cells. AFP is the most widely used serological test for HCC. Reliance on AFP levels to detect HCC, however, is confounded by the fact that AFP may be elevated in individuals with chronic HBV or HCV infection and hepatic cirrhosis. Most studies have adopted a cutoff value of 20 ng/mL for AFP, with a sensitivity ranging from 49 to 71% and specificity from 49 to 86% in HCCs [40–43]. Limitations in the sensitivity and specificity of AFP in the surveillance of high-risk populations have led to the use of US as an additional method for the detection of HCC. The sensitivity and specificity of AFP for diagnosing HCC vary with the population studied, and the cutoff value above which AFP is considered positive. These values have ranged from 52 to 80% and 90 to 98%, respectively [44].

Des-Gamma-Carboxyprothrombin

Des-gamma-carboxyprothrombin (DCP), also known as prothrombin induced by vitamin K absence-II (PIVKA-II), is an abnormal prothrombin protein that is increased in the serum of HCC patients. DCP has been recognized as not only a highly specific marker for HCC but also a predictor of prognosis of HCC patients [41, 43, 45, 46]. The sensitivity and specificity of DCP at the time of diagnosis of HCC has been reported as 74 and 86%, respectively, at a cutoff of 40 mAU/mL and 43 and 100%, respectively, at a cutoff of 150 mAU/mL [46]. A high DCP level is an important prognostic factor for recurrence, even in the case of a small HCC before histological invasion of the tumor such as vascular invasion becomes obvious. Patients who have a high DCP level can expect the expression of future vascular invasion and early tumor recurrence extrahepatically after resection [47, 48].

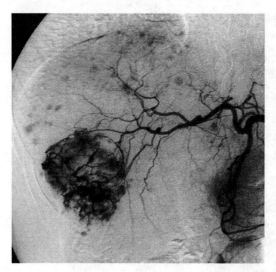

Fig. 10.8 Hepatic angiography. Celiac angiogram showed the presence of multiple hypervascular tumor staining mainly at the right hepatic lobe

Alpha-Fetoprotein Lens Culinaris Agglutinin 3

Measurement of an AFP glycoform may prove to be clinically superior to the measurement of AFP. Alpha-fetoprotein lens culinaris agglutinin 3 (AFP-L3) is a fucosylated variant of AFP that reacts with lens culinaris agglutinin A and can differentiate an increase in AFP due to HCC from that in patients with benign liver disease [49–51]. AFP-L1 does not bind to lens culinaris agglutinin (LCA) and is the major glycoform found in individuals with nonmalignant hepatopathy (e.g., cirrhosis or chronic HBV infection). AFP-L2 has an intermediate LCA binding capacity and is primarily produced by yolk sac tumors. AFP-L3 is produced by malignant liver cells, binds to LCA with high affinity, and is the major glycoform found in individuals with HCC. The sensitivity and specificity, and positive likelihood ratio of AFP-L3 in HCC smaller than 5 cm in diameter ranged from 22 to 33%, and 93 to 94%, respectively, with a cutoff value of 10% and 21–49%, and 94–100%, respectively, with a cutoff value of 15% [52]. Malignant liver cells that produce AFP-L3 have an increased tendency for rapid growth, early invasion, and intrahepatic metastasis, thus making AFP-L3 an indicator of poor prognosis in affected individuals [53].

Staging Systems

The prognosis of solid tumors is generally related to tumor stage at presentation. Tumor stage also guides treatment decisions. However, in HCC patients, the prediction of prognosis is more complex because the underlying liver function also affects prognosis. Most major trials of HCC therapy have chosen the BCLC staging system. The BCLC staging system was developed based on a combination of data from several independent studies representing different disease stages and/or treatment modalities and can define patient groups for therapies across the continuum of disease extent seen with HCC [11, 54, 55] (Fig. 10.9). The main advantage of the BCLC staging system is that it links staging with treatment modalities and with an estimation of life expectancy that is based on published response rates to the various treatments.

Treatment

Surgical Resection

This is the treatment of choice for HCC in non-cirrhotic patients, who account for just 5% of the cases in Western countries and about 40% in Asia. These patients will tolerate major resections with low morbidity, but in cirrhosis, candidates for resection have to be carefully selected in order to diminish the risk of postoperative liver failure with increased risk of death. Hepatic resection for HCC is associated with a hospital mortality rate of less than 5% in major centers; however, the complication rate remains high, around 30–40% in large series [56–58]. At present, serious complications such as liver failure, postoperative bleeding, and bile leak occur nowadays in less than 5% of patients after hepatectomy [56–58]. The 5-year survival after resection is 35–50% in recent large cohort studies [59–61]. For patients with tumors less than 5 cm in diameter, the 5-year survival rate is about 70% [62].

Endoscopic surgery, a rapidly adopted minimally invasive surgery, has been applied to the treatment of HCC. There have been reports of

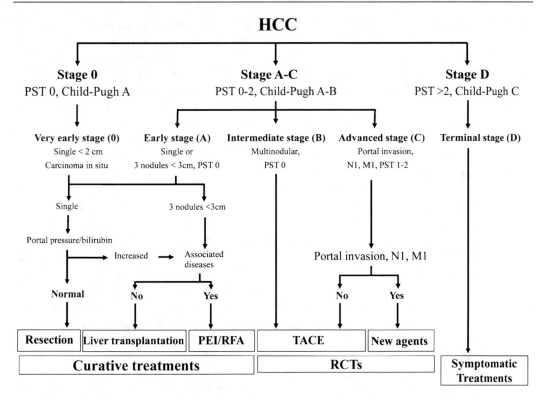

Fig. 10.9 BCLC staging. The BCLC system integrates liver function and tumor features into a classification that is useful for selecting appropriate treatment options. BCLC stage A patients are those suitable for surgical/ablative therapy and transplant, BCLC B patients are suitable for regional therapy such as embolization, and BCLC C patients are those best suited for systemic therapies or clinical trials

laparoscopic right and left lobectomy [63–65], and laparoscopic surgery has also been applied to left lateral segmentectomy of the living donor's liver for transplant [66]. Laparoscopic hepatectomy can avoid the disadvantages of standard hepatectomy and is beneficial for patient QOL due to its minimal invasiveness.

Chemoembolization of the tumor prior to resection offers no benefit [67]. The same is true for the general use of portal vein embolization of the hepatic lobe hosting the tumor to induce compensatory liver growth and functional capacity in the nonaffected lobe prior to major resection [68, 69]. Clearly, large RCTs are needed to define the benefits and risks of these procedures.

Liver Transplantation

The liver transplant procedure involves replacing a part or whole of the diseased liver with a healthy donor liver. When the diseased liver is removed from the patient's body and a new healthy liver is transplanted, the procedure is referred as orthotopic liver transplant. In this procedure, the donor is a person who has died recently. Orthotopic liver transplantation is recommended in the cases of total liver failure [11].

Live donor liver transplantation is a procedure in which a living person donates a portion of his or her liver to another and has several potential benefits, most importantly a reduction in waiting time and risk of death prior to a cadaveric liver transplantation. Other advantages are the scheduling of an elective liver transplantation, allowing time to optimize the medical condition of the recipient, and use a better quality organ coming from a healthy donor with a smaller chance of potential injury based on the shorter time in preservation solution. The risks of live donor liver transplantation to the recipient are generally identical to those following cadaveric liver transplantation, especially for biliary problems. In addition, there are significant donor complications and death rates, estimated to be 10–20% and 0.2–0.5%, respectively. The Milan criteria, which include solitary HCC with a less than 5 cm or fewer than three tumor nodules each of size less than 3 cm and without radiological evidence of venous invasion or distant metastasis, are widely used for the selection of HCC patients for liver transplantation based on the achievement of a 4-year survival rate of up to 75%, with a recurrence rate lower than 15% [70]. Liver transplantation is a particularly effective treatment for patients with early HCC but advanced Child-Pugh class B or C cirrhosis when other effective treatments cannot be offered.

The lack of sufficient liver donation is the major limitation of liver transplantation. There is always a waiting period between listing and transplantation. This varies among programs, but if the wait is prolonged, the tumor will grow and develop major contraindications (vascular invasion, extrahepatic spread) to transplantation [71]. The rate of exclusion on the waiting list may be as high as 25% if the waiting list is longer than 12 months [71, 72]. Obviously, if patients with more advanced tumors are included as a result of expanded listing criteria, the dropout rate will be higher, and this will translate into poor survival figures on an intention-to-treat analysis.

Percutaneous Local Ablation

Image-guided percutaneous local ablation therapies, such as percutaneous ethanol injection [73, 74], microwave coagulation [75], and radiofrequency ablation [76–78] have been widely performed on patients with small HCC, generally for those with Child A or B cirrhosis with three or fewer tumors each 3 cm or less in diameter. These procedures are potentially curative, minimally invasive, and easily repeatable for recurrence. Percutaneous ethanol injection was first reported in the early 1980s. Percutaneous microwave coagulation, in which the cancer tissue is ablated by dielectric heat produced by microwave energy emitted from a bipolar-type electrode, was intro-

duced into clinical practice in the 1990s and reported to improve local tumor control. Since the introduction of radiofrequency ablation in the 1990s, there has been a drastic shift from ethanol injection and microwave coagulation to radiofrequency ablation. RCTs proved that radiofrequency ablation is superior to ethanol injection in the treatment of small HCCs in terms of treatment response, recurrence, and overall survival [78–80].

Percutaneous ablation therapy is recommended particularly for HCC nodules with a maximum diameter of 3 cm in patients with no more than three tumors who are contraindicated for surgery. In radiofrequency ablation, survival rates have been reported to be 39.9–68.5% at 5 years [81–85] and local tumor progression rates to be 2.4–16.9% [81–83, 86]. Mortality and morbidity rates of RFA have been reported to be 0.9–7.9% and 0–1.5%, respectively [82–87].

A recent trial comparing the combination of chemoembolization and radiofrequency ablation suggested that this approach offered an improvement in survival compared to chemoembolization or ablation alone [88]. In addition, the use of a laparoscopic or open approach allows repeated placement of radiofrequency electrodes at multiple sites to ablate larger tumors.

Transcatheter Arterial Chemoembolization

Catheterization of the hepatic artery via the femoral artery and celiac axis allows embolization of the blood supply to the tumor. By such route, chemotherapeutic agents may be delivered in high concentration to the target tissue. Transcatheter arterial chemoembolization (TACE) has been widely accepted as an effective measure not only for the palliative treatment of unresectable or recurrent HCC but also for the management of resectable small HCC. Treatment-related mortality is less than 5% [89]. Untreated patients at an intermediate stage have a median survival of 16 months, whereas TACE increases the median survival of these patients to 19–20 months and is considered the standard of care

10 Hepatocellular Carcinoma

[90, 91]. In two RCTs, 1-, 2-, and 3-year survival rates for Asian patients and for European patients were 57% versus 96%, 31% versus 77%, and 26% versus 47%, respectively [92–94].

Systemic Chemotherapy

Sorafenib inhibits the kinase activity of Raf-1, wild-type B-Raf, and oncogenic B-Raf V600E. In addition, sorafenib inhibits vascular endothelial growth factor receptors (VEGFR), platelet-derived growth factor receptors (PDGFR), c-kit, Flt-3, and RET [95]. Therefore, both antiproliferative and antiangiogenic mechanisms may account for the antitumor effects. Sorafenib prolongs time to progression and overall survival in patients with advanced HCC [96, 97]. Patients with a more advanced stage or who fail TACE are candidates for sorafenib provided they remain in Child-Pugh class A status with a good performance status.

Prevention

Prevention of HBV infection can successfully reduce the incidence of HCC [98]. The hepatitis B vaccine is the first example of a cancer-preventive vaccine in humans, which proves that prevention of infection by an infectious agent can prevent its related cancer. Moreover, the meta-analysis indicated that long-term nucleotide analogue therapy for adults with chronic hepatitis B prevents or delays the development of long-term complications including decompensated cirrhosis, chronic hepatitis B-related death and chronic hepatitis B-related HCC [99]. Patients who need to take antiviral drugs should receive such therapy as soon as possible. During monotherapy, when lamivudine resistance occurs, lamivudine should be combined with other antiviral drugs without cross-resistance to lamivudine because it is still more benefited than not providing any treatment. However, so far, there is no convincing evidence that interferon therapy for chronic hepatitis B reduces the incidence of HCC [11, 100].

With HCV-related HCC, recurrence is particularly frequent, and a substantial proportion of recurrence in the late phase is thought to represent de novo, or multicentric, hepatocarcinogenesis [101–103]. Therefore, it could be reasonably assumed that antiviral therapy would reduce the overall incidence of recurrence by preventing de novo carcinogenesis. Indeed, several small RCTs performed in Japan and Taiwan have shown that the incidence of recurrence was reduced in HCV-related HCC by interferon therapy subsequent to initial HCC treatment [104, 105].

References

1. Jemal A, Siegel R, Xu J, Ward E. Cancer statistics, 2010. CA Cancer J Clin. 2010;60(5):277–300.
2. Ferenci P, Fried M, Labrecque D, et al. World Gastroenterology Organization. Hepatocellular carcinoma (HCC): a global perspective. J Clin Gastroenterol. 2010;44(4):239–45.
3. Llovet JM, Burroughs A, Bruix J. Hepatocellular carcinoma. Lancet. 2003;362(9399):1907–17.
4. Gomaa AI, Khan SA, Toledano MB, Waked I, Taylor-Robinson SD. Hepatocellular carcinoma: epidemiology, risk factors and pathogenesis. World J Gastroenterol. 2008;14(27):4300–8.
5. El-Serag HB. Hepatocellular carcinoma: an epidemiologic view. J Clin Gastroenterol. 2002;35(5 Suppl 2):S72–8.
6. Calvaruso V, Craxi A. Fibrosis in chronic viral hepatitis. Best Prac Res Clin Gastroenterol. 2011;25(2): 219–30.
7. Kawada N, Imanaka K, Kawaguchi T, et al. Hepatocellular carcinoma arising from non-cirrhotic nonalcoholic steatohepatitis. J Gastroenterol. 2009; 44(12):1190–4.
8. Kowdley KV. Iron, hemochromatosis, and hepatocellular carcinoma. Gastroenterology. 2004;127(5 Suppl 1):S79–86.
9. Zhang Q, Cao G. Genotypes, mutations, and viral load of hepatitis B virus and the risk of hepatocellular carcinoma. Hepat Mon. 2011;11(2):86–91.
10. Birrer RB, Birrer D, Klavins JV. Hepatocellular carcinoma and hepatitis virus. Ann Clin Lab Sci. 2003;33(1):39–54.
11. Bruix J, Sherman M. Management of hepatocellular carcinoma: an update. Hepatology. 2011;53(3): 1020–2.
12. Omata M, Lesmana LA, Tateishi R, et al. Asian Pacific Association for the Study of the Liver consensus recommendations on hepatocellular carcinoma. Hepatol Int. 2010;4(27):439–74.
13. Fattovich G, Stroffolini T, Zagni I, Donato F. Hepatocellular carcinoma in cirrhosis: incidence and

risk factors. Gastroenterology. 2004;127(5 Suppl 1): S35–50.

14. Hessheimer AJ, Forner A, Varela M, Bruix J. Metabolic risk factors are a major comorbidity in patients with cirrhosis independent of the presence of hepatocellular carcinoma. Eur J Gastroenterol Hepatol. 2010;22(10):1239–44.

15. Bugianesi E, Leone N, Vanni E, et al. Expanding the natural history of nonalcoholic steatohepatitis: from cryptogenic cirrhosis to hepatocellular carcinoma. Gastroenterology. 2002;123(1):134–40.

16. Sanyal AJ, Yoon SK, Lencioni R. The etiology of hepatocellular carcinoma and consequences for treatment. Oncologist. 2010;15 Suppl 4:14–22.

17. Kudo M, Han KH, Kokudo N, et al. Liver Cancer Working Group report. Jpn J Clin Oncol. 2010;40 Suppl 1:i19–27.

18. Okuda K, Nakashima T, Kojiro M, Kondo Y, Wada K. Hepatocellular carcinoma without cirrhosis in Japanese patients. Gastroenterology. 1989;97(1): 140–6.

19. Kojiro M. Histopathology of liver cancers. Best Pract Res Clin Gastroenterol. 2005;19(1):39–62.

20. Roncalli M, Park YN, Di Tommaso L. Histopathological classification of hepatocellular carcinoma. Dig Liver Dis. 2010;42 Suppl 3:S228–34.

21. Burrel M, Llovet JM, Ayuso C, et al. MRI angiography is superior to helical CT for detection of HCC prior to liver transplantation: an explant correlation. Hepatology. 2003;38:1034–42.

22. Yu JS, Kim KW, Kim EK, Lee JT, Yoo HS. Contrast enhancement of small hepatocellular carcinoma: usefulness of three successive early image acquisitions during multiphase dynamic MR imaging. AJR Am J Roentgenol. 1999;173:597–604.

23. Forner A, Vilana R, Ayuso C, et al. Diagnosis of hepatic nodules 20 mm or smaller in cirrhosis: Prospective validation of the noninvasive diagnostic criteria for hepatocellular carcinoma. Hepatology. 2008;47:97–104.

24. Minami Y, Kudo M. Hepatic malignancies: correlation between sonographic findings and pathological features. World J Radiol. 2010;2(7):249–56.

25. Makuuchi M, Hasegawa H, Yamazaki S, Bandai Y, Watanabe G, Ito T. Ultrasonic characteristics of the small hepatocellular carcinoma. Ultrasound Med Biol. 1983;2:489–91.

26. Matsui O. Detection and characterization of small hepatocellular carcinoma. J Gastroenterol Hepatol. 2004;19:S266–9.

27. Solbiati L, Tonolini M, Cova L, Goldberg SN. The role of contrast-enhanced ultrasound in the detection of focal liver lesions. Eur Radiol. 2001;11:E15–26.

28. Konopke R, Bunk A, Kersting S. The role of contrast-enhanced ultrasound for focal liver lesion detection: an overview. Ultrasound Med Biol. 2007;33(10):1515–26.

29. Efremidis SC, Hytiroglou P. The multistep process of hepatocarcinogenesis in cirrhosis with imaging correlation. Eur Radiol. 2002;12(4):753–64.

30. Yamanaka J, Saito S, Fujimoto J. Impact of preoperative planning using virtual segmental volumetry on liver resection for hepatocellular carcinoma. World J Surg. 2007;31(6):1249–55.

31. Subramanian N, Pichon E, Solomon SB. Automatic registration using implicit shape representations: applications in intraoperative 3D rotational angiography to preoperative CTA registration. Int J Comput Assist Radiol Surg. 2009;4(2):141–6.

32. Oi H, Murakami T, Kim T, Matsushita M, Kishimoto H, Nakamura H. Dynamic MR imaging and early-phase helical CT for detecting small intrahepatic metastases of hepatocellular carcinoma. AJR Am J Roentgenol. 1996;166(2):369–74.

33. Noguchi Y, Murakami T, Kim T, et al. Detection of hepatocellular carcinoma: comparison of dynamic MR imaging with dynamic double arterial phase helical CT. AJR Am J Roentgenol. 2003;180(2): 455–60.

34. Tanimoto A, Kuribayashi S. Application of superparamagnetic iron oxide to imaging of hepatocellular carcinoma. Eur J Radiol. 2006;58(2):200–16.

35. Reimer P, Tombach B. Hepatic MRI with SPIO: detection and characterization of focal liver lesions. Eur Radiol. 1998;8(7):1198–204.

36. Reimer P, Rummeny EJ, Daldrup HE, et al. Enhancement characteristics of liver metastases, hepatocellular carcinomas, and hemangiomas with Gd-EOB-DTPA: preliminary results with dynamic MR imaging. Eur Radiol. 1997;7(2):275–80.

37. Vogl TJ, Kümmel S, Hammerstingl R, et al. Liver tumors: comparison of MR imaging with Gd-EOB-DTPA and Gd-DTPA. Radiology. 1996;200(1):59–67.

38. Ueda K, Matsui O, Kawamori Y, et al. Hypervascular hepatocellular carcinoma: evaluation of hemodynamics with dynamic CT during hepatic arteriography. Radiology. 1998;206(1):161–6.

39. Matsui O, Takashima T, Kadoya M, et al. Dynamic computed tomography during arterial portography: the most sensitive examination for small hepatocellular carcinomas. J Comput Assist Tomogr. 1985; 9:19–24.

40. Oka H, Tamori A, Kuroki T, Kobayashi K, Yamamoto S. Prospective study of alpha-fetoprotein in cirrhotic patients monitored for development of hepatocellular carcinoma. Hepatology. 1994;19(1):61–6.

41. Volk ML, Hernandez JC, Su GL, Lok AS, Marrero JA. Risk factors for hepatocellular carcinoma may impair the performance of biomarkers: a comparison of AFP, DCP, and AFP-L3. Cancer Biomark. 2007;3(2):79–87.

42. Di Bisceglie AM. Issues in screening and surveillance for hepatocellular carcinoma. Gastroenterology. 2004;127(5 Suppl 1):S104–7.

43. Marrero JA, Feng Z, Wang Y, et al. Alpha-fetoprotein, des-gamma carboxyprothrombin, and lectin-bound alpha-fetoprotein in early hepatocellular carcinoma. Gastroenterology. 2009;137(1):110–8.

44. Lopez JB, Thambyrajah V, Balasegaram M, et al. Appropriate cut-off levels for serum alpha-fetoprotein

in hepatocellular carcinoma. Diagn Oncol. 1994–1995;4:287–91.

45. Weitz IC, Liebman HA. Des-gamma-carboxy (abnormal) prothrombin and hepatocellular carcinoma: a critical review. Hepatology. 1993;18(4): 990–7.

46. Lok AS, Sterling RK, Everhart JE, HALT-C Trial Group, et al. Des-gamma-carboxy prothrombin and alpha-fetoprotein as biomarkers for the early detection of hepatocellular carcinoma. Gastroenterology. 2010;138(2):493–502.

47. Koike Y, Shiratori Y, Sato S, et al. Des-gamma-carboxy prothrombin as a useful predisposing factor for the development of portal venous invasion in patients with hepatocellular carcinoma: a prospective analysis of 227 patients. Cancer. 2001;91: 561–9.

48. Hagiwara S, Kudo M, Kawasaki T, et al. Prognostic factors for portal venous invasion in patients with hepatocellular carcinoma. J Gastroenterol. 2006;41: 1214–9.

49. Toyoda H, Kumada T, Kaneoka Y, et al. Prognostic value of pretreatment levels of tumor markers for hepatocellular carcinoma on survival after curative treatment of patients with HCC. J Hepatol. 2008;49(2):223–32.

50. Sato Y, Nakata K, Kato Y, et al. Early recognition of hepatocellular carcinoma based on altered profiles of alpha-fetoprotein. N Engl J Med. 1993;328:1802–6.

51. Li D, Mallory T, Satomura S. AFP-L3: a new generation of tumor marker for hepatocellular carcinoma. Clin Chim Acta. 2001;313:15–9.

52. Tateishi R, Yoshida H, Matsuyama Y, Mine N, Kondo Y, Omata M. Diagnostic accuracy of tumor markers for hepatocellular carcinoma: a systematic review. Hepatol Int. 2008;2:17–30.

53. Toyoda H, Kumada T, Kiriyama S, et al. Prognostic significance of simultaneous measurement of three tumor markers in patients with hepatocellular carcinoma. Clin Gastroenterol Hepatol. 2006;4:111–7.

54. Forner A, Reig ME, Rodrigruez de Lope C, Bruix J. Current strategy for staging and treatment: the BCLC update and future prospects. Semin Liver Dis. 2010;30:61–74.

55. Bruix J, Llovet JM. Prognostic prediction and treatment strategy in hepatocellular carcinoma. Hepatology. 2002;35:519–24.

56. Torzilli G, Makuuchi M, Inoue K, et al. No-mortality liver resection for hepatocellular carcinoma in cirrhotic and noncirrhotic patients: is there a way? A prospective analysis of our approach. Arch Surg. 1999;134:984–92.

57. Poon RT, Fan ST, Lo CM, et al. Improving perioperative outcome expands the role of hepatectomy in management of benign and malignant hepatobiliary diseases: analysis of 1222 consecutive patients from a prospective database. Ann Surg. 2004;240: 698–708.

58. Asiyanbola B, Chang D, Gleisner AL, et al. Operative mortality after hepatic resection: are literature-based rates broadly applicable? J Gastrointest Surg. 2008; 12:842–51.

59. Grazi GL, Ercolani G, Pierangeli F, et al. Improved results of liver resection for hepatocellular carcinoma on cirrhosis give the procedure added value. Ann Surg. 2001;234:71–8.

60. Poon RT, Fan ST, Lo CM, et al. Improving survival results after resection of hepatocellular carcinoma: a prospective study of 377 patients over 10 years. Ann Surg. 2001;234:63–70.

61. Capussotti L, Muratore A, Amisano M, Polastri R, Bouzari H, Massucco P. Liver resection for hepatocellular carcinoma on cirrhosis: analysis of mortality, morbidity and survival—a European single center experience. Eur J Surg Oncol. 2005;31: 986–93.

62. Poon RT, Fan ST, Lo CM, Liu CL, Wong J. Difference in tumor invasiveness in cirrhotic patients with hepatocellular carcinoma fulfilling the Milan criteria treated by resection and transplantation: impact on long-term survival. Ann Surg. 2007;245:51–8.

63. Chequi D, Husson E, Hammond R, et al. Laparoscopic liver resection: a feasibility study in 30 patients. Ann Surg. 2000;232:753–62.

64. Descottes B, Lachachi F, Sodji M, et al. Early experience with laparoscopic approach for solid liver tumors: initial 16 cases. Ann Surg. 2000;232: 641–5.

65. Gigot JF, Glineur D, Santiago AJ, et al. Laparoscoic liver resection for malignant liver tumors: preliminary results of a multicenter European study. Ann Surg. 2002;236:90–7.

66. Chequi D, Soubarane O, Husson E, et al. Laparoscopic living donor hepatectomy for liver transplantation in children. Lancet. 2002;359:392–6.

67. Yamasaki S, Hasegawa H, Kinoshita H, et al. A prospective randomized trial of the preventive effect of pre-operative transcatheter arterial embolization against recurrence of hepatocellular carcinoma. Jpn J Cancer Res. 1996;87:206–11.

68. Farges O, Belghiti J, Kianmanesh R, et al. Portal vein embolization before right hepatectomy: prospective clinical trial. Ann Surg. 2003;237:208–17.

69. Tanaka H, Hirohashi K, Kubo S, Shuto T, Higaki I, Kinoshita H. Preoperative portal vein embolization improves prognosis after right hepatectomy for hepatocellular carcinoma in patients with impaired hepatic function. Br J Surg. 2000;87:879–82.

70. Mazzaferro V, Regalia E, Doci R, et al. Liver transplantation for the treatment of small hepatocellular carcinomas in patients with cirrhosis. N Engl J Med. 1996;334:693–9.

71. Yao FY, Bass NM, Nikolai B, et al. Liver transplantation for hepatocellular carcinoma: analysis of survival according to the intention-to-treat principle and dropout from the waiting list. Liver Transpl. 2002;8:873–83.

72. Freeman RB, Mithoefer A, Ruthazer R, et al. Optimizing staging for hepatocellular carcinoma before liver transplantation: A retrospective analysis

of the UNOS/OPTN database. Liver Transpl. 2006;12:1504–11.

73. Livraghi T, Festi D, Monti F, Salmi A, Vettori C. US-guided percutaneous alcohol injection of small hepatic and abdominal tumors. Radiology. 1986;161: 309–12.

74. Bartolozzi C, Lencioni R. Ethanol injection for the treatment of hepatic tumours. Eur Radiol. 1996;6:682–96.

75. Seki T, Wakabayashi M, Nakagawa T, et al. Ultrasonically guided percutaneous microwave coagulation therapy for small hepatocellular carcinoma. Cancer. 1994;74:817–25.

76. Cho YK, Kim JK, Kim WT, Chung JW. Hepatic resection versus radiofrequency ablation for very early stage hepatocellular carcinoma: a Markov model analysis. Hepatology. 2010;51:1284–90.

77. Minami Y, Kudo M. Radiofrequency ablation of hepatocellular carcinoma: current status. World J Radiol. 2010;2(11):417–24.

78. Shiina S, Teratani T, Obi S, et al. A randomized controlled trial of radiofrequency ablation with ethanol injection for small hepatocellular carcinoma. Gastroenterology. 2005;129:122–30.

79. Lencioni RA, Allgaier HP, Cioni D, et al. Small hepatocellular carcinoma in cirrhosis: randomized comparison of radio-frequency thermal ablation versus percutaneous ethanol injection. Radiology. 2003;228:235–40.

80. Lin SM, Lin CJ, Lin CC, Hsu CW, Chen YC. Radiofrequency ablation improves prognosis compared with ethanol injection for hepatocellular carcinoma B4 cm. Gastroenterology. 2004;127:1714–23.

81. Machi J, Bueno RS, Wong LL. Long-term follow-up outcome of patients undergoing radiofrequency ablation for unresectable hepatocellular carcinoma. World J Surg. 2005;29:1364–73.

82. Lencioni R, Cioni D, Crocetti L, et al. Early-stage hepatocellular carcinoma in patients with cirrhosis: long-term results of percutaneous image-guided radiofrequency ablation. Radiology. 2005;234:961–7.

83. Tateishi R, Shiina S, Teratani T, et al. Percutaneous radiofrequency ablation for hepatocellular carcinoma. An analysis of 1000 cases. Cancer. 2005;103: 1201–9.

84. Cabassa P, Donato F, Simeone F, Grazioli L, Romanini L. Radiofrequency ablation of hepatocellular carcinoma: long-term experience with expandable needle electrodes. AJR Am J Roentgenol. 2006;186:S316–21.

85. Livraghi T, Meloni F, Di Stasi M, et al. Sustained complete response and complications rates after radiofrequency ablation of very early hepatocellular carcinoma in cirrhosis: is resection still the treatment of choice? Hepatology. 2008;47:82–9.

86. Yan K, Chen MH, Yang W, et al. Radiofrequency ablation of hepatocellular carcinoma: long-term outcome and prognostic factors. Eur J Radiol. 2008;67:336–47.

87. Kasugai H, Osaki Y, Oka H, Kudo M, Seki T. Severe complications of radiofrequency ablation therapy for hepatocellular carcinoma: an analysis of 3,891 ablations in 2,614 patients. Oncology. 2007;72 Suppl 1:72–5.

88. Hsu YS, Chien RN, Yeh CT, et al. Long-term outcome after spontaneous HBeAg seroconversion in patients with chronic hepatitis B. Hepatology. 2002;35:1522–7.

89. El-Serag HB, Marrero JA, Rudolph L, Reddy KR. Diagnosis and treatment of hepatocellular carcinoma. Gastroenterology. 2008;134:1752–63.

90. Llovet JM, Bruix J. Systematic review of randomized trials for unresectable hepatocellular carcinoma: chemoembolization improves survival. Hepatology. 2003;37:429–42.

91. Bruix J, Sherman M, Llovet JM, et al. Clinical management of hepatocellular carcinoma. Conclusions of the Barcelona-2000 EASL Conference. European Association for the Study of the Liver. J Hepatol. 2001;35:421–30.

92. Staunton M, Dodd JD, McCormick PA, Malone DE. Finding evidence-based answers to practical questions in radiology: which patients with inoperable hepatocellular carcinoma will survive longer after transarterial chemoembolization? Radiology. 2005; 237:404–13.

93. Lo CM, Ngan H, Tso WK, et al. Randomized controlled trial of transarterial lipiodol chemoembolization for unresectable hepatocellular carcinoma. Hepatology. 2002;35:1164–71.

94. Llovet JM, Real MI, Montana X, et al. Arterial embolisation or chemoembolisation versus symptomatic treatment in patients with unresectable hepatocellular carcinoma: a randomised controlled trial. Lancet. 2002;359:1734–9.

95. Wilhelm S, Carter C, Lynch M, et al. Discovery and development of sorafenib: a multikinase inhibitor for treating cancer. Nat Rev Drug Discov. 2006;5: 835–44.

96. Llovet JM, Ricci S, Mazzaferro V, et al. Sorafenib in advanced hepatocellular carcinoma. N Engl J Med. 2008;359:378–90.

97. Cheng AL, Kang YK, Chen Z, et al. Efficacy and safety of sorafenib in patients in the Asia-Pacific region with advanced hepatocellular carcinoma: a phase III randomised, double-blind, placebo-controlled trial. Lancet Oncol. 2009;10:25–34.

98. Chang MH, Hepatitis B. virus and cancer prevention. Recent Results Cancer Res. 2011;188:75–84.

99. Zhang QQ, An X, Liu YH, et al. Long-term nucleos(t) ide analogues therapy for adults with chronic hepatitis B reduces the risk of long-term complications: a meta-analysis. Virol J. 2011;8:72.

100. Baffis V, Shrier I, Sherker AH, Szilagyi A. Use of interferon for prevention of hepatocellular carcinoma in cirrhotic patients with hepatitis B or hepatitis C virus infection. Ann Intern Med. 1999;131(9): 696–701.

101. Kumada T, Nakano S, Takeda I, et al. Patterns of recurrence after initial treatment in patients with small hepatocellular carcinoma. Hepatology. 1997; 25:87–92.
102. Poon RT, Fan ST, Ng IO, Lo CM, Liu CL, Wong J. Different risk factors and prognosis for early and late intrahepatic recurrence after resection of hepatocellular carcinoma. Cancer. 2000;89:500–7.
103. Sakon M, Umeshita K, Nagano H, et al. Clinical significance of hepatic resection in hepatocellular carcinoma: analysis by disease-free survival curves. Arch Surg. 2000;135:1456–9.
104. Ikeda K, Arase Y, Saitoh S, et al. Interferon beta prevents recurrence of hepatocellular carcinoma after complete resection or ablation of the primary tumor—a prospective randomized study of hepatitis C virus-related liver cancer. Hepatology. 2000;32: 228–32.
105. Kubo S, Nishiguchi S, Hirohashi K, et al. Effects of long-term postoperative interferon-alpha therapy on intrahepatic recurrence after resection of hepatitis C virus-related hepatocellular carcinoma. A randomized, controlled trial. Ann Intern Med. 2001; 134:963–7.

Biomarkers for Prognosis and Molecularly Targeted Therapy in Renal Cell Carcinoma

11

Laura S. Schmidt

Introduction

Kidney cancer or renal cell carcinoma (RCC) comprises about 3% of all adult malignancies, and its incidence has been steadily rising at a rate of ~2–3% per decade but now appears to be leveling off or even declining in some US and European registries due in part to diagnosis of RCC at earlier stage and smaller size [1, 2]. Limited symptoms often result in late diagnosis in advanced stages frequently by incidental radiography for another health problem. Surgical resection of primary RCC can be effective as treatment of localized advanced tumors. However, approximately 25% of cases will be metastatic upon diagnosis [3], and since metastatic RCC is notoriously refractory to chemotherapy and only moderately responsive to immunotherapy, these distant metastases remain the primary cause of cancer-related deaths. Therefore, there is a critical need for validated biomarkers of RCC as prognostic indicators of local and advanced disease and as predictors of tumor response to therapy. Importantly, the identification of biotargets for the development of effective molecularly targeted

L.S. Schmidt, Ph.D. (✉)
Urologic Oncology Branch, National Cancer Institute, National Institutes of Health, Bldg 10/CRC/Rm 1-3961, 10 Center Drive MSC 1107, Bethesda, MD 20892, USA

Basic Science Program, SAIC-Frederick, Inc.,
NCI-Frederick, Frederick, MD 21702, USA
e-mail: schmidtl@mail.nih.gov

therapies personalized to the patient is of the highest priority and a major focus of current research efforts in the field today.

Epidemiology

It was estimated that approximately 209,000 new cases of RCC arose in 2006 worldwide with nearly 103,000 deaths [3, 4]. RCC affects men and women in the sixth and seventh decades of life, although earlier age of onset is associated with inherited renal cancer syndromes. Known risk factors that contribute to the development of RCC include cigarette smoking, obesity (body mass index), hypertension, male gender, and a first-degree relative with kidney cancer [2]. Evidence is accumulating to suggest that end-stage renal disease, parity in women, alcohol consumption (inverse), reduced physical activity, and occupational exposure to trichloroethylene may also contribute to overall risk for RCC while a diet rich in fruits and vegetables may be protective [2].

Classification of RCC: Diagnostic and Prognostic Implications

Histologic Subtypes and Characteristic Cytogenetics

RCC is not a single entity but is a diverse group of epithelial tumors classified according to histology into the following major subtypes which can occur in both sporadic cases and inherited RCC syndromes: clear cell, papillary type 1 and type 2, chromophobe, and collecting duct renal carcinomas. Renal oncocytoma is a benign neoplasm that can occur in these settings, progress to large size, and compromise renal function [5, 6] (Table 11.1). Renal medullary carcinoma, a rare tumor associated with sickle cell trait, and renal angiomyolipoma, a benign renal lesion consisting of fat, blood vessels, and smooth muscle, which is associated with the inherited multisystem disorder tuberous sclerosis complex (TSC), will not be discussed here.

Clear Cell RCC

Clear cell renal carcinomas (ccRCC) account for approximately 75% of RCC and are named for the clear cytoplasmic regions that remain when lipids and glycogen dissolve during histologic processing. Clear cell renal tumors arise from the proximal tubule, are generally solitary and unifocal (except in a familial setting), and are characterized cytogenetically by loss of chromosome 3 at three separate regions (3p25-26, 3p21-22, 3p13-14), gains of chromosomes 5q22-ter, 7, and 17, and, less frequently, loss of chromosomes 9p, 10q, 13q, and 14q, which are associated with poor prognosis and/or high histologic grade [7–9]. Sarcomatoid features are also associated with poor outcome and rapid progression to metastasis. Approximately 60–90% of clear cell renal tumors show loss of heterozygosity (LOH) on chromosome 3p that includes the *von Hippel–Lindau* (*VHL*) tumor suppressor gene locus at 3p25-26 [10, 11]. In a recent large retrospective study, 91% of sporadic clear cell renal tumors demonstrated mutational inactivation of the *VHL* allele by sequence alteration or hypermethylation [12], underscoring a conclusive role for *VHL* inactivation in the vast majority of sporadic clear cell renal tumors. Clear cell tumors are the only histologic subtype found in patients with the inherited renal cancer syndrome, VHL disease, and families with constitutional translocations involving chromosome 3. They also occur with lower frequency in Birt–Hogg–Dubé syndrome, familial renal cancer associated with *succinate dehydrogenase* (*SDH*)

mutations, and rarely in patients with TSC (see "Familial RCC Syndromes: Causative Genes and Their Pathways as Potential Biotargets").

Papillary RCC

Papillary renal tumors, which arise from the proximal tubules, comprise 10% of renal carcinomas and may be further subdivided histologically into type 1 and type 2 [7]. Type 1 tumors have delicate papillae with small tumor cells containing scant cytoplasm arranged in a single layer on the papillary basement membrane and often contain aggregates of foamy macrophages. Type 1 tumors tend to be multifocal, bilateral, and less aggressive compared to clear cell tumors. Type 2 tumors are characterized by higher nuclear grade with eosinophilic cytoplasm and pseudostratified nuclei on papillary cores and are most often solitary, unilateral, and more frequently metastasize due to their aggressive growth pattern [7, 8]. Type 1 tumors are usually associated with lower stage and grade than type 2 tumors and therefore are linked to longer patient survival and better prognosis [13]. Cytogenetic studies of papillary renal tumors have shown characteristic trisomies/tetrasomies of chromosome 7 and 17, and loss of Y, but only infrequent loss of 3p [9]. In two studies, trisomies of 7 and 17 were infrequent in type 2 papillary tumors suggesting two distinct morphologic and genetic subgroups [13, 14]. Trisomies of 12, 16, and 20 are also frequent and may be associated with tumor progression, with LOH at 9p13 significantly more frequent in type 2 corresponding to shorter patient survival [13, 15]. Additional regions of loss reported in papillary renal tumors include 1p, 4q, 6q, 13q, and X [9]. Papillary type 1 renal tumors are the only histologic variant that arises in the inherited renal cancer syndrome, hereditary papillary renal carcinoma (HPRC), whereas type 2 papillary renal tumors are the most frequent tumors found in the inherited RCC syndrome, hereditary leiomyomatosis and renal cell carcinoma (HLRCC) (see "Familial RCC Syndromes: Causative Genes and Their Pathways as Potential Biotargets"). Clear cell tumors not only with papillary architecture but also with granular eosinophilic cytoplasm develop in patients with a somatic

Table 11.1 Classification of RCC by histology, characteristic cytogenetics, and diagnostic immunoprofiles

Tumor type	Chromosome	Potential gene involved	Alteration	Other genetic alterations	Diagnostic immunomarkers
Clear cell RCC	3p13-14 3p21-22 3p25-26	*FHIT* *RASSF1A* *VHL*	Loss Loss Loss, mutation, methylation	+5q22-ter, +7, +17 (more freq); −9q, −13p, −17p, −14q (less freq); −8p, −9p, −10q, −13q, −14q (poor prognosis)	RCC marker+, CD10+, vimentin+, CAIX+, CD117−, KS-cadherin−, parvalbumin−
Papillary RCC, type 1	7q31 7 17 Y	*MET* *MET?* Unknown Unknown	Mutation or gain Gain Gain Loss	+8, +12q, +16q, +20q, (more freq); −1p, −4q, −6q, −9p, −11p, −13q,−14q,−18, −21q, −X (less freq)	RCC marker+, CD10+, vimentin+, CK7+, AMACR+, CD117−, KS-cadherin−, parvalbumin−
Papillary RCC, type 2	9p13	Unknown	Loss	+7, +17 (less freq than type 1)	More variable profile than type 1
Chromophobe RCC	Multiple complex losses	Unknown	Loss	−1, −2, −6, −10, −13q, −17, −21, −X	RCC marker−,CD10−, vimentin−, CAIX−, AMACR−, CD117+, KS-cadherin+, parvalbumin+, CK7+, S100A1−, CD82+
Oncocytoma	Few alterations reported	Unknown	Loss	Less complex pattern of loss than chromophobe RCC; −1, −14q, rearr. 11q13	Similar to chromophobe but S100A1+, CD82−
Collecting duct RCC	Rare, not well studied	Unknown	Loss	−1q32, −6p, −8p, −13q, −21q	RCC marker−, CD10−, CK7+, PAX2/8+
RCC associated with Xp11.2 translocation	Xp11.2	ASPL-TFE3 PRCC-TFE3 PSF-TFE3 NONO-TFE3 CLTC-TFE3 ?-TFE3	t(X;17)(p11.2;q25) t(X;1)(p11.2;q21) t(X;1)(p11.2;p34) inv(X)(p11.2;q12) t(X;17)(p11.2;q23) t(X;3)(p11.2;q23)	None	TFE3+, RCC marker+, CD10+

CD10, membrane metallo-endopeptidase; *RCC*, renal cell carcinoma; *RASSF1A*, Ras association (RalGDS/AF-6) domain family member 1; *FHIT*, fragile histidine triad gene; *AMACR*, α-methylacyl coenzyme A racemase; *CAIX*, carbonic anhydrase IX; *CD117*, c-kit oncogene; *CK7*, cytokeratin 7; *KS-cadherin*, kidney-specific cadherin; *VHL*, von Hippel–Lindau; *MET*, hepatocyte growth factor receptor; *TFE3*, transcription factor 3; *ASPL*, alveolar soft part sarcoma chromosomal region candidate gene1; *PRCC*, papillary renal cell carcinoma; *PSF*, splicing factor proline/glutamine rich; *NONO*, non-Pou domain containing, octamer-binding; *CLTC*, clathrin, heavy chain; *PAX*, paxillin; *?*, unknown or not confirmed

translocation involving chromosome Xp11.2 resulting in gene fusions with *transcription factor E3 gene, TFE3,* and at least six gene partners, one of which is unknown (*PRCC, ASPL, NONO, PSF, CLTC*). They are fairly indolent in children but aggressive in adults where they are rare, and can be distinguished by nuclear immunohistochemical staining for TFE3 [16].

Chromophobe RCC

Chromophobe renal tumors, which are thought to arise from intercalated cells of the collecting duct, account for about 5% of cases and are a distinct subtype that tend to have a better prognosis than clear cell or type 2 papillary RCC [9]. Histologically, chromophobe tumors are characterized by large polygonal cells with transparent slightly reticulated cytoplasm and prominent cell membranes, irregular often wrinkled nuclei, small nucleoli, and characteristic perinuclear halos. They stain positively with Hale's colloidal iron stain, which is one distinguishing feature from renal oncocytomas [7]. As with clear cell RCC, sarcomatoid phenotype in chromophobe RCC is associated with aggressive tumor growth and metastases. Chromophobe RCC is characterized by extensive chromosomal losses, most frequently chromosomes 1, 2, 6, 10, 13q, 17, and 21 with a low chromosomal number ranging between 32 and 39 [7–9]. Rare sporadic composite chromophobe/oncocytoma tumors have been described termed "oncocytosis," raising the possibility that the two types of tumors might be related [17]. "Oncocytic" hybrid tumors have been described as the predominant tumor type in the inherited renal cancer disorder, Birt–Hogg–Dubé syndrome (see "Familial RCC Syndromes: Causative Genes and Their Pathways as Potential Biotargets").

Collecting Duct (Bellini Duct) RCC

This tumor, thought to be derived from the principal cells of the collecting duct of Bellini, occurs very rarely (<1%), has poor prognosis, and is often metastatic at presentation. Mortality is high and two-thirds of patients die of their disease within 2 years of diagnosis [7]. Histologically, collecting duct tumors have a tubular/papillary growth pattern containing inflamed fibrous stroma, desmoplasia, with hobnail appearance and are of high nuclear grade [7, 8]. Very few tumors of this rare entity have been evaluated, but in one study, loss of multiple chromosomal arms was documented including 1q32, 6p, 8p, 13q, and 21q, while another study suggested that 8p LOH might be associated with poor patient prognosis [7]. Collecting duct tumors are infrequently associated with the familial RCC syndrome, HLRCC (see "Familial RCC Syndromes: Causative Genes and Their Pathways as Potential Biotargets").

Renal Oncocytoma

Renal oncocytoma is a benign renal neoplasm originating from the intercalated cells of the collecting system comprising about 5% of all renal neoplasms [7]. Histologically, these neoplasms have round to polygonal cells with densely granular eosinophilic cytoplasm arranged in nests and, on low power, give the appearance of an island, a characteristic feature of oncocytomas. Ultrastructurally, they contain many mitochondria with predominantly lamellar cristae [8]. They are generally solitary except in a familial setting, asymptomatic with excellent prognosis, and may be distinguished from malignant chromophobe RCC by the fact that the latter has a more complex karyotype in addition to loss of chromosome 1. In a few oncocytomas, translocation of t(5;11)(q35;q13) was detected, and in some cases, partial or complete loss of chromosomes 1 and 14 was described [7, 8]. Regions of "oncocytosis" containing large numbers of oncocytic lesions with a spectrum of morphologic features, sometimes including chromophobe or hybrid features, have been described in sporadic oncocytomas [17], rare families with familial renal oncocytomas [18], and the familial RCC disorder Birt–Hogg–Dubé syndrome (see "Familial RCC syndromes: Causative Genes and Their Pathways as Potential Biotargets").

Diagnostic Immunomarkers

In addition to the characteristic histology generally diagnostic for each subtype of RCC, a number of immunomarkers have been identified that have proven useful for diagnostic purposes in several contexts. Immunohistochemistry using these markers has become essential for differentiating renal from nonrenal neoplasms that they may resemble, subtyping RCCs to accurately determine the subtype variant since it may affect choice of therapy regimens, and diagnosing rare types of renal neoplasms or metastatic RCC at a distant site in small biopsy specimens.

The following immunomarkers are considered to have good diagnostic utility (reviewed in Truong et al.): (1) cytokeratins including CK18, CK7, and high-molecular-weight CKs [34βE12+]; (2) vimentin, a mesenchymal marker, expressed almost exclusively by RCC and not many other cancers; (3) α-methylacyl coenzyme A racemase (AMACR), a mitochondrial enzyme important in fatty acid oxidation; (4) carbonic anhydrase IX, a transmembrane enzyme involved in maintenance of cellular pH; (5) PAX2 and PAX8, nuclear transcription factors involved in fetal kidney development; (6) RCC marker, an antibody that detects a glycoprotein in the brush border of proximal renal tubule cells; (7) CD10, a glycoprotein enzyme involved in cellular response to peptide hormones and located in the proximal tubule brush border; (8) E-cadherin/kidney-specific cadherin important for cell–cell interactions and located in distal convoluted and collecting duct cells; (9) parvalbumin, a calcium-binding protein involved in calcium homeostasis located in the distal tubule and collecting duct cells; (10) claudins 7 and 8, tight cell junction proteins expressed in the distal tubule and collecting duct cells; (11) S100A1 expressed throughout the kidney; (12) CD82, a known metastasis suppressor gene, expressed in the distal nephron; (13) c-kit (CD117), a proto-oncogene mutated in several cancers and a potential therapeutic target; and (14) TFE3, a transcription factor involved in Xp11.2 translocation renal cancers [19]. The immunoprofiles of the major histologic subtypes of RCC are extremely valuable for diagnosing renal neoplasms in problematic settings or to distinguish metastases from primaries in distant organs. Clear cell RCC is usually positive for vimentin, AE1/AE3 keratins, CD10, RCC marker, and CAIX and negative for CD117, kidney-specific cadherin,

and parvalbumin. Papillary type 1 RCC is also often positive for vimentin, AE1/AE2 keratins, CD10, and RCC marker, but unlike clear cell RCC, it is also positive for CK7 and AMACR. Similar to clear cell RCC, papillary type 1 RCC is usually negative for CD117, kidney-specific cadherin, and parvalbumin. Papillary type 2 RCC has a more variable immunoprofile. Since chromophobe RCC arises from the distal nephron, its immunoprofile is distinctly different from clear cell and papillary renal tumors. Chromophobe RCC is positive for kidney-specific cadherin, parvalbumin, CD117, AE1/AE3 keratin, CK7, and claudins 7 and 8 (limited data) but negative for vimentin, CAIX, and AMACR. Benign renal oncocytoma which also arises from the distal nephron shares a similar immunoprofile with chromophobe RCC, but in two studies oncocytomas were distinguished from chromophobe RCC by positive expression of S100A1 and negative expression for CD82. Conversely, chromophobe RCC was S100A1 negative and CD82 positive [20, 21]. Collecting duct carcinoma is negative for the common RCC markers, CD10 and RCC marker, and positive for CK7, PAX2, and PAX8. Tumors that develop in Xp11.2 translocation patients are distinguished by markers for clear cell RCC (CD10, RCC marker) and positive nuclear staining for TFE3 protein (Table 11.1).

Prognostication of Histologic Subtype

Of the main histologic types of RCC, patients with chromophobe RCC were found to have excellent prognosis and overall survival that was superior to the other histologic types in two independent series [22, 23]. In a third study, chromophobe and papillary RCC patients were associated with improved progression-free survival following nephrectomy compared with clear cell RCC; however, only chromophobe RCC was retained as prognostic after multivariate analyses [24]. In a recent retrospective series of 2,446 nephrectomy patients, clear cell RCC was a predictor of metastasis and cancer-specific death (HR 2.76 and 1.77, respectively; $p < 0.001$) relative to papillary and chromophobe RCC in multivariate analyses [25]. Teloken et al. reported that chromophobe and papillary histologies were also significantly associated with better outcome compared with clear cell histology in a multivariate analysis of 1,863 postnephrectomy patients (HR 0.40 vs. 0.62; $p=0.014$) [26]. On the other hand, in a multicenter study of 4,063 patients with clear cell, papillary and chromophobe RCC who underwent nephrectomy, Eastern Cooperative Oncology Group (ECOG) performance, TNM stage, and Fuhrman grade but not histology were retained as independent prognostic variables in multivariate analysis [27]. Higher expression of VEGFR-2 and VEGFR-3, loss of chromosome 1p, 3p, or 9p, and absence of trisomy 17 were all associated with poor prognosis. In several series, papillary type 2 RCC was associated with worse prognosis. Klatte et al. evaluated 51 papillary type 1 and 107 papillary type 2 RCC patients and found type 2 patients to have worse ECOG performance status, higher stage and grade, increased nodal and distant metastases, and worse survival although type was not retained as prognostic on multivariate analysis [28]. The question of whether histologic subtypes predict different survival outcomes needs additional validation, but in the majority of reported studies, patients with clear cell RCC demonstrated worse prognosis than other histologic subtypes. The prognosis for papillary type 2 RCC patients is consistently worse than papillary type 1 patients.

Familial RCC Syndromes: Causative Genes and Their Pathways as Potential Biotargets

Although familial renal cancers comprise only 4% of all RCC, our current understanding of the genetics of renal carcinoma has come almost exclusively from studies of families with rare inherited renal cancer syndromes (Table 11.2) [6]. The discovery of each of the predisposing renal cancer genes — *VHL, MET, FH, SDH, FLCN* — came from linkage analysis in these RCC families. Elucidation of the function of these genes in normal cells has provided clues to how loss-of-function (*VHL, FH, SDH, FLCN*) or activation (*MET*) of these genes leads to renal

tumor development. In the following sections, the clinical presentation and causative gene for each major renal cancer syndrome will be presented followed by functional consequences of each gene mutation. Finally, molecular targets identified from among the pathway components will be discussed in light of their diagnostic, prognostic, and predictive utility. The potential of several of these novel biotargets for molecularly targeted therapy will be considered.

Inherited Clear Cell RCC: VHL Disease

VHL disease is an autosomal dominantly inherited multisystem disorder in which patients develop tumors in a number of organ systems including central nervous system hemangioblastomas, retinal angiomas, pheochromocytomas, endolymphatic sac, and pancreatic islet cell tumors, as well as multiple cysts in the kidney and pancreas. About 25–45% of VHL patients will develop bilateral multifocal clear cell renal tumors during the second to fourth decade with 70% penetrance by age 60 [29]. Patients with VHL disease inherit a germline mutation in the *VHL* tumor suppressor gene located on chromosome 3p25-26 [30] with subsequent loss of the wild-type *VHL* allele in the kidney cell, priming it to progress to tumor. In fact, *VHL* biallelic inactivation occurs in microfoci of RCC as well as preneoplastic renal cysts in kidneys of VHL patients confirming this as an early event in *VHL*-associated tumor progression [31, 32]. Over 1,000 germline *VHL* mutations in 945 VHL families located throughout the gene (with the exception of the 35 residue acidic domain) have been reported worldwide [33]. VHL subclasses based upon the predisposition to develop pheochromocytomas and high/low risk of RCC have established functionally related genotype–phenotype associations [29].

Inherited Clear Cell RCC: Chromosome 3p Translocation Families

A family with a constitutional t(3;8)(p14;q24) balanced translocation was described in which

Table 11.2 Inherited RCC syndromes and predisposing genes: basis for molecularly targeted therapy

Inherited syndrome	Chromosomal locus	Gene[a]	Function	Renal manifestations	Other manifestations
von Hippel–Lindau disease (VHL)	3p25	VHL	Tumor suppressor (loss of function)	Clear cell RCC	Retinal and central nervous system hemangioblastomas, pheochromocytomas, pancreatic cysts and neuroendocrine tumors, endolymphatic sac tumors, epididymal and broad ligament cystadenomas
Hereditary papillary renal carcinoma (HPRC)	7q31	MET	Oncogene (gain of function)	Papillary RCC, type 1	None
Hereditary leiomyomatosis and renal cell carcinoma (HLRCC)	1q42-43	FH	Tumor suppressor (loss of function)	Papillary RCC type 2, collecting duct carcinoma	Uterine and cutaneous leiomyomas, leiomyosarcomas
SDH-associated familial renal carcinoma and hereditary paraganglioma	1p36 11q23	SDHB SDHD	Tumor suppressor (loss of function)	Clear cell RCC (often early onset), rarely chromophobe RCC	Pheochromocytomas, head and neck paragangliomas, extra-adrenal pheochromocytomas
Birt–Hogg–Dubé syndrome (BHD)	17p11.2	FLCN	Tumor suppressor (loss of function)	Hybrid oncocytic renal tumors, chromophobe RCC, clear cell RCC, oncocytomas, cysts	Cutaneous papules (fibrofolliculomas), lung cysts, spontaneous pneumothoraces, colon polyps
Tuberous sclerosis complex (TSC)	9q34 16p13	TSC1 TSC2	Tumor suppressor (loss of function)	Cysts, angiomyolipomas, rarely clear cell RCC	Facial angiofibromas, giant cell astrocytomas, cardiac rhabdomyoma, lymphangioleiomyomatosis
Constitutional chromosome 3 translocation	3p	VHL	Tumor suppressor (loss of function)	Clear cell RCC	None

VHL, von Hippel–Lindau; MET, hepatocyte growth factor receptor; FH, fumarate hydratase; SDHB, succinate dehydrogenase subunit B; SDHD, succinate dehydrogenase subunit D; FLCN, folliculin; TSC, tuberous sclerosis; RCC, renal cell carcinoma

bilateral multifocal clear cell renal tumors coseg-regated with the chromosomal translocation [34]. Loss of the derivative chromosome carrying the 3p25 segment followed by acquisition of different somatic *VHL* mutations in the remaining alleles was identified in tumors from this family leading to a proposed three-step tumorigenesis model in which an individual inherits the constitutional translocation, the derivative chromosome 3 is lost, and a *VHL* mutation occurs in the remaining copy of the gene [35]. A number of chromosome 3 translocation families have been described in which *VHL* inactivation through loss of the derivative chromosome and *VHL* somatic mutation contributes to clear cell renal tumors [36].

Inherited Clear Cell RCC: *SDH* Mutation-Associated Early Onset Renal Cancer

Bilateral multifocal renal tumors with early onset (<40 years of age) have been reported in the setting of hereditary head and neck paragangliomas (HPGL) and adrenal/extra-adrenal pheochromocytomas [37]. Most frequently, clear cell RCC develops; however, chromophobe RCC, papillary type 2 RCC, and renal oncocytoma have been described [38, 39]. Loss-of-function germline mutations in the genes encoding subunits B and D of the Krebs cycle enzyme SDH (SDHB, SDHD) are responsible for the RCC, HPGL, and/or pheochromocytoma phenotypes in these families [39–43] (see "Inherited Papillary Type 2 RCC: Functional Consequence of Krebs Cycle Enzyme Mutations").

Inherited Clear Cell RCC: Function of the *VHL* Gene

Although new roles for pVHL are continuing to be discovered, the most well-understood function for the pVHL tumor suppressor protein is to serve as the substrate recognition site for the transcription factor family, hypoxia-inducible factor α [HIF-α]. HIF-α is targeted for proteasomal degradation by an E3 ubiquitin ligase complex containing pVHL, elongin B, elongin C, cullin-2 and Rbx

1 [44–47]. When cells are exposed to normal oxygen levels, a family of HIF prolyl hydroxylases (PHDs) that require 2-oxoglutarate, molecular oxygen, ascorbic acid, and iron as cofactors act to hydroxylate HIF-α on critical prolines [48, 49]. pVHL then binds to hydroxylated HIF-α through its β-domain, targeting HIF-α for ubiquitylation by the E3 ligase complex and subsequent proteasomal degradation [50]. However, under hypoxic conditions when PHDs cannot function or when pVHL is mutated and unable to bind HIF-α or elongin C, HIF-α evades pVHL-facilitated degradation and stabilizes. Accumulated HIF-α then complexes with its partner HIF-β in the nucleus and transcriptionally upregulates genes important in angiogenesis (*EPO*, *VEGF*), cell proliferation [*PDGFβ*, *TGFα*], and glucose metabolism (*GLUT 1*) (Fig. 11.1) [44, 51]. HIF-α-dependent upregulation of proangiogenic factors accounts for the highly vascular nature of *VHL*-deficient clear cell renal tumors. Germline *VHL* mutations frequently occur in the pVHL binding domains for HIF-α and elongin C [52]. Stabilization of HIF-2α, rather than HIF-1α, appears to be critical for renal tumor development [53, 54], possibly through HIF-2α-mediated upregulation of c-Myc and its targets, driving tumor cell proliferation and enabling tumor cells to escape DNA damage-activated checkpoints [55].

Inherited Papillary Type 1 RCC: Hereditary Papillary Renal Carcinoma

In contrast to VHL disease, affected individuals with the rare autosomal dominant familial cancer syndrome, HPRC, develop bilateral, multifocal renal tumors of papillary type 1 histology with no other manifestations [56, 57]. HPRC develops in the fifth and sixth decades of life with an age-dependent penetrance of 67% by the age of 60 [58]; however, early age of onset HPRC families have been reported [59]. Fewer than 40 HPRC families have been reported worldwide underscoring the rare nature of this disorder. Affected individuals with HPRC inherit activating mutations in the *MET proto-oncogene* located on chromosome 7q31 [60]. To date, all HPRC-associated

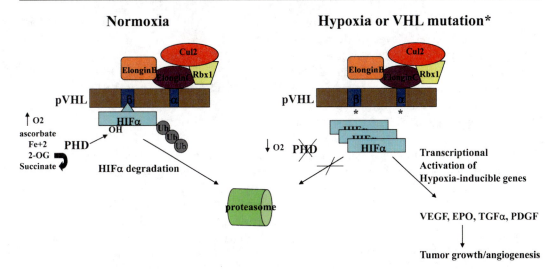

Fig. 11.1 pVHL targets HIFα for degradation. Under normoxic conditions, HIF prolyl hydroxylase (PHD), with cofactors 2-oxoglutarate (2-OG), Fe^{+2}, and ascorbate, hydroxylates HIFα on critical prolines enabling its recognition by pVHL. pVHL, in complex with elongins C and B, Cul2, and Rbx1, targets HIFα for ubiquitin-mediated degradation. When oxygen is low and PHD is unable to hydroxylate HIFα, or when VHL is mutated (*) in sporadic clear cell RCC or tumors from VHL patients, HIFα is not recognized by pVHL and accumulates, resulting in transcriptional activation of genes that stimulate tumor growth (*PDGF*, *TGFα*) and neovascularization (*VEGF*, *EPO*) [from Schmidt LS, Pavlovich CP. et al. Hereditary Renal Cell Carcinoma Syndromes. In: *Cancer Hereditario*, 2nd Edition. Segura, PP (ed). Sociedad Espanola de Oncologia Medica (SEOM), Madrid 2010, with permission]

MET mutations are missense that exchange the amino acid and are located in the tyrosine kinase (TK) domain of the Met protein [56]. The frequency of *MET* mutations in sporadic papillary type 1 tumors is low ranging from 12.5 to 13% in several reported studies [61, 62], suggesting that sporadic PRC may arise by a Met-independent pathway as well.

Inherited Papillary Type 1 RCC: Functional Consequence of *MET* Mutations

The *MET* gene encodes the hepatocyte growth factor/scatter factor (HGF/SF) receptor tyrosine kinase, Met. HGF/SF ligand binding triggers Met autophosphorylation on two critical tyrosines in the intracellular kinase domain that activates Met kinase activity. Subsequent phosphorylation of two additional tyrosines in the carboxyterminal docking site results in the recruitment of a variety of intracellular effectors or adaptor proteins that link HGF/Met signaling to downstream cascades regulating cell proliferation, branching morphogenesis, differentiation, and "invasive growth" [63]. Among the many genes upregulated by HGF/Met signaling is the receptor itself, and Met overexpression has been demonstrated in a number of epithelial cancers including RCC [64]. HPRC was the first cancer syndrome in which germline *MET* mutations were identified, all of which are constitutively activating, display oncogenic potential in animal and cell-based assays [65, 66], and are predicted to stabilize Met kinase in the active conformation [67]. Nonrandom duplication of the chromosome 7 bearing the mutant *MET* allele was demonstrated in papillary renal tumors from HPRC patients [68–70], suggesting that duplication of mutant *MET* may give kidney cells a proliferative growth advantage and represent the second step in HPRC tumor pathogenesis. Targeting the MET signaling pathway has great therapeutic potential for treatment of both inherited and sporadic papillary renal tumors. Moreover, *MET* has been identified as a

HIFα target gene. Hypoxia was shown to activate *MET* transcription, increase levels of Met protein, amplify HGF signaling and induce invasion [71]. Therefore, Met signaling is a likely contributor to *VHL*-deficient clear cell renal cancer and an important biotarget for therapy in clear cell RCC. Finally, *MET* was also shown to be transcriptionally upregulated by the strongly activating TFE3 fusion proteins produced in renal cancer associated with Xp11.2 translocations and may contribute to the mechanism of tumorigenesis in these tumors (see "Papillary RCC") [72].

Inherited Papillary Type 2 RCC: Hereditary Leiomyomatosis and Renal Cell Carcinoma

Initially referred to as multiple cutaneous and uterine leiomyomatosis (MCUL) [73], this autosomal dominantly inherited syndrome was renamed HLRCC upon the identification of renal tumors in association with skin and uterine leiomyomata in affected individuals [74]. The skin leiomyomas (benign smooth muscle tumors) and uterine leiomyomas (fibroids) are the most penetrant manifestations in HLRCC whereas renal tumors develop in 15–62% of affected individuals [75, 76]. They tend to be solitary and unilateral and develop with an early age of onset. Unlike papillary tumors that develop in the setting of HPRC, HLRCC tumors are highly aggressive and can metastasize causing death within 5 years of diagnosis. HLRCC renal tumors are most often papillary type 2 histology, but several reports of tumors with collecting duct histology have appeared [76, 77]. Affected individuals with HLRCC inherit germline mutations in the gene that encodes the Krebs cycle enzyme fumarate hydratase (*FH*) [78, 79]. *FH* mutations identified in HLRCC include missense, protein truncating, and partial and complete gene deletions occurring in most coding exons but without clear genotype–phenotype associations [75, 80]. *FH* acts as a classic tumor suppressor gene with loss or somatic mutation of the wild-type *FH* allele at high frequency in renal tumors, and skin and uterine leiomyomata found in the setting of HLRCC [76], but rarely in sporadic counterpart tumors [81].

Inherited Papillary Type 2 RCC: Functional Consequence of Krebs Cycle Enzyme Mutations

HLRCC-associated *FH* mutations reduce enzyme activity to varying degrees depending on mutation type [77, 78, 82]. Reduced FH activity causes fumarate accumulation and stalling of the Krebs cycle [83, 84] resulting in stabilization of HIF-1α. Fumarate acts as a competitive inhibitor of the PHD cosubstrate, 2-oxoglutarate [84], releasing HIF-1α from proline hydroxylation and VHL-mediated proteasomal degradation. This "pseudohypoxia" drives transcriptional activation of HIF-target genes that promote increased microvessel density in the HLRCC-associated leiomyomas [85] (*VEGF, EPO*), aggressive growth of papillary type 2 renal tumors (*TGF-α, PDGF-β*), and rapid glucose uptake that drives aerobic glycolysis (*GLUT 1, HK2*), known as "the Warburg effect," in HLRCC-associated renal cancer (Fig. 11.2) [84, 86]. Elevated reactive oxygen species (ROS) levels, a known consequence of HIF-1α stabilization and high glucose levels, were observed in an HLRCC-derived renal tumor cell line [87]; however, in another study elevated ROS levels were not detected in HLRCC tumors and *FH*-deficient mouse cysts [88], suggesting that HIF-1α stabilization was a direct result of fumarate accumulation which was shown to occur even in the presence of disrupted mitochondrial energy metabolism. Resolution of the mechanism by which fumarate accumulation drives HIF stabilization and aerobic glycolysis awaits further investigation. In a manner analogous to mutational inactivation of *FH*, *SDH* mutations lead to reduced SDH enzyme activity and accumulation of succinate in renal tumors. Consequently, accumulation of succinate competitively inhibits 2-oxoglutarate and blocks PHD activity [84, 85], resulting in HIF-α stabilization and transcriptional activation of HIF α target genes driving tumor development in *SDH* mutation-associated familial renal cancer.

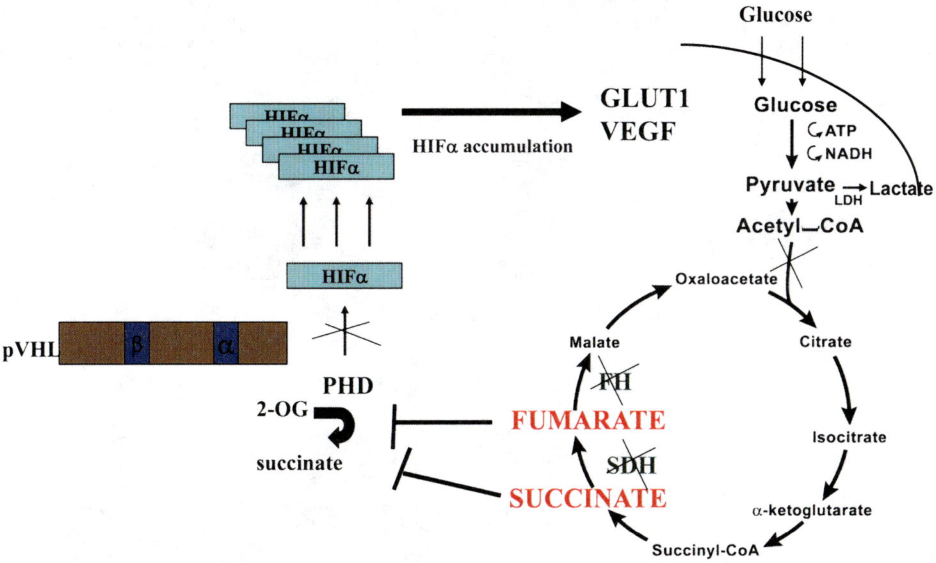

Fig. 11.2 Molecular mechanism of *FH* and *SDH* mutation-driven renal tumorigenesis. Mutations in the genes encoding Krebs cycle enzymes fumarate hydratase (FH) or succinate dehydrogenase subunit B or D (SDH) lead to reduced enzyme activity and elevated levels of fumarate or succinate, which in turn competitively inhibit HIF prolyl hydroxylase (PHD) cosubstrate 2-oxoglutarate (2-OG), and impair PHD function. Consequently, HIFα cannot be hydroxylated for recognition by the pVHL-E3 ubiquitin ligase and HIFα accumulates resulting in transcriptional upregulation of HIF-target genes such as *VEGF* and the glucose transporter *GLUT 1*. "Pseudohypoxia" appears to be the driving force for development of FH-deficient or SDH-deficient renal tumors, which are completely dependent upon aerobic glycolysis, not oxidative phosphorylation, for energy production. Elevated lactic dehydrogenase (LDH) expression in tumor cells catalyzes reduction of pyruvate to lactate and acidifies the cancer cell microenvironment [from Schmidt LS, Pavlovich CP. Hereditary Renal Cell Carcinoma Syndromes. In: *Cancer Hereditario*, 2nd Edition. Segura, PP (ed). Sociedad Espanola de Oncologia Medica (SEOM), Madrid 2010, with permission]

Inherited Chromophobe RCC: Birt–Hogg–Dubé Syndrome

Similar to HLRCC, Birt–Hogg–Dubé syndrome is a rare autosomal dominantly inherited dermatologic disorder that predisposes affected individuals to develop benign hair follicle tumors (fibrofolliculomas), lung cysts and, spontaneous pneumothorax [89] with high penetrance (>85%) [90]. The cosegregation of renal tumors with BHD cutaneous lesions in several renal cancer kindreds confirmed that renal neoplasia was part of the phenotypic spectrum of BHD syndrome [91], which increases risk for renal neoplasia by seven-fold compared with unaffected siblings [92]. Bilateral, multifocal renal tumors with variable histologies will develop in about one-third of BHD patients but rarely metastasize [90, 93, 94]. Chromophobe RCC, clear cell RCC, and a hybrid oncocytic tumor with features of oncocytoma and chromophobe RCC were reported in 34, 9 and 50% of cases, respectively, with areas of microscopic "oncocytosis" observed in normal kidney parenchyma of some BHD patients [95]. Germline mutations in the *BHD* or *folliculin* (*FLCN*) gene located on chromosome 17p11.2 were identified in affected individuals with BHD syndrome [96] including protein truncating mutations [93, 97, 98] and rare missense mutations [99] that occur in nearly all exons with no conclusive genotype–phenotype correlations. Inactivation of the remaining copy of *FLCN* by somatic mutation or loss of chromosome 17p sequences in renal tumors from BHD patients [100], and homozygous loss of *FLCN* in kidney tumors from *Flcn* knockout mice [101] confirm a tumor suppressor role for *FLCN*. *FLCN* is infrequently mutated in sporadic chromophobe or clear cell RCC, or renal oncocytomas [102–104].

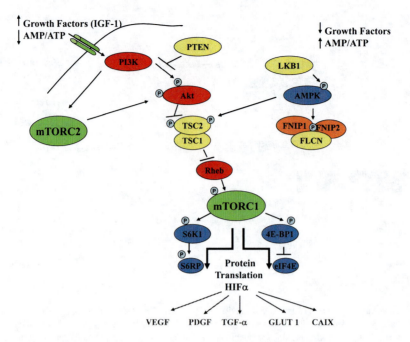

Fig. 11.3 Akt–mTOR pathway dysregulation promotes renal tumorigenesis. Growth factor stimulation (i.e., insulin and insulin-like growth factors IGF-1) of receptor tyrosine kinases activates the PI3K–Akt–mTOR pathway driving mRNA translation through release of 4E-BP1 inhibition of eIF-4E and phosphorylation of S6 kinase 1. mTOR kinase exists in two complexes—mTORC1, which promotes mRNA translation of a number of genes that drive tumor growth including HIF-1α, and mTORC2, which phosphorylates and activates Akt, further driving the Akt–mTORC1 signaling axis and promoting cell survival through inhibition of apoptotic signals. Negative regulation of mTORC1 is exerted by 5′-AMP-activated protein kinase (AMPK), which is phosphorylated by its upstream kinase LKB1 in response to nutrient or energy deficit. AMPK then phosphorylates and activates TSC2, which in complex with TSC1 phosphorylates and defuses GTP-bound Rheb that is necessary for mTORC1 activation. This negative regulation of mTORC1 by TSC2 through Rheb can be inhibited by Akt phosphorylation of TSC2 at a different site. FLCN through its binding partners FNIP1 and FNIP2 complexes with AMPK and is thought to be important for mTOR regulation since *FLCN* mutational inactivation leads to mTOR dysregulation and renal cancer. Mutational inactivation of other tumor suppressor genes on the pathway (*LKB1*, *PTEN*, *TSC1*, *TSC2*) also results in dysregulation of PI3K–Akt–mTOR signaling and development of cancer and/or hamartomas.

Inherited Chromophobe RCC: Functional Consequences of *FLCN* Mutation

Folliculin (FLCN) encoded by the *FLCN* gene is a novel protein of unknown function and under intense investigation in a number of laboratories. The discovery of two folliculin-interacting proteins, FNIP1 [105] and FNIP2/L [106, 107], has led to the finding that a third protein, 5′AMP-activated protein kinase (AMPK), interacts with FLCN through FNIP1/2 [105]. AMPK functions in pathways that sense cellular nutrient and/or energy deficit but, importantly, also serves as a negative regulator of mammalian target of rapamycin (mTOR), the master controller of protein translation and cell growth, through phosphorylation of TSC2 (Fig. 11.3). Inappropriate activation of mTOR through mutation of tumor suppressor genes in the LKB1–AMPK–TSC1/2-mTOR pathway (*TSC1/2*, *LKB1*, *PTEN*) can lead to the development of a number of cancer syndromes [108, 109]. Accumulating evidence suggests that the FLCN/FNIP complex may participate in the regulation of the mTOR pathway through its association with AMPK and that *FLCN* mutations may dysregulate mTOR resulting in the hair follicle tumors and renal neoplasia associated with BHD. However, conflicting data supporting both mTOR activation [101, 110] and mTOR inhibition [111, 112] as a consequence of *FLCN* inactivation have led to the suggestion that the mechanism by which FLCN interacts with and modulates mTOR is context dependent [113]. Recently, elevated levels of HIF-1α and its target genes were demonstrated in a *FLCN*-null renal tumor cell line, in BHD-associated chromophobe tumors, and in cells with *FLCN* knockdown with higher dependency upon glycolysis, suggesting that the "Warburg effect" supports the growth of renal tumors in BHD syndrome [114]. Clarification of FLCN function awaits further experimentation.

Biomarkers of Renal Cell Carcinoma: Lessons Learned from Familial RCC Syndromes

Traditionally, stage, grade, and performance status have been used as predictors of outcome in RCC [115]. However, molecular markers have the potential to profoundly impact the ability to correctly diagnose RCC subtypes, identify tumors at high risk for recurrence and/or metastasis, predict response to available therapeutic treatments for RCC, and enable the development of new, more effective targeted therapies for RCC patients. In recent years, the discoveries uncovered by studying families with inherited renal cancer syndromes have significantly contributed to our understanding of the molecular basis of renal carcinoma, revealing important biochemical pathways involved in the pathogenesis of RCC that provide opportunities for molecularly targeted therapies. The VHL–HIF pathway is dysregulated in the majority of RCC and most extensively investigated for therapeutic biotargets. Recent progress elucidating the complexities of the Akt–mTOR axis has confirmed roles for components of this pathway in renal tumorigenesis, underscoring this pathway as critical for biotarget discovery. The HGF/Met signaling cascade has also been widely implicated in both familial and sporadic RCC and intensely explored for therapeutic drug development. Finally, the genes and pathways uniquely involved in cancer cell metabolism have offered new potential biotargets for therapy.

The next sections will highlight important validated and novel diagnostic, prognostic, and predictive biomarkers, and review potential biotargets for molecularly targeted therapy of RCC (Table 11.3).

Table 11.3 Biomarkers for RCC for diagnosis, prognosis, and predicted response to therapy

Biomarker	Diagnostic	Prognostic	Predictive for therapeutic response
VHL mutation	For clear cell RCC	↑RCC in VHL patients with truncating vs. missense mutations ↑RCC in VHL patients with partial vs. whole gene deletions Inconclusive for clear cell RCC	For VEGF therapy: inconclusive
HIF-1α	Not specific for histology	Inconclusive for survival	ND
VEGF/VEGFR	For clear cell and papillary, not chromophobe	↓tVEGFR-3, ↑mets, ↓survival ↓sVEGF, ↑survival (2) ↑VEGFR-2,↓survival in pap2 vs. pap1RCC	↑VEGF/VEGFR — not predictive for sorafenib ↓sVEGFC/↓sVEGFR-3, better response to sunitinib ↑sVEGF/↓sVEGFR-2,-3 post therapy, good response to sunitinib ↑sVEGF isoforms, good response to sunitinib ↓sVEGFR-2 post therapy, good response to pazopanib

(continued)

Table 11.3 (continued)

Biomarker	Diagnostic	Prognostic	Predictive for therapeutic response
CAIX	For clear cell RCC, not chromophobe RCC or oncocytoma	↑CAIX, low tumor grade/stage, ↑survival ↓CAIX, ↓survival	↑CAIX, good response to IL-2 therapy (2)
phospho-S6	Not specific for histology	↑phospho-S6, high grade/stage, ↑mets, ↓survival	↑phospho-S6, good response to temsirolimus therapy
Met	For papillary, collecting duct, less for clear cell RCC, not for chromophobe or oncocytoma	↑Met expression in clear cell RCC, high grade/stage Met mutation in pap 1	ND for Met-targeted therapy
NOX4	For clear cell RCC	↑NOX4, poor prognosis	ND; therapeutics in development
LDH-A	ND	↑LDH-A, poor prognosis	ND; therapeutics in development
FASN	For clear cell RCC	↑FASN, high grade/stage, mets, poor prognosis	ND; therapeutics in development
B7H1, B7x	ND	↑B7H1/B7x, high grade/stage, mets, poor prognosis, ↓survival	ND; therapeutics in development
IMP3	Not specific for histology	↑IMP3, high grade/stage, metastasis, poor prognosis, ↓survival	ND; therapeutics in development
AQP1	For clear cell and papillary RCC, not chromophobe or oncocytoma	↓AQP1, high grade/stage, poor prognosis, ↓survival ↑AQP1, low grade/stage, good prognosis, ↑survival	Decreased levels in urine following nephrectomy
ADFP	For clear cell and lesser extent papillary RCC	↑ADFP, low grade/stage, good prognosis, ↑survival	Decreased levels in urine following nephrectomy

ND, not determined

Biomarkers and Molecular Targets in the HIF–VHL Pathway

VHL Mutation

Biallelic inactivation of *VHL* is the underlying event responsible for the vast majority of sporadic RCC [12]. Stabilization of HIF-α and upregulation of HIF-target genes involved in angiogenesis and proliferation as a consequence of *VHL* mutation contribute to the highly vascular and invasive characteristics of clear cell renal tumors (see "Inherited Clear Cell RCC: Function of the VHL Gene"). *VHL* mutation status may predict outcome of patients with clear cell RCC and has been investigated as a prognostic biomarker for RCC.

VHL Mutation as Prognostic Indicator

VHL disease has been subclassified according to the presence or absence of RCC or adrenal tumors (pheochromocytoma) [116, 117], and results from

genotype-phenotype studies have suggested that *VHL* mutation type and functional consequence may be prognostic for sporadic clear cell RCC. Genotype–phenotype correlations in large VHL cohorts demonstrated that patients with truncating mutations or large rearrangements predicted to interfere with elongin C or HIF binding developed RCC more frequently than those with missense mutations [118, 119]. Furthermore, Maranchie et al. observed a lower prevalence of RCC clinically in VHL patients with complete germline deletion of *VHL*, and in an age-adjusted comparison of 123 VHL patients, they found a higher prevalence of RCC in patients with partial deletions relative to complete deletions (48.9% vs. 22.6%, $p=0.007$) [120]. An even greater correlation was seen when a 30-kb region telomeric to *VHL* containing the *HSPC300* gene was retained, suggesting that a neighboring gene might be critical for RCC development, and this observation was confirmed in another VHL cohort of 127 patients [121].

Many studies over the last few years have investigated *VHL* mutation as a prognostic and predictive biomarker for clear cell RCC with conflicting results. In a series of 227 sporadic clear cell RCC, Brauch et al. found *VHL* mutations in 45% of clear cell RCC with 3p loss in 93% and a significant association with pT3 stage ($p=0.009$). Few to no *VHL* mutations were found in papillary RCC, chromophobe RCC, or oncocytomas [122]. Schraml et al. identified loss-of-function *VHL* mutations in 34% of 113 clear cell RCC that correlated with worse prognosis in univariate analysis ($p=0.02$) but without correlation to stage, grade, proliferation index, or microvessel density [123]. Conversely, in 187 Japanese patients with clear cell RCC who had undergone radical nephrectomy, Yao et al. found strong association of *VHL* alteration [mutation (52%) or hypermethylation (5.3%)] with better cancer-free survival and cancer-specific survival for patients with stage I–III but not stage IV tumors [124]. Additionally, in a series of 100 clear cell RCC patients that had undergone radical nephrectomy, Patard et al. evaluated *VHL* mutation and expression of the HIF target, CAIX (see section "CAIX") and found mutations in 58% of patients that predicted longer progression-free survival ($p=0.037$). Low CAIX expression and absence of *VHL* mutations were correlated with more advanced tumors that had higher stage and more frequent metastases [125]. Further, in a large case–control study of clear cell RCC, Nickerson et al. reported that nonsense mutations in *VHL* were significantly associated with high Fuhrman nuclear grade, lymph node positivity, and metastases [12]. However, several reports have not shown any association between the presence or absence of *VHL* mutations and prognosis for patient outcome and survival [126–128]. It seems apparent that determination of the prognostic value of *VHL* mutations in predicting patient outcome must await further investigation with additional large cohorts. The diagnostic value of *VHL* mutations for clear cell RCC, however, remains undisputed.

VHL Mutation as a Predictor of Therapeutic Response

A number of studies have also evaluated *VHL* mutation as a predictor of response to therapies that target the VHL–HIF pathway. In a study of 123 metastatic clear cell RCC patients who had received VEGF-targeted therapy, Choueiri et al. investigated *VHL* mutation status relative to response rate. Patients with *VHL* mutations that abrogated function had a 52% response rate compared with a 31% response in patients with wild-type *VHL* ($p=0.04$) but no differences in progression-free or overall survival. On multivariate analysis, the presence of a *VHL* loss-of-function mutation was an independent prognostic factor associated with better response [129]. In a study of 43 patients treated with VEGF therapy, those with *VHL* methylation or a mutation predicted to truncate or shift the reading frame had a time to tumor progression that was significantly longer than patients without *VHL* mutation ($p=0.06$) [130]. Three other studies attempted to correlate *VHL* mutation status with response to therapy—a small study of patients on immunotherapy[131], another evaluation of patients on axitinib that targets VEGF receptors [132], and a third small study looking at patients treated with temsirolimus therapy that targets the mTOR pathway [133], but no association was observed. Given the conflicting results, additional large prospective studies are necessary to confirm any association.

HIF-1α and HIF-2α

HIF-1α vs. HIF-2α as Distinct Molecular Targets

HIF1α stabilization and transcriptional activation of HIF-target genes are important contributors to VHL-deficient clear cell renal tumorigenesis. Although HIF-1α and HIF-2α regulate overlapping target genes involved in angiogenesis and extracellular matrix remodeling, they each have unique targets that reflect their different functional roles in a variety of cellular pathways. HIF-1α plays a role in regulating genes involved in glycolytic metabolism and apoptosis, while HIF-2α was shown to induce stem cell factor *Oct 4* and the gene for erythropoietin, *EPO* [134, 135]. They seem to have opposing roles in regulation of c-Myc with HIF-2α acting as an agonist promoting c-Myc-mediated cell-cycle progression in the setting where HIF-1α acts to antagonize c-Myc [136]. Convincing evidence is mounting to support the concept that HIF-2α, rather than HIF-1α, is the driving force for *VHL*-deficient renal tumorigenesis. Studies in *VHL*-deficient cell lines and in vivo mouse models have demonstrated that high levels of HIF-2α but not HIF-1α can override tumor suppression by wild-type pVHL in nude mice [53, 54], and have shown that downregulation of HIF-2α is sufficient to abrogate *VHL*-deficient renal tumor growth in vivo [137]. To determine if these observations in *VHL*-deficient mouse models and in vitro culture would extend to ccRCC in patients, Gordan et al. evaluated 162 sporadic clear cell RCC tumors for *VHL* mutation status, HIF-1α/HIF-2α expression, and c-Myc activity [55]. Tumors were grouped as *VHL* wild-type (VHL WT) tumors with no detectable HIF-1α or HIF-2α expression, *VHL*-mutated tumors with HIF-1α and HIF-2α expression (H1H2 tumors), and *VHL*-mutated tumors with HIF-2α expression alone (H2 tumors). H2 tumors displayed greater c-Myc activity and cell proliferation (Ki-67 staining) than H1H2 or *VHL* WT tumors. H2 tumors demonstrated elevated levels of c-Myc-target genes involved in G1/S cell-cycle transition and genes involved in DNA damage repair by mRNA expression profiling with less accumulated DNA damage and fewer genomic copy number changes. On the other hand, H1H2 and *VHL* WT tumors (but not H2 tumors) showed activation of the Akt/mTOR and ERK/MAPK1 growth factor signaling pathways by immunohistochemistry and elevated levels of HIF-1α target genes involved in glycolysis by mRNA expression profiling. The results of this study reinforce the important differences in functional roles of HIF-1α and HIF-2α in clear cell RCC and their potential as biomarkers in renal cancer, and underscore the critical need to characterize tumors by both HIF-1α and HIF-2α expression prior to initiating therapeutic treatment options for a patient. Topotecan is a topoisomerase 1 inhibitor that represses HIF-1α transcriptional activity through inhibition of HIF-1α translation [138] and is being evaluated in clinical trials in patients whose tumors express HIF-1α. Small molecule inhibitors of HIF-2α that may be useful in treating patients with *VHL*-deficient tumors expressing HIF-2α are in the early stages of development [139]. Drugs which target the translation

of both HIF-1α and HIF-2α through inhibition of mTORC1 and mTORC2 are in clinical trials (see section "Biomarkers and Molecular Targets in the mTOR Pathway").

HIF-1α and HIF-2α as Prognostic Biomarkers

Given the functional similarities as well as differences between the two HIF transcription factors, an important consideration is whether HIF-1α or HIF-2α might predict outcome in clear cell RCC. In 92 RCC tumor samples examined for HIF-1α levels by immunohistochemistry, Lidgren et al. found highest expression in clear cell RCC compared with papillary and chromophobe RCC or normal kidney and reported that high HIF-1α levels were an independent prognostic marker for better overall survival ($p = 0.024$) [140]. These results were replicated by the same group using a tissue microarray (TMA) containing 216 RCC samples. A trend toward a prolonged survival ($p = 0.055$) was seen in clear cell RCC with high HIF-1α staining but no differences in papillary RCC [141]. Conflicting findings were reported by two other groups. Klatte et al. evaluated 308 clear cell RCC tumors by TMAs and found that high HIF-1α expression was correlated with poor survival when compared with low HIF-1α expression (13.5 months vs. 24 months; $p = 0.005$) [142]. Dorevic et al. examined 94 clear cell RCC samples again by TMA and found nuclear HIF-1α expression correlated with good prognosis whereas high cytoplasmic expression of HIF-1α correlated with a more aggressive subtype and poor prognosis [143]. Given these inconclusive results, determination of the prognostic value of HIF-1α in RCC awaits validation in larger studies. To date, no studies of prognostic significance of HIF-2α in RCC have been reported.

VEGF and VEGFR

VEGF and VEGFR as Biotargets for Therapy

Angiogenesis, the physiological process that involves the growth of new blood vessels from preexisting blood vessels, is an early and essential

11 Biomarkers for Prognosis and Molecularly Targeted Therapy in Renal Cell Carcinoma

Table 11.4 Biotargets for molecularly targeted RCC therapies in clinical trials

Biotarget	Therapeutic agent	Mechanism of inhibition	FDA approved
VEGF	Bevacizumab	Monoclonal antibody against VEGF-A	For advanced RCC
VEGFR	Sunitinib Sorafenib Pazopanib Axitinib	Small molecule inhibitors of tyrosine kinase receptor activity	All for advanced RCC
PDGFR-β	Sunitinib Sorafenib Axitinib	Small molecule inhibitors of tyrosine kinase receptor activity	All for advanced RCC
Raf kinase	Sorafenib	Small molecule inhibitor of tyrosine kinase receptor activity	For advanced RCC
mTORC1	Temsirolimus Everolimus	Binds to FKBP12 in mTORC1 complex	Both for advanced RCC
mTORC1 and mTORC2	AZD8055	Targets both mTORC1 and mTORC2	No
Met	Foretinib	Small molecule inhibitor of the Met tyrosine kinase	No

event for tumor growth and metastasis. The vascular endothelial growth factor (VEGF) family of proteins, VEGF-A, VEGF-B, VEGF-C, and VEGF-D, are HIF targets upregulated in *VHL*-deficient RCC. The VEGF ligands signal through three VEGF tyrosine kinase receptors, VEGFR-1, VEGFR-2, and VEGFR-3, to activate downstream signaling pathways leading to endothelial cell activation, proliferation, migration, and survival to promote angiogenesis and lymphangiogenesis [144]. In the context of renal tumor angiogenesis, VEGF-A and VEGFR-2 are the main signaling partners. Blocking VEGF/VEGFR signaling to inhibit tumor angiogenesis and growth through molecularly targeted therapies has shown great promise for treatment of metastatic RCC. Inhibitors currently in phase II and/or phase III trials for treatment of RCC include sorafenib, a small molecule inhibitor that targets the VEGFR family, PDGFR-β, and Raf kinase; sunitinib, which inhibits the VEGFR family and PDGFR-β; axitinib, which inhibits VEGFR-1, VEGFR-2, VEGFR-3, and PDGFR-β at low dose; pazopanib, which inhibits the VEGF family and c-kit; and bevacizumab, a monoclonal antibody that neutralizes VEGF-A (Table 11.4) [145].

VEGF as a Prognostic Indicator

A number of studies have evaluated the prognostic value of VEGF in clear cell RCC but with conflicting results. Lam et al. used a TMA of 340 RCC specimens and associated clinical data to determine the correlation between the VEGF family of ligands/receptors and prognosis, and determined that low endothelial expression of VEGFR-3 was an independent predictor of lymph node metastasis and poor disease-free survival on multivariate analysis [146]. In another study, Jacobsen et al. measured VEGF levels in serum of RCC patients prior to surgery and found a correlation with grade and stage of tumor in multivariate analysis. Serum VEGF levels were significantly higher for RCC patients than for control patients with benign renal masses, similar for clear cell and papillary RCC, but lower for chromophobe RCC. Patients with VEGF levels below median value (343.5 pg/mL) had significantly longer survival time than those with higher VEGF levels ($p=0.001$), but significance was lost upon multivariate analysis [147]. Similarly, no differences in VEGF expression levels using VEGF immunostaining on TMAs were seen in the different histologic subtypes of RCC in a follow-up study by the same group; however, there was significant correlation between VEGF expression and tumor size and stage [148]. Higher expression levels of VEGFR-2 and VEGFR-3 were associated with poor prognosis in papillary type 2 RCC ($n=107$) but not papillary type 1 RCC ($n=51$) as part of a study to identify distinguishing molecular and chromosomal alterations between the two subtypes [28].

VEGF as a Predictor of Response to VEGF-Targeted Therapy

Reports from several clinical studies have presented data evaluating serum or tumor VEGF expression as a predictor of response to VEGF therapy. In a large phase III trial (TARGET) comparing sorafenib with placebo, high baseline levels of VEGF measured in 712 patients with advanced RCC were prognostic for poor outcome, correlating with high Memorial Sloan-Kettering Cancer Center (MSKCC) score indicating poor prognosis, and high ECOG performance status, reflecting poor performance. In the placebo arm, patients with high baseline VEGF levels had shorter progression-free survival times and lower overall survival than those with low baseline VEGF levels on univariate analysis [149]. However, in the TARGET trial, VEGF levels had no predictive value as patients with both low and high levels of VEGF had a response to sorafenib therapy [150]. On the other hand, in a phase II study of bevacizumab-refractory metastatic RCC patients treated with sunitinib, patients with baseline levels of sVEGFR-3 and VEGF C below the median baseline had longer progression-free survival with sunitinib treatment than patients with levels greater than the median (36.7 and 46.1 weeks vs. 19.4 and 21.9 weeks, respectively) [151]. Finally, in a phase II study of 63 cytokine-refractory metastatic RCC patients treated with sunitinib, Deprimo et al. evaluated plasma levels of four VEGF and VEGFR proteins to measure patient response to therapy. Patients with objective tumor response had significantly greater increases in serum VEGF levels and decreases in sVEGFR-2 and sVEGFR-3 levels than patients with stable disease or no response [152]. Similarly, high tumor expression of VEGF isoforms ($VEGF_{121}$ and $VEGF_{165}$) were significantly correlated with response to sunitinib therapy in 23 metastatic RCC patients [153], and in a phase II trial of pazopanib in RCC patients, decreases in plasma sVEGFR-2 were significantly correlated with tumor response [154]. Taken together, these studies strongly support a role for VEGF/VEGFR levels as a biomarker for response to VEGF-targeted therapy.

CAIX

Carbonic anhydrase IX (CAIX, CA9, G250) was first described as an antigen detected by the monoclonal antibody G250 specifically in RCC but not in normal kidney tissue [155]. Subsequently, G250 antigen was cloned and identified as a transmembrane glycoprotein identical to the tumor-associated antigen MN/CAIX [156]. CAIX, the ninth member of the family of carbonic anhydrase enzymes, catalyzes the reversible reaction that hydrates carbon dioxide with the production of bicarbonate and the release of a proton. In cancer cells that are hypoxic, anaerobic reduction of pyruvate to lactic acid can occur, and acidosis may result. In cooperation with anion exchangers and sodium/bicarbonate cotransporters, CAIX facilitates a transmembrane proton–bicarbonate transfer that neutralizes the intracellular pH enabling cancer cells to survive and grow in an acidic microenvironment [157, 158]. CAIX is a HIF-1α [but not HIF-2α] target gene upregulated in *VHL*-mutated clear cell RCC [44, 159].

CAIX as a Diagnostic and Prognostic Biomarker

CAIX expression is the most robust and reliable biomarker currently known for RCC displaying strong specificity for clear cell tumors both by immunohistochemical staining and RT-PCR, negative expression in oncocytoma and chromophobe RCC, and no expression in normal kidney or benign cysts [160–162]. Furthermore, in a study of 49 clear cell RCC, levels of *CAIX* mRNA expression in tumors of low clinical stage (I and II) measured by RT-PCR was significantly higher than those of high clinical stage (III and IV), and Kaplan–Meier survival analyses indicated a correlation between high *CAIX* expression and good patient outcome [161]. Several additional studies investigating prognostic value of CAIX have been reported. Sandlund et al. evaluated CAIX expression in 228 tumors using TMA and found that patients with tumors with 0–11% CAIX expression had a significantly poorer disease-specific survival (DSS) rate than patients whose tumors expressed CAIX at greater levels [163].

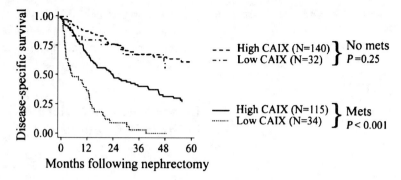

Fig. 11.4 Kaplan–Meier curves showing high CAIX expression correlated with longer survival in metastatic RCC patients. Using a staining cutoff of 85%, patients with metastatic RCC and high CAIX staining (>85%) of tumor tissue core biopsies were associated with longer disease-specific survival than patients with low CAIX (≤85%) staining tumors (24.8 months vs. 5.5 months, $p<0.001$) (adapted and reprinted by permission from the American Association for Cancer Research, Bui et al. [164])

Bui et al. evaluated 321 RCC cases on TMAs, and using a cutoff of 85% CAIX expression, they found that low CAIX staining (≤85%) was an independent poor prognostic factor for survival for metastatic RCC patients (Fig. 11.4). Overall expression of CAIX decreased with progression with lower CAIX expression in the metastatic lesions relative to the primary tumor from the same patient [164]. Leibovich et al. attempted to replicate these results in 730 cases of clear cell RCC by immunohistochemistry, but reported data indicating that although low CAIX expression was correlated with increased risk of death from RCC relative to high expression in univariate analysis, this association was lost after adjusting for nuclear grade or necroses [165]. However, in a later series of 100 ccRCC that also evaluated *VHL* mutation status, high CAIX expression was correlated with longer DSS [125]. In all of these studies, the diagnostic value of CAIX for clear cell RCC was validated, and a correlation between low CAIX expression and poor prognosis (shorter survival, higher grade/stage, metastases) was most often observed.

CAIX as a Predictive Biomarker for Response to Therapy

Although treatment strategies have changed with the implementation of angiogenesis inhibitors, immunotherapy still plays a role in treatment of metastatic RCC. CAIX has been evaluated as a predictor of response to IL-2 therapy by a number of groups. One study evaluated 86 RCC patients who underwent IL-2-based immunotherapy for metastatic RCC, and when stratified according to CAIX expression levels, all complete responders (8%) to IL-2 therapy were in the high CAIX expression group, and overall response rate was greater in the high CAIX group (27%) than in the low CAIX group (14%) (Table 11.5) [164]. Atkins et al. evaluated 66 tumor specimens from RCC patients previously treated with IL-2 therapy and found that 78% (21/27) of responders had high CAIX (>85%) expression compared with 51% (30/39) of nonresponders ($p=0.04$). Median survival was prolonged and survival >5 years was associated only with those patients with high CAIX expression [166]. Interestingly, a recent report described the identification of a single nucleotide polymorphism rs12553173 in the *CAIX* gene and correlation of the synonymous C-allele variant with improved overall survival in 54 metastatic clear cell RCC patients (median 27.3 months vs. 13.6 months, $p=0.0431$) and a trend to better response to IL-2 therapy (57% vs. 22%; $p=0.081$) [167]. The affect of this SNP on the function of CAIX awaits additional experimentation, but *CAIX* genotyping might be considered in the evaluation of clear cell RCC patients who are being considered for IL-2 therapy. Taken together, the evidence supports a role for CAIX as a

Table 11.5 Response of patients with CAIX-expressing RCC to IL-2 therapy

IL-2 therapy ($n=86$)	CAIX	
	Low ($\leq 85\%$, $n=14$)	High ($>85\%$, $n=72$)
Overall response $n=22$	2	20
Complete response $n=7$	0	7
No response	7	20
Stable response	4	23
Not evaluable	1	2

Based on data from reference [164]

diagnostic, prognostic, and predictive biomarker for clear cell RCC with a significantly better response to IL-2 therapy among patients with tumors with high CAIX expression.

CAIX as a Biotarget for Therapy

Besides its utility as a diagnostic and prognostic marker, CAIX has also proven useful as a therapeutic target due to several important properties of this protein—its cell surface location, antigenicity, and specific expression in RCC with low to no expression in normal kidney parenchyma. In a recent clinical trial, Bleumer et al. evaluated 35 patients with progressive clear cell RCC who were treated with the chimeric monoclonal CAIX antibody WX-G250 in combination with low dose IL-2 therapy. A durable benefit was achieved in 23% (8/35) of patients including three with a partial response and five with stabilization and a mean survival of 22 months [168]. An international phase III trial known as ARISER is in progress to evaluate the effect of the WX-G250 antibody as adjuvant therapy for patients with high-risk localized RCC. A second approach to therapy is through the use of a vaccination that stimulates the host immune response to generate cytotoxic T-lymphocytes targeting CAIX. Uemura et al. have shown safety and efficacy in a clinical trial investigating CAIX-derived peptide vaccination in HLA-A24-matched progressive metastatic RCC patients. Patients developed CAIX-peptide-specific cytotoxic T-lymphocytes and more importantly, among the patients with lung metastases, three gave partial response and six were stable for greater than 6 months [169]. Additional innovative approaches to CAIX-targeted vaccines that take advantage of this highly promising molecular biomarker and therapeutic target for clear cell RCC are in progress.

Biomarkers and Molecular Targets in the mTOR Pathway

The cascade of biologic events that ensue following loss of VHL function in a renal cell also directly impacts the PI3K (phosphatidylinositol-3-kinase)–Akt–mTOR pathway. Through nutrient-activated growth factor signaling, mTOR serves as a nutrient- and energy-sensing master switch for protein translation and cell growth in nonneoplastic cells. However, mTOR dysregulation occurs in the context of inherited cancer syndromes involving loss-of-function mutations in *LKB1*, *PTEN*, and *TSC1/2* tumor suppressor genes, and as a consequence of mutational activation of upstream components of the pathway (Akt, PI3K) promoting tumor growth and invasion (Fig. 11.3) [109]. Important for prognosis and treatment of RCC is the fact that activation of mTOR also leads to increased HIF-α protein levels through cap-dependent translation of certain mRNAs including *HIF-α*, *VEGF*, *survivin*, and cell-cycle regulators *cyclin D1* and *c-Myc* [170, 171]. mTOR exists in two complexes that are differentially sensitive to rapamycin—mTORC1 that regulates cell growth and protein translation in response to growth factors, amino acids, nutrients, energy, and cell stress factors, and mTORC2 that regulates actin cytoskeleton organization and activates the Akt–mTORC1 pathway in response to growth factors [109]. In vitro knockdown experiments have revealed that whereas HIF-1α expression is dependent on both mTORC1 and mTORC2, HIF-2α expression depends only on mTORC2 [172]. The mTOR-dependent increase in HIF-α protein levels in renal cells, which lack *VHL*-mediated HIF-α degradation, promotes the HIF-α-driven angiogenic and proliferation programs that support tumor growth and progression underscoring the importance of mTOR as a biotarget in RCC.

Phospho-S6 as Prognostic Marker

mTOR activation has been demonstrated in clear cell RCC by immunostaining of pathway components. Robb et al. confirmed phospho-S6 immunoreactivity, a downstream effector of mTOR, in 59% of 29 ccRCC and demonstrated phospho-mTOR staining in the majority of the tumors [173]. Pantuck et al. evaluated mTOR pathway biomarkers for prognostic value in 375 nephrectomy-treated patients using TMA immunostaining. Strong phospho-S6 staining was significantly correlated with high stage and grade, metastasis, and worse DSS compared with weakly staining tumors (13.6 months vs. 20.2 months; $p = 0.002$) [174].

mTOR as a Biotarget for Therapy

Temsirolimus and everolimus belong to a class of rapamycin analogue drugs that inactivate mTOR in one of its two complexes, mTORC1 (Table 11.4). These drugs have been approved by the FDA for treatment of RCC and have shown encouraging response in phase II/III clinical trials for patients with advanced RCC [175, 176]. A promising biomarker for predicting response rate to these drugs is phospho-S6. Cho et al. evaluated pretreatment tumor tissues from 20 patients with advanced RCC in a phase II trial of temsirolimus by immunostaining and found a positive association of phospho-S6 expression and a trend toward positive phospho-Akt expression ($p = 0.07$) with response to temsirolimus ($p = 0.02$) [133]. New drugs such as AZD8055 [177] that target both mTOR1 and mTORC2 with the potential to down regulate both HIF-1α and HIF-2α in clear cell kidney cancer are predicted to be more effective than the rapamycin analogue drugs alone and are currently being evaluated in clinical trials.

Additional *VHL*-independent mechanisms of mTOR activation in renal cancer have been uncovered through studies of inherited syndromes that give rise to renal neoplasia. Loss-of-function mutations in the *TSC1* and *TSC2* tumor suppressor genes in the setting of the multisystem disorder TSC, in which patients develop benign angiomyolipomas and rarely RCC, result in loss of TSC1/2-mediated negative regulation of mTOR (Fig. 11.3) [178]. Results from studies with preclinical models of Birt–Hogg–Dubé syndrome and immunohistochemical staining of BHD renal tumors suggest that inactivation of the *FLCN* tumor suppressor gene leads to dysregulation of the mTOR pathway (see "Inherited chromophobe RCC: Functional Consequences of FLCN Mutation") [101, 112, 113]. Therefore, mTOR has emerged as an important biotarget for directed-therapy in advanced clear cell RCC and may hold promise as a therapeutic target for renal tumors that arise in the setting of BHD and TSC.

Biomarkers and Molecular Targets in the HGF/MET Pathway

Hepatocyte Growth Factor Receptor, Met

Met as a Prognostic Indicator

HPRC is caused by germline-activating mutations in the *MET* proto-oncogene that predispose to papillary type 1 tumors in HPRC affected patients (see "Inherited Papillary RCC: Hereditary Papillary Renal Carcinoma") [60]. However, although Met mutations are infrequently found in sporadic papillary RCC (up to 13%) [61, 62], Met overexpression is consistently observed in sporadic papillary RCC and in some clear cell renal tumors. In an evaluation of 55 tumors, Sweeney et al. identified Met protein expression in the cytoplasm and cell membrane of 80 and 56% of these cases, respectively, that correlated with higher tumor stage ($p = 0.004$) and trended toward lower survival ($p = 0.07$) [179]. In a larger study of 145 RCC cases, Met expression was diffusely and strongly expressed in 90% of papillary RCC and all collecting duct tumors but no or focally positive staining was seen in clear cell RCC, chromophobe RCC, and oncocytomas. Met expression in clear cell tumors was associated with aggressive behavior [180].

Met as a Therapeutic Biotarget for Papillary RCC

Met overexpression is common in many cancers including RCC and leads to activation of HGF/Met signaling that drives tumor growth, invasion, and metastasis [63, 64]. Targeting the HGF/Met signaling pathway is an area of critical importance, and a number of approaches to inhibit Met are in development or in clinical trials including small molecule inhibitors of Met tyrosine kinase activity, and antibodies to Met and its ligand HGF (Table 11.4) [181]. A multicenter phase II clinical trial is underway in sporadic and hereditary papillary RCC patients to determine the therapeutic effect of foretinib (XL-880; GSK1363089), a receptor tyrosine kinase inhibitor of both MET and VEGF-2 receptors with interim reporting indicating promise for this approach to treat RCC with activated Met [182].

Biomarkers and Molecular Targets in Cancer Cell Metabolism

NOX4

The familial renal cancer syndromes HLRCC and *SDHB/D* mutation-associated early onset familial renal cancer are caused by mutations in Krebs cycle enzymes that effectively block the cancer cells from using oxidative phosphorylation for energy production (see "Familial RCC Syndromes: Causative Genes and Their Pathways as Potential Biotargets") [87]. In both familial renal cancers, the accumulation of the Krebs cycle intermediates leads to inactivation of HIF PHD and stabilization of HIFα subunits. Additionally, ROS has been found to accumulate in *FH*-deficient renal tumor cells due to abnormal electron transport chain function [87]. The family of NADPH oxidases (NOX) is a major source of ROS generation in cancer cells that contributes to neoplastic growth. NOX4 is a novel NADPH oxidase that is highly expressed in renal tubules and found to be critical for HIF-2α transcriptional activity in *VHL*-deficient cells [183, 184]. NOX4 forms a heterodimer with p22^{phox} subunits to facilitate ROS generation. Block et al. have recently shown that NOX4 and p22^{phox} are important for the maintenance of HIF-2α expression and are upregulated in *VHL*-deficient cell lines and human clear cell RCC compared to normal kidney [185]. Their results support a major role for p22^{phox}-dependent NADPH oxidase as a dominant positive regulator of a translational signaling pathway responsible for HIF-2α expression in *VHL*-deficient renal cancer. They found that p22^{phox}-dependent NADPH oxidases, through ROS generation, facilitate the inhibition of the gene product of *TSC2*, tuberin, through Akt phosphorylation, resulting in downstream phosphorylation of mTOR targets and mTOR-dependent HIF-2α translation. Pharmacological inhibition of NOX4 would reduce ROS and abrogate this mechanism for HIF-2α translational signaling strongly supporting NOX4 as a novel molecular target for treatment of *VHL*-deficient RCC.

LDH-A

As mentioned above, HIF-1α stabilization in HLRCC- and *SDHB/D* mutation-associated renal tumors leads to the upregulation of HIF-target genes including the glucose transporter *GLUT1* that promotes increased glucose uptake to support the shift to aerobic glycolysis, the "Warburg effect." Subsequent fermentation of pyruvate to lactate by lactate dehydrogenase-A (LDH-A) is necessary for ATP and NAD+ production. *LDH-A* is also a HIF-1α target gene, and LDH-A expression levels were found to be high in *VHL*-deficient clear cell renal tumors [186] and associated with poor prognosis in advanced RCC [187]. In an in vitro system, knockdown of *LDH-A* resulted in increased ROS production, leading to apoptosis of the *FH/LDH-A*-deficient cells, thereby reducing their tumorigenic properties in mice compared with the *FH*-deficient cells that expressed LDH-A [186]. These data strongly support the idea that targeting LDH-A may be a viable strategy for treating HLRCC-associated *FH*-deficient renal tumors as well as *VHL*-deficient clear cell renal tumors with elevated levels of LDH-A. LDH-A inhibitors are currently being developed for this exciting new approach to RCC therapy.

FASN

Another classic feature of tumor cells in addition to the switch to aerobic glycolysis is a dramatic increase in de novo fatty acid synthesis, which generates phospholipids to support membrane production for rapidly proliferating tumor cells. Acetyl coenzyme A (acetyl CoA) generated from pyruvate through glycolysis is condensed with malonyl CoA by fatty acid synthase (FASN), the main biosynthetic enzyme catalyzing the first step in fatty acid synthesis [188]. Although most normal tissues acquire fatty acids from the circulation and therefore have low FASN levels and very little de novo lipogenesis [188], overexpression and increased activity of FASN is one of the most common features of cancer cells and has been the focus of efforts to develop pharmacologic agents to block FASN activity [189].

FASN was recently shown to be a prognostic indicator in clear cell RCC. A recent study by Horiguchi et al. evaluated FASN in 120 renal tumors from patients with RCC by immunohistochemistry. Of the 120 tumors, 15% showed positive FASN expression that was significantly associated with more advanced tumor stage and grade, lymph node involvement, and metastasis, and on multivariate analysis, was shown to be an independent predictor of short cancer-specific survival (HR 3.7, $p = 0.036$) [190]. In vitro and in vivo studies by the same group evaluated the effects of the fatty acid synthase inhibitor C75 on a number of RCC cell lines, and found that C75 significantly reduced RCC cell invasion, induced cell-cycle arrest at G2/M, and reduced tumor volume in an RCC-induced xenograft mouse model [191]. FASN may be a novel biotarget in certain RCC tumors in which a block of FASN activity with a pharmacologic inhibitor could be an effective strategy for treatment of RCC.

Biomarkers of the Immune Response

B7-H1 and B7x

B7-H1 and B7x as Immune Regulators

The fate of immune responses is determined by T-cell costimulatory molecule signaling. B7-H1 (PD-L1), and B7x (B7-H4) glycoproteins are members of the B7 family of inhibitory T-cell costimulatory molecule ligands that signal through their respective receptors to inhibit T-cell function and diminish T-cell survival in order to protect against hyperactivation of the immune response and development of autoimmune disease. Normally, the expression of these glycoproteins is restricted to the surface of macrophage-lineage cells where they regulate T-cell activation with little or no expression seen in normal kidney tissues [192]. However, aberrant expression of these ligands by tumor cells has been well documented and shown to downregulate tumor-specific immune response by inhibiting activated or memory T-cells through tumor-specific T-cell apoptosis, impaired cytokine production, and reduced cytotoxicity of activated T-cells [192, 193]. Several of these molecules have been explored as potential prognostic markers for RCC.

B7-H1 as a Prognostic Indicator

Thompson et al. was the first to report elevated expression of B7-H1 in RCC tumors and RCC tumor-infiltrating lymphocytes [194]. In a series of 196 fresh-frozen clear cell RCC tumors using immunohistochemistry, they found that patients with tumors expressing high levels of B7-H1 due either to tumor or infiltrating lymphocytes exhibited more aggressive tumors and were 4.5 times more likely to die from their disease than patients with low B7-H1-expressing tumors on univariate analysis (RR 4.53; 95% confidence interval 1.94–10.56; $p < 0.001$). Using a cutoff of 10%, patients with tumors showing ≥10% B7-H1 immunostaining were significantly more likely to die from cancer-specific disease on univariate analysis (RR 2.91; $p = 0.005$), which was further supported on multivariate analysis after adjusting for stage, metastases, or size. A follow-up study a year later [195] found 66.3% of the 196 RCC tumors had aberrant tumor-associated B7-H1 expression and included eight more cancer-related deaths. Patients with high B7-H1 tumor expression had a relative risk for cancer-related death of 3.52 ($p=0.010$) in multivariate analyses adjusted for the Mayo Clinic SSIGN stage, size, grade, and necrosis score. In a 10-year follow-up study of 306 clear cell RCC patients by the same group, 23.9% had tumors with B7-H1 expression, and those patients were at increased risk of both cancer-specific death (RR 3.92; $p<0.001$) and overall mortality (RR 2.37; $p<0.001$) [196]. Five-year cancer-specific survival rates were 41.9 and 82.9% for patients with and without tumor B7-H1 expression, respectively, and B7-H1 tumor expression was associated with cancer-related death (RR 2.0; $p=0.003$) even after adjusting for TNM stage, grade, and performance. In a subgroup of 268 patients with localized disease, tumor B7-H1 expression was significantly associated with metastasis (RR 3.46; $p<0.001$) and cancer-related death (RR 4.13; $p<0.001$), even after adjusting for TNM status.

B7x as a Prognostic Indicator

In a retrospective study, elevated expression of a second inhibitory costimulatory molecule B7x, also known as B7-H4, was reported in 59.1% of 259 RCC tumors from nephrectomy by immunohistochemistry and was associated with advanced tumor size, grade, and stage [197]. The relative risk of death from RCC was 3.05 in patients with B7-H4 expressing tumors compared with those lacking B7-H4 expression ($p=0.002$). Patients whose tumors were positive for both B7-H1 and B7-H4 had significantly lower cancer-specific survival rates ($p<0.001$) and were four times more likely to die from RCC than those with negative or singly positive tumors ($p<0.001$). Using a serum-based ELISA assay in 101 clear cell RCC cases and matched normal controls, Thompson et al. found significantly higher levels of B7-H4(B7x) in serum of 53 of 101 RCC patients compared with 18 of 101 controls

(14.4 ng/mL vs. 2.7 ng/mL), and higher B7-H4 levels in RCC patients were significantly correlated with positive lymph nodes, distant metastases, and trended toward significance with higher grade tumors [198].

Future Potential of B7-H1 and B7x as Biotargets for Therapy

Based on convincing studies from a single institution, B7-H1 and B7x(B7-H4) are potentially important biomarkers for clear cell RCC associated with high grade and advanced tumors that await further validation in additional studies from other clinical centers. An in vivo blockade of tumor-associated B7-H1 has been shown to potentiate antitumor T-cell responses against B7-H1-expressing tumors in mice [4] and may represent a promising approach to therapeutic treatment of B7-H1- and B7-H4-expressing RCC tumors in patients.

Biomarker for Metastasis

IMP3

IMP3 as a Prognostic Indicator for RCC

Insulin-like growth-factor-II mRNA-binding protein 3 (IMP3) is a member of a family of three IGF-II mRNA-binding proteins. IMP3 is an oncofetal protein with biphasic expression during embryogenesis but rarely in the adult [199]. IMP3 functions in RNA shuttling and translational control during embryogenesis [200] but has been found to be reexpressed in a variety of malignancies [201, 202] and may have a role in cell migration and adhesion, leading to tumor invasion and metastasis [203]. In an effort to identify biomarkers for metastatic RCC, Jiang et al. evaluated 501 primary and metastatic RCC tumors for IMP3 mRNA and protein expression and correlated the results with survival in a subset of patients. IMP3 expression was high in metastatic tumors as well as predictive for localized tumors that went on to metastasize [204]. Patients with IMP3-positive localized tumors had a much lower 5-year metastasis-free survival and overall survival than those with IMP3-negative localized tumors (stage I, 32% vs. 89% with HR of 6.44; stage III, 14% vs. 58% with HR of 3.46) and was retained on multivariate analysis. These results were validated in an independent study by Hoffman et al. who performed IMP3 immunostaining of a large series of 716 clear cell RCC and found IMP3 expression was associated with advanced stage and grade of primary tumors as well as tumor necrosis and sarcomatoid features [205]. In that study, IMP3 expression was associated with a fivefold increased risk of distant metastases (HR, 4.71; $p < 0.001$). In a subsequent study of 317 localized papillary and chromophobe RCC cases, Jiang et al. were able to demonstrate a tenfold increased risk of progression to distant metastases in both papillary and chromophobe RCC with high expression of IMP3 compared to IMP3-negative tumors (RR, 13.45; $p < 0.001$) [206]. Taken together, these results confirm that IMP3 is an independent prognostic marker for patients with high potential to develop metastasis and who might benefit from early systemic treatment. A new system has been proposed combining quantitative IMP3 and tumor stage for predicting metastasis for patients with localized RCC which has been validated in only a single study to date [207].

Urine Biomarkers for RCC Diagnosis: Potential for Noninvasive Screening

Since renal carcinoma often presents with mild or no clinical manifestations until the tumor mass has reached substantial size and advanced grade and stage, nearly 25% of renal tumors have already metastasized at time of diagnosis. Early diagnosis of RCC would provide the opportunity for early intervention, minimally invasive nephron-sparing surgery to conserve kidney function, and early and appropriate treatment for improved patient prognosis and survival. Identification of biomarkers for RCC that are detectable in urine would enable noninvasive population screening and early diagnosis and would greatly improve overall survival for RCC patients. Unfortunately, there are no existing urine

biomarkers for renal cancer diagnosis at present, but several good candidates have been evaluated in large tumor series with encouraging results.

Aquaporin-1 as a Prognostic Indicator

Aquaporin-1 (AQP1) is a water channel protein that is expressed in the proximal tubule and descending thin limb of the kidney. AQP1 molecules form a homotetramer through the cell membrane lipid bilayer creating a selective water permeability channel [208]. AQP1 is also highly expressed in cells with rapid gas (O_2/CO_2) turnover such as erythrocytes and microvessel endothelium, and a recent study in lung cancer cells has suggested that AQP1 may be involved in O_2 homeostasis and facilitate transmembrane O_2 transport [209]. Aquaporins are expressed in a variety of tumor types, especially in organs that rely on water permeability for function such as the kidney [210], and may be upregulated in response to hypoxia in tumor microenvironments. Based on these research findings and the well-established "pseudohypoxic response" of HIFα stabilization in *VHL*-deficient clear cell RCC, a number of researchers have investigated the potential for AQP1 as both diagnostic and prognostic in RCC. *AQP1* mRNA expression was originally investigated due to its role in kidney differentiation by Takenawa et al. in 66 RCC tumors using Northern blot and in situ hybridization [211]. They found that low *AQP1* expression along with low *CAIX* expression correlated with poor prognosis, with shorter overall survival, and with nonclear RCC relative to high *AQP1* expression. In a TMA study of 202 renal neoplasms, AQP1 expression was diagnostic for clear and papillary RCC (tumors arising from the proximal tubule) but not for collecting duct carcinoma, chromophobe RCC, or oncocytoma (neoplasms arising from the distal nephron) [212]. Again, high AQP1 expression was associated with low grade in clear cell (but not papillary) RCC. In a larger study of 559 sporadic RCC from nephrectomy patients, Huang et al. evaluated *AQP1* mRNA expression by RT-PCR and found that clear and papillary RCCs expressed AQP1 at significantly higher levels compared with other histologic types [213]. Consistent with the earlier studies, they found a significant correlation between higher AQP1 expression and lower tumor size and grade in both clear cell and papillary RCC. Patients with high AQP1 expression in clear cell renal tumors had longer cancer-specific and cancer-free survival compared with patients whose tumors expressed low levels of AQP1, which was retained on multivariate analysis. Taken together, these results support a role for AQP1 in predicting patient outcome in clear cell and papillary RCC.

Adipose Differentiation-Related Protein as a Prognostic Indicator

Adipose differentiation-related protein (ADFP; adipophilin) is important for fatty acid uptake by cells and involved in the stabilization of lipid storage droplets [214]. Clear cell RCC is characterized by abundant lipids and cholesterol, which are lost during histologic processing to produce "clear cells." Moreover, *ADFP* is a HIFα-target gene that is upregulated in *VHL*-deficient renal tumors [215]. Finally, several gene expression microarray studies have identified ADFP as upregulated in RCC [216]. In a later study to identify prognostic and diagnostic biomarkers of RCC by gene expression microarray, ADFP was also identified as upregulated in RCC by Yao et al. [217]. They validated their microarray results by evaluating *ADFP* mRNA and ADFP protein expression in 151 RCC using RT-PCR and immunohistochemistry, and found a strong correlation of ADFP expression with clear cell RCC and to a lesser extent papillary RCC compared with other histologic types. Importantly, patients with high levels of ADFP expression had better cancer-specific survival than patients with low ADFP expression ($p=0.011$) on both univariate and multivariate analyses [217]. In a follow-up study of 432 patients with sporadic clear cell RCC by the same group [218], ADFP expression was high in tumors from patients who were asymptomatic, had low grade/stage tumors, or

carried *VHL* mutations compared with low ADFP expressing cases, and patients with high ADFP expression tumors had better outcome than patients with low ADFP expression in both cancer-free and cancer-specific survival. These results taken together support a role for ADFP as a prognostic indicator in RCC and diagnostic for tumors from the proximal tubule. Interestingly, Schmidt et al. have identified several ADFP peptides as major histocompatibility class I ligands, one of which was shown to induce an antigen-specific cytotoxic T-lymphocyte response, and suggested ADFP peptides might be potential candidates for targeted cancer vaccine development [219]. These experimental results support the concept of ADFP as a biotarget for RCC therapy.

AQP1 and ADFP as Urine Biomarkers for Noninvasive Screening for RCC

As mentioned above, biomarkers for noninvasive screening for RCC are critically needed to identify asymptomatic RCC patients for early detection, diagnosis, and intervention. Based on the published reports that tumor tissue expression levels of AQP1 and ADFP were elevated in RCC, Morrissey et al. examined prenephrectomy and postnephrectomy urine samples from 42 patients with incidental radiographically discovered renal mass and presumed presurgical diagnosis of RCC. They evaluated these proteins by Western blot analysis and found that presurgery levels of AQP1 and ADFP (76 ± 29 and 117 ± 74 units, respectively) were significantly greater in patients whose resected tumor had a diagnosis of clear cell or papillary RCC compared with patients with nonproximal origin tumors or control/healthy patients (0.1 ± 0.1 and 1.0 ± 1.6 units, respectively; $p < 0.001$) [220]. Importantly, urine concentrations of AQP1 and ADFP decreased 88–97% in available postnephrectomy patients. Although these results will require independent validation in subsequent series, AQP1 and ADFP appear to be promising candidates for the long-sought urine biomarkers for early diagnosis of RCC.

Novel Approaches to Identify Biomarkers: Molecular Expression Profiling

Molecular expression profiling is a novel approach for the identification of new genes that are important for the pathogenesis of renal carcinoma and may have potential as biotargets for therapeutic intervention. In addition, investigators are searching for a gene expression signature that can be diagnostic for distinguishing histologic subtypes of RCC and aggressive from nonaggressive tumors, prognostic for patient outcome and overall survival, and predictive for response to therapy.

One of the earliest gene expression studies profiled clear cell RCC using cDNA microarrays and identified a 40 gene set that could distinguish aggressive from nonaggressive clear cell RCC that was validated in a clinical sample set [216]. Subsequent studies have produced independent gene profiles predictive of aggressive vs. nonaggressive or metastatic vs. nonmetastatic clear cell RCC that were validated within studies by additional sample sets [221–224]. However, little overlap was observed when comparing the different gene profiles in part due to differences in experimental design, reagents, and methods of data analysis. Two reports have identified gene expression patterns that can distinguish histologic subtypes of RCC with a very low error rate [225, 226]. One challenge has been to distinguish benign renal oncocytoma from chromophobe RCC, which is often difficult by histology alone and critical for clinical management of these patients. Gene expression profiling [227] alone or in combination with high density SNP arrays for detection of small copy number variations [228, 229] has been utilized to distinguish oncocytoma from chromophobe RCC, and within each of these studies, validation was reported in a second series, although little or no overlap of gene sets was observed across studies. It will be important to prospectively validate these findings using standardized experimental methods in larger sample sets with additional molecular methodologies (RT-PCR, immunohistochemistry, proteomics).

A new and exciting application of molecular profiling microarray technology is the search for RCC-associated microRNAs (miRNA), which are small, noncoding RNA molecules that regulate gene expression through translational repression, can act as tumor suppressors or oncogenes, and have been implicated in cancer pathogenesis [230]. A number of investigations have reported miRNA expression signatures that identified specific miRNAs that were up- or downregulated in clear cell RCC, although overlap of only a single miRNA was observed among the studies [231–233]. miRNA expression profiling has the potential to identify novel biotargets for therapeutic intervention in RCC.

Conclusion

Renal carcinoma is not a single entity, but a heterogeneous group of tumors, each associated with characteristic histology, cytogenetic changes, and molecular genetics, and each associated with a different clinical course and outcome. We have gained great insight into the causative genes and their molecular pathways from family studies of inherited RCC syndromes, most notably the VHL–HIF axis, and it is from this pathway that the most promising biotargets for molecularly targeted therapy have come (VEGF, VEGFR, CAIX) (Fig. 11.5). Recent discoveries contributing to our understanding of mechanisms leading to RCC pathogenesis have focused on biotargets in the Akt–mTOR and HGF–Met pathways (mTORC1, Met) and pathways dysregulated in cancer cell metabolism for therapeutic intervention. Molecular expression profiling in RCC holds great promise for further elucidation of the underlying pathogenic mechanisms of renal carcinogenesis and has great potential for novel biotarget discovery.

Acknowledgments This research was supported in part by the Intramural Research Program of the NIH, National Cancer Institute, Center for Cancer Research. This project has been funded in whole or in part with Federal funds from the National Cancer Institute, National Institutes of Health (NIH), under contract HHSN261200800001E. The content of this publication does not necessarily reflect the

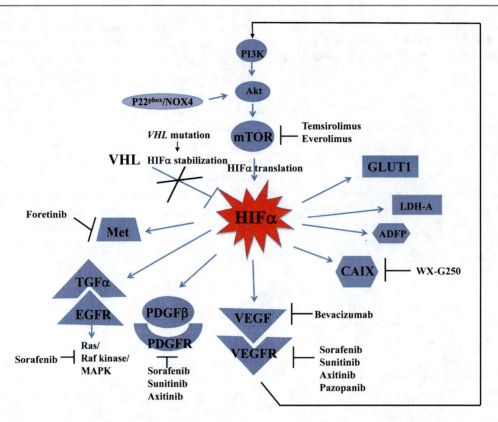

Fig. 11.5 Activation of HIF α target genes is the driving force for renal tumorigenesis and affords promising biotargets for molecularly targeted RCC therapy. HIF α stabilization resulting from *VHL* inactivation or increased HIF α translation through Akt–mTOR activation leads to transcriptional activation of HIF α target genes [*VEGF, TGFα, CAIX, PDGFβ, GLUT1, MET, LDH-A, ADFP*] driving tumor angiogenesis, cell growth and proliferation, and cancer cell survival. Therapeutic intervention with agents that target these HIFα-driven pathways has shown great promise for molecularly targeted therapy for RCC (mTOR-targeted therapy: temsirolimus, everolimus; VEGF-targeted therapy: bevacizumab; VEGFR, PDGFRβ, and Raf-targeted therapy: sorafenib, sunitinib, axitinib, pazopanib; Met-targeted therapy: foretinib; CAIX-targeted therapy: WX-G250)

views or policies of the Department of Health and Human Services, nor does mention of trade names, commercial products, or organizations imply endorsement by the US Government.

References

1. Chow WH, Devesa SS, Warren JL, et al. Rising incidence of renal cell cancer in the United States. JAMA. 1999;281:1628–31.
2. Chow WH, Dong LM, Devesa SS. Epidemiology and risk factors for kidney cancer. Nat Rev Urol. 2010;7:245–57.
3. Rini BI, Campbell SC, Escudier B. Renal cell carcinoma. Lancet. 2009;373:1119–32.
4. Gupta K, Miller JD, Li JZ, et al. Epidemiologic and socioeconomic burden of metastatic renal cell carcinoma (mRCC): a literature review. Cancer Treat Rev. 2008;34:193–205.
5. Kovacs G, Akhtar M, Beckwith BJ, et al. The Heidelberg classification of renal cell tumours. J Pathol. 1997;183:131–3.
6. Linehan WM, Srinivasan R, Schmidt LS. The genetic basis of kidney cancer: a metabolic disease. Nat Rev Urol. 2010;7:277–85.
7. Eble JN, Sauter G, Epstein JI, et al. editors. Pathology and genetics of tumours of the urinary system and male genital organs. World Health Organization, International Agency for Research on Cancer, International Academy of Pathology, IARC Press: Lyon; Oxford University Press (distributor): Oxford; 2004.
8. van den Berg E, Storkel S. Kidney: renal cell carcinoma. Atlas Genet Cytogenet Oncol Haematol. 2003. http://AtlasGeneticsOncology.org/Tumors/Renal CellCarcinID5021.html.

9. Moch H, Mihatsch MJ. Genetic progression of renal cell carcinoma. Virchows Arch. 2002;441:320–7.
10. Shuin T, Kondo K, Torigoe S, et al. Frequent somatic mutations and loss of heterozygosity of the von Hippel-Lindau tumor suppressor gene in primary human renal cell carcinomas. Cancer Res. 1994;54: 2852–5.
11. Gnarra JR, Tory K, Weng Y, et al. Mutations of the VHL tumour suppressor gene in renal carcinoma. Nat Genet. 1994;7:85–90.
12. Nickerson ML, Jaeger E, Shi Y, et al. Improved identification of von Hippel-Lindau gene alterations in clear cell renal tumors. Clin Cancer Res. 2008;14: 4726–34.
13. Sanders ME, Mick R, Tomaszewski JE, et al. Unique patterns of allelic imbalance distinguish type 1 from type 2 sporadic papillary renal cell carcinoma. Am J Pathol. 2002;161:997–1005.
14. Jiang F, Richter J, Schraml P, et al. Chromosomal imbalances in papillary renal cell carcinoma: genetic differences between histologic subtypes. Am J Pathol. 1998;153:1467–73.
15. Schraml P, Müller D, Bednar R, et al. Allelic loss at the D9S171 locus on chromosome 9p13 is associated with progression of papillary renal cell carcinoma. J Pathol. 2000;190:457–61.
16. Armah HB, Parwani AV. Xp11.2 translocation renal cell carcinoma. Arch Pathol Lab Med. 2010;134: 124–9.
17. Tickoo SK, Reuter VE, Amin MB, et al. Renal oncocytosis: a morphologic study of fourteen cases. Am J Surg Pathol. 1999;23:1094–101.
18. Weirich G, Glenn G, Junker K, et al. Familial renal oncocytoma: clinicopathological study of 5 families. J Urol. 1998;160:335–40.
19. Truong LD, Shen SS. Immunohistochemical diagnosis of renal neoplasms. Arch Pathol Lab Med. 2011;135:92–109.
20. Yusenko MV, Zubakov D, Kovacs G. Gene expression profiling of chromophobe renal cell carcinomas and renal oncocytomas by Affymetrix GeneChip using pooled and individual tumours. Int J Biol Sci. 2009;5:517–27.
21. Kauffman EC, Barocas DA, Chen YT, et al. Differential expression of KAI1 metastasis suppressor protein in renal cell tumor histological subtypes. J Urol. 2009;181:2305–11.
22. Amin MB, Amin MB, Tamboli P, et al. Prognostic impact of histologic subtyping of adult renal epithelial neoplasms: an experience of 405 cases. Am J Surg Pathol. 2002;26:281–91.
23. Moch H, Gasser T, Amin MB, et al. Prognostic utility of the recently recommended histologic classification and revised TNM staging system of renal cell carcinoma: a Swiss experience with 588 tumors. Cancer. 2000;89:604–14.
24. Beck SD, Patel MI, Snyder ME, et al. Effect of papillary and chromophobe cell type on disease-free survival after nephrectomy for renal cell carcinoma. Ann Surg Oncol. 2004;11:71–7.

25. Leibovich BC, Lohse CM, Crispen PL, et al. Histological subtype is an independent predictor of outcome for patients with renal cell carcinoma. J Urol. 2010;183:1309–15.
26. Teloken PE, Thompson RH, Tickoo SK, et al. Prognostic impact of histological subtype on surgically treated localized renal cell carcinoma. J Urol. 2009;182:2132–6.
27. Patard JJ, Leray E, Rioux-Leclercq N, et al. Prognostic value of histologic subtypes in renal cell carcinoma: a multicenter experience. J Clin Oncol. 2005;23:2763–27671.
28. Klatte T, Pantuck AJ, Said JW, et al. Cytogenetic and molecular tumor profiling for type 1 and type 2 papillary renal cell carcinoma. Clin Cancer Res. 2009;15: 1162–9.
29. Maher ER. von Hippel-Lindau disease. Curr Mol Med. 2004;4:833–42.
30. Latif F, Tory K, Gnarra J, et al. Identification of the von Hippel-Lindau disease tumor suppressor gene. Science. 1993;260:1317–20.
31. Walther MM, Lubensky IA, Venzon D, et al. Prevalence of microscopic lesions in grossly normal renal parenchyma from patients with von Hippel-Lindau disease, sporadic renal cell carcinoma and no renal disease: clinical implications. J Urol. 1995;154: 2010–5.
32. Lubensky IA, Gnarra JR, Bertheau P, et al. Allelic deletions of the VHL gene detected in multiple microscopic clear cell renal lesions in von Hippel-Lindau disease patients. Am J Pathol. 1996;149: 2089–94.
33. Nordstrom-O'Brien M, van der Luijt RB, van Rooijen E, et al. Genetic analysis of von Hippel-Lindau disease. Hum Mutat. 2010;31:521–37.
34. Cohen AJ, Li FP, Berg S, et al. Hereditary renal-cell carcinoma associated with a chromosomal translocation. N Engl J Med. 1979;301:592–5.
35. Schmidt L, Li F, Brown RS, et al. Mechanism of tumorigenesis of renal carcinomas associated with the constitutional chromosome 3;8 translocation. Cancer J Sci Am. 1995;1:191–5.
36. Bodmer D, van den Hurk W, van Groningen JJ, et al. Understanding familial and non-familial renal cell cancer. Hum Mol Genet. 2002;11:2489–98.
37. Vanharanta S, Buchta M, McWhinney SR, et al. Early-onset renal cell carcinoma as a novel extraparaganglial component of SDHB-associated heritable paraganglioma. Am J Hum Genet. 2004;74: 153–9.
38. Henderson A, Douglas F, Perros P, et al. SDHB-associated renal oncocytoma suggests a broadening of the renal phenotype in hereditary paragangliomatosis. Fam Cancer. 2009;8:257–60.
39. Ricketts C, Woodward ER, Killick P, et al. Germline SDHB mutations and familial renal cell carcinoma. J Natl Cancer Inst. 2008;100:1260–2.
40. Astuti D, Douglas F, Lennard TW, et al. Germline SDHD mutation in familial pheochromocytoma. Lancet. 2001;357:1181–2.

41. Pawlu C, Bausch B, Neumann HPH. Mutations of the SDHB and SDHD genes. Fam Cancer. 2005;4:49–54.
42. Astuti D, Latif F, Dallol A, et al. Gene mutations in the succinate dehydrogenase subunit SDHB cause susceptibility to familial pheochromocytoma and to familial paraganglioma. Am J Hum Genet. 2001;69: 49–54.
43. Ricketts CJ, Forman JR, Rattenberry E, et al. Tumor risks and genotype-phenotype-proteotype analysis in 358 patients with germline mutations in SDHB and SDHD. Hum Mutat. 2010;31:41–51.
44. Kaelin Jr WG. The von Hippel-Lindau tumor suppressor protein: O2 sensing and cancer. Nat Rev Cancer. 2008;8:865–73.
45. Duan DR, Pause A, Burgess WH, et al. Inhibition of transcriptional elongation by the VHL tumor suppressor protein. Science. 1995;269:1402–6.
46. Pause A, Lee S, Worrell RA, et al. The von Hippel–Lindau tumor-suppressor gene product forms a stable complex with human CUL-2, a member of the Cdc53 family of proteins. Proc Natl Acad Sci USA. 1997;94:2156–61.
47. Kibel A, Iliopoulos O, DeCaprio JA, et al. Binding of the von Hippel-Lindau tumor suppressor protein to Elongin B and C. Science. 1995;269:1444–6.
48. Ivan M, Kondo K, Yang H, et al. HIFα targeted for VHL-mediated destruction by proline hydroxylation: implications for O2 sensing. Science. 2001;292:464–8.
49. Jaakkola P, Mole DR, Tian YM, et al. Targeting of HIF-alpha to the von Hippel-Lindau ubiquitylation complex by O2-regulated prolyl hydroxylation. Science. 2001;292:468–72.
50. Maxwell P, Wiesener MS, Chang GW, et al. The von Hippel–Lindau gene product is necessary for oxgyen-dependent proteolysis of hypoxia-inducible factor-α subunits. Nature. 1999;399:271–5.
51. Semenza G. Regulation of mammalian O2 homeostasis by hypoxia-inducible factor 1. Annu Rev Cell Dev Biol. 1999;15:551–78.
52. Stebbins CE, Kaelin Jr WG, et al. Structure of the VHL-ElonginC-ElonginB complex: implications for VHL tumor suppressor function. Science. 1999;284:455–61.
53. Kondo K, Kico J, Nakamura E, et al. Inhibition of HIF is necessary for tumor suppression by the von Hippel-Lindau protein. Cancer Cell. 2002;1:237–46.
54. Maranchie JK, Vasselli JR, Riss J, et al. The contribution of VHL substrate binding and HIF1-alpha to the phenotype of VHL loss in renal cell carcinoma. Cancer Cell. 2002;1:247–55.
55. Gordan JD, Lal P, Dondeti VR, et al. HIF-α effects on c-Myc distinguish two subtypes of sporadic *VHL*-deficient clear cell renal carcinoma. Cancer Cell. 2008;14:435–46.
56. Dharmawardana PG, Giubellino A, Bottaro DP. Hereditary papillary renal carcinoma type I. Curr Mol Med. 2004;4:855–68.
57. Zbar B, Glenn G, Lubensky I, et al. Hereditary papillary renal cell carcinoma: clinical studies in 10 families. J Urol. 1995;153:907–12.
58. Schmidt L, Junker K, Weirich G, et al. Two North American families with hereditary papillary renal carcinoma and identical novel mutations in the MET proto-oncogene. Cancer Res. 1998;58:1719–22.
59. Schmidt LS, Nickerson ML, Angeloni D, et al. Early onset hereditary papillary renal carcinoma: germline missense mutations in the tyrosine kinase domain of the met proto-oncogene. J Urol. 2004;172:1256–61.
60. Schmidt L, Duh FM, Chen F, et al. Germline and somatic mutations in the tyrosine kinase domain of the MET proto-oncogene in papillary renal carcinomas. Nat Genet. 1997;16:68–73.
61. Schmidt L, Junker K, Nakaigawa N, et al. Novel mutations of the MET proto-oncogene in papillary renal carcinomas. Oncogene. 1999;18:2343–50.
62. Salvi A, Marchina E, Benetti A, et al. Germline and somatic c-met mutations in multifocal/bilateral and sporadic papillary renal carcinomas of selected patients. Int J Oncol. 2008;33:271–6.
63. Gentile A, Trusolino L, Comoglio PM. The Met tyrosine kinase receptor in development and cancer. Cancer Metastasis Rev. 2008;27:85–94.
64. Birchmeier C, Birchmeier W, Gherardi E, et al. Met, metastasis, motility and more. Nat Rev Mol Cell Biol. 2003;4:915–25.
65. Jeffers M, Schmidt L, Nakaigawa N, et al. Activating mutations in the met tyrosine kinase receptor in human cancer. Proc Natl Acad Sci USA. 1997;94: 11445–50.
66. Jeffers M, Fiscella M, Webb CP, et al. The mutationally activated Met receptor mediates motility and metastasis. Proc Natl Acad Sci USA. 1998;95: 14417–22.
67. Miller M, Ginalski K, Lesyng B, et al. Structural basis of oncogenic activation caused by point mutations in the kinase domain of the MET proto-oncogene: modeling studies. Proteins. 2001;44:32–43.
68. Kovacs G, Fuzesi L, Emanual A, et al. Cytogenetics of papillary renal cell tumors. Genes Chromosomes Cancer. 1991;3:249–55.
69. Zhuang Z, Park WS, Pack S, et al. Trisomy 7: harboring non-random duplication of the mutant MET allele in hereditary papillary renal carcinomas. Nat Genet. 1998;20:66–9.
70. Fischer J, Palmedo G, von Knobloch R, et al. Duplication and overexpression of the mutant allele of the MET proto-oncogene in multiple hereditary papillary renal cell tumours. Oncogene. 1998;17:733–9.
71. Pennacchietti S, Michieli P, Galluzzo M, et al. Hypoxia promotes invasive growth by transcriptional activation of the met protooncogene. Cancer Cell. 2003;3:347–61.
72. Tsuda M, Davis IJ, Argani P, et al. TFE3 fusions activate MET signaling by transcriptional up-regulation, defining another class of tumors as candidates for therapeutic MET inhibition. Cancer Res. 2007;67: 919–29.
73. Alam NA, Bevan S, Churchman M, et al. Localization of a gene (MCUL1) for multiple cutaneous leiomyomata and uterine fibroids to chromosome 1q42.3-q43. Am J Hum Genet. 2001;68:1264–9.

74. Launonen V, Vierimaa O, Kiuru M, et al. Inherited susceptibility to uterine leiomyomas and renal cell cancer. Proc Natl Acad Sci USA. 2001;98:3387–92.

75. Kiuru M, Launonen V. Hereditary leiomyomatosis and renal cell cancer (HLRCC). Curr Mol Med. 2004;4:869–75.

76. Wei MH, Toure O, Glenn GM, et al. Novel mutations in FH and expansion of the spectrum of phenotypes expressed in families with hereditary leiomyomatosis and renal cell cancer. J Med Genet. 2006;43:18–27.

77. Alam NA, Rowan AJ, Wortham NC, et al. Genetic and functional analyses of FH mutations in multiple cutaneous and uterine leiomyomatosis, hereditary leiomyomatosis and renal cancer, and fumarate hydratase deficiency. Hum Mol Genet. 2003;12:1241–52.

78. Tomlinson IP, Alam NA, Rowan AJ, et al. Germline mutations in FH predispose to dominantly inherited uterine fibroids, skin leiomyomata and papillary renal cell cancer. Nat Genet. 2002;30:406–10.

79. Toro JR, Nickerson ML, Wei MH, et al. Mutations in the fumarate hydratase gene cause hereditary leiomyomatosis and renal cell cancer in families in North America. Am J Hum Genet. 2003;73:95–106.

80. Bayley JP, Launonen VP, Tomlinson IP. The FH mutation database: an online database of fumarate hydratase mutations involved in the MCUL (HLRCC) tumor syndrome and congenital fumarase deficiency. BMC Med Genet. 2008;9:20.

81. Kiuru M, Lehtonen R, Arola J, et al. Few FH mutations in sporadic counterparts of tumor types observed in hereditary leiomyomatosis and renal cell cancer families. Cancer Res. 2002;62:4554–7.

82. Pithukpakorn M, Wei MH, Toure O, et al. Fumarate hydratase enzyme activity in lymphoblastoid cells and fibroblasts of individuals in families with hereditary leiomyomatosis and renal cell cancer. J Med Genet. 2006;43:755–62.

83. Pollard PJ, Briere JJ, Alam NA, et al. Accumulation of Krebs cycle intermediates and over-expression of HIF1alpha in tumours which result from germline FH and SDH mutations. Hum Mol Genet. 2005;14:2231–9.

84. Isaacs JS, Jung YJ, Mole DR, et al. HIF overexpression correlates with biallelic loss of fumarate hydratase in renal cancer: novel role of fumarate in regulation of HIF stability. Cancer Cell. 2005;8:143–53.

85. Pollard P, Wortham N, Barclay E, et al. Evidence of increased microvessel density and activation of the hypoxia pathway in tumours from the hereditary leiomyomatosis and renal cell cancer syndrome. J Pathol. 2005;205:41–9.

86. Warburg O. On the origin of cancer cells. Science. 1956;123:309–14.

87. Sudarshan S, Sourbier C, Kong HS, et al. Fumarate hydratase deficiency in renal cancer induces glycolytic addiction and hypoxia-inducible transcription factor 1alpha stabilization by glucose-dependent generation of reactive oxygen species. Mol Cell Biol. 2009;29:4080–90.

88. O'Flaherty L, Adam J, Heather LC, et al. Dysregulation of hypoxia pathways in fumarate hydratase-deficient cells is independent of defective mitochondrial metabolism. Hum Mol Genet. 2010;19:3844–51.

89. Birt AR, Hogg GR, Dube WJ. Hereditary multiple fibrofolliculomas with trichodiscomas and acrochordons. Arch Dermatol. 1977;113:1674–7.

90. Schmidt LS, Nickerson ML, Warren MB, et al. Germline BHD-mutation spectrum and phenotype analysis of a large cohort of families with Birt-Hogg-Dube syndrome. Am J Hum Genet. 2005;76: 1023–33.

91. Toro JR, Glenn GM, Duray PH, et al. Birt-Hogg-Dube syndrome: a novel marker of kidney neoplasia. Arch Dermatol. 1999;135:1195–202.

92. Zbar B, Alvord WG, Glenn GM, et al. Risk of renal and colonic neoplasms and spontaneous pneumothorax in the Birt-Hogg-Dube syndrome. Cancer Epidemiol Biomarkers Prev. 2002;11:393–400.

93. Toro JR, Wei MH, Glenn GM, et al. BHD mutations, clinical and molecular genetic investigations of Birt-Hogg-Dubé syndrome: a new series of 50 families and a review of published reports. J Med Genet. 2008;45:321–31.

94. Menko FH, van Steensel MA, Giraud S, et al. Birt-Hogg-Dubé syndrome: diagnosis and management. Lancet Oncol. 2009;10:1199–206.

95. Pavlovich CP, Walther MM, Eyler RA, et al. Renal tumors in the Birt-Hogg-Dube syndrome. Am J Surg Pathol. 2002;26:1542–52.

96. Nickerson ML, Warren MB, Toro JR, et al. Mutations in a novel gene lead to kidney tumors, lung wall defects, and benign tumors of the hair follicle in patients with the Birt-Hogg-Dube syndrome. Cancer Cell. 2002;2:157–64.

97. Leter EM, Koopmans AK, Gille JJ, et al. Birt-Hogg-Dubé syndrome: clinical and genetic studies of 20 families. J Invest Dermatol. 2008;128:45–9.

98. Kluger N, Giraud S, Coupier I, et al. Birt-Hogg-Dubé syndrome: clinical and genetic studies of 10 French families. Br J Dermatol. 2010;162:527–37.

99. Lim DH, Rehal PK, Nahorski MS, et al. A new locus-specific database (LSDB) for mutations in the folliculin (FLCN) gene. Hum Mutat. 2010;31: E1043–51.

100. Vocke CD, Yang Y, Pavlovich CP, et al. High frequency of somatic frameshift BHD gene mutations in Birt-Hogg-Dube-associated renal tumors. J Natl Cancer Inst. 2005;97:931–5.

101. Hasumi Y, Baba M, Ajima R, et al. Homozygous loss of BHD causes early embryonic lethality and kidney tumor development with activation of mTORC1 and mTORC2. Proc Natl Acad Sci USA. 2009;106: 18722–7.

102. Gad S, Lefevre SH, Khoo SK, et al. Mutations in BHD and TP53 genes, but not in HNF1beta gene, in a large series of sporadic chromophobe renal cell carcinoma. Br J Cancer. 2007;96:336–40.

103. Khoo SK, Kahnoski K, Sugimura J, et al. Inactivation of BHD in sporadic renal tumors. Cancer Res. 2003;63:4583–7.
104. Nagy A, Zoubakov D, Stupar Z, et al. Lack of mutation of the folliculin gene in sporadic chromophobe renal cell carcinoma and renal oncocytoma. Int J Cancer. 2004;109:472–5.
105. Baba M, Hong SB, Sharma N, et al. Folliculin encoded by the BHD gene interacts with a binding protein, FNIP1, and AMPK, and is involved in AMPK and mTOR signaling. Proc Natl Acad Sci USA. 2006;103:15552–7.
106. Hasumi H, Baba M, Hong SB, et al. Identification and characterization of a novel folliculin-interacting protein FNIP2. Gene. 2008;415:60–7.
107. Takagi Y, Kobayashi T, Shiono M, et al. Interaction of folliculin (Birt-Hogg-Dubé gene product) with a novel Fnip1-like (FnipL/Fnip2) protein. Oncogene. 2008;27:5339–47.
108. Inoki K, Corradetti MN, Guan KL. Dysregulation of the TSC-mTOR pathway in human disease. Nat Genet. 2005;37:19–24.
109. Zoncu R, Efeyan A, Sabatini DM. mTOR: from growth signal integration to cancer, diabetes and ageing. Nat Rev Mol Cell Biol. 2011;12:21–35.
110. Baba M, Furihata M, Hong SB, et al. Kidney-targeted Birt-Hogg-Dube gene inactivation in a mouse model: Erk1/2 and Akt-mTOR activation, cell hyperproliferation, and polycystic kidneys. J Natl Cancer Inst. 2008;100:140–54.
111. van Slegtenhorst M, Khabibullin D, Hartman TR, et al. The Birt-Hogg-Dube and tuberous sclerosis complex homologs have opposing roles in amino acid homeostasis in Schizosaccharomyces pombe. J Biol Chem. 2007;282:24583–90.
112. Hartman TR, Nicolas E, Klein-Szanto A, et al. The role of the Birt-Hogg-Dubé protein in mTOR activation and renal tumorigenesis. Oncogene. 2009;28:1594–604.
113. Hudon V, Sabourin S, Dydensborg AB, et al. Renal tumor suppressor function of the Birt-Hogg-Dube syndrome gene product folliculin. J Med Genet. 2009;47:182–9.
114. Preston RS, Philp A, Claessens T, et al. Absence of the Birt-Hogg-Dube´ gene product is associated with increased hypoxia-inducible factor transcriptional activity and a loss of metabolic flexibility. Oncogene. 2011;30(10):1159–73.
115. Zisman A, Pantuck AJ, Dorey F, et al. Improved prognostication of renal cell carcinoma using an integrated staging system. J Clin Oncol. 2001;19:1649–57.
116. Zbar B, Kishida T, Chen F, et al. Germline mutations in the von Hippel-Lindau disease (VHL) gene in families from North America, Europe, and Japan. Hum Mutat. 1996;8:348–57.
117. Frierich CA. Genotype-phenotype correlation in von Hippel-Lindau syndrome. Hum Mol Genet. 2001;10:763–7.
118. Clifford SC, Cockman ME, Smallwood AC, et al. Contrasting effects on HIF-1alpha regulation by disease-causing pVHL mutations correlate with patterns of tumourigenesis in von Hippel-Lindau disease. Hum Mol Genet. 2001;10:1029–38.
119. Gallou C, Chauveau D, Richard S, et al. Genotype-phenotype correlation in von Hippel-Lindau families with renal lesions. Hum Mutat. 2004;24:215–24.
120. Maranchie JK, Afonso A, Albert PS, et al. Solid renal tumor severity in von Hippel Lindau disease is related to germline deletion length and location. Hum Mutat. 2004;23:40–6.
121. McNeill A, Rattenberry E, Barber R, et al. Genotype-phenotype correlations in VHL exon deletions. Am J Med Genet A. 2009;149A:2147–51.
122. Brauch H, Weirich G, Brieger J, et al. VHL alterations in human clear cell renal cell carcinoma: association with advanced tumor stage and a novel hot spot mutation. Cancer Res. 2000;60:1942–8.
123. Schraml P, Struckmann K, Hatz F, et al. VHL mutations and their correlation with tumour cell proliferation, microvessel density, and patient prognosis in clear cell renal cell carcinoma. J Pathol. 2002;196:186–93.
124. Yao M, Yoshida M, Kishida T, et al. VHL tumor suppressor gene alterations associated with good prognosis in sporadic clear-cell renal carcinoma. J Natl Cancer Inst. 2002;94:1569–75.
125. Patard JJ, Fergelot P, Karakiewicz PI, et al. Low CAIX expression and absence of VHL gene mutation are associated with tumor aggressiveness and poor survival of clear cell renal cell carcinoma. Int J Cancer. 2008;123:395–400.
126. Kondo K, Yao M, Yoshida M, et al. Comprehensive mutational analysis of the VHL gene in sporadic renal cell carcinoma: relationship to clinicopathological parameters. Genes Chromosomes Cancer. 2002;34:58–68.
127. Smits KM, Schouten LJ, van Dijk BA, et al. Genetic and epigenetic alterations in the von Hippel-Lindau gene: the influence on renal cancer prognosis. Clin Cancer Res. 2008;14:782–7.
128. Baldewijns MM, van Vlodrop IJ, Smits KM, et al. Different angiogenic potential in low and high grade sporadic clear cell renal cell carcinoma is not related to alterations in the von Hippel-Lindau gene. Cell Oncol. 2009;31:371–82.
129. Choueiri TK, Vaziri SA, Jaeger E, et al. von Hippel-Lindau gene status and response to vascular endothelial growth factor targeted therapy for metastatic clear cell renal cell carcinoma. J Urol. 2008;180:860–5.
130. Rini BI, Jaeger E, Weinberg V, et al. Clinical response to therapy targeted at vascular endothelial growth factor in metastatic renal cell carcinoma: impact of patient characteristics and von Hippel-Lindau gene status. BJU Int. 2006;98:756–62.
131. Kim JH, Jung CW, Cho YH, et al. Somatic VHL alteration and its impact on prognosis in patients

with clear cell renal cell carcinoma. Oncol Rep. 2005;13:859–64.

132. Gad S, Sultan-Amar V, Meric J, et al. Somatic von Hippel-Lindau (VHL) gene analysis and clinical outcome under angiogenic treatment in metastatic renal cell carcinoma: preliminary results. Target Oncol. 2007;2:3–6.

133. Cho D, Signoretti S, Dabora S, et al. Potential histologic and molecular predictors of response to temsirolimus in patients with advanced renal cell carcinoma. Clin Genitourin Cancer. 2007;5:379–85.

134. Rankin EB, Giaccia AJ. The role of hypoxia-inducible factors in tumorigenesis. Cell Death Differ. 2008;15:678–85.

135. Raval RR, Lau KW, Tran MG, et al. Contrasting properties of hypoxia-inducible factor 1 (HIF-1) and HIF-2 in von Hippel-Lindau-associated renal cell carcinoma. Mol Cell Biol. 2005;25:5675–86.

136. Gordan JD, Bertout JA, Hu CJ, et al. HIF-2alpha promotes hypoxic cell proliferation by enhancing c-myc transcriptional activity. Cancer Cell. 2007;11:335–47.

137. Kondo K, Kim WY, Lechpammer M, et al. Inhibition of HIF2alpha is sufficient to suppress pVHL-defective tumor growth. PLoS Biol. 2003;1:E83.

138. Rapisarda A, Uranchimeg B, Sordet O, et al. Topoisomerase I-mediated inhibition of hypoxia-inducible factor 1: mechanism and therapeutic implications. Cancer Res. 2004;64:1475–82.

139. Zimmer M, Ebert BL, Neil C, et al. Small-molecule inhibitors of HIF-2alpha translation link its 5′UTR iron-responsive element to oxygen sensing. Mol Cell. 2008;32:838–48.

140. Lidgren A, Hedberg Y, Grankvist K, et al. The expression of hypoxia-inducible factor 1 alpha is a favorable independent prognostic factor in renal cell carcinoma. Clin Cancer Res. 2005;11:1129–35.

141. Lidgren A, Hedberg Y, Grankvist K, et al. Hypoxia-inducible factor 1 alpha expression in renal cell carcinoma analyzed by tissue microarray. Eur Urol. 2006;50:1272–7.

142. Klatte T, Seligson DB, Riggs SB, et al. Hypoxia-inducible factor 1 alpha in clear cell renal cell carcinoma. Clin Cancer Res. 2007;13:7388–93.

143. Dorević G, Matusan-Ilijas K, Babarović E, et al. Hypoxia inducible factor-1 alpha correlates with vascular endothelial growth factor A and C indicating worse prognosis in clear cell renal cell carcinoma. J Exp Clin Cancer Res. 2009;28:40.

144. Grothey A, Galanis E. Targeting angiogenesis: progress with anti-VEGF treatment with large molecules. Nat Rev Clin Oncol. 2009;6:507–18.

145. Rini BI. Vascular endothelial growth factor-targeted therapy in metastatic renal cell carcinoma. Cancer. 2009;115:2306–12.

146. Lam JS, Leppert JT, Figlin RA, et al. Role of molecular markers in the diagnosis and therapy of renal cell carcinoma. Urology. 2005;6:1–9.

147. Jacobsen J, Rasmuson T, Grankvist K, et al. Vascular endothelial growth factor as prognostic factor in renal cell carcinoma. J Urol. 2000;163:343–7.

148. Jacobsen J, Grankvist K, Rasmuson T, et al. Expression of vascular endothelial growth factor protein in human renal cell carcinoma. BJU Int. 2004;93:297–302.

149. Peña C, Lathia C, Shan M, et al. Biomarkers predicting outcome in patients with advanced renal cell carcinoma: results from sorafenib phase III treatment approaches in renal cancer global evaluation trial. Clin Cancer Res. 2010;16:4853–63.

150. Escudier B, Eisen T, Stadler WM, et al. Sorafenib for treatment of renal cell carcinoma: final efficacy and safety results of the phase III treatment approaches in renal cancer global evaluation trial. J Clin Oncol. 2009;27:3312–8.

151. Rini BI, Michaelson MD, Rosenberg JE, et al. Antitumor activity and biomarker analysis of sunitinib in patients with bevacizumab-refractory metastatic renal cell carcinoma. J Clin Oncol. 2008;26:3743–8.

152. Deprimo SE, Bello CL, Smeraglia J, et al. Circulating protein biomarkers of pharmacodynamic activity of sunitinib in patients with metastatic renal cell carcinoma: modulation of VEGF and VEGF-related proteins. J Transl Med. 2007;5:32.

153. Paule B, Bastien L, Deslandes E, et al. Soluble isoforms of vascular endothelial growth factor are predictors of response to sunitinib in metastatic renal cell carcinomas. PLoS One. 2010;5:e10715.

154. Hutson TE, Davis ID, Machiels JH, et al. Biomarker analysis and final efficacy and safety results of a phase II renal cell carcinoma trial with pazopanib (GW786034), a multikinase angiogenesis inhibitor. J Clin Oncol. 2008;26:5046s.

155. Oosterwijk E, Ruiter DJ, Hoedemaeker PJ, et al. Monoclonal antibody G250 recognizes a determinant present in renal-cell carcinoma and absent from normal kidney. Int J Cancer. 1986;38:489–96.

156. Grabmaier K, Vissers JLM, De Weuert MCA, et al. Molecular cloning and immunogenicity of renal cell carcinoma-associated antigen G250. Int J Cancer. 2000;85:865–70.

157. Ivanov S, Liao SY, Ivanova A, et al. Expression of hypoxia-inducible cell-surface transmembrane carbonic anhydrases in human cancer. Am J Pathol. 2001;158:905–19.

158. Pastorekova A, Ratcliffe PJ, Pastorek J. Molecular mechanisms of carbonic anhydrase IX-mediated pH regulation under hypoxia. BJU Int. 2008;101 Suppl 4:8–15.

159. Grabmaier K, A de Weijert MC, Verhaegh GW, et al. Strict regulation of CAIX(G250/MN) by HIF-1alpha in clear cell renal cell carcinoma. Oncogene. 2004;23:5624–31.

160. Liao SY, Aurelio ON, Jan K, et al. Identification of the MN/CA9 protein as a reliable diagnostic

biomarker of clear cell carcinoma of the kidney. Cancer Res. 1997;57:2827–31.

161. Murakami Y, Kanda K, Tsuji M, et al. *MN/CA9* gene expression as a potential biomarker in renal cell carcinoma. BJU Int. 1999;83:743–7.

162. McKiernan JM, Buttyan R, Bander NH, et al. Expression of the tumor-associated gene MN: a potential biomarker for human renal cell carcinoma. Cancer Res. 1997;57:2362–5.

163. Sandlund J, Oosterwijk E, Grankvist K, et al. Prognostic impact of carbonic anhydrase IX expression in human renal cell carcinoma. BJU Int. 2007;100:556–60.

164. Bui MH, Seligson D, Han KR, et al. Carbonic anhydrase IX is an independent predictor of survival in advanced renal clear cell carcinoma: implications for prognosis and therapy. Clin Cancer Res. 2003;9: 802–11.

165. Leibovich BC, Sheinin Y, Lohse CM, et al. Carbonic anhydrase IX is not an independent predictor of outcome for patients with clear cell renal cell carcinoma. J Clin Oncol. 2007;25:4757–64.

166. Atkins M, Regan M, McDermott D, et al. Carbonic anhydrase IX expression predicts outcome of interleukin 2 therapy for renal cancer. Clin Cancer Res. 2005;11:3714–21.

167. de Martino M, Klatte T, Seligson DB, et al. CA9 gene: single nucleotide polymorphism predicts metastatic renal cell carcinoma prognosis. J Urol. 2009;182:728–34.

168. Bleumer I, Oosterwijk E, Oosterwijk-Wakka JC, et al. A clinical trial with chimeric monoclonal antibody WX-G250 and low dose interleukin-2 pulsing scheme for advanced renal cell carcinoma. J Urol. 2006;175:57–62.

169. Uemura H, Fujimoto K, Tanaka M, et al. A phase I trial of vaccination of CA9-derived peptides for HLA-A24-positive patients with cytokine-refractory metastatic renal cell carcinoma. Clin Cancer Res. 2006;12:1768–75.

170. Laughner E, Taghavi P, Chiles K, et al. HER2 (neu) signaling increases the rate of hypoxia-inducible factor 1alpha (HIF-1alpha) synthesis: novel mechanism for HIF-1-mediated vascular endothelial growth factor expression. Mol Cell Biol. 2001;21: 3995–4004.

171. Fingar DC, Richardson CJ, Tee AR, et al. mTOR controls cell cycle progression through its cell growth effectors S6K1 and 4E-BP1/eukaryotic translation initiation factor 4E. Mol Cell Biol. 2004;24:200–16.

172. Toschi A, Lee E, Gadir N, et al. Differential dependence of hypoxia-inducible factors 1 alpha and 2 alpha on mTORC1 and mTORC2. J Biol Chem. 2008;283:34495–9.

173. Robb VA, Karbowniczek M, Klein-Szanto AJ, et al. Activation of the mTOR signaling pathway in renal clear cell carcinoma. J Urol. 2007;177:346–52.

174. Pantuck AJ, Seligson DB, Klatte T, et al. Prognostic relevance of the mTOR pathway in renal cell carcinoma: implications for molecular patient selection for targeted therapy. Cancer. 2007;109:2257–67.

175. Hudes G, Carducci M, Tomczak P, Global ARCC Trial, et al. Temsirolimus, interferon alfa, or both for advanced renal-cell carcinoma. N Engl J Med. 2007;356:2271–81.

176. Motzer RJ, Escudier B, Oudard S, RECORD-1 Study Group, et al. Phase 3 trial of everolimus for metastatic renal cell carcinoma: final results and analysis of prognostic factors. Cancer. 2010;116:4256–65.

177. Chresta CM, Davies BR, Hickson I, et al. AZD8055 is a potent, selective, and orally bioavailable ATP-competitive mammalian target of rapamycin kinase inhibitor with in vitro and in vivo antitumor activity. Cancer Res. 2010;70:288–98.

178. Crino PB, Nathanson KL, Henske EP. The tuberous sclerosis complex. N Engl J Med. 2006;355: 1345–56.

179. Sweeney P, El-Naggar AK, Lin SH, et al. Biological significance of c-met over expression in papillary renal cell carcinoma. J Urol. 2002;168:51–5.

180. Choi JS, Kim MK, Seo JW, et al. MET expression in sporadic renal cell carcinomas. J Korean Med Sci. 2006;21:672–7.

181. Cecchi F, Rabe DC, Bottaro DP. Targeting the HGF/Met signalling pathway in cancer. Eur J Cancer. 2010;46:1260–70.

182. Srinivasan R, Linehan WM, Vaishampayan U, et al. A phase II study of two dosing regimens of GSK 1363089 (GSK089), a dual MET/VEGFR2 inhibitor, in patients (pts) with papillary renal carcinoma (PRC). J Clin Oncol. 2009;27(15S post-meeting addition):5103.

183. Maranchie JK, Zhan Y. Nox4 is critical for hypoxia-inducible factor 2-alpha transcriptional activity in von Hippel-Lindau-deficient renal cell carcinoma. Cancer Res. 2005;65:9190–3.

184. Block K, Gorin Y, Hoover P, et al. NAD(P)H oxidases regulate HIF-2alpha protein expression. J Biol Chem. 2007;282:8019–26.

185. Block K, Gorin Y, New DD, et al. The NADPH oxidase subunit p22phox inhibits the function of the tumor suppressor protein tuberin. Am J Pathol. 2010;176:2447–55.

186. Xie H, Valera VA, Merino MJ, et al. LDH-A inhibition, a therapeutic strategy for treatment of hereditary leiomyomatosis and renal cell cancer. Mol Cancer Ther. 2009;8:626–35.

187. Motzer RJ, Bacik J, Mazumdar M. Prognostic factors for survival of patients with stage IV renal cell carcinoma: Memorial Sloan-Kettering Cancer Center experience. Clin Cancer Res. 2004;10(18 Pt2): 6302S–3.

188. Menendez JA, Lupu R. Fatty acid synthase and the lipogenic phenotype in cancer pathogenesis. Nat Rev Cancer. 2007;7:763–77.

189. Kridel SJ, Lowther WT, Pemble 4th CW. Fatty acid synthase inhibitors: new directions for oncology. Expert Opin Investig Drugs. 2007;16:1817–29.

190. Horiguchi A, Asano T, Asano T, et al. Fatty acid synthase over expression is an indicator of tumor aggressiveness and poor prognosis in renal cell carcinoma. J Urol. 2008;180:1137–40.

191. Horiguchi A, Asano T, Asano T, et al. Pharmacological inhibitor of fatty acid synthase suppresses growth and invasiveness of renal cancer cells. J Urol. 2008;180:729–36.

192. Thompson RH, Kwon ED, Allison JP. Inhibitors of B7-CD28 costimulation in urologic malignancies. Immunotherapy. 2009;1:129–39.

193. Seliger B, Marincola FM, Ferrone S, et al. The complex role of B7 molecules in tumor immunology. Trends Mol Med. 2008;14:550–9.

194. Thompson RH, Gillett MD, Cheville JC, et al. Costimulatory B7-H1 in renal cell carcinoma patients: indicator of tumor aggressiveness and potential therapeutic target. Proc Natl Acad Sci USA. 2004;101:17174–9.

195. Thompson RH, Webster WS, Cheville JC, et al. B7-H1 glycoprotein blockade: a novel strategy to enhance immunotherapy in patients with renal cell carcinoma. Urology. 2005;66(5 Suppl):10–4.

196. Thompson RH, Kuntz SM, Leibovich BC, et al. Tumor B7-H1 is associated with poor prognosis in renal cell carcinoma patients with long-term follow-up. Cancer Res. 2006;66:3381–5.

197. Krambeck AE, Thompson RH, Dong H, et al. B7-H4 expression in renal cell carcinoma and tumor vasculature: associations with cancer progression and survival. Proc Natl Acad Sci USA. 2006;103:10391–6.

198. Thompson RH, Zang X, Lohse CM, et al. Serum-soluble B7x is elevated in renal cell carcinoma patients and is associated with advanced stage. Cancer Res. 2008;68:6054–8.

199. Nielsen FC, Nielsen J, Christiansen J. A family of IGF-II mRNA binding proteins (IMP) involved in RNA trafficking. Scand J Clin Lab Invest Suppl. 2001;234:93–9.

200. Yaniv K, Yisraeli JK. The involvement of a conserved family of RNA binding proteins in embryonic development and carcinogenesis. Gene. 2002;287:49–54.

201. Schaeffer DF, Owen DR, Lim HJ, et al. Insulin-like growth factor 2 mRNA binding protein 3 (IGF2BP3) overexpression in pancreatic ductal adenocarcinoma correlates with poor survival. BMC Cancer. 2010;10:59.

202. Ikenberg K, Fritzsche FR, Zuerrer-Haerdi U, et al. Insulin-like growth factor II mRNA binding protein 3 (IMP3) is overexpressed in prostate cancer and correlates with higher Gleason scores. BMC Cancer. 2010;10:341.

203. Vikesaa J, Hansen TV, Jønson L, et al. RNA binding IMPs promote cell adhesion and invadopodia formation. EMBO J. 2006;25:1456–68.

204. Jiang Z, Chu PG, Woda BA, et al. Analysis of RNA-binding protein IMP3 to predict metastasis and prognosis of renal-cell carcinoma: a retrospective study. Lancet Oncol. 2006;7:556–64.

205. Hoffmann NE, Sheinin Y, Lohse CM, et al. External validation of IMP3 expression as an independent prognostic marker for metastatic progression and death for patients with clear cell renal cell carcinoma. Cancer. 2008;112:1471–9.

206. Jiang Z, Lohse CM, Chu PG, et al. Oncofetal protein IMP3: a novel molecular marker that predicts metastasis of papillary and chromophobe renal cell carcinomas. Cancer. 2008;112:2676–82.

207. Jiang Z, Chu PG, Woda BA, et al. Combination of quantitative IMP3 and tumor stage: a new system to predict metastasis for patients with localized renal cell carcinomas. Clin Cancer Res. 2008;14:5579–84.

208. Nielsen S, Frøkiaer J, Marples D, et al. Aquaporins in the kidney: from molecules to medicine. Physiol Rev. 2002;82:205–44.

209. Echevarría M, Muñoz-Cabello AM, Sánchez-Silva R, et al. Development of cytosolic hypoxia and hypoxia-inducible factor stabilization are facilitated by aquaporin-1 expression. J Biol Chem. 2007;282:30207–15.

210. Magni F, Chinello C, Raimondo F, et al. AQP1 expression analysis in human diseases: implications for proteomic characterization. Expert Rev Proteomics. 2008;5:29–43.

211. Takenawa J, Kaneko Y, Kishishita M, et al. Transcript levels of aquaporin 1 and carbonic anhydrase IV as predictive indicators for prognosis of renal cell carcinoma patients after nephrectomy. Int J Cancer. 1998;79:1–7.

212. Mazal PR, Stichenwirth M, Koller A, et al. Expression of aquaporins and PAX-2 compared to CD10 and cytokeratin 7 in renal neoplasms: a tissue microarray study. Mod Pathol. 2005;18:535–40.

213. Huang Y, Murakami T, Sano F, et al. Expression of aquaporin 1 in primary renal tumors: a prognostic indicator for clear-cell renal cell carcinoma. Eur Urol. 2009;56:690–8.

214. Bickel PE, Tansey JT, Welte MA. PAT proteins, an ancient family of lipid droplet proteins that regulate cellular lipid stores. Biochim Biophys Acta. 2009;1791:419–40.

215. Saarikoski ST, Rivera SP, Hankinson O. Mitogen-inducible gene 6 (MIG-6), adipophilin and tuftelin are inducible by hypoxia. FEBS Lett. 2002;530:186–90.

216. Takahashi M, Rhodes DR, Furge KA, et al. Gene expression profiling of clear cell renal cell carcinoma: gene identification and prognostic classification. Proc Natl Acad Sci USA. 2001;98:9754–9.

217. Yao M, Tabuchi H, Nagashima Y, et al. Gene expression analysis of renal carcinoma: adipose differentiation-related protein as a potential diagnostic and prognostic biomarker for clear-cell renal carcinoma. J Pathol. 2005;205:377–87.

218. Yao M, Huang Y, Shioi K, et al. Expression of adipose differentiation-related protein: a predictor of cancer-specific survival in clear cell renal carcinoma. Clin Cancer Res. 2007;13:152–60.

219. Schmidt SM, Schag K, Müller MR, et al. Induction of adipophilin-specific cytotoxic T lymphocytes using a novel HLA-A2-binding peptide that mediates tumor cell lysis. Cancer Res. 2004;64:1164–70.

220. Morrissey JJ, London AN, Luo J, et al. Urinary biomarkers for the early diagnosis of kidney cancer. Mayo Clin Proc. 2010;85:413–21.

221. Vasselli JR, Shih JH, Iyengar SR, et al. Predicting survival in patients with metastatic kidney cancer by

221. gene-expression profiling in the primary tumor. Proc Natl Acad Sci USA. 2003;100:6958–63.
222. Kosari F, Parker AS, Kube DM, et al. Clear cell renal cell carcinoma: gene expression analyses identify a potential signature for tumor aggressiveness. Clin Cancer Res. 2005;11:5128–39.
223. Zhao H, Ljungberg B, Grankvist K, et al. Gene expression profiling predicts survival in conventional renal cell carcinoma. PLoS Med. 2006;3:e13.
224. Yao M, Huang Y, Shioi K, et al. A three-gene expression signature model to predict clinical outcome of clear cell renal carcinoma. Int J Cancer. 2008;123:1126–32.
225. Sültmann H, von Heydebreck A, Huber W, et al. Gene expression in kidney cancer is associated with cytogenetic abnormalities, metastasis formation, and patient survival. Clin Cancer Res. 2005;11(2 Pt 1): 646–55.
226. Jones J, Otu H, Spentzos D, et al. Gene signatures of progression and metastasis in renal cell cancer. Clin Cancer Res. 2005;11:5730–9.
227. Rohan S, Tu JJ, Kao J, et al. Gene expression profiling separates chromophobe renal cell carcinoma from oncocytoma and identifies vesicular transport

228. and cell junction proteins as differentially expressed genes. Clin Cancer Res. 2006;12:6937–45.
228. Tan MH, Wong CF, Tan HL, et al. Genomic expression and single-nucleotide polymorphism profiling discriminates chromophobe renal cell carcinoma and oncocytoma. BMC Cancer. 2010;10:196.
229. Yusenko MV, Kuiper RP, Boethe T, et al. High-resolution DNA copy number and gene expression analyses distinguish chromophobe renal cell carcinomas and renal oncocytomas. BMC Cancer. 2009; 9:152.
230. Kent OA, Mendell JT. A small piece in the cancer puzzle: microRNAs as tumor suppressors and oncogenes. Oncogene. 2006;25:6188–96.
231. Gottardo F, Liu CG, Ferracin M, et al. Micro-RNA profiling in kidney and bladder cancers. Urol Oncol. 2007;25:387–92.
232. Chow TF, Youssef YM, Lianidou E, et al. Differential expression profiling of microRNAs and their potential involvement in renal cell carcinoma pathogenesis. Clin Biochem. 2010;43:150–8.
233. Juan D, Alexe G, Antes T, et al. Identification of a microRNA panel for clear-cell kidney cancer. Urology. 2010;75:835–41.

Bladder Cancer

12

Andrea Tubaro, Daniele Santini, Cosimo De Nunzio, Alice Zoccoli, and Michele Iuliano

Abbreviations

ALA	5-Aminolaevulinic acid
ATP	Adenosine triphosphate
BCG	Bacillus Calmette-Guerin
BTA	Bladder tumor antigen test
GC	Gemcitabine/cisplatin
GC	Gemcitabine, Cisplatin
GCS	Gemcitabine, cisplatin, and sunitinib
CGA	Comprehensive geriatric assessment
CIS	Carcinoma in situ
CISCA	Cisplatin, cyclophosphamide, adriamycin
CT	Computerized tomography
EBRT	External beam radiotherapy
ECOG	Eastern Cooperative Oncology Group
EGFR	Epidermal growth factor receptor
EORTC	European Organization for Research and Treatment of Cancer
ESMO	European Society of Medical Oncology
FDA	Food and Drug Administration
FGF	Fibroblast growth factor
FISH	Fluorescence in situ hybridization
FLT-3	FMS-like tyrosine kinase-3 receptor
5-FU	5-Fluorouracil
GFR	Glomerular filtration rate
HAL	Hexaminolevulinic acid
HD	High dose
HER	Human epidermal growth factor receptor
HIF	Hypoxia-inducible factor-1
IHC	Immunohistochemistry
KIT	stem cell growth factor receptor or proto-oncogene c-Kit or tyrosine-protein kinase Kit
M-CAVI	Methotrexate, carboplatin, and vinblastine
MIBC	Muscle-invasive bladder cancer
MRI	Magnetic resonance imaging
MSKCC	Memorial Sloan-Kettering Cancer Center
MVAC	Methotrexate, vinblastine, doxorubicin, cisplatin
MVD	Microvessel density
NMIBC	Non-muscle-invasive bladder cancer
NPP22	Nuclear matrix protein test
PDGFR	Platelet-derived growth factor
PFS	Progression-free survival
PS	Performance status
PUNLMP	Papillary urothelial neoplasm of low malignant potential
QLQ-BLM	Quality of life questionnaire on muscle-invasive bladder cancer
RC	Radical cystectomy
RCC	Renal cell carcinoma
RTK	Receptor tyrosine kinase
TCC	Transitional cell carcinoma
TKI	Tyrosine kinase inhibitor
TUR	Transurethral resection

A. Tubaro, M.D., F.E.B.U. (✉) • C. De Nunzio, M.D.
Department of Urology, Sant'Andrea Hospital,
"La Sapienza" University of Rome,
Via di Grottarossa 1035, Rome 00198, Italy
e-mail: andrea.tubaro@mac.com

D. Santini, M.D. • A. Zoccoli, M.D. • M. Iuliano, M.D.
Department of Medical Oncology, Campus Bio-Medico
University, Rome, Italy

TURB	Transurethral resection of the bladder
UUT	Upper urinary tract
VEGF	Vascular endothelial growth factor
WHO	World Health Organization

Introduction

Bladder cancer is the most common malignancy of the urinary tract, and it scores fourth among the most common neoplasms of the adult male. An incidence of 330,000 new cases/year with 130,000 deaths/year has been calculated. A male to female ratio of 3:1 has been described with a decreasing ratio due to the increase of cigarette smoking in the female population. Incidence of the disease may vary significantly within a single continent (27.1:4.1 male to female in Southern Europe versus 14.7:2.2 male to female in Eastern Europe) [1].

In the majority of cases (75–85%), the disease is not invasive but limited to either the urothelium or the submucosa.

Bladder cancer is staged according to the TNM (2002) system according to the following criteria.

TNM

T-Primary Tumor

TX Primary tumor cannot be assessed

T0 No evidence of primary tumor

Ta Noninvasive papillary carcinoma

Tis Carcinoma in situ: "flat tumor"

T1 Tumor invades subepithelial connective tissue

T2 Tumor invades muscle

T2a Tumor invades superficial muscle (inner half)

T2b Tumor invades deep muscle (outer half)

T3 Tumor invades perivesical tissue

T3a Microscopically

T3b Macroscopically (extravesical mass)

T4 Tumor invades any of the following: prostate, uterus, vagina, pelvic wall, abdominal wall

T4a Tumor invades prostate, uterus, or vagina

T4b Tumor invades pelvic wall or abdominal wall

Table 12.1 1973 and 2004 WHO grading system

1973 WHO grading	2004 WHO grading
Urothelial papilloma	Urothelial papilloma
Grade 1: well differentiated	Papillary urothelial neoplasm of low malignant
Grade 2: moderately differentiated	Potential (PUNLMP)
Grade 3: poorly differentiated	Low-grade papillary urothelial carcinoma
	High-grade papillary urothelial carcinoma

N-Lymph Nodes

NX Regional lymph nodes cannot be assessed

N0 No regional lymph node metastasis

N1 Metastasis in a single lymph node 2 cm or less in greatest dimension

N2 Metastasis in a single lymph node more than 2 cm but not more than 5 cm in greatest dimension, or multiple lymph nodes, none more than 5 cm in greatest dimension

N3 Metastasis in a lymph node more than 5 cm in greatest dimension

M-Distant Metastasis

MX Distant metastasis cannot be assessed

M0 No distant metastasis

M1 Distant metastasis

Tumor grading has been updated from the WHO 1973 classification into a new grading system that only applies to Ta and T1 tumors [2, 3] (Table 12.1).

Although the implementation of the WHO 2004 classification is highly recommended, most published evidences still rely on the 1973 classification. In the new one, a new item is introduced represented by the papillary urothelial neoplasm of low malignant potential (PUNLMP) which is characterized by normal urothelial cells in papillary configuration; this entity is not completely benign, has a minimal risk for progression but with a tendency to recur.

Although Ta, T1, and CIS are grouped under the same term of non-muscle invasive tumors, they are very different in terms of malignancy and tendency to progress. Notwithstanding careful

Risk Factors

Chemical carcinogenesis plays an important role in bladder cancer, and both smoking and professional exposure to carcinogens are considered of importance. Smoking is considered to be responsible for 50–65% of cases in men and for 20–30% of cases in women [4]. Different carcinogens including arylamines have been considered to be of importance in tobacco smoking. The risk of developing bladder cancer is directly related to duration and amount of cigarette smoking with starting smoking at a young age increasing the risk [5]. The risk decreases rapidly after smoke cessation (risk decreases from 2.77 to 1.72) with a 40% reduction after 1–4 years and a 60% decrease after 25 years [5–7].

Occupational risk accounts for 20–25% of cancers. At risk industry includes industrial painting, aluminum and iron processing, and gas and tar manufacturing. Involved carcinogens include benzene derivatives and arylamines [8]. Because of the strict regulations in western countries, the occupational risk of bladder cancer has decreased [6, 9, 10].

An increased risk for bladder cancer has been observed following external beam radiotherapy (e.g., EBRT for prostate cancer) [11]. There is no clear relation between dietary factors and bladder cancer although vegetable and fruit intake is considered to be protective [12]. Although the link between schistosomiasis and squamous cell carcinoma of the bladder is well established, the risk seems to be significantly reduced in countries like Egypt over the last decades [13]. Acrolein, a metabolite of cyclophosphamide, is considered to be responsible for the increased occurrence of bladder cancer in patients receiving cyclophosphamide for lymphoproliferative disorders [14, 15].

Involvement of the upper urinary tract is not uncommon in patients with bladder cancer. Patients with multiple bladder neoplasms or tumors of the trigone have a 69% and 41% chance of UUT involvement [16]. Upper and lower urinary tract diseases are rarely synchronous and more often metachronous.

Women are more frequently diagnosed with muscle-invasive disease than men (85 versus 51%) and are diagnosed at an older age [17]. The postmenopausal status is associated with an increased risk of bladder cancer suggesting a possibly protective role of estrogens in the carcinogenesis.

Diagnosis

Diagnosis of bladder cancer relies on hematuria, which is the most common sign of the disease, although urgency, dysuria, and frequency deriving from bladder irritation can be reported and should trigger evaluation for bladder cancer if not resolved by pharmacological treatment. Pelvic pain may be referred in more advanced tumors.

Physical Examination

Bladder cancer is usually not diagnosed on physical examination of the lower abdomen although a palpable mass can be found in locally advanced tumors. Bimanual palpation can be performed at the time of TUR to assess whether the mass is fixed to the pelvic wall.

Imaging

Diagnosis of bladder cancer may be occasionally performed while imaging the urinary bladder with ultrasound during abdominal or pelvic ultrasonography, in patients reporting symptoms and signs that are compatible with bladder cancer. Intravenous urography, once the mainstay of bladder cancer diagnosis, is now rarely performed since uroCT (uro Computerized Tomography) and uroMRI (uro Magnetic Resonance Imaging) have been developed [18–20]. When a bladder mass is imaged, it must be confirmed by histology (confirmation on diagnostic endoscopy may be superfluous).

Urine Cytology

The diagnosis of bladder cancer with urine cytology is limited by the need for cell shedding to obtain valuable urine samples and by the

Table 12.2 Sensitivity and specificity for bladder cancer diagnosis of urine biomarkers

	UroVysion®	Microsatellite analysis	Gene microarray	ImmunoCyt/ uCyt+™	NMP22	BTA stat	BTA trak
Sensitivity	30–72	58	80–90	76–85	49–68	57–83	53–91
Specificity	63–95	73	62–65	63–75	85–87.5	68–85	28–83
Sensitivity for high-grade tumors	66–70	90	80	67–92	75–83	61–5	77

Modified from Babjuk M, Oosterlinck W, Sylvester R, et al. Guidelines on Non-muscle invasive Bladder Cancer (TaT1 and CIS). 2011. http://www.uroweb.org/?id=217&tyid=1. Accessed 10 May 2011. With permission from European Association of Urology

confounding presence of erythrocytes and inflammatory urothelial cells that may coexists with the bladder neoplasm or be responsible for symptoms and signs of it. In experienced hands, urine cytology may yield a 90% specificity [21].

Urine Markers

A number of urine markers have been described over the years, although none of the involved molecules and diagnostic tests reached adequate levels of sensitivity and specificity to be recommended in daily practice [22–28] (Table 12.2).

The following three markers are of interest: NMP22, UroVysion, and ImmunoCyt [25, 28–33]. The BTA test provides a quantitative detection of human complement factor H-related protein, but it suffers a high false-positive rate and a low sensitivity for low-grade tumors although its sensitivity and specificity for pTis is high [34, 35]. Measurement of the nuclear matrix protein NMP22 showed a high false-positive rate and a sensitivity higher than urine cytology; the good negative predictive value can be used to delay cystoscopy in follow-up protocols [29, 31, 36–38]. ImmunoCyt is an immunocytological fluorescence assay based on three monoclonal antibodies, two are directed to a mucin-like antigen located in the urine on exfoliated tumor cells and one binds to a high-molecular-weight glycosylated form of carcinoembryonic antigen; notwithstanding a high sensitivity for low-grade tumors, the 60% detection rate makes it inadequate to substitute cystoscopy [33, 39]. UroVysion is a multitarget fluorescence in situ hybridization (FISH) assay that can be useful in the follow-up of high-grade tumors in alternative to urine cytology [32, 40, 41]. Microsatellite analysis is a promising test to predict recurrence of low-grade tumor, but its sensitivity is low [42–44].

From a clinical standpoint, urine cytology and biomarkers can be used to screen populations at high risk for bladder cancer provided cost-effectiveness is proven, to investigate patients with hematuria or symptoms suggestive of bladder cancer and to follow-up non-muscle-invasive bladder cancer reducing the number of unnecessary cystoscopies; unfortunately, none of the proposed biomarkers can yet replace cystoscopy.

Cystoscopy

Diagnosis of bladder cancer is based on diagnostic endoscopy and pathological evaluation of resected specimens although the diagnosis of in situ carcinoma may require urine cytology and pathological evaluation of bladder biopsies on top of cystoscopy [46]. When bladder cancer is imaged on ultrasonography, CT, or MRI, diagnostic endoscopy may be superfluous.

Treatment of Non-muscle-Invasive Bladder Cancer

Transurethral Resection

The goal of transurethral resection (TUR) of superficial bladder tumors is to make a histological diagnosis to stage the disease locally, and to remove the neoplasm/s entirely when possible. For staging purposes, the resection should be deep enough to sample a layer of tissue that is free of tumor. Submucosal tissue should be available to diagnose pTa tumors, superficial muscle should be sampled to diagnose pT1, and deep muscle layers should be available to diagnose a pT2 neoplasm. Small lesions can be sampled in en bloc; in larger tumors, the exophytic part, the bladder wall, and the lesion margins should be provided separately. Each bladder lesion should be placed in a separate container. Bladder tissue resection is not trivial surgery, and proper tissue sampling is crucial for correct diagnosis and optimal patient management.

Bladder biopsies using a cold cup forceps or a resection loop may be taken when suspicious (reddish or velvetlike) areas are observed. In patients with positive urine cytology and negative cystoscopy, random biopsies are usually obtained from the bladder trigone, lateral, posterior, and anterior wall to diagnose CIS. Random bladder biopsies are not recommended in patients with papillary neoplasm. Biopsies of prostatic urethra are recommended in the presence of suspicious areas; carcinoma of prostatic urethra and ducts are more frequently diagnosed in association with CIS, multiple neoplasms, tumors of the bladder trigone, and neck.

The use of fluorescence cystoscopy with 5-aminolaevulinic acid (ALA) or hexaminolevulinic acid (HAL) has been proposed for its superior ability in identifying malignant tumors and CIS [47–51]. Notwithstanding some preliminary experience suggesting a 15.8–27% and 12–15% higher rate of recurrence-free survival at 12 and 24 months, respectively, one large study reported no additional benefit with ALA fluorescence cystoscopy, and a 9% lower recurrence rate was found in another large study using HAL fluorescence-guided TUR. In consideration of the costs involved in the examination and the false-positive rate following BCG treatment, the use of fluorescence-guided cystoscopy could be limited in the diagnosis of patients with positive urine cytology and negative endoscopy and in the follow-up of high-grade bladder tumors.

Clinical experience suggests that persistent tumor can be observed after initial resection of pT1 disease in 33–53% of cases and the disease can be understaged in 4–25% of patients [52–58]. Indications for a second resection include incomplete resection of multiple or large neoplasms, absence of muscle tissue in the pathological specimen, and diagnosis of high-grade or pT1 tumor in the first resection.

To evaluate the risk of local recurrence and progression, the following parameters are of importance: number of tumors, tumor size, prior recurrence rate, T category, concomitant CIS, and tumor grade. For clinical purposes, a risk calculator (http://eortc.be/tools/bladdercalculator/) has been developed by the genitourinary group of the EORTC, and patients with low, intermediate, and high risk for local recurrence and progression can be derived (Fig. 12.1).

In patients with CIS, disease progression to muscle-invasive disease is observed in about 54% of cases; multiple CIS and association with pT1 disease are associated with poor prognosis [59]. Response to BCG treatment is an important prognostic factor as 10–20% of responders progress to muscle-invasive disease compared to 66% of nonresponders [60–62].

Imaging in Histologically Verified Bladder Cancer

Since the management of muscle-invasive bladder cancer strongly depends on staging, CT or MRI imaging may be required to evaluate local tumor invasion, lymph node involvement, and the presence of distant metastases. Local staging aims at diagnosing T3b disease as microscopic invasion cannot be detected. MR imaging has been proposed because using fast dynamic contrast-enhanced sequences, tumor enhancement may occur earlier than in the normal bladder wall. Staging accuracy ranges from 73% to 96% and score higher than observed for CT. CT has been considered to have lower sensitivity but higher specificity compared to MR imaging for the diagnosis of perivesical invasion since mild inflammation may mimic perivesical invasion on MR imaging. Sensitivity of CT and MR imaging for nodal involvement is relatively low as it is only based on node enlargement (48–87%). There is no current role for PET scan in staging bladder cancer.

CT and MR urography are the gold standard techniques to diagnose and stage urothelial cancer

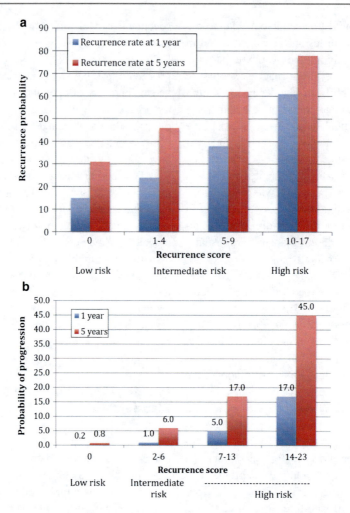

Fig. 12.1 The relation between probability of tumor recurrence and recurrence risk (**a**) and tumor progression and progression risk (**b**) according to the EORTC calculator (http://www.eortc.be/tools/bladdercalculator/) (**a**) Recurrence risk according to the EORTC calculator. (**b**) Tumor progression risk according to the EORTC calculator

of the upper urinary tract although the radiation exposure in CT imaging is not negligible.

Metastases from bladder cancer usually involve lungs and liver and rarely comprise brain and bones; imaging for brain and bone metastases is therefore performed only when symptoms or signs suggest involvement of such districts.

Adjuvant Treatment

Although bladder resection may suffice in managing Ta and T1 disease, data from the peer-reviewed literature suggest that tumors recur locally in a high percentage of patients and more rarely progress. Adjuvant treatment may therefore be required based on the amount of risk that patients are willing to accept; the choice of the optimal treatment is not necessary and only based on the degree of risk.

A single postoperative instillation of chemotherapeutic agents is able to reduce the absolute and relative risk of recurrence by 11.7% and 24.2%, respectively [63]. Although these data mostly refer to patients with single lesions, the benefit seems to be even greater for those with multiple tumors [64, 65]. Adjuvant single instillation is considered to work through the destruction of tumor cells circulating in the urinary bladder following TUR and ablation on tumor cells remaining in the resection site. In order to be effective, the instillation should be given within 24 h, possibly within the same day of surgery and even as early as in the surgical theater or recovery room. Mitomycin C, epirubicin, and doxorubicin were shown to be equally effective [64]. Early single instillation is recommended in patients with low risk of progression; in patients with intermediate risk, an early treatment can be used in association with subsequent adjuvant intravesical treatment [66]. In patients at high risk, early instillation is an option although the superior efficacy of BCG adjuvant treatment should also be considered. Early instillation should not be performed in case of bladder perforation and bleeding that requires irrigation, but it remains feasible in the majority of patients.

In patients with intermediate or high risk of recurrence and progression, adjuvant intravesical chemotherapy or immunotherapy is required beyond an early single instillation. The choice between chemo- and immunotherapy is based on the desired effect: chemotherapy is known to reduce recurrence but not progression that is only influenced by immunotherapy with BCG, but the duration of the adjuvant treatment is questionable although no additional benefit is considered to exist beyond 1 year of treatment.

There is strong evidence that adjuvant treatment with BCG is superior to TUR alone and TUR plus adjuvant treatment with intravesical chemotherapy in reducing the recurrence rate in intermediate- and high-risk patients [67–70]. A 32% reduction in the risk of recurrence can be expected with BCG compared to chemotherapy, and BCG maintenance cycles are recommended [71]. BCG treatment with maintenance cycles is also considered to reduce the risk of tumor progression by 27% in both TaT1 and CIS patients [72, 73]. Although the optimal frequency and duration of maintenance BCG cycles is unknown, it is considered to provide a 37% reduction in the risk of progression [70–73].

Reduced BCG dosages have been investigated to reduce local and systemic toxicity while maintaining the therapeutic effect. A dose of 1/3 of the standard one seems to maintain a good therapeutic effect with a lower incidence of side effects although the incidence of severe systemic adverse events was not reduced [74, 75]. It has been suggested that the standard dose is more efficacious in patients with multifocal disease [74, 75]. One-third of the standard dose seems to be the minimum efficacious dose in the management of patients with intermediate risk; the use of a lower dose (1/6 of the standard one) resulted in a lower efficacy with no improvement in side effects [76].

BCG side effects occur in less than 5% of patients [77]. The more severe side effects (sepsis) occur following systemic absorption of BCG, and instillations should not be done within 2 weeks for TUR, in case of hematuria or traumatic catheterization. BCG-induced cystitis and allergic reactions may also occur. BCG should not be instilled in immunocompromised patients [78]. Proper management of BCG side effects may require high-dose fluoroquinolones and antibiotic regimens for the treatment of tuberculosis. Recommendations for management of BCG complications can be found by Witjes JA, Palou J, Soloway M, et al. Clinical practice recommendations for the prevention and management of intravesical therapy-associated adverse events [79].

The choice between intravesical chemotherapy and BCG is based on the relative cost-benefit ratio of the two treatments. Patients at high risk of progression who would otherwise be scheduled for radical cystectomy should receive BCG treatment with a 1-year maintenance. Patients at intermediate or high risk of recurrence and intermediate risk of progression can receive either intravesical chemotherapy or immunotherapy taking into consideration that BCG is more efficacious and has more side effects.

There is no clear guidance for the management of CIS. When CIS is diagnosed in association with muscle-invasive disease, treatment is dictated by the muscle-invasive tumor. When CIS is associated with TaT1 disease, patients are at high risk of progression, and treatment should be performed accordingly. Isolated CIS can either be treated with BCG or with immediate cystectomy; this latter approach provides excellent disease-specific survival rates, but up to one in two patients may be overtreated. Complete response of 48 and 72–93% has been described following intravesical chemotherapy or BCG treatment, respectively, but up to 50% of responders may recur locally or progress [59, 80–84]. Randomized trials of BCG versus intravesical chemotherapy showed a 59% reduction in the risk of failure with BCG; long-term benefit of BCG treatment with maintenance has been confirmed (OR: 57%) [85]. A 35% decrease in the risk of progression has been shown in patients receiving BCG treatment compared with intravesical instillation [45].

Attention should be paid to the possible CIS involvement of the upper urinary tract that makes patients' survival worse. CIS may also involve prostatic urethra in which case standard BCG treatment is required, but if the prostatic ducts are involved by CIS, radical surgery should be considered likewise when the prostate stroma in involved [86].

In the management of TUR failures, patients with local recurrences following intravesical chemotherapy may benefit from BCG treatment, and in patients with a local recurrence 3 months after a BCG course, a second course can achieve a complete response in 50% of cases although the risk of progression is increased [87, 88]. Following BCG failure, radical surgery is recommended as any other therapeutic approach remains investigational [60, 88, 89].

Follow-Up for TaT1 and CIS

Follow-up is aimed at the early diagnosis of tumor progression versus muscle-invasive disease, and we know that results of a 3-month cystoscopy are a prognostic factor for both recurrence and progression. In low-grade tumors, if the 3-month cystoscopy is negative, a second one can be performed at 12 months and then yearly as these tumors tend to recur locally but not to progress. In high-risk disease, endoscopy and urine cytology should be performed 3-monthly for 2 years, 6-monthly for the following 3 years, and then yearly. In patients with intermediate risk, the follow-up schedule can be adapted to individual factors [45].

Radical Surgery for TaT1 Bladder Cancer

Immediate radical cystectomy can be offered even for non-muscle-invasive disease in case of multiple recurrent high-grade tumors, in case of high-grade T1 lesions, and in the presence of high-grade tumors associated with CIS. A 5-year disease-free survival rate of 80% or greater has been observed when radical cystectomy is performed in patients with non-muscle-invasive disease [90–94].

Notwithstanding a 34% staging error in recurrent TaT1 tumors, mostly associated with CIS, the 10-year survival in T1 and T2 tumors undergoing radical cystectomy is similar, suggesting that previous TUR is not a negative predictive factor.

There are no clear indications as to the management of BCG failures as data from the peer-reviewed literature differ in terms of BCG treatment and maintenance schedule and definition of failure. We know that 80% of patients with a local recurrence at 3 months will develop muscle-invasive disease and that tumor persistence at 9 months is associated with 30% chance of invasive disease and death. It is therefore reasonable to offer radical surgery in case of tumor persistence at 9 months after BCG treatment as additional BCG can offer a 27–51% response of unknown duration.

Treatment of Muscle-Invasive Bladder Cancer

Neoadjuvant Treatment

Provided the gold standard treatment of muscle-invasive bladder cancer is radical cystectomy, 5-year survival does not exceed 50%, and strategies to improve results have been explored [90, 95–98]. Neoadjuvant chemotherapy is one of such strategies although pros and cons have to be considered. On the positive side, patients are considered to tolerate chemotherapy better before than after surgery, and the burden of micrometastases is supposed to be low; on the negative side, chemotherapy delays surgery, and since staging

12 Bladder Cancer

accuracy does not exceed 70%, overtreatment may occur [99, 100]. On average, about 70% of patients are expected to receive a full neoadjuvant treatment with a total of 78% receiving any treatment [101]. Preoperative anemia and neuropathy can be expected [102]. The question whether neoadjuvant chemotherapy improves survival remains open. A first meta-analysis published in 2003 suggested a 5% improvement in overall survival (from 45 to 50%) [103, 104]. Similar results were obtained in a second meta-analysis (2004) with overall survival improving from 50 to 55%. Another meta-analysis published in 2005 confirmed a 5% benefit although studies from the Nordic group achieved an 8% survival benefit with 11% benefit in T3 disease [105]. Nevertheless, data suggest that perioperative chemotherapy is used in only 11.6% of patients enrolled in the National Cancer Data Base in the USA suggesting a low degree of integration of guideline's recommendations into clinical practice.

Radical Surgery

Radical cystectomy is the standard treatment for recurrent NMIBC and muscle-invasive disease, although there is an interest in organ-sparing treatment such as radio- and chemotherapy [90, 106]. We know that preoperative conditions and pathological state are related to survival following radical surgery, and therefore careful counseling is advised [107] (Table 12.3). Evaluation of series in patients older than 80 years suggest increased postoperative morbidity but not mortality. In older patients, an ileal conduit is generally preferred [108].

Timing of surgery is essential, and a delay of 90 days has been considered to increase the chance of extravesical disease from 52% to 81% and the type of surgery to be executed [109]. The average time to surgery is in fact shorter for orthotopic neobladder compared to ileal conduits [110].

Indications for radical cystectomy include BCG resistant Tis and T1G3, papillary tumors that cannot be managed with TUR, and muscle-invasive disease (T2-T4a, N0-X, M0) [106].

Patients who do not respond to conservative treatment and patients with nonurothelial cancers, intractable fistulas, or hematuria may undergo salvage cystectomy.

The standard surgical technique involves removal of prostate gland together with the urinary bladder. Attempts to spare part of the prostate gland have been made, but no randomized trials are available [111, 112]. Overall, between 1 in 4 and 1 in 3 of patients undergoing radical cystectomy have no involvement of the prostate gland; in fact, a 32–33% of patients have urothelial cancer in the prostate gland, and prostate cancer is found in 23–54% of cases [113–115].

Radical cystectomy includes removal of lymph nodes draining the urinary bladder although a standard template has not been defined yet. In retrospective analysis, an extended template including the aortic bifurcation was associated with improved survival [116]. Retrospective analysis indicates that removal of 15 lymph nodes is sufficient for a correct staging and to improve patient survival [117–119]. Evaluation of ureteral margins should be performed in case of CIS, and urethrectomy is recommended when positive urethral margins are found, in case of extensive tumors at the bladder neck or urethra in women and prostatic involvement in men.

Laparoscopic and robotic-assisted cystectomy should be considered as investigational techniques since they have been tested in relative small series only [120, 121].

Different types of diversions can be used in which urine is drained through an abdominal opening with or without interposition of a continent or incontinent intestinal segment (ureterocutaneostomy, ileal conduit, colonic conduit continent ileal pouch, etc.), orthotopic continent pouches, and diversions to the sigma and rectum [122]. Although orthotopic diversions are preferred for the maintenance of an intact body image, contraindications to complex reconstructions drive from short life expectancy, liver and renal dysfunction, TCC of surgical margins or urethra, and neurological and psychiatric disorders. Previous radiation therapy that compromised both the ileum and colon segments may prevent the confection of an intestinal pouch, and

Table 12.3 Disease and overall survival after radical cystectomy

Author	Disease-free survival		Disease-specific survival		Overall survival		Comments
	5 yrs	10 yrs	5 yrs	10 yrs	5 yrs	10 yrs	
Shariat et al. [145]	58%		66%		66%		
Stein et al. [90]	68%	60%			66%	43%	
Gschwend et al. [146]			72.9%		49.1%		Organ-confined disease
			33.3%		22.8%		Non-organ-confined disease
			27.7%		20.9%		N + disease

severe urethral stenosis may contraindicate an orthotopic reconstruction.

Ureterocutaneostomy

This is the simplest form of diversion that is generally used in patients with severe comorbidities [123, 124]. Postoperative complications are considered to be low although stenosis of the anastomosis with the abdominal skin and retrograde infection of the upper urinary tract are reported [125].

Ileal Conduit

Although this is one of the most commonly used types of diversion, it is not free of complications that seem to increase with longer follow-up reaching a prevalence of 94% at 15 years [126]. Upper urinary tract deterioration and problems with the stoma have been described [126–128].

Continent Cutaneous Diversions

Ileal and colonic intestinal segments can be used to construct a continent pouch that is attached to the abdominal skin (usually the umbilicus) using either the appendix or an intussuscepted ileal loop. The pouch is emptied by self-catheterization. Satisfactory continence rate can be achieved (>90%), although stomal problems, stone formation, and incontinence have been reported [129–135].

Ureterosigmoidostomy

This is the most common form of anastomosis between the ureters and the colon; notwithstanding antireflux techniques for ureteric reimplantation, infection of the upper urinary tract is frequently observed, and the technique is now rarely used; a risk of colon carcinogenesis has also been described [136, 137].

Orthotopic Diversions

There is now a large experience with the confection of orthotopic neobladders consisting of detubularized ileal segments arranged in a more or less spherical shape in which both ureters are anastomosed and that is connected to the remaining urethral stump. Voiding is achieved with a combination of pelvic floor relaxation and abdominal straining. Daytime and nighttime continence is possible provided timed voiding is implemented to compensate for increased urine volume due to osmotic diuresis. Ileal segments are most frequently used compared to colonic or sigmoid segments. Complications are not unusual and include stenosis of the ureteric and urethral anastomoses, stone formation, urinary retention, and urethral recurrence [138, 139]. The type of urinary diversion does not seem to influence the oncological outcome [140].

In general, there is no consensus as to the type of diversion that offers the best quality of life [141–143]. No particular type of diversion can be recommended, and the choice is left to surgeon's experience and patient preference. Radical cystectomy is not void of complications with 3% mortality and 28% of complications [95, 144]. Morbidity and mortality rates seem to be related to surgeon's experience.

Flow Chart for the Management of MIBC

1. Diagnosis
   (a) Pathological staging by TURB with biopsy of proximal (females) or prostatic urethra (males)
   (b) UUT staging by CT/RM
   (c) Staging of the chest and abdomen by CT/RM

12 Bladder Cancer

2. Treatment
   (a) In pT2,N0,M0 tumors, bladder sparing techniques may be considered in selected patients.
   (b) In pT2-3,N0,M0 tumors:
       • Neoadjuvant chemotherapy can be considered with 5–7% survival benefit at 5 years.
       • Radical cystectomy.
       • No adjuvant chemotherapy is indicated after cystectomy.

Neoadjuvant Radiotherapy

The effect of preoperative radiotherapy has been investigated in various trials. They suggest a tumor downstaging in T3 patients [147, 148] with improved local control in pT3b and improvement of overall survival from 40% to 52%. A dose of 40 Gy proved to be efficacious with reduced risk of local recurrence and improved survival (from 21% to 63%) [149].

Overall, preoperative radiotherapy followed by radical cystectomy results in tumor downstaging, reduced risk of local recurrence, and improved survival [147–155]. Pathological complete response is associated with increased survival [156–158]. Preoperative radiotherapy is not associated with increased toxicity [158], but a meta-analysis of prospective randomized trials of preoperative radiotherapy failed to confirm a survival advantage [159, 160].

Bladder-Sparing Treatment for Locally Advanced Disease

In selected cases, a bladder-sparing approach can be proposed provided risks and benefits are properly discussed with the patient.

TURB

Patients with MIBC diagnosed at *trans*urethral resection may present with either pT0 or pT1 status at the re-TURB, about half of them will end up with a radical cystectomy, and a cancer-specific survival rate <50% has been described. A negative TURB is considered to be essential in planning bladder-sparing management of these patients in selected cases when the initial disease in ≤pT2 or when the patient is unfit for radical surgery.

Radiotherapy

External beam radiotherapy is associated with severe morbidity and a tumor-free rate <5%. The 5-year survival rate of MIBC treated with external beam radiotherapy is 30–60% with cancer-specific survival of 20–50% [161–165]. Meta-analysis from the Cochrane Collaboration suggests a survival benefit of radical cystectomy over radiotherapy [160]. Radiotherapy remains a viable option in those unfit for radical surgery with an expected control and survival rates of 56% and 36% at 3 years [166].

Chemotherapy

Complete (12–50% for MVAC and 12–22% for gemcitabine/cisplatin) and partial responses have been reported in patients with MIBC treated with neoadjuvant chemotherapy [102, 167–177]. A bladder-spring approach with TURB followed by i.v. chemotherapy can be proposed in selected cases, and it may allow survival with an intact bladder, although there is a risk of a staging error and recurrent or metastatic disease.

Multiple Modality Bladder-Sparing Treatment

A combination of TURB followed by external beam radiotherapy and i.v. chemotherapy can be proposed in selected cases of small T2 neoplasms with no CIS. In the presence of a complete response (70–80% with cisplatin), radical cystectomy can be avoided although the risk of local recurrence is high [178]. No comparative data exist versus radical cystectomy although survival

Patient characteristics	First line		Second line	
Performance status 0-1 GFR ≥60 ml/min	GC/MVAC/HD MVAC		Progression >6-12 months after 1st line Normal GFR	a. Re-exposition to 1st line b. Clinical trial
		PS 0-1	Progression >6-12 months after 1st line Impaired GFR	a. Vinflunine b. Clinical trial
			Progression <6-12 months after 1st line	a. Vinflunine b. Clinical trial
Performance status 2 GFR <60 ml/min	Carboplatin-based combination chemotherapy			
Performance status ≥2 GFR <60 ml/min	Clinical trials Single agent, non-CISplatin chemotherapy Best supportive care	PS ≥2		a. Best supportive care b. Clinic al trial

Fig. 12.2 Management of metastatic bladder cancer

rates seem comparable. Patients who then end up with radical surgery (30–40%) have a poor prognosis, and a 20–50% survival at 5 years has been described [178, 179]. Patients undergoing bladder sparing multimodality treatment should be aware of the required intense follow-up schedule and the possibility of multiple TURBs [178–182].

Adjuvant Chemotherapy

Chemotherapy can be used after radical surgery in patients with locally advanced or node-positive disease. There is limited evidence available as to the outcome of this adjuvant approach [183–189] to support its use in daily practice. Patients with extravesical disease or positive lymph nodes can be considered for adjuvant chemotherapy, provided they are fully informed of the limited evidence available. There is no evidence to prefer adjuvant chemotherapy to chemotherapy upon evidence of disease recurrence. Long-term survival has been described in patients with positive nodes and good performance [173, 190, 191].

Metastatic Disease

A minority of patients presents with distant metastases at diagnosis. The majority of patients with metastases are relapses following radical cystectomy for MIBC [192]. In the absence of chemotherapy, survival is not beyond 6 months [193].

Trials on chemotherapy of metastatic bladder cancer have identified two major prognostic factors for clinical response: Karnofsky performance status and visceral metastases, PS of 80% or less, visceral disease, elevated LDH levels, and more than three sites of disease were found to be associated with reduced survival [171, 175, 190, 194–196]; ECOG PS2-3 and hemoglobin levels <10 mg/dl have also been associated with poor survival [197]. The presence of comorbidities is also considered of importance for mortality [198–201]. Patients with PS of 3–4 are considered not to benefit from chemotherapy (Fig. 12.2).

A number of conditions including reduced GFR, poor performance status, neuropathy and

Table 12.4 Response rates to single-agent chemotherapy

Agent	Response rate	Reference
Cisplatin	12	[171]
Carboplatin	12%	[203]
Paclitaxel	425	[204]
Docetaxel	31	[205]
Methotrexate	29	[206, 207]
Adriamycin	19%	[206, 207]
Epirubicin	15%	[206, 207]
Mitomycin C	13%	[206, 207]
5-FU	35%	[206, 207]
Vinblastine	14%	[206, 207]
Ifosfamide	29%	[206, 207]
Cyclophosphamide	8%	[206, 207]
Gemcitabine	25%	[208–214]

severe presbycusis, cardiovascular disease, and congestive heart failure have been considered of importance in precluding or cautioning the use of chemotherapy and particularly of cisplatin. It is generally considered that one in two patients with metastatic bladder cancer is unfit for chemotherapy. Although the comprehensive geriatric assessment (CGA) has been considered of importance to better evaluate patients' performance status, its use in clinical practice remains marginal [202].

Different drugs have been evaluated as single agents in metastatic bladder cancer, and variable response rates have been described (Table 12.4).

Single-agent chemotherapy is rarely used because of the absence of complete responses and the short life of the observed responses with a mean survival of less than 9 months.

First-Line Combination Chemotherapy

Current therapeutic regimens are based on cisplatin-containing chemotherapy. MVAC and the combination of gemcitabine and cisplatin proved to be effective (14.8 and 13.8 months survival) and more efficacious than CISCA and cisplatin/docetaxel [168, 215–217]. MVAC and GC appear to be equally effective with 46% and 49% of response rates, respectively, although GC is better tolerated. The use of high-dose-intensity MVAC supplemented with GCSF seems to offer 2-year survival with reduced toxicity compared to standard MVAC [218, 219]. Lymph node metastases respond better to MVAC or HD-MVAC compared to extranodal disease (66% and 77% response versus 29 and 33%, respectively) and 20.9% versus 6.8% survival at 5 years.

The use of carboplatin-containing regimens resulted in lower response rate and shortened survival; therefore, it has been abandoned [220, 221].

Non-cisplatin-containing regimens such as gemcitabine/docetaxel have been used with response rates of 36–60%, but no comparative data with cisplatin-containing cocktails are available, and these regimens are not currently used in patients with good prognostic factors [214, 222–224].

In patients with poor PS, renal impairment, or other comorbidities (about one in two patients with metastatic bladder cancer), non-cisplatin-containing regimens have been investigated such as carboplatin/gemcitabine and M-CAVI with 42% and 30% response rate, respectively. Subanalyses suggested that patients with PS2 and renal insufficiency do not benefit much from chemotherapy [225].

Second-Line Chemotherapy

Different prognostic factors have been considered for clinical response to second-line treatment, but no consensus has been reached, and there is no standard regimen.

Good response rates have been observed with gemcitabine chemotherapy, but most patients already received this drug as first line [208, 211–214]. Response rates from 0% to 13% have been described with agents including paclitaxel, docetaxel, oxaliplatin, ifosfamide, topotecan, lapatinib, gefitinib, and bortezomib [226–230]. The combination of paclitaxel and gemcitabine has been used with variable response (38–60%) depending on pretreatment response and indication for prior chemotherapy, but further randomized trials are required [193, 223].

A new vinca alkaloid, vinflunine, proved to be efficacious in second-line treatment of patients relapsing after cisplatin-containing regimens, although the response rate is modest (<10%), a survival benefit could be observed.

In selected cases, postchemotherapy surgery has been advocated considering the high degree of complete responses and long-term survival in about 20% of patients in which the disease is limited to lymph nodes [176, 231, 232].

In case of bone metastases, which occur in 30–40% of patients with metastatic and advanced disease, i.v. bisphosphonate treatment is required to reduce the frequency of and delay skeletal-related events such as pain, need for external beam radiotherapy, bone fractures, and need for bone surgery, the occurrence of which is associated with reduced survival. Direct evidence of the benefit of zoledronic acid treatment in patients with bone metastases from bladder cancer is limited, but this regimen is supported by a large body of evidence from studies on solid tumors [233].

Biomarkers

Retrospective analysis of study cohorts has been looking at the possible prognostic value of different biomarkers although no sufficient evidence could be found to support their use in our daily practice. Investigated markers include multidrug resistance genes, circulating tumor cells, thrombospondin-1, urinary and tissue fibroblast growth factor receptor-3, urinary and tissue basic fibroblast growth factor, serum vascular endothelial growth factor, p53 expression, and microvessel density [234–240].

What the Future Holds

Having reviewed the current standards in the management of bladder cancer, let us have a look at the current research and possible future developments. Although the current management of bladder cancer is fundamentally surgical, recently there has been a growing interest in multimodal combination therapy in various clinical scenarios to improve outcomes, also due to the high "distant and local" failure rate in both superficial and invasive disease. Advances in tumor biology have led to the identification of new molecular targets in bladder cancer and the development of specific therapies for bladder cancer. To ensure translation of research from bench to bedside, it is now required to drive into clinical practice these promising therapies.

Nowadays, the interest is mainly focused in developing novel therapeutic agents that specifically target growth factor pathways that are deregulated in tumor cells. Among the molecular therapies for bladder cancer treatment, we will focus on those that are currently in a most advanced phase of clinical development such as the study of agents that target EGFR and angiogenesis pathways.

Targeting EGFR Pathway

The epidermal growth factor receptor (EGFR) is a 170-kDa transmembrane receptor tyrosine kinase expressed on the surface of epithelial cells. The EGFR family of RTKs consists of four closely related type I transmembrane receptors: the EGFR, HER2 (ErbB2/neu), HER3 (ErbB3), and HER4 (ErbB4). EGFR regulates important processes in carcinogenesis, including cell survival, cell cycle progression, tumor invasion, and angiogenesis. Ligands including epidermal growth factor (EGF) bind to EGFR-activating signal transduction pathways that upregulate transcription factors, leading to growth stimulation. EGFR was first characterized in invasive and superficial bladder cancer in 1989 [241]. Abnormal expression of the urothelial EGFR and/or altered excretion of EGF may well precede overt manifestations of transitional cell carcinoma (TCC) and thus may serve as an early marker of the invasive phenotype; the degree of EGFR overexpression in bladder tumors has been shown to correlate with tumor stage and grade [242]. Laboratory investigations have shown that stimulation of the EFGR pathway both increases proliferation and the migration of bladder cancer cells [243]. Work to identify the predictive markers for the response of bladder cancer cells to EGFR inhibition is underway, using a broad spectrum of bladder cancer cell lines [244]. Surprisingly, there is no correlation between expression of EGF, the ligand of EGFR, and the activity of EGFR inhibitors in bladder cancer cells [244]. Activating mutations of EGFR, a key predictive marker for the activity of EGFR inhibitors in non-small-cell lung cancer [245], are uncommon in TCC of the bladder [246]. Similarly, increased ErbB2 expression has been associated with worse disease-specific survival [247]. Therefore, the EGFR pathway represents a potential therapeutic target in bladder cancer.

Two groups of EGFR-targeting agents are currently approved for clinical use in some solid tumors today: the monoclonal antibody-mediated blockade of the extracellular ligand-binding domain (cetuximab and trastuzumab) and small-molecule inhibition of the intracellular tyrosine kinase domain (gefitinib, erlotinib, and lapatinib) [248].

Gefitinib
Gefitinib (Iressa; AstraZeneca, London, UK) is an orally bioavailable small, reversible TKI that blocks the ATP-binding domain of EGFR that has demonstrated antiproliferative effects on bladder tumour cells in vitro and in vivo [249–251].

Despite these preclinical evidences, Gefitinib combined with gemcitabine and cisplatin in a phase II trial involving in 55 chemotherapy-naive patients with locally advanced or metastatic failed to improve first-line therapy response rates compared with historic controls achieving a response rate of 51% and a median overall survival of 14.4 months, which were very similar to those obtained with GC alone [252].

Erlotinib
Erlotinib (Tarceva; Genentech, South San Francisco, CA) is another EGFR-targeting TKI and was approved in 2004 for treatment of patients with NSCLC and in 2005 for use in combination with gemcitabine for pancreatic cancer. Erlotinib reversibly inhibits the tyrosine kinase function of wild-type EGFR and also show a slight inhibitory effect on the mutant EGFRvIII tyrosine kinase activity [253]. The M.D. Anderson Cancer Center recently conducted a phase II

study on 20 patients (15 men) with histologically confirmed muscle-invasive bladder carcinoma (clinical stage T2) that examined the value of neoadjuvant erlotinib. All patients received treatment with 150 mg daily of erlotinib orally for 4 weeks before a radical cystectomy. Results of operative pathology showed that five (25%) of 20 patients had a complete response (pT0) at the time of RC, and seven (35%) and 15 (75%) had pathological downstaging (≤pT1N0) and organ-confined disease (≤pT2N0), respectively. Interestingly, one patient was found to have microscopic lymph node-positive disease but no residual primary tumor (pT0, N1) at the time of RC [254].

Cetuximab
Cetuximab (Erbitux; ImClone, New York, NY) is a recombinant human/murine monoclonal antibody (IgG1) that binds to subdomain III on the EGFR. It is one of two monoclonal antibodies against EGFR that has been licensed for clinical use. It was approved in February 2004 for treatment of EGFR-positive late-stage chemorefractory colorectal cancer and in December 2005 for treatment of squamous cell carcinoma of the head and neck in combination with irradiation.

The EGFR antibody cetuximab has been investigated also in a human urothelial carcinoma cell line and in a mouse model with human bladder carcinoma. Cetuximab was found to inhibit tumorigenesis and metastatic progression in vivo and in vitro by means of suppression of angiogenesis and simultaneous induction of apoptosis [255]. There are currently two ongoing studies of cetuximab in metastatic bladder cancer: a randomized phase II study of first-line treatment with gemcitabine and cisplatin +/− Erbitux (NCT00645593) [256] and a randomized phase II study of second-line treatment with Erbitux +/− Paclitaxel [256].

Trastuzumab
Trastuzumab (Herceptin; Genentech, South San Francisco, CA) is the first recombinant humanized monoclonal antibody directed against the HER2. The HER2 gene located on chromosome 17q encodes a transmembrane ligand orphan

receptor tyrosine kinase that amplifies the signal provided by other members of the HER family (HER1/EGFR, HER3, and HER4) by forming heterodimers with them. HER2 activation and dimerization causes alterations in several complex downstream-signaling cascades that are involved in regulation of cell growth, proliferation, migration, adhesion, and survival and thus has been implicated in oncogenesis. A phase II trial that treated 44 patients with HER2-positive (protein overexpression by immunohistochemistry [IHC] or gene amplification by fluorescence in situ hybridization [FISH]) in the primary or metastatic site) advanced urothelial carcinoma with a combination of trastuzumab, paclitaxel, carboplatin, and gemcitabine showed 31 (70%) responding patients, including 5 complete and 26 partial responses. Median time to progression and survival were 9.3 and 14.1 months, respectively. However, the study lacked appropriate controls, given the same chemotherapy without trastuzumab. Trastuzumab is also being evaluated in combination with paclitaxel and radiotherapy for bladder conservation [257].

Lapatinib

Lapatinib (GW572016, Tykerb) is a dual synthetic reversible inhibitor of EGFR and HER2 tyrosine kinases and has been demonstrated to inhibit significantly the proliferation of cancer cells, evidencing EGFR and/or HER2 overexpression both in vitro and in vivo [258]. At the intracellular level, lapatinib binds reversibly to the cytoplasmic ATP-binding site of the kinase, thereby preventing receptor phosphorylation. Lapatinib blocks ligand-activated signaling from multiple receptor combinations, including omo- and heterodimers of EGFR and HER2. Lapatinib daily as monotherapy was tested in patient with advanced bladder cancer and evidence of EGFR and/or ErbB2 overexpression by IHC who progressed after cisplatin-based first-line chemotherapy, showing possibly efficacy (median survival for strong expression 30.3 weeks compared with 10.6 for weak expression) [259]. Ongoing studies of lapatinib include a first-line trial in combination with GC (NCT00623064) [256] and as maintenance after response or stable disease

following treatment with GC for patients with HER1 or HER2 overexpression in their tumors (NCT00949455) [256].

Targeting Angiogenesis

Angiogenesis is required for tumor growth and metastasis [260]. Blood vessels are built to supply the tumor with nutrients and oxygen, failing which central necrosis occurs in tumor implants bigger than 3 mm^3 in vitro [261]. If hypoxia ensues, the cellular response to low oxygen tension involves stabilization of the hypoxia-inducible factor-1 (HIF-1) transcriptional complex that promotes cell survival and tumor invasion. This induces the formation of new blood vessels.

It has been demonstrated that in the neoplastic bladder, both VEGF mRNA and protein are overexpressed compared with normal urothelium [262, 263]. In addition to its pro-angiogenic properties, recent in vitro experiments also suggest a role for VEGF signaling as an autocrine and paracrine growth factor to directly promote bladder cancer growth [264].

Moreover, clinical studies have suggested that elevated MVD, a surrogate marker for angiogenic activity, has been demonstrated to be a predictive marker of vascular invasion, lymph node involvement, tumor recurrence, and poor survival in invasive TCC, while levels of VEGF and bFGF are inversely associated with prognosis [265, 266]. Finally, retrospective evaluation of serum VEGF levels in the metastatic setting suggests a correlation of high levels with poor disease-free survival [267]. Baseline VEGF mRNA expression levels and microvessel density were found to be independent prognostic factors for recurrence and metastasis in 51 patients treated with neoadjuvant MVAC chemotherapy preceding cystectomy [268].

Based on these findings, recently, strategies to block serum VEGF or its signal through RTKs were pursued. A number of agents with these features have entered clinical trials in urothelial cell carcinoma, including bevacizumab (Avastin; Genentech), a monoclonal antibody against VEGF that has been registered in other solid tumor types including colon, lung, and breast cancers, and aflibercept (VEGF Trap; Regeneron Pharmaceuticals), a fully humanized, soluble decoy VEGF receptor generated by fusing the extracellular domains of VEGFR-1 and VEGFR-2 to the Fc portion of human IgG1 and several RTK inhibitors including sunitinib (Sutent, Pfizer), which has VEGFR, PDGFR, and KIT activity, and sorafenib (Nexavar), which has VEGFR, RAF, PDGFR, and Kit TKI activities.

Sorafenib

Sorafenib (Nexavar; Bayer, Leverkusen, Germany) is an orally active, small-molecule multikinase inhibitor that targets wild-type and mutant b-Raf and c-Raf kinase isoforms in vitro but also inhibits angiogenesis via inhibition of VEGFR-2, VEGFR-3, and/or platelet-derived growth factor receptor-beta (PDGFR-β) [269]. In a phase II trial, sorafenib as a single agent showed minimal activity in patients with advanced urothelial cancer in the second-line setting, with no objective responses and a median overall survival of only 6.8 months [256].

Similar results were obtained in first-line setting in which none of 14 evaluable patients had an objective response.

Sunitinib

Sunitinib malate (Sutent; Pfizer, New York, NY, USA) is a multitargeted receptor tyrosine kinase inhibitor that acts on vascular endothelial growth factor (VEGF) receptor 1, 2, and 3; platelet-derived growth factor (PDGF) receptor; KIT; and FMS-like tyrosine kinase-3 receptor (FLT3): its antitumor activity has been demonstrated in various tumors, including renal cell carcinoma (RCC), gastrointestinal stromal tumor, non-small-cell lung cancer, and colorectal cancer.

Sunitinib activity has been evaluated in phase II trials (in a 6-week cycle, patients received sunitinib 50 mg daily for 4 weeks) as frontline or salvages therapy for metastatic TCC.

Leading to partial response or stable disease in 33 of 77 patients (43%), the median PFS was 2.4 months and median survival was 6.9 months. In a frontline trial, patients unsuitable for cisplatin with creatinine clearance between 30 and 60 mL/min and ECOG performance status of 1 or higher received sunitinib 50 mg daily for 4 weeks in a 6-week cycle. Sunitinib produced a partial response in 2 of 16 patients, and an additional 50% (8 of 16 patients) had stable disease [256].

Sunitinib is being evaluated in phase II study of GCS (gemcitabine, cisplatin, and sunitinib) as neoadjuvant chemotherapy in patients with muscle-invasive urothelial carcinoma of the bladder [256].

Pazopanib

Pazopanib (GW786034) is a second-generation multitargeted tyrosine kinase inhibitor against VEGFR-1, -2, and -3; platelet-derived growth factor receptor-α; platelet-derived growth factor receptor-β; and c-kit. Pazopanib was approved for use in advanced renal cell carcinoma (RCC) by the Food and Drug Administration in the USA in October of 2009. An ongoing phase II trial pazopanib for metastatic urothelial cancer has generated promising but very preliminary early results, reported in ESMO 2010. Patients received pazopanib 800 mg once daily until their disease progressed or they experienced unacceptable toxicity. Tumor shrinkage has occurred in 4 of 18 patients, and necrotic evolution of metastatic lesion was observed in 12 of 18 patients, by monthly computed tomography and positron emission tomography scans [256].

Bevacizumab

Bevacizumab (Avastin; Genentech, South San Francisco, CA), a humanized IgG1 murine monoclonal antibody that binds all VEGF isoforms, was the first VEGF inhibitor to be approved by the FDA. Bevacizumab neutralizes the ability of VEGF to bind to the VEGF receptor (VEGFR), primarily VEGF-1 (fit-l) and VEGF-2 (KDWflk-1), on the surface of endothelial cells. VEGFR-1 and VEGFR-2 are membrane-bound tyrosine kinase receptors responsible for specific downstream survival and proliferation pathways. Bevacizumab was tested as first line, in a phase II trial in combination with GC for metastatic UC showing promising overall response rate of 72% with a median overall survival of 20.4 months [270]. Based on these promising results, CALGB has begun a first-line phase III trial comparing

GC with GC plus bevacizumab. Another phase II trial at MSKCC is assessing the combination of carboplatin, gemcitabine, and bevacizumab for cisplatin-ineligible patients [256].

Aflibercept

Aflibercept (VEGF Trap; Regeneron, Tarrytown, NY) is a fully humanized, soluble decoy VEGF receptor generated by fusing the extracellular domains of VEGFR-1 and VEGFR-2 to the Fc portion of human IgG1. Like bevacizumab, this agent binds and inactivates VEGF. However, this molecule may also bind other VEGF family members such as placental growth factor and VEGF-B. In addition, its binding affinity for VEGF is similar to that of the high-affinity VEGFR-1, resulting in binding that is potentially 100-fold tighter than is achieved with bevacizumab [271]. These unique features differentiate this agent from other anti-VEGF strategies. Aflibercept has demonstrated a limited efficacy as single agent with a response rate of 4.5% and median progression-free survival of 3.5 months.

Conclusions

The current treatment of advanced bladder cancer relies heavily on traditional cytotoxic agents, despite the tumor expression of many targets of emerging biologic agents currently available. Current regimens yield suboptimal outcomes in the frontline setting, and there is no proven and effective second-line regimen.

Bladder cancer is a biologically intriguing disease. Its molecular pathogenesis is now increasingly understood, and the identification of potential therapeutical targets is under way. The translation of these evidences into the clinical treatment of patients with urothelial cancer is however still at the beginning. Some agents seem to be more promising than others, but the lack of reliable predictive factors that are able to identify the patients more likely to benefit from a targeted therapy approach still limit the clinical use of such drugs.

The challenge for the future remains how to integrate all the increasing knowledge incoming from preclinical setting and to translate them in data useful to achieve biologic profile of individual patient tumors.

The information contained in the current review clearly points at the absolute need for a strict collaboration between urologists, medical oncologists, and radiotherapists in the management of locally advanced and metastatic bladder cancer. Shared care is undoubtedly the primary quality parameter in the management this condition.

Quality of Life

Bladder cancer has a relevant impact on psychological, physical, emotional, and social function as any other tumor, but radical cystectomy may modify patient's body image, result in impotence and incontinence, and impact on patient's sexual life. The use of a urine bag always raises concern about the possible odor from contained urine. These and other issues are often neglected in retrospective studies on quality of life in patients with bladder cancer and are more properly investigated in specific questionnaires such as the EORTC-QLQ-BLM (muscle-invasive bladder cancer module) [272].

There is no consensus on the type of urinary diversion that results in the best quality of life for bladder cancer patients. Although most patients would rather prefer orthotopic neobladders, some studies failed to prove an advantage in patients' quality of life [273–276], but more recent studies are pointing in a different direction and suggest that a better quality of life is associated with orthotopic reconstruction [272, 277–280]. Health quality of life is an important issue in oncology as it is an independent prognostic factor for survival [281].

Follow-Up

Pelvic recurrences following radical cystectomy are observed in 5–15% of patients, and metastases develop in about 50% of patients. Although disease recurrence is most frequently observed within the first 2 years, pelvic recurrences may occur up to 5 years after surgery and distant disease may become manifest even after 10 years.

Patients with pelvic recurrences have a short survival (months) even when treatment is applied (surgery, radiotherapy, chemotherapy). Bladder cancer may recur in the upper urinary tract (usually in the first 3 years after cystectomy), and it may metastasize to the liver, lungs, and bones [282–285].

Tumor recurrence in the urethra occurs in 5–17% of patients within 1–3 years from surgery particularly when tumor invasion of the prostatic stroma is found in the pathology specimen of the radical cystectomy in men and when bladder cancer involves the bladder neck in women [286–289]. A lower rate of urethral recurrence is observed after orthotopic diversions compared to non-orthotopic ones [286, 290–292].

In Synthesis

The management of non-muscle-invasive bladder cancer has not changed significantly since BCG was introduced by Morales in 1986, but the management of muscle-invasive disease is a rapidly evolving area. Surgical reconstruction of an orthotopic neobladder is becoming less invasive by laparoscopic and robotic-assisted techniques, and chemotherapeutic treatment of locally advanced and metastatic disease is facing a new era with targeted treatments. Multidisciplinary management of bladder cancer patients is a feature without which proper management of urothelial tumors is no longer possible.

References

1. Ploeg M, Aben KK, Kiemeney LA. The present and future burden of urinary bladder cancer in the world. World J Urol. 2009;27(3):289–93.
2. Epstein JI, Amin MB, Reuter VR, Mostofi FK. The World Health Organization/International Society of Urological Pathology consensus classification of urothelial (transitional cell) neoplasms of the urinary

bladder. Bladder Consensus Conference Committee. Am J Surg Pathol. 1998;22(12):1435–48.
3. Sauter G, Algaba F, Amin M, et al. Tumours of the urinary system: non-invasive urothelial neoplasias. In: Eble JN, Sauter G, Epstein JL, Sesterhenn I, editors. WHO classification of tumours of the urinary system and male genital organs. Lyon: IARCC Press; 2004. p. 29–34.
4. IARC Working Group on the Evaluation of Carcinogenic Risks to Humans. Tobacco smoke and involuntary smoking. IARC Monogr Eval Carinog Risks Hum. 832004:1–1438.
5. Bjerregaard BK, Raaschou-Nielsen O, Sorensen M, et al. Tobacco smoke and bladder cancer–in the European prospective investigation into cancer and nutrition. Int J Cancer. 2006;119(10):2412–6.
6. Zeegers MP, Swaen GM, Kant I, Goldbohm RA, van den Brandt PA. Occupational risk factors for male bladder cancer: results from a population based case cohort study in the Netherlands. Occup Environ Med. 2001;58(9):590–6.
7. Puente D, Hartge P, Greiser E, et al. A pooled analysis of bladder cancer case-control studies evaluating smoking in men and women. Cancer Causes Control. 2006;17(1):71–9.
8. Pashos CL, Botteman MF, Laskin BL, Redaelli A. Bladder cancer: epidemiology, diagnosis, and management. Cancer Pract. 2002;10(6):311–22.
9. McCahy PJ, Harris CA, Neal DE. The accuracy of recording of occupational history in patients with bladder cancer. Br J Urol. 1997;79(1):91–3.
10. Samanic CM, Kogevinas M, Silverman DT, et al. Occupation and bladder cancer in a hospital-based case-control study in Spain. Occup Environ Med. 2008;65(5):347–53.
11. Chrouser K, Leibovich B, Bergstralh E, Zincke H, Blute M. Bladder cancer risk following primary and adjuvant external beam radiation for prostate cancer. J Urol. 2005;174(1):107–10. discussion 110–101.
12. Steinmaus CM, Nunez S, Smith AH. Diet and bladder cancer: a meta-analysis of six dietary variables. Am J Epidemiol. 2000;151(7):693–702.
13. Gouda I, Mokhtar N, Bilal D, El-Bolkainy T, El-Bolkainy NM. Bilharziasis and bladder cancer: a time trend analysis of 9843 patients. J Egypt Natl Canc Inst. 2007;19(2):158–62.
14. Kaldor JM, Day NE, Kittelmann B, et al. Bladder tumours following chemotherapy and radiotherapy for ovarian cancer: a case-control study. Int J Cancer. 1995;63(1):1–6.
15. Travis LB, Curtis RE, Glimelius B, et al. Bladder and kidney cancer following cyclophosphamide therapy for non-Hodgkin's lymphoma. J Natl Cancer Inst. 1995;87(7):524–30.
16. Azemar MD, Comperat E, Richard F, Cussenot O, Roupret M. Bladder recurrence after surgery for upper urinary tract urothelial cell carcinoma: frequency, risk factors, and surveillance. Urol Oncol. 2011;29(2):130–6.
17. Vaidya A, Soloway MS, Hawke C, Tiguert R, Civantos F. De novo muscle invasive bladder

cancer: is there a change in trend? J Urol. 2001;165(1):47–50. discussion 50.

18. Goessl C, Knispel HH, Miller K, Klan R. Is routine excretory urography necessary at first diagnosis of bladder cancer? J Urol. 1997;157(2):480–1.

19. Palou J, Rodriguez-Rubio F, Huguet J, et al. Multivariate analysis of clinical parameters of synchronous primary superficial bladder cancer and upper urinary tract tumor. J Urol. 2005;174(3): 859–61. discussion 861.

20. Holmang S, Hedelin H, Anderstrom C, Holmberg E, Johansson SL. Long-term followup of a bladder carcinoma cohort: routine followup urography is not necessary. J Urol. 1998;160(1):45–8.

21. Raitanen MP, Aine R, Rintala E, et al. Differences between local and review urinary cytology in diagnosis of bladder cancer. An interobserver multicenter analysis. Eur Urol. 2002;41(3):284–9.

22. Lokeshwar VB, Habuchi T, Grossman HB, et al. Bladder tumor markers beyond cytology: International consensus panel on bladder tumor markers. Urology. 2005;66(6 Suppl 1):35–63.

23. Glas AS, Roos D, Deutekom M, Zwinderman AH, Bossuyt PM, Kurth KH. Tumor markers in the diagnosis of primary bladder cancer. A systematic review. J Urol. 2003;169(6):1975–82.

24. Lotan Y, Roehrborn CG. Sensitivity and specificity of commonly available bladder tumor markers versus cytology: results of a comprehensive literature review and meta-analyses. Urology. 2003;61(1):109–18. discussion 118.

25. Vrooman OP, Witjes JA. Urinary markers in bladder cancer. Eur Urol. 2008;53(5):909–16.

26. Lotan Y, Shariat SF, Schmitz-Drager BJ, et al. Considerations on implementing diagnostic markers into clinical decision making in bladder cancer. Urol Oncol. 2010;28(4):441–8.

27. Van Rhijn BW, van der Poel HG, van der Kwast TH. Urine markers for bladder cancer surveillance: a systematic review. Eur Urol. 2005;47(6):736–48.

28. Van Rhijn BW, van der Poel HG, van der Kwast TH. Cytology and urinary markers for the diagnosis of bladder cancer. Eur Urol Suppl. 2009;8:536–41.

29. Grossman HB, Messing E, Soloway M, et al. Detection of bladder cancer using a point-of-care proteomic assay. JAMA. 2005;293(7):810–6.

30. Lotan Y, Svatek RS, Malats N. Screening for bladder cancer: a perspective. World J Urol. 2008;26(1): 13–8.

31. Grossman HB, Soloway M, Messing E, et al. Surveillance for recurrent bladder cancer using a point-of-care proteomic assay. JAMA. 2006;295(3): 299–305.

32. Hajdinjak T. UroVysion FISH test for detecting urothelial cancers: meta-analysis of diagnostic accuracy and comparison with urinary cytology testing. Urol Oncol. 2008;26(6):646–51.

33. Mowatt G, Zhu S, Kilonzo M, et al. Systematic review of the clinical effectiveness and cost-effectiveness of photodynamic diagnosis and urine bio-

markers (FISH, ImmunoCyt, NMP22) and cytology for the detection and follow-up of bladder cancer. Health Technol Assess. 2010;14(4):1–331. iii-iv.

34. Babjuk M, Soukup V, Pesl M, et al. Urinary cytology and quantitative BTA and UBC tests in surveillance of patients with pTapT1 bladder urothelial carcinoma. Urology. 2008;71(4):718–22.

35. Raitanen MP. The role of BTA stat test in follow-up of patients with bladder cancer: results from FinnBladder studies. World J Urol. 2008;26(1): 45–50.

36. Shariat SF, Marberger MJ, Lotan Y, et al. Variability in the performance of nuclear matrix protein 22 for the detection of bladder cancer. J Urol. 2006;176(3):919–26. discussion 926.

37. Lotan Y, Shariat SF. Impact of risk factors on the performance of the nuclear matrix protein 22 point-of-care test for bladder cancer detection. BJU Int. 2008;101(11):1362–7.

38. Nguyen CT, Jones JS. Defining the role of NMP22 in bladder cancer surveillance. World J Urol. 2008;26(1):51–8.

39. Schmitz-Drager BJ, Beiche B, Tirsar LA, Schmitz-Drager C, Bismarck E, Ebert T. Immunocytology in the assessment of patients with asymptomatic microhaematuria. Eur Urol. 2007;51(6):1582–8. discussion 1588.

40. Schlomer BJ, Ho R, Sagalowsky A, Ashfaq R, Lotan Y. Prospective validation of the clinical usefulness of reflex fluorescence in situ hybridization assay in patients with atypical cytology for the detection of urothelial carcinoma of the bladder. J Urol. 2010;183(1):62–7.

41. Bergman J, Reznichek RC, Rajfer J. Surveillance of patients with bladder carcinoma using fluorescent in-situ hybridization on bladder washings. BJU Int. 2008;101(1):26–9.

42. van der Aa MN, Zwarthoff EC, Steyerberg EW, et al. Microsatellite analysis of voided-urine samples for surveillance of low-grade non-muscle-invasive urothelial carcinoma: feasibility and clinical utility in a prospective multicenter study (cost-effectiveness of follow-up of urinary bladder cancer trial [CEFUB]). Eur Urol. 2009;55(3):659–67.

43. de Bekker-Grob EW, van der Aa MN, Zwarthoff EC, et al. Non-muscle-invasive bladder cancer surveillance for which cystoscopy is partly replaced by microsatellite analysis of urine: a cost-effective alternative? BJU Int. 2009;104(1):41–7.

44. Roupret M, Hupertan V, Yates DR, et al. A comparison of the performance of microsatellite and methylation urine analysis for predicting the recurrence of urothelial cell carcinoma, and definition of a set of markers by Bayesian network analysis. BJU Int. 2008;101(11):1448–53.

45. Babjuk M, Oosterlinck W, Sylvester R, et al. Guidelines on non-muscle invasive bladder cancer (TaT1 and CIS). 2011; http://www.uroweb.org/?id= 217&tyid=1. Accessed 10 May 2011.

46. Hong YM, Loughlin KR. Economic impact of tumor markers in bladder cancer surveillance. Urology. 2008;71(1):131–5.

47. Daniltchenko DI, Riedl CR, Sachs MD, et al. Long-term benefit of 5-aminolevulinic acid fluorescence assisted transurethral resection of superficial bladder cancer: 5-year results of a prospective randomized study. J Urol. 2005;174(6):2129–33. discussion 2133.

48. Kausch I, Sommerauer M, Montorsi F, et al. Photodynamic diagnosis in non-muscle-invasive bladder cancer: a systematic review and cumulative analysis of prospective studies. Eur Urol. 2010;57(4):595–606.

49. Draga RO, Grimbergen MC, Kok ET, Jonges TN, van Swol CF, Bosch JL. Photodynamic diagnosis (5-aminolevulinic acid) of transitional cell carcinoma after bacillus Calmette-Guerin immunotherapy and mitomycin C intravesical therapy. Eur Urol. 2010;57(4):655–60.

50. Babjuk M, Soukup V, Petrik R, Jirsa M, Dvoracek J. 5-aminolaevulinic acid-induced fluorescence cystoscopy during transurethral resection reduces the risk of recurrence in stage Ta/T1 bladder cancer. BJU Int. 2005;96(6):798–802.

51. Denzinger S, Burger M, Walter B, et al. Clinically relevant reduction in risk of recurrence of superficial bladder cancer using 5-aminolevulinic acid-induced fluorescence diagnosis: 8-year results of prospective randomized study. Urology. 2007;69(4):675–9.

52. Brausi M, Collette L, Kurth K, et al. Variability in the recurrence rate at first follow-up cystoscopy after TUR in stage Ta T1 transitional cell carcinoma of the bladder: a combined analysis of seven EORTC studies. Eur Urol. 2002;41(5):523–31.

53. Miladi M, Peyromaure M, Zerbib M, Saighi D, Debre B. The value of a second transurethral resection in evaluating patients with bladder tumours. Eur Urol. 2003;43(3):241–5.

54. Brauers A, Buettner R, Jakse G. Second resection and prognosis of primary high risk superficial bladder cancer: is cystectomy often too early? J Urol. 2001;165(3):808–10.

55. Schips L, Augustin H, Zigeuner RE, et al. Is repeated transurethral resection justified in patients with newly diagnosed superficial bladder cancer? Urology. 2002;59(2):220–3.

56. Grimm MO, Steinhoff C, Simon X, Spiegelhalder P, Ackermann R, Vogeli TA. Effect of routine repeat transurethral resection for superficial bladder cancer: a long-term observational study. J Urol. 2003;170(2 Pt 1):433–7.

57. Divrik RT, Yildirim U, Zorlu F, Ozen H. The effect of repeat transurethral resection on recurrence and progression rates in patients with T1 tumors of the bladder who received intravesical mitomycin: a prospective, randomized clinical trial. J Urol. 2006;175(5):1641–4.

58. Jahnson S, Wiklund F, Duchek M, et al. Results of second-look resection after primary resection of T1 tumour of the urinary bladder. Scand J Urol Nephrol. 2005;39(3):206–10.

59. Lamm DL. Carcinoma in situ. Urol Clin North Am. 1992;19(3):499–508.

60. Solsona E, Iborra I, Dumont R, Rubio-Briones J, Casanova J, Almenar S. The 3-month clinical response to intravesical therapy as a predictive factor for progression in patients with high risk superficial bladder cancer. J Urol. 2000;164(3 Pt 1):685–9.

61. van Gils-Gielen RJ, Witjes WP, Caris CT, Debruyne FM, Witjes JA, Oosterhof GO. Risk factors in carcinoma in situ of the urinary bladder. Dutch South East Cooperative Urological Group. Urology. 1995;45(4):581–6.

62. Hudson MA, Herr HW. Carcinoma in situ of the bladder. J Urol. 1995;153(3 Pt 1):564–72.

63. Sylvester RJ, Oosterlinck W, van der Meijden AP. A single immediate postoperative instillation of chemotherapy decreases the risk of recurrence in patients with stage Ta T1 bladder cancer: a meta-analysis of published results of randomized clinical trials. J Urol. 2004;171(6 Pt 1):2186–90. quiz 2435.

64. Berrum-Svennung I, Granfors T, Jahnson S, Boman H, Holmang S. A single instillation of epirubicin after transurethral resection of bladder tumors prevents only small recurrences. J Urol. 2008;179(1):101–5. discussion 105–106.

65. Gudjonsson S, Adell L, Merdasa F, et al. Should all patients with non-muscle-invasive bladder cancer receive early intravesical chemotherapy after transurethral resection? The results of a prospective randomised multicentre study. Eur Urol. 2009;55(4):773–80.

66. Kaasinen E, Rintala E, Hellstrom P, et al. Factors explaining recurrence in patients undergoing chemoimmunotherapy regimens for frequently recurring superficial bladder carcinoma. Eur Urol. 2002;42(2):167–74.

67. Shelley MD, Kynaston H, Court J, et al. A systematic review of intravesical bacillus Calmette-Guerin plus transurethral resection vs transurethral resection alone in Ta and T1 bladder cancer. BJU Int. 2001;88(3):209–16.

68. Han RF, Pan JG. Can intravesical bacillus Calmette-Guerin reduce recurrence in patients with superficial bladder cancer? A meta-analysis of randomized trials. Urology. 2006;67(6):1216–23.

69. Shelley MD, Wilt TJ, Court J, Coles B, Kynaston H, Mason MD. Intravesical bacillus Calmette-Guerin is superior to mitomycin C in reducing tumour recurrence in high-risk superficial bladder cancer: a meta-analysis of randomized trials. BJU Int. 2004;93(4):485–90.

70. Bohle A, Jocham D, Bock PR. Intravesical bacillus Calmette-Guerin versus mitomycin C for superficial bladder cancer: a formal meta-analysis of comparative studies on recurrence and toxicity. J Urol. 2003;169(1):90–5.

71. Malmstrom PU, Sylvester RJ, Crawford DE, et al. An individual patient data meta-analysis of the

71. long-term outcome of randomised studies comparing intravesical mitomycin C versus bacillus Calmette-Guerin for non-muscle-invasive bladder cancer. Eur Urol. 2009;56(2):247–56.

72. Bohle A, Bock PR. Intravesical bacille Calmette-Guerin versus mitomycin C in superficial bladder cancer: formal meta-analysis of comparative studies on tumor progression. Urology. 2004;63(4):682–6. discussion 686–687.

73. Sylvester RJ, van der MA, Lamm DL. Intravesical bacillus Calmette-Guerin reduces the risk of progression in patients with superficial bladder cancer: a meta-analysis of the published results of randomized clinical trials. J Urol. 2002;168(5):1964–70.

74. Martinez-Pineiro JA, Flores N, Isorna S, et al. Long-term follow-up of a randomized prospective trial comparing a standard 81 mg dose of intravesical bacille Calmette-Guerin with a reduced dose of 27 mg in superficial bladder cancer. BJU Int. 2002;89(7):671–80.

75. Martinez-Pineiro JA, Martinez-Pineiro L, Solsona E, et al. Has a 3-fold decreased dose of bacillus Calmette-Guerin the same efficacy against recurrences and progression of T1G3 and Tis bladder tumors than the standard dose? Results of a prospective randomized trial. J Urol. 2005;174(4 Pt 1):1242–7.

76. Ojea A, Nogueira JL, Solsona E, et al. A multicentre, randomised prospective trial comparing three intravesical adjuvant therapies for intermediate-risk superficial bladder cancer: low-dose bacillus Calmette-Guerin (27 mg) versus very low-dose bacillus Calmette-Guerin (13.5 mg) versus mitomycin C. Eur Urol. 2007;52(5):1398–406.

77. van der Meijden AP, Sylvester RJ, Oosterlinck W, Hoeltl W, Bono AV. Maintenance Bacillus Calmette-Guerin for Ta T1 bladder tumors is not associated with increased toxicity: results from a European Organisation for Research and Treatment of Cancer Genito-Urinary Group Phase III Trial. Eur Urol. 2003;44(4):429–34.

78. Lamm DL, van der Meijden PM, Morales A, et al. Incidence and treatment of complications of bacillus Calmette-Guerin intravesical therapy in superficial bladder cancer. J Urol. 1992;147(3):596–600.

79. Witjes JA, Palou J, Soloway M, et al. Clinical practice recommendations for the prevention and management of intravesical therapy-associated adverse events. Eur Urol Suppl. 2008;7(10):667–74.

80. Losa A, Hurle R, Lembo A. Low dose bacillus Calmette-Guerin for carcinoma in situ of the bladder: long-term results. J Urol. 2000;163(1):68–71. discussion 71–62.

81. Griffiths TR, Charlton M, Neal DE, Powell PH. Treatment of carcinoma in situ with intravesical bacillus Calmette-Guerin without maintenance. J Urol. 2002;167(6):2408–12.

82. Takenaka A, Yamada Y, Miyake H, Hara I, Fujisawa M. Clinical outcomes of bacillus Calmette-Guerin instillation therapy for carcinoma in situ of urinary bladder. Int J Urol. 2008;15(4):309–13.

83. Lamm DL, Blumenstein BA, Crissman JD, et al. Maintenance bacillus Calmette-Guerin immunotherapy for recurrent TA, T1 and carcinoma in situ transitional cell carcinoma of the bladder: a randomized Southwest Oncology Group Study. J Urol. 2000; 163(4):1124–9.

84. Gofrit ON, Pode D, Pizov G, et al. The natural history of bladder carcinoma in situ after initial response to bacillus Calmette-Guerin immunotherapy. Urol Oncol. 2009;27(3):258–62.

85. Sylvester RJ, van der Meijden AP, Witjes JA, Kurth K. Bacillus calmette-guerin versus chemotherapy for the intravesical treatment of patients with carcinoma in situ of the bladder: a meta-analysis of the published results of randomized clinical trials. J Urol. 2005;174(1):86–91. discussion 91–82.

86. van der Meijden AP, Sylvester R, Oosterlinck W, et al. EAU guidelines on the diagnosis and treatment of urothelial carcinoma in situ. Eur Urol. 2005; 48(3):363–71.

87. Sylvester RJ, van der Meijden A, Witjes JA, et al. High-grade Ta urothelial carcinoma and carcinoma in situ of the bladder. Urology. 2005;66(6 Suppl 1): 90–107.

88. Herr HW, Dalbagni G. Defining bacillus Calmette-Guerin refractory superficial bladder tumors. J Urol. 2003;169(5):1706–8.

89. Lerner SP, Tangen CM, Sucharew H, Wood D, Crawford ED. Failure to achieve a complete response to induction BCG therapy is associated with increased risk of disease worsening and death in patients with high risk non-muscle invasive bladder cancer. Urol Oncol. 2009;27(2):155–9.

90. Stein JP, Lieskovsky G, Cote R, et al. Radical cystectomy in the treatment of invasive bladder cancer: long-term results in 1,054 patients. J Clin Oncol. 2001;19(3):666–75.

91. Hautmann RE, Gschwend JE, de Petriconi RC, Kron M, Volkmer BG. Cystectomy for transitional cell carcinoma of the bladder: results of a surgery only series in the neobladder era. J Urol. 2006;176(2):486–92. discussion 491–482.

92. Ghoneim MA, Abdel-Latif M, El-Mekresh M, et al. Radical cystectomy for carcinoma of the bladder: 2,720 consecutive cases 5 years later. J Urol. 2008;180(1):121–7.

93. Madersbacher S, Hochreiter W, Burkhard F, et al. Radical cystectomy for bladder cancer today—a homogeneous series without neoadjuvant therapy. J Clin Oncol. 2003;21(4):690–6.

94. Shariat SF, Palapattu GS, Amiel GE, et al. Characteristics and outcomes of patients with carcinoma in situ only at radical cystectomy. Urology. 2006;68(3):538–42.

95. Stein JP, Skinner DG. Radical cystectomy for invasive bladder cancer: long-term results of a standard procedure. World J Urol. 2006;24(3):296–304.

96. Dalbagni G, Genega E, Hashibe M, et al. Cystectomy for bladder cancer: a contemporary series. J Urol. 2001;165(4):1111–6.

97. Bassi P, Ferrante GD, Piazza N, et al. Prognostic factors of outcome after radical cystectomy for bladder cancer: a retrospective study of a homogeneous patient cohort. J Urol. 1999;161(5):1494–7.

98. Ghoneim MA, el-Mekresh MM, el-Baz MA, el-Attar IA, Ashamallah A. Radical cystectomy for carcinoma of the bladder: critical evaluation of the results in 1,026 cases. J Urol. 1997;158(2):393–9.

99. Sternberg CN, Pansadoro V, Calabro F, et al. Can patient selection for bladder preservation be based on response to chemotherapy? Cancer. 2003;97(7):1644–52.

100. Herr HW, Scher HI. Surgery of invasive bladder cancer: is pathologic staging necessary? Semin Oncol. 1990;17(5):590–7.

101. Sherif A, Holmberg L, Rintala E, et al. Neoadjuvant cisplatinum based combination chemotherapy in patients with invasive bladder cancer: a combined analysis of two Nordic studies. Eur Urol. 2004;45(3):297–303.

102. Grossman HB, Natale RB, Tangen CM, et al. Neoadjuvant chemotherapy plus cystectomy compared with cystectomy alone for locally advanced bladder cancer. N Engl J Med. 2003;349(9):859–66.

103. Neoadjuvant chemotherapy in invasive bladder cancer: a systematic review and meta-analysis. Advanced Bladder Cancer Meta-analysis Collaboration. Lancet. 2003;361(9373):1927–1934.

104. Winquist E, Kirchner TS, Segal R, Chin J, Lukka H. Neoadjuvant chemotherapy for transitional cell carcinoma of the bladder: a systematic review and meta-analysis. J Urol. 2004;171(2 Pt 1):561–9.

105. Neoadjuvant chemotherapy in invasive bladder cancer: update of a systematic review and meta-analysis of individual patient data advanced bladder cancer (ABC) meta-analysis collaboration. Advanced Bladder Cancer Meta-analysis Collaboration. Eur Urol. 2005;48(2):202–205; discussion 205–206.

106. Hautmann RE, Abol-Enein H, Hafez K, et al. Urinary diversion. Urology. 2007;69 Suppl 1:17–49.

107. Miller DC, Taub DA, Dunn RL, Montie JE, Wei JT. The impact of co-morbid disease on cancer control and survival following radical cystectomy. J Urol. 2003;169(1):105–9.

108. Figueroa AJ, Stein JP, Dickinson M, et al. Radical cystectomy for elderly patients with bladder carcinoma: an updated experience with 404 patients. Cancer. 1998;83(1):141–7.

109. Chang SS, Hassan JM, Cookson MS, Wells N, Smith Jr JA. Delaying radical cystectomy for muscle invasive bladder cancer results in worse pathological stage. J Urol. 2003;170(4 Pt 1):1085–7.

110. Hautmann RE, Paiss T. Does the option of the ileal neobladder stimulate patient and physician decision toward earlier cystectomy? J Urol. 1998;159(6):1845–50.

111. Vallancien G, Abou El Fettouh H, Cathelineau X, Baumert H, Fromont G, Guillonneau B. Cystectomy with prostate sparing for bladder cancer in 100 patients: 10-year experience. J Urol. 2002;168(6):2413–7.

112. Muto G, Bardari F, D'Urso L, Giona C. Seminal sparing cystectomy and ileocapsuloplasty: long-term followup results. J Urol. 2004;172(1):76–80.

113. Shen SS, Lerner SP, Muezzinoglu B, Truong LD, Amiel G, Wheeler TM. Prostatic involvement by transitional cell carcinoma in patients with bladder cancer and its prognostic significance. Hum Pathol. 2006;37(6):726–34.

114. Revelo MP, Cookson MS, Chang SS, Shook MF, Smith Jr JA, Shappell SB. Incidence and location of prostate and urothelial carcinoma in prostates from cystoprostatectomies: implications for possible apical sparing surgery. J Urol. 2004;171(2 Pt 1):646–51.

115. Pettus JA, Al-Ahmadie H, Barocas DA, et al. Risk assessment of prostatic pathology in patients undergoing radical cystoprostatectomy. Eur Urol. 2008;53(2):370–5.

116. Poulsen AL, Horn T, Steven K. Radical cystectomy: extending the limits of pelvic lymph node dissection improves survival for patients with bladder cancer confined to the bladder wall. J Urol. 1998;160(6 Pt 1):2015–9. discussion 2020.

117. Leissner J, Hohenfellner R, Thuroff JW, Wolf HK. Lymphadenectomy in patients with transitional cell carcinoma of the urinary bladder; significance for staging and prognosis. BJU Int. 2000;85(7):817–23.

118. Fleischmann A, Thalmann GN, Markwalder R, Studer UE. Extracapsular extension of pelvic lymph node metastases from urothelial carcinoma of the bladder is an independent prognostic factor. J Clin Oncol. 2005;23(10):2358–65.

119. Studer UE, Collette L. Morbidity from pelvic lymphadenectomy in men undergoing radical prostatectomy. Eur Urol. 2006;50(5):887–9. discussion 889–892.

120. Hautmann RE. The oncologic results of laparoscopic radical cystectomy are not (yet) equivalent to open cystectomy. Curr Opin Urol. 2009;19(5):522–6.

121. Ng CK, Kauffman EC, Lee MM, et al. A comparison of postoperative complications in open versus robotic cystectomy. Eur Urol. 2010;57(2):274–81.

122. Stenzl A. Bladder substitution. Curr Opin Urol. 1999;9(3):241–5.

123. Deliveliotis C, Papatsoris A, Chrisofos M, Dellis A, Liakouras C, Skolarikos A. Urinary diversion in high-risk elderly patients: modified cutaneous ureterostomy or ileal conduit? Urology. 2005;66(2):299–304.

124. Kilciler M, Bedir S, Erdemir F, Zeybek N, Erten K, Ozgok Y. Comparison of ileal conduit and transureteroureterostomy with ureterocutaneostomy urinary diversion. Urol Int. 2006;77(3):245–50.

125. Pycha A, Comploj E, Martini T, et al. Comparison of complications in three incontinent urinary diversions. Eur Urol. 2008;54(4):825–32.

126. Madersbacher S, Schmidt J, Eberle JM, et al. Long-term outcome of ileal conduit diversion. J Urol. 2003;169(3):985–90.

127. Wood DN, Allen SE, Hussain M, Greenwell TJ, Shah PJ. Stomal complications of ileal conduits are significantly higher when formed in women with intractable urinary incontinence. J Urol. 2004;172 (6 Pt 1):2300–3.

128. Neal DE. Complications of ileal conduit diversion in adults with cancer followed up for at least five years. Br Med J (Clin Res Ed). 1985;290(6483):1695–7.

129. Benson MC, Olsson CA. Continent urinary diversion. Urol Clin North Am. 1999;26(1):125–47. ix.

130. Jonsson O, Olofsson G, Lindholm E, Tornqvist H. Long-time experience with the Kock ileal reservoir for continent urinary diversion. Eur Urol. 2001; 40(6):632–40.

131. Gerharz EW, Kohl UN, Melekos MD, Bonfig R, Weingartner K, Riedmiller H. Ten years' experience with the submucosally embedded in situ appendix in continent cutaneous diversion. Eur Urol. 2001; 40(6):625–31.

132. Wiesner C, Stein R, Pahernik S, Hahn K, Melchior SW, Thuroff JW. Long-term followup of the intussuscepted ileal nipple and the in situ, submucosally embedded appendix as continence mechanisms of continent urinary diversion with the cutaneous ileocecal pouch (Mainz pouch I). J Urol. 2006;176(1): 155–9. discussion 159–160.

133. Wiesner C, Bonfig R, Stein R, et al. Continent cutaneous urinary diversion: long-term follow-up of more than 800 patients with ileocecal reservoirs. World J Urol. 2006;24(3):315–8.

134. Thoeny HC, Sonnenschein MJ, Madersbacher S, Vock P, Studer UE. Is ileal orthotopic bladder substitution with an afferent tubular segment detrimental to the upper urinary tract in the long term? J Urol. 2002;168(5):2030–4. discussion 2034.

135. Leissner J, Black P, Fisch M, Hockel M, Hohenfellner R. Colon pouch (Mainz pouch III) for continent urinary diversion after pelvic irradiation. Urology. 2000;56(5):798–802.

136. Azimuddin K, Khubchandani IT, Stasik JJ, Rosen L, Riether RD. Neoplasia after ureterosigmoidostomy. Dis Colon Rectum. 1999;42(12):1632–8.

137. Gerharz EW, Turner WH, Kalble T, Woodhouse CR. Metabolic and functional consequences of urinary reconstruction with bowel. BJU Int. 2003;91(2): 143–9.

138. Stein JP, Dunn MD, Quek ML, Miranda G, Skinner DG. The orthotopic T pouch ileal neobladder: experience with 209 patients. J Urol. 2004;172(2):584–7.

139. Abol-Enein H, Ghoneim MA. Functional results of orthotopic ileal neobladder with serous-lined extramural ureteral reimplantation: experience with 450 patients. J Urol. 2001;165(5):1427–32.

140. Yossepowitch O, Dalbagni G, Golijanin D, et al. Orthotopic urinary diversion after cystectomy for bladder cancer: implications for cancer control and patterns of disease recurrence. J Urol. 2003;169(1): 177–81.

141. Gerharz EW, Mansson A, Hunt S, Skinner EC, Mansson W. Quality of life after cystectomy and urinary diversion: an evidence based analysis. J Urol. 2005;174(5):1729–36.

142. Hobisch A, Tosun K, Kinzl J, et al. Life after cystectomy and orthotopic neobladder versus ileal conduit urinary diversion. Semin Urol Oncol. 2001;19(1): 18–23.

143. Porter MP, Penson DF. Health related quality of life after radical cystectomy and urinary diversion for bladder cancer: a systematic review and critical analysis of the literature. J Urol. 2005;173(4):1318–22.

144. Stein JP, Skinner DG. Results with radical cystectomy for treating bladder cancer: a "reference standard" for high-grade, invasive bladder cancer. BJU Int. 2003;92(1):12–7.

145. Shariat SF, Karakiewicz PI, Palapattu GS, et al. Outcomes of radical cystectomy for transitional cell carcinoma of the bladder: a contemporary series from the Bladder Cancer Research Consortium. J Urol. 2006;176(6 Pt 1):2414–22. discussion 2422.

146. Gschwend JE, Dahm P, Fair WR. Disease specific survival as endpoint of outcome for bladder cancer patients following radical cystectomy. Eur Urol. 2002;41(4):440–8.

147. Pollack A, Zagars GK, Dinney CP, Swanson DA, von Eschenbach AC. Preoperative radiotherapy for muscle-invasive bladder carcinoma. Long term follow-up and prognostic factors for 338 patients. Cancer. 1994;74(10):2819–27.

148. Cole CJ, Pollack A, Zagars GK, Dinney CP, Swanson DA, von Eschenbach AC. Local control of muscle-invasive bladder cancer: preoperative radiotherapy and cystectomy versus cystectomy alone. Int J Radiat Oncol Biol Phys. 1995;32(2):331–40.

149. Spera JA, Whittington R, Littman P, Solin LJ, Wein AJ. A comparison of preoperative radiotherapy regimens for bladder carcinoma. The University of Pennsylvania experience. Cancer. 1988;61(2): 255–62.

150. Pollack A, Zagars GK, Cole CJ, Dinney CP, Swanson DA, Grossman HB. Significance of downstaging in muscle-invasive bladder cancer treated with preoperative radiotherapy. Int J Radiat Oncol Biol Phys. 1997;37(1):41–9.

151. Chougule P, Aygun C, Salazar O, Young Jr J, Prempree T, Amin P. Radiation therapy for transitional cell bladder carcinoma. A ten-year experience. Urology. 1988;32(2):91–5.

152. Batata MA, Chu FC, Hilaris BS, Whitmore WF, Kim YS, Lee MZ. Bladder cancer in men and women treated by radiation therapy and/or radical cystectomy. Urology. 1981;18(1):15–20.

153. Fossa SD, Ous S, Berner A. Clinical significance of the "palpable mass" in patients with muscle-infiltrating bladder cancer undergoing cystectomy after preoperative radiotherapy. Br J Urol. 1991;67(1): 54–60.

154. Gilloz A, Heritier P. Comparative study of actuarial survival rates in P3 P4 (N+ Mo) transitional cell carcinoma of bladder managed by total cystectomy alone or associated with preoperative radiotherapy

and pelvic lymphadenectomy. Prog Clin Biol Res. 1984;162B:15–9.

155. Smith Jr JA, Batata M, Grabstald H, Sogani PC, Herr H, Whitmore Jr WF. Preoperative irradiation and cystectomy for bladder cancer. Cancer. 1982;49(5):869–73.

156. Gospodarowicz MK, Quilty PM, Scalliet P, et al. The place of radiation therapy as definitive treatment of bladder cancer. Int J Urol. 1995;2 Suppl 2:41–8.

157. Gospodarowicz MK, Hawkins NV, Rawlings GA, et al. Radical radiotherapy for muscle invasive transitional cell carcinoma of the bladder: failure analysis. J Urol. 1989;142(6):1448–53. discussion 1453–1444.

158. Shipley WU, Zietman AL, Kaufman DS, Althausen AF, Heney NM. Invasive bladder cancer: treatment strategies using transurethral surgery, chemotherapy and radiation therapy with selection for bladder conservation. Int J Radiat Oncol Biol Phys. 1997; 39(4):937–43.

159. Tonoli S, Bertoni F, De Stefani A, et al. Radical radiotherapy for bladder cancer: retrospective analysis of a series of 459 patients treated in an Italian institution. Clin Oncol (R Coll Radiol). 2006;18(1): 52–9.

160. Shelley MD, Barber J, Wilt T, Mason MD. Surgery versus radiotherapy for muscle invasive bladder cancer. Cochrane Database Syst Rev. 2002(1): CD002079

161. Pollack A, Zagars GZ. Radiotherapy for stage T3b transitional cell carcinoma of the bladder. Semin Urol Oncol. 1996;14(2):86–95.

162. De Neve W, Lybeert ML, Goor C, Crommelin MA, Ribot JG. Radiotherapy for T2 and T3 carcinoma of the bladder: the influence of overall treatment time. Radiother Oncol. 1995;36(3):183–8.

163. Mameghan H, Fisher R, Mameghan J, Brook S. Analysis of failure following definitive radiotherapy for invasive transitional cell carcinoma of the bladder. Int J Radiat Oncol Biol Phys. 1995;31(2): 247–54.

164. Herskovic A, Martz K, al-Sarraf M, et al. Combined chemotherapy and radiotherapy compared with radiotherapy alone in patients with cancer of the esophagus. N Engl J Med. 1992;326(24):1593–8.

165. Naslund I, Nilsson B, Littbrand B. Hyperfractionated radiotherapy of bladder cancer. A ten-year follow-up of a randomized clinical trial. Acta Oncol. 1994;33(4):397–402.

166. Piet AH, Hulshof MC, Pieters BR, Pos FJ, de Reijke TM, Koning CC. Clinical results of a concomitant boost radiotherapy technique for muscle-invasive bladder cancer. Strahlenther Onkol. 2008;184(6): 313–8.

167. Neoadjuvant cisplatin, methotrexate, and vinblastine chemotherapy for muscle-invasive bladder cancer: a randomised controlled trial. International collaboration of trialists. Lancet. 1999;354(9178):533–540.

168. Sternberg CN, Yagoda A, Scher HI, et al. M-VAC (methotrexate, vinblastine, doxorubicin and cisplatin) for advanced transitional cell carcinoma of the urothelium. J Urol. 1988;139(3):461–9.

169. Logothetis CJ, Dexeus FH, Finn L, et al. A prospective randomized trial comparing MVAC and CISCA chemotherapy for patients with metastatic urothelial tumors. J Clin Oncol. 1990;8(6):1050–5.

170. Latta D, Finnamore VP, Dalton K, Allman S. An open, randomized comparative study of a low-strength frusemide/amiloride combination and bumetanide/potassium chloride in the treatment of mild congestive cardiac failure. J Int Med Res. 1990;18 Suppl 2:10B–6.

171. Loehrer Sr PJ, Einhorn LH, Elson PJ, et al. A randomized comparison of cisplatin alone or in combination with methotrexate, vinblastine, and doxorubicin in patients with metastatic urothelial carcinoma: a cooperative group study. J Clin Oncol. 1992;10(7):1066–73.

172. Kaufman D, Raghavan D, Carducci M, et al. Phase II trial of gemcitabine plus cisplatin in patients with metastatic urothelial cancer. J Clin Oncol. 2000;18(9):1921–7.

173. Stadler WM, Hayden A, von der Maase H, et al. Long-term survival in phase II trials of gemcitabine plus cisplatin for advanced transitional cell cancer. Urol Oncol. 2002;7(4):153–7.

174. Moore MJ, Winquist EW, Murray N, et al. Gemcitabine plus cisplatin, an active regimen in advanced urothelial cancer: a phase II trial of the National Cancer Institute of Canada Clinical Trials Group. J Clin Oncol. 1999;17(9):2876–81.

175. Bajorin DF, Dodd PM, Mazumdar M, et al. Long-term survival in metastatic transitional-cell carcinoma and prognostic factors predicting outcome of therapy. J Clin Oncol. 1999;17(10):3173–81.

176. Herr HW, Donat SM, Bajorin DF. Post-chemotherapy surgery in patients with unresectable or regionally metastatic bladder cancer. J Urol. 2001;165(3):811–4.

177. von der Maase H, Andersen L, Crino L, Weinknecht S, Dogliotti L. Weekly gemcitabine and cisplatin combination therapy in patients with transitional cell carcinoma of the urothelium: a phase II clinical trial. Ann Oncol. 1999;10(12):1461–5.

178. Rodel C, Grabenbauer GG, Kuhn R, et al. Combined-modality treatment and selective organ preservation in invasive bladder cancer: long-term results. J Clin Oncol. 2002;20(14):3061–71.

179. Zietman AL, Grocela J, Zehr E, et al. Selective bladder conservation using transurethral resection, chemotherapy, and radiation: management and consequences of Ta, T1, and Tis recurrence within the retained bladder. Urology. 2001;58(3):380–5.

180. Housset M, Maulard C, Chretien Y, et al. Combined radiation and chemotherapy for invasive transitional-cell carcinoma of the bladder: a prospective study. J Clin Oncol. 1993;11(11):2150–7.

181. Chung PW, Bristow RG, Milosevic MF, et al. Long-term outcome of radiation-based conservation therapy for invasive bladder cancer. Urol Oncol. 2007; 25(4):303–9.

182. Weiss C, Wittlinger M, Engehausen DG, et al. Management of superficial recurrences in an irradiated bladder after combined-modality organ-preserving therapy. Int J Radiat Oncol Biol Phys. 2008;70(5):1502–6.

183. Sylvester R, Sternberg C. The role of adjuvant combination chemotherapy after cystectomy in locally advanced bladder cancer: what we do not know and why. Ann Oncol. 2000;11(7):851–6.

184. Johnson D, Arriagada R, Barthelemy N, et al. Postoperative adjuvant therapy for non-small-cell lung cancer. Lung Cancer. 1997;17 Suppl 1:S23–5.

185. Freiha F, Reese J, Torti FM. A randomized trial of radical cystectomy versus radical cystectomy plus cisplatin, vinblastine and methotrexate chemotherapy for muscle invasive bladder cancer. J Urol. 1996;155(2):495–9. discussion 499–500.

186. Stockle M, Meyenburg W, Wellek S, et al. Adjuvant polychemotherapy of nonorgan-confined bladder cancer after radical cystectomy revisited: long-term results of a controlled prospective study and further clinical experience. J Urol. 1995;153(1):47–52.

187. Studer UE, Bacchi M, Biedermann C, et al. Adjuvant cisplatin chemotherapy following cystectomy for bladder cancer: results of a prospective randomized trial. J Urol. 1994;152(1):81–4.

188. Skinner DG, Daniels JR, Russell CA, et al. Adjuvant chemotherapy following cystectomy benefits patients with deeply invasive bladder cancer. Semin Urol. 1990;8(4):279–84.

189. Adjuvant chemotherapy in invasive bladder cancer: a systematic review and meta-analysis of individual patient data. Advanced Bladder Cancer (ABC) Meta-analysis Collaboration. Eur Urol. 2005;48(2):189–199; discussion 199–201.

190. von der Maase H, Sengelov L, Roberts JT, et al. Long-term survival results of a randomized trial comparing gemcitabine plus cisplatin, with methotrexate, vinblastine, doxorubicin, plus cisplatin in patients with bladder cancer. J Clin Oncol. 2005;23(21):4602–8.

191. Sternberg CN. Perioperative chemotherapy in muscle-invasive bladder cancer to enhance survival and/or as a strategy for bladder preservation. Semin Oncol. 2007;34(2):122–8.

192. Rosenberg JE, Carroll PR, Small EJ. Update on chemotherapy for advanced bladder cancer. J Urol. 2005;174(1):14–20.

193. Sternberg CN, Vogelzang NJ. Gemcitabine, paclitaxel, pemetrexed and other newer agents in urothelial and kidney cancers. Crit Rev Oncol Hematol. 2003;46(Suppl):S105–15.

194. Sengelov L, Kamby C, von der Maase H. Metastatic urothelial cancer: evaluation of prognostic factors and change in prognosis during the last twenty years. Eur Urol. 2001;39(6):634–42.

195. Bajorin D. The phase III candidate: can we improve the science of selection? J Clin Oncol. 2004;22(2):211–3.

196. Bellmunt J, Albanell J, Paz-Ares L, et al. Pretreatment prognostic factors for survival in patients with advanced urothelial tumors treated in a phase I/II trial with paclitaxel, cisplatin, and gemcitabine. Cancer. 2002;95(4):751–7.

197. Bamias A, Efstathiou E, Moulopoulos LA, et al. The outcome of elderly patients with advanced urothelial carcinoma after platinum-based combination chemotherapy. Ann Oncol. 2005;16(2):307–13.

198. Charlson M, Szatrowski TP, Peterson J, Gold J. Validation of a combined comorbidity index. J Clin Epidemiol. 1994;47(11):1245–51.

199. Inouye SK, Peduzzi PN, Robison JT, Hughes JS, Horwitz RI, Concato J. Importance of functional measures in predicting mortality among older hospitalized patients. JAMA. 1998;279(15):1187–93.

200. Lee SJ, Lindquist K, Segal MR, Covinsky KE. Development and validation of a prognostic index for 4-year mortality in older adults. JAMA. 2006;295(7):801–8.

201. Walter LC, Brand RJ, Counsell SR, et al. Development and validation of a prognostic index for 1-year mortality in older adults after hospitalization. JAMA. 2001;285(23):2987–94.

202. Balducci L, Yates J. General guidelines for the management of older patients with cancer. Oncology (Williston Park). 2000;14((11A)):221–7.

203. Bellmunt J, Albanell J, Gallego OS, et al. Carboplatin, methotrexate, and vinblastine in patients with bladder cancer who were ineligible for cisplatin-based chemotherapy. Cancer. 1992;70(7):1974–9.

204. Roth BJ, Dreicer R, Einhorn LH, et al. Significant activity of paclitaxel in advanced transitional-cell carcinoma of the urothelium: a phase II trial of the Eastern Cooperative Oncology Group. J Clin Oncol. 1994;12(11):2264–70.

205. de Wit R, Kruit WH, Stoter G, de Boer M, Kerger J, Verweij J. Docetaxel (Taxotere): an active agent in metastatic urothelial cancer; results of a phase II study in non-chemotherapy-pretreated patients. Br J Cancer. 1998;78(10):1342–5.

206. Yagoda A. Chemotherapy of urothelial tract tumors. Cancer. 1987;60 Suppl 3:574–85.

207. Roth BJ, Bajorin DF. Advanced bladder cancer: the need to identify new agents in the post-M-VAC (methotrexate, vinblastine, doxorubicin and cisplatin) world. J Urol. 1995;153(3 Pt 2):894–900.

208. von der Maase H. Gemcitabine in transitional cell carcinoma of the urothelium. Expert Rev Anticancer Ther. 2003;3(1):11–9.

209. Moore MJ, Tannock IF, Ernst DS, Huan S, Murray N. Gemcitabine: a promising new agent in the treatment of advanced urothelial cancer. J Clin Oncol. 1997;15(12):3441–5.

210. Stadler WM, Kuzel T, Roth B, Raghavan D, Dorr FA. Phase II study of single-agent gemcitabine in previously untreated patients with metastatic urothelial cancer. J Clin Oncol. 1997;15(11):3394–8.

211. Pollera CF, Ceribelli A, Crecco M, Calabresi F. Weekly gemcitabine in advanced bladder cancer: a

preliminary report from a phase I study. Ann Oncol. 1994;5(2):182–4.

212. Lorusso V, Pollera CF, Antimi M, et al. A phase II study of gemcitabine in patients with transitional cell carcinoma of the urinary tract previously treated with platinum. Italian Co-operative Group on Bladder Cancer. Eur J Cancer. 1998;34(8):1208–12.

213. Gebbia V, Testa A, Borsellino N, et al. Single agent 2′,2′-difluorodeoxycytidine in the treatment of metastatic urothelial carcinoma: a phase II study. Clin Ter. 1999;150(1):11–5.

214. Albers P, Siener R, Hartlein M, et al. Gemcitabine monotherapy as second-line treatment in cisplatin-refractory transitional cell carcinoma—prognostic factors for response and improvement of quality of life. Onkologie. 2002;25(1):47–52.

215. Bamias A, Aravantinos G, Deliveliotis C, et al. Docetaxel and cisplatin with granulocyte colony-stimulating factor (G-CSF) versus MVAC with G-CSF in advanced urothelial carcinoma: a multicenter, randomized, phase III study from the Hellenic Cooperative Oncology Group. J Clin Oncol. 2004;22(2):220–8.

216. Sternberg CN, Yagoda A, Scher HI, et al. Methotrexate, vinblastine, doxorubicin, and cisplatin for advanced transitional cell carcinoma of the urothelium. Efficacy and patterns of response and relapse. Cancer. 1989;64(12):2448–58.

217. von der Maase H, Hansen SW, Roberts JT, et al. Gemcitabine and cisplatin versus methotrexate, vinblastine, doxorubicin, and cisplatin in advanced or metastatic bladder cancer: results of a large, randomized, multinational, multicenter, phase III study. J Clin Oncol. 2000;18(17):3068–77.

218. Sternberg CN, de Mulder PH, Schornagel JH, et al. Randomized phase III trial of high-dose-intensity methotrexate, vinblastine, doxorubicin, and cisplatin (MVAC) chemotherapy and recombinant human granulocyte colony-stimulating factor versus classic MVAC in advanced urothelial tract tumors: European Organization for Research and Treatment of Cancer Protocol no. 30924. J Clin Oncol. 2001;19(10): 2638–46.

219. Sternberg CN, de Mulder P, Schornagel JH, et al. Seven year update of an EORTC phase III trial of high-dose intensity M-VAC chemotherapy and G-CSF versus classic M-VAC in advanced urothelial tract tumours. Eur J Cancer. 2006;42(1):50–4.

220. Petrioli R, Frediani B, Manganelli A, et al. Comparison between a cisplatin-containing regimen and a carboplatin-containing regimen for recurrent or metastatic bladder cancer patients. A randomized phase II study. Cancer. 1996;77(2):344–51.

221. Bellmunt J, Ribas A, Eres N, et al. Carboplatin-based versus cisplatin-based chemotherapy in the treatment of surgically incurable advanced bladder carcinoma. Cancer. 1997;80(10):1966–72.

222. Sternberg CN, Calabro F, Pizzocaro G, Marini L, Schnetzer S, Sella A. Chemotherapy with an every-2-week regimen of gemcitabine and paclitaxel in patients with transitional cell carcinoma who have received prior cisplatin-based therapy. Cancer. 2001;92(12):2993–8.

223. Meluch AA, Greco FA, Burris 3rd HA, et al. Paclitaxel and gemcitabine chemotherapy for advanced transitional-cell carcinoma of the urothelial tract: a phase II trial of the Minnie pearl cancer research network. J Clin Oncol. 2001;19(12): 3018–24.

224. Calabro F, Lorusso V, Rosati G, et al. Gemcitabine and paclitaxel every 2 weeks in patients with previously untreated urothelial carcinoma. Cancer. 2009;115(12):2652–9.

225. De Santis M, Bellmunt J, Mead G, et al. Randomized phase II/III trial assessing gemcitabine/ carboplatin and methotrexate/carboplatin/vinblastine in patients with advanced urothelial cancer "unfit" for cisplatin-based chemotherapy: phase II-results of EORTC study 3098. J Clin Oncol. 2009;27(33): 5634–9.

226. Vaughn DJ, Broome CM, Hussain M, Gutheil JC, Markowitz AB. Phase II trial of weekly paclitaxel in patients with previously treated advanced urothelial cancer. J Clin Oncol. 2002;20(4):937–40.

227. Papamichael D, Gallagher CJ, Oliver RT, Johnson PW, Waxman J. Phase II study of paclitaxel in pre-treated patients with locally advanced/metastatic cancer of the bladder and ureter. Br J Cancer. 1997;75(4):606–7.

228. McCaffrey JA, Hilton S, Mazumdar M, et al. Phase II trial of docetaxel in patients with advanced or metastatic transitional-cell carcinoma. J Clin Oncol. 1997;15(5):1853–7.

229. Witte RS, Manola J, Burch PA, Kuzel T, Weinshel EL, Loehrer Sr PJ. Topotecan in previously treated advanced urothelial carcinoma: an ECOG phase II trial. Invest New Drugs. 1998;16(2):191–5.

230. Witte RS, Elson P, Bono B, et al. Eastern Cooperative Oncology Group phase II trial of ifosfamide in the treatment of previously treated advanced urothelial carcinoma. J Clin Oncol. 1997;15(2):589–93.

231. Sweeney P, Millikan R, Donat M, et al. Is there a therapeutic role for post-chemotherapy retroperitoneal lymph node dissection in metastatic transitional cell carcinoma of the bladder? J Urol. 2003;169(6): 2113–7.

232. Siefker-Radtke AO, Walsh GL, Pisters LL, et al. Is there a role for surgery in the management of metastatic urothelial cancer? The M. D. Anderson experience. J Urol. 2004;171(1):145–8.

233. Rosen LS, Gordon D, Tchekmedyian NS, et al. Long-term efficacy and safety of zoledronic acid in the treatment of skeletal metastases in patients with nonsmall cell lung carcinoma and other solid tumors: a randomized, Phase III, double-blind, placebo-controlled trial. Cancer. 2004;100(12):2613–21.

234. Youssef RF, Mitra AP, Bartsch Jr G, Jones PA, Skinner DG, Cote RJ. Molecular targets and targeted therapies in bladder cancer management. World J Urol. 2009;27(1):9–20.

235. Shariat SF, Youssef RF, Gupta A, et al. Association of angiogenesis related markers with bladder cancer outcomes and other molecular markers. J Urol. 2010;183(5):1744–50.

236. Song S, Wientjes MG, Gan Y, Au JL. Fibroblast growth factors: an epigenetic mechanism of broad spectrum resistance to anticancer drugs. Proc Natl Acad Sci U S A. 2000;97(15):8658–63.

237. Gomez-Roman JJ, Saenz P, Molina M, et al. Fibroblast growth factor receptor 3 is overexpressed in urinary tract carcinomas and modulates the neoplastic cell growth. Clin Cancer Res. 2005;11 (2 Pt 1):459–65.

238. Ioachim E, Michael MC, Salmas M, et al. Thrombospondin-1 expression in urothelial carcinoma: prognostic significance and association with p53 alterations, tumour angiogenesis and extracellular matrix components. BMC Cancer. 2006;6:140.

239. Gallagher DJ, Milowsky MI, Ishill N, et al. Detection of circulating tumor cells in patients with urothelial cancer. Ann Oncol. 2009;20(2):305–8.

240. Hoffmann AC, Wild P, Leicht C, et al. MDR1 and ERCC1 expression predict outcome of patients with locally advanced bladder cancer receiving adjuvant chemotherapy. Neoplasia. 2010;12(8):628–36.

241. Smith K, Fennelly JA, Neal DE, Hall RR, Harris AL. Characterization and quantitation of the epidermal growth factor receptor in invasive and superficial bladder tumors. Cancer Res. 1989;49(21):5810–5.

242. Chow NH, Liu HS, Lee EI, et al. Significance of urinary epidermal growth factor and its receptor expression in human bladder cancer. Anticancer Res. 1997;17((2B)):1293–6.

243. Messing EM. Growth factors and bladder cancer: clinical implications of the interactions between growth factors and their urothelial receptors. Semin Surg Oncol. 1992;8(5):285–92.

244. Black PC, Brown GA, Inamoto T, et al. Sensitivity to epidermal growth factor receptor inhibitor requires E-cadherin expression in urothelial carcinoma cells. Clin Cancer Res. 2008;14(5):1478–86.

245. Lynch TJ, Bell DW, Sordella R, et al. Activating mutations in the epidermal growth factor receptor underlying responsiveness of non-small-cell lung cancer to gefitinib. N Engl J Med. 2004;350(21): 2129–39.

246. Blehm KN, Spiess PE, Bondaruk JE, et al. Mutations within the kinase domain and truncations of the epidermal growth factor receptor are rare events in bladder cancer: implications for therapy. Clin Cancer Res. 2006;12(15):4671–7.

247. Kruger S, Weitsch G, Buttner H, et al. Overexpression of c-erbB-2 oncoprotein in muscle-invasive bladder carcinoma: relationship with gene amplification, clinicopathological parameters and prognostic outcome. Int J Oncol. 2002;21(5):981–7.

248. Rocha-Lima CM, Soares HP, Raez LE, Singal R. EGFR targeting of solid tumors. Cancer Control. 2007;14(3):295–304.

249. Nutt JE, Lazarowicz HP, Mellon JK, Lunec J. Gefitinib ("Iressa", ZD1839) inhibits the growth response of bladder tumour cell lines to epidermal growth factor and induces TIMP2. Br J Cancer. 2004;90(8):1679–85.

250. Dominguez-Escrig JL, Kelly JD, Neal DE, King SM, Davies BR. Evaluation of the therapeutic potential of the epidermal growth factor receptor tyrosine kinase inhibitor gefitinib in preclinical models of bladder cancer. Clin Cancer Res. 2004;10(14): 4874–84.

251. Nutt JE, Foster PA, Mellon JK, Lunec J. hEGR1 is induced by EGF, inhibited by gefitinib in bladder cell lines and related to EGF receptor levels in bladder tumours. Br J Cancer. 2007;96(5):762–8.

252. Philips G, Sanford B, Halabi S, Bajorin D, Small EJ. Phase II study of cisplatin (C), gemcitabine (G), and gefitinib for advanced urothelial carcinoma (UC): Analysis of the second cohort of CALGB 90102. Paper presented at: ASCO Annual Meeting2006; Atlanta, GA

253. Zureikat AH, McKee MD. Targeted therapy for solid tumors: current status. Surg Oncol Clin N Am. 2008;17(2):279–301. vii-viii.

254. Clinical trials. 2008. http://www.clinicaltrials.gov. Accessed 2 Jul 2011

255. Perrotte P, Matsumoto T, Inoue K, et al. Anti-epidermal growth factor receptor antibody C225 inhibits angiogenesis in human transitional cell carcinoma growing orthotopically in nude mice. Clin Cancer Res. 1999;5(2):257–65.

256. Hussain MH, Study of gemcitabine and cisplatin with or without cetuximab in urothelial cancer. 2008. http://clinicaltrials.gov/ct2/show/NCT00645593. Accessed 2 Jul 2011

257. Hussain MH, MacVicar GR, Petrylak DP, et al. Trastuzumab, paclitaxel, carboplatin, and gemcitabine in advanced human epidermal growth factor receptor-2/neu-positive urothelial carcinoma: results of a multicenter phase II National Cancer Institute trial. J Clin Oncol. 2007;25(16):2218–24.

258. Nelson MH, Dolder CR. Lapatinib: a novel dual tyrosine kinase inhibitor with activity in solid tumors. Ann Pharmacother. 2006;40(2):261–9.

259. Wulfung C, Michiels JP, Richel DJ, et al. EGF20003: a single arm, multicentre, open-label phase II study of roally administered lapatinib (GW572016) as single-agent, second-line treatment of patients with locally advanced or metastatic transitional cell carcinoma of the urothelial tract: Wnal analysis. Ann Oncol. 2005;15 Suppl 3:41.

260. Folkman J. Angiogenesis in cancer, vascular, rheumatoid and other disease. Nat Med. 1995;1(1): 27–31.

261. Folkman J, Hochberg M. Self-regulation of growth in three dimensions. J Exp Med. 1973;138(4): 745–53.

262. Yang CC, Chu KC, Yeh WM. The expression of vascular endothelial growth factor in transitional cell

carcinoma of urinary bladder is correlated with cancer progression. Urol Oncol. 2004;22(1):1–6.

263. Crew JP, Fuggle S, Bicknell R, Cranston DW, de Benedetti A, Harris AL. Eukaryotic initiation factor-4E in superficial and muscle invasive bladder cancer and its correlation with vascular endothelial growth factor expression and tumour progression. Br J Cancer. 2000;82(1):161–6.

264. Wu W, Shu X, Hovsepyan H, Mosteller RD, Broek D. VEGF receptor expression and signaling in human bladder tumors. Oncogene. 2003;22(22): 3361–70.

265. Canoglu A, Gogus C, Beduk Y, Orhan D, Tulunay O, Baltaci S. Microvessel density as a prognostic marker in bladder carcinoma: correlation with tumor grade, stage and prognosis. Int Urol Nephrol. 2004;36(3):401–5.

266. Goddard JC, Sutton CD, Furness PN, O'Byrne KJ, Kockelbergh RC. Microvessel density at presentation predicts subsequent muscle invasion in superficial bladder cancer. Clin Cancer Res. 2003;9(7): 2583–6.

267. Bernardini S, Fauconnet S, Chabannes E, Henry PC, Adessi G, Bittard H. Serum levels of vascular endothelial growth factor as a prognostic factor in bladder cancer. J Urol. 2001;166(4):1275–9.

268. Inoue K, Kamada M, Slaton JW, et al. The prognostic value of angiogenesis and metastasis-related genes for progression of transitional cell carcinoma of the renal pelvis and ureter. Clin Cancer Res. 2002;8(6):1863–70.

269. Adnane L, Trail PA, Taylor I, Wilhelm SM. Sorafenib (BAY 43-9006, Nexavar), a dual-action inhibitor that targets RAF/MEK/ERK pathway in tumor cells and tyrosine kinases VEGFR/PDGFR in tumor vasculature. Methods Enzymol. 2006;407:597–612.

270. Osai WE, Ng CS, Pagliaro LC. Positive response to bevacizumab in a patient with metastatic, chemotherapy-refractory urothelial carcinoma. Anticancer Drugs. 2008;19(4):427–9.

271. Dupont J, Bienvenu B, Aghajanian C, et al. Phase I and pharmacokinetic study of the novel oral cell-cycle inhibitor Ro 31-7453 in patients with advanced solid tumors. J Clin Oncol. 2004;22(16): 3366–74.

272. Sogni F, Brausi M, Frea B, et al. Morbidity and quality of life in elderly patients receiving ileal conduit or orthotopic neobladder after radical cystectomy for invasive bladder cancer. Urology. 2008;71(5): 919–23.

273. Autorino R, Quarto G, Di Lorenzo G, et al. Health related quality of life after radical cystectomy: comparison of ileal conduit to continent orthotopic neobladder. Eur J Surg Oncol. 2009;35(8):858–64.

274. Mansson A, Davidsson T, Hunt S, Mansson W. The quality of life in men after radical cystectomy with a continent cutaneous diversion or orthotopic bladder substitution: is there a difference? BJU Int. 2002;90(4):386–90.

275. Wright JL, Porter MP. Quality-of-life assessment in patients with bladder cancer. Nat Clin Pract Urol. 2007;4(3):147–54.

276. Hedgepeth RC, Gilbert SM, He C, Lee CT, Wood Jr DP. Body image and bladder cancer specific quality of life in patients with ileal conduit and neobladder urinary diversions. Urology. 2010;76(3):671–5.

277. Dutta SC, Chang SC, Coffey CS, Smith Jr JA, Jack G, Cookson MS. Health related quality of life assessment after radical cystectomy: comparison of ileal conduit with continent orthotopic neobladder. J Urol. 2002;168(1):164–7.

278. Hara I, Miyake H, Hara S, et al. Health-related quality of life after radical cystectomy for bladder cancer: a comparison of ileal conduit and orthotopic bladder replacement. BJU Int. 2002;89(1):10–3.

279. Stenzl A, Sherif H, Kuczyk M. Radical cystectomy with orthotopic neobladder for invasive bladder cancer: a critical analysis of long term oncological, functional and quality of life results. Int Braz J Urol. 2010;36(5):537–47.

280. Philip J, Manikandan R, Venugopal S, Desouza J, Javle PM. Orthotopic neobladder versus ileal conduit urinary diversion after cystectomy–a quality-of-life based comparison. Ann R Coll Surg Engl. 2009;91(7):565–9.

281. Roychowdhury DF, Hayden A, Liepa AM. Health-related quality-of-life parameters as independent prognostic factors in advanced or metastatic bladder cancer. J Clin Oncol. 2003;21(4):673–8.

282. Malkowicz SB, van Poppel H, Mickisch G, et al. Muscle-invasive urothelial carcinoma of the bladder. Urology. 2007;69 Suppl 1:3–16.

283. Bochner BH, Montie JE, Lee CT. Follow-up strategies and management of recurrence in urologic oncology bladder cancer: invasive bladder cancer. Urol Clin North Am. 2003;30(4):777–89.

284. Sanderson KM, Cai J, Miranda G, Skinner DG, Stein JP. Upper tract urothelial recurrence following radical cystectomy for transitional cell carcinoma of the bladder: an analysis of 1,069 patients with 10-year followup. J Urol. 2007;177(6):2088–94.

285. Stenzl A, Bartsch G, Rogatsch H. The remnant urothelium after reconstructive bladder surgery. Eur Urol. 2002;41(2):124–31.

286. Freeman JA, Tarter TA, Esrig D, et al. Urethral recurrence in patients with orthotopic ileal neobladders. J Urol. 1996;156(5):1615–9.

287. Hardeman SW, Soloway MS. Urethral recurrence following radical cystectomy. J Urol. 1990;144(3): 666–9.

288. Levinson AK, Johnson DE, Wishnow KI. Indications for urethrectomy in an era of continent urinary diversion. J Urol. 1990;144(1):73–5.

289. Stenzl A, Draxl H, Posch B, Colleselli K, Falk M, Bartsch G. The risk of urethral tumors in female bladder cancer: can the urethra be used for orthotopic reconstruction of the lower urinary tract? J Urol. 1995;153(3 Pt 2):950–5.

290. Huguet J, Palou J, Serrallach M, Sole Balcells FJ, Salvador J, Villavicencio H. Management of urethral recurrence in patients with Studer ileal neobladder. Eur Urol. 2003;43(5):495–8.
291. Nieder AM, Sved PD, Gomez P, Kim SS, Manoharan M, Soloway MS. Urethral recurrence after cystoprostatectomy: implications for urinary diversion and monitoring. Urology. 2004;64(5):950–4.
292. Varol C, Thalmann GN, Burkhard FC, Studer UE. Treatment of urethral recurrence following radical cystectomy and ileal bladder substitution. J Urol. 2004;172(3):937–42.

Biomarkers in Prostate Cancer

13

Mauro Bologna and Carlo Vicentini

Abbreviations

BPH	Benign prostatic hyperplasia
CaPSURE	Cancer of Prostate Strategic Urologic Research Endeavor
CRPC	Castration-resistant prostate cancer
CTC	Circulating tumor cells
DMAB	(3,2′-Dimethyl-4-aminobiphenyl)
DRE	Digital rectal examination
ETS	Erythroblastosis virus E26 transforming sequence: a family of transcription factors
GRP	Gastrin-releasing peptide
GSTP1	Glutathione S-transferase
HDAC	Histone deacetylase
hK2	Human glandular kallikrein-2
HRPCa	Hormone-resistant prostate cancer
LH	Luteinizing hormone
LHRH	Luteinizing hormone-releasing hormone
MMPs	Matrix metalloproteases
NE	Neuroendocrine
NET	Neuroendocrine transdifferentiation
NSE	Neuron-specific enolase

PAP	Prostatic acid phosphatase
PCa	Prostate cancer
PCA3	Prostate cancer gene 3
PIN	Prostatic intraepithelial neoplasia
PSA	Prostate-specific antigen
PSMA	Prostate-specific membrane antigen
PSP94	Prostate secretory protein-94
TMPRSS2	Prostate-specific gene transmembrane protease serine 2
uPA	Urokinase-type plasminogen activator
VPA	Valproic acid

Introduction

After a systematic description of pathological and clinical features of prostate cancer (PCa), the most recent concepts regarding PCa biomarkers are reviewed in this chapter, based on current scientific reports and some of the most advanced research programs which are ongoing.

Biomarkers are essential elements to determine early diagnosis, define prognosis of single cases of disease, and possibly also to represent targets for molecular therapies, which are gaining great momentum in the present era of individualized therapy strategies. All the above goals are of relevant importance in the field of PCa in which a large number of diagnosed cases [due to the wide use of prostate-specific antigen (PSA) testing] have enhanced the percentage of early diagnosed cases, most of which have modest

M. Bologna, M.D. (✉)
Department of Experimental Medicine, University of L'Aquila, Via Vetoio, Coppito-2, L'Aquila 67100, Italy
e-mail: mauro.bologna@univaq.it

C. Vicentini, M.D.
Department of Urology, University Hospital of Teramo, L'Aquila, Italy

M. Bologna (ed.), *Biotargets of Cancer in Current Clinical Practice*, Current Clinical Pathology,
DOI 10.1007/978-1-61779-615-9_13, © Springer Science+Business Media, LLC 2012

clinical relevance but hard-to-predict prognostic perspective. Very difficult is the decision to opt in the first line for the "watchful waiting" (active surveillance) strategy that should be appropriate for most but not all PCa-diagnosed patients.

So, dependable biomarkers are absolutely needed in the clinical management of PCa and are extremely useful in the daily medical practice for optimal patient treatment and outcomes, in particular for the early determination of the many indolent, slow progression cases (low-risk PCa) and of the few aggressive, rapid progression cases (high-risk PCa).

Biomarkers must be considered in two broad categories: tissue-specific markers and disease-specific markers.

The major current biomarker of PCa is the PSA, which is used both as a screening tool, before the disease is diagnosed, and as an instrument to monitor the disease extension and progression, once PCa presence has been ascertained and possibly treated with a first-line therapy (surgery, radiotherapy, or their combination). PSA is, however, only a tissue-specific marker and not a disease-specific one; therefore, many caveats exist in the interpretation of PSA testing.

Several other markers are being actively studied and discussed in this chapter.

For a very quick summary, besides classical biomarkers like PSA, specific sections discuss prostate cancer gene 3 (PCA3), gene fusions, prostate secretory proteins, circulating tumor cells (CTCs), and neuroendocrine markers [1]. Further paragraphs discuss current research issues concerning future biomarkers under active investigation.

Epidemiology of Prostate Cancer

Prostate cancer (PCa) is the top-ranking cancer cause for men and the second cancer-death cause for males in the USA and in many industrialized countries [2, 3]; it affects one in six men (more than 210,000 cases per year) and claims more than 30,000 deaths each year in the USA [3, 4]. Every day, about 600 men are given the diagnosis of PCa in that country. Although PCa incidence is slightly decreasing in the USA in recent times [3], it is, however, still on the rise in many other geographical areas, and its mortality rate accounts for a large proportion of male cancer death statistics.

The decrease in PCa incidence rates in the USA (by 2.4% per year from 2000 to 2006) can reflect recent stabilization of PSA antigen testing, resulting in a decreased detection or a decreased number of undiagnosed cases [5].

Comprehensible and updated epidemiological data can also be found, together with extensive clinical discussion, in a very useful publication recently issued and devoted to the general public of the USA, with the title "Report to the Nation on Prostate Cancer," published in 2005 by the Prostate Cancer Foundation of Santa Monica, California, USA [4]. It covers all aspects of the matter, starting from epidemiology and extending then mostly to the major questions raised in the general public by this pervasive and worrisome health problem becoming a widespread social issue in populations with a progressively increasing proportion of aging citizens.

The most heavily interested population stratus interested by PCa is indeed that of elderly males (but includes obviously their families), since it affects mostly the advanced age classes [3], while the race affected the most is that of African-Americans, having an incidence considerably higher and a mortality rate more than double as compared to that of American whites [3].

Another striking element emerging from the most recent statistical evaluations published for the USA is the figures concerning the probability of developing an invasive form of PCa for an American male at different ages, which is precisely 1 in 9,400 (birth to 39 years of age), 1 in 41 (40–59 years of age), 1 in 16 (60–69 years of age), 1 in 8 (70–79 years of age), and 1 in 6 (birth to death) [3].

In 1990, PCa surpassed lung cancer as the most frequently diagnosed malignant neoplasm in North American men, due both to the reduction of lung cancer frequency and to the increase of PCa diagnosis attributed at least in part to the wide use of PSA serum testing introduced in 1980 by Papsidero and coworkers [6]. PSA had a

13 Biomarkers in Prostate Cancer

long and still-debated discovery story (see below at the paragraph entitled "A Brief Story of the Discovery of PSA").

Recent European data (Eurostat 2008) reveal a death rate for PCa of 21.9 deaths per 100,000 inhabitants (EU-27 cumulative statistics), with generally higher rates in northern European countries (37.1, Latvia; 36.3, Lithuania; 35.4, Denmark; 35.3, Iceland; 34.1, Norway; 34.4, Sweden; 33.3, Estonia), intermediate rates for central Europe (29.0, Belgium; 25.4, the UK; 26.6, the Netherlands; 26.4, Czech Republic; 25.9, Switzerland; 22.3, Austria and Hungary; 23.8, France; 21.2, Germany), and lower rates for southern Europe (18.8, Italy; 18.0, Spain; 16.4, Bulgaria; 15.3, Romania), with some notable geographical exceptions (33.9, Slovenia; 26.4, Finland) [7].

The reported incidence of PCa in Europe makes it the most common malignancy in men in such geographical area [8].

PCa is very rare before the age of 50 and is mostly a disease of aged men, since 75% of the diagnosed cases are aged between 60 and 80 years. In the USA, the cases younger than 50 years are less than 1% of all the PCa cases. At the age 50, the probability to develop a clinically evident PCa in the rest of life is 10% in American males.

Autopsy studies have revealed that the real frequency of PCa is much higher than that of the clinical disease. Most cases (70–90%) are only accidental autopsy evidences or histological findings of small microscopic tumor foci in the context surgical specimens of benign prostatic hyperplasia (BPH). Autoptic frequency of PCa increases with age, being less than 10% in subjects aged 40–50 years, but reaching levels even up to 50–70% in subjects aged more than 80 years [2, 9].

Some data infer a future increase in PCa incidence in the USA, since the epidemiological stratum named "the baby boomers" [indicating the category of increased births in the economic boom period (see the description of "Baby Boom Generation" in Wikipedia, where the term is related in extended manner to the people born during the middle part of the twentieth century)] will become aged people in the next years and may bring PCa incidence to new cancer cases to 300,000 in 2015

and even to 400,000 in 2035, according to Peter Carroll in a recent Web conference (http://www.medscape.org/viewprogram/3398).

Considerable geographical differences exist in the age-related incidence and mortality rates of PCa. Highest frequencies are recorded in the USA (69 cases every 100,000 men) and in the northern European countries (Scandinavia), while the lowest rates have been recorded in Mexico, Greece, and Japan (3–4 cases every 100,000 men). Most central European countries are at intermediate rates. The highest rates are recorded in black Americans, as already mentioned, with frequency almost double compared to whites [2]. Migration studies have demonstrated that second-generation emigrants to the USA coming from Japan have higher rates of PCa compared to their nationals in the country of origin; in parallel, rates in American blacks are higher than that of blacks in Africa. Hereditary factors and dietary factors (high-lipid-content diet) have also been implied in PCa risk. Familial cases are about one-tenth of all cases, with a risk significantly higher in first-degree relatives of ascertained PCa cases [9]. In particular, if a male subject has a first-degree relative with PCa, its lifelong risk of having PCa is double, compared to general population of males without relatives affected, and if a male subject has two first-degree relatives with PCa, its lifelong risk of having PCa is even five times higher with respect to familial history-negative subjects [2].

Data from CaPSURE (Cancer of Prostate Strategic Urologic Research Endeavor) have revealed that the percentage of cases having a low-risk PCa (according to published criteria) [10] has increased from 31% in 1989–1990 to 47% in 2001–2002. In contrast, the incidence of the high-risk disease has decreased from 41 to 15% [11]. This trend has enormously expanded the proportion of men diagnosed as having PCa at early stages, and posing the question whether all patients should be treated anyway or if a substantial proportion of them, being affected only by a slowly progressing disease that does not need any invasive treatment, should be simply followed though a "watchful waiting" strategy (or active surveillance). Some recent review papers have addressed exactly these points, focusing on how to avoid PCa overdiagnosis and how to best recognize aggressive cases, deserving immediate treatment, through the appropriate use of biomarkers [1].

Genetics and Causes of Prostate Cancer

As mentioned in the above paragraph on epidemiology, a quote of PCa cases is detected in family clusters, mostly in first-degree relatives of index cases. This observation did not allow, so far, the identification of a specific set of genes univocally related to PCa pathogenesis. However, several indications point to the existence of gene combinations constituting a higher risk for the disease in some families and in some young-onset sporadic cases.

The genetic basis of cancer is recognized as due to the accumulation of several genetic defects in time in the same cells, giving origin to neoplasia. The substantial identity of frequency for subclinical (sporadic) form of PCa in both high clinical case populations (USA) and low clinical case populations (Japan) supports the idea that the probability of acquiring further mutations is lower in Asian populations and that in "western life-style" populations, such probability is instead considerably higher. All this is in keeping with the demonstrated higher rate seen in populations migrated from low-risk areas to high-risk areas and with increased trends in time spent in the high-risk areas characterized by a "westernized" lifestyle [2].

Androgen receptor (AR) gene mutations have been extensively studied, but they may play a significant role only in a minority of cases of PCa. Gene amplification events involving AR genes may, however, play a role in androgen sensitivity of PCa. Among various gene alterations studied in PCa, a susceptibility gene was mapped in chromosome 1 (1q24–25), together with several other chromosomic areas [12].

Onco-suppressor genes which are lost in several PCa samples involve genetic loci of 8p, 10q, 13q, and 16q chromosomal regions. In most cases, the identity of such genes is still under investigation and seems to be mostly relevant during metastatic disease. This allows to retain that involvement of well-known genes like TP53 happens only late during the biological history of the multi-hit genetic pathways leading to invasive and highly malignant forms of PCa. Further data have implicated the genes PTEN and KAI1 and the loss of cell-surface molecules like E-cadherin and CD-44 [2]. Moreover, the EGF pathway which is significantly involved in the pathogenesis of several invasive carcinomas has been studied in PCa (overexpression of her-2/neu in cancer, like breast cancer and other malignant epithelial neoplasms), together with GSTP1 (glutathione S-transferase), localized in chromosome 11q13, and related to rare cases of PCa characterized by very aggressive behavior [13].

Further gene studies have indicated possible roles in PCa susceptibility at locations 11q25 (RNASEL or PRCA1) [14], 8p22 (MSR1 or SCARA1) [15], 3p26 (OGG1) [16], and 6q25 (SOD2 or MnSOD) [17]. The last two are notably related to oxidant detoxification and repair (see below, at the paragraph entitled "Pathogenesis of PCa").

Moreover, some inflammation-related genes may be involved with PCa pathogenesis and are currently studied: at locations 19p13 (GDF15) [18], 9q32–33 (TLR4), 4q13–21 (IL8), and 1q31–32 (IL10) [19, 20].

A very recent and promising report indicated in PTEN, SMAD4, cyclin D1, and SPP1 a four-gene combination able to predict the aggressive behavior of PCa cases, starting with a demonstration in mouse PTEN-negative models and extending the experience to human cases [21]. The results of this kind of research allow to envision the future possibility of identifying, through genetic analysis of tumor cells, which PCa cases may rapidly progress to become aggressive, lethal forms of disease (and therefore deserve aggressive, radical therapy) and which ones instead (not having the genetic traits of fast progressive cases) may have high probability of progressing slowly: these will be better treated by watchful waiting strategies and avoiding useless costs and distressing treatments. The function of these genes are described in further detail in section "Current Research Issues and Discovery on New Biomarkers of Prostate Cancer."

One more of the gene alterations currently under investigation is a gene fusion between prostate-specific gene transmembrane protease, serine 2 (TMPRSS2), and members of the erythroblastosis virus E26 transforming sequence (ETS) family of transcription factors [1]. A more detailed description of these research findings are discussed in section "Gene Fusions."

In high-risk subjects (having first-degree relatives affected at young age), clinical controls are recommended even starting at age 40: this is probably the population which may benefit the most from early detection efforts through detailed genetic analysis [2].

Causes of PCa are still largely unknown. But many are the ascertained factors connecting with PCa risk: age-related frequency, race-related factors, geographical differences, and diet-related factors. Among diet influences, there are both negative factors (hypercaloric and particularly hyperlipidic composition of diet) and positive factors (high vegetable consumption, substantial lycopene assumption with tomatoes and tomato-derived products, [22] vitamins, selenium, soy derivatives, etc.).

Conclusive evidences in the genetic studies of PCa are, however, still lacking. The available data, which concern not few but many different genes, confirm the paradigm that a genetic approach to the solution of cancer management is still vague and not easily at reach, requiring complex and multigene further investigation.

Pathology of Prostate Cancer

Pathological features of PCa have been extensively studied and have led to a relevant amount of knowledge on the morphological and biomolecular aspects of the disease, although the original cause of prostatic adenocarcinoma remains elusive. A clear endocrine dependence of early stages of the disease is, however, well established [2].

The prostate gland anatomy is well known, and PCa insurgence takes place in most cases in the posterior lobes of the gland (Fig. 13.1), where a nodule with increased hardness may be detected through a classical urological procedure named

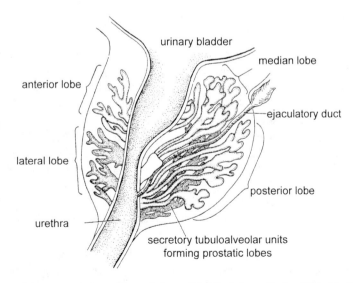

Fig. 13.1 Drawing of the anatomical structure of the prostate gland, with indication of the various lobes. The posterior lobe, where most cases of PCa occur, is adjacent to the rectum and may be palpated by digital rectal exam. [Modified from Spring-Mills E. Krall A. Functional Anatomy of the Prostate. In: Hafez ESE. Spring-Mills E (eds). Prostatic Carcinoma: Biology and Diagnosis. Martinus NiJhoff. The Hague; 1981: 5–12]

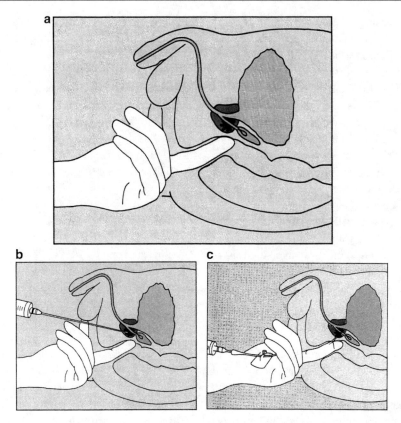

Fig. 13.2 Digital rectal exam, by which the urologist can appreciate by palpation across the rectal mucosa the presence of nodules in the adjacent posterior lobe of the prostate gland (**a**) and, if judged necessary, perform a bioptic sample collection, either *trans*-perineally (core biopsy) (**b**) or *trans*-rectally (fine-needle aspiration biopsy) (**c**)

digital rectal exam (DRE), consisting in a palpatory exploration of the anterior surface of the rectal mucosa, which is closely adjacent to the posterior lobes of the prostate. During DRE, it is possible to perform needle biopsies of the suspect nodules and to obtain histological samples of that area for histo-microscopic examination (Fig. 13.2).

Pathogenesis of PCa

The hormone dependence of prostate gland growth and development, under androgenic control, and the response of prostate carcinoma to castration or to exogenously administered estrogen molecules confirm a clear implication of male sexual hormones in PCa growth and progression.

In patients with PCa, however, androgen levels were never demonstrated to be consistently higher than normal. Although several reports have pointed to the detection of higher than average urinary ratios of estrone/testosterone, this parameter never reached significant adoption as a biomarker for PCa diagnosis or screening.

Experimental induction of PCa was obtained with chemical carcinogens, like DMAB (3,2'-dimethyl-4-aminobiphenyle) and other mutagens (tumor inducers, as charred meat polycyclic compounds like phenylimidazopyridines, PIPs) [23], with a secondary role played by androgenic hormones (tumor promotion effect).

In the PCa carcinogenesis experiments, a clear inhibitory effect is played by some antioxidants, like isothiocyanates (sulforaphane) in cruciferous vegetables and lycopene (a vegetable

13 Biomarkers in Prostate Cancer

alpha-carotenoid), abundant in tomatoes. Therefore, to counteract carcinogenetic events active in the prostatic epithelium, it is widely accepted that a diet rich in antioxidants and particularly in cruciferous vegetables and tomatoes may be highly recommended [24–26].

There are no demonstrations of a possible origin of prostate adenocarcinoma from nodules of BPH although this hypothesis has been evaluated extensively and for long time. High scientific interest is devoted, however, to nodules of dysplastic intraductal foci (PIN, often detected incidentally in BPH surgical samples or in prostatic biopsy samples), which consists of native prostatic ducts lined by secretory layer cells which are cytologically atypical and by a scarcity of basal cells. Today, PIN foci are considered, based on extensive studies, true preneoplastic lesions able to progress toward prostatic adenocarcinoma. These lesions precede by 20 years the appearance of invasive PCa and their frequency and degree of atypical features increases with age [27].

Morphological evidence linking PIN to PCa includes (a) prevalence of peripheral localization in the prostate gland for both lesions, (b) cytological similarity of high-grade PIN cells with invasive PCa, and (c) the close topographical proximity of high-grade PIN with PCa in many specimens. Moreover, PIN lesions are found with the highest frequency in prostates carrying also PCa nodules, as compared to prostates negative for PCa nodules. Some markers are similar in high-grade PIN and in invasive PCa, namely, aneuploidy, TGF-alpha, type IV collagenase, and oncogene expression (*bcl-2* and *c-erb-B2*).

High-grade PIN, when present in biopsy specimens, is therefore an important marker for the possible presence of PCa. Many patients showing only high-grade PIN in their initial biopsies develop in following samples evidence of PCa, within weeks or months of follow-up.

Morphology of PCa

Prostatic adenocarcinomas, constituting 98% of all primitive prostate tumors, are usually multicentric in their distribution and localized most frequently in the peripheral areas of the prostate gland. The cut surface of a prostate with PCa shows irregular nodules, white to yellowish in color, of higher consistency, and having mostly a subcapsular localization.

Prostatic Intraepithelial Neoplasia

Low-grade PIN is characterized by crowding and overlapping of secretory cells showing wide variability in nuclear dimensions. Nucleoli are often present but normal sized. Basal cells are present. On the contrary, *high-grade PIN* shows a denser crowding of cells, a more pronounced nuclear enlargement, and prominent, abnormally sized nucleoli [27, 28].

A smaller number of basal cells can be demonstrated with immunohistochemical staining methods for high-molecular-weight cytokeratins. Atypical cells in ducts with PIN have a flat, papillary, or cribriform aspect. Basal layer prostatic cells can be recognized through several immunohistochemical methods for numerous immunological markers of such cells. Recently, also cDNA microarray methods have been introduced but can help only in conjunction with accurate standard histological methods [29].

All the available evidences support the concept that PIN is an intermediate lesion between normal prostatic epithelium and prostate adenocarcinoma [2, 27].

Invasive Carcinoma Features

Most prostatic adenocarcinoma samples derive from acinar cells and are composed by small to mid-size glands with irregular organization and invading the surrounding stroma. Well-differentiated tumors show uniform glands with small or mid-sized acini, lined by a single layer of neoplastic epithelial cells. The most widely used morphological criterion to diagnose microscopically the PCa specimens is indeed the presence of a single layer of cuboidal cells lining the neoplastic glands. Progressive loss of differentiation in prostatic adenocarcinoma is characterized by

(a) increasing variability of gland dimensions and distribution; (b) papillary and cribriform architecture; and (c) formation of rudimental glands, having only infiltrating cell cords. Only rarely PCa is formed by small undifferentiated cells growing singularly or in layers without any structural tissue organization (see below, "Grading of PCa").

Cytology and Grading of PCa

In PCa microscopic samples, polymorphic and hyperchromatic nuclei are very variable: nuclei tend to have most frequently one or two prominent nucleoli in a dense chromatin context, close to the nuclear membrane. Moderately eosinophilic cytoplasm can be sometimes markedly vacuolated and resemble clear cell carcinoma of the kidney. Cell borders are evident in well-differentiated tumors, but are less marked in poorly differentiated cases.

The most widely used and best clinically recognized biomarker of PCa is the morphological grading system refined by Gleason [30] (Fig. 13.3).

PCa grading is executed traditionally in keeping with the *Gleason grading system,* based on five histological aspects concerning gland architecture and infiltration features evident in low-power optical microscopy. In order to take in consideration the very heterogeneous and mixed tumor foci, the *Gleason score* is used, which is the sum of the grades (1–5) related to the primary tumoral component, that is, more prevalent (more represented in the sample) and the secondary tumoral component (less represented). Therefore, the well-differentiated PCa cases have a Gleason score of 2 (1+1), while the very undifferentiated PCa cases have a Gleason score of 10 (5+5). Most cases, however, have intermediate scores, ranging from 4 to 7 (2+2 to 3+4 or 4+3). A PCa sample characterized by a very homogeneous tissue pattern (i.e., without a more prevalent and a less prevalent pattern) is given a Gleason score of 2× the value corresponding to its differentiation pattern. According to this principle, the more differentiated tumors are of grades 2–4, the intermediate tumors have grades of 5–6, and the most undifferentiated tumors have grades 7–10. Although some

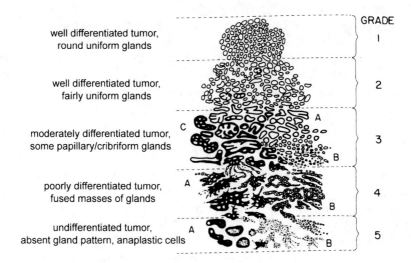

Fig. 13.3 PCa histological tumor grading system, according to Gleason. The final grading is obtained by the sum of the two predominant gland patterns in each sample. The five basic patterns are illustrated, with variants A, B, C existing in the more anaplastic and less differentiated samples. 3A, irregular glands, medium to large in size; 3B, irregular glands, small to minute in size, not fused or "chained"; 3C, cribriform pattern or papillary nodules, with rounded outer margins; 4A, irregular masses of confluent epithelial tissue, with single tumor cells in the stroma; 4B, same as before, with large clear cells; 5A, Uniform, cribriform, or solid masses, often with necrosis-like comedocarcinoma; 5B, anaplastic carcinoma with vacuoles and glands suggesting adenocarcinoma, invading the stroma

authors have described the possibility of a clinical case to become less differentiated with time, usually the Gleason score remains unaltered for several years and neoplasias with the highest scores tend to be untreatable [9].

Together with tumor clinical stage, Gleason score has a prognostic value: the lower the score, the better is the prognosis of the single PCa case [30]. Some authors even consider the tertiary histological component, if it is less differentiated but, however, present since it may in time progress and overcome the more differentiated components.

Other Rare Forms of Prostatic Neoplasms

Prostatic adenocarcinoma is by far the most frequent form of PCa. However, a few rare forms of different tumors exist in the prostate, like ductal carcinoma (with symptoms similar to urothelial tumors: hematuria and urinary obstruction), squamous carcinoma, and mucinous carcinoma. The most aggressive and rare form of tumor is the small-cell carcinoma [31, 32].

Occasionally, also mesenchymal tumors (leiomyoma, sarcomas) may grow in the prostate [2, 33, 34].

Natural History of Human Prostate Cancer and Metastatic Spreading Routes

Several PCa cases are discovered during the histological exam of prostate glands surgically removed during standard therapeutic procedures for BPH. The malignant neoplastic disease within the prostate is mostly asymptomatic and not rare are the cases in which PCa is discovered when already in progression phase, that is, when tumor cells have already crossed the anatomical barriers of the gland capsule and have established distant metastases.

Prostate capsule invasion is frequent in PCa, also due to the prevalent subcapsular localization of the primary tumor. Also frequent is the perineural invasion within the prostate and the spreading toward the adjacent tissues. Since peripheral nerves do not have lymphatic vessels, perineural invasion is considered a local contiguity spreading in a space anatomically constituting a reduced resistance site.

Seminal vesicles are very often involved in PCa spreading. Less frequent is the urinary bladder involvement, which can, however, occur in advanced stages. Early metastasis of PCa can take place in lymph nodes of the obturator and periaortic regions. Further lymphatic or venous spreading localizations may be represented by pulmonary metastases (through thoracic duct or inferior vena cava). Of particular frequency and gravity are bone metastases, mostly at the lumbar spine, the ribs, and the pelvic bones, where pathological fractures can occur and markedly complicate the clinical situation. Hip fractures tend to be the most common, although the most significant complication from PCa bone metastases is spinal cord compression due to vertebral fractures and nerve compression consequences causing intense pain, severe nerve damage, and possibly, paralysis (if not managed immediately). All these possibilities deserve special treatment and intense care efforts.

Major Clinical Features of Prostate Cancer: Open Issues

Current screening programs of PCa are based on DRE (rectal exploration) and PSA serum measurement: they are useful to detect the malignant tumor in most cases. Patients having high levels of serum PSA are studied further with needle biopsies of the prostate (see Fig. 13.2). PSA levels prior to surgery have been related to tumor volume. Very rare is the development of urinary flow obstruction for advanced PCa.

Most new PCa cases are diagnosed at an early stage, since over 80% of the patients are diagnosed with localized or locally advanced disease (T1 or T2 stage; see below "Staging of Prostate Cancer," and Fig. 13.4).

Symptoms of PCa are rare, since most cases of PCa are today found before the disease can cause

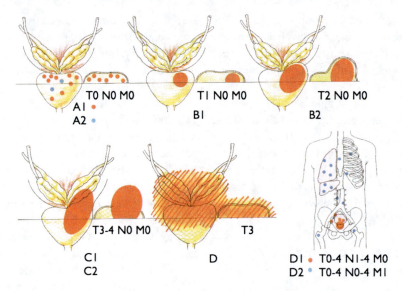

Fig. 13.4 PCa staging. Intracapsular tumors (*upper row*) and extracapsular tumors (*lower row*) are illustrated, with the corresponding classifications according to the ABCD (American Urological Association) and the TNM (UICC) grading systems. See also Table 13.2

symptoms. Most of the symptoms are, however, very aspecific, since they can be associated not only with prostate cancer but most of the times mainly with non-cancerous conditions.

Here is a list of possible symptoms: urinary hesitancy (delayed or slowed start of urinary stream), urinary dripping, especially immediately after urinating, urinary retention, pain with urination, pain with ejaculation, lower back pain, pain with bowel movement. Additional symptoms may be associated with PCa, like excessive urination at night, incontinence, bone pain or tenderness, hematuria (blood in the urine), abdominal pain, anemia, weight loss, lethargy, and hemospermia. None of the above-mentioned symptoms is, however, particularly significant, nor in any case specific for PCa or prostate disease.

To determine primitive tumor in cases diagnosed at the metastatic stage, prostatic histological biomarkers (PSA and prostatic acid phosphatase, cytokeratins, racemase) are useful in bioptic samples of the metastatic sites. These markers are evaluated also in the blood stream (serum) of PCa patients. PSA is considered useful as a screening method for presence of PCa disease and for therapy response since it is generally proportional to the secretory prostatic tissue mass within the body (normal and pathological tissue growth). Prostate-specific acid phosphatase is instead present in the serum only in cases with PCa metastatic to bone, particularly in relation with bone metastases of the osteoblastic type.

Biomarkers of Diagnosis

In addition to DRE-discovered palpable mass in the anatomical area of dorsal prostate, measurement of serum PSA is the most useful biomarker for the early detection of prostate cancer. Concerning PSA biochemical and historical information, see also the following section entitled "A Brief Story of Discovery of PSA."

Prostatic cytology (microscopic exam of exfoliated cells in the urine or seminal fluid, derived from epithelial lining of prostatic acini and ducts) is nowadays mostly of historical value, although it has been at the basis of some experimental and clinical comparison research, [35] but is still of clinical interest in conjunction with modern molecular techniques.

A very extensive literature is available about all aspects of PSA testing. However, its usefulness for screening activities of the tumor is still very much debated and widely unagreed. Urinary symptoms are very rare in PCa, since the tumor tends to emerge in peripheral areas of the gland, far from the urethra; therefore, urinary symptoms emerge only in very late clinical stages. Still many cases, unfortunately, come to clinical attention only in a stage of advanced metastatic disease because of low back pain in relation to secondary localizations of PCa to vertebral bone. Transrectal ultrasound analysis can add some objective evidence to an accurate DRE procedure, but the most dependable confirmation test remains the transrectal or transperineal needle biopsy of the prostate gland, sometimes ecographically guided. On the contrary, computed tomography (CT) scans and magnetic resonance imaging (MRI) analysis of the prostatic gland are only rarely of particular importance in diagnostics although multimodal MRI with endorectal coil can produce the best images of prostate and may, through spectroscopy, reveal different levels of metabolites in cancer tissue. This procedure may be of some usefulness for early diagnosis of suspect lesions.

Serum PSA levels represent essentially a measure of prostate cell activity: highly concentrated in the cytoplasm of the prostatic epithelium, PSA is normally secreted in the prostatic fluid and not backward in the blood. If present in the blood in measurable amounts, PSA concentrations indicate that some causes may have diverted some secretion to the blood: this is the case of prostatic inflammation (prostatitis) and prostatic manipulation (palpation, like DRE, even recent ejaculation, or neoplastic disease causing a disarray of PSA secretion by PCa cells anywhere in the body, at primary site or metastasis).

PSA is therefore used in diagnosis and monitoring of PCa, but many caveats must be set. Being a product of normally functioning prostatic epithelium, PSA is regularly secreted in the seminal fluid. In the normal subject, and in absence of the above-mentioned conditions, only very small amounts of PSA are present in the serum. On the opposite, high levels of serum PSA may be found in cases of extensive PCa growth, both localized and metastatic.

In most laboratories a threshold value of 4 ng/ml of PSA in the serum is considered a "cut-off"

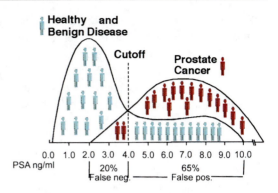

Fig. 13.5 PSA test dependability. A blood sample positive for PSA (assuming a cut-off value of 4.0 ng/ml) is characterized by a substantial proportion of false-negative results (about 20%) and an even more substantial proportion of false-positive results (about 65%), including many different pathological conditions like prostatitis, vascular accidents (prostatic infarcts), and benign prostatic hyperplasia (BPH). Therefore, sensitivity and specificity of PSA test are too low to be generally reliable. This test, however, remains a mainstay of PCa diagnosis

value between normal and pathological results. To rely confidently on such cut-off value is, however, simplistic; every case deserves instead a very careful clinical evaluation, in particular regarding time trends of such values and accurate single patient evaluation.

Estimates of positive predictive value of PSA > 4 ng/ml for the presence of a PCa is 33–47%, in various case series. A PSA serum level between 4 and 10 ng/ml gives a 20–40% probability of presence of PCa, while a PSA value > 10 ng/ml gives a probability of PCa between 50 and 70%.

This situation (see Fig. 13.5) creates a high uncertainty area (so-called gray area) for PSA serum values between 4 and 10 ng/ml, in which repeated determinations and prostate biopsy may be recommended.

PSA, at the best, is an organ-specific marker and not a tumor-specific marker: it may be found elevated in many prostatic diseases, including prostatitis, prostatic vascular accidents like infarcts, and the very prevalent affection named BPH. Even instrumental manipulation of the prostate and ejaculation may increase serum PSA levels within minutes and for the duration of hours to days.

Refinements of serum PSA evaluations have included ratios between measured serum PSA and gland volume (*PSA density*), curves of serum PSA variations in time (*PSA velocity*), the use of specific reference values according to age, and the ratio between free and bound PSA in the blood. PSA density allows to better distinguish BPH from PCa, but serum PSA evaluation is not sufficient to diagnose PCa with high confidence anyway.

With older age, the prostate gland is naturally enlarged, and therefore, serum PSA levels increase. For this simple reason, threshold "cut-off" values of serum PSA should be age-adjusted, namely, around 2.5 ng/ml for subjects aged 40–49; 3.5 ng/ml for subjects aged 50–59; 4.5 ng/ml for subjects aged 60–69; and 6.5 ng/ml for subjects aged 70–79 [36].

Moreover, PCa patients have serum PSA variations more rapid than normal aging male subjects: therefore, a normal increase in time of serum PSA levels should not exceed 0.75 ng/ml per year, while higher variations may be suspect for the presence of a possible neoplasia of prostatic origin [2].

Some studies revealed that serum immunoreactive PSA (the antigen is currently measured with immunological laboratory methods) belongs to two different molecular species: a larger fraction which is bound to alpha-1-antichymotrypsin and beta-2-macroglobulin, with a smaller unbound (free PSA) fraction [37]. The bound fraction represents 80–90% of total PSA, with the bound form being generally higher in case of PCa presence. The ratio between free and bound PSA is therefore usually smaller in men with PCa respect to men without the disease or to men with BPH, since both proteins are produced in higher quantities by cancer cells [38]. Moreover, it appears that the free-to-bound PSA ratio is more sensitive in the "gray zone" of total PSA values comprised between 4 and 10 ng/ml [39]. In these cases, if free PSA is higher than 25%, neoplastic risk is apparently low; meanwhile, if free PSA is below 10%, neoplastic risk is considerably higher.

Even with such improvements, however, serum PSA evaluations cannot be used as a single biomarker for early diagnosis of PCa and are not suitable for dependable screening programs.

In case of suspect PCa (anomalous DRE findings, elevated serum PSA and transrectal ultrasound with dubious findings), a prostatic biopsy is indicated if the patient can benefit from any available treatment and in particular in young subjects with potentially long life span ahead.

Some other biomarkers of diagnosis of PCa have been studied in the past, like prostate-specific acid phosphatase, lately considered without major clinical significance.

One of them is human glandular kallikrein 2 (hK2), a trypsin-like serine protease expressed predominantly in the prostate epithelium. hK2 has proven to be a useful marker that can be used in combination with PSA for screening and diagnosis of prostate cancer. But further developments have led to a reduction in the clinical interest on this marker [40, 41]. However, some claims indicate its usefulness in discriminating stage and grade of PCa cases [42].

Another biomarker of PCa of some success has been the prostate-specific membrane antigen (PSMA): analog to PSA, but membrane-bound, it can be useful to detect circulating PCa cells, and has been related to the identification of patients with progressing disease and in research of immunotherapeutic agents able to attach upon and destroy cells carrying such membrane-bound prostate-specific molecules although with limited success and no practical clinical application yet [43, 44]. Research in this field is, however, still in progress and may have important developments in the future [45, 46].

A Brief Story of the Discovery of PSA

PSA is a 237-amino-acid glycosylated protein, present both in the prostatic epithelial cells and in the seminal fluid: because of its multiple location, it has been discovered in different times by various researchers and given different names, in the years 1960–1980, before being recognized as a single proteic species. PSA is a protein with proteolytic enzyme activity: it is a member of the kallikrein sub family of trypsin proteases. PSA is

13 Biomarkers in Prostate Cancer

Table 13.1 The chronology of the discovery of PSA

Year	Person	Discovery
1960	Rubin H. Flocks	Species-specific prostate antigens
1964	Mitsuwo Hara	Unique antigen in the semen
1970	Richard J. Ablin	Prostate-specific antigen
1971	Mitsuwo Hara	Gamma-seminoprotein
1973	Tien Shun Li Carl G. Beling	Purification of E1 antigen
1978	George Sensabaugh	P30
1979	Ming C. Wang	Prostate antigen from prostate tissue
1980	Lawrence C. Papsidero	Prostate-specific antigen from blood

[Reprinted from Rao AR, Motiwala HG, Karim OM. The discovery of prostate-specific antigen. *BJU Int.* Jan 2008;101(1):5-10. With permission from John Wiley & Sons, Inc.]

produced by the prostatic secretory epithelium in the acini of the gland, reversed in the prostatic fluid which mixes during ejaculation with the spermatozoa originated in the testicles. PSA role in seminal fluid is mostly that of semen fluidification, after ejaculation, by hydrolyzing the high-molecular-mass seminal vesicle protein (responsible of seminal coagulum), to favor sperm mobility and their capacity to fertilize ovocytes during sexual intercourse. PSA protein production is under androgenic control. Minimal amounts of PSA are produced also by periurethral glands (in both sexes) and in other organs (pancreas, salivary glands, perianal glands) and in some chronic inflammatory conditions.

Some of the different names given in time to the same biological entity, now generally indicated as PSA, include: gamma-seminoprotein, semen p30 protein, E1 protein, kallikrein 3 (KLK3), prostate antigen, and, finally, PSA.

A chronology table may be useful in this respect. A recent review article delineates accurately this historical timeline [6] (Table 13.1).

In 1960, Flocks was the first to search for antigens in the prostate, but only 10 years later, Ablin described precipitation antigen experiences in the prostate. In 1971, there was the first biochemical characterization of a protein in the seminal fluid,

by Hara, given the name of gamma-seminoprotein. Afterward, the E1 protein isolated from the human semen by Li and Beling was studied in the context of human fertility manipulation and control. In 1978, the description of semen-specific protein p30 by Sensabaugh added further biochemical information and still another name to the same proteic species. In 1979, Wang purified a tissue-specific antigen from the prostate and named it "prostate antigen." PSA quantitative measurement in the blood was first performed by Papsidero in 1980, with Stamey carrying out the initial work on the clinical use of PSA as a marker of PCa. A huge amount of literature ever since has been dealing with PSA and its clinical meaning, raising many controversies. Worth mentioning is also the fact that early work on PSA was aimed at using it as a forensic marker for ascertaining sexual rape victims.

There is no doubt that serum PSA determination revolutionized the diagnosis and the management of benign and malignant diseases of the prostate, with great consequences on clinical management of PCa cases.

Its clinical usefulness became rapidly evident, soon after the introduction of the clinical laboratory test for its serum-level measurement [47]. PSA testing increased by far the number of diagnosed cases, bringing to the present high rate of early case detection, but in parallel to the high numbers of patients with clinically insignificant disease that would have better fared without this worrisome knowledge.

PSA is currently the most widely used marker in the diagnosis and follow-up of any type of cancer [48]. Only very recently, a slight decline of its clinical use has been described, mostly in oldest men, at least in the USA: but probably, this finding is not generalizable [49].

Staging of Prostate Cancer

Clinical staging criteria for PCa, according to the widely accepted TNM classification, are listed in Table 13.2 and illustrated in Fig. 13.4.

At the initial discovery, 10% of PCa cases are at stage T1. Nonpalpable tumors represent a

Table 13.2 Staging Systems of PCa: American AUC system and TNM systems compared

AUC	TNM
Stage A: accidental discovery A1 focal; A2 diffuse	$T_0N_0M_0$: not palpable tumor, not clinically evident T_0 undetected tumor, focal or diffuse
Stage B: tumor confined to the prostate gland B1: small- or medium-size nodule; B2: large nodule or multiple nodules	$T_1\ N_0M_0$: clinically unapparent lesion (not palpable tumor, imaging negative) T_1: intracapsular tumor surrounded by normal gland upon palpation (discovered at biopsy or after surgery for BPH) T_{1a}: involving less than 5% of resected tumor tissue T_{1b}: involving more than 5% of resected tumor tissue T^{1c}: tumor diagnosed by needle biopsy (after elevated PSA values) T_2: palpable, intracapsular tumor with nodules protruding and deforming the gland surface T_{2a}: involving less than 5% of resected tumor tissue in a single lobe of the gland T_{2b}: involving more than 5% of resected tumor tissue in a single lobe of the gland T_{2c}: involving both lobes of the gland
Stage C: tumor localized in the peri-prostatic area C1: seminal vesicles not involved; <70 g C2: seminal vesicles involved; >70 g	$T_{3-4}\ N_0M_0$: local or extraprostatic extension T_3: tumor diffused beyond the prostate capsule, with or without seminal vesicles involvement T_{3a}: extra capsular extension T_{3b}: seminal vesicle invasion T_4 firm, solid tumor infiltrating the surrounding structures, like urinary bladder neck, rectum, perianal muscles
Stage D: metastatic disease D1: pelvic lymph node metastasis or ureteral obstruction D2: bone metastasis or regional lymph node metastasis or soft tissue iuxtaregional metastases	$T_{0-4}N_{1-4}M_0 - T_{0-4}N_{0-4}M_1$ N_{1-3}: regional lymph node metastasis N_4: iuxtaregional lymph node metastasis M_0: no distant metastasis M_1: distant metastasis detected M_{1a}: distant lymphnode metastasis detected M_{1b}: skeleton (bone) metastasis detected M_{1c}: other sites of metastasis detected

(See also Fig. 13.4). Note that the A-B-C-D staging system according to AUC organization is now widely dismissed and is recorded here mostly for historical interest

particular clinical challenge [50]. Among the T2 cases (palpable prostate-organ confined tumors), 60% demonstrate microscopic evidence of capsule invasion or lymph node invasion (T3).

Metastatic localization frequency is highest in lymph nodes, followed by bones, bone marrow, lungs, and liver. The final stage of the disease (PCa carcinomatosis) is characterized by terminal pneumonia, anemia, and sepsis, which ultimately causes death.

Biomarkers of Follow-Up in Prostate Cancer

While serum PSA levels are not the "gold standard" for diagnosing a subclinical PCa case, serial measurements of serum PSA are instead a very useful biomarker to monitor response to therapy in already diagnosed cases. For instance, a rise in serum PSA after radical prostatectomy or after radiotherapy applied for a localized PCa is an indication of a relapse of the disease. Moreover, immunohistochemical localization of the PSA can allow the pathologist to determine if a metastasis may be of prostatic origin [51].

After prostatectomy or radiotherapy of localized PCa, serum PSA levels drop to "undetectable levels," typically below 0.1 ng/ml. If this does not happen, the surgical removal of neoplastic prostatic tissue may not have been radical or distant metastases, already present, were not revealed. Ideally, PSA levels remain close to zero (undetectable levels) until a possible recurrence of PCa, that is, the formation of new colonies of PCa cells possibly escaped from the initial site before primary treatment. Such regrowth of PCa may be detected by a new rise in serum PSA levels, which are considered significant in these patients, when they reach levels above 0.2 ng/ml after prostatectomy or 1.0–1.5 ng/ml after radiotherapy. This event takes place usually between 1 and 2 years after initial treatment. The rate at which PSA levels rise after initial treatment (prostatectomy or radiation therapy) can be a very significant factor in determining how aggressive the single PCa case is.

A measure of this is the PSA doubling time, that is, the time frame in which a significantly elevated PSA value doubles. This velocity (or doubling time) may moreover vary with time and be related to further progression of malignity of the tumor (usually progressively reducing doubling time in following serial evaluations). This indeed is a bad prognostic parameter. The most aggressive tumors end up having a serum PSA doubling time of less than three months.

Prognosis of Prostate Cancer

Despite the work of hundreds of researchers in the PCa field, there is still currently no exact method to ascertain how each single PCa case will evolve, in which time frame and how it will respond to any particular treatment or intervention. At diagnosis, it is important to establish if the disease had already progressed, or not, outside the anatomical limits of the prostate gland, how aggressive the disease looks (objective evaluation done by the Gleason score), and if surgery was performed, was it really radical (i.e., able to remove entirely the cancerous tissue)?

Five-year survival of PCa depends on clinical stage of the disease, at diagnosis, and on the Gleason grade of the histological evaluation. According to the clinical stage, T1 and T2 stages have a 5-year survival of 90%, with a progression very slow, of the order of 10 or more years [2]; T3 stage has a 5-year survival of 40% and T4 stage has a 5-year survival of only 10%.

Some special attention must be given to young diagnosed cases of early stage, for their long life expectancy and for the usefulness of an early

therapy in case of progression (effectively adopted watchful waiting strategy).

Therefore, receiving a diagnosis of PCa raises in so many male subjects an important series of concerns and questions that need to be resolved, with the help of expert and available physicians and urologists. "Can I be cured?" and "What is my prognosis?" are fundamental questions that need urgent and possibly clear-cut answers, which are, however, difficult to provide quickly and clearly enough to fulfill patient expectations in most cases [4].

Prognostic biomarkers may better define the situation: to discover and validate better and dependable biomarkers is the goal that all the involved researchers and clinicians must pursue. The contact with single patients should be managed by a team of physicians to discuss at their best the various aspects of the problem with the patient. The urologist mostly for the surgical options, a radiation oncologist for the radiotherapeutic options and a medical oncologist about drug therapy options, with a need of a continuous intercommunication between the patient and them and between them as a clinical team: all this is easy to describe in theory but certainly elaborate to realize and sometimes difficult to obtain in real life.

Pathological and clinical findings able to predict tumor behavior have been extensively studied and allow to establish that clinically insignificant tumors (low-risk PCa) may be defined as a small volume lesion (0.2–0.5 ml), entirely confined within the prostate gland, and with a Gleason score up to 6. This lesion may be either unpalpable (occasionally found at biopsy for BPH, stage T1) or palpable (stage T2). The early data published on this issue by Epstein [50] have been validated in subsequent studies, both in the USA [52, 53] and in Europe [54]. However, the Epstein criteria, applied retrospectively to a large case series, have revealed to be inaccurate in 24% of the cases with "insignificant tumors," in which a radical prostatectomy performed according to previous clinical criteria revealed histologically the presence of a Gleason 7–10 PCa and even non-organ-confined disease [54].

Further developments of research in the area led to the publication of nomograms by Kattan (prognostic models) aiming at the prediction of the pathological extent of PCa, through a combination of PSA values, clinical stage, and Gleason score [55] These instruments have been refined in time and are still actively revised and validated [56, 57].

However, the search for dependable and high-sensitivity new biomarkers is still very much needed in PCa.

Therapy of Prostate Cancer

PCa can be treated with surgery, radiotherapy, and hormone therapy, or combinations of them. More than 90% of patients undergoing such therapies can have a life expectancy of 15 years or more [2].

Therapy options of PCa are, however, dependent on clinical stage at diagnosis. Patients at stages T1 and T2 are best treated with radical prostatectomy or with radiotherapy. In T3 PCa cases, radiation therapy is the treatment of choice, having clear that these patients have occult metastases in pelvic nodes and probably also further systemic dissemination sites and cannot, therefore, be cured by surgery. Improvements of the surgical technique aimed at limiting blood loss during the intervention, avoiding postsurgical incontinence and/or impotence (nerve-sparing techniques) have led to much better results than before. Analysis of surgical sample margins, performed systematically at the pathological evaluation of each surgical PCa sample, added further to the efficacy and completeness of treatment, by recommending postsurgical radiotherapy in case of presence of residual tumor tissue at the surgical margin, in periprostatic area where the surgical radicality may be impossible or unadvisable by the presence of vital nerve and vascular elements fundamental for urinary continence and sexual function.

Three very different treatments are available for localized PCa: active surveillance (also named "watchful waiting"), surgery, and radiation therapy. Surgery and radiation therapy have both shown positive outcomes in this situation: they can result in "cure" (defined as disease-free case for 5 years) in more than 90% of men with localized PCa. The slow-growing cancers actually may not need aggressive treatment: so, active surveillance is an option.

But which are the cases truly having a slow growth (constantly in time)? Will these cases really reach death for other reasons eventually (arriving therefore at the end of their life "with" a PCa and not "because" of a PCa)? When is a good time to start a treatment in a diagnosed PCa patient, judged initially to have and indolent form of disease inducing to adopt only an active surveillance strategy? Men older than 65 years and those with low-grade tumors are the best candidates for this approach: active surveillance means vigilant monitoring, with frequent PSA and DRE evaluations, is the best current option in such cases. But better future biomarkers of progression and dependable biomarkers of prognosis may change this current clinical standard which is widely agreed upon.

Another issue to consider is how healthy is the patient overall, because if he is affected by other major illnesses like heart disease, long-standing high blood pressure, and poorly controlled diabetes, there is the solid possibility that a major clinical treatment like radical prostatectomy or intense radiotherapy may have potential complications that may be avoided, in view of the limited survival benefit that could be expected from them, overall.

So it is never enough to remember that every man's circumstances are unique and that only a full discussion between the patient and his clinical team of experts can reach the best treatment strategy [4].

Radical prostatectomy is aimed at enucleating the entire prostate gland, with its organ-confined PCa tissue, and to remove it. In doing so, other structures may be involved, like vascular and nervous bundles around the gland, essential to other important functions like erectile function. Therefore, to save such functions, more delicate surgical techniques have been adopted in recent times, and namely the "nerve sparing" prostatectomy procedure, which preserves the peripros tatic nerve bundles.

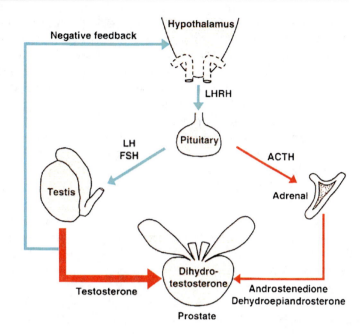

Fig. 13.6 Hormonal regulation of prostate gland growth and function. Androgen-dependence of the prostate gland is a basic feature of its physiology. Prostatic tumors, at least in the early stages, maintain androgen-dependence and can be inhibited by antiandrogens, by castration (removal of testes), and by several hormonal manipulations affecting the hypothalamus-pituitary-adrenal feedback relationships in a complex variety of ways

Radiation therapy aims at killing the cancer cells where they live, in the prostate, and possibly around it: but the prostate is located next to other two important internal structures, the urinary bladder and the rectum, which may receive radiation damage. This damage may cause significant urinary and bowel problems, which may worsen over time (even after 3 years) as radiation effects accumulate. So also this therapy is not devoid of potential undesired effects.

In patients with clinical progression or having regional or distant metastases at the time of diagnosis, the main therapy is hormone-based. Hormonal therapy comprises orchiectomy or the administration of hypophyseal luteinizing hormone (LH) antagonists or luteinizing hormone-releasing hormone (LHRH) agonists. In both cases, the goal is the androgenic ablation effect, capable to reduce the growth stimulation exerted by androgens on PCa cells which are androgen responsive, due to the presence and activity of androgen receptor (AR) in them. Long-term LHRH agonist administration (after an initial transient increase of LH secretion) inhibits LH release and determines a so-called chemical castration. The principles of hormone therapy of PCa are delineated in the Fig. 13.6.

It is worth mentioning the concept that hormone therapy is essential in men with documented metastatic PCa, particularly if they have symptomatic disease. However, for most men, the hardest part of hormone therapy is the side effects.

Although antiandrogenic therapy induces remission of PCa, some androgen-insensitive clones may emerge in the progression steps of the neoplasia and hesitate in hormone-unresponsive disease which almost inevitably progresses to further invasion and metastasis. A rising serum PSA value despite hormone therapy (even with estrogens) is an early warning sign that the tumor is becoming less sensitive to the changes of testosterone concentration. So in parallel to hormone therapy, other options should be considered in such cases.

Chemotherapy options in PCa are limited, in contrast with the situation of most other types of cancer, in which chemotherapy is a mainstay of treatment. This has not been the case for PCa, in which most classical chemotherapy regimens have provided only modest results. In recent years, however, taxanes have produced some appreciable outcomes and are currently considered a valid therapeutic option with or without concurrent hormonal treatment in advanced PCa, especially in combination and aiming at different biotargets at the same time [58].

So, in conclusion to this brief review of therapeutic concepts for PCa, we may stress how it is of particular importance to tailor treatment to each single patient. By evaluating the extent of the tumor (cancer spread beyond the prostate capsule or not), the overall health situation of the subject (heart disease, respiratory diseases like emphysema or asthma, blood clotting problems, hypertension, diabetes), and the age of the subject (younger men usually fare better with surgical treatment, while older men fare better with radiation therapy) clinicians decide together with the patient the best treatment option. In subjects older than 65 years, usually, the best solution is watchful waiting (active surveillance) [4]. New precise biomarkers may help considerably in taking the right choices, based on the biological features of each PCa case.

One of the most important goals is to preserve the quality of life after initial treatment since prostatectomy and radiotherapy may affect urinary function, bowel function, erectile function, and fertility, all deserving great attention and measures to preserve them or to recover them after a transient perturbation.

Current Research Issues and Discovery of New Biomarkers in Prostate Cancer

Great interest is receiving the strategy of targeted therapy in all forms of cancer. Targeting a special key biological passage to interfere with the way cancer cells grow and interact with each other or with the way the immune system attacks cancer cells is a very attractive perspective being actively pursued in all possible biological pathways.

Growth factors, cell surface receptors sensitive to growth factors, cytoplasmic messaging networks transporting the activation signal to the nucleus and conducing to the decision of the cell to undergo proliferation are among the major targets of potentially interfering pharmaceutical actions that can be of high value in cancer therapy. Some of these approaches have produced

exceedingly positive results, like the protein-kinase inhibitor approach at the basis of new drugs like imatinib (Gleevec) in leukemia and other forms of rare cancers (like GIST, gastrointestinal stromal tumor). Other approaches are targeting angiogenesis: some anti-angiogenetic factors and drugs are currently in use and may show further relevant promise, at least in the form of combination therapies, in many cancers, including PCa. Among these we may cite bevacizumab and thalidomide, under evaluation.

In addition, for metastatic disease a very promising approach involving a specific biological target is that against the endothelin receptor activity, of particular importance on osteoblasts, and involved in PCa growth in the bone metastases. Atrasentan is a new drug being evaluated, since it has the ability to block the endothelin receptor, with a slowing of growth of bone metastases in PCa [59, 60].

The research group active in our team at the University of L'Aquila (Italy) since 1978 has developed over time a series of strategies and results comprised within this broad field of biomarker research in PCa and the identification of better diagnostic, prognostic, and therapeutic strategies based on biological parameters obtained from tumor cells of single patients, through in vitro evaluations. An early cell biology approach allowed to refine a tissue culture score able to correlate with prognosis of single cases: this evaluation has been used for some time to corroborate the clinical decisions but failed to gain prompt international recognition although still gives important and objective parameters in vitro in our local clinical experience [61]. An extension of the method allowed an early detection of PCa cases through culture of exfoliated cells [35]. Further search for diagnostic markers led us to consider the presence of neuroendocrine markers in PCa cells, with the significant action of neuropeptides like bombesin [62].

A following line of research involved the detection of proteases to establish a prognosis evaluation in terms of tissue invasion and metastatic potential: also in this case, the clinical correlations were found, and the method contributed to extend the biological data available on the PCa cells obtained from each single patient in our clinical case series [63, 64].

Prostate Cancer Gene 3

Prostate cancer gene 3 (PCA3, DD3) is a recently discovered noncoding, prostate-specific mRNA highly overexpressed in PCa cases, as compared to benign tissue [65]. Similarly to PSA, it is not a tumor-specific marker, but can be useful in evaluating presence and extension of neoplastic disease. A new urinary test for PCA3 has been developed in 2002, with encouraging results [66]. Briefly, the procedure of the test requires a digital rectal massage of the prostate, to favor prostate epithelial cell shedding from acinar and ductal sites (where cancer foci are particularly prone to shed loosely bound cancer cells) [35], their passage into the prostatic urethra and following collection of the first stream of urine (about 20 ml). Amplification of PSA and PCA3 mRNAs is performed by molecular biology techniques and a PCA3 score is calculated, in the form of the ratio between PCA3 mRNA to PSA mRNA $\times 10^3$ [67].

A significant correlation has been demonstrated between PCA3 score and tumor volume [68], so that in some centers, this parameter has been included in pre-operative nomograms, also in view of its potential ability to predict capsular extension of PCa cases [69].

PCA3 test alone, however, does not seem to have a better role as compared to PSA alone, nor enough sensitivity, to allow prediction of extra capsular extension of PCa [1]. The diagnostic performance of the PCA3 test is being evaluated: it is clear, however, that it may be improved by the combination with other molecular markers of PCa [70, 71].

Gene Fusions

Because of chromosomal translocations or deletions of genomic segments, gene fusions may take place in DNA. Therefore, two normally distinct gene transcripts may happen to become a single protein and may determine a trigger point of oncogenesis [72].

A significant gene fusion has been evidentiated in PCa involving the prostate-specific gene transmembrane protease, serine 2 (TMPRSS2), and members of the ETS family of transcription factors [73, 74].

There are different genetic events by which a gene fusion involving TMPRSS2 gene can be determined in PCa cases. Two different mechanisms have been evidentiated so far and are illustrated in the Fig. 13.7.

Current research involving the evaluation of TMPRSS2 gene fusion is in progress, with the aim of relating changes of fusion protein expression and PCA3 levels under therapy in locally advanced or metastatic PCa subjects (Triptocare study) [1].

Very recent developments of this research produced indeed extremely promising results [71, 75]. It was demonstrated indeed that it is possible to predict, via a urine test, the presence of PCa and improve the precision of diagnosing such cancer in the future. Evidence of TMPRSS2:ERG fusion gene transcript, PCA3 positivity, and a noncoding RNA (PCAT-1) may confirm the presence of PCa, avoid an enormous number of unnecessary prostate biopsies, and may potentially save considerable amounts of health expenses in the ever-growing population of subjects with high blood levels of PSA. The high proportion of false-positive subjects can be understood through the graph in Fig. 13.5.

Further Genetic Studies

Genetic studies have produced many interesting results. Among the most recent ones, there is the discovery of a series of genetic variants able to predict aggressive forms of PCa. Indeed, a major problem in the field is to predict which limited number of cases, among the many subjects with PCa, which is often an indolent neoplasm, carry instead aggressive tumors. Five genetic variants have been identified which are strongly associated with aggressive, lethal PCa [76].

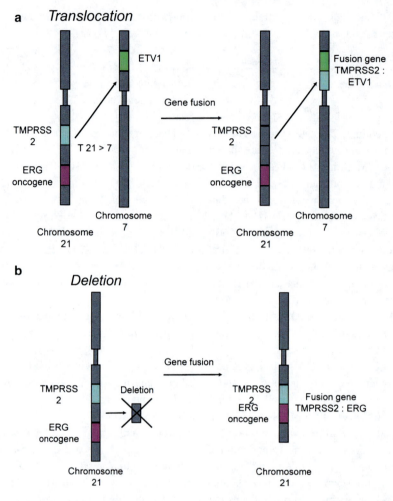

Fig. 13.7 Gene fusions described in PCa. Tomlins et al. described in 2005 a series of recurrent fusions of genes detected in PCa cases. The TMPRSS2: ETV1 fusion on chromosome 7 (occurring in 1–10% of cases) (*panel A*) and the TMPRSS2: ERG fusion in chromosome 21 (occurring in about 50% of cases) (*panel B*). [Reprinted from Martinez-Pineiro L. Personalised Patient Diagnosis and Prognosis in Prostate Cancer: What are the future perspectives? *Eur Urol Supplements.* 2010;9:794–789. With permission from Elsevier]

These are five single nucleotide polymorphisms (SNPs) which have been validated as being related to PCa-specific mortality:

- *LEPR*, the strongest marker associated with prostate cancer mortality in the study, is a cytokine receptor that is highly expressed in normal and malignant prostate tissue. The binding of leptin to its receptor leads to several downstream effects that may affect prostate carcinogenesis, including stimulation of tissue growth, inflammation, angiogenesis, and bone mass regulation. The latter effect, according to the study's authors, makes *LEPR* an interesting candidate for disease progression because the primary metastatic site for prostate cancer is the bone and bony metastases are predictive of fatal prostate cancer.
- *CRY1*, the cryptochrome 1 gene, is in the circadian rhythm pathway, and circadian clock genes regulate androgen levels, which are known to affect prostate cancer progression and may also function as tumor suppressors through regulation of cell proliferation, apoptosis, and response to DNA damage.
- *RNASEL* is associated with hereditary prostate cancer and is associated with apoptosis,

inflammation, and cell proliferation and adhesion.

- *IL4* plays a role in cancer via activation of the Stat6 transcription factor.
- *ARVCF* is a member of the p120 catenin family of proteins, and increased expression has been shown to disrupt cell adhesion, which may facilitate cancer progression.

Patients with 4–5 at-risk genotypes had a 50% higher risk for prostate cancer-specific mortality than patients who had only 2 or fewer of these genotypes. After adjusting for clinicopathological factors known to affect prognosis, the risk for mortality increased with the number of at-risk genotypes (P for trend = 0.001).

Although confirmation studies are always necessary, these findings may open very important perspectives in the elucidation of PCa prognosis of single cases.

Viruses and Prostate Cancer

In 2006, a new finding indicated the possible implication of viruses in the pathogenesis of PCa [77]. Analogous findings happened also earlier in time, without practical consequences and probably only in conjunction with occasional viral infections. The constant and reproducible presence of a viral entity in PCa would represent an important element under the point of view of biomarkers and also of potential new therapy, but unfortunately this does not appear to be the case, according to the available data.

More recent research, however, indicated a possible role of XMRV (xenotropic murine leukemia virus-related virus) in PCa, new human gammaretrovirus identified in prostate cancer tissue from patients homozygous for a reduced-activity variant of the antiviral enzyme RNase L. Neither a causal relationship between XMRV infection and prostate cancer nor a mechanism of tumorigenesis has been established, but a potential biological interaction consistent with a model in which XMRV may contribute to tumorigenicity via a paracrine mechanism [78].

However, a demonstration that appears to offer nearly conclusive evidence, in this respect, reaches the conclusion that, after testing nearly 800 PCa samples, using a combination of real-time PCR and immunohistochemistry, no evidence for XMRV in PCa was obtained. By discussing possible explanations for the discrepancies in the results from different laboratories, it is possible that XMRV is not actually circulating in the human population; even if this is the case, the data do not seem to support a causal role for this virus in PCa [79]. A final demonstration identified in a laboratory sample contamination the origin of XMRV hypothesis and seems therefore to have said the last word on the issue, by excluding the viral origin of PCa [80].

Circulating Tumor Cells

One more of the currently investigated biomarkers in PCa involves the detection of CTCs in blood samples. CTCs are evidently a marker of ongoing metastatic process although we know from experimental data that tumor cells in circulation are only half way through their successful metastatic journey. This procedure of CTC detection is not new, since it has been described and used in several forms of cancer [81], without particularly advantageous results in the clinical setting.

In PCa, however, recent data have indicated that there is a correlation between the number of CTCs and survival in castration-resistant PCa (CRPC) [82, 83]. Further studies, some of which are in progress, will give more data in this approach, to establish how good this evaluation can be as a general biomarker of prognosis in PCa.

Prostatic Secretory Protein-94

Prostatic secretory protein-94 (PSP94), also known as beta-microseminoprotein or prostatic inhibin-like protein, is a small peptide, nonglycosylated, and formed by 94 amino acids [84]. It is one of the major secretory proteins of the prostate gland and, together with PSA and PAP (prostate acid phosphatase), among the three most abundant proteins in seminal fluid. Studies have demonstrated that PSP94 levels decrease with progression of PCa, from a hormone-dependent to a hormone-refractory state. In highly advanced and metastatic PCa cases, PSP94 production is almost null, and therefore, its serum levels are extremely low. PSP94 can therefore be a good prognostic marker in the identification of tumor progression and to recognize the most aggressive forms of PCa. Serum and seminal plasma levels of PSP94 are linked; therefore, its serum measurement may reflect prostate secretory function.

Some recent developments in this field have also indicated the possible function of the PSP94 gene as a tumor suppressor in PCa [85], and even the feasibility of pharmaceutical interventions through the anti-metastatic function of this molecule [86].

Neuroendocrine Markers in PCa

Neuroendocrine (NE) phenotype in PCa is generally related to a rapid progression of disease and androgen independence; therefore NE features are considered a bad prognostic marker. NE differentiation parameters include, among others, neuron-specific enolase (NSE), serotonin, calcitonin, various neuronal peptides such as GRP (gastrin-releasing peptide), bombesin, and chromogranin-A.

The NE differentiation of PCa cases was further investigated in our laboratory, both to find new biomarkers and to evaluate the efficacy of new anticancer therapies; we tried to ascertain that neuroendocrine transdifferentiation (NET) induced by valproic acid (VPA) in PCa cells is mediated by PPARgamma activation and confers resistance to antiblastic therapy. VPA is a promising anticancer agent assigned to the class of histone deacetylase (HDAC) inhibitors. However, molecular mechanisms underlying VPA action in PCa cells are largely unknown and further experimental validation to prove its potential application in clinic practice is needed. We showed that VPA is a potent inducer of NET in androgen receptor null PCa cells, both in vitro and in vivo.

NET was an early event detectable through the expression of neuroendocrine (NE) markers within 72 h after VPA treatment, and it was associated to a reduction in the overall cell proliferation. When we interrupted VPA treatment, we observed the recovery in residual cells of the basal proliferation rate both in vitro and in a xenograft model. The NET process was related to Bcl-2 over-expression in non-NE PCa cells and to the activation of PPARgamma in NE cells. The use of specific PPARgamma antagonist was able to reduce significantly the expression of NE markers induced by VPA. The use of VPA as monotherapy in PCa has to be considered with extreme caution, since it may induce an unfavorable NET. In order to counteract the VPA-induced NET, the inhibition of PPARgamma may represent a suitable adjuvant treatment strategy and awaits further experimental validation [87].

Progression and Metastasis Markers in PCa

Some molecules involved in the metastatic process of PCa have been studied. Some are related in particular to the interplay between PCa cells and bone cells, where PCa preferentially establishes secondary colonies. Among these, proteolytic enzymes (like uPA, and matrix metalloproteases, MMPs) have been studied and found in good correlation with disease stage and grade.

Other molecules of interest are TGF-beta, PDGF, VEGF, endothelin, and also osteopontin, a normal non-collagenous component of bone matrix, found in bone matrix but also present in human milk, and active on PCa cells [88].

For a review of many of those factors, explaining why PCa metastases to bone are frequently osteoblastic rather than osteolytic, see in particular the extensive review by Logothetis and Lin, published in 2005 [89].

Moreover, special aspects of metastasis are illustrated in Chap. 19, with abundant and updated literature references on the metastatic process in many different malignancies, including PCa.

Conclusions

Although established solutions for PCa like radical prostatectomy and radiotherapy continue to reveal optimization in their use, with a very important late study demonstrating how prostatectomy is the best solution for early-stage PCa cases younger than 65 years [90, 91], new and better use of established biomarkers remains an imperative need in PCa, as clearly underlined in other recent review articles on the subject [92].

In particular, notwithstanding the increase of biomarker discovery in recent years, their translation into clinical utility has been limited because of the lack of suitable validation conditions and the need for the adoption not of single biological markers but of panels for them to be evaluated at once in selected patient populations.

Many clinical decisions are made with less-than ideal biomarkers and therefore many situations show the need for biomarker discovery and validation, with a clear roadmap inserting them in the major clinical issues of cancer detection, staging, grading, and clinical significance, which is so important in PCa, a disease with many "low-risk" cases which would end up their lives at advanced age "with" cancer and not "because" of cancer.

As nicely underlined in a recent editorial [93], with time, the prognosis of PCa has changed remarkably, from a first era (around 1980) when most PCa cases were detected as advanced and incurable disease cases, through a second era (in the mid-1980s) with the advent of PSA testing, leading to a doubling of incidence rates and a higher fraction of cases diagnosed with curable disease, and finally, to a third era (today) when most PCa cases are detected as smaller lesions of lower grade. So at present, even among patients with low-grade, low-volume cancer, more than 90% receive surgery or radiation therapy. Unnecessary for many, these treatments may reduce the quality of life, while in subjects above 65 years of age, several data stress the clear advantage of active surveillance as the most valid initial treatment approach [94].

References

1. Martinez-Pineiro L. Personalised patient diagnosis and prognosis in prostate cancer: what are the future perspectives? Eur Urol Suppl. 2010;9:794–89.
2. Kumar V, Abbas AA, Fausto N. Robbins and Cotran—pathologic basis of disease. New York: Elsevier; 2005.
3. Jemal A, Siegel R, Xu J, Ward E. Cancer statistics, 2010. CA Cancer J Clin. 2010;60(5):277–300.
4. Carroll PR, Carducci MA, Zietman AL, Rothaermel JM. Report to the nation on prostate cancer. Santa Monica, CA, USA: Prostate Cancer Foundation; 2006.
5. Farwell WR, Linder JA, Jha AK. Trends in prostate-specific antigen testing from 1995 through 2004. Arch Intern Med. 2007;167(22):2497–502.
6. Rao AR, Motiwala HG, Karim OM. The discovery of prostate-specific antigen. BJU Int. 2008;101(1):5–10.
7. Eurostat Cancer Death rates. European Commission—Health and Consumers Directorate-General; 2008. Accessed Jan 2011
8. Ferlay J, Autier P, Boniol M, Heanue M, Colombet M, Boyle P. Estimates of the cancer incidence and mortality in Europe in 2006. Ann Oncol. 2007;18(3):581–92.
9. Rubin E, Gorstein F, Rubin R, Schwartig R, Strayer D. Rubin's pathology: clinicopathologic foundations of medicine. Philadelphia, USA: Lippincott Williams & Wilkins; 2005.
10. D'Amico AV, Whittington R, Malkowicz SB, et al. Biochemical outcome after radical prostatectomy, external beam radiation therapy, or interstitial radiation therapy for clinically localized prostate cancer. JAMA. 1998;280(11):969–74.
11. Cooperberg MR, Lubeck DP, Mehta SS, Carroll PR. Time trends in clinical risk stratification for prostate cancer: implications for outcomes (data from CaPSURE). J Urol. 2003;170(6 Pt 2):S21–5. discussion S26-27.
12. DeMarzo AM, Nelson WG, Isaacs WB, Epstein JI. Pathological and molecular aspects of prostate cancer. Lancet. 2003;361(9361):955–64.
13. Rhodes DR, Sanda MG, Otte AP, Chinnaiyan AM, Rubin MA. Multiplex biomarker approach for determining risk of prostate-specific antigen-defined recurrence of prostate cancer. J Natl Cancer Inst. 2003;95(9):661–8.
14. Carpten J, Nupponen N, Isaacs S, et al. Germline mutations in the ribonuclease L gene in families showing linkage with HPC1. Nat Genet. 2002;30(2):181–4.
15. Xu J, Zheng SL, Komiya A, et al. Germline mutations and sequence variants of the macrophage scavenger receptor 1 gene are associated with prostate cancer risk. Nat Genet. 2002;32(2):321–5.
16. Xu J, Zheng SL, Turner A, et al. Associations between hOGG1 sequence variants and prostate cancer susceptibility. Cancer Res. 2002;62(8):2253–7.
17. Woodson K, Tangrea JA, Lehman TA, et al. Manganese superoxide dismutase (MnSOD) polymorphism,

17. alpha-tocopherol supplementation and prostate cancer risk in the alpha-tocopherol, beta-carotene cancer prevention study (Finland). Cancer Causes Control. 2003;14(6):513–8.

18. McCarron SL, Edwards S, Evans PR, et al. Influence of cytokine gene polymorphisms on the development of prostate cancer. Cancer Res. 2002;62(12):3369–72.

19. Lindmark F, Zheng SL, Wiklund F, et al. H6D polymorphism in macrophage-inhibitory cytokine-1 gene associated with prostate cancer. J Natl Cancer Inst. 2004;96(16):1248–54.

20. Zheng SL, Augustsson-Balter K, Chang B, et al. Sequence variants of toll-like receptor 4 are associated with prostate cancer risk: results from the cancer prostate in Sweden study. Cancer Res. 2004;64(8): 2918–22.

21. Ding Z, Wu CJ, Chu GC, et al. SMAD4-dependent barrier constrains prostate cancer growth and metastatic progression. Nature. 2011;470(7333):269–73.

22. Giovannucci E. Tomatoes, tomato-based products, lycopene, and cancer: review of the epidemiologic literature. J Natl Cancer Inst. 1999;91(4):317–31.

23. Salmon CP, Knize MG, Panteleakos FN, Wu RW, Nelson DO, Felton JS. Minimization of heterocyclic amines and thermal inactivation of Escherichia coli in fried ground beef. J Natl Cancer Inst. 2000;92(21): 1773–8.

24. Nelson CP, Kidd LC, Sauvageot J, et al. Protection against 2-hydroxyamino-1-methyl-6-phenylimidazo [4,5-b] pyridine cytotoxicity and DNA adduct formation in human prostate by glutathione S-transferase P1. Cancer Res. 2001;61(1):103–9.

25. Gupta S. Prostate cancer chemoprevention: current status and future prospects. Toxicol Appl Pharmacol. 2007;224(3):369–76.

26. Barber NJ, Zhang X, Zhu G, et al. Lycopene inhibits DNA synthesis in primary prostate epithelial cells in vitro and its administration is associated with a reduced prostate-specific antigen velocity in a phase II clinical study. Prostate Cancer Prostatic Dis. 2006;9(4):407–13.

27. Bostwick DG, Liu L, Brawer MK, Qian J. High-grade prostatic intraepithelial neoplasia. Rev Urol. 2004; 6(4):171–9.

28. Montironi R, Mazzucchelli R, Santinelli A, Scarpelli M, Beltran AL, Bostwick DG. Incidentally detected prostate cancer in cystoprostatectomies: pathological and morphometric comparison with clinically detected cancer in totally embedded specimens. Hum Pathol. 2005;36(6):646–54.

29. Rubin MA, Zhou M, Dhanasekaran SM, et al. alpha-Methylacyl coenzyme A racemase as a tissue biomarker for prostate cancer. JAMA. 2002;287(13):1662–70.

30. Gleason DF, Mellinger GT. Prediction of prognosis for prostatic adenocarcinoma by combined histological grading and clinical staging. J Urol. 1974; 111(1):58–64.

31. Tetu B, Ro JY, Ayala AG, Johnson DE, Logothetis CJ, Ordonez NG. Small cell carcinoma of the prostate. Part I. A clinicopathologic study of 20 cases. Cancer. 1987;59(10):1803–9.

32. Ro JY, Tetu B, Ayala AG, Ordonez NG. Small cell carcinoma of the prostate. II. Immunohistochemical and electron microscopic studies of 18 cases. Cancer. 1987;59(5):977–82.

33. Gaudin PB, Rosai J, Epstein JI. Sarcomas and related proliferative lesions of specialized prostatic stroma: a clinicopathologic study of 22 cases. Am J Surg Pathol. 1998;22(2):148–62.

34. Cheville JC, Dundore PA, Nascimento AG, et al. Leiomyosarcoma of the prostate. Report of 23 cases. Cancer. 1995;76(8):1422–7.

35. Bologna M, Vicentini C, Festuccia C, et al. Early diagnosis of prostatic carcinoma based on in vitro culture of viable tumor cells harvested by prostatic massage. Eur Urol. 1988;14:474–6.

36. Oesterling JE, Jacobsen SJ, Chute CG, et al. Serum prostate-specific antigen in a community-based population of healthy men. Establishment of age-specific reference ranges. JAMA. 1993;270(7):860–4.

37. Catalona WJ. Clinical utility of measurements of free and total prostate-specific antigen (PSA): a review. Prostate Suppl. 1996;7:64–9.

38. Stenman UH, Leinonen J, Alfthan H, Rannikko S, Tuhkanen K, Alfthan O. A complex between prostate-specific antigen and alpha 1-antichymotrypsin is the major form of prostate-specific antigen in serum of patients with prostatic cancer: assay of the complex improves clinical sensitivity for cancer. Cancer Res. 1991;51(1):222–6.

39. Catalona WJ, Smith DS, Wolfert RL, et al. Evaluation of percentage of free serum prostate-specific antigen to improve specificity of prostate cancer screening. JAMA. 1995;274(15):1214–20.

40. Cloutier SM, Chagas JR, Mach JP, Gygi CM, Leisinger HJ, Deperthes D. Substrate specificity of human kallikrein 2 (hK2) as determined by phage display technology. Eur J Biochem. 2002;269(11):2747–54.

41. Martin BJ, Finlay JA, Sterling K, et al. Early detection of prostate cancer in African-American men through use of multiple biomarkers: human kallikrein 2 (hK2), prostate-specific antigen (PSA), and free PSA (fPSA). Prostate Cancer Prostatic Dis. 2004;7(2):132–7.

42. Stephan C, Jung K, Nakamura T, Yousef GM, Kristiansen G, Diamandis EP. Serum human glandular kallikrein 2 (hK2) for distinguishing stage and grade of prostate cancer. Int J Urol. 2006;13(3):238–43.

43. Aggarwal S, Ricklis RM, Williams SA, Denmeade SR. Comparative study of PSMA expression in the prostate of mouse, dog, monkey, and human. Prostate. 2006;66(9):903–10.

44. Wolf P, Gierschner D, Buhler P, Wetterauer U, Elsasser-Beile U. A recombinant PSMA-specific single-chain immunotoxin has potent and selective toxicity against prostate cancer cells. Cancer Immunol Immunother. 2006;55(11):1367–73.

45. Fortmuller K, Alt K, Gierschner D, et al. Effective targeting of prostate cancer by lymphocytes redirected

by a PSMA×CD3 bispecific single-chain diabody. Prostate. 2010;71(6):588–96.

46. Wolf P, Freudenberg N, Buhler P, et al. Three conformational antibodies specific for different PSMA epitopes are promising diagnostic and therapeutic tools for prostate cancer. Prostate. 2010;70(5):562–9.

47. Catalona WJ, Richie JP, Ahmann FR, et al. Comparison of digital rectal examination and serum prostate specific antigen in the early detection of prostate cancer: results of a multicenter clinical trial of 6,630 men. J Urol. 1994;151(5):1283–90.

48. Hernandez J, Thompson IM. Prostate-specific antigen: a review of the validation of the most commonly used cancer biomarker. Cancer. 2004;101(5):894–904.

49. Zeliadt SB, Hoffman RM, Etzioni R, Gore JL, Kessler LG, Lin DW. Influence of publication of US and European prostate cancer screening trials on PSA testing practices. J Natl Cancer Inst. 2011;103(6):520–3.

50. Epstein JI, Walsh PC, Carmichael M, Brendler CB. Pathologic and clinical findings to predict tumor extent of nonpalpable (stage T1c) prostate cancer. JAMA. 1994;271(5):368–74.

51. Epstein JI. PSA and PAP as immunohistochemical markers in prostate cancer. Urol Clin North Am. 1993;20(4):757–70.

52. Bastian PJ, Mangold LA, Epstein JI, Partin AW. Characteristics of insignificant clinical T1c prostate tumors. A contemporary analysis. Cancer. 2004; 101(9):2001–5.

53. Carter HB, Kettermann A, Warlick C, et al. Expectant management of prostate cancer with curative intent: an update of the Johns Hopkins experience. J Urol. 2007;178(6):2359–64. discussion 2364–2355.

54. Jeldres C, Suardi N, Walz J, et al. Validation of the contemporary epstein criteria for insignificant prostate cancer in European men. Eur Urol. 2008;54(6):1306–13.

55. Partin AW, Kattan MW, Subong EN, et al. Combination of prostate-specific antigen, clinical stage, and Gleason score to predict pathological stage of localized prostate cancer. A multi-institutional update. JAMA. 1997;277(18):1445–51.

56. Kattan MW, Eastham JA, Wheeler TM, et al. Counseling men with prostate cancer: a nomogram for predicting the presence of small, moderately differentiated, confined tumors. J Urol. 2003;170(5): 1792–7.

57. Chun FK, Haese A, Ahyai SA, et al. Critical assessment of tools to predict clinically insignificant prostate cancer at radical prostatectomy in contemporary men. Cancer. 2008;113(4):701–9.

58. Bologna M, et al. Cancer multitarget pharmacology in prostate tumors: tyrosine kinase inhibitors and beyond. Curr Med Chem. 2011;18:2827–35.

59. Lassiter LK, Carducci MA. Endothelin receptor antagonists in the treatment of prostate cancer. Semin Oncol. 2003;30(5):678–88.

60. Nelson JB, Love W, Chin JL, et al. Phase 3, randomized, controlled trial of atrasentan in patients with nonmetastatic, hormone-refractory prostate cancer. Cancer. 2008;113(9):2478–87.

61. Bologna M, Vicentini C, Festuccia C, Muzi P, Angeletti PU, Miano L. Human prostatic carcinoma in tissue culture - correlations between histological diagnosis and in vitro parameters. Eur Urol. 1985;11: 330–3.

62. Bologna M, Festuccia C, Muzi P, Biordi L, Ciomei M. Bombesin stimulates growth of human prostatic cancer cells in vitro. Cancer. 1989;63(9):1714–20.

63. Festuccia C, Vincentini C, di PA, et al. Plasminogen activator activities in short-term tissue cultures of benign prostatic hyperplasia and prostatic carcinoma. Oncol Res. 1995;7(3–4):131–8.

64. Festuccia C, Guerra F, D'Ascenzo S, Giunciuglio D, Albini A, Bologna M. In vitro regulation of pericellular proteolysis in prostatic tumor cells treated with bombesin. Int J Cancer. 1998;75:418–31.

65. Bussemakers MJ, van Bokhoven A, Verhaegh GW, et al. DD3: a new prostate-specific gene, highly overexpressed in prostate cancer. Cancer Res. 1999; 59(23):5975–9.

66. Hessels D, Klein Gunnewiek JM, van Oort I, et al. DD3(PCA3)-based molecular urine analysis for the diagnosis of prostate cancer. Eur Urol. 2003;44(1): 8–15. discussion 15–16.

67. Marks LS, Fradet Y, Deras IL, et al. PCA3 molecular urine assay for prostate cancer in men undergoing repeat biopsy. Urology. 2007;69(3):532–5.

68. Nakanishi H, Groskopf J, Fritsche HA, et al. PCA3 molecular urine assay correlates with prostate cancer tumor volume: implication in selecting candidates for active surveillance. J Urol. 2008;179(5):1804–9. discussion 1809–1810.

69. Whitman EJ, Groskopf J, Ali A, et al. PCA3 score before radical prostatectomy predicts extracapsular extension and tumor volume. J Urol. 2008;180(5):1975–8. discussion 1978–1979.

70. Lee GL, Dobi A, Srivastava S. Prostate cancer: diagnostic performance of the PCA3 urine test. Nat Rev Urol. 2011;8(3):123–4.

71. Tomlins SA, Aubin SM, Siddiqui J, et al. Urine TMPRSS2:ERG fusion transcript stratifies prostate cancer risk in men with elevated serum PSA. Sci Transl Med. 2011;3(94):94ra72.

72. Mitelman F, Johansson B, Mertens F. The impact of translocations and gene fusions on cancer causation. Nat Rev Cancer. 2007;7(4):233–45.

73. Morris DS, Tomlins SA, Montie JE, Chinnaiyan AM. The discovery and application of gene fusions in prostate cancer. BJU Int. 2008;102(3):276–82.

74. Tomlins SA, Rhodes DR, Perner S, et al. Recurrent fusion of TMPRSS2 and ETS transcription factor genes in prostate cancer. Science. 2005;310(5748): 644–8.

75. Prensner JR, Iyer MK, Balbin OA, et al. Transcriptome sequencing across a prostate cancer cohort identifies PCAT-1, an unannotated lincRNA implicated in disease progression. Nat Biotechnol. 2011;29(8):742–9.

76. FitzGerald LM, Kwon EM, Conomos MP, et al. Genome-wide association study identifies a genetic variant associated with risk for more aggressive prostate cancer. Cancer Epidemiol Biomarkers Prev. 2011;20(6):1196–203.
77. Urisman A, Molinaro RJ, Fischer N, et al. Identification of a novel Gammaretrovirus in prostate tumors of patients homozygous for R462Q RNASEL variant. PLoS Pathog. 2006;2(3):e25.
78. Kim S, Kim N, Dong B, et al. Integration site preference of xenotropic murine leukemia virus-related virus, a new human retrovirus associated with prostate cancer. J Virol. 2008;82(20):9964–77.
79. Aloia AL, Sfanos KS, Isaacs WB, et al. XMRV: a new virus in prostate cancer? Cancer Res. 2010;70(24):10028–33.
80. Garson JA, Kellam P, Towers GJ. Analysis of XMRV integration sites from human prostate cancer tissues suggests PCR contamination rather than genuine human infection. Retrovirology. 2011;8:13.
81. Allard WJ, Matera J, Miller MC, et al. Tumor cells circulate in the peripheral blood of all major carcinomas but not in healthy subjects or patients with non-malignant diseases. Clin Cancer Res. 2004;10(20):6897–904.
82. de Bono JS, Scher HI, Montgomery RB, et al. Circulating tumor cells predict survival benefit from treatment in metastatic castration-resistant prostate cancer. Clin Cancer Res. 2008;14(19):6302–9.
83. Scher HI, Jia X, de Bono JS, et al. Circulating tumour cells as prognostic markers in progressive, castration-resistant prostate cancer: a reanalysis of IMMC38 trial data. Lancet Oncol. 2009;10(3):233–9.
84. Kumar M, Jagtap DD, Mahale SD, et al. Crystallization and preliminary X-ray diffraction analysis of human seminal plasma protein PSP94. Acta Crystallogr Sect F Struct Biol Cryst Commun. 2009;65(Pt 4):389–91.
85. Beke L, Nuytten M, Van Eynde A, Beullens M, Bollen M. The gene encoding the prostatic tumor suppressor PSP94 is a target for repression by the Polycomb group protein EZH2. Oncogene. 2007;26(31):4590–5.
86. Annabi B, Bouzeghrane M, Currie JC, et al. Inhibition of MMP-9 secretion by the anti-metastatic PSP94-derived peptide PCK3145 requires cell surface laminin receptor signaling. Anticancer Drugs. 2006;17(4):429–38.
87. Angelucci A, Muzi P, Cristiano L, et al. Neuroendocrine transdifferentiation induced by VPA is mediated by PPARgamma activation and confers resistance to antiblastic therapy in prostate carcinoma. Prostate. 2008;68(6):588–98.
88. Angelucci A, Festuccia C, Gravina GL, et al. Osteopontin enhances the cell proliferation induced by the epidermal growth factor in human prostate cancer cells. Prostate. 2004;59(2):157–66.
89. Logothetis CJ, Lin SH. Osteoblasts in prostate cancer metastasis to bone. Nat Rev Cancer. 2005;5(1):21–8.
90. Bill-Axelson A, Holmberg L, Ruutu M, et al. Radical prostatectomy versus watchful waiting in early prostate cancer. N Engl J Med. 2011;364(18):1708–17.
91. Smith MR. Effective treatment for early-stage prostate cancer–possible, necessary, or both? N Engl J Med. 2011;364(18):1770–2.
92. Oon SF, Pennington SR, Fitzpatrick JM, Watson RW. Biomarker research in prostate cancer-towards utility, not futility. Nat Rev Urol. 2011;8(3):131–8.
93. Thompson IM, Klotz L. Active surveillance for prostate cancer. JAMA. 2010;304(21):2411–2.
94. Hayes JH, Ollendorf DA, Pearson SD, et al. Active surveillance compared with initial treatment for men with low-risk prostate cancer: a decision analysis. JAMA. 2010;304(21):2373–80.

Ovarian Cancer

14

Jessica Wangui Oribabor, Allison Ambrosio,
Cesar M. Castro, and Michael J. Birrer

Introduction

Each year, ovarian cancer leads to the most fatalities among gynecologic malignancies [1]. For perspective, breast cancers are 90% more common yet display disproportionately better survival rates as most are diagnosed at early stage — within the optimal window for curative intervention. Since early detection is the exception and not the rule for ovarian cancers, strategies to improve screening should promote better outcomes given the marked differences in survival rates (30% vs. 90% for advanced and early stages, respectively).

Screening biotargets represent ideal candidates to identify preclinical and localized disease thereby dramatically improving survival. The current modalities of using CA-125 and transvaginal ultrasound are ineffective. As will be described later, a clear need exists for developing other biotargets to impact incidence rates.

Following a diagnosis of new onset or recurrent ovarian cancer, most clinicians grapple with (1) whether to offer chemotherapy at all in the early-stage settings or (2) in advanced settings, which subsequent line treatment to pursue that could offer the most clinical benefit. The standard first-line regimen for advanced-stage ovarian cancer is a combination of carboplatin or cisplatin with paclitaxel. Clearly, one or multiple biotargets signaling aggressive tumor biology and, hence, unfavorable outcomes could justify the addition of chemotherapy to surgical resection. Eighty-five percent of epithelial ovarian cancer patients respond to first-line platinum-based therapies, yet despite this high response rate, 50–75% of patients will recur and require subsequent treatment to manage their disease [1]. Patients who are diagnosed with recurrent disease are classified (refractory, resistant, or sensitive) by their response to a platinum-based regimen. Clinicians use this information to plan which therapies to use to treat recurrent disease. The growing appreciation for the heterogeneity of ovarian cancers has spurred development of therapies targeted toward specific pathways involved in cell-death and cell growth of such tumors. It is anticipated that their concurrent use with accepted standard treatments will improve overall response and survival. This enthusiasm has brought along multiple candidate agents to investigate in the context clinical trials [2]. Along with the myriad other advanced line chemotherapies available to clinicians, a priori information that can accurately predict tumor response to a particular therapeutic class could help shift the side effect/benefit pendulum toward benefit and help achieve personalized medicine.

J.W. Oribabor, B.S. • A. Ambrosio, B.A.
• M.J. Birrer, M.D., Ph.D. (✉)
Gillette Center for Women's Cancers, Massachusetts
General Hospital, Yawkey 9-072, 55 Fruit Street,
Boston, MA 02114, USA
e-mail: mbirrer@partners.org

C.M. Castro, M.D., M.M.Sc.
Department of Medicine, Massachusetts General
Hospital, Boston, MA, USA

M. Bologna (ed.), *Biotargets of Cancer in Current Clinical Practice*, Current Clinical Pathology,
DOI 10.1007/978-1-61779-615-9_14, © Springer Science+Business Media, LLC 2012

Screening Biotargets: The Challenge

The presenting symptoms associated with ovarian cancer typically result from metastatic disease to the abdomen. Early detection biotargets, readily sampled in urine or blood, with selectivity for ovarian cancers and demonstrated efficacy in the asymptomatic phase are therefore a highly unmet clinical need.

Ovarian cancer is a low incidence disease in the general population with an incidence of 40 per 100,000 per year. Essential criteria for any ovarian cancer screening test includes very high specificity and moderate to high sensitivity for preclinical disease to avoid unnecessary surgery for false-positive screening results while still identifying a clinically meaningful amount of early-stage ovarian cancers. Specifically, an acceptable ovarian cancer screening method needs a minimum positive predictive value (PPV) of 10% (i.e., for every true positive case surgically confirmed, there must be no more than nine false-positive surgeries). With an incidence of 40/100,000, a true screening program must have a 99.6% overall annual specificity. All in all, this is considered a high standard by any screening metric.

Single Biotargets

CA-125

The first screening biotarget for ovarian cancer, Cancer Antigen 125 or CA-125, was discovered three decades ago yet is still intimately linked with ovarian cancer management today. CA-125 is a surface glycoprotein that circulates in blood at elevated levels in the presence of ovarian cancer cells. Eighty percent of all serous epithelial ovarian cancers have elevated levels [3]. Of these 80%, only 50% of stage I disease patients have elevated levels. CA-125 is also found at elevated levels in benign gynecologic conditions such as fibroids or endometriosis, T-cell lymphoma, pancreatic, lung, colon, and even breast cancer metastatic to the peritoneum, and physiological conditions such as pregnancy and menstruation [3].

Since elevated levels are not always specific to ovarian cancer, CA-125 screening has a false-positive rate if used as the sole test, and should therefore be used as a first-line test to determine who warrants additional testing and monitoring.

A prospective study focused on the likelihood of detecting early-stage disease from pre-diagnostic CA-125 values in the general population [4]. From a single serum bank, 20,305 serum samples collected were compared to 11,009 peripheral blood samples collected the following year from the same population of women. Ages ranged from 11 to 98 years old, with most between 55 and 64 years old. The patients were followed from 1975 to 1989 with annual CA-125 evaluations. Ultimately, 37 cases of ovarian cancer, 89% from epithelial origin, were detected and only 23 displayed CA-125 levels at or above 35 U/mL (57% sensitivity). These data showed little difference in CA-125 levels in ovarian cancer cases across cell type, extent of disease, or year of diagnosis. One case of stage IV ovarian cancer was found in the first 3 years of follow-up with a CA-125 of 270 U/mL. Control group analyses demonstrated one stage I endometrial cancer, one unknown primary cancer with liver metastatic disease, and one case of colon cancer; all had CA-125 levels below the reference level. Of those patients who developed ovarian cancer during the study, the data suggested that a pre-diagnostic serum value as low 10 U/mL was associated with an elevated risk of ovarian cancer (estimated risk 3.4; 95% confidence interval 1.3–8.8). Four of seven patients diagnosed with ovarian cancer within the first 3 years had significantly higher pre-diagnostic CA-125 levels greater than 35 U/mL while none of the controls had levels above 35 U/ml (i.e., 57% sensitivity and 100% specificity). CA-125 may thus have limited promise for screening early-stage disease, although the data did indicate that a woman was three times more likely to develop ovarian cancer within 15 years if CA-125 levels hovered at greater than 10 U/mL. The obvious drawback to using a lower reference level for screening would be falsely classifying a high percentage of women as high risk who were truly not.

The JANUS project, an ongoing large serum banking effort, examined various biochemical, immunological, or chemical changes in the

14 Ovarian Cancer

Table 14.1 FIGO staging for ovarian cancer

Stage I	Growth limited to the ovaries
IA	Growth limited to one ovary; no ascites; no tumor on the external surface; capsule intact
IB	Growth limited to both ovaries; no ascites; no tumor on the external surfaces; capsules intact
IC	Growth either stage 1A or 1B, but with tumor on surface of one or both ovaries, or with capsule rupture, or with ascites present containing malignant cells, or with positive peritoneal washings
Stage II	Growth involving one or both ovaries with pelvic extension
IIA	Extension and/or metastases to the uterus and/or tubes
IIB	Extension to other pelvic tissues
IIC	Tumor either stage IIA or IIB, but with tumor on surface of one or both ovaries; or with capsules rupture, or with ascites present containing malignant cells or with positive peritoneal washings
Stage III	Tumor involving one or both ovaries with histologically confirmed peritoneal implants outside the pelvis and/or positive retroperitoneal or inguinal nodes; presence of superficial liver metastases, tumor is limited to the true pelvis, but with histologically proven malignant extension to small bowel or omentum
IIIA	Tumor grossly limited to the true pelvis, with negative nodes, but with histologically confirmed microscopic seeding of abdominal peritoneal surfaces or histologically proven malignant extension to small bowel or mesentery
IIIB	Tumor of one or both ovaries with histologically confirmed implants; peritoneal metastasis of abdominal peritoneal surfaces not exceeding 2 cm in diameter; nodes are negative
IIIC	Peritoneal metastasis beyond the pelvis greater than 2 cm in diameter and/or positive retroperitoneal or inguinal nodes
Stage IV	Growth involving one or both ovaries with distant metastases; if pleural effusion is present, there must be positive cytology to a lot a case to stage IV; parenchymal liver metastasis is present

pre-morbid sera potentially suggestive of early-stage cancer [5]. Samples from 105 women with subsequent ovarian cancer were compared with 323 matched healthy controls. The entire collection-to-diagnosis interval ranged from 1 to 143 months. The median CA-125 collected 24–60 months prior to diagnosis for the controls was 10.9 and 18 U/mL for the cases. Half of the cases had a CA-125 greater than 30 U/mL within 18 months of being diagnosed with one-third demonstrating CA-125 values of 65 or greater. All elevations in the cases were eventually diagnosed with localized or advanced-stage disease. It is unclear from the data the precise stages of disease found because it was not a primary endpoint of the initial study. Of interest, 25% of women with eventual ovarian cancer had elevated CA-125 levels five years or more prior to diagnosis, showing a long CA-125 lead time for a substantial fraction of cases. At the very least, these efforts illustrate the value and need for appropriately handled and properly stored specimens with robust clinical annotation when seeking to validate novel biotargets.

While CA-125 remains the most extensively studied biotarget, it is clear that, as a single marker, it is not a panacea. Other markers and combinations thereof have been the focus of active inquiry especially over the past decade.

HE4

A more recently discovered serum-based biotarget tested as a single modality for screening is Human Epididymis protein, a protease inhibitor from the whey acidic protein family also known as WFDC2. HE4 was initially thought to be a prognostic biomarker in endometrial cancer alone, but recent studies demonstrated upregulation in malignant serous ovarian carcinomas [6]. Data shows that it is expressed in 32% of ovarian cancers without CA-125 elevations [7]. In 2008, HE4 testing was FDA approved for monitoring (not diagnosing) women with known epithelial ovarian cancer under the premise of equivalence to CA-125 performance.

Fujirebio Diagnostics conducted the largest HE4 preclinical study (>1,100 samples) and examined the distribution of elevated HE4 values across various cancers, benign conditions, and healthy pre- and postmenopausal women to test its screening potential [8]. The results in Table 14.2

Table 14.2 An overview of representative ovarian cancer screening trials

Study	Sample size	Population characteristics	(+) Screening tests	Sensitivity	Specificity	Outcomes
CA-125						
Jacobs et al. (1988)	1,010	Postmenopausal	31 (3.2%)	–	97%	1/31 women had stage 1A ovarian cancer
Einhorn et al. (1992)	5,550	Age 40+	175 (3.1%)	–	98.5% for 50+ years old/94.5% for 40–49 years old	6/175 had ovarian cancer; 4/6 had advanced-stage disease; 3 with normal CA-125 developed ovarian cancer
Heizisouer et al. (1993)[a]	20,305	Asymptomatic Women	–	24%	96%	37/20,305 developed ovarian cancer within 15 years of study
Skates et al. (1995)[b]	3,554	Age 50+ and stored serum samples from Stockholm Study	–	83%	99.80%	6 confirmed cases of ovarian cancer
TVUS						
Campbell et al. (1989) [9][c]	5,550	–	388	–	–	5 (1.5%) stage I ovarian cancer cases
van Nagell et al. (1991)	1,300	–	33	–	–	2 (6%) stage I ovarian cancer cases, had normal pelvic exam and CA-125 <35 U/mL at the time of diagnosis
Bourne et al. (1991)	1,601	Self-referred women, 88% with at least 1 first-degree relative with ovarian cancer	61 and required surgical exploration	–	–	6/61 had ovarian cancer; 5 stage I; 1 stage III; 3 were borderline tumors
van Nagell et al. (1995)	8,500	Postmenopausal, age 50+ and age 25+ with immediate relative with ovarian cancer	121	–	–	8 cases of ovarian cancer; 6 stage I; 1 stage IIC; 1 stage IIIB; 1 false-negative
CA-125 + TVUS						
Jacobs et al. (1993)[d]	22,000	Postmenopausal and asymptomatic	340 (1.5%) had abnormal CA-125; 41 (0.2%) had tested abnormal and underwent surgical exploration	78.6% at 1 year/59.5% at 2 years	99.90%	1 ovarian cancer, 3 with early-stage disease and 8 with both normal tests developed ovarian cancer
van Nagell et al. (2000) [10][e]	14,469	Postmenopausal, age 50+ and age 30+ with family history ovarian cancer	180 required surgical exploration	81%	98.90%	17 had ovarian cancer over 12 years; 11 stage I; 3 stage II; 3 stage III; 4 ovarian/peritoneal cancers found in pts with normal US

[a] Used stored serum samples
[b] Developed model to predict ovarian cancer risk using CA-125
[c] Transabdominal ultrasound
[d] If elevated CA-125, followed with ultrasound
[e] After abnormal TVUS, repeat with morphology/Doppler and CA-125

show that 95% of healthy women had an HE4 value below the reference level of 150 pmol (72/76 and 97/103 for pre- and postmenopausal women, respectively). For the 127 ovarian cancer samples, 27 were below the reference level and 82 demonstrated values above 300 pmol. Of the latter samples, 61 were above 500 pmol.

HE4 serum levels fluctuate less in the setting of benign gynecologic processes, making it a potentially more useful test in the premenopausal setting. Specifically, HE4 has a greater sensitivity for its given specificity than CA-125 in premenopausal women and equivalent sensitivity in postmenopausal women [6]. In at least a third of patients with epithelial ovarian cancers that fail to overexpress CA-125, HE4 serum levels are elevated [7]. Indeed, studies investigating the clinical performance of the two markers combined have occurred and will be discussed later.

Ultrasound

Ultrasonography is another modality studied as first-line screening for ovarian cancer. Transvaginal ultrasonography (TVU) is a type of pelvic ultrasound used as a noninvasive tool to evaluate and detect ovarian abnormalities. Mainly, it can detect both morphological abnormalities and changes in ovarian volume—potential indications of disease. TVU provides a higher image quality of the ovary compared to transabdominal ultrasounds, and a morphology index is typically used to distinguish a unilocular cyst with a low risk of malignancy versus a complex ovarian cyst with a significant risk. To date, there have been several studies evaluating TVU as single modality detection for early-stage ovarian cancer followed by scans every 4–6 weeks for women with initial positive scans. Repetitive scans have been found to reduce the number of false-positive cases.

One representative prospective study using transabdominal ultrasound, enrolled 5,479 healthy women, most over 45 years of age, to undergo single modality ultrasound for ovarian cancer screening [9]. Of those women, 338 had positive screens resulting in 326 exploratory laparotomies

that would not have been clinically indicated outside the context of a research trial. Five subjects had stage I disease, three harbored a borderline histology, and four cases were detected with advanced disease. The odds of detecting a primary ovarian malignancy using this modality were 1 in 67.

A similar, yet larger study was conducted from 1987 to 1999 involving nearly 14,500 women older than 50 years or with a family history of ovarian cancer [10]. This study examined the efficacy of annual screening TVU evaluations. An abnormal sonogram in this study was defined as an enlarged ovarian volume greater than 10 cm for postmenopausal women or greater than 20 cm for premenopausal women. TVUs were repeated every 4–6 weeks from the initial abnormal scan. Women with consistently abnormal secondary scans were followed with CA-125, Doppler flow sonography, and then recommended for surgery. One hundred and eight patients met criteria for exploratory laparoscopy or laparotomy and 17 ovarian cancers were detected: one stage I, three stage III, and three stage IV. Only three stage I cancers were detected by clinical exam alone. In the study, four patients developed cancer within less than 12 months of a normal TVU; specifically, two stage II and two stage III disease. Another set of patients developed disease beyond 12 months of a normal TVU, all presenting clinically with stage III disease. TVU screening displayed 81% sensitivity, 98.9% specificity, and a PPV 9.4% [10]. The results highlight the potential for annual TVU to identify early-stage disease.

To improve upon TVU alone, studies have investigated whether addition of functional imaging modalities such as color-flow Doppler imaging that can measure blood flow patterns, can better distinguish malignant from benign conditions. Spontaneous new blood vessel development called neo-angiogenesis is characteristic of some fast-growing tumors that may lead to irregular blood flow or resistance. Color-flow Doppler may theoretically pick up on these abnormalities better than standard ultrasound. To evaluate this prospectively, Guerriero et al. led a study comparing the performance of these two imaging modalities in the evaluation of an adnexal mass prior to surgery [11]. In total, 2,148 masses were evaluated. Color Doppler conferred better specificity (94% vs. 89%, $P=0.001$) and equal sensitivity (95% vs. 98%, $P=0.44$) than standard ultrasound. The pretest probability that an adnexal mass was an ovarian malignancy rose from 22 to 82% when evaluated with color Doppler imaging. This study demonstrated the potential benefit of combining TVU with color Doppler sonography for screening.

Various limitations and concerns still exist with using TVU as a single modality. TVU leads to many false-negatives—instances where results are normal yet patients still present with advanced-stage disease. Moreover, there are doubts as to whether the addition of Doppler would impact the management of an adnexal mass. In other words, it remains unclear whether enough confidence exists in the readouts to render decisions on who can forego surgery and who can be managed conservatively. Due to the high cost of operation and low incidence of this disease in the general population, TVU may also not be fiscally practical as a screening modality. Indeed, insurers still consider them experimental tests and will not reimburse them as a screening tool.

Proteomics

Proteomics reflect the large-scale study of protein structure and function. New proteomic technologies have provided extraordinary opportunities for the identification of novel serum- or plasma-based biotargets. Matrix-associated laser desorption/ionization time-of-flight (MALDI-TOF) technology, a technique used in mass spectrometry, can analyze and identify protein patterns or "fingerprint" from serum or plasma samples. Surface-enhanced laser desorption and ionization time-of-flight (SELDI-TOF) is a lower cost version of this technology that has also generated enthusiasm for biotarget discovery. Correlogic systems, Inc. developed an assay named OvaCheck using SELDI-TOF to detect early ovarian cancer from human serum samples [12]. Specifically, proteomic patterns in serum samples from 50 patients with epithelial

ovarian cancer were compared with serum from 50 healthy women. Additionally 63 of 66 non-cancers were correctly identified as benign. These data indicate that SELDI-TOF analysis conferred 100% sensitivity and 95%. specificity. Although the preliminary data are highly encouraging, the company has not identified the specific proteins corresponding to the spectral peaks used to differentiate cases from controls in this study. Moreover, many have questioned its validity and methodology and wait for independent studies to be conducted and for results to be replicated. The Correlogic case illustrates the barriers proteomic technologies encounter from both a regulatory and scientific perspective. From a regulation standpoint, the tension lies between balancing a patient's desire to tap into cutting edge diagnostics with efficacy and appropriate clinical use of a test. Scientifically, the metric of success for a diagnostic lies in reproducibility within and outside the laboratory of origin, clinical performance (sensitivity, specificity, accuracy), and clinical adoption (is it user friendly and feasible to conduct?) among other factors [13].

There are additional challenges with using serum proteomic technology as a cancer screening tool. For example, it may be difficult to identify subtle changes in the proteome or generate enough sensitivity to detect low-abundant proteins present in early preclinical cancers. Nevertheless, serum proteomic technology still holds potential for facilitating biotarget discovery. If it reliably identifies biotargets shed into the blood circulation by subclinical disease, then profiling their expression within longitudinal patient specimens could enhance our understanding of temporality.

Novel Uses of Biotargets: Combination Modalities

Due to the complexities appreciated in the presentation and behavior of ovarian carcinoma, the screening field has shifted focus toward multiple serum biotargets (i.e., multiplexing) or combination modalities with hopes of increasing early detection sensitivities. An ambitious study interrogating the screening performance of a panel of serum tumor markers (CA-125, HER-2/*neu*, UGP, LASA, and DM/70K) has been attempted [14]. Over 6 years, serum samples were collected from 1,257 asymptomatic pre- and postmenopausal women with a first or second-degree relation or family history of breast, gynecologic, or colon cancer. The findings supported differences in multiplexed values according to menopausal status. For instance, in postmenopausal women the mean CA-125 level and HER-2/*neu* levels were significantly lower and the mean UGP, DM/70K, and LASA levels significantly higher than their premenopausal counterparts. Two percent of postmenopausal women had CA-125 values above the upper-limit of normal (defined as 35 U/mL) compared to 15% of premenopausal women. Overall, CA-125 had a specificity of 98% and HER-2/neu a specificity of 95% but when combined, did not prove any superior than CA-125 alone.

Unlike single-marker comparisons, multiple-marker screening analyses require partnerships with experienced statisticians and bioinformatics personnel since determining threshold values to discriminate between malignant or benign lesions is not trivial.

CA-125 Plus TVU

The Prostate, Lung, Colorectal and Ovarian Trial (PLCO), a large screening study sponsored by the National Cancer Institute, enrolled 78,216 healthy women ages 55–74 to be screened annually for 6 years with a 13-year maximum follow-up. Subjects were randomized to either standard of care or TVU and CA-125. If either TVU or CA-125 were positive, referral to a gynecologist would occur. Recently, the final analyses from this ambitious study were announced to the medical community. Unfortunately, combined modality screening did not confer a survival advantage. Moreover, in women with false-positive results in whom screening led to surgical intervention, 15% sustained at least one serious complication underscoring the need for improved screening tools. The investigators of this major study will explore other screening options either in addition or in lieu of CA-125 and TVU.

CA-125: Risk of Ovarian Cancer Algorithm

Although studies fail to support CA-125 as a screening tool, it still remains the most characterized screening biotarget available and provides the best indication of disease presence. In an attempt to improve the sensitivity of CA-125, the utility of serial tests has been explored. The philosophy behind the approach is establishing a baseline reference value for each woman as opposed to a global reference and monitoring the relative fluctuations from the internal value. Repetitive samples over a given time that generate statistically significant elevations above an individual's baseline are hypothesized to indicate early disease [15]. This is similar to how CA-125 is used to monitor chemotherapy response. Researchers have hypothesized that the serial approach will increase sensitivity without losing specificity and hence personalize the interpretation of CA-125 values.

ROCA or Risk of Ovarian Cancer Algorithm was developed from statistical models of serial CA-125 values [15]. ROCA incorporates age and individual CA-125 values to assess incremental increase of recent values compared to priors. The computerized algorithm was derived by applying Bayes theorem and comparing an individual's serial CA-125 values to two sets of patterns, the first set based on patterns observed in women without a diagnosis in screening studies (controls), and the second set based on CA-125 patterns observed in women subsequently diagnosed with ovarian cancer (cases). The more the serial collection behaves like the known cases' profiles, the greater the risk of ovarian cancer; for example, a ROC of 2% suggests a 1 in 50 risk for an individual to develop cancer, which is high relative to the initial risk of 1 in 2,500 for postmenopausal women. ROCA was designed to capture a better snapshot of cases than using a single elevated cut point. A CA-125 rule using a single reference value when screening asymptomatic women will miss cases with low CA-125 levels, whereas ROCA can detect those cases with prompt interval changes even though they may still remain below the reference level [15]. Also, ROCA can rule out women with consistently elevated but stable CA-125 values above the reference level. Multiple studies are under way examining whether ROCA followed by ultrasound in high-risk women, as determined by ROCA, can be combined to improve screening techniques and whether that translates into reduced ovarian cancer mortality.

ROCA + TVU

The combination of ROCA with TVU in postmenopausal women has been investigated prospectively [16]. Conducted over 9 years and including 3,238 postmenopausal women ages 50–74 years old without any familial risk of disease, every new CA-125 result was used to calculate risk. Based on this, participants were triaged into three risk arms depending on baseline ROCA scores: a woman with low risk was referred to the next annual CA-125 evaluation, a woman with intermediate risk was referred to CA-125 evaluations repeated every 3 months, and a woman with high risk was referred for TVU and consult with a gynecologic oncologist. Overall, 2.6% of women were classified as high risk and in need of TVU. Eight women from the study had surgery, and five cases were diagnosed with ovarian cancer; three were high-grade epithelial tumors and two borderline. Of the three cases of ovarian cancers that were detected, two had stage IC and one had stage IIB. All three had low-risk annual ROCA scores before their values rose. Two had exponential rises after years of normal levels and one doubled (from 10 to 22 U/mL) after an annual evaluation. ROCA had a PPV of 37.5% (95% confidence interval [CI]. 8.5–75.5%) and when combined with TVU a specificity of 99.7% (95% CI, 99.5–99.9%). These results demonstrate the high potential for sensitivity improvements even when combining familiar clinical tools such as CA-125 with TVU for screening purposes.

UKCTOCS

To build upon the promising ROCA with TVU results, an on-going study in the UK addresses their impact on a much larger population of women. The study, called United Kingdom Collaborative Trial of Ovarian Cancer Screening (UKCTOCS), enrolled over 200,000 postmenopausal women with average risk of disease and randomized them into three arms: standard of care, annual TVU, or annual CA-125 using ROCA and TVU for those at elevated risk. In this final group, if the CA-125 rose significantly over the baseline as measured by an intermediate or elevated ROCA risk, enhanced surveillance was implemented with either a 3-month CA-125 evaluation (intermediate risk) or TVU (elevated risk). Interim analyses reveal that about 50% of cancers in both screening arms were detected at early stage compared to the 25% detected, based on FIGO alone [17]. There were significantly less needed surgeries in the ROCA arm (CA-125 followed by TVU) versus the TVU arm; with PPVs of 35% (ROCA) and 3% (TVU). These data are encouraging for ROCA (a combination tool using serial CA-125 tests, a risk calculation, followed by TVU for women at elevated risk) as an ovarian cancer screening tool. This study will end in 2015 and should provide enough mature data to investigate its impact on mortality. Table 14.2 shows an overview of representative ovarian cancer screening trials.

CA-125 + HE4

To move beyond the limitations of CA-125 and TVU, combined HE4 and CA-125 has been evaluated. One preclinical study analyzed 65 various proteins in patients with adnexal masses to find patterns that would discriminate benign from malignant cases [18]. As single markers, CA-125 had the greatest significance between benign and malignant cases while HE4 had the greatest significance for late-stage disease. Biotargets were then tested in sets of two, three, and four, with CA-125 and HE4 performing the best via 83% sensitivity and 85% specificity in early-stage disease and 74.2% and 91.7%, respectively, for late stage disease. In another recent but small prospective clinical study, combining HE4 with CA-125 did not translate into appreciable improvement in detecting early-stage cancers [19].

Another recent study compared CA-125, HE4, and a symptom index as ovarian cancer screening modalities to determine which one independently or in combination offered the best diagnostic accuracy [20]. Seventy-four cases were collected from women with an undefined mass prior to surgery and were compared to 137 healthy, age-matched controls. A positive test in the serum panel needed to have a threshold for positivity in the 95th percentile. Of the 74 cancer cases, there were 50 serous carcinomas, 7 endometrioid, 6 clear cell, and 5 adenocarcinoma cancers; with 31 early-stage cases and 41 advanced stage. In high-risk patients, HE4 had the highest sensitivity at 95% and specificity at 100%. Its other commonly used counterpart, CA-125, had a 95% sensitivity and 81% specificity, identifying 79% of the high-risk and 68% of the early-stage cases. The symptom index alone demonstrated a sensitivity of 64% and specificity of 88%. In this study, HE4 and CA-125, either independently or in combination, performed better than the symptom index. HE4 slightly outperformed CA-125 (100% vs. 79% sensitivities and similar 95% specificities) in high-risk women, the population of greatest interest because it is the only group for whom screening is currently strongly recommended.

Diagnostics

The Risk of Ovarian Malignancy Algorithm (ROMA) provides a mathematical calculation to predict malignancy risk based on menopausal status. Its initial study combined serum HE4 and CA-125 levels to assess the risk of developing epithelial ovarian cancer in patients with an ovarian cyst or pelvic mass [21]. Given that ROMA is a feasible and relatively low-cost approach, other groups have readily investigated its performance prospectively. The area under the curve (AUC) is widely recognized as the measure of a diagnostic test's discriminatory capability. A value of 1.0 indicates a perfect test (100% sensitive and 100% specific) while a value of 0.5 indicated no discriminatory value (essentially random). Van Gorp

et al. evaluated preoperative HE4 and CA-125 levels in 389 women [22]. The diagnostic performance of each marker, as well as that of ROMA, was examined. Of those malignant tumors, ROMA's AUC of 0.89 was equivalent to CA-125's AUC of 0.88 although slightly better than HE (AUC=0.86). In postmenopausal women, ROMA offered a 91% sensitivity and a specificity of 66%. In all, the Belgium group concluded that HE4 and ROMA offered no improvement beyond CA-125 alone. Also recently, a U.S. group published their results from a prospective, multi-center blinded trial of 472 women presenting to their health-care provider (across specialties) with an adnexal mass [23]. Preoperative serum HE4, CA-125, and ROMA were analyzed. Pathology deemed 89 women as harboring a malignant mass with 39 of them being epithelial ovarian cancers. In the postmenopausal women, ROMA had a sensitivity of 92% and a specificity of 76% compared to 100% and 74%, respectively for their pre-menopausal counterparts. Considering all comers, ROMA offered 94% sensitivity, 75% specificity, and a negative predictive value of 99%. The authors concluded that in this study examining real life clinical scenarios (i.e., greater external validity), ROMA can be supported as a tool to triage women to gynecologic oncologists.

In 2009, Vermillion, Inc developed Oval, an assay to detect malignancy in a pelvic mass and claiming to measure the levels of five proteins in blood (CA-125, transferrin, transthyretin, apo AI, and beta-2 microglobulin) to derive a single numerical value between 0 and 10; where 10 reflects the highest level of probability for malignancy [24]. The algorithm used to arrive at a score remains proprietary. Recently, a study involving nearly 600 women compared the clinical performance of Oval relative to CA-125 [25]. Both in early and late-stage ovarian malignancies, the multiplexed analyses outperformed CA-125. For instance, the assay detected 75% of malignancies missed by CA-125 alone and when combined with physician assessment, sensitivity improved to 86%. Increased sensitivity occurred at the expense of decreased specificity, resulting in nearly twice as many false-positives as CA-125 alone. While this may not be so problematic in women already undergoing surgery for suspicious masses, concerns heighten in the context of general screening of large numbers of asymptomatic women.

Prognostic Biotargets

Predicting prognosis for individuals with ovarian cancer and identifying predictive factors that can guide therapy that will impact the course of the disease remain some of the most important goals in the management of the most fatal of all gynecologic malignancies. The current "gold standard" for prognosis uses patient, surgical, and tumor characteristics. The most powerful predictors of outcome likely reflect intrinsic biology and include tumor grade, histologic subtype, size, debulkability (size of tumor leaving the operating room), and stage (the extent to which the disease has spread). Prognostic factors are notoriously inaccurate as inevitably some patients with the most favorable prognostic features die of recurrent disease (10% of stage I and 25% of stage II), while we can still cure 25% of patients with advanced metastatic and bulky tumors with poor prognostic features.

This prognostic uncertainty and the drive to identify predictive factors by which we can select novel and targeted therapy drive researchers to look beyond traditional markers and test and validate molecular and genomic biomarkers, which are anticipated to soon complement or even eclipse traditional factors, further clarifying prognosis and treatment selection.

Traditional Prognostic Biotargets

A surgical diagnosis remains the standard of care for all ovarian cancer patients. Surgery serves to establish the diagnosis and accurately determine clinical and pathological prognostic variables. A proper staging laparotomy includes a total abdominal hysterectomy, bilateral salpingo-oophorectomy, node dissection, multiple peritoneal biopsies, exploration, and peritoneal lavage

Table 14.3 Traditional prognostic factors in ovarian cancer

FIGO stage
Tumor grade
Histologic subtype
Age
Performance status
Presence of ascites
Residual disease following cytoreductive surgery

with cytology. Pathologic evaluation of these specimens defines stage. The stage classification of patients is based upon the FIGO system and correlates well with a 5-year survival at the time of diagnosis. It is important to note, however, that there are major differences in survival reported for patients within the same FIGO stage [1] Table 14.1. This variability and lack of continuity highlights the inadequacy of stage as a prognostic factor, yet nonetheless is highly regarded as the most dependable means of prognosis and the management of treatment.

Aside from staging, the laparotomy also allows the surgeon to physically remove as much tumor as possible, and the volume of residual disease following their cytoreductive surgery is highly prognostic [26]. Optimal cytoreduction is arbitrarily defined as less than 1 cm of residual tumor remaining after surgery, typically associated with a nearly 2-year (22-month) improvement in median survival, compared with patients who have less than optimum (suboptimal) resection [1]. The Gynecological Oncology Group (GOG) reported a 37-month median survival for patients with residual disease less than 1 cm, whereas patients that have residual disease between 1 and 2 cm, had a median survival that was 31 months, and patients with disease greater than 2 cm had a mean survival of only 21 months [27].

All epithelial ovarian cancers are assigned a tumor grade depending on the degree of differentiation of the tumor cells (grades 1–3), correlated with patient prognosis. Epithelial ovarian cancers are classified by their pathologic appearance into histologic subtypes, and include serous (most common), endometrioid, and less commonly, clear cell, transitional, squamous, mucinous, mixed, and undifferentiated subtypes. These subtypes have substantial clinical differences and reflect different origins, and molecular drivers that impact presentation and prognosis [1]. Approximately 75% of papillary serous carcinomas of the ovary are diagnosed at an advanced stage while only approximately 40% of mucinous, endometrioid and clear cell carcinomas are diagnosed in the advanced stages [28]. When controlling for stage, in multivariate analysis, histologic grade (1 well, 2 moderately, and 3 poorly differentiated) and subtype remain important prognostic factors. Early-stage, patients with endometrioid and mucinous tumors have a 10-year disease-specific survival of 85 and 79%, respectively, while those patients with clear cell and high-grade serous tumors have a 10-year disease-specific survival of 70% and 57%, respectively [29]. In addition, clear cell and mucinous tumors have a dramatically poorer prognosis compared to endometrial and serous tumors when diagnosed in late-stage disease.

Universally important prognostic factors also used in ovarian cancer are performance status and age Table 14.3. Based on 2,000 patients enrolled in six different phase III trials, the GOG identified age and performance status as two of the three major prognostic factors, with the third being volume of residual disease [30]. When taking into account all FIGO stages, women younger than 45 years at diagnosis have a 5-year survival rate as high as 67% compared to 12% for patients older than 80 years [31]. Overall, reproducible independent factors that prolong survival include younger age, early-stage, low-tumor grade and residual tumor volume, and rapid rate of tumor response.

CA-125

CA-125 was the 125th, and is still the best-characterized serum marker for ovarian cancer. Initial CA-125, the rate of fall on chemotherapy, and the final value are all prognostic factors in patients with advanced epithelial cancer [32–34]. Patients with persistently elevated levels of CA-125 (chemotherapy refractory disease) have a dismal prognosis. Multiple investigators have suggested

important thresholds for preoperative CA-125 concentration (>65 U/L or >500 U/mL associated with a worse prognosis) or post-chemotherapy values associated with a greater change of cure (<35, <20, <15, <12, and <10 U/mL) [35]. The rate of decline of the CA-125 marker is perhaps the most important dynamic prognostic indicator during chemotherapy with a 50% decline in less than 20 days was associated with significantly improved survival (28 months vs. 19 months) as compared to greater than 20 days [36], and the time to complete marker remission (<35 U/mL) consistently predictive of survival [37].

Molecular Prognostic Biotargets

Ploidy

Aneuploidy is defined as an abnormal number of chromosomes. Cells that compose a tumor may be described in terms of their overall DNA content as compared to that of normal tissue. When this distribution is not in balance, aneuploidy occurs, and is believed to occur in approximately 70% of human tumors [1]. Ploidy studies of epithelial ovarian cancer have detected aneuploidy in 0–34% of borderline tumors (grade 0) and in 50% or more of invasive carcinomas [38]. Many ploidy studies that have included advanced-stage disease have also reported a significant adverse association between aneuploidy and median time to recurrence or long-term survival [38]. Unfortunately, ploidy status as a prognostic biomarker lacks significant substantiated evidence. As such, the characterization and quantification of ploidy has been difficult and a number of studies have not confirmed its prognostic value [39].

TP53

Mutations in p53 are the most frequent genomic abnormality in human cancers, including ovarian cancer [40]. p53 is a major cell cycle regulator and mediates the cell response to DNA damage. The prognostic value of TP53 mutation in ovarian cancer has provided conflicting prognostic

Table 14.4 Studies relating p53 immunostaining to survival

References	Antibody	Positive staining (%)	Sample size	Univariate analysis	Multivariate analysis
[43]	D07	72	54 (stages II and IV only)	NS	NS
[44]	CM1, PAb240, PAb1801	52	61	NS	NS
[45]	D01 PAb1801 D07 RSP53 Bp53-12	Quantitative	73	Worse prognosis	Worse prognosis
[46]	D07, BP53-12	53.7	82	Worse prognosis	NS
[47]	PAb1801	Quantitative	83	Worse prognosis	Worse prognosis
[48]	CM1	45	89	Worse prognosis	NS
[49]	D07	47	90	NS	NS
[50]	D07	47	93	Not conducted	NS
[51]	D07	44	105	NS	NS
[52]	D07	48.6	107	NS	NS
[53]	PAb1801	50	107	NS	Not conducted
[54]	D07	59	134	Worse prognosis	NS alone
[55]	D07	52	162	NS	Not conducted
[56]	D07	48.5	171	NS	NS
[57]	D01	49	185	Worse prognosis	Worse prognosis
[58]	D07	14	187	Worse prognosis	Not conducted
[59]	PAb1801	62	284	Worse prognosis	NS
[60]	D07	53	783	Worse prognosis	NS

results, which may result in part from differences in assessment including the utilization of different antibodies, genomic analysis and more recent technologies [41]. To date, there have been approximately 30 studies analyzing the prognostic value of mutated p53 for ovarian cancer. Eighteen of these studies utilize immmunohistochemical staining, while 12 determined the genomic status of p53. Two separate studies reported that positive immunostaining with the D01 antibody was an independently poor prognostic variable, while another study reached the same conclusion utilizing the PAb1801 antibody. While these data are sufficient to suggest that, utilizing p53 immunohistochemistry, one can detect an adverse prognostic factor in univariate analysis, only few studies have yielded significant results in a multivariate model [41]. Unfortunately, only two studies have shown a mutation in TP53 to be an adverse prognostic factor after a multivariate analysis, and to date, there is no consistent evidence suggesting that TP53 mutation alone is an independent adverse prognostic factor in ovarian cancer. A more recent comprehensive analysis of p53 has yielded another possible reason for the lack of substantiated data concerning the prognostic value of mutated p53. The mutation rate of p53 for serous tumors has been as high as 97% [42]. These data suggest that all of these cancers have disruption of the p53 pathway. However, important remaining issues include the possibly differential impact of specific mutation types (missense, deletion, or truncation), on clinical behavior [43–69] (Tables 14.4 and 14.5).

P53 and MDM2

Recent studies have also looked to MDM2, a (murine double minute-2) gene that is a proto-oncogene encoding a nuclear protein that

14 Ovarian Cancer

Table 14.5 Studies relating TP53 mutation by direct sequencing to survival

References	Method	Exons	Mutation rate (%)	Sample size	Univariate analysis	Multivariate analysis
[61]	SSCP/direct	5–8	63	27 (endometrioid histologies only)	Worse prognosis	Worse prognosis
[62]	SSCP	4–8	41.9	31	NS	Not conducted
[63]	DGGE	2–11	64.4	45	NS	Not conducted
[64]	Direct	2–11	32	68 (early-stage cancers only)	Worse prognosis	Not conducted
[65]	SSCP/direct	5–8	44	73	NS	Not conducted
[66]	SSCP/direct	5–8	39	82	NS	Not conducted
[40]	Direct	2–11	74	109	Improved prognosis in short term, lost in long term	Not conducted
[68]	TTGE/direct	2–11	73.4	109	NS	Not conducted
[56]	SSCP/direct	2–11	57.3	171	Null-worse prognosis	Null-worse prognosis
[67]	TTGE/direct	2–11	28.9	178 (early-stage cancers only)	NS	Not conducted
[69]	SSCP/direct	2–11	55.6	178	Worse prognosis	NS
[41]	SSCP/direct	4–10	47	267	NS	Not conducted

negatively regulates the transcriptional activating function of p53. The MDM2 protein can bind to and interfere with the p53 protein, suggesting that overexpression of MDM2 results in a biological effect similar to the mutational inactivation of p53 [70]. IHC evaluation of tumor specimens from 82 patients treated with the same regimen indicates that 54 and 33% of the cases stained positive for p53 and MDM2, respectively. Since p53 expression is associated with serous type, higher grade, positive cytology, residual tumor, and stage of disease, it supplemented the MDM2 expression predicted of chemosensitivity related with higher grade. The co-expression of p53 and MDM2 was also associated with poor outcome [46]. After conducting a multivariate analysis, it was revealed that FIGO stage, MDM2 expression, response to chemotherapy, and optimal cytoreduction were significant independent prognostic factors of survival.

BRCA 1/2

The majority of families with multiple cases of ovarian cancer and breast cancer have inherited mutations in the BRCA 1/2 genes. BRCA 1/2 play important roles in the repair of DNA via homologous recombination. As such, cells carrying defects in BRCA 1 or BRCA 2 produce error-prone cells with high levels of damage that compromise the viability of the cell. Of interest, recent research has also suggested that patients with mutations at BRCA 1 and BRCA 2 sites may have a better prognosis [71]. Multiple studies have reported that the survival of patients with BRCA-associated ovarian cancer is better when compared to the survival in women with sporadic ovarian cancer. The mechanism underlying the improved survival of these patients is under intense debate. Whether BRCA-associated tumors respond better to current therapies or if it is due to the natural history of ovarian cancer in the two subgroups remains unclear. A study of consecutive cases of ovarian cancers, which compared BRCA-associated ovarian cancers to sporadic ovarian cancers at the same institution, found that BRCA mutation status was a favorable and independent predictor of survival for women with advanced disease [71]. More specifically, Cass et al. reported that BRCA 1 mutation carriers with ovarian cancer had a higher response rate to primary therapy than did matched noncarriers. Carrier patients with advanced disease had better overall survival, with 91 months for BRCA1 carriers versus 54 months for noncarriers of the

Table 14.6 Summary of studies reporting survival in ovarian cancer cases with a germline mutation in BRCA1/2 compared with noncarriers

References	Population	Carriers	Sporadic	Survival results	P for Carriers vs. Noncarriers
[73]	Consecutive cases; BRCA1: stages III–IV; matched controls by age, stage, grade and histology	43	NA	Median survival	<0.001
[74]	High-risk families; BRCA1	13	29	5-year survival: BRCA1 carriers, 78.6%; controls, 30.3%	<0.05
[75]	Familial BRCA1 carriers; age- and stage-matched controls	38	97	Hazard ratio = 1.2; 95% Cl, 0.5–2.8	NS
[76]	High-risk families; sporadic cases	151	119	5-year survival: BRCA1 carriers, 21%; BRCA2 carriers, 25%; noncarriers, 19%	NS
[77]	Consecutive cases; BRCA ½ tissues; Jewish Origin	88	101	5-year survival: BRCA ½ carriers, ~47%; noncarriers, ~22%	BRCA 1/2 vs. noncarriers, P=0.004; BRCA1 vs. noncarriers, P=0.008; BRCA2 vs. noncarriers, P=0.09
[78]	Familial cases; BRCA 1/2	23	17	5-year survival: BRCA ½ carriers, ~40%; noncarriers, ~46%	NS
[79]	Consecutive cases; Jewish origin; BRCA 1/2	27	71	Median survival: BRCA 1 carriers, 52 months; BRCA 2 carriers, 49 months; noncarriers, 35 months	NS
[80]	Incidence cases; Jewish origin; BRCA 1/2	229	549	3-year survival: BRCA ½ carriers, 65.8%; noncarriers, 51.9%	<0.001
[81]	Incidence cases: BRCA 1 carriers; stage-matched noncarriers	24	24	Medial survival: BRCA1 carriers, 4.5 years; noncarriers, 4.6 years	NS
[82]	Consecutive cases, BRCA 1/2; Jewish Ashkenazi; stages III–IV	29	25	Median survival: BRCA ½ carriers, 91 months; noncarriers, 54 months	0.046
[83]	Familial cases: BRCA 1	30	100	5-year survival: BRCA1 carriers, 33%; noncarriers, 23%	NS
[84]	Population-based sample, BRCA 1/2	32	200	4-year survival: BRCA 1 carriers, 37%; BRCA 2 carriers, 87%; noncarriers, 12%	BRCA1 vs. noncarriers, P=0.17; BRCA2 vs. noncarriers, P=0.013

BRCA1 mutation [72]. Further, women with BRCA1 mutations were diagnosed with ovarian cancer at a younger average age of 52.6 years, compared to 58.8 years for carriers of BRCA 2 mutations and 57.3 years for the nonhereditary cases. If diagnosed at a younger age, patients are more likely to have a favorable prognosis (Table 14.6).

Cyclin-E

Cyclins are proteins that are key regulators of the cell cycle movement. They bind to and activate cyclin-dependent kinases to push the cell through the cell cycle by raising or lowering the level of specific cyclin members D, E, A, and B. Cyclin E, in particular, binds cyclin-dependent kinases to move the cell through mitosis. Over expression of cyclin E has been shown to ascribe a poor prognosis in advanced-stage ovarian cancer. Immunohistochemical expression of cyclin E was evaluated in 139 suboptimally debulked epithelial ovarian cancer specimens from patients enrolled in a prospective randomized clinical trial. High cyclin E expression (greater than or equal to 40% cyclin E-positive tumor cells) was seen in 45% of the suboptimally debulked advanced ovarian cancer patients [42]. Expression of cyclin E was not associated with age, race, stage, grade, cell type, or amount of residual disease. High versus low cyclin E expression was associated with a shorter mean survival of 29 months versus 35 months and worse overall survival [42].

Angiogenesis Markers and VEGF

Vascular endothelial growth factor (VEGF) is the best understood of the angiogenic growth factors and their receptors and has been identified as an important regulator of angiogenesis. VEGF expression can be detected in all stages of ovarian cancer and has been found to be associated with a poor prognosis and a shorter survival. The VEGF family of peptides and their receptors play a pivotal role in the process that stimulates the formation of new blood vessels of cancerous tumors. Furthermore, VEGF is an important autocrine growth factor in ovarian cancer, influencing the tumor directly by protecting the cancer cells from apoptosis [85]. Several studies reported an association between high VEGF levels and prognostic markers such as disease stage, grade, and it is prognostic for disease-free survival time (DFS), and cancer-related death (OS) [85]. Numerous studies have reported high VEGF levels in ovarian cancer patients associated with advanced tumor stage, metastasis, poor disease-free survival, and shortened overall survival [86]. Additionally, overexpression is directly associated with the production of ascites. When VEGF pathways are inhibited, ascites formation is disrupted [85]. Frustratingly, no antiangiogenic parameter has been confirmed to be predictive of

benefit from bevacizumab, the monoclonal antibody against VEGF [87].

Maspin

Maspin (mammary serine protease inhibitor) is a member of the serine protease inhibitor superfamily. Multiple studies indicate that maspin suppresses tumor growth, angiogenesis, invasion, and metastasis. Interestingly, maspin has been shown to be over expressed in ovarian cancer compared to normal human ovarian tissue [88]. Maspin is upregulated in borderline tumors and the early stages of ovarian carcinoma and then significantly downregulated with malignant transformation. Paradoxically, high expression may promote the invasion and metastasis of ovarian carcinomas, therefore rendering low expression levels of maspin as an indicator of longer survival [88]. In other studies focusing on advanced-stage epithelial ovarian cancer, non-detectable maspin is associated with suboptimally debulked disease and may be an independent predictor of an increased risk of progression and death [72]. Further studies are needed to validate these exploratory claims, and the prognostic relevance of maspin expression remains controversial.

Signal Transduction Molecules: EGF and HER Signaling

The EGF family of peptides and their receptors are implicated in tumor development and progression via effects on the cell cycle, apoptosis, angiogenesis, tumor cell motility and metastasis [89]. The EGFR superfamily (counting several members) is overexpressed and/or dysregulated in numerous cases of epithelial ovarian cancer. A poor prognostic factor and expression of EGF and EGFR were found to be significantly higher in patients with mucinous cystadenocarcinomas than in mucinous LMP tumors [90]. Further, in a series of 226 patients with early-stage epithelial ovarian cancer, EGFR (ERB1) status was a significant independent prognostic factor with regard to disease-free survival.

The c-erbB-2 oncogene expresses a transmembrane protein, p185, also known as HER-2/NEU. In ovarian cancer, 9–38% of patients have elevated levels of p105, the extracellular domain of the HER-2/NEU protein [91]. While other reports have asserted that the measurement of HER-2/NEU alone or in combination with CA-125 is not useful for differentiating benign from malignant ovarian tumors [92], elevation of p105 in serum or the overexpression immunohistochemically of HER-2/NEU in tumors has correlated with an aggressive tumor type, advanced clinical stages, and poor clinical outcome [93].

Meden et al. were some of the first to investigate the prognostic value of EGFR (c-erbB-1), comparing it to the overexpression of the c-erbB-2 oncogene product p185 in ovarian cancer. These data, unfortunately, yielded results that questioned the value of EGFR as a reliable prognostic biomarker. The study was conducted on 266 newly diagnosed ovarian cancer patients with FIGO stage I through IV disease that had yet to embark on any treatment regimen. The EGFR and c-erbB-2 oncogene product p185 were evaluated using immunohistochemistry. EGFR was detected in 13% of the patients while the c-erB-2 oncogene product p185 was detected in 18% of primary tumors. EGFR showed no significant impact on the survival time, whereas c-erbB-2 oncogene product p185-positive patients had a significantly worse prognosis compared to p185 negative cases. In the multivariate analysis, p185, like tumor stage, histological grade, and age, was found to be a significant prognostic factor [94]. These data confirm the prognostic importance of the c-erbB-2 oncogene product p185 in ovarian cancer at the time of primary surgery, while EGFR does not seem to hold any prognostic relevance.

Conversely, Nicholson et al. examined the relationship between EGFR expression and cancer prognosis based on literature compiled on PubMed between 1985 and 2000. More than 200 studies were identified that analyzed progression-free-interval or survival data directly in relation to EGFR levels in over 20,000 patients. Analysis of these data showed that ten cancer types, including ovarian cancer, express elevated levels of EGFR relative to normal tissues. The EGFR was found to act as a strong prognostic indicator in head and neck, ovarian, cervical, bladder and esophageal cancers. In these cancers, increased EGFR expression was associated with reduced recurrence-free or overall survival rates in 70% of studies [95]. Frustratingly, the prognostic significance is inconsistently reported [96], and the expected predictive benefit of anti-HER-2/neu therapy, such as trastuzumab, has been very disappointing [97]. However, novel antibodies such as MM-121 and pertuzumab are being investigated, as HER-3 down regulation may reflect HER-2 drive to tumor [98].

Aurora-A

Aurora kinase A (Aurora-A) is a gene known to affect genomic instability and tumorigenesis through cell cycle dysregulation and BRCA2 suppression. Its over-expression is thought to contribute to the extensive aneuploidy seen in epithelial ovarian cancers. Aurora-A protein expression is strongly linked with poor patient outcome and aggressive disease characteristics. Further, over expression of Aurora-A predicted poor overall and disease-free survival [99]. Further studies using independent sets of tumors will need to be performed in order to accurately assess the value of Aurora-A expression as a prognostic factor.

Genomic Profiles

The genomic revolution has provided new technologies, which can detail the molecular signature of many tumors. These studies have utilized a broad number of genomic platforms including cGH, gene expression profiling, and methylation patterns. The results of these studies have provided investigators with a variety of potential new and novel prognostic biomarkers. These signatures could potentially stratify patients according to prognosis. Such biomarkers may identify patients with advanced-stage disease in whom standard therapeutic interventions are likely to be ineffective, thus identifying potential candidates for experimental treatments.

Tothill et al. attempted to identify novel molecular subtypes of ovarian cancer by gene expression profiling with linkage to clinical and pathologic features. Using high-density expression oligonucleotide microarrays for profiling 285 well-annotated serous and endometrioid invasive ovarian, fallopian, and peritoneal cancers, they found six potential subsets of ovarian cancer. These tumor subsets had different activated biochemical pathways and patient survival. Two subtypes represented predominantly serous low malignant potential and low-grade endometrioid subtypes. The remaining four subtypes represented higher grade and advanced-stage cancers of serous and endometrioid morphology. Among their discoveries was a novel subtype of high-grade serous cancers reflecting a mesenchymal cell, with overexpression of N-cadherin and P-cadherin and low expression of differentiation markers, including CA 125 and MUC1. A reactive stroma gene expression signature defined a poor prognosis subtype, correlating with extensive desmoplasia. Each subtype also displayed distinct levels and patterns of immune cell infiltration. Class prediction identified similar subtypes in an independent dataset with similar prognostic trends [42]. The precise clinical value of these subsets remains to be defined.

Conversely, another large-scale genomic study by Bonome et al. used gene expression profiling to identify a prognostic signature accounting for the distinct clinical outcomes associated with ovarian cancer. They analyzed a series of advanced stage, high-grade ovarian cancer specimens using the Affymetrix human U133S gene chip oligonucleotide expression array. No clear subsets of these tumors were identified [100]. Although the algorithm successfully identified a validated signature for suboptimal tumors, it was unable to do so for optimally debulked patients. The expression of these genes significantly affects the survival of this particular patient group by defining tumor biology and as such, clinicians could use these genes to serve as possible targets to determine individualized therapeutic intervention, not only facilitating management of the disease, but also identifying optimal therapeutic targets.

Mok et al. identified and confirmed a gene expression signature correlating with poor survival in microdissected advanced serous ovarian tumors. They performed expression profiling on a series of late-stage, high-grade papillary serous ovarian adenocarcinomas to identify a prognostic gene signature, using similar methods employed by Bonome et al., with an independent evaluation to confirm the association of a prognostic gene microfibril-associated glycoprotein 2 (MAGP2) with poor prognosis. MAGP2 promotes tumor epithelial cell survival as well as stimulates endothelial cell motility and survival. Their work managed to develop a prognostic gene signature of biological significance, where increased MAGP2 expression correlated with microvessel density suggesting a proangiogenic role in vivo, indicating poor prognosis, and identifying MAGP2 as a possible ovarian cancer target [101].

Conclusion

Progress in the treatment of ovarian cancer over the past 20 years has resulted in prolongation of patients' survival, without an equal improvement in the rate of cured patients. Through the use of genomic, proteomic, and transcriptional profiling methods on DNA, RNA, and protein levels in tumors, blood, and urine, scientists are looking to identify tumor markers with acceptable sensitivity and specificity. It is clear that detection of a greater fraction of ovarian cancers in the early stage might significantly affect survival. While promising leads have been made in this regard, statistical evidence of a single and reliable biomarker has proved to be elusive. There are no fully validated, clinically relevant prognostic markers for ovarian cancer currently available. Of course, the absence of evidence is not evidence of the absence. There is an urgent need for new and more sensitive tumor markers, and as technology advances in the field of genetics and proteomics, it is highly likely that several new tumor markers will be discovered. Conceptually, there are many limitations in attempting to detect biomarkers as a dependent prognostic factor. Current discovery efforts are highly variable, not only in methods of marker identification, but also in study design and patient selection. Moreover, there is the danger of bias and problems of overfitting the data, as well as the handling and storing of clinical specimens. There is also great hardship in distinguishing studies that are looking for new biomarkers for disease and studies seeking to validate a new biomarker. Nonetheless, these studies need to undergo rigorous validation to assess their clinical value.

References

1. Fleming GF, Ronnett BM, Seidman J, Zaino RJ, Rubin SC. Epithelial Ovarian Cancer. In: Markman M, Barakat RR, Randall ME, editors. Principles and practice of gynecologic oncology. 5th ed. Baltimore: Lippincott Williams & Wilkins; 2009. p. 763–835.
2. Bast Jr RC, Hennessy B, Mills GB. The biology of ovarian cancer: new opportunities for translation. Nat Rev Cancer. 2009;9:415–28.
3. Hennessy BT, Coleman RL, Markman M. Ovarian cancer. Lancet. 2009;374:1371–82.
4. Helzlsouer KJ, Bush TL, Alberg AJ, Bass KM, Zacur H, Comstock GW. Prospective study of serum CA-125 levels as markers of ovarian cancer. JAMA. 1993;269:1123–6.
5. Jellum E, Andersen A, Lund-Larsen P, Theodorsen L, Orjasaeter H. Experiences of the Janus Serum Bank in Norway. Environ Health Perspect. 1995;103 Suppl 3:85–8.
6. Hellstrom I, Raycraft J, Hayden-Ledbetter M, et al. The HE4 (WFDC2) protein is a biomarker for ovarian carcinoma. Cancer Res. 2003;63:3695–700.
7. Rosen DG, Wang L, Atkinson JN, et al. Potential markers that complement expression of CA125 in epithelial ovarian cancer. Gynecol Oncol. 2005;99:267–77.
8. Fujirebio Diagnostics I. HE4 EIA [package insert]. Malvern, PA; 2008.
9. Campbell S, Bhan V, Royston P, Whitehead MI, Collins WP. Transabdominal ultrasound screening for early ovarian cancer. BMJ. 1989;299:1363–7.
10. Van Nagell Jr JR, DePriest PD, Reedy MB, et al. The efficacy of transvaginal sonographic screening in asymptomatic women at risk for ovarian cancer. Gynecol Oncol. 2000;77:350–6.
11. Guerriero S, Alcazar JL, Ajossa S, et al. Transvaginal color Doppler imaging in the detection of ovarian cancer in a large study population. Int J Gynecol Cancer. 2010;20:781–6.
12. Petricoin EF, Ardekani AM, Hitt BA, et al. Use of proteomic patterns in serum to identify ovarian cancer. Lancet. 2002;359:572–7.
13. Giljohann DA, Mirkin CA. Drivers of biodiagnostic development. Nature. 2009;462:461–4.
14. Cane P, Azen C, Lopez E, Platt LD, Karlan BY. Tumor marker trends in asymptomatic women at risk for ovarian cancer: relevance for ovarian cancer screening. Gynecol Oncol. 1995;57:240–5.
15. Skates SJ, Menon U, MacDonald N, et al. Calculation of the risk of ovarian cancer from serial CA-125 values for preclinical detection in postmenopausal women. J Clin Oncol. 2003;21:206s–10.
16. Lu KH, Skates SJ, Bevers TB, et al. A prospective U.S. ovarian cancer screening study using the risk of ovarian cancer algorithm (ROCA). J Clin Oncol. 2010;28(suppl). abstr 5003.
17. Menon U, Gentry-Maharaj A, Hallett R, et al. Sensitivity and specificity of multimodal and ultrasound screening for ovarian cancer, and stage distribution of detected cancers: results of the prevalence screen of the UK Collaborative Trial of Ovarian Cancer Screening (UKCTOCS). Lancet Oncol. 2009;10:327–40.
18. Nolen B, Velikokhatnaya L, Marrangoni A, et al. Serum biomarker panels for the discrimination of benign from malignant cases in patients with an adnexal mass. Gynecol Oncol. 2010;117:440–5.
19. Jacob F, Meier M, Caduff R, et al. No benefit from combining HE4 and CA125 as ovarian tumor markers in a clinical setting. Gynecol Oncol. 2011;121:487–91.
20. Andersen MR, Goff BA, Lowe KA, et al. Use of a Symptom Index, CA125, and HE4 to predict ovarian cancer. Gynecol Oncol. 2010;116:378–83.
21. Moore RG, Miller MC, Disilvestro P, et al. Evaluation of the diagnostic accuracy of the risk of ovarian malignancy algorithm in women with a pelvic mass. Obstet Gynecol. 2011;118:280–8.
22. Van Gorp T, Cadron I, Despierre E, et al. HE4 and CA125 as a diagnostic test in ovarian cancer: prospective validation of the Risk of Ovarian Malignancy Algorithm. Br J Cancer. 2011;104:863–70.
23. Moore RG, McMeekin DS, Brown AK, et al. A novel multiple marker bioassay utilizing HE4 and CA125 for the prediction of ovarian cancer in patients with a pelvic mass. Gynecol Oncol. 2009;112:40–6.
24. Zhang Z, Chan DW. The road from discovery to clinical diagnostics: lessons learned from the first FDA-cleared in vitro diagnostic multivariate index assay of proteomic biomarkers. Cancer Epidemiol Biomarkers Prev. 2010;19:2995–9.
25. Ueland FR, Desimone CP, Seamon LG, et al. Effectiveness of a multivariate index assay in the preoperative assessment of ovarian tumors. Obstet Gynecol. 2011;117:1289–97.
26. Holschneider C, Berek J. Ovarian cancer: epidemiology, biology and prognostic factors. Semin Surg Oncol. 2000;19(1):3–10.
27. Bristow RE, Puri I, Chi DS. Cytoreductive surgery for recurrent ovarian cancer: a meta-analysis. Gynecol Oncol. 2009;112:265–74.
28. Kaku T, Ogawa S, Kawano Y, et al. Histological classification of ovarian cancer. Med Electron Microsc. 2003;36:9–17.

29. Kobel M, Kalloger SE, Santos JL, Huntsman DG, Gilks CB, Swenerton KD. Tumor type and substage predict survival in stage I and II ovarian carcinoma: insights and implications. Gynecol Oncol. 2010;116:50–6.

30. Thigpen T, Brady MF, Omura GA, et al. Age as a prognostic factor in ovarian carcinoma. The Gynecologic Oncology Group experience. Cancer. 1993;71:606–14.

31. Omura GA, Brady MF, Homesley HD, et al. Long-term follow-up and prognostic factor analysis in advanced ovarian carcinoma: the Gynecologic Oncology Group experience. J Clin Oncol. 1991;9:1138–50.

32. Cooper BC, Sood AK, Davis CS, et al. Preoperative CA 125 levels: an independent prognostic factor for epithelial ovarian cancer. Obstet Gynecol. 2002;100:59–64.

33. Gadducci A, Cosio S, Fanucchi A, Negri S, Cristofani R, Genazzani AR. The predictive and prognostic value of serum CA 125 half-life during paclitaxel/platinum-based chemotherapy in patients with advanced ovarian carcinoma. Gynecol Oncol. 2004;93:131–6.

34. Rustin GJ. The clinical value of tumour markers in the management of ovarian cancer. Ann Clin Biochem. 1996;33(Pt 4):284–9.

35. Meyer T, Rustin GJ. Role of tumour markers in monitoring epithelial ovarian cancer. Br J Cancer. 2000;82:1535–8.

36. Verheijen RH, von Mensdorff-Pouilly S, van Kamp GJ, Kenemans P. CA 125: fundamental and clinical aspects. Semin Cancer Biol. 1999;9:117–24.

37. Riedinger JM, Wafflart J, Ricolleau G, et al. CA 125 half-life and CA 125 nadir during induction chemotherapy are independent predictors of epithelial ovarian cancer outcome: results of a French multicentric study. Ann Oncol. 2006;17:1234–8.

38. Diaz-Montes TaB, RE. Clinical predictors of outcome in epithelial ovarian carcinoma. In: Levenback C, Sood, AK, Lu, KH, Coleman, R, editors. Prognostic and predictive factors in gynecologic cancers. Houston, TX: Informa; 2007. p. 9.

39. Skirnisdottir I, Sorbe B, Karlsson M, Seidal T. Prognostic importance of DNA ploidy and p53 in early stages of epithelial ovarian carcinoma. Int J Oncol. 2001;19:1295–302.

40. Havrilesky L, Darcy M, Hamdan H, et al. Prognostic significance of p53 mutation and p53 overexpression in advanced epithelial ovarian cancer: a Gynecologic Oncology Group Study. J Clin Oncol. 2003;21:3814–25.

41. Rose SL. TP53/p53 as a prognostic factor. In: Levenback C, Sood AK, Lu KH, Coleman R, editors. Prognostic and predictive factors in gynecologic cancers. Houston, TX: Informa; 2007. p. 45–61.

42. Tothill RW, Tinker AV, George J, et al. Novel molecular subtypes of serous and endometrioid ovarian cancer linked to clinical outcome. Clin Cancer Res. 2008;14:5198–208.

43. Goff BA, Ries JA, Els LP, Coltrera MD, Gown AM. Immunophenotype of ovarian cancer as predictor of clinical outcome: evaluation at primary surgery and second-look procedure. Gynecol Oncol. 1998;70:378–85.

44. Allan LA, Campbell MK, Milner BJ, et al. The significance of p53 mutation and over-expression in ovarian cancer prognosis. Int J Gynecol Cancer. 1996;6:483–90.

45. Tachibana M, Watanabe J, Matsushima Y, et al. Independence of the prognostic value of tumor suppressor protein expression in ovarian adenocarcinomas: a multivariate analysis of expression of p53, retinoblastoma, and related proteins. Int J Gynecol Cancer. 2003;13:598–606.

46. Dogan E, Saygili U, Tuna B, et al. p53 and mdm2 as prognostic indicators in patients with epithelial ovarian cancer: a multivariate analysis. Gynecol Oncol. 2005;97:46–52.

47. Geisler JP, Geisler HE, Wiemann MC, Givens SS, Zhou Z, Miller GA. Quantification of p53 in epithelial ovarian cancer. Gynecol Oncol. 1997;66:435–8.

48. van der Zee AG, Hollema H, Suurmeijer AJ, et al. Value of P-glycoprotein, glutathione S-transferase pi, c-erbB-2, and p53 as prognostic factors in ovarian carcinomas. J Clin Oncol. 1995;13:70–8.

49. Sagarra RA, Andrade LA, Martinez EZ, Pinto GA, Syrjanen KJ, Derchain SF. P53 and Bcl-2 as prognostic predictors in epithelial ovarian cancer. Int J Gynecol Cancer. 2002;12:720–7.

50. Sheridan E, Silcocks P, Smith J, Hancock BW, Goyns MH. P53 mutation in a series of epithelial ovarian cancers from the U.K., and its prognostic significance. Eur J Cancer. 1994;30A:1701–4.

51. Mano Y, Kikuchi Y, Yamamoto K, et al. Bcl-2 as a predictor of chemosensitivity and prognosis in primary epithelial ovarian cancer. Eur J Cancer. 1999;35:1214–9.

52. Hashiguchi Y, Tsuda H, Inoue T, Nishimura S, Suzuki T, Kawamura N. Alteration of cell cycle regulators correlates with survival in epithelial ovarian cancer patients. Hum Pathol. 2004;35:165–75.

53. Marks JR, Davidoff AM, Kerns BJ, et al. Overexpression and mutation of p53 in epithelial ovarian cancer. Cancer Res. 1991;51:2979–84.

54. Bali A, O'Brien PM, Edwards LS, Sutherland RL, Hacker NF, Henshall SM. Cyclin D1, p53, and p21Waf1/Cip1 expression is predictive of poor clinical outcome in serous epithelial ovarian cancer. Clin Cancer Res. 2004;10:5168–77.

55. Ferrandina G, Fagotti A, Salerno MG, et al. p53 overexpression is associated with cytoreduction and response to chemotherapy in ovarian cancer. Br J Cancer. 1999;81:733–40.

56. Shahin MS, Hughes JH, Sood AK, Buller RE. The prognostic significance of p53 tumor suppressor gene alterations in ovarian carcinoma. Cancer. 2000;89:2006–17.

57. Baekelandt M, Kristensen GB, Nesland JM, Trope CG, Holm R. Clinical significance of apoptosis-related factors p53, Mdm2, and Bcl-2 in advanced ovarian cancer. J Clin Oncol. 1999;17:2061.

58. Marx D, Meden H, Ziemek T, Lenthe T, Kuhn W, Schauer A. Expression of the p53 tumour suppressor gene as a prognostic marker in platinum-treated patients with ovarian cancer. Eur J Cancer. 1998;34:845–50.

59. Hartmann LC, Podratz KC, Keeney GL, et al. Prognostic significance of p53 immunostaining in epithelial ovarian cancer. J Clin Oncol. 1994;12:64–9.

60. Nielsen JS, Jakobsen E, Holund B, Bertelsen K, Jakobsen A. Prognostic significance of p53, Her-2, and EGFR overexpression in borderline and epithelial ovarian cancer. Int J Gynecol Cancer. 2004;14:1086–96.

61. Okuda T, Otsuka J, Sekizawa A, et al. p53 mutations and overexpression affect prognosis of ovarian endometrioid cancer but not clear cell cancer. Gynecol Oncol. 2003;88:318–25.

62. Niwa K, Itoh M, Murase T, et al. Alteration of p53 gene in ovarian carcinoma: clinicopathological correlation and prognostic significance. Br J Cancer. 1994;70:1191–7.

63. Smith-Sorensen B, Kaern J, Holm R, Dorum A, Trope C, Borresen-Dale AL. Therapy effect of either paclitaxel or cyclophosphamide combination treatment in patients with epithelial ovarian cancer and relation to TP53 gene status. Br J Cancer. 1998;78:375–81.

64. Leitao Jr MM, Boyd J, Hummer A, et al. Clinicopathologic analysis of early-stage sporadic ovarian carcinoma. Am J Surg Pathol. 2004;28:147–59.

65. Fallows S, Price J, Atkinson RJ, Johnston PG, Hickey I, Russell SE. P53 mutation does not affect prognosis in ovarian epithelial malignancies. J Pathol. 2001;194:68–75.

66. Schuyer M, van der Burg ME, Henzen-Logmans SC, et al. Reduced expression of BAX is associated with poor prognosis in patients with epithelial ovarian cancer: a multifactorial analysis of TP53, p21, BAX and BCL-2. Br J Cancer. 2001;85:1359–67.

67. Wang Y, Helland A, Holm R, et al. TP53 mutations in early-stage ovarian carcinoma, relation to long-term survival. Br J Cancer. 2004;90:678–85.

68. Wang Y, Kringen P, Kristensen GB, et al. Effect of the codon 72 polymorphism (c.215G>C, p.Arg72Pro) in combination with somatic sequence variants in the TP53 gene on survival in patients with advanced ovarian carcinoma. Hum Mutat. 2004;24:21–34.

69. Reles A, Wen WH, Schmider A, et al. Correlation of p53 mutations with resistance to platinum-based chemotherapy and shortened survival in ovarian cancer. Clin Cancer Res. 2001;7:2984–97.

70. Bai L, Zhu WG. p53: Structure, Function and Therapeutic Applications. J Cancer Mol. 2006;2:141–53.

71. Chu CS, Rubin SC. Influence of BRCA1 and BRCA2 on Ovarian Cancer Survival. In: Levenback C, Sood AK, Lu KH, Coleman R, editors. Prognostic and predictive factors in gynecologic cancers. Houston, TX: Informa; 2007. p. 15–23.

72. Secord AA, Lee PS, Darcy KM, et al. Maspin expression in epithelial ovarian cancer and associations with poor prognosis: a Gynecologic Oncology Group study. Gynecol Oncol. 2006;101:390–7.

73. Rubin SC, Benjamin I, Behbakht K, et al. Clinical and pathological features of ovarian cancer in women with germ-line mutations of BRCA1. N Engl J Med. 1996;335:1413–6.

74. Aida H, Takakuwa K, Nagata H, et al. Clinical features of ovarian cancer in Japanese women with germ-line mutations of BRCA1. Clin Cancer Res. 1998;4:235–40.

75. Johannsson OT, Ranstam J, Borg A, Olsson H. Survival of BRCA1 breast and ovarian cancer patients: a population-based study from southern Sweden. J Clin Oncol. 1998;16:397–404.

76. Pharoah PD, Easton DF, Stockton DL, Gayther S, Ponder BA. Survival in familial, BRCA1-associated, and BRCA2-associated epithelial ovarian cancer. United Kingdom Coordinating Committee for Cancer Research (UKCCCR) Familial Ovarian Cancer Study Group. Cancer Res. 1999;59:868–71.

77. Boyd J, Sonoda Y, Federici MG, et al. Clinicopathologic features of BRCA-linked and sporadic ovarian cancer. JAMA. 2000;283:2260–5.

78. Zweemer RP, Verheijen RH, Coebergh JW, et al. Survival analysis in familial ovarian cancer, a case control study. Eur J Obstet Gynecol Reprod Biol. 2001;98:219–23.

79. Ramus SJ, Fishman A, Pharoah PD, Yarkoni S, Altaras M, Ponder BA. Ovarian cancer survival in Ashkenazi Jewish patients with BRCA1 and BRCA2 mutations. Eur J Surg Oncol. 2001;27:278–81.

80. Ben David Y, Chetrit A, Hirsh-Yechezkel G, et al. Effect of BRCA mutations on the length of survival in epithelial ovarian tumors. J Clin Oncol. 2002;20:463–6.

81. Buller RE, Shahin MS, Geisler JP, Zogg M, De Young BR, Davis CS. Failure of BRCA1 dysfunction to alter ovarian cancer survival. Clin Cancer Res. 2002;8:1196–202.

82. Cass I, Baldwin RL, Varkey T, Moslehi R, Narod SA, Karlan BY. Improved survival in women with BRCA-associated ovarian carcinoma. Cancer. 2003;97:2187–95.

83. Kringen P, Wang Y, Dumeaux V, et al. TP53 mutations in ovarian carcinomas from sporadic cases and carriers of two distinct BRCA1 founder mutations; relation to age at diagnosis and survival. BMC Cancer. 2005;5:134.

84. Pal T, Permuth-Wey J, Kapoor R, Cantor A, Sutphen R. Improved survival in BRCA2 carriers with ovarian cancer. Fam Cancer. 2007;6:113–9.

85. Banerjee S, Gore M. The future of targeted therapies in ovarian cancer. Oncologist. 2009;14:706–16.

86. Lose F, Nagle CM, O'Mara T, et al. Vascular endothelial growth factor gene polymorphisms and ovarian cancer survival. Gynecol Oncol. 2011;119:479–83.

87. Horowitz NS, Penson RT, Duda DG, et al. Safety, efficacy, and biomarker exploration in a phase II study of bevacizumab, oxaliplatin, and gemcitabine in recurrent Mullerian carcinoma. Clin Ovarian Cancer Other Gynecol Malig. 2011;4:26–33.

88. Sood AK, Fletcher MS, Gruman LM, et al. The paradoxical expression of maspin in ovarian carcinoma. Clin Cancer Res. 2002;8:2924–32.

89. Mackay HJ, Oza AM. Other new targets. Int J Gynecol Cancer. 2009;19 Suppl 2:S49–54.

90. Shen GH, Ghazizadeh M, Kawanami O, et al. Prognostic significance of vascular endothelial growth factor expression in human ovarian carcinoma. Br J Cancer. 2000;83:196–203.

91. Meden H, Fattahi-Meibodi A, Marx D. ELISA-based quantification of p105 (c-erbB-2, HER2/neu) in serum of ovarian carcinoma. Methods Mol Med. 2001;39:125–33.

92. Cheung TH, Wong YF, Chung TK, Maimonis P, Chang AM. Clinical use of serum c-erbB-2 in patients with ovarian masses. Gynecol Obstet Invest. 1999;48:133–7.

93. Hellstrom I, Goodman G, Pullman J, Yang Y, Hellstrom KE. Overexpression of HER-2 in ovarian carcinomas. Cancer Res. 2001;61:2420–3.

94. Meden H, Marx D, Raab T, Kron M, Schauer A, Kuhn W. EGF-R and overexpression of the oncogene c-erbB-2 in ovarian cancer: immunohistochemical findings and prognostic value. J Obstet Gynaecol (Tokyo 1995). 1995;21:167–78.

95. Nicholson RI, Gee JM, Harper ME. EGFR and cancer prognosis. Eur J Cancer. 2001;37 Suppl 4:S9–15.

96. Elie C, Geay JF, Morcos M, et al. Lack of relationship between EGFR-1 immunohistochemical expression and prognosis in a multicentre clinical trial of 93 patients with advanced primary ovarian epithelial cancer (GINECO group). Br J Cancer. 2004;91:470–5.

97. Bookman MA, Darcy KM, Clarke-Pearson D, Boothby RA, Horowitz IR. Evaluation of monoclonal humanized anti-HER-2 antibody, trastuzumab, in patients with recurrent or refractory ovarian or primary peritoneal carcinoma with overexpression of HER-2: a phase II trial of the Gynecologic Oncology Group. J Clin Oncol. 2003;21:283–90.

98. Engelman JA, Zejnullahu K, Mitsudomi T, et al. MET amplification leads to gefitinib resistance in lung cancer by activating ERBB3 signaling. Science. 2007;316:1039–43.

99. Lassus H, Staff S, Leminen A, Isola J, Butzow R. Aurora-A overexpression and aneuploidy predict poor outcome in serous ovarian carcinoma. Gynecol Oncol. 2011;120:11–7.

100. Bonome T, Levine DA, Shih J, et al. A gene signature predicting for survival in suboptimally debulked patients with ovarian cancer. Cancer Res. 2008;68:5478–86.

101. Mok SC, Bonome T, Vathipadiekal V, et al. A gene signature predictive for outcome in advanced ovarian cancer identifies a survival factor: microfibril-associated glycoprotein 2. Cancer Cell. 2009;16:521–32.

Uterine Cancer: The Influence of Genetics and Environment on Cell Cycling Pathways in Cancer

15

Annekathryn Goodman, Leslie S. Bradford, and Leslie A. Garrett

Introduction

An estimated 43,470 women in the USA developed endometrial cancer in 2010 [1]. Historically, endometrial cancer has been categorized by histology, demographics, and behavior into low risk (type I) and high risk (type II) [2]. Over the last 25 years, there has been an explosion of information about the relationship between disruption of cellular controls and the development of cancer. The categorization of endometrial cancer as type I and II continues to be used to describe the histology of endometrial cancers, its behavior clinically, and to evaluate prognostic information. Type I cancers comprise about 80% of endometrial cancers and are believed to be associated with a favorable prognosis. Type I cancers are associated with unopposed estrogen, obesity, and metabolic syndrome. They are associated with the premalignant histological field defect of endometrial hyperplasia and have an endometrioid histology. Type II cancers, on the other hand, are associated with older age, higher grade, and lack of estrogen receptors, and are predominantly serous histology. Type II cancers either present at late stage or are associated with a high likelihood of recurrence despite diagnosis at an early stage.

This chapter reviews current knowledge of genetic and molecular mechanisms of malignancy and its implication for strategies at prevention and treatment in endometrial cancer.

Categorization of Endometrial Cancer

Endometrial cancer has been further classified by the knowledge derived from the available scientific tools of each decade. Originally, this cancer was described both by the symptoms and characteristics of the women who suffered from it. With improving surgical techniques, endometrial cancer became classified by a surgical staging system.

As the field of pathology evolved, histologic subsets of endometrial cancer were identified. Immunohistochemistry and a knowledge of hormone receptors led to the addition of receptor status. With the advent of analytic methods to quantitate DNA and chromosomal analysis, ploidy status and chromosomal shifts were discovered.

Genetic associations for endometrial cancer were first described by family trees. With loss of heterozygosity studies, actual gene mutations were mapped [3]. By the 1990s, with the identification of tumor suppressor genes, loss and amplifications of certain genes were linked with various types of endometrial cancers. For instance,

A. Goodman, M.D. (✉) • L.A. Garrett, M.D.
Department of Obstetrics and Gynecology,
Massachusetts General Hospital, Yawkey 9E Women's
Cancer Center, 55 Fruit Street, Boston, MA 02114, USA
e-mail: agoodman@partners.org

L.S. Bradford, M.D.
Division of Gynecologic Oncology,
Massachusetts General Hospital, Boston, MA, USA

M. Bologna (ed.), *Biotargets of Cancer in Current Clinical Practice*, Current Clinical Pathology,
DOI 10.1007/978-1-61779-615-9_15, © Springer Science+Business Media, LLC 2012

loss of heterozygosity studies identified the p53 mutation on chromosome 17p in endometrial cancer [4]. Currently, knowledge about the cell signaling pathways that control the processes of cell growth and death have helped identify key pathways that, when altered, lead to malignant transformation.

Symptoms

Abnormal bleeding is the single most important symptom. Any postmenopausal bleeding, regardless of quantity, should be evaluated by tissue sampling to rule out a malignancy. Forty percent of endometrial cancers occur before menopause, and 5% occur before age 40 years. Intermenstrual bleeding or excessive and changing menses may be hallmarks of malignant or premalignant changes within the endometrium and should also be evaluated by biopsy.

Table 15.1 lists possible presenting symptoms for endometrial cancer. As the cancer grows, involving surrounding organs, additional symptoms such as urinary frequency, pelvic and back pain, and leg swelling from compression of pelvic vessels, occur. However, endometrial cancers may have no other symptoms beyond a change in the bleeding pattern. Some women may have developed cervical stenosis either from atrophy or scarring from prior surgical procedures. In the setting of cervical stenosis, they may not have any bleeding and may present with hematometria, or a blood-filled uterus.

Table 15.1 Symptoms and signs of endometrial cancer

Bleeding
Menorrhagia
Intermenstrual bleeding
Postmenopausal bleeding
Watery vaginal discharge
Pelvic pain
Urinary frequency
Back pain
Leg swelling
Uterine mass
Adnexal masses

Clinical Characteristics

Clinical features of women who develop endometrial cancer are usually those associated with type I cancers. Table 15.2 summarizes these features. Comorbid conditions include hypertension, osteoarthritis, metabolic syndrome, type 2 diabetes, and abdominal obesity [5]. The majority are associated with either exogenous or endogenous excessive or unopposed estrogen stimulation. Obesity is found in up to 93% of patients and leads to high estrone levels. Obesity is an increasing problem in industrialized countries. In the USA, 71% of Americans were classified as obese in 2007 [6]. This is up from 61% in 1999 [7]. The USA, however, is not alone in facing this epidemic of obesity and the subsequent increased rates of endometrial cancer. In Japan, for instance, endometrial cancer has had the fastest growing cancer incidence over the past decade [8].

Hormonal hypotheses may provide some explanation for this. Anovulation due to excessive weight and polycystic ovarian syndrome are also associated with a high estradiol levels and the absence of opposing progesterone. Estrogen is thought to be the most important environmental factor in the development of endometrial cancer. Estrogen induces the expression of TGF-alpha (transforming growth factor alpha) and its receptor. This leads to progression through the cell cycle and subsequent cell proliferation. Intracellular signaling pathways are directly activated independently by estrogen via the nuclear estrogen receptor [8].

Dietary hypotheses have also been presented as an explanation for the increasing rates of endometrial cancer. Accumulation of adipose tissue has been identified as an associated risk factor

Table 15.2 Clinical characteristics in endometrial cancer

Obesity
Anovulation
Polycystic ovarian syndrome
Hypertension
Diabetes
Metabolic syndrome

for cancer. Both type I and type II endometrial cancers (described in further detail below) are associated with subcutaneous adipose accumulation. The correlation appears to be stronger for type I endometrial cancer [9]. A 1997 case–control study in Hawaii provides additional evidence for the important role of diet in the development of endometrial cancer. The authors examined role of dietary soy and fiber on the risk of developing endometrial cancer. High fat intake had a positive association with risk of endometrial cancer (OR 1.6), whereas a high fiber intake was associated with a 29–46% reduction in risk. High consumption of soy was also associated with a decrease in risk (OR 0.46). Similar risk reductions were noted with other phytoestrogens, such as whole grains, vegetables, fruits, and seaweeds [10]. A 2009 meta-analysis of soy intake and endocrine-related tumors, including endometrial and ovarian cancers, confirms the protective effect of a soy diet, with an OR of 0.71 for endometrial cancer [11].

The strong association between obesity and endometrial cancer has been well studied. Diabetes has been shown to be an independent risk factors for endometrial cancer. New information about molecular mechanisms for tumorigenesis suggests that insulin resistance plays a role in altering the cell signaling pathways [12, 13]. The term "insulin resistance" encompasses overt diabetes as well as varying degrees of hyperglycemia and prediabetes. An insulin-resistant state is highly prevalent among women with endometrial cancer. In both obese and nonobese patients, rates of insulin resistance have been reported as high as 66% [14]. In addition, preclinical studies have demonstrated that insulin resistance accompanied by high circulating levels of insulin further potentiates the effect of estrogen on endometrial proliferation [15].

The insulin-like growth factor (IGF) is a complex system of peptide hormones, cell-surface receptors, and circulating binding proteins. Specifically, IGF-1 and -2, two of the peptide hormones, are mitogens and function to regulate cell proliferation, differentiation, and apoptosis. Their effects are mediated through the insulin-like growth factor receptor, type 1 (IGF-R1). At any level in this signaling pathway, disruptions can lead to the development and progression of various cancers. IGF ligands and IGF-R1 appear to be the most influential players; when disrupted, they act as potent oncogenes. High serum concentrations of IGF-1 and IGF-2 are associated with an increased risk of cancers, such as breast, prostate, colorectal, and lung. IGF-R1 is commonly disturbed in many gastric, lung, and endometrial cancers. In contrast, IGF-R2 is considered to act as a tumor suppressor gene [12–14].

Surgical Staging

Surgical staging of endometrial cancer has become the standard of care as up to 25% of women with apparent stage I cancers have metastatic disease at surgery. Optimal definitive therapy requires knowledge of the true extent of disease at diagnosis [16]. The New FIGO surgical staging of endometrial cancer is shown in Table 15.3 [17]. Staging information is obtained during surgery after the removal of the uterus, adnexa, pelvic, and *para*aortic lymph nodes.

Histology

Endometrial cancer can be classified by its morphologic appearance, the architectural and nuclear organization, and the presence of preinvasive precursors. These cancers arise from the endometrial glands of the lining of the uterus [18]. Table 15.4 lists the various histological variants

Table 15.3 Endometrial cancer staging

IA	Tumor confined to the uterus, no or <½ myometrial invasion
IB	Tumor confined to the uterus, >½ myometrial invasion
II	Cervical stromal invasion, but not beyond uterus
IIIA	Tumor invades serosa or adnexa
IIIB	Vaginal and/or parametrial involvement
IIIC1	Pelvic node involvement
IIIC2	*Para*aortic involvement
IVA	Tumor invasion bladder and/or bowel mucosa
IVB	Distant metastases including abdominal metastases and/or inguinal lymph nodes

Table 15.4 Histologic subtypes of endometrial cancer

Association with clinical type I or II

Histology	Type
Endometrioid	I
Villoglandular	I
Secretory	I
Endometrioid with squamous differentiation	I
Mucinous	I
Serous	II
Clear cell	II
Squamous cell	?
Undifferentiated	I

and their association with either type I or type II classification.

The preinvasive phase of type I endometrial cancer has historically been called complex atypical hyperplasia based on the complexity of the architecture and the presence of nuclear atypia. The term, endometrial intraepithelial neoplasia (EIN), has also been used to define this premalignant lesion. EIN is reported as an intrinsically proliferative monoclonal lesion that arises focally and confers an elevated risk of adenocarcinoma [19]. Atypical hyperplasia shares genomic alterations with endometrioid cancers [20]. Type II endometrial cancers have been postulated to have a precursor lesion, endometrial intraepithelial carcinoma (EIC). EIC frequently coexists with serous papillary endometrial carcinomas and is hypothesized to be its precursor lesion [21].

Connected with the histologic classification is grade, a descriptive strategy dividing adenocarcinomas into three distinct groups based on the degree of architectural and nuclear disorganization. A grade 1 tumor contains less than 5% of a solid nonsquamous growth pattern. A grade 2 cancer manifests a range from 6 to 50% solid pattern, and grade 3 tumors contain over 50% solid pattern. Increasing disorganization within the tumor architecture as described by grade is directly correlated with an increase in invasiveness, risk or metastases, and recurrence [22]. Figure 15.1 demonstrates the various grades of endometrioid histology. Figure 15.2 demonstrates clear cell and serous histologies.

Immunohistochemistry

Immunohistochemistry has been used to study the expression of different biomarkers in endometrial cancer. Hormone receptor status (ER, PR), proliferation-associated indices, tumor suppressor gene products (i.e., p53 protein), cell cycle-related proteins (i.e., cyclin D1), antiapoptotic proteins (i.e., bcl-2), and adhesion molecules (i.e., CD44s) are just some of the biomarkers that have been investigated. Each has been shown to be involved in tumorigenesis. These biomarkers also appear to be correlated with tumor differentiation and myometrial invasion and thus provide another tool for better understanding the biological behavior of endometrial carcinogenesis [23].

Human endometrium expresses estrogen (ER) and progesterone (PR) receptors (Fig. 15.3). The expression of ER and PR and their distribution pattern play a role in both normal endometrial function and pathogenesis. Positive progesterone receptor status correlates with better grade and lower risk of recurrence of the cancer. Hormone receptors are less likely to be present in grade 3 cancers and in the histological subtypes associated with type II cancers — serous and clear cell [18].

Family History

Endometrial cancers are presumed to develop after a series of genetic alterations. Inherited mutations in DNA repair genes associated with the clinical familial syndrome, hereditary nonpolyposis colon cancer (HNPCC), are associated with 5% of endometrial cancers [24]. HNPCC syndrome, also known as Lynch syndrome, presents as an autosomal dominant pattern of colon and endometrial cancers. Clinically, women with HNPCC present with endometrial cancers at least 10 years earlier than those with sporadic cancers, with 49 years being the average age at diagnosis. The histologic appearance of HNPCC cancers is similar to type I cancers with well-differentiated, early-stage endometrioid adenocarcinoma being the most common [25].

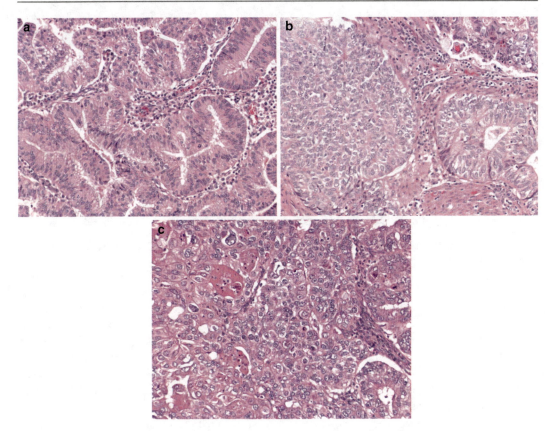

Fig. 15.1 Histology of type I endometrial cancers. (**a**) Grade I endometrioid endometrial cancer; >95% greater gland forming. (**b**) Grade 2 endometrioid endometrial cancer; 50–95% gland forming. (**c**) Grade 3 endometrioid endometrial cancer; >50% solid elements [Courtesy of Dr. Rosemary Tambouret; Department of Pathology; Massachusetts General Hospital]

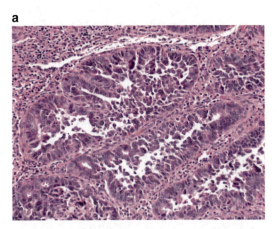
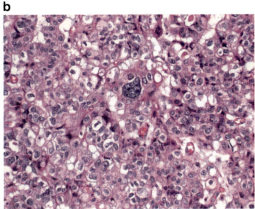

Fig. 15.2 Histology of type II endometrial cancers. (**a**) Serous endometrial cancer; all serous carcinomas are high grade. (**b**) Clear cell endometrial cancer; all clear cell carcinomas are high grade [Courtesy of Dr. Rosemary Tambouret; Department of Pathology; Massachusetts General Hospital]

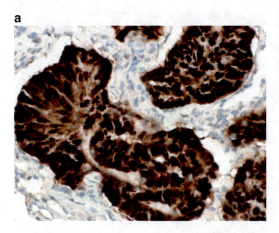 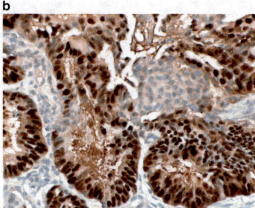

Fig. 15.3 Immunohistochemistry of endometrial cancer [Courtesy of Dr. Rosemary Tambouret; Department of Pathology; Massachusetts General Hospital]

Unlike the familial cluster associated with HNPCC, a cohort of 289 Ashkenazi Jewish women diagnosed with endometrial cancer were screened for BRCA mutations—mutations linked to the most common familial breast and ovarian cancer syndrome. Despite the known relationship between Ashkenazi heritage and BRCA mutation, there did not appear to be an association among this population of endometrial cancer with BRCA 1 or 2 mutations [26].

Gene Mutations

For the clinical family syndrome, HNPCC, genetic alterations occur in MSH2, MSH6, MLH1, PMS1, and PMS2 genes that are important for DNA mismatch repair [27, 28]. Loss of mismatch repair causes genetic mutations to accumulate throughout the genome. Microsatellites are repetitive DNA sequences in the noncoding areas of the genome and within genes. Microsatellite mutations secondary to DNA mismatch repair gene mutations lead to microsatellite instability (MSI) [29]. This is believed to cause inactivation of tumor suppressor genes and thus lead to malignant transformation.

MSI can occur from DNA methylation as a somatic epigenetic cause [30, 31]. In sporadic endometrial cancer, reported rates of MSI range from 10 to 43% [32]. MSI with DNA methylation has been analyzed in premenopausal versus postmenopausal women with endometrial cancer. In a group of 101 women younger than age 50 years and 112 older women, MSI in the absence of DNA methylation identified 13% of the younger cohort and 5% of the older group as having true germ line mutation found in HNPCC [33]. While MSI due to replication error repair appears common in endometrial cancer, especially earlier-stage disease, its prognostic implications are not fully understood [34, 35].

MSI was first described in patients with HNPCC, and mutational analysis of DNA mismatch repair genes is currently the standard for diagnosis. MSI confers a survival advantage in sporadic and hereditary colorectal cancer but may carry a poorer prognosis in breast cancer [36, 37]. It has also been noted that there is an increased incidence of ovarian cancer in women with HNPCC. However, while MSI in HNPCC related endometrial cancer is caused by the loss of DNA mismatch repair genes, for those HNPCC patients with simultaneous ovarian cancers, the ovarian cancers do not carry a MSI mechanism for malignant transformation [38].

Another novel cause of HNPCC (Lynch syndrome) was identified with a germ line mutation in the EPCAM gene. The deletion leads to transcriptional errors and epigenetic silencing of the neighboring MSH2 gene. In this cohort, those with deletions extending close to the MSH2 promoter showed an increased development of endometrial cancer [39].

Eighty percent of endometrial cancers have a normal diploid DNA content. Aneuploidy occurs in the remaining 20% and is associated with advanced stage, high grade, nonendometrioid histology, and poor survival [40]. For sporadic type I cancers, the most common sites of chromosomal gain are 1q, 8q, 10p, and 10q. Chromosomal losses are also observed [41, 42].

Using cDNA microarray analysis, normal endometrial tissue was compared to malignant tissue. In malignancies, the 100 hormonally regulated genes found in normal tissue become expressed in a disorderly manner in endometrial cancers [43]. Distinct gene expression profiles have been associated with different histologic types of endometrial cancer. Specifically, Maxwell and colleagues described 160 genes differentially expressed among endometrioid versus papillary serous cancers [44]. In another microarray study, 31 genes were upregulated in endometrioid carcinomas, and a different 35 genes were overexpressed in serous and clear cell carcinomas [45]. Retrospective evaluation by gene expression profiles have shown that genes most associated with risk of recurrence could be used to further stratify an intermediate risk group of endometrial cancers into high risk and low risk for recurrence [46]. In another study using microarray technology, 117 genes distinguished endometrial cancer specimens from normal endometrium. An additional 10 genes were only differentially regulated in late-stage cancer compared to early stage [47].

The microarray technology of the last decade has identified the complexity of genetic alterations in a quantitative manner. It was not within the domain of this technology to explore the actual molecular and subcellular alterations leading to malignant transformation but has led to some important information regarding classification and risk stratification within histological subtypes of endometrial cancer.

Table 15.5 summarizes the gene mutation findings in endometrial cancer.

Table 15.5 Summary of gene mutation studies in endometrial cancer

Germ line mutation in DNA mismatch repair genes leads to hereditary risk of endometrial cancer
–80% of endometrial cancers are diploid and are associated with type I cancers
Aneuploid tumors correlate with type II endometrial cancers
Multiple chromosomal depletions and additions are associated with malignant phenotype
cDNA microarray identifies between 60 and 160 genes associated with malignant phenotype

Cell Signaling Pathways

Table 15.6 is a glossary of cell cycle genes, cell surface receptors, and signaling pathways.

Intracellular signaling pathways stimulated by individual receptors on the cell membrane induce various cellular functions such as cell proliferation, differentiation, and apoptosis. Figures 15.4 and 15.5 demonstrate current knowledge of these cell signaling pathways. Apoptosis is a normal regulatory system for homeostasis and is dictated by mitochondria dependent on the death receptor system. A thorough understanding of these signaling pathways provides insight into mechanisms of disease, resistance to chemotherapy, and promising targets for future therapies. While a consistent pattern of pathway mutations for targeted therapies has been difficult to identity in ovarian cancer, endometrial cancer presents a host of therapeutic targets.

For instance, receptor tyrosine kinases play an important role in regulation of cellular proliferation and differentiation. The epidermal growth factor receptor (EGFR) family consists of four tyrosine kinase cell-surface receptors (EGFR (erbB-1), HER-2/neu (ErbB-2), Her-3 (ErbB-3), and Her-4 (ErbB-4)) [48]. Following binding to EGF growth factor, the intracellular tyrosine kinase domain is activated. This leads to cellular proliferation. Both type I and type II endometrial cancers can overexpress EGFR. This overexpression is correlated to tumor grade, depth of myometrial invasion, and poor survival [49]. Her-2/neu overexpression

Table 15.6 Glossary of cell genes, cell-surface receptors, and signaling pathways

Akt serine-threonine kinase

ATM—ataxia telangiectasia mutated gene

EGFR—epidermal growth factor receptor

EPCAM gene—codes for epithelial cell adhesion molecule which is a membrane protein expressed in all carcinomas

HER-2/neu (ErbB-2)—EGFR tyrosine kinase

IGFs—insulin-like growth factors

IGFBPs—IGF—binding proteins

KIT—receptor tyrosine kinase

K-ras—y-Ki-ras2 Kirsten rat sarcoma 2 viral oncogene homolog

MAPK—mitogen-activated protein kinase

MLH1—DNA mismatch repair genes

MSH2—DNA mismatch repair genes

MSH6—DNA mismatch repair genes

MSI—microsatellite instability

mTOR—mammalian target of rapamycin

PARP—poly-ADP ribose polymerase

Pathways

  PI3K/PTEN/Akt/mTOR

  ATM/p53—promotes DNA repair

  Raf-MEK-ERK

PI3K—phosphatidylinositol 3-kinase

PMS1—DNA mismatch repair genes

PMS2—DNA mismatch repair genes

PTEN—phosphatase and tensin homologue on chromosome 10 gene a tumor suppressor gene

SNPs—single nucleotide polymorphisms

TGF-alpha—transforming growth factor alpha: may play a role in tumor angiogenesis

TP53—tumor suppressor gene

occurs in about 10% of endometrial cancers and is more likely associated with serous papillary tumors [49–53].

K-ras (y-Ki-ras2 Kirsten rat sarcoma 2 viral oncogene homolog) mutations are identified in approximately 11–26% of type I and 2% of type II endometrial cancers [54–57]. c-Kit, a tyrosine-protein kinase, is a protein is encoded by the Kit gene and is a cytokine receptor expressed on the cell surface. Unlike K-ras, the immunohistochemical KIT expression and mutational status of the KIT gene was studied in 30 primary and 15 recurrent endometrial cancers. These cases did not show KIT gene mutations [58].

Tumor suppressor gene products such as TP53 and PTEN have a regulatory effect on the cell cycle and promote apoptosis. The ATM/p53 signaling pathway promotes DNA repair after damage from radiation. Ataxia telangiectasia mutated gene (ATM) phosphoylates p53. P53 causes growth arrest of the cell to allow DNA damage repair. P53 also causes the cell to undergo apoptosis if the damage is too severe.

The inactivation of TP53 tumor suppressor gene is the most common genetic event in endometrial cancer. Overexpression of mutant p53 gene product, seen in 20% of cancers, is also associated with other poor prognostic factors [59]. TP53 mutations occur in approximately 20% of type I cancers but are found in almost 90% of type II endometrial cancers [56, 60, 61]. Overexpression of p53 protein occurs in cancers with missense mutations causing amino acid substitutions in the gene product [62]. This is thought to be a late event in endometrial cancer formation. TP53 mutation and p53 protein overexpression are present in most papillary serous tumors and are rarely described in endometrioid tumors of their precursors [61].

TP53 mutations rarely occur in endometrial intraepithelial neoplasia (EIN); however, PTEN mutations (phosphatase and tensin homologue on chromosome 10 gene), a tumor suppressor gene, have been reported in 20% of endometrial hyperplasias [43, 54]. PTEN loss in the setting of EIN on endometrial biopsies has been used to predict the existence of endometrial cancer [63].

PTEN mutations occur with 30–50% of endometrial cancers [64]. PTEN loss of function is much more common in type I endometrial cancers [65, 66]. The PTEN tumor suppressor gene regulates the oncogenic phosphatidylinositol 3-kinase (PI3K) signaling pathway that is involved in carcinogenesis. The PTEN gene encodes a phosphatase that opposes the activity of cellular kinases [67, 68]. The phosphatase activity of PTEN is crucial for its role in tumorigenesis. Downstream of the PI3K pathway is Akt, a serine-threonine kinase, that is regulated by PI3K and influences apoptosis and cell proliferations. Mammalian target of rapamycin

15 Uterine Cancer: The Influence of Genetics and Environment on Cell Cycling Pathways in Cancer 411

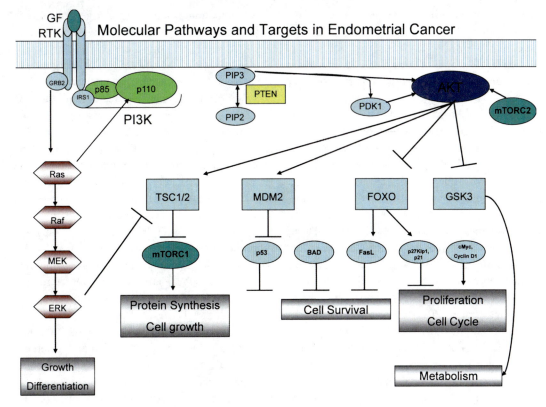

Fig. 15.4 Molecular pathways and targets in endometrial cancer: implications for synthetic function

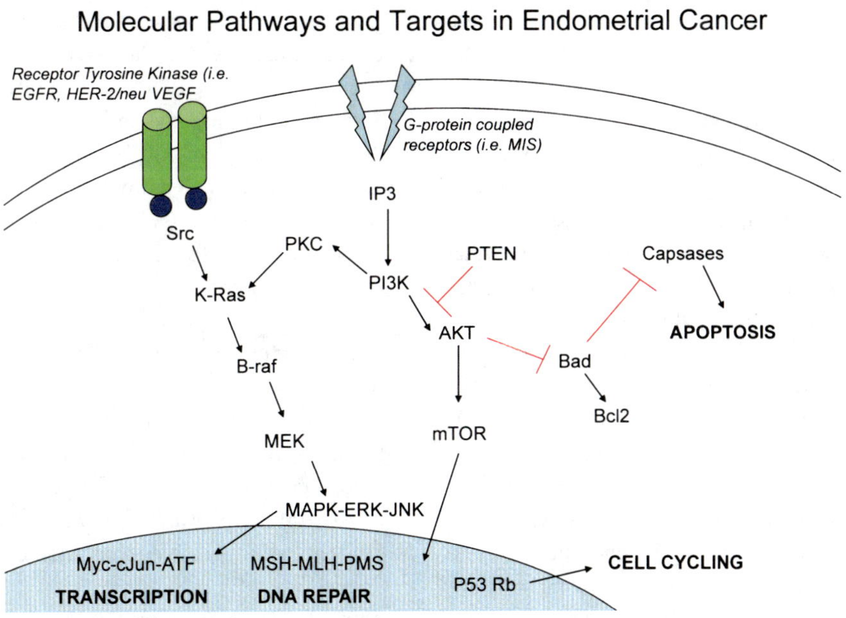

Fig. 15.5 Molecular pathways and targets in endometrial cancer: nuclear targets

(mTOR) is also a serine/threonine protein kinase which integrates signals from nutrients, growth factors, hormones, cellular energy stores, and oxygen levels to control critical cellular processes such as growth, differentiation, transcription, and mRNA translation [68].

The PI3K-Akt-mTOR pathway plays a major role in regulating cell proliferation, growth, and survival. Alterations in the PTEN-PI3K-Akt pathways are noted in hormone-related tumors of the endometrium. Molecular alterations in AKT are rare, but both type I and type II endometrial cancers demonstrate a high rate of mutations in the PI3KCA gene, which encodes PI3K [69]. These are seen in 20–30% of endometrial cancers [70–72]. Amplification of the PI3KCA gene, however, is much more common in type II endometrial cancer, with a prevalence of about 46% [72]. PTEN antagonizes PI3K function and negatively regulates Akt activities, mainly cell survival and apoptosis. Loss of PTEN in endometrial cancers is associated with increased activity of the PI3k with resultant phosphorylation of its downstream substrate Akt [73]. In turn, Akt upregulates mTOR activity. Hyperactivation of mTOR signaling increases translation of mRNAs encoding growth factors, cell cycle regulators, survival proteins, and angiogenic factors. Dysregulation of the PI3K/Akt/mTOR pathway as a result of genetic mutations and amplifications is thought to be a conduit for carcinogenesis [74].

The PI3K-Akt-mTOR pathway has been shown to be active in many solid tumors and plays a key role in maintaining a tumorigenic state [67, 75, 76]. Preclinical studies suggest that such interactions may affect resistance to chemotherapy in endometrial cell lines.

In a case–control study of 417 women with endometrial cancer and 407 matched controls, common genetic variations in PTEN, PIK3CA, AKT1, MLH1, and MSH2 were not statistically significantly associated with endometrial cancer [77]. Other studies have found PTEN gene mutations to be associated with endometrioid histology, early stage, and favorable clinical behavior [66]. Interestingly, in a study of uterine carcinosarcomas, comparative evaluation of the carcinomatous and sarcomatous elements showed a similar mutation profile. Forty-six percent of the 52 patients had cancer gene mutations with TP53, PIK3CA, and KRAS mutations dominating [78].

The location of the Akt activity is important in the behavior of the cancer. The nuclear p-Akt L1 was significantly higher in grade 1 than in grade 3 cancers and was associated with estrogen receptor (ER-alpha) expression. Higher nuclear p-Akt levels were associated with worse prognosis in grade 1 endometrial cancers allowing for even further subclassification of similar grade tumors [8]. Conversely, cytoplasmic p-Akt expression was higher in grade 3 cancers.

PTEN also plays a role in cellular signaling by inhibiting the MAP kinase pathway. The MAPK pathway is another major intracellular signaling cascade by which signals are transmitted through phosphorylation by tyrosine kinase-type receptors on cell membranes.

The mitogen-activated protein kinase (MAPK) pathway involves cell proliferation and differentiation via Raf-MEK-ERK. MAPK is activated by growth factors and their receptors upstream of functional cascades. An autonomous and constitutive activation of MAPK signal transduction is induced by the overexpression of growth factors and their receptors in cancer cells [48].

Other growth factor pathways play roles in carcinogenesis. The IGF pathway plays a critical role in the growth and development of the uterus. IGFs are potent mitogenic and antiapoptotic molecules which regulate cell proliferation and steroid actions in the endometrium. Increased amounts of unbound IGF may lead to uncontrolled cellular proliferation in the uterus [12].

One case–control study investigated the association between 44 polymorphisms within IGFs and IGF binding proteins (IGFBPs) with endometrial cancer risk; 692 cases of endometrial cancer and 1,723 control cases were analyzed, and the authors found an inverse relation between certain polymorphisms and cancer risks. Specifically, variation with IGF-2 and IGFP-3 may influence endometrial cancer risk in Caucasians [12].

Table 15.7 summarizes the molecular alterations detected in type I and type II endometrial cancers.

Table 15.7 Molecular alterations in endometrial cancer

Alteration	Prevalence type I (%)	Prevalence type II (%)
PIK3CA mutation [60, 70–72]	~30	~20
PIK3CA amplification [72]	2–14	46
KRAS mutation [56, 57]	11–26	2
AKT mutation [69]	3	0
PTEN loss of function [65, 66]	83	5
Microsatellite instability [32, 35]	20–45	0–5
TP53 mutation [56, 60, 61]	~20	~90
HER2 overexpression [49, 53]	3–10	32
HER2 amplification [52]	1	17

Translational Implications for Therapy

In the past 25 years, our understanding of signaling pathways regulating cellular growth, cell cycle, and apoptosis has evolved. This molecular insight has led to the investigation of numerous cell cycle signaling targets as therapeutic agents. Studies to date begin to unpack the complexity and variability of genetic alterations in malignant transformation and also the variable cell signaling pathways that are blocked, suppressed, or amplified when mutations lead to malignancies. While we still divide endometrial cancers into type I and II based on clinical and histological factors, gene profiling and gene mutational analysis reveal a vast heterogeneity within both groups.

Molecular profiling of tumors to identify targeted therapy is being explored for many solid tumors. Figure 15.6 identifies several points in the cell cycle for therapeutic targets. In an early pilot study of 86 patients, 27% had response from therapy identified by molecular profiling [79]. Gene expression profiles have been used to target therapy in leukemia, lung cancer, and gastrointestinal cancers. Breast and ovarian cancers are now evaluated for BRCA1/2 mutations with the advent of poly-ADP ribose polymerase (PARP) inhibitors [80]. However, due to the great genetic heterogeneity, some have endorsed therapy selection to become individualized by single gene mutations [81].

Traditional chemotherapy continues to play a major role in the treatment of endometrial cancer. However, for recurrent endometrial cancers, pooled response rates from multiple trials range from 17 to 42%. For patients receiving second-line chemotherapy, response rates drop to 4–27% [82]. There is much hope that targeted therapy will provide a novel approach to treating the formidable problem of endometrial cancer recurrence.

The best established targeted therapy in endometrial cancer is hormone therapy with agents that bind to estrogen and progesterone receptors. Progesterone has a 70% response rate when used as primary, fertility-sparing therapy in early-stage disease. However, up to 30% of patients have resistance to progesterone [83].

Metformin has been evaluated in vitro and shown to reverse progesterone resistance. It has also shown to enhance progesterone-induced cell proliferation inhibition, and induced apoptosis in vitro [84]. Loss of PTEN has been associated with progesterone refractory endometrial hyperplasia [85].

Despite promising preclinical studies using a targeted approach to anticancer therapy, early human trials have been somewhat disappointing. A review of the nine Gynecologic Oncology Group (GOG) studies focused on recurrent or advanced endometrial cancer summarizes progression free survivals ranging from 5 to 7 months for traditional chemotherapies. Temsirolimus, an mTor inhibitor; thalidomide, an antiangiogenesis inhibitor; and the VEGF inhibitor, bevicizumab, reveal progression free survival rates of 1.7–3 months [48]. Additionally, GOG #181 reported there was no significant activity for trastuzumab, an EGFR inhibitor, in women with advanced or recurrent endometrial cancer [86]. GOG #188, a study of Faslodex, an estrogen receptor downregulator approved for use in ER-positive breast cancer, was equally disappointing when testing in women with endometrial cancer [87].

PI3K pathway inhibitors have been aggressively developed as novel cancer therapies [75, 87]. From a therapeutic perspective, the complex regulation of mTORC1 is important. Inhibition of mTOR with sirolimus in endometrial cancer has shown some response [74]. Some PI3K

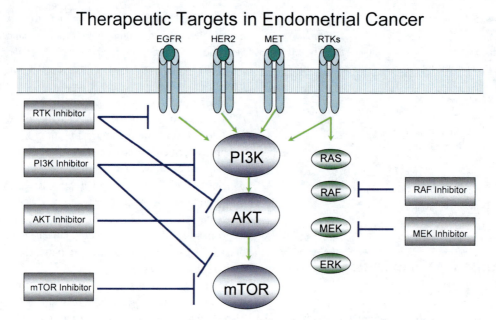

Fig. 15.6 Therapeutic targets in endometrial cancer

inhibitors in clinical trials directly block both PI3K and mTOR, whereas others inhibit only PI3K. Dual PI3K–mTOR inhibitors might offer a therapeutic advantage in cancers in which PI3K is not the primary regulator of mTORC1 [76].

To date, none of the targeted therapies response rates approach comparable responses to progesterone or conventional chemotherapy. It is not surprising that single therapeutic interventions at the cell signaling pathway may not be useful given the cDNA microarray data from the last decade that suggest that hundreds of genes are involved with carcinogenesis. Careful study of how to selectively target multiple cancer related pathways while preserving the pathways of normal cells will be the work of the next decade.

References

1. Jamal A, Siegel R, Xu J, et al. Cancer statistics 2010. CA Cancer J Clin. 2010;60:277–300.
2. Deligdisch L, Holinka CF. Endometrial carcinoma: two diseases? Cancer Detect Prev. 1987;10:237–46.
3. Lin WM, Forgacs E, Warshal DP, Yeh T, Martin JS, Ashfaq R, Muller CY. Loss of heterozygosity and mutational analysis of the PTEN/MMAC1 gene in synchronous endometrial and ovarian carcinomas. Clin Cancer Res. 1998;4:2577–83.
4. Okamoto A, Sameshima Y, Yamada Y, Teshima SI, Terashima Y, Terada M, Yokota J. Allelic loss on chromosome 17p and p53 mutations in human endometrial carcinoma of the uterus. Cancer Res. 1991;51:5632–5.
5. von Gruenigen VE, Waggoner SE, Frasure HE, Kavanagh MB, Janata JW, Rose PG, Courneya KS, Lerner E. Lifestyle challenges in endometrial cancer survivorship. Obstet Gynecol. 2011;117(1):93–9.
6. Lauren Streib. World's FastestCountries. http://www.forbes.com/2007/02/07/worlds-fattest-countries-forbeslife-cx_ls_0208worldfat_2.html Accessed 1 Mar 2011.
7. The Surgeon General's Call to Action to Prevent and Decrease Overweight and Obesity. http://www.surgeongeneral.gov/topics/obesity/ Accessed 1 Mar 2011.
8. Abe N, Watanabe J, Tsunoda S, Kuramoto H, Okayasu I. Significance of nuclear p-Akt in endometrial carcinogenesis. Int J Gynecol Cancer. 2011;21(2):194–202.
9. Nakmura K, Hongo A, Kodama J, Hiramatsu Y. Fat accumulation in adipose tissues as a risk factor for the development of endometrial cancer. Oncol Rep. 2011 Jul;26(1):65–71.
10. Goodman MT, Wilkens LR, Hankin JH, Lyu LC, Wu AH, Kolonel LN. Association of soy and fiber consumption with the risk of endometrial cancer. Am J Epidemiol. 1997;146(4):294–306.
11. Myung SK, Ju W, Choi HJ, Kim SC. Soy intake and risk of endocrine-related gynaecological cancer: a meta-analysis. Br J Obstet Gynaecol. 2009;116(13):1697–705.
12. McGrath M, Lee IM, Buring J, De Vivo I. Common genetic variation within IGFI, IGFII, IGFPB-1, and IGFBP-3 and endometrial cancer risk. Gynecol Oncol. 2011;120:174–8.

13. Maki RG. Small is beautiful: insulin-like growth factors and their role in growth, development, and cancer. J Clin Oncol. 2010;28(33):4985–95.

14. Burzawa JK, Schmeler KM, Soliman PT, Meyer LA, Bevers MW, Pustilnik TL, Anderson ML, Ramondetta LM, Tortolero-Luna G, Urbauer DL, Chang S, Gershenson DM, Brown J, Lu KH. Prospective evaluation of insulin resistance among endometrial cancer patients. Am J Obstet Gynecol. 2011 Apr;204(4):355.

15. Zhang Q, Shen Q, Celestino J. Enhanced estrogen-induced proliferation in obese rat endometrium. Am J Obstet Gynecol. 2009;200:186.e1–e8.

16. Creasman WT, DeGeest K, DiSaia PJ, Zaino RJ. Significance of true surgical pathologic staging: A Gynecologic Oncology Group study. Am J Obstet Gynecol. 1999;181:31–4.

17. Pecorelli S. Revised FIGO staging for carcinoma of the vulva, cervix, and endometrium. Int J Gynaecol Obstet. 2009;105(2):103–4.

18. Kurman RJ, Zaino RJ, Norris HJ. Endometrial carcinoma. In: Kurman RJ, editor. Blaustein's pathology of the female genital tract. 4th ed. New York: Springer; 1994. p. 439–86.

19. Mutter GL. Endometrial intraepithelial neoplasia (EIN): will it bring order to chaos? The endometrial Collaborative group. Gynecol Oncol. 2000;76:287.

20. Baloglu H, Cannizzaro LA, Jones J, Koss LG. Atypical endometrial hyperplasia shares genomic abnormalities with endometrioid carcinoma by comparative genomic hybridization. Human Pathol. 2001;32(6):615–22.

21. Soslow RA, Pirog E, Isacson C. Endometrial intraepithelial carcinoma with associated peritoneal carcinomatosis. Am J Surg Pathol. 2000;24(5):726–32.

22. Pecorelli S, Benedet JL, Creasman WT, et al. FIGO staging of gynecologic cancer 1994–1997. Int J Gynaecol Obstet. 1999;65(3):243–9.

23. Iochin E. Immunohistochemical tumour markers in endometrial carcinoma. Eur J Gynaecol Oncol. 2005;26(4):363–71.

24. Lynch HT, Lynch J. Lynch syndrome: genetics, natural history, genetic counseling, and prevention. J Clin Oncol. 2000;18:19S–31.

25. Boks DES, Trujillo AP, Voogd AC, Morreau H, Kenter GG, Vasen HFA. Survival analysis of endometrial carcinoma associated with hereditary nonpolyposis colorectal cancer. Int J Cancer. 2002;102:198–200.

26. Barak F, Milgrom R, Laitman Y, Gemer O, Rabinovich A, Piura B, Anteby E, Ben Baruch G, Korach J, Friedman E. The rate of the predominant Jewish mutations in the BRCA 1, BRCA2, MSH2, and MSH6 genes in unselected Jewish endometrial cancer patients. Gynecol Oncol. 2010;119:511–5.

27. Service RF. Stalking the start of colon cancer. Science. 1994;263:1559–60.

28. Thibodeau SN, French AJ, Roche PC, Cunningham JM, Tester DJ, Lindor NM, Moslein G, Baker SM, Liskay M, Burgart LJ, Honchel R, Halling KC. Altered expression of hMSH2 and hMLH1 in tumors with microsatellite instability and genetic alterations in mismatch repair genes. Cancer Res. 1996;56:4836–40.

29. Peltomaki P, Lothe RA, Aaltonen LA, Pylkkanen L, Nystrom-Lahti M, Seruca R, David L, Holm R, Ryberg D, Haugen A, Brogger A, Borresen AL, de la Chapelle A. Microsatellite Instability is associated with tumors that characterize the hereditary non-polyposis colorectal carcinoma syndrome. Cancer Res. 1993;53:5853–5.

30. Kanaya T, Kyo S, Maida Y, Yatabe N, Tanaka M, Nakamura M, Inoue M. Frequent hypermethylation of MLH1 promoter in normal endometrium of patients with endometrial cancers. Oncogene. 2003;22:2352–60.

31. Hirasaw A, Aoki D, Inoue J, Imoto I, Susumu N, Sugano K, Nozawa S, Inazawa J. Unfavorable prognostic factors associated with high frequency of microsatellite instability and comparative genomic hybridization analysis in endometrial cancer. Clin Cancer Res. 2003;9:5675–82.

32. MacDonald ND, Salvesen HB, Ryan A. Frequency and prognostic impact of microsatellite instability in a large population-based study of endometrial carcinomas. Cancer Res. 2000;60:1750–2.

33. Zauber NP, Denehy TR, Taylor RR, Ongcapin EH, Marotta SP, Saabbath-Solitaire M, Kulkarni R, Pradham TS, Hermelin D, Bishop DT. Microsatellite instability and DNA methylation of endometrial tumors and clinical features in young women compared to older women. Int J Gynecol Cancer. 2010;20:1549–56.

34. Caduff RF, Johnston DM, Svoboda-Newman SM, Poy EL, Merajver SD, Frank TS. Clinical and pathological significance of microsatellite instability in sporadic endometrial carcinoma. Am J Pathol. 1996;148:1671–8.

35. Basil JB, Goodfellow PJ, Rader JS, Mutch DG, Herzog TJ. Clinical significance of microsatellite instability in endometrial carcinoma. Cancer. 2000;89:1758–64.

36. Lynch HT, Smyrk TC, Watson P, Lanspa SJ, Lynch JF, Lynch PM, Cavalieri J, Boland CR. Genetics, natural history, tumor spectrum and pathology of hereditary nonpolyposis colorectal cancer: an updated review. Gastroenterology. 1993;104:1535–49.

37. Paulson TG, Wright FA, Parker BA, Russack V, Wahl GM. Microsatellite instability correlates with reduced survival and poor disease prognosis in breast cancer. Cancer Res. 1996;56:4021–6.

38. Shannon C, Kirk J, Barnetson R, Evans J, Schnitzler M, Quinn M, Hacker N, Crandon A, Harnett P. Incidence of microsatellite instability in synchronous tumors of the ovary and endometrium. Clin Cancer Res. 2003;9:1387–92.

39. Kempers MJE, Kuiper RP, Ockeloen CW, Chappuis PO, Hutter P, Rahner N, Schackert HK, Steinke V, Holinski-Feder E, et al. Risk of colorectal and endometrial cancers in EPCAM deletion-positive Lynch syndrome: a cohort study. Lancet Oncol. 2011;12:49–55.

40. Lukes AS, Kohler MF, Pieper CF, Kerns BJ, Bentley R, Rodriguez GC, Soper JT, Clarke-Pearson DL, Bast RC, Berchuk A. Multivariable analysis of DNA ploidy, p53, and HER-2/neu as prognostic factors in endometrial cancer. Cancer. 1994;73(9):2380–5.

41. Kiechle M, Hinrichs M, Jacobsen A, Luttges J, Pfisterer J, Kommoss F, Arnold N. Genetic imbalances in precursor lesions of endometrial cancer detected by comparative genomic hybridization. Am J Pathol. 2000;156(6):1827–33.
42. Shah NK, Curries JL, Rosenshein N, Campbell J, Long P, Abbas F, Griffin CA. Cytogeneic and FISH analysis of endometrial carcinoma. Cancer Genet Cytogenet. 1994;73:142–6.
43. Mutter GL, Baak JPA, Fitzgerald JT, Gray R, Neuberg D, Kust GA, Gentleman R, Gullans SR, Wei LJ, Wilcox M. Global expression changes of constitutive and hormonally regulated genes during endometrial neoplastic transformation. Gynecol Oncol. 2001;83:177–85.
44. Maxwell GL, Chandramouli GVR, Dainty L, Litzi TJ, Berchuk A, Barrett JC, Risinger JI. Microarray analysis of endometrial carcinomas and mixed mullerian tumors reveals distinct gene expression profiles associated with different histologic types of uterine cancer. Clin Cancer Res. 2005;11:4056–66.
45. Moreno-Bueno G, Fernandez-Marcos PJ, Collado M, Tendero MI, Rodriguez-Pinilla SM, Garcia-Cao I, Hardisson D, Diaz-Meco MT, Moscat J, Serrano M, Palacios J. Inactivation of the candidate tumor suppressor par-4 in endometrial cancer. Cancer Res. 2007;67:1927–34.
46. Ferguson SE, Olshen AB, Viale A, Barakat RB, Boyd J. Stratification of intermediate-risk endometrial cancer patients into groups at high risk or low risk for recurrence based on tumor gene expression profiles. Clin Cancer Res. 2005;11:2252–7.
47. Wong YF, Cheung TH, Lo KWK, Yim SF, Siu NSS, Chan SCS, Ho TWF, Wong KWY, Yu MY, Wang VW, Li C, Gardner GJ, Bonome T, Johnson WB, Smith DI, Chung TKH, Birrer MJ. Identification of molecular markers and signaling pathway in endometrial cancer in Hong Kong Chinese women by genomic-wide gene expression profiling. Oncogene. 2007;26:1971–82.
48. Gehrig PA, Bae-Jump VL. Promising novel therapies for treatment of endometrial cancer. Gynecol Oncol. 2010;116:187–94.
49. Morrison C, Zanagnolo V, Ramirez N, Cohn DE, Kelbick N, Copeland L, Maxwell LG, Fowler JM. Her-2 is an independent prognostic factor in endometrial cancer: association with outcome in a large cohort of surgically staged patients. J Clin Oncol. 2006;24(15):2376–85.
50. Santin AD, Bellone S, van Stedum S, Bushen W, de las Casas LE, Korourian S, Tiam E, Roman JJ, Burnett A, Pecorelli S. Determination of HER2/neu status in uterine serous papillary carcinoma: comparative analysis of immunohistochemistry and fluorescence in situ hybridization. Gynecol Oncol. 2005;98:24–30.
51. Slomovitz BM, Lu KH, Johnston T, Coleman RL, Munsell M, Broaddus RR, Walker C, Ramondetta LM, Burke TW, Gershenson DM, Wolf J. A phase 2 study of the oral mammalian target of rapamycin inhibitor, Everolimus, in patients with recurrent endometrial carcinoma. Cancer. 2010;116:5415–9.
52. Konecny GE, Santos L, Winterhoff B, Hatmal M, Keeney GL, Mariani A, Jones M, Neuper C, Thomas B, Muderspach L, Riehle D, Wang HJ, Dowdy S, Podratz KC, Press MF. HER2 gene amplification and EGFR expression in a large cohort of surgically staged patients with nonendometrioid (type II) endometrial cancer. Br J Cancer. 2009;100(1):89–95.
53. Fadare O, Zheng W. Insights into endometrial serous carcinogenesis and progression. Int J Clin Exp Pathol. 2009;2(5):411–32.
54. Enomoto T, Inoue M, Perantoni AO, Terakawa N, Tanizawa O, Rice JM. K-ras activation in neoplasms of the human female reproductive tract. Cancer Res. 1990;50:6139–45.
55. Duggan BD, Felix JC, Muderspach LI, Tsao JL, Shibata DK. Early mutational activation of the c-Ki-ras oncogene in endometrial carcinoma. Cancer Res. 1994;54:1604–7.
56. Lax SF, Kendall B, Tashiro H, Slebos RJ, Hedrick L. The frequency of p53, K-ras mutations, and microsatellite instability differs in uterine endometrioid and serous carcinoma: evidence of distinct molecular genetic pathways. Cancer. 2000;88(4):814–24.
57. Koul A, Willén R, Bendahl PO, Nilbert M, Borg A. Distinct sets of gene alterations in endometrial carcinoma implicate alternate modes of tumorigenesis. Cancer. 2002;94(9):2369–79.
58. Vandenput I, Debiec-Rychter M, Capoen A, Verbist G, Vergote I, Moerman P, Amant F. Kit gene in endometrial carcinoma. Int J Gynecol Cancer. 2011;21:203–5.
59. Kohler MF, Berchuk A, Davidoff AM, Humphrey PA, Dodge RK, Iglehart JD, Soper JT, Clarke-Pearson DL, Bast RC, Marks JR. Overexpression and mutation of p53 in endometrial carcinoma. Cancer Res. 1992;52:1622–7.
60. Catasus L, Gallardo A, Cuatrecasas M, Prat J. PIK3CA mutations in the kinase domain (exon 20) of uterine endometrial adenocarcinomas are associated with adverse prognostic parameters. Mod Pathol. 2008;21:131–9.
61. Jia L, Liu Y, Yi X, Miron A, Crum CP, Kong B, Zheng W. Endometrial glandular dysplasia with frequent p53 gene mutation: a genetic evidence supporting its precancer nature for endometrial serous carcinoma. Clin Cancer Res. 2008;14:2263–9.
62. Enomoto T, Fujita M, Inoue M, Rice JM, Nakajima R, Tanizawa O, Nomura T. Alterations of the p53 tumor suppressor gene and its association with activation of the c-K-ras-2 proto-oncogene in premalignant and malignant lesions of the human uterine endometrium. Cancer Res. 1993;53:1883–8.
63. Pavlakis K, Messini I, Vrekoussis T, Panoskaltsis T, Chrissanthakis D, Yiannou P, Stathopoulos EN. PTEN-loss and nuclear atypia of EIN in endometrial biopsies can predict the existence of a concurrent endometrial carcinoma. Gynecol Oncol. 2010;119:516–9.
64. Kong D, Suzuki A, Zou TT, Sakurada A, Kemp LW, Wakatsuki S, Yokoyama T, Yamakawa H, Furukawa T, Sato M, Ohuchi N, Sato S, Yin J, Wang S, Abraham

JM, Souza RF, Smolinski KN, Meltzer SJ, Horii A. PTEN1 is frequently mutated in primary endometrial carcinomas. Nature genetics. 1997;17:143–4.

65. Mutter GL, Lin MC, Fitzgerald JT, Kum JB, Baak JP, Lees JA, Weng LP, Eng C. Altered PTEN expression as a diagnostic marker for the earliest endometrial precancers. J Natl Cancer Inst. 2000;92(11):924–30.

66. Risinger JI, Hayes K, Maxwell GL, Carney ME, Dodge RK, Barrett JC, Berchuk A. PTEN Mutation in endometrial cancers is associated with favorable clinical and pathological characteristics. Clin Cancer Res. 1998;4:3005–10.

67. Engelman JA, Chen L, Tan X, Crosby K, Guimaraes AR, Upadhyay R, Maira M, McNamara K, Perera SA, Song Y, Chirieac LR, Kaur R, Lightbown A, Simendinger J, Li T, Padera RF, Garcia-Echeverria C, Weissleder R, Mahmood U, Cantley LC, Wong KK. Effective use of PI3K and MEK inhibitors to treat mutant K-ras G12D and PIK3CA H1047R murine lung cancers. Nat Med. 2008;14(12):1351–6.

68. Brachmann SM, Hofmann I, Schnell C, Fritsch C, Wee S, Lane H, Wang S, Garcia-Echeverria C, Maira SM. Specific apoptosis induction by the dual PI3K/mTor inhibitor NVP-BEZ235 in HER2 amplified and PIK3CA mutant breast cancer cells. Proc Natl Acad Sci U S A. 2009;106(52):22299–304.

69. Shoji K, Oda K, Nakagawa S, Hosokawa S, Nagae G, Uehara Y, Sone K, Miyamoto Y, Hiraike H, Hiraike-Wada O, Nei T, Kawana K, Kuramoto H, Aburatani H, Yano T, Taketani Y. The oncogenic mutation in the pleckstrin homology domain of AKT1 in endometrial carcinomas. Br J Cancer. 2009;101(1):145–8.

70. Oda K, Stokoe D, Taketani Y, McCormick F. High frequency of coexistent mutations of PIK3CA and PTEN genes in endometrial carcinoma. Cancer Res. 2005;65(23):10669–73.

71. Hayes MP, Douglas W, Ellenson LH. Molecular alterations of EGFR and PIK3CA in uterine serous carcinoma. Gynecol Oncol. 2009;113(3):370–3.

72. Miyake T, Yoshino K, Enomoto T, Takata T, Ugaki H, Kim A, Fujiwara K, Miyatake T, Fujita M, Kimura T. PIK3CA gene mutations and amplifications in uterine cancers, identified by methods that avoid confounding by PIK3CA pseudogene sequences. Cancer Lett. 2008;261(1):120–6.

73. Kanamori Y, Kigawa J, Itamochi H, Himada M, Takahashi M, Kamazawa S, Sato S, Akeshima R, Terakawa N. Correlation between loss of PTEN expression and AKT phosphorylation in endometrial carcinoma. Clin Cancer Res. 2001;7:892–5.

74. Dowling RJO, Pollak M, Sonenberg N. Current status and challenges associated with targeting mTOR for cancer therapy. Biodrugs. 2009;23(2):77–91.

75. Maira SM, Staauffer F, Schnell C, Garcia-Escheverria C. PI3K inhibitors for cancer treatment: where do we stand? Biochem Soc Trans. 2009;37:265–72.

76. Lui TJ, Koul D, LaFortune T, Tiao N, Shen RJ, Maira SM, Garcia-Echevrria C, Yung WK. NVP-BEZ235, a novel dual phosphatidylinositol 3-kinase/mammalian target of rapamycin inhibitor, elicits multifaceted antitumor activities in human gliomas. Mol Cancer Ther. 2009;8(8):2204–10.

77. Lacey JV, Yang H, Gaudet MM, Dunning A, Lissowska J, Sherman ME, Peplonska B, Brinton LA, Healey CS, Ahmed S, Pharoah P, Easton D, Chanock S, Garcia-Closas M. Endometrial cancer and genetic variation in PTEN, PIK3CA, AKT1, MLH1, and MSH2 within a population-based case–control study. Gynecol Oncol. 2011;120:167–73.

78. Growdon WB, Roussel BN, Scialabba VL, Foster R, Dias-Santagata D, Iafrate AJ, Ellisen LW, Tambouret RH, Rueda BR, Borger DR. Tissue-specific signature of activating PIK3CA and RAS mutations in carcinosarcomas of gynecologic origin. Gynecol Oncol. 2011 Apr;121(1):212–7.

79. Von Hoff DD, Stephenson JJ, Rosen P, Loesch DM, Borad MJ, Anthony S, Jameson G, Brown S, Cantafio N, Richards DA, Fitch TR, Wasserman E, Fernandez C, Green S, Sutherland W, Bittner M, Alarcon A, Mallery D, Penny R. Pilot study using molecular profiling of patients' tumors to find potential targets and select treatments for their refractory cancers. J Clin Oncol. 2010;28(33):4877–83.

80. McDermott U, Downing JR, Stratton MR. Genomics and the continuum of cancer care. N Engl J Med. 2011;364(4):340–50.

81. Doroshow JH. Selecting Systemic Cancer therapy one patient at a time: Is there a role for molecular profiling of individual patients with advanced solid tumors? J Clin Oncol. 2010;28(33):4869–71.

82. Moxley KM, McMeekin DS. Endometrial carcinoma: a review of chemotherapy, drug resistance, and the search for new agents. Oncologist. 2010;13:1026–33.

83. Hahn HS, Yoon SG, Hong JS, et al. Conservative treatment with progestin and pregnancy outcomes in endometrial cancer. Int J Gynecol Cancer. 2009;19:1068–73.

84. Zhang Z, Dong L, Sui L, Yang Y, Liu X, Yu Y, Zhu Y, Feng Y. Metformin reverses progestin resistance in endometrial cancer cells by downregulating Glol expression. Int J Gynecol Cancer. 2011;21:213–21.

85. Milam MR, Soliman PT, Chung LH, Schmeler KM, Bassett RL, Broaddus RR, Lu KH. Loss of phosphatase and tensin homologue deleted on chromosome 10 and phosphorylation of mammalian target of rapamycin are associated with progesterone refractory endometrial hyperplasia. Int J Gyn Cancer. 2008;18:146–51.

86. Fleming GI, Sill MW, Darcy KM, McMeekin DS, Thigpen JT, Adler LM, Berek JS, Chapman JA, DiSilvestro PA, Horowitz IR, Fiorica JV. Phase II trial of trastuzumab in women with advanced or recurrent, HER2-positive endometrial carcinoma: A Gynecologic Oncology Group Study. Gynecol Oncol. 2010;116:15–20.

87. Covens AL, Filiaci V, Gersell D, Lutman CV, Bonebrake A, Lee YC. Phase II study of fulvestrant in recurrent/metastatic endometrial carcinoma: a Gynecologic Oncology Group Study. Gynecol Oncol. 2011;120:185–8.

Biotargets in Sarcomas: The Past, Present, and a Look into the Future

16

Vivek Subbiah and Razelle Kurzrock

Introduction

Sarcoma (derived from the Greek word sarkos—flesh) is an umbrella term for more than 50 diverse solid neoplastic subtypes. They are broadly divided into bone and soft tissue sarcomas. Sarcomas originate from the mesenchyme, which comprises a large proportion of body mass that includes skeletal and smooth muscles, nerves, blood vessels, connective tissue, bone, tendons, ligaments, and joints [1, 2]. Sarcomas occur very commonly in all mammals except for man, with an incidence of only 1% of all human cancers. Even so, more than 13,000 cases, primary or metastatic, are diagnosed in the USA annually and are responsible for more than 5,000 estimated deaths [3]. In this regard, they are similar to leukemias, also mesodermal in origin, in that their biological significance is disproportionate to their frequency and incidence. Sarcomas occur across the age spectrum, affecting children, adolescents, and young adults, as well as the geriatric population. Some sarcomas, like Ewing's sarcoma and

osteosarcoma, are more common in young people, whereas leiomyosarcoma and liposarcoma are seen in older individuals. Although they universally arise from the mesenchyme, there is considerable heterogeneity in the biology of various sarcomas, which is reflected by differences in clinical behavior, prognosis, drug responsiveness, and, consequently, optimal management [4]. This chapter outlines the past history of sarcomas, explores current challenges, and highlights future opportunities for developmental therapeutics aimed at novel biotargets.

Sarcomas: The Past

Historically, sarcomas have played a significant role in understanding the biology of cancer. In the early 1900s, Rous successfully transferred spindle cell sarcoma from one chicken to another, heralding the field of tumor virology. It was later discovered that a gene designated V-SRC was the transforming region of the Rous sarcoma virus. This observation, together with the first demonstration of its tyrosine kinase activity, launched a new and fertile field of investigation [1]. In the 2000s, the responsiveness of the sarcoma subtype gastrointestinal stromal tumor (GIST) to imatinib created a paradigm for the promise of molecular targeted therapy in solid tumors.

A major therapeutic landmark in treating bone sarcoma occurred in the 1960s when it was first noted that total amputation was not a curative solution, and many patients eventually died of

V. Subbiah, M.D. (✉)
Division of Cancer Medicine, The University of Texas MD Anderson Cancer Center, 1515 Holcombe Blvd, Unit 463, Houston, TX 77030, USA
e-mail: vsubbiah@mdanderson.org

R. Kurzrock, M.D.
Department of Investigational Cancer Therapeutics, MD Anderson Cancer Center, Houston, TX, USA

M. Bologna (ed.), *Biotargets of Cancer in Current Clinical Practice*, Current Clinical Pathology,
DOI 10.1007/978-1-61779-615-9_16, © Springer Science+Business Media, LLC 2012

metastatic disease. Subsequently, adding chemotherapy to the treatment regimen dramatically improved patient outcomes in this subtype of bone sarcomas in young patients and led to the fundamental belief that most, if not all, sarcoma patients have micrometastatic disease at diagnosis.

The Present and Future

Unfortunately, therapeutic options for sarcomas have essentially remained unchanged, with cytotoxic regimens reaching a therapeutic plateau in their potential. However, rapid strides have been made in the neoadjuvant and the adjuvant settings in the "pediatric bone sarcomas" (osteosarcoma and Ewing's sarcoma). Recent advances in the ability to molecularly characterize individual patient tumors leading to the consequent personalization of chemotherapy have further broadened research in this area.

The successful translation of a compound targeting c-kit receptors in GIST with imatinib and recent identification of insulin-like growth factor 1 receptor (IGF1R) as a potential target for Ewing's sarcoma demonstrate the benefit that can be derived from targeted agents in sarcoma patients. Because most sarcomas are driven by a translocation or mutation, the need to identify targeted agents for these anomalies has become apparent. Most patients with sarcoma should ideally receive treatment in specialty or tertiary care centers that employ a multidisciplinary approach that combines surgery, radiation therapy, and chemotherapy. If available, newer agents in rationally designed clinical studies based on molecularly "targeted therapy" will also become an integral component of this armamentarium.

The adult sarcomas comprising the heterogenous soft tissue sarcomas (STS) have historically been grouped together in clinical trials. Consequently, responses in subtypes with their particular histologies combined with the rarity of their occurrence could not be evaluated even if they had excellent responses in early phase trials.

Classification

Broadly, sarcomas are divided into soft tissue and bone sarcomas. Histopathologically, STS are classified based on the soft tissue cell of origin. The exponential increase of cytogenetic information has led to reclassification and regrouping of subtypes. Genome sequencing technologies may further refine and redefine these subgroups in the future. The current WHO classification below takes into account such detailed genetic and histologic data (Table 16.1).

Table 16.1 WHO classification of soft tissue tumors

Adipocytic tumors
Benign
Lipoma 8850/0[a]
Lipomatosis 8850/0
Lipomatosis of nerve 8850/0
Lipoblastoma/lipoblastomatosis 8881/0
Angiolipoma 8861/0
Myolipoma 8890/0
Chondroid lipoma 8862/0
Extrarenal angiomyolipoma 8860/0
Extra-adrenal myelolipoma 8870/0
Spindle cell 8857/0
Pleomorphic lipoma 8854/0
Hibernoma 8880/0
Intermediate (locally aggressive)
Atypical lipomatous tumor/well-differentiated liposarcoma 8851/3
Malignant
Dedifferentiated liposarcoma 8858/3
Myxoid liposarcoma 8852/3
Round cell liposarcoma 8853/3
Pleomorphic liposarcoma 8854/3
Mixed-type liposarcoma 8855/3
Liposarcoma, not otherwise specified 8850/3
Fibroblastic/myofibroblastic tumors
Benign
Nodular fasciitis
Proliferative fasciitis
Proliferative myositis
Myositis ossificans fibro-osseous pseudotumor of digits
Ischemic fasciitis
Elastofibroma 8820/0
Fibrous hamartoma of infancy
Myofibroma/myofibromatosis 8824/0
Fibromatosis colli
Juvenile hyaline fibromatosis
Inclusion body fibromatosis
Fibroma of tendon sheath 8810/0

(continued)

16 Biotargets in Sarcomas: The Past, Present, and a Look into the Future

Desmoplastic fibroblastoma 8810/0
Mammary-type myofibroblastoma 8825/0
Calcifying aponeurotic fibroma 8810/0
Angiomyofibroblastoma 8826/0
Cellular angiofibroma 9160/0
Nuchal-type fibroma 8810/0
Gardner fibroma 8810/0
Calcifying fibrous tumor
Giant cell angiofibroma 9160/0

Intermediate (locally aggressive)

Superficial fibromatoses (palmar/plantar)
Desmoid-type fibromatoses 8821/1
Lipofibromatosis

Intermediate (rarely metastasizing)

Solitary fibrous tumor 8815/1 and hemangiopericytoma
9150/1 (incl. lipomatous hemangiopericytoma)
Inflammatory myofibroblastic tumor 8825/1
Low-grade myofibroblastic sarcoma 8825/3
Myxoinflammatory
Fibroblastic sarcoma 8811/3
Infantile fibrosarcoma 8814/3

Malignant

Adult fibrosarcoma 8810/3
Myxofibrosarcoma 8811/3
Low-grade fibromyxoid sarcoma 8811/3
Hyalinizing spindle cell tumor
Sclerosing epithelioid fibrosarcoma 8810/3

So-called fibrohistiocytic tumors

Benign

Giant cell tumor of tendon sheath 9252/0
Diffuse-type giant cell tumor 9251/0
Deep benign fibrous histiocytoma 8830/0

Intermediate (rarely metastasizing)

Plexiform fibrohistiocytic tumor 8835/1
Giant cell tumor of soft tissues 9251/1

Malignant

Pleomorphic "MFH"/undifferentiated
Pleomorphic sarcoma 8830/3
Giant cell "MFH"/undifferentiated
Pleomorphic sarcoma
With giant cells 8830/3
Inflammatory "MFH"/undifferentiated
Pleomorphic sarcoma with
Prominent inflammation 8830/3

Smooth muscle tumors
Angioleiomyoma 8894/0
Deep leiomyoma 8890/0
Genital leiomyoma 8890/0
Leiomyosarcoma (excluding skin) 8890/3

Pericytic (perivascular) tumors
Glomus tumor (and variants) 8711/0
Malignant glomus tumor 8711/3
Myopericytoma 8713/1

Skeletal muscle tumors

Benign

Rhabdomyoma 8900/0

Adult type 8904/0
Fetal type 8903/0
Genital type 8905/0

Malignant

Embryonal rhabdomyosarcoma 8910/3 (incl. spindle
cell, 8912/3 botryoid, anaplastic) 8910/3
Alveolar rhabdomyosarcoma (incl. solid, anaplastic)
8920/3
Pleomorphic rhabdomyosarcoma 8901/3

Vascular tumors

Benign

Hemangiomas
Subcut/deep soft tissue 9120/0
Capillary 9131/0
Cavernous 9121/0
Arteriovenous 9123/0
Venous 9122/0
Intramuscular 9132/0
Synovial 9120/0
Epithelioid hemangioma 9125/0
Angiomatosis
Lymphangioma 9170/0

Intermediate (locally aggressive)

Kaposiform hemangioendothelioma 9130/1

Intermediate (rarely metastasizing)

Retiform hemangioendothelioma 9135/1
Papillary intralymphatic angioendothelioma 9135/1
Composite hemangioendothelioma 9130/1
Kaposi sarcoma 9140/3

Malignant

Epithelioid hemangioendothelioma 9133/3
Angiosarcoma of soft tissue 9120/3

Chondro-osseous tumors
Soft tissue chondroma 9220/0
Mesenchymal chondrosarcoma 9240/3
Extraskeletal osteosarcoma 9180/3

Tumors of uncertain differentiation

Benign

Intramuscular myxoma 8840/0 (incl. cellular variant)
Juxta-articular myxoma 8840/0
Deep ("aggressive") angiomyxoma 8841/0
Pleomorphic hyalinizing
Angiectatic tumor
Ectopic hamartomatous thymoma 8587/0

Intermediate (rarely metastasizing)

Angiomatoid fibrous histiocytoma 8836/1
Ossifying fibromyxoid tumor 8842/0 (incl. atypical/
malignant)
Mixed tumor/8940/1
Myoepithelioma/8982/1
Parachordoma 9373/1

Malignant

Synovial sarcoma 9040/3
Epithelioid sarcoma 8804/3
Alveolar soft part sarcoma 9581/3
Clear cell sarcoma of soft tissue 9044/3

(continued)

(continued)

Table 16.1 (continued)

Extraskeletal myxoid chondrosarcoma 9231/3
("chordoid" type)
PNET/extraskeletal Ewing's tumor
pPNET 9364/3
Extraskeletal Ewing's tumor 9260/3
Desmoplastic small round cell tumor 8806/3
Extrarenal rhabdoid tumor 8963/3
Malignant mesenchymoma 8990/3
Neoplasms with perivascular epithelioid cell
differentiation (PEComa)
Clear cell myomelanocytic tumor
Intimal sarcoma 8800/3

Adapted from Fletcher CDM, Unni KK, Mertens F, World Health Organization, International Agency for Research on Cancer. Pathology and genetics of tumours of soft tissue and bone. Lyon: IARC Press; 2002
[a]Morphology code of the international classification of diseases for oncology (ICD-O) {} and the systematized nomenclature of medicine (http://snomed.org)

Grouping

Although traditionally, sarcomas have been broadly grouped into bone and STS, this now seems oversimplified in view of their diverse biology and intrasubtype and intersubtype heterogeneity.

Other classification schemes divide sarcomas into:

1. Translocation-positive versus translocation-negative sarcomas
2. Adult-type sarcomas versus pediatric type sarcomas
3. Chemosensitive versus chemoresistant types

In a cumulative compendium of current knowledge of histology, clinical features, and specific molecular events that define tumor subtypes, Nielson et al. recently devised a classification that groups sarcomas into four categories [2] shown in Table 16.2 and Fig. 16.1.

Table 16.2 Clinical, pathologic, molecular classes of sarcoma. Adapted with permission from [2]

Group	Definition	Examples
1	Nonpleomorphic histology and known pathognomonic molecular events	GIST with activating *KIT* mutations, dermatofibrosarcoma protuberans and pigmented villonodular synovitis where translocations fuse collagen promoters to growth factors, and sarcomas bearing fusion transcription factor translocations including Ewing family of tumors
2	Affect younger patients and generally have nonpleomorphic histology and karyotypes of limited complexity, but pathognomonic molecular events, which are likely to exist, have yet to be identified	Adamantinoma, chordoma
3	Seen mostly in adult populations and show pleomorphic histology, but on a background of complex changes, do include consistently identified molecular events	Dedifferentiated liposarcoma with *CDK4/MDM2* amplifications, malignant peripheral nerve sheath tumor with *NF1* deletions, myxoinflammatory fibroblastic sarcoma with recently recognized t(1;10) and 3p amplifications11
4	This group is most common in adult populations. They have complex karyotypes, pleomorphic histology, and lack consistently identifiable molecular events	Undifferentiated pleomorphic sarcoma/malignant fibrous histiocytoma, leiomyosarcoma, pleomorphic lipo- and rhabdomyosarcomas, angiosarcoma, osteosarcoma, myxofibrosarcoma, myofibroblastic sarcoma

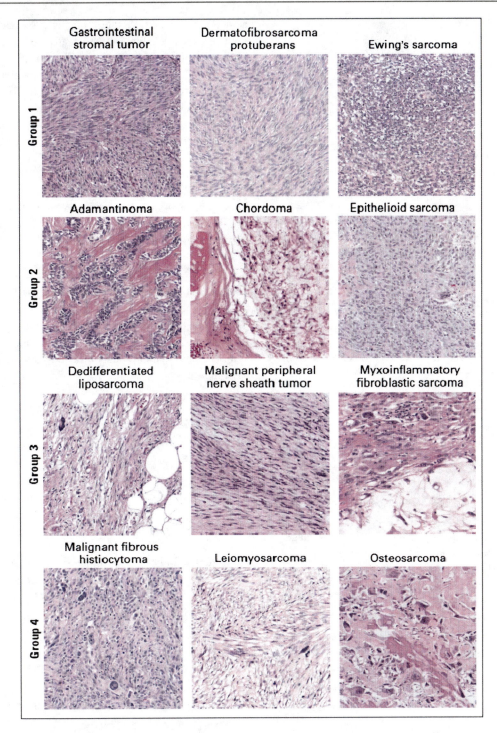

Fig. 16.1 Clinical, pathologic, molecular classes of sarcoma. Group 1: nonpleomorphic tumors with pathognomonic molecular events. Group 2: nonpleomorphic tumors for which pathognomonic molecular events have yet to be identified. Group 3: sarcomas with pleomorphic histology and some defined molecular events alongside complex karyotypic changes. Group 4: pleomorphic sarcomas with complex karyotypes and expression profiles. Adapted with permission from [2]

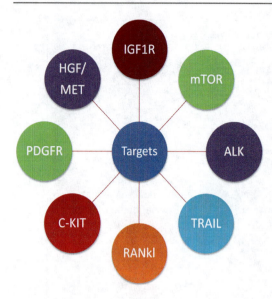

Fig. 16.2 Targeted therapies in sarcomas: This illustrates some specific opportunities for targeted therapies in sarcomas. *IGF1R* insulin-like growth factor 1 receptor, *mTOR* mammalian target of rapamycin, *ALK* anaplastic lymphoma kinase, *TRAIL* TNF-related apoptosis-inducing ligand, *RANKL* receptor activator of NF-κB ligand *PDGFR* platelet-derived growth activating factor, *HGF/MET* hepatocyte growth factor/mesenchymal-epithelial transition factor pathway

Genetic Aberrations/Translocations

Many sarcomas harbor specific genetic events/aberrations that are often diagnostic and sometimes confer a prognostic and therapeutic advantage.

The exclusive genomic events include:
1. Aberrant transcription factors that lead to unique genetic rearrangements
2. Constitutively active receptor tyrosine kinases (RTKs)
3. Constitutively active growth factors

These exclusive events as shown in Fig. 16.2 may be amenable to targeted therapies. Table 16.3 catalogs the known translocations/genetic events.

TET-Family Genetic Rearrangements

TET gene families are so-named using the first letters of *TLS/FUS*, *EWSR1*, and *TAFII68* genes. TET-family proteins possess a unique 87-amino acid RNA recognition motif that is associated with protein-RNA binding and that participates in transcription and RNA metabolism [6, 7]. More than 50% of these fusion proteins are associated with many sarcomas and are thought to be primordial events in sarcomagenesis [7].

Each of these family members may be intermixed, generating a sarcoma subtype. For instance, EWSR1-ERG as well as some FUS-ERG fusions are associated genotypically with Ewing's sarcoma, and these may be phenotypically impossible to tell apart [6]. Likewise, EWSR1-DDIT3 and FUS-DDIT3 are found in myxoid liposarcoma and are phenotypically alike.

Major Sarcoma Subtypes: Key Points

The complete epidemiology of the several types of sarcoma is beyond the scope of this chapter. Below are the salient points of the most common sarcoma subtypes.

Group 1 Sarcomas

Gastrointestinal Stromal Tumors

- GISTs are the most common among the gastrointestinal sarcomas.
- Most frequently occur in the 40–60-year age group.
- More than three-fourths of patients with GIST harbor activating mutations of the *c-kit* gene. The *c-kit* gene encodes the tyrosine kinase receptor for stem cell ligand.

Dermatofibrosarcoma Protuberans

- This very rare sarcoma presents near the body surface; surgical resection is the primary modality of therapy.
- The hallmark of DFSP is rearrangement of chromosomes 17 and 22 (17q22 and 22q13).
- There is constitutive production of the platelet-derived growth factor B ligand (PDGFB), leading to autostimulation in

Table 16.3 Genetic translocations in sarcomas

Sarcomas with fusion genes

Fusion genes involving TET genes

	Gene (N-C)	Chromosomal location	Clinical significance	Proposed function of gene product	Detection method
Ewing's/PNET	*EWSR1-FLI1 EWSR1-ERG EWSR1-ETV1 EWSR1-ETV4 EWSR1-FEV FUS-ERG FUS-FEV EWSR1-ZSG*	t(11;22)(q24;q12) t(21;22) (q22;q12) t(7;22)(p22;q12) t(17;22)(q12;q12) t(2;22) (q33;q12) t(16;21)(p11;q22) t(2;16) inv (22)	Diagnosis	Overexpression of oncogene, e.g., *MYC, ID2, CCND1, IGF1*	IHC (FLI1) karyotype FISH (EWSR1 break apart probe), RT-PCR
Desmoplastic small round cell tumor	*EWSR1-WT1 EWSR1-ERG*	t(11;22)(p13;q12) t(21;22) (q22;q12)	Diagnosis, therapeutic (PDGF inhibitors)	Upregulates oncogenic factors, e.g., *PDGF, IL2Rβ, BAIALP3, TALLA1,MLF1*	IHC (WT1) FISH (EWSR1 break-apart probe) karyotype
Clear cell sarcoma (CCS)	*EWSR1-ATF1 EWSR1-CREB1*	t(12;22)(q13;q12) t(2;22) (q33;q12)	Diagnosis	Upregulation of *ARNT2, ATM, GPP34, MITF* gene	FISH (EWSR1 break-apart probe), PCR
Angiomatoid fibrous histiocytoma	*FUS-ATF1 EWSR1-ATF1 EWSR1-CREB1*	t(12;16)(q13;p11) t(12;22) (q13;q12) t(2;22)(q33;q12)	Diagnosis		FISH
Extraskeletal myxoid chondrosarcoma	*EWSR1-NR4A3 TAF2N-NR4A3 TCF12-NR4A3 TFG-NR4A3*	t(9;22)(q22;q12) t(9;17) (q22;q11) t(9;15)(q22;q21) t(9;22)(q22;q15)	Diagnosis		FISH, RT-PCR (NR3A3-EWS fusion)
Myxoid/round cell liposarcoma	*FUS-DDIT3 (CHOP) EWSR1-DDIT3 (CHOP)*	t(12;16)(q13;p11) t(12;22) (q13;q12)	Diagnosis, potential therapeutic	Overexpression of MDM2, CDK4,*MET. PDGFα*	FISH (FUS break-apart probe)
Low-grade fibromyxoid sarcoma/HSCT	*FUS-CREB3L2 FUS-CREB3L1*	t(7;16)(q33;p11) t(11;16) (p11;p11)	Diagnosis		FISH (FUS break-apart probe), RT-PCR

Fusion genes involving RTK genes

	Gene (N-C)	Chromosomal location	Clinical significance	Proposed function of gene product	Detection method
Congenital mesoblastic nephroma	*ETV6-NTRK3*	t(12;15)(p13;q25)	Diagnosis		FISH, RT-PCR
Congenital fibrosarcoma	*ETV6-NTRK3*	t(12;15)(p13;q25)	Diagnosis		FISH, RT-PCR
Inflammatory myofibroblastic tumor	*TPM3-ALK TPM4-ALK CLTC-ALK RANBP2-ALK*	t(1;2)(q25;q23) t(2;19) (q23;q13) t(2;17)(q23;q23) t(2;2)(p23;q13)	Diagnosis		IHC (ALK protein) FISH, RT-PCR

(continued)

Table 16.3 (continued)

Sarcomas with fusion genes

Fusion genes involving TET genes

	Gene (N-C)	Chromosomal location	Clinical significance	Proposed function of gene product	Detection method
Fusion genes involving chromatin remodeling genes					
Synovial sarcoma	SS18-SSX1 SS18-SSX2 SS18-SSX4 SS18L1-SSX1 TLE1 gene	t(X;18)(p11;q11) t(X;18)(p11;q11) t(X;18)(p11;q13) t(x;20)(p11;q13)	Diagnosis, better prognosis of SS18-SSX2		FISH (SYT probe), RT-PCR, IHC (TLE1 protein)
Endometrial stromal sarcoma	JAZF1-SUZ12 JAZF1-PHF1 EPC1-PHF1	t(7;17)(p15;q21) t(6;7)(p21;p15) t(6;10)(p21;p11)	Diagnosis		RT-PCR
Fusion genes involving growth factors genes					
Dermatofibrosarcoma protuberans	COL1A1-PDGFB	t(17;22)(q22;q13)	Diagnosis, therapeutic (Gleevec responsive)	Upregulate the expression of *PDGFR*	FISH, RT-PCR
Giant cell fibroblastoma	COL1A1-PDGFB	t(17;22)(q22;q13)	Diagnosis		FISH, RT-PCR
Other type of fusion genes					
Alveolar rhabdomyosarcoma	PAX3-FOXO1A PAX7-FOXO1A PAX3-MLLT7 PAX3-NCOA1	t(2;13)(q35;q14) t(1;13)(q36;q14) T(2;X)(p35;q13) T(2;2)(q35;q23)	Diagnostic better prognosis with PAX7-FOXO1A		FISH (*FOXO1A* break-apart probe), karyotype, RT-PCR
Alveolar soft part sarcoma	ASPSL-TFE3	t(X;17)(p11;q25)	Diagnosis		IHC (TFE3), RT-PCR
Aneurysmal bone cyst	CDH11-USP6 THRAP3-USP6 CNBP-USP6 OMD-USP6 COL1A1-USP6	t(16;17) t(1;17) t(3;17) t(9;17) t(17;17)	Diagnosis		FISH, RT-PCR
Tenosynovial giant cell tumor	CSF1-COL6A3	t(1;2)	Diagnosis		
Hemangiopericytoma		t(12;19)	Diagnosis		
Pericytoma	*ACTB-GLI1*	t(7;12)	Diagnosis		
Sarcomas with specific oncogenic mutation					
Gastrointestinal stromal tumors	KIT or PGDFRA	Occult 4q12	Diagnosis, c-kit Gleevec responsive	Activation tyrosine kinase receptor	IHC (c-kit), PCR
Rhabdcid tumor	SMARCB1	del 22q11.22	Diagnosis	LOH	IHC (loss of INI1)
Atypical lipomatous tumor/well-differentiated liposarcoma	Giant marker and in *Micatio3*		Cyclin-dependent kinase	FISH (*MDM2, CDK4* amplification)	
Fibromatosis	APC inactivation	Trisomies 8 and 20 Deletion of 5q	Diagnosis		IHC(β-catenin)

Adapted from Jain S, Xu R, Prieto VG, Lee P. Molecular classification of soft tissue sarcomas and its clinical applications. Int J Clin Exp Pathol 2010;3:416–28

Synovial Sarcoma

- Monophasic synovial sarcoma (spindle cell morphology) and biphasic (both spindle + epithelioid morphology) are two subtypes within this type.
- Possess a pathognomonic t(X,18) translocation (p11.2;q11.2). This leads to the apposition of the *SS18* (also known as *SYT*) gene on chromosome 18 with one of three closely related genes (*SSX1*, *SSX2*, and *SSX4*) on the X chromosome. The fusion product is associated with sarcomagenesis.
- Surgery, chemotherapy, and radiation are used, and it is a high-grade sarcoma. The SYT-SSX fusion protein that results from the X,18 translocation may be a druggable target. Other overexpressed proteins are bcl-2, EGFR, and HER2/neu which may also be targets.

Group 2 Sarcomas

Adamantinoma

- Adamantinoma is a very rare low-grade malignant bone tumor with males more prone to develop it than females.
- Surgery, which is the mainstay of treatment, includes wide tumor excision, amputation, or limb salvage reconstruction surgery.
- It is radiotherapy and chemotherapy resistant.

Chordoma

- The most common primary malignant tumor of the spine and sacrum.
- Causes significant morbidity through local aggressiveness, leading to neurologic compromise and lytic destruction of bone.
- Surgery is the mainstay of treatment and is relatively radiotherapy and chemotherapy resistant.
- Recent studies show activity of PDGFR inhibitors, and EGFR inhibitors of both EGFR (HER1) and HER2/neu, and as inhibitors of mTOR.

sarcomagenesis. This has been demonstrated preclinically and has important clinical implications.

- Imatinib blocks the PDGF receptor PDGFB in addition to its ABL and KIT kinase activity and has been used in advanced DFSP.

Pigmented Villonodular Synovitis

- Benign tumor associated with proliferation of giant cells in the synovium.
- The hallmark is a t(1;2) translocation involving a collagen gene and *CSF1*, the gene for macrophage colony-stimulating factor (M-CSF).
- Occurs in young and older adults.
- Open synovectomy is the standard treatment with arthroscopic synovectomy in some patients. Radiation therapy may also be used.
- Recently, there has been some success with imatinib mesylate for the treatment of locally advanced and/or metastatic pigmented villonodular synovitis/tenosynovial giant cell tumor (GCT). Imatinib also seems to inhibit the M-CSF receptor in addition to its c-kit and PDGFR activity.

Ewing's Sarcoma

- Second most common bone cancer in children, adolescents, and young adults.
- Incidence is around 250–700/year.
- Nonmetastatic disease has 70% 5-year survival.
- Metastatic and recurrent disease confer less than a 20% chance of survival.
- Relatively highly chemosensitive to standard cytotoxic agents.
- Hallmark is EWS-FLI1 translocation. There are other subtypes with EWS fusing with translocation partners other than FLI1.
- Recent studies have shown IGF1R/mTOR pathway activity in Ewing's sarcoma.

Group 3 Sarcomas

Dedifferentiated Liposarcoma

- Liposarcoma comprises the most common soft tissue sarcoma in the USA.
- Well-differentiated liposarcoma/dedifferentiated liposarcoma, myxoid liposarcoma, round cell liposarcoma, and pleomorphic liposarcoma are the various histopathologic subtypes and differ in their clinical presentation.
- Considerable heterogeneity in clinical behavior as in well-differentiated liposarcoma/dedifferentiated liposarcoma has a low metastatic potential, in contrast to the round cell (RC) variants of MLPS or PLPS that have a high propensity to metastasize.
- Treatment is surgery with or without radiotherapy and chemotherapy for aggressive disease.
- There is an oncogenic *MDM2, CDK4, HMGA2,* and *TSPAN31* in well-differentiated liposarcoma/dedifferentiated liposarcoma sarcoma subtypes. This is of significance as MDM2 inhibitors are in clinical development.

Malignant Peripheral Nerve Sheath Tumor with *NF1* Deletions

- Malignant peripheral nerve sheath tumor (MPNST) includes tumors that were previously called malignant schwannoma, neurogenic sarcoma, and neurofibrosarcoma.
- This commonly affects adults and older adults, and more than half of these tumors are in patients with neurofibromatosis type 1 (NF1).
- This is a common autosomal dominant disorder with a prevalence of ~1:3,000–3,500 individuals worldwide.
- Highly aggressive nature confers a grave prognosis.
- There is a role for the HGF/MET autocrine loop in this disease which may be amenable to targeted therapy.

Group 4 Sarcomas

Undifferentiated Pleomorphic Sarcoma/ Malignant Fibrous Histiocytoma

- The term malignant fibrous histiocytoma has undergone a lot of name changes and has been classified and reclassified.
- MFH can be subdivided into five subtypes: storiform-pleomorphic (most common; up to 70%), myxoid (myxofibrosarcoma) (10–20%), giant cell (malignant GCT of soft parts), inflammatory, and angiomatoid.
- Gene expression profiling points to MFH having a mesenchymal stem cell origin.

Leiomyosarcoma

- Leiomyosarcoma is another very common sarcoma subtype.
- Uterine leiomyosarcomas are the most common. However, leiomyosarcoma may occur in extrauterine sites.
- The gene expression signatures of uterine and extrauterine leiomyosarcomas are different.
- Aberrations in *TP53* and *MDM2* expression and overexpression of cyclin-dependent kinase inhibitor 2A (*CDKN2A*) are seen commonly with this sarcoma.

Rhabdomyosarcomas

- Most common pediatric sarcoma and very rare in the older population.
- Is a relatively chemosensitive sarcoma with VAC-based therapies, surgery, and radiation conferring more than a 70% 5-year survival.
- Potential targets include IGF1R and mTOR. Preclinical studies show expression of ALK, FGF receptor 4, and the hepatocyte growth factor receptor in some cases of rhabdomyosarcoma which may be amenable to targeted therapy. Also, c-Met and MET expression are

associated with the PAX3-FKHR fusion and in patients with metastatic disease. CDK4 inhibitors might be particularly valuable in RMS as some subsets have CDK4 expression.

Angiosarcoma

- Very rare subtype. Occurs in scalp and facial areas.
- Some cases are seen in postradiotherapy planes.
- Recently, VEGF-based therapies have shown some clinical benefit.

Osteosarcoma

- The most common primary bone cancer, with approximately 1,000 cases occurring annually in the USA.
- Three-fourths of the patients with osteosarcoma are younger than 25 years.
- A second peak incidence of osteosarcoma occurs in patients older than 50 years of age.
- In the younger age group, it is mostly de novo (>95%) compared to the older age group in which more than 50% of patients have predisposing factors such as a prior history of radiotherapy or Paget's disease. A genetic predisposition to osteosarcoma is found in patients with hereditary retinoblastoma, characterized by mutation of the retinoblastoma gene RB1 on chromosome 13q14; Rothmund–Thomson syndrome, an autosomal recessive disorder with mutation in the RECQL4 gene in a subset of cases; and also in Li-Fraumeni syndrome, an autosomal dominant disorder. It is associated with a germline mutation of *p53*, a suppressor gene. A second recessive *p53* oncogene on chromosome 17p13.1 may also play a role in the development and progression of osteosarcoma.

Current Therapy for Sarcomas

As with most solid tumors, surgery remains the mainstay of therapy for localized STS. In addition, neoadjuvant chemotherapy and radiotherapy are employed for Stage II and beyond [8]. Bone sarcomas and STS are approached differently. Guidelines for the upfront management and treatment of soft tissue and bone sarcomas, including principles of biopsy, surgery, radiotherapy, and chemotherapy, are provided by the National Comprehensive Cancer Network (NCCN) and published in The Journal of the National Comprehensive Cancer Network (JCCN) [9, 10]. For that reason, it will only be touched upon and is not the primary purpose of this chapter.

In short, ifosfamide and Adriamycin are the two most widely accepted agents for the treatment of advanced STS. When they are administered in combination up to their full doses as upfront therapy, an overall response rate of 64% has been seen [11]. Bone tumors are treated with cisplatin and methotrexate in addition to ifosfamide and Adriamycin [12]. Accepted second-line agents include gemcitabine and docetaxel. These agents are also outlined in the NCCN guidelines [10] and are listed in Table 16.4 for STS and Table 16.5 for bone sarcomas.

Opportunity for Current and Future Targeted Therapy of Sarcomas

New drug development encompasses new cytotoxic chemotherapies, immunotherapies, and molecularly targeted treatments, which include both monoclonal antibodies and small molecule inhibitors of various targets and agonists. The current treatment paradigm in STS is a "one-size-fits-all" approach for sarcomas that are resistant to a particular accepted first-line therapy. Figure 16.3 illustrates the paradigm for targeted therapies. The challenge in that setting is how to design studies in single rare disease sarcoma subtypes. It is important to acknowledge that trials of targeted agents in sarcoma may be reporting low response rates as a group, which may overshadow the higher responses in some specific sarcoma subtypes. As illustrated in Fig. 16.4, while common relatively homogeneous cancers such as breast cancer are increasingly being divided by their molecular phenotype, it is still unfortunate that different types of sarcomas, though biologically distinct, are grouped together in clinical trials.

Table 16.4 Systemic therapy agents and regimens with activity in soft tissue sarcoma

Extremity, retroperitoneal, intra-abdominal sarcomas

Combination regimens AD (doxorubicin, dacarbazine), AIM (doxorubicin, ifosfamide, mesna), MAID (mesna, doxorubicin, ifosfamide, dacarbazine), ifosfamide, epirubicin, mesna, gemcitabine and docetaxel, gemcitabine and vinorelbine

Single agents doxorubicin, ifosfamide, epirubicin, gemcitabine, dacarbazine, liposomal doxorubicin, temozolomide

Angiosarcoma

Paclitaxel, docetaxel, vinorelbine, sorafenib, sunitinib, bevacizumab

Desmoid tumors (fibromatosis)

Sulindac or other nonsteroidal anti-inflammatory drugs including celecoxib[a], tamoxifen, toremifene, methotrexate, and vinblastine. Low-dose interferon, doxorubicin-based regimens, imatinib mesylate

GIST

Imatinib, sunitinib, sorafenib, nilotinib, dasatinib

Solitary fibrous tumor/hemangiopericytoma

Bevacizumab and temozolomide, sunitinib

Pigmented villonodular synovitis/tenosynovial giant cell tumor (PVNS/TGCT)

Imatinib

PEComa, recurrent angiomyolipoma, lymphangioleiomyomatosis

Sirolimus

Alveolar soft part sarcoma (ASPS)

Sunitinib

Chordoma

Combination regimens: erlotinib and cetuximab, imatinib and cisplatin, imatinib and sirolimus

Single agents: erlotinib, imatinib, and sunitinib

Adapted from Demetri GD, Antonia S, Benjamin RS, et al. Soft tissue sarcoma. J Natl Compr Canc Netw 2010;8:630–74

[a]The risk for cardiovascular events may be increased in patients receiving celecoxib. Physicians prescribing celecoxib should consider this information when weighing the benefits against risks for individual patients

It would be beneficial for protocols to include tumor tissue banking for correlative studies and biomarker development. At present, despite the less than fully developed approaches to sarcoma treatment as with the algorithm for neoadjuvant therapy for STS, sarcomas that have a definite translocation and those that express specific aberrant receptors and/or mutations are exciting tumors for targeted therapy.

Fusion Transcription Factors

Hypothetically, the fusion proteins in translocation-positive sarcomas are likely to become the molecular targets with the greatest promise. Fusion proteins are present only in tumor, not in normal tissue, and are primarily associated with survival, pathogenesis, metastasis, and progression and, hence, may be amenable to targeting. Agents directed against fusion proteins themselves

would be the preferred choice, although other opportunities may be their downstream targets. For instance, in the case of Ewing's sarcoma, abrogating EWS-FLI1 fusion protein expression in cell lines and nude mice models by oligodeoxynucleotides (ODNs), antisense RNA, and siRNA delivery via nanoparticles inhibited tumor growth and produced disease regression. While based on this preclinical success, targeting EWS-FLI1 may be the best approach, but translating these findings to real patients has not been possible. Hopefully, future advances in technology such as nanotechnology will allow translation of successful laboratory advancements in to clinical benefit.

Another approach would be to understand the transcription factors' downstream effects. For instance, EWS FLI1 binds to the insulin like growth factor binding protein 3 (IGFBP3) promoter and downregulates it. A secondary effect

16 Biotargets in Sarcomas: The Past, Present, and a Look into the Future

Table 16.5 Systemic therapy agents and regimens with activity in bone sarcoma. Adapted from [9]

Chondrosarcoma

Conventional chondrosarcoma (grades 1–3) has no known standard chemotherapy options

Mesenchymal chondrosarcoma: follow Ewing's regimens

Dedifferentiated chondrosarcoma: follow osteosarcoma regimens

Ewing's sarcoma

First-line therapy (primary/neoadjuvant/adjuvant)[a]

VAC/IE (vincristine, doxorubicin, and cyclophosphamide alternating with ifosfamide and etoposide)

VAI (vincristine, doxorubicin, and ifosfamide)

VIDE (vincristine, ifosfamide, doxorubicin, and etoposide)

Primary therapy for metastatic disease at initial presentation

CVD (cyclophosphamide, vincristine, and doxorubicin)

VAC/IE (vincristine, doxorubicin, and alternating with ifosfamide and etoposide) VAI (vincristine, doxorubicin, and ifosfamide)

VIDE (vincristine, ifosfamide, doxorubicin, and etoposide)

Second-line therapy (relapsed or refractory disease)[b]

Cyclophosphamide and topotecan

Temozolomide and irinotecan

Ifosfamide and etoposide

Ifosfamide, carboplatin, and etoposide

Docetaxel and gemcitabine

Osteosarcoma

First-line therapy

Cisplatin and doxorubicin MAP (high-dose methotrexate, cisplatin, and doxorubicin)

Doxorubicin, cisplatin, ifosfamide, and high-dose methotrexate ifosfamide and etoposide ifosfamide, cisplatin, and epirubicin

Second-line therapy (relapsed or refractory disease) docetaxel and gemcitabine cyclophosphamide and etoposide cyclophosphamide and topotecan gemcitabine ifosfamide and etoposide ifosfamide, carboplatin, and etoposide high-dose methotrexate, etoposide, and ifosfamide

MFH of bone

Follow osteosarcoma regimens

[a]Dactinomycin can be substituted for doxorubicin for concerns regarding cardiotoxicity
[b]Vincristine may be added to any of the regimens below

of a decrease binding protein might be an increase in insulin-like growth factor and activation of IGF1R machinery. This phenomenon may explain the striking activity of IGF1R inhibitors in some patients with Ewing's sarcoma.

Pathways and Specific Targeted Therapies

Cellular signaling pathways, cell surface adhesion molecules, RTKs, and growth factors are overexpressed in various sarcoma subtypes. Developments in genomics and proteomics have elucidated several of these pathways with a role in sarcomas as well as some plausible druggable targets as detailed below.

Insulin-Like Growth Factor/Akt/mTOR

IGF1 and its receptor, IGF1R, are components of a hormone system (which includes insulin and its receptor) whose activity is driven by binding to a tyrosine kinase cell surface receptor, thereby activating a series of intracellular signaling pathways that include the MAPK kinase pathway and the Akt pathway. This activation results in increased cell proliferation and resistance to apoptosis. IGF1R/PI3K/Akt and mTOR pathway activation have been shown to be critical for sarcoma tumor oncogenesis, proliferation, and survival across histologic subtypes both in preclinical studies and in retrospective review of patient specimens.

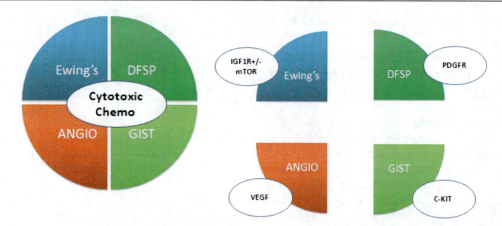

Fig. 16.3 Classical cytotoxic chemotherapy versus novel targeted therapeutics. A one-size-fits-all approach with the cytotoxic chemotherapeutics in large groups of patients represents the old paradigm in contrast to the novel targeted therapeutics approach, viz., imatinib mesylate for activated c-kit in GISTs or IGF1R inhibitors in Ewing's sarcoma

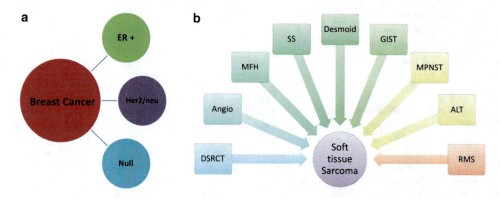

Fig. 16.4 Tumor subclassification homogeneous cancer type versus rare and diverse cancer/legend: common relatively homogeneous cancers such as breast cancer are increasingly being divided by their molecular phenotype (**a**) for purposes of treatment and clinical trials; conversely, STS subtypes, given their rarity, are often grouped together (**b**). *STS* soft tissue sarcomas, *SS* synovial sarcoma, *LMS* leiomyosarcoma, *ALT* atypical lipomatous tumor, *Angio* angiosarcoma, *MPNST* malignant peripheral nerve sheath tumor or neurofibrosarcoma, *MFH* malignant fibrous histiocytoma, *GIST* gastrointestinal stromal tumor, *RMS* rhabdomyosarcoma, *DSRCT* desmoplastic small round blue cell tumor. Adapted from [8]

Agents directed at these pathways have the potential to play an important role in the future of sarcoma developmental therapeutics. Other than mTOR inhibitors (rapamycin, temsirolimus, everolimus), which are FDA approved, the rest in other classes of agents (IGF1R inhibitors, Akt inhibitors) are in different stages of clinical and preclinical development.

Because the IGF1R signaling pathway has been implicated in the cancer biology of many different sarcoma subtypes, several associated clinical studies have enrolled advanced sarcoma patients [13]. In particular, IGF1R inhibitors have demonstrated early potential in the Ewing's sarcoma family of tumors. Three different IGF1R-antibody-based (R1507, AMG479, CP-751, 871) phase I trials [14–17] have been recently published showing activity even as monotherapy. In a phase I study of R1507 (Roche, Nutley, NJ), two patients with Ewing's sarcoma achieved partial responses (PR), with one patient achieving a near complete response (CR) for more than 26 months [14] (Fig. 16.5). In another study using AMG479 or ganitumab (Amgen, Thousand Oaks, CA), one patient achieved a CR and one had a PR [16]. In another phase I study using figitumumab, or CP-751, 871, (New York, NY) exclusively in 29 sarcoma patients, out of 16

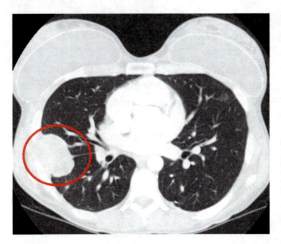 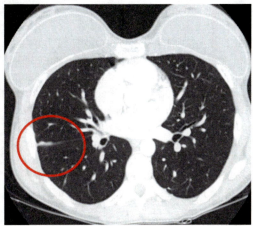

Fig. 16.5 Imaging responses in a patient with Ewing's sarcoma showing benefit to molecularly targeted IGF1R therapy. CT of the thorax in patient with Ewing's sarcoma showing response to IGF1R antibody (R1507) alone [14]. *Left panel* shows pretreatment CT scan of the thorax showing metastatic Ewing's sarcoma in the lung. *Right panel*: 6 weeks after IGF1R antibody (R1507) therapy shows regression of tumor

Ewing's sarcoma patients, one patient had a CR, one patient had a PR, and six patients had stable disease (SD) (range 4–16 months) [15]. Using different antibodies targeting different epitopes of the receptor, significant responses, albeit in only a subset of patients, have been seen in patients with advanced Ewing's sarcoma who had been refractory to multiple lines of earlier treatment.

The combination of IGF1R and mammalian target of rapamycin (mTOR), although using a different antibody (IMC-A12/cixutumumab and temsirolimus), also demonstrated responses [18, 19]. In the latter study, two patients who initially responded to an IGF1R inhibitor but later showed progression achieved a response to the combination, suggesting that mTOR inhibition helped overcome IGF1R resistance [19]. Furthermore, morphoproteomic analysis of tissue at the time of development of resistance to the IGF1R antibody confirmed upregulation of mTOR.

Preclinical studies have also shown that IGF1R-based agents may be efficacious in sarcomas such as alveolar rhabdomyosarcoma. Alveolar rhabdomyosarcoma harbors a PAX3-FOXOA1 translocation. IGF1R is a direct target of the oncogenic gene product. It may also have activity in other IGF2 secreting sarcomas, such as in patients with solitary fibrous tumors and those with GIST. These patients may present with symptomatic hypoglycemia as well as tumor, which is known as Doege–Potter syndrome. In fact, in an early-phase translational study using combined mTOR and IGF1R inhibition (everolimus and figitumumab) in patients with advanced sarcomas, PR was seen in a patient with massive solitary fibrous tumor. [20] Overexpression and activation of IGF1R have been shown in wild-type GIST but have not yet been translated into clinical benefit.

mTOR

Activation of the Akt/mammalian target of rapamycin (mTOR) pathway is associated with cell growth, metabolism, and angiogenesis. Growth factors like IGF1R control cell functions via the P13K pathway. The tumor suppressor phosphatase and tensin homolog (PTEN) is also very closely responsible for the functional signaling of mTOR. There has been an exponential growth in knowledge about the mTOR signaling pathway and associated aberrations in various sarcomas. Two complexes, mTOR complex 1 (TORC1) and mTOR complex 2 (TORC2), together orchestrate mTOR signaling. Rapalogs is the name given to rapamycin (sirolimus) and its analogs temsirolimus and everolimus, which are now available commercially. These agents have been shown to selectively target mTORC1 and have demonstrated preclinical and clinical activity in various types of sarcomas. A new generation of mTOR inhibitors with both mTORC1 and mTORC2 activity has been recently in clinical development. Other known drugs like metformin and also natural agents like curcumin, caffeine, and resveratrol have been shown to inhibit this pathway. Most recently, a new mTOR inhibitor AP23573 (deforolimus) has been through phase I, II, and III (NCT00093080, NCT00538239) in advanced sarcomas and from preliminary data seems promising. Final results of this trial are expected soon.

The Platelet-Derived Growth Factor Receptor Pathway

The platelet-derived growth factor group of signaling molecules and its receptor PDGFs and PDGFRs play a major role in angiogenesis, regulation of tumor growth, and also as transforming growth factors associated with cell cycle progression and evading apoptosis. The PDGF/PDGFR pathway has been shown to be active and expressed in many sarcoma subtypes, including GIST, osteosarcoma rhabdomyosarcoma, dermatofibrosarcoma protuberans, Ewing's sarcoma, desmoplastic small round cell tumor, MPNST, and uterine sarcomas.

In addition to KIT activity, imatinib is active against several other tyrosine kinase-containing cell surface receptors. The sarcoma subtype dermatofibrosarcoma protuberans possesses a unique PDGFB-COL1A1 translocation, which is ultimately processed into wild-type PDGF beta, which is a secreted signaling protein that binds to the PDGFR. The use of imatinib has resulted in dramatic activity in this disease, although other tumors like Ewing's sarcoma and osteosarcoma that express PDGFR yielded dismal results.

Death Receptor/TRAIL

Recombinant human apoptosis ligand 2/tumor necrosis factor-related apoptosis-inducing ligand (rhu Apo2L/TRAIL) (ligand for the death receptor), or dulanermin, is a proapoptotic receptor agonist that binds both death receptors 4 and 5 (also known as TRAIL 1 and 2, respectively) [21]. Binding

triggers cell death independently of the p53 pathway by activating the extrinsic pathway [21].

In a phase I study of rhu Apo2L/TRAIL in 71 advanced cancer patients, two chondrosarcoma patients had significant PRs, including one patient with a durable response over 5 years [21]. These results offer hope to patients with advanced chondrosarcoma who generally are relatively chemotherapy and radiotherapy resistant. It is unclear why chondrosarcoma patients in particular responded, and underlying mechanisms of response and resistance remain to be elucidated.

Anaplastic Lymphoma Kinase

Approximately 50% of cases of inflammatory myofibroblastic tumor harbor rearrangements of the anaplastic lymphoma kinase (*ALK*) locus on chromosome 2p23, causing aberrant ALK expression [22]. Recently, a sustained PR to the ALK (and c-Met) inhibitor crizotinib (PF-02341066, Pfizer, New York, NY) was reported as a part of a phase I study in a patient with *ALK*-translocated tumor. There was no activity in another patient with the same type of tumor but with no ALK translocation [22]. These divergent results in such a rare chemoresistant tumor demonstrate that ALK-mediated signaling contributes to tumorigenesis in a subgroup of patients with this disease and support the theory and hypothesis underlying successful translation of a molecularly targeted therapy.

Vascular Endothelial Growth Factor Receptor

Like many solid tumors, several sarcoma subtypes produce VEGF and/or express VEGFR, aberrations associated with growth, migration, and metastases.

The recombinant human monoclonal antibody bevacizumab (Avastin) has been shown to have some modest activity in refractory sarcoma subtypes. A 12% objective response rate was reported in angiosarcoma [23] In addition, several of the other VEGFR-2 small molecule inhibitors like sunitinib, sorafenib, and pazopanib are in different stages of clinical trials for sarcoma subtypes.

Cediranib (Recentin, AZD2171, AstraZeneca Pharmaceuticals, Wilmington, DE) is an orally bioavailable small molecule that potently inhibits the tyrosine kinase activity of vascular endothelial growth factor receptor 1 (VEGFR-1; Flt-1), VEGFR-2 (KDR), and VEGFR-3 (Flt-4), which mediate angiogenesis and lymphangiogenesis. In a pediatric phase I study, objective responses were seen in Ewing's sarcoma, synovial sarcoma, and osteosarcoma patients with pulmonary metastases [24]. A patient with alveolar soft part sarcoma (ASPS) had disease stabilization. In fact, cedarinib demonstrated promising activity in phase II studies in patients with ASPS (ClinicalTrials.gov number: NCT00942877), which is considered a chemoresistant sarcoma. Combination phase I studies using other anti-VEGF agents such as bevacizumab (Avastin, Genentech/Roche, and CA) are underway (ClinicalTrials.gov number: NCT00458731).

Receptor Activator of NF-κB Ligand

Osteoblasts and osteoclasts are required for normal bone physiology and are the primary cells associated with bone growth, modeling, and remodeling. The receptor activator of the NF-κB (RANK) pathway is a prerequisite for the differentiation of osteoclasts. Also required is the ligand of RANK known as RANKL. Preclinical models have demonstrated that loss of function of alleles in RANK and/or its ligand RANKL is associated with osteopetrosis. Interestingly, in one of the sarcoma subtypes, the GCT RANKL was overexpressed in a subpopulation of stromal cells, which comprise the tumor in addition to giant cells. These stromal elements may ultimately be incriminated as contributors to the bony destruction and resultant pathology seen in this sarcoma subtype. Although most commonly benign, these tumors may undergo malignant transformation. Surgery and radiation have thus far been the only options in the absence of systemic treatments. Denosumab (now approved by the FDA for osteoporosis), a monoclonal antibody to RANKL, was studied in GCT patients with clinical benefit achieved in as many as 86% of patients. The exact role of denosumab in the treatment algorithm remains to be defined, and several trials are exploiting this rational strategy.

Macrophage Colony-Stimulating Factor 1

Recurrent aberrations in the macrophage colony-stimulating factor (M-CSF 1) are seen in pigmented villonodular synovitis or tenosynovial GCT (PVNS/TGCT). In a similar fashion to GCT of the bone, which expresses RANKL, these tumors show overexpression of CSF1 receptors. Interestingly, KIT inhibitors like imatinib, nilotinib, and/or dasatinib may inhibit CSF1R in addition to KIT and PDGFR. Although this tumor is benign and does not cause mortality, it causes significant pain and morbidity as it attacks the tendons and joints. Clinically, imatinib was shown to demonstrate some activity in this tumor type. Studies using second-generation KIT inhibitors are in clinical trials.

p53 Pathway/MDM2 Pathway

Well-differentiated liposarcoma/dedifferentiated liposarcoma are associated with a similar genetic abnormality, typified by 12q14–15 amplification involving the MDM2 gene [25–27]. Preclinical studies have demonstrated that intact wild-type p53 together with MDM2 amplification can predict susceptibility to MDM2 inhibitor targeted therapy [25]. Two different MDM2 antagonists, RO5045337 [RG7112, Hoffmann-La Roche] (NCT00559533) and JNJ-26854165 [Ortho Biotech; Johnson & Johnson] (NCT00676910), are in phase I studies. Results in patients with advanced well-differentiated liposarcoma and dedifferentiated liposarcomas are awaited.

Hepatocyte Growth Factor/ Mesenchymal-Epithelial Transition Factor Pathway

Hepatocyte growth factor mediates cell survival, similar to other growth factors. This activity is mediated through the mesenchymal-epithelial transition factor (MET), which is an RTK. Several c-Met inhibitors are in various phases of preclinical and clinical development as activating mutations are seen in the more common cancers such as lung and gastric tumors. Mutations in the MET pathway have not yet been reported in sarcomas. However, several sarcoma subtypes like ASPS, clear cell sarcoma, some osteosarcoma subtypes, and alveolar rhabdomyosarcoma express MET. This may be a potential strategy that can be exploited in these sarcoma subtypes.

Other Targets and Early Clinical Trials for Sarcomas

Sarcoma patients are sometimes offered enrollment in early clinical trials using targeted or nontargeted agents after failing multiple lines of standard of care therapy. These trials establish the maximum tolerated dose in the case of cytotoxic agents and/or the optimal biologic dose of targeted agents for further phase II studies. Increasingly, eliciting response signals has become an important objective of these trials. Phase I trials represent the most critical step in translating findings from the bench to the bedside, especially for many novel first-in-human studies. Sarcomas that have a definite translocation and express aberrant receptors or specific mutations hold particular promise for deriving clinical benefit from targeted therapy [28]. Although many published preclinical studies with novel targets and agents have provided a rationale for using this approach in a clinical setting, actually translating these study findings to the bedside is difficult given the rarity and heterogeneity of sarcomas. On the other hand, clinically evaluating investigational agents, especially novel targeted therapies in sarcoma patients enrolled in phase I trials, may enlighten basic science researchers and clinical trialists about novel potential pathway involvement [29]. Such discoveries can delineate various subpopulations of sarcomas based on their pharmacodynamic and clinical responses. A list of such potential agents in development and potential sarcoma are shown in the Table 16.6.

Table 16.6 Specific targets and opportunities for enrollment of sarcoma patients in molecularly targeted phase 1 trials

Target/pathway	Potential target-specific sarcoma
Insulin-like growth factor 1 receptor (IGF1R)	Ewing's sarcoma, desmoplastic small round cell tumor, rhabdomyosarcoma, wild-type GIST
Mammalian target of rapamycin (mTOR)	Ewing's sarcoma, desmoplastic small round cell tumor, malignant peripheral nerve sheath tumor (MPNST), PEComa
Apoptosis ligand 2/tumor necrosis factor-related apoptosis-inducing ligand (Apo2L/TRAIL)	Chondrosarcoma, osteosarcoma
Receptor activator of NF-κB and ligand (RANKL)	Giant cell tumor of bone, other bone sarcomas, bone mets
Macrophage colony-stimulating factor 1 (M-CSF 1)	Pigmented villonodular synovitis and tenosynovial giant cell tumor
Retinoblastoma (RB gene)—CDK4	Well- and dedifferentiated liposarcoma
p53/mouse double minute (MDM2) inhibitor	Well- and dedifferentiated liposarcoma, malignant peripheral nerve sheath tumors and osteosarcomas, Ewing's sarcoma
Vascular endothelial growth factor receptor	All sarcomas in combination with chemo, angiosarcoma, alveolar soft part sarcoma, hemangioendothelioma
c-Met	Clear cell sarcoma, alveolar soft part sarcoma, alveolar rhabdomyosarcoma, MPNST, and osteosarcoma
PI 3 kinase/Akt/mTOR	Ewing's sarcoma, neurofibrosarcoma, chondrosarcoma
Aurora kinase	Ewing's sarcoma, liposarcoma
Histone deacetylases (HDAC)	Osteosarcoma, dedifferentiated chondrosarcoma, and liposarcoma
Chemokine receptor type 4 (CXCR-4)	Rhabdomyosarcoma, synovial sarcoma, Ewing's sarcoma
Her2/neu	Osteosarcoma, synovial sarcoma, and sarcoma expressing Her2/neu

(continued)

Table 16.6 (continued)

Target/pathway	Potential target-specific sarcoma
Nerve growth factor receptor NGFR	Neurogenic sarcoma
Platelet-derived growth factor receptors (PDGFR)	Ewing's sarcoma, dermatofibrosarcoma protuberans, hemangiopericytoma, GIST, desmoplastic small round cell tumor
Neurotrophin-3 receptor (NTRK3)	Congenital fibrosarcoma
BRAF	Gastrointestinal stromal tumor (refractory to imatinib)
RAF kinase	All types of sarcoma
Osteoclast/mevalonate	Bone sarcomas
Cell cycle inhibition/poly (ADP-ribose) polymerase (PARP)	Any type of sarcoma
Hedgehog	Ewing's sarcoma, bone sarcomas
Notch/gamma secretase inhibition	Osteosarcoma, liposarcoma
Anaplastic lymphoma kinase-1(ALK-1)	Inflammatory myofibroblastic tumor
SRC-kinase	Undifferentiated pleomorphic sarcoma, all sarcoma subtypes in combination with cytotoxics
c-kit/PDGFR	Gastrointestinal stromal tumor (refractory to imatinib), dermatofibrosarcoma protuberans
Proteasome	Liposarcoma, Ewing's sarcoma
Estrogen receptor	Desmoid

Conclusion

The recent molecular characterization of biotargets in sarcomas offers a tantalizing array of opportunities for targeted therapy, especially in those sarcomas that have a definite translocation and those that express specific receptor aberration. So far, the targeted agents used to address these aberrations have demonstrated mixed results. The challenge is identifying biomarkers predictive of response/resistance and matching them with a specific patient's histology.

References

1. Skubitz KM, D'Adamo DR. Sarcoma. Mayo Clin Proc. 2007;82:1409–32.
2. Nielsen TO, West RB. Translating gene expression into clinical care: sarcomas as a paradigm. J Clin Oncol. 2010;28:1796–805.
3. Jemal A, Siegel R, Xu J, Ward E. Cancer statistics, 2010. CA Cancer J Clin. 2010;60:277–300.
4. Chugh R, Baker LH. Pharmacotherapy of sarcoma. Expert Opin Pharmacother. 2009;10:1953–63.
5. Fletcher CDM, Unni KK, Mertens F. World Health Organization, International Agency for Research on Cancer. Pathology and genetics of tumours of soft tissue and bone. Lyon: IARC Press; 2002.
6. Jain S, Xu R, Prieto VG, Lee P. Molecular classification of soft tissue sarcomas and its clinical applications. Int J Clin Exp Pathol. 2010;3:416–28.
7. Riggi N, Cironi L, Suva ML, Stamenkovic I. Sarcomas: genetics, signalling, and cellular origins. Part 1: the fellowship of TET. J Pathol. 2007;213:4–20.
8. Reynoso D, Subbiah V, Trent JC, et al. Neoadjuvant treatment of soft-tissue sarcoma: a multimodality approach. J Surg Oncol. 2010;101:327–33.
9. Biermann JS, Adkins DR, Benjamin RS, et al. Bone cancer. J Natl Compr Canc Netw. 2010;8:688–712.
10. Demetri GD, Antonia S, Benjamin RS, et al. Soft tissue sarcoma. J Natl Compr Canc Netw. 2010;8:630–74.
11. Patel SR, Vadhan-Raj S, Burgess MA, et al. Results of two consecutive trials of dose-intensive chemotherapy with doxorubicin and ifosfamide in patients with sarcomas. Am J Clin Oncol. 1998;21:317–21.
12. Patel SR, Vadhan-Raj S, Papadopolous N, et al. High-dose ifosfamide in bone and soft tissue sarcomas: results of phase II and pilot studies–dose-response and schedule dependence. J Clin Oncol. 1997;15:2378–84.
13. Rodon J, DeSantos V, Ferry Jr RJ, Kurzrock R. Early drug development of inhibitors of the insulin-like growth factor-I receptor pathway: lessons from the first clinical trials. Mol Cancer Ther. 2008;7:2575–88.
14. Kurzrock R, Patnaik A, Aisner J, et al. A phase I study of weekly R1507, a human monoclonal antibody insulin-like growth factor-I receptor antagonist, in patients with advanced solid tumors. Clin Cancer Res. 2010;16:2458–65.

15. Olmos D, Postel-Vinay S, Molife LR, et al. Safety, pharmacokinetics, and preliminary activity of the anti-IGF-1R antibody figitumumab (CP-751,871) in patients with sarcoma and Ewing's sarcoma: a phase 1 expansion cohort study. Lancet Oncol. 2010;11:129–35.

16. Tolcher AW, Sarantopoulos J, Patnaik A, et al. Phase I, pharmacokinetic, and pharmacodynamic study of AMG 479, a fully human monoclonal antibody to insulin-like growth factor receptor 1. J Clin Oncol. 2009;27:5800–7.

17. Subbiah V, Anderson P, Lazar AJ, Burdett E, Raymond K, Ludwig JA. Ewing's sarcoma: standard and experimental treatment options. Curr Treat Options Oncol. 2009;10:126–40.

18. Subbiah V, Benjamin RS, Naing A, et al. Novel phase I clinical trials in sarcoma patients: the MD Anderson Cancer Center experience. J Clin Oncol (Meeting Abstracts). 2010;28:e13111.

19. Subbiah V NA, Brown RE, Robert Benjamin, Anderson PM, Kurzrock R. Targeted morphoproteomic profiling of Ewing's sarcoma treated with insulin-like growth factor 1 receptor (IGF1R) inhibitor: response and resistance signatures. In: Connective Tissue Oncology Society Proceedings. Paris, France; 2010.

20. Quek R, Wang Q, Morgan JA, et al. Combination mTOR and IGF-1R inhibition: phase I trial of everolimus and figitumumab in patients with advanced sarcomas and other solid tumors. Clin Cancer Res. 2011;17:871–9.

21. Herbst RS, Eckhardt SG, Kurzrock R, et al. Phase I dose-escalation study of recombinant human Apo2L/TRAIL, a dual proapoptotic receptor agonist, in patients with advanced cancer. J Clin Oncol. 2010;28:2839–46.

22. Butrynski JE, D'Adamo DR, Hornick JL, et al. Crizotinib in ALK-rearranged inflammatory myofibroblastic tumor. N Engl J Med. 2010;363:1727–33.

23. Judson I. Targeted therapies in soft tissue sarcomas. Ann Oncol. 2010;21:vii277–80.

24. Fox E, Aplenc R, Bagatell R, et al. A phase 1 trial and pharmacokinetic study of cediranib, an orally bioavailable pan-vascular endothelial growth factor receptor inhibitor, in children and adolescents with refractory solid tumors. J Clin Oncol. 2010;28(35):5174–81. Epub 2010 Nov 8.

25. Conyers R, Young S, Thomas DM. Liposarcoma: molecular genetics and therapeutics. Sarcoma. 2011;2011:483154.

26. Italiano A, Bianchini L, Gjernes E, et al. Clinical and biological significance of CDK4 amplification in well-differentiated and dedifferentiated liposarcomas. Clin Cancer Res. 2009;15:5696–703.

27. Coindre JM, Pedeutour F, Aurias A. Well-differentiated and dedifferentiated liposarcomas. Virchows Arch. 2010;456:167–79.

28. Wardelmann E, Schildhaus HU, Merkelbach-Bruse S, et al. Soft tissue sarcoma: from molecular diagnosis to selection of treatment. Pathological diagnosis of soft tissue sarcoma amid molecular biology and targeted therapies. Ann Oncol. 2010;21 Suppl 7:vii265–9.

29. Thomas DM, Wagner AJ. Specific targets in sarcoma and developmental therapeutics. J Natl Compr Canc Netw. 2010;8:677–85. quiz 86.

Melanoma and Other Skin Cancers

17

Kim H.T. Paraiso, Jobin K. John,
and Keiran S.M. Smalley

Melanoma and Skin Cancers: An Introduction

Skin cancers are the most common of all cancers. The incidence of skin cancer continues to increase year on year, with nearly 50% of all Americans reaching the age of 65 expected to have skin cancer at some point in their lives. Skin cancers are broadly categorized according to their cell of origin. The two most common forms of skin cancer, basal cell carcinoma (BCC) and squamous cell carcinoma (SCC), derive from the keratinocytes and are generally less deadly. In contrast, melanoma arises from the malignant transformation of melanocytes and is responsible for the majority of skin cancer deaths. Although exposure to solar ultraviolet radiation is the major risk factor for all skin cancers, keratinocyte- and melanocyte-derived cancers have distinct biological behavior, follow different clinical courses, and require different therapeutic management. In this chapter, we discuss the latest information on the epidemiological and molecular characteristics of both melanoma and nonmelanoma skin cancers and will describe how new information about the genetic mutations that drive these tumors can both dictate the prognosis and help guide therapy selection.

K.H.T. Paraiso, M.S. • J.K. John, M.D.
• K.S.M. Smalley, Ph.D. (✉)
Department of Molecular Oncology, The Moffitt Cancer Center, 12902 Magnolia Drive, Tampa, FL 33612, USA
e-mail: keiran.smalley@moffitt.org

Melanoma: Incidence, Epidemiology, and Risk Factors

Melanoma is the most aggressive, therapy resistant, and deadly form of skin cancer. Approximately 68,130 new cases of melanoma and 46,770 cases of melanoma in situ, resulting in 8,700 deaths, are estimated for the USA in 2010 [1]. Whereas overall rates of cancer death continue to decrease, risk of death from melanoma—particularly in male patients—continues to rise and showed a 7% increase during the period 1990–2006 [1]. The incidence of melanoma is both gender- and age-related, with melanoma frequencies being higher in women than men <40 years of age and then significantly higher in men than women above 40 years of age [2, 3]. Melanoma rates in men aged 75 years are currently three times higher than those of age-matched women [3]. Of particular concern, recent years have seen a dramatic increase (a 2.7% increase per year) in new melanoma diagnoses in women aged 15–39, thought to result in part through the increased use of sun tanning beds [4].

Risk factors for melanoma development include ultraviolet (UV) radiation exposure (e.g., sunlight and the use of tanning beds), family history of melanoma, skin type, numbers of nevi, age, ethnicity, and occupation [3]. UV radiation is a potent carcinogen and is known to damage genomic DNA leading to acquisition of mutations. There are good correlations between average annual UV exposure and melanoma risk,

M. Bologna (ed.), *Biotargets of Cancer in Current Clinical Practice*, Current Clinical Pathology,
DOI 10.1007/978-1-61779-615-9_17, © Springer Science+Business Media, LLC 2012

with similar correlations also existing between latitude and melanoma risk (with UV radiation being most intense at the equator) and altitude (where UV exposures are also greater) and melanoma risk [5]. Epidemiological studies have also shown that the age at which UV exposure occurs is also an important factor in determining melanoma risk. It is known that persons born in Australia have a higher lifetime incidence of melanoma development than those individuals who migrated to Australia after 10 years of age [6]. However, this is unlikely to be the only determinant of risk with other studies showing that prolonged UV exposure in later life also leads to increased melanoma incidence [7]. The causative role of UV exposure in melanoma development is further supported by the findings that individuals with a poor tanning response (such as those with fair skin and a tendency to freckle), and a presumably higher rate of UV-induced DNA damage in their skin, have the highest risk of melanoma development [3]. Support for these epidemiological studies also comes from whole genome-sequencing studies that have shown the presence of multiple UV-signature mutations in human melanoma cell lines [8]. Reduction of UV exposure through regular use of sunscreens significantly reduces melanoma development. A recent randomized trial of 1,621 people in Queensland, Australia, who were followed for 14 years, showed daily sunscreen use to reduce melanoma development by 50% [9].

A clear relationship exists between family history and risk of melanoma development with ~10% of all melanomas occurring in family clusters [3]. So far, two high-penetrance genes, encoding for the cyclin-dependent kinase inhibitor 2A (CDKN2A: p16) and cyclin-dependent kinase 4 (CDK4), respectively, have been associated with the development of hereditary melanoma [10, 11]. Of these, the incidence of CDKN2A mutation is more prevalent and is thought to account for 20–40% of all familial melanomas [10]. In comparison, CDK4 mutations have only been identified in 15 families worldwide, making them relatively rare [11].

Another predictive factor for melanoma development is the presence of large numbers of nevi [12]. Common acquired nevi are melanocytic proliferations that typically develop on areas of sun-exposed skin [13]. Although most nevi are benign, they can, in rare cases, develop into melanoma. There is a good correlation between nevus number and melanoma development, with individuals harboring >120 nevi having a 20-fold increased risk of melanoma [13, 14].

Melanoma Diagnosis and Prognosis: The Role of Biomarkers

Accepted markers for melanoma prognosis are vertical tumor (Breslow) thickness, invasion (Clark) level, the mitotic rate (measured as the number of mitoses per mm^2), the presence of ulceration, and the degree of lymph node involvement [15]. Breslow thickness (in millimeter) is measured from the granular layer of the epidermis down to the deepest point of invasion [16] (Fig. 17.1). Clark level describes the level of anatomical invasion of the melanoma in the skin (epidermis, papillary dermis, reticular dermis, subcutis) [17]. The current version of the AJCC melanoma staging and classification defines mitotic rate and ulceration as the most powerful predictors of survival in patients with localized melanomas (stages I and II) [15, 18]. The number of metastatic nodes, tumor burden, and presence or absence of melanoma ulceration are the most powerful predictors of survival in patients with nodal metastases (stage III), and the anatomic site of distant metastases was the most significant predictor of survival in patients with distant metastases (stage IV) [15].

The risk of metastasis to lymph nodes is directly related to the Breslow thickness and the number of mitoses in the primary melanoma [19, 20]. Metastases are rare for thin melanomas (<0.75 mm), and the risk for tumors 0.76–1.0-mm thick is about 5%. Melanomas that have an intermediate thickness (1–4 mm) have a risk that starts at about 8% for 1-mm tumors; this rises steadily to 30% with increasing depth. In addition to a high risk of systemic spread, melanomas thicker than 4 mm have a risk of approximately 40% for nodal involvement, in addition to a high

17 Melanoma and Other Skin Cancers

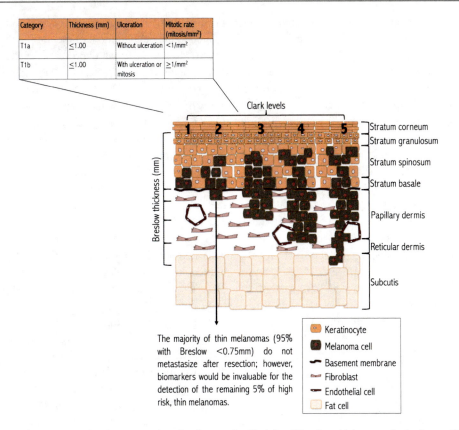

Fig. 17.1 Schematic showing the progression of melanoma by Clark level Breslow thickness and mitotic rate. Diagram shows the layers of the skin and its constituent cells

risk of systemic spread. A sentinel lymph node is one that receives lymphatic drainage directly from the primary tumor site. Although the survival benefit of sentinel lymph node dissection is highly debated, the sentinel lymph node status provides accurate prognostic information for disease-free and overall survival for melanomas stage T1b or greater [15, 21–23].

Although most melanomas can be adequately diagnosed through histological criteria, there remain subsets of melanoma that are difficult to distinguish from benign melanocytic nevi. Specific examples of these difficult diagnoses include certain types of nevi, such as dysplastic nevi and Spitz nevi, as these share overlapping histopathological features with melanomas. Diagnosis of these cases is especially difficult as none of the histochemical or immunohistochemical markers used in routine diagnosis can adequately differentiate between nevi and melanoma [24–26]. The one exception to this is the marker HMB45, which, in benign and dysplastic nevi, shows a gradient of strong staining in the superficial cells and weak-to-negative staining in the deeper tumor cells; in melanoma, HMB45 shows strong staining in the deep tumor cells. As misdiagnosis can have potentially grave consequences, there have been a number of attempts to develop diagnostic markers that allow the differentiation of benign and malignant melanocytic lesions. In a recent study, Kashani-Sabet et al. [27] defined a panel of five molecular markers that included developmental WNT pathway member-2 (WNT-2), fibronectin (FN1), actin-related protein 2/3 complex subunit 2 (ARPC2), secreted phosphoprotein-1 (SPP1), and regulator of G-protein signaling 1 (RGS1). Using a sample set of 693 melanocytic lesions (composed of Spitz nevi, melanomas, nevi, and misdiagnosed melanomas), the authors successfully used their marker panel to differentiate benign melanocytic lesions from melanoma with a specificity of 95% and a sensitivity of 91% [27].

The diagnosis of amelanotic melanomas can also be difficult. In these instances, the approach of choice is the immunohistochemical staining of lesions for components of the pigmentation machinery including the S100 protein, gp100 (HMB-45 antigen), and melanoma antigen recognized by T-cell one (MART-1; Melan-A protein). MART-1/Melan-A, S100, and gp100/HMB-45 show high sensitivity for melanoma (75–92%, 97–100%, 69–93%). As all of these markers are also found in melanocytic nevi, their specificity to distinguishing melanoma from nevi is low [24–26]. MART-1/Melan-A and S100 strongly stain both benign and malignant melanocytic neoplasms.

As melanomas frequently metastasize early, it is therefore critical to identify patients who are at risk for relapse and dissemination. Although biomarker strategies have been used successfully for prognostic and diagnostic purposes in other tumor types, no reliable biomarkers have yet been identified that are both highly sensitive and melanoma specific [28]. A recent meta-analysis of the literature identified over 515 publications [29] that described novel melanoma biomarkers. As yet, none of these have found their way into routine clinical practice for either diagnostic or prognostic purposes. The reasons for this lack of translation were manifold and included the lack of statistical power in the sample size and inadequate validation techniques. Of the initial 515 studies under consideration, only 37 of these were judged to be worth of analysis. The molecules identified in this subset of publications included melanoma cell adhesion molecule (Mel-CAM), matrix metalloproteinase-2 (MMP-2), the proliferation markers Ki67 and proliferating cell nuclear antigen (PCNA), and the tumor suppressor locus p16^{INK4A} [29]. The interested reader is directed to a series of excellent review articles that examine each of these biomarkers in detail [28–31].

The Ki-67 protein is expressed at all stages of the cell cycle except for the G0 quiescent phase and is considered to be a sensitive marker of cell proliferation. Expression of dermal Ki-67 is related to the development of melanoma metastases, with high dermal expression of Ki-67 of >20% being demonstrated to be an independent prognostic factor [32]. A 10-year retrospective study of 396 patients with thin melanomas stained for Ki-67 identified two groups with high risk of metastasis: the first consisted of men and women with a dermal mitotic rate of >0 and a dermal Ki-67 positivity of >20% and the second group consisted of men with a mitotic rate of >0 and a dermal Ki-67 of <20%, with 10-year metastasis rate of 39% and 20%, respectively [32].

The increased invasive potential of melanoma cells compared to melanocytes is due in part to altered expression of cell–cell and cell–matrix proteins, and a number of these molecules have been investigated as potential prognostic biomarkers for melanoma. Melanoma cells are known to express increased levels of receptors of the immunoglobulin gene superfamily of cell adhesion molecules (CAMs), such as melanoma cell adhesion molecule (MCAM, Mel-CAM, MUC18, CD146), L1 cell adhesion molecule (L1-CAM, CD171), activated leukocyte cell adhesion molecule (ALCAM, CD166), vascular cell adhesion molecule 1 (VCAM-1, CD106), intercellular cell adhesion molecule 1 (ICAM-1, CD54), and carcinoembryonic antigen-related cell adhesion molecule 1 (CEACAM1, CD66a) reviewed in [33]. Of these, Mel-CAM is required for homologous and heterologous interactions between melanoma cells and endothelial cells, respectively, via a heterophilic Ca^{2+}-independent adhesion to a currently unidentified ligand [34–36]. In melanocytic cells, expression of Mel-CAM is initially found in nevi, when the cells have separated from the epidermal keratinocytes and have migrated into the dermis [37, 38]. As the tumor progresses, Mel-CAM expression gradually increases and is at its highest in melanoma metastases [37, 39–42]. Two recent studies ($n = 76$ and $n = 170$, respectively) have shown Mel-CAM expression to independently predict for development of lymph node metastases [43] and worse overall survival (after adjustment for age, Breslow index, and Clark level) [44]. It was noted that Mel-CAM-negative patients had a 5-year survival of 92% compared to 40% for patients who were Mel-CAM positive [43]. One further study, on a larger cohort of patients ($n=340$) showed Mel-CAM expression to predict for disease-free and overall survival in a univariate analysis but not when multivariate analysis was performed. The discrepancy between this and the two previous studies was suggested to be a consequence of differences in the antibodies used and the methods of sample preservation [45].

L1-CAM is a neuronal cell adhesion molecule that is also detected in melanoma [46, 47]. It mediates adhesion both via homophilic (L1-CAM–L1-CAM) and heterophilic (L1-CAM–$\alpha_v\beta_3$ integrin) mechanisms [48] and allows for melanoma/melanoma cell and melanoma/endothelial cell interactions through its binding to $\alpha_v\beta_3$ integrin [49]. The interaction of L1-CAM and $\alpha_v\beta_3$ integrin plays an important role in transendothelial migration of melanoma cells [50] whereas overexpression of L1-CAM promotes conversion from radial to vertical growth phase melanoma without upregulation of $\alpha_v\beta_3$ integrin expression [51]. L1-CAM immunoreactivity is known to be increased in melanoma compared to nevi [52]. A study that systematically identified novel melanoma-specific genes confirmed L1-CAM not to be expressed in normal skin and melanocytic nevi but was highly and differentially expressed in primary melanoma tissues and melanoma lymph node metastases [53]. A recent study, evaluating 12 nevi, 67 primary melanomas, 40 sentinel lymph nodes and 35 distant metastases, showed L1-CAM to be a highly sensitive (90–93%) and specific (100%) diagnostic marker for melanoma [26]. A 10-year retrospective biomarker study, evaluating 100 melanoma specimens, showed the expression of L1-CAM in human primary cutaneous melanoma to be associated with metastatic spread and an independent predictor for metastasis [47].

Intercellular adhesion molecule (ICAM)-1 binds to integrin $\alpha_L\beta_2$ (lymphocyte function-associated antigen 1, LFA-1) and Mac1 on lymphocytes [54]. Its expression is known to correlate with melanoma progression and the increased risk of metastasis [55]. Increases in ICAM-1 expression parallel the transition from nevi to melanoma metastasis and correlate with Breslow index in primary melanomas [56–59]. The observation that stage I patients with ICAM-1-positive melanomas had a significantly shorter disease-free interval and overall survival than those with ICAM-1 negative tumors [57] and that the suppression of ICAM-1 in an animal model reduced the metastatic capacity [60] supported the role of ICAM-1 in melanoma progression and metastasis. However, the exact role of ICAM-1 in melanoma progression remains obscure with contradictory reports showing both that ICAM-1 promotes the aggregation of melanoma cells with leukocytes that enhances survival of tumor cells in the vascular system [61] and that ICAM-1 is shed from melanoma cells [62]—possibly in a form that inhibits lymphocyte–tumor cell interactions [63].

CEACAM1, CD66a, is a member of the immunoglobin family of cellular adhesion molecules involved in intercellular adhesion. In epithelial cells, CEACAM1 acts as a growth suppressor with its expression being either lost or significantly down- or dysregulated in carcinomas of liver, prostate, endometrium, breast, and colon reviewed in [33]. CEACAM1 interacts with the β_3 integrin subunit via the CEACAM1 cytoplasmic domain and colocalizes at the tumor–stroma interface, suggesting a role for the CEACAM1–integrin β_3 interaction in melanoma cell migration and invasion [64] and the development of metastases [65]. Forced overexpression of CEACAM1 in CEACAM1-negative melanocytic cells and melanoma cell lines leads to increased migratory and invasive growth potentials in vitro [66], supporting the role of CEACAM1 in melanoma progression and metastasis. An evaluation of 12 nevi, 67 primary melanomas, 40 sentinel lymph nodes, and 35 distant metastases showed CEACAM1 to be a highly sensitive (93–97%) and specific (63%) diagnostic marker for melanoma [26].

E-cadherin is expressed on the cell surface of both keratinocytes and melanocytes and is the major adhesion molecule mediating the interaction between these two cell types in the epidermis [67, 68]. In cell culture, melanoma cells lose their expression of E-cadherin and undergo a cadherin switch that favors an increase in N-cadherin expression that allows the melanoma cells to associate with fibroblasts and vascular endothelial cells [67]. Although experimental studies confirm that E-cadherin loss is critical to melanoma progression (reviewed in [69, 70]), the clinical data are conflicting and show that E-cadherin expression is not decreased in many cases of advanced melanoma [71–73]. A recent study evaluating 144 primary melanomas, 53 metastases, and 8 nevi reported E-cadherin expression to be significantly correlated with primary tumor depth, but this was not predictive of patient outcome [74]. Interestingly, when the E-cadherin expression data was combined with that of the calcium-binding protein S100A4, a stronger significant correlation between high E-cadherin-expressing and S100A4-negative biopsies and increased disease-free survival was revealed [74]. Another recent study evaluating 115 melanoma samples (55% of which were acral lentiginous melanomas) and 4–285-month follow-up (median 69 months) reported that 91% of the tumors showed reduced E-cadherin expression; however, there was no significant correlation between the level of E-cadherin expression and patient survival [75].

Molecular Subtypes of Melanoma: Personalizing Therapy

Currently, there are few effective treatments for disseminated melanoma, and the median survival from the disease is 6–10 months. Although primary melanoma is curable through surgery, treatment of advanced disease remains a challenge, and therapeutic strategies employed over the past 30 years have not significantly improved cure rates. Until very recently, all major chemotherapy drugs, immunotherapies, and radiotherapies failed to prolong survival when tested in large-scale phase III clinical trials [76]. The past decade has seen breakthroughs in personalized cancer medicine, where new targeted therapies are being developed that inhibit cellular proliferation and survival in tumors with certain specific oncogenic mutations. Use of these new agents, such as imatinib mesylate (Gleevec) in chronic myeloid leukemia (CML) and

gastrointestinal stromal tumors (GIST), represents a major advance in cancer therapy [77–79]. It is becoming clear that melanoma constitutes a heterogeneous group of tumors, with different patterns of oncogenic mutation, overexpression, and genomic amplification [80–82]. There are now encouraging signs that the deadlock in the therapeutic management of disseminated melanoma may be broken and that therapeutic strategies designed to specifically target the genetic mutations required for melanoma initiation and progression may allow for better levels of response. In the next sections, we outline the major molecular subtypes of melanoma and review the latest progress in matching small molecule targeted therapies with genotypes.

BRAF Mutant Melanoma

A significant advance in our understanding of melanoma initiation and progression was the discovery of activating mutations in *BRAF* in over 50% of melanomas [83, 84]. Rapidly growing fibrosarcoma (derived from Raf) proteins constitute a three member family of serine/threonine kinases (ARAF, BRAF, and CRAF) with closely overlapping functions [85]. So far, over 50 distinct mutations in *BRAF* have been identified [86]. Of these, the *BRAF* V600E mutation, resulting from a valine to glutamic acid substitution, is by far the most common and accounts for over 80% of all reported *BRAF* mutations [83, 87]. Most of the transforming activity of the *BRAF* V600E mutation is thought to result from the stimulation of the MAPK pathway [83] (Fig. 17.2). Constitutive activity in the Ras/Raf/MEK/ERK MAPK pathway contributes to the oncogenic phenotype of melanoma through its effects on cell proliferation, invasion, and survival [88] (Fig. 17.3). Of these, the best characterized role for MAPK signaling in melanoma is in the regulation of cell growth, particularly at the G1 cell-cycle checkpoint (Fig. 17.2). Progression through the G1 restriction point into S-phase is driven by cyclin-dependent kinases (CDK) 4 and 6 which interact with cyclin D1, as well as by CDK2 which interacts with cyclins A/E [89] (Fig. 17.3). Constitutive MAPK activity

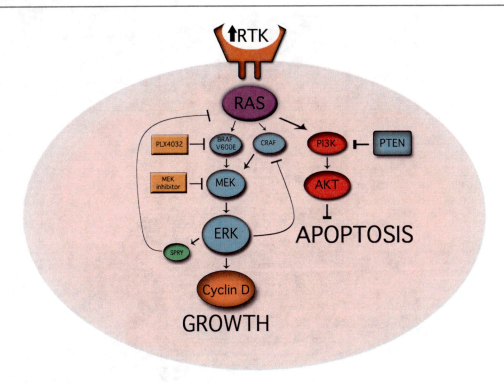

Fig. 17.2 Cell signaling scheme of pathways activated in melanoma cells through either receptor tyrosine kinases (RTKs), Ras, and BRAF. Irrespective of the activating oncogenic mutation, nearly all melanoma cells are known to have constitutive signaling in the BRAF/MEK/ERK and PI3K/AKT pathways. Together, these pathways drive the uncontrolled growth of melanoma cells and prevent the induction of apoptosis

increases cyclin D1 and downregulates p27 expression in melanoma cells [90]. Inhibition of either BRAF or MEK in melanoma cell lines using siRNA strategies and pharmacological inhibitors leads to a profound G1 phase cell-cycle arrest. In experimental systems, the role of mutated *BRAF* in melanoma is convincing. In vitro studies have shown that V600E mutant *BRAF* is an oncogene in immortalized mouse melanocytes [91] and that selective downregulation of the V600E-mutated *BRAF* using RNAi leads to reversal of the melanoma phenotype [92]. Increased BRAF activity also suppresses the activity of the melanocyte-specific transcription factor microphthalmia (MITF), diverting the melanoma cells from a differentiated state into one of rapid proliferation [93].

Acquisition of the *BRAF* V600E mutation appears to be an early event in melanoma development with a high percentage of nevi found to be BRAF V600E mutation positive [94]. In line with observations that nevi only rarely develop into melanoma, the presence of a *BRAF* V600E mutation alone is not sufficient to oncogenically transform primary human melanocytes into melanoma and instead leads to an irreversible growth arrest—characteristic of senescence [95]. Clinical studies have confirmed these findings and have shown that most nevi are growth-arrested and stain positively for the senescence marker β-galactosidase [95]. This phenomenon, which is termed "oncogene-induced senescence" is an important mechanism by which cells protect themselves from oncogenic transformation by activating pathways leading to irreversible cell-cycle exit, such as the ARF/p53/p21 axis and the cyclin-dependent kinase inhibitor p16^{INK4A} [96]. As silencing of and mutation of the p16 gene is a common event in some inherited forms of melanoma, *BRAF* mutations were initially thought to occur in tandem with p16 inactivation [97]. Interestingly, this seems not to be the case with the introduction of mutated *BRAF* leading to a rather irregular pattern of p16 induction [95].

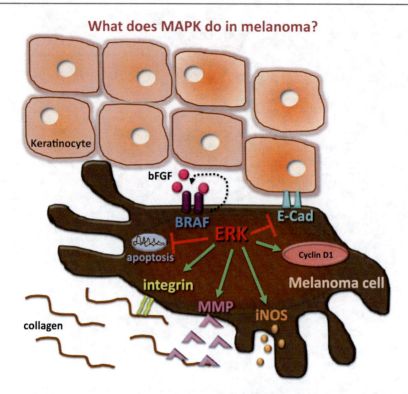

Fig. 17.3 Constitutive MAPK signaling plays a key role in the oncogenic behavior of melanoma cells. Increased activity in the MAPK pathway is known to decrease control by local skin keratinocytes by downregulating E-cadherin expression. Pathway activity also stimulates melanoma growth by increasing cyclin D1 expression and invasion through the modulation of integrin expression and increased matrix metalloproteinase (MMP) release

Further, in vitro studies confirmed the clinical findings and showed that siRNA knockdown of p16 in melanocytes did not lead to malignant transformation when combined with the *BRAF* V600E mutation [95]. Nor was the introduction of *BRAF* V600E alone found to activate the ARF/p53/p21 axis [95].

A wealth of evidence now supports the idea that multiple signaling pathways must be activated to drive melanoma development. The other major signal transduction cascade known to contribute to melanoma initiation and development is the phosphoinositide-3-kinase (PI3K)/protein kinase B (AKT) pathway. Activation of PI3K/AKT signaling occurs via multiple mechanisms, and in *BRAF* V600E, mutated melanoma arises through loss/inactivation of PTEN, activating mutations in AKT3, or increased AKT3 expression [98–100]. The strongest supporting evidence for the dual requirement of BRAF and PI3K/AKT signaling in melanoma initiation comes from mouse modeling studies showing that introduction of mutant *BRAF* alone leads to the development of melanocytic hyperplasia; development of melanoma only occurs when BRAF is introduced in concert with inactivation of PTEN [101].

NRAS Mutant Melanoma

The first activating oncogenic mutation to be reported in melanoma was in *NRAS* [102, 103]. *NRAS* mutant melanomas constitute the most significant group of *BRAF* wild-type melanomas identified so far. RAS proteins are a large family of low molecular weight GTP-binding proteins (or GTPases). Three of the RAS family members, *NRAS*, *HRAS,* and *KRAS,* are often mutated in human cancers, and >20% of all tumors harbor activating mutations in one of their *RAS* genes [104].

Mutations in *NRAS* have since been identified in 15–20% of all melanomas and are most commonly the result of a point mutation leading to the substitution of leucine to glutamine at position 61 [83, 105]. *NRAS* mutations have also been reported at positions 12 and 13 [106]. Mechanistically, the acquisition of point mutations in *NRAS* leads to impaired GTPase activity, so that the GTP-bound NRAS is more abundant than GDP-bound NRAS. This facilitates the recruitment of adapter proteins leading to an increase in intracellular signaling (Fig. 17.2). In addition to NRAS, 1–2% of melanomas have *KRAS* mutations, and 2% are *HRAS* mutant [83, 105]. Although it is unclear why NRAS mutations predominate in melanoma, there are suggestions that this may result from NRAS being overexpressed in melanocytes relative to the other Ras isoforms. It is also possible that NRAS possesses distinct signaling properties over the other Ras isoforms that favors melanocyte transformation [107]. In agreement with this, it is known that although both mutated KRAS and NRAS stimulate Raf signaling in mouse melanocytes and increase their anchorage-independent growth in vitro, NRAS has greater transforming activity than KRAS in mouse melanoma models [108].

In its GTP-bound state, RAS binds to and activates a number of effector signaling pathways involved in proliferation. The best characterized of these is the serine/threonine kinase RAF (discussed in more depth under the BRAF section above) [109]. Most of the oncogenic activity of RAF is mediated through activation of the mitogen-activated protein kinase (MAPK) cascade, which regulates the cell-cycle entry through control of cyclin D1 expression [110] (Fig. 17.3). RAS is also known to activate the phosphoinositide-3-kinase (PI3K)/AKT pathway, which contributes to tumor progression via the modulation of growth and survival of transformed cells [110] (Fig. 17.2). In addition to MAPK and PI3K/AKT, mutant *NRAS* can also activate other intracellular signaling pathways important for malignant transformation with recent studies demonstrating the importance of Ral guanine nucleotide exchange factors (Ral-GEFs) in the anchorage-independent

growth observed following the *NRAS*-mediated melanocytes transformation [111]. The relative importance of each RAS effector pathway in driving the malignant phenotype has not yet been determined.

Although *BRAF* and *NRAS* mutant melanomas tend to show constitutive activation of their RAF/MEK/ERK and PI3K/AKT signaling, there are important differences in how these pathways are regulated. Melanomas harboring activating *NRAS* mutations are different from melanomas with *BRAF* mutations in that they rely upon CRAF to induce their MAPK pathway activity [112]. In normal melanocytes, receptor tyrosine kinase (RTK)-induced activation of RAS leads to the stimulation of both BRAF and CRAF [112]. Under these conditions, activation of the MAPK pathway only proceeds via BRAF, as constitutive protein kinase A (PKA) activity leads to the phosphorylation and inactivation of CRAF. In melanomas with *NRAS* mutations, the cyclic AMP/PKA system is deregulated, so that PKA no longer suppresses CRAF, allowing CRAF-mediated MAPK activation to occur [112].

c-KIT Mutant Melanoma

Melanomas on sites with little UV exposure, such as the skin on the palms of the hands, the soles of the feet or subungual sites (acral melanomas), and on mucous membranes (mucosal melanomas), have a very low incidence of *BRAF* mutations [80]. *BRAF* mutations are also known to be rare on skin that exhibits signs of chronic sun damage (as shown by increased solar elastosis). The incidence of acral and mucosal melanomas is uniform across all racial groups. A landmark study by Bastian and colleagues in 2006 made the observation that 21% of mucosal melanomas, 11% of acral melanomas, and 17% of melanomas arising on sun-damaged skin harbor activating mutations in *c-KIT*, with most of these occurring at the imatinib-sensitive juxtamembrane position [80]. The *KIT* gene was originally identified as the viral oncogene *v-KIT*, derived from the feline sarcoma virus HZ 4-FeSV, and then subsequently as the proto-oncogene form *c-KIT*. c-KIT is an

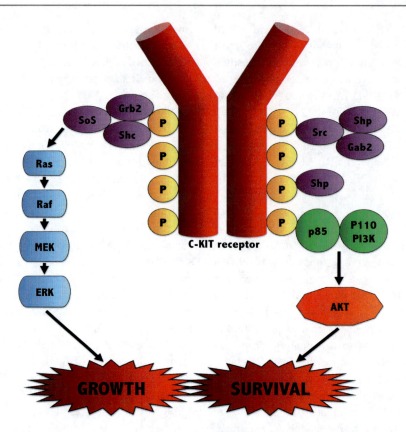

Fig. 17.4 Structure of the c-KIT receptor and signaling pathways activated downstream of KIT. Upon phosphorylation, the KIT receptor stimulates the MAPK pathway (Ras/Raf/MEK/ERK) through recruitment of an adaptor complex consisting of Grb2/Sos/Shc. Other phosphorylation sites on the KIT receptor are also known to recruit Src family kinases and the p85 subunit of PI3K. Activation of all of these pathways leads to increased growth and survival of melanoma cells

RTK member of the platelet-derived growth factor (PDGF) family. Structurally, it is composed of five immunoglobin-like motifs in the extracellular portion and a hydrophilic kinase insert domain that forms the intracellular portion (Fig. 17.4). Its ligand is the glycoprotein stem cell factor (SCF), which is also known under a variety of other names including mast cell growth factor and steel factor (SF). SCF activates c-KIT through binding and the induction of a process that leads to receptor dimerization and autophosphorylation.

Sequencing of *c-KIT* exons 11, 13, 17, and 18 revealed the most prevalent mutations in melanoma to be K642E, L576P, D816H, and V559A [113]. It was also shown that the presence of a *c-KIT* mutation is typically accompanied by an increase in KIT gene copy number and genomic amplification as identified by array comparative genomic hybridization (a-CGH) [80]. There were also instances where c-KIT was amplified in the absence of a mutation, and thus, it was reported that a total number of c-KIT aberrations (either amplification and/or mutation) were 39% for mucosal, 36% for acral, and 28% for melanomas arising on sun-damaged skin [80]. Subsequent studies have shown that c-KIT is expressed in 88% of oral mucosal melanomas and that at least 22% of these harbored activating mutations [114]. Another recent paper also reported the presence of the activating L576P mutation in *c-KIT* in 15% of anal melanomas, a mutation that the authors showed to be imatinib sensitive in vitro [115]. It should be noted that acral lentiginous and mucosal melanomas are relatively rare and, when combined, account for only about 4% of all melanomas [113]. The numbers of melanoma patients presenting with activating mutations in *c-KIT* are likely to be quite low.

A further subset of melanomas that lacked *BRAF* mutations but expressed high levels of c-KIT and cyclin-dependent kinase (CDK) 4 was also recently identified [116]. These melanoma cell lines lacked activating *c-KIT* mutations and showed no evidence of an SCF/c-KIT autocrine loop. They were, however, found to have constitutive c-KIT receptor signaling as shown by the presence of high-level phospho-c-KIT expression, suggesting that the signaling activity may have arisen as a consequence of very high receptor expression levels leading to spontaneous dimerization. Similar findings have been reported in non-small cell lung cancer where very high epidermal growth factor (EGF) receptor expression levels lead to constitutive signaling activity [117].

The role of SCF/c-KIT in melanocyte biology is quite well studied, and it is known that SCF stimulates the migratory behavior of melanocytes grown on fibronectin by increasing their expression of pro-invasive integrins [118, 119]. The likely source of SCF during this process is the tissue microenvironment of the neural crest/skin, with both dermal fibroblasts and human epidermal keratinocytes being shown to express SCF. Consistent with these findings, the *c-KIT* and *SCF* genes are located at genetic loci associated with pigmentary defects, with *c-KIT* being located at the *W* (white spotting) locus on human chromosome 4 and mouse chromosome 5 [120] and *SCF* being located at the steel locus on human chromosome 12 and mouse chromosome 10 [121]. Naturally occurring inactivating mutations at either of these loci leading to impaired c-KIT signaling are associated with depigmented patches of skin/fur characteristic of piebaldism in humans and white spotting in mice [122]. In these instances, c-KIT signaling appears to be critical at the level of the melanocyte precursor and promotes the survival and proliferation of c-KIT-positive neural crest-derived cells, where it works in concert with other soluble factors such as endothelin 3 (ET-3) [123]. Although c-KIT signaling is essential for melanocyte development, recent

work has shown that it may in fact be dispensable for the survival/proliferation of mature pigmented melanocytes. The forced expression of a constitutively active c-KIT (D814Y) mutant into mouse melanocytes led to decreased pigmentation and an increase in migration [124]. Mechanistically, this seems to occur as a result of increased degradation of the melanocyte-specific transcription factor microphthalmia-associated transcription factor (MITF) following the c-KIT-mediated Ser-73/Ser-409 phosphorylation of MITF leading to its proteasomal degradation [125]. This study further showed that constitutive levels of c-KIT signaling led to increased N-cadherin expression in the melanocytes, a finding consistent with both increased motile behavior and increased oncogenic potential in melanoma cells [126]. The lack of proliferation seen in the *c-KIT*-mutated melanocytes was unexpected but is likely to be a consequence of *c-KIT* constituting only one oncogenic "hit." These data suggest that *c-KIT* can only oncogenically transform melanocytes when accompanied by genetic lesions in other pathways. In agreement with this, recent studies have shown that the expression of mutated c-KIT in melanocytes grown under hypoxic conditions, or in concert with the overexpression of hypoxia-inducible factor (HIF)-1α, leads to anchorage-independent growth in soft agar [127]. Here, it appears that hypoxia is required for the activation of MAPK signaling in the c-KIT mutant cells, as this was not observed in the melanocytes expressing wild-type c-KIT [127]. Taken together, these results point to the fact that melanocytes derived from different skin locations may inhabit different microenvironmental conditions and may therefore follow different paths to oncogenic transformation.

For a long time the possible involvement of c-KIT/SCF signaling in melanoma progression was mostly discounted. This stemmed from immunohistochemical studies showing that c-KIT receptor expression was progressively lost during local melanoma growth and invasion [128, 129] and the finding that >70% of melanoma cell lines and tumor samples lacked any c-KIT expression [129]. On the basis of these results, it was assumed that c-KIT was primarily a regulator of melanocyte behavior and therefore dispensable for melanoma growth. Some studies went even further and showed that overexpression of c-KIT in previously metastatic melanoma cell lines led to significant reductions in tumor growth and suppression of metastasis [130, 131]. It was also demonstrated that the exposure of c-KIT-expressing melanoma cells to the c-KIT ligand SCF led to the induction of apoptosis. Mechanistically, it was shown that loss of the AP-2 transcription factor was the likely mechanism underlying the downregulation of c-KIT receptor expression [131].

Other Subgroups of Melanoma

A minor subgroup of melanomas have been identified with *BRAF* mutations in positions other than 600. Many of the non-V600 *BRAF* mutants tend to show impaired BRAF kinase activation in isolated kinase assays (hence, the name "low-activity" *BRAF* mutants) and required the presence of CRAF to transactivate their MAPK signaling [87]. Analysis of a large panel of melanoma cell lines and tissues revealed that ~1% of melanoma cell lines had either D594G or G469E mutation in *BRAF*, respectively, and that 1% of melanoma specimens harbored a G469A mutation in *BRAF* [132]. These "low-activity" *BRAF*-mutated cell lines differed in their signaling from the *BRAF* V600E mutants and showed high levels of phospho-ERK, low levels of phospho-MEK, and resistance to MEK inhibition [132]. Interestingly, these "low-activity" *BRAF* mutants seem to form part of a broader subgroup of melanoma cell lines, including some that are *BRAF* wild type and *BRAF* V600K-mutated, that are reliant upon CRAF for their survival [133]. Studies from two independent groups have now demonstrated that shRNA knockdown of CRAF in the CRAF-dependent melanoma groups leads to MEK-independent effects upon BAD phosphorylation and Bcl-2 expression, leading in turn to apoptosis and impaired tumor growth in a mouse xenograft model [132].

There also exists a group of *BRAF/NRAS* wild-type melanoma for which the initiating oncogenic event is currently unknown. This group is likely to account for ~30% of all melanomas. Efforts are currently underway to study this potentially significant subgroup of melanomas.

Distinct Pathological and Prognostic Features of Melanomas with Different Activating Mutations

Both *NRAS* and *BRAF* mutant melanomas are found on sun-exposed skin, whereas c-KIT mutant melanomas arise on sun-protected sites [81, 134]. Evidence is emerging that the duration and frequency of sun exposure may also determine the nature of initiating oncogenic event, with *BRAF* mutant melanomas tending to occur in younger patients with a lower cumulative UV exposure and *NRAS* mutant melanomas more likely to develop in older patients with a more sustained history of sun exposure [135]. Careful pathological examination of large numbers of *BRAF*, *NRAS*, and *c-KIT* mutant melanoma specimens has revealed significantly different mutation-specific biological behavior [136]. It was found that *BRAF*-mutated melanomas had an increased tendency to upward migration and nest formation and gave rise to larger, rounded, and more pigmented tumor cells [136]. In contrast, *NRAS*-mutated melanomas were not found to exhibit these morphological and phenotypic characteristics [136]. With regard to the possible prognostic value of mutation status, there is some suggestion that that *NRAS* mutant primary melanomas may pose a higher risk of metastasis, as they tend to be more deeply invasive at the time of initial diagnosis than *BRAF*-mutated melanomas and tend to have a higher mitotic rate. The effects of the different initiating mutations upon melanoma prognosis and biological behavior remain an area of intense study. As things stand, the available evidence suggests that both *BRAF* and *NRAS* mutant melanomas ultimately follow a similar clinical course, with little differences in overall survival noted [137].

Targeted Therapy for Melanoma: Matching Therapies with Genotypes: Targeting Mutant BRAF

Since the discovery of activating BRAF mutations in melanoma, a number of BRAF inhibitors have been developed and subjected to extensive in vitro testing [138–142]. The most thoroughly studied of these is the kinase inhibitor sorafenib (BAY43-9006, Nexxavar®) [142]. Although originally developed as a CRAF inhibitor, sorafenib was also found to inhibit BRAF with moderate potency and was evaluated as the potentially first proof-of-concept for BRAF inhibition in melanoma [143]. In animal studies, sorafenib treatment led to limited regression of BRAF V600E-mutated melanoma xenografts and was associated with only minor levels of apoptosis induction [132, 143]. Extension preclinical investigations have now shown sorafenib to be a relatively weak inhibitor of BRAF, with many off-target effects (including inhibition of VEGFR, PDGFR, and p38 MAP kinase [142, 144]); it is likely that any antimelanoma activity of sorafenib is independent of its putative effects upon BRAF inhibition [145].

Since the evaluation of sorafenib, a new generation of BRAF inhibitors has been developed. These drugs show higher potency against mutated BRAF and have fewer off-target effects; the list of those currently under preclinical investigation includes SB590885, GSK2118436, PLX4032/4720 (RG704), AZ628, XL281, and GDC-0879 [138, 139, 146–152]. PLX4032 (and its analogue PLX4720) are ATP-competitive RAF inhibitors (wt BRAF IC50 100 nM, mutated BRAF 31 nM) that selectively inhibit growth in melanoma cell lines harboring the BRAF V600E mutation both in vitro and in vivo mouse in xenograft models [139, 151, 153]. Another BRAF inhibitor currently exciting much interest in both the preclinical and clinical arenas is GSK2118436, an ATP-competitive inhibitor of BRAF V600E/ D/K, wild-type BRAF, and CRAF [154]. The compound has been shown to have promising activity in preclinical models of melanoma and is now the subject of clinical evaluation [155].

Responses to PLX4032 in melanoma xenograft models were BRAF V600E specific and highly potent, with either partial or complete responses observed in all cases [151, 153]. Interestingly, not all BRAF-mutated melanoma cell lines were similarly sensitive to PLX4032 and PLX4720, with a significant proportion showing varying degrees of intrinsic resistance [146, 149, 150]. Current data suggests that PLX4032/4720 induces both cell-cycle arrest and apoptosis in the most sensitive cell lines and cell-cycle arrest only in less sensitive cell lines [146, 150]. A recent genetic study, looking for patterns of mutation and genomic amplification between PLX4032-sensitive and PLX4032-resistant cell lines, was unable to identify any unifying differences between the two groups [150]. More recent studies have suggested that increased cyclin D1 expression (in ~17% of BRAF-mutated melanomas) allows for cell-cycle entry when BRAF and MAPK signaling is abrogated [156, 157]. Studies from our own lab identified loss of the tumor suppressor PTEN, observed in >10% of melanoma specimens, as being responsible for increased PI3K/AKT signaling when BRAF was inhibited. It was noted that recovery of AKT signaling impaired apoptosis when BRAF was inhibited through the suppression of BIM and BAD expression [158]. In addition to changes in PTEN and cyclin D1, it is also known that BRAF V600E-mutated melanomas show alterations in CDK2, CDK4, MITF, and AKT3 [82, 159]. How the expression and mutational status of these genes impacts upon biological behavior and future therapy selection remains to be determined.

The mechanisms by which BRAF inhibition leads to melanoma regression are not fully understood. The best characterized role for BRAF/ MAPK signaling in melanoma is in the regulation of cell growth, with constitutive BRAF/ MAPK activity being shown to increase cyclin D1 expression [90]. Inhibition of either BRAF or MEK in melanoma cell lines using pharmacological inhibitors leads to a profound G1 phase cell-cycle arrest. Indeed, the BRAF inhibitors SB590885 [138], AZ628 [148], and PLX4720 [139] as well as the MEK inhibitors U0126 [160], CI-1040 [141], PD0325901, and AZD6244 [140], all have cytostatic effects upon melanoma cell lines harboring the *BRAF* V600E mutation. The role of *BRAF* in melanoma survival is less clear, with both pharmacological inhibitors and siRNA knockdown of BRAF being relatively weak apoptosis inducers [138, 139]. There is, however, evidence implicating *BRAF* in the control of anoikis, with siRNA studies showing a link between mutated *BRAF* and regulation of the pro-apoptotic BH3-family (Bcl-2 family) proteins BIM, BAD, and Mcl-1 [161–163].

Clinically, the most highly studied of the new class of BRAF-specific inhibitors is PLX4032 or RG7204 (vemurafenib) (Fig. 17.2). In the recent phase I clinical trial, 80% of melanoma patients ($n = 32$) selected for the presence of the *BRAF* V600E mutation responded to RG7204 (960 mg/kg BID) and showed significant levels of tumor regression [164]. Pharmacodynamic studies suggested that >80% BRAF inhibition was required for clinical activity to be observed [153]. RG7204 was well tolerated with the most common side effects being rash, arthralgia, photosensitivity, and fatigue. Intriguingly, >23% of patients rapidly (mostly <12 weeks of treatment) developed SCCs of the keratoacanthoma type [164]. These tumors were removed surgically and did not recur. Although the exact cause of these carcinomas is not known, there is evidence showing that SCC often harbor mutations in *HRAS*, and it is known that inhibition of BRAF in RAS-mutant cell lines leads to the paradoxical increase in cell growth following the transactivation of CRAF [147, 165, 166]. In the phase II BRAF in melanoma (BRIM)-2 trial, 132 patients were recruited and received 960 mg of RG7204 BID. The primary end point was best overall response, with duration of response, progression free survival, overall response, and safety as the secondary end points. Results from the trial showed that 52.3% ($n = 69$) had a complete (2.3%) or partial response (50%), 29.5% ($n = 39$) had stable disease, and 13.6% ($n = 18$) had progressive disease. Average duration of response was 6.8 months, and progression free survival was 6.2 months. Like the phase I trial, 24.2% of the patients developed low-grade SCC. A phase III trial of RG7204 (BRIM-3) has now completed accrual. In it, a proposed 680 patients were randomized 1:1 against dacarbazine with the primary endpoint being overall survival. Data from this trial have been submitted to the FDA for possible regulatory approval.

Although very encouraging, the responses seen to RG7204 were not durable in most patients, with the median progression free survival from the phase I and II trials being ~7 months. These observations mirror the pattern of response seen to targeted therapy in CML, GIST [77, 78], and most recently medulloblastoma [167, 168], where an initial period of tumor regression is later followed by relapse. The current model for drug resistance to targeted therapy suggests that secondary mutations are acquired in drug-target proteins. In CML and GIST, imatinib resistance emerges via the acquisition of secondary mutations at sites within the kinase's ATP binding site that prevent the binding of the drug to the hydrophobic pocket at so-called "gatekeeper" residues [78, 169, 170]. Although BRAF gatekeeper mutants that confer drug resistance have been generated in vitro, similar drug-insensitive *BRAF* mutations have not yet been observed in melanoma patients [145]. Analysis of tumor samples from patients failing RG7204 therapy using both deep and ultra-deep sequencing was unable to identify de novo mutations in *BRAF*, suggesting that the acquisition of a gatekeeper mutation is not the mechanism of resistance [171]. Further studies, where the BRAF kinase was immunoprecipitated from in vitro cultures of RG7204, resistant melanoma specimens showed the BRAF to retain its sensitivity to RG7204, again suggesting the absence of secondary *BRAF* mutations [171]. Instead, it currently appears that resistance is mediated by signals arising upstream of mutated *BRAF*. In support of this, recent data from two independent groups have shown BRAF inhibitor resistance to be mediated through increased RTK signaling (PDGFRβ and IGF1R, respectively) [154, 171] (Fig. 17.5). In the case of IGFR1, downstream MAPK signaling was reactivated following the rerouting of signaling from mutated *BRAF* to ARAF and CRAF [154] (Fig. 17.5). In those melanomas with increased PDGFR-β expression, the nature of the rebound signaling is

Pathway Switching

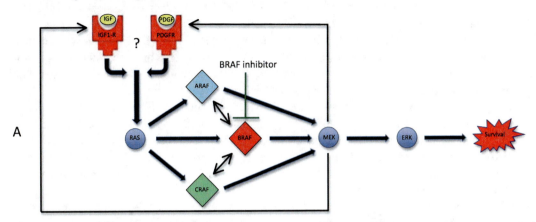

Fig. 17.5 Putative mechanisms of acquired resistance to the BRAF inhibitor PLX4032. *BRAF* V600E melanoma cells chronically treated with BRAF inhibitors acquire drug resistance via switching between the three isoforms of RAF to activate the MAPK pathway. Establishment of IGFR1 and PDGFR signaling may also allow mutated *BRAF* to be bypassed

currently unclear [171]. The observation that melanoma cells quickly compensate for the lack of a mutated *BRAF* signal is also supported by studies showing that MAPK signaling recovers very rapidly (often within 48 h) following treatment with BRAF inhibitors [146, 172, 173]. There is now a growing list of mechanisms by which melanoma cells can reactivate their MAPK signaling when BRAF is inhibited. Another recent study demonstrated that increased COT (MAP3K8) expression drives BRAF inhibitor resistance through the RAF-independent activation of ERK [174]. The clinical relevance of increased COT expression in the resistance phenotype was confirmed in a limited number of melanoma samples from patients failing BRAF and MEK inhibitor treatment [172, 174]. These data fit with earlier preclinical studies showing that exogenously added growth factors and cytokines rescued melanoma cells from cell death following siRNA-induced knockdown of BRAF by reactivating MAPK signaling [175, 176]. These findings provide the rationale for how BRAF inhibitor resistance could potentially be managed, with a number of groups now suggesting that dual BRAF/MEK inhibition may prevent or delay the onset of resistance [146, 174, 177]. This hypothesis is currently being evaluated clinically in a phase I/II clinical trial of the BRAF inhibitor GSK2118436 in combination with the MEK inhibitor GSK1120212 in *BRAF* V600E-mutated melanoma patients who are treatment naïve (NCT01072175).

NRAS

NRAS is a small GTPase and therefore a difficult target for conventional drug discovery [104]. The only class of drugs to be developed so far specifically designed to inhibit RAS signaling is the farnesyltransferase inhibitors (FTIs) [178]. This strategy is predicated on the fact that RAS family proteins require farnesylation to form complexes with their effectors at the cell membrane. Although inhibition of farnesylation was shown in vitro to deplete the pool of RAS available to drive downstream signaling, many proteins require farnesylation to function effectively, making FTIs nonspecific inhibitors of RAS signaling. Despite being evaluated in many tumor types, these compounds have shown little single-agent activity, even in colorectal carcinoma where ~40% of the tumors have activating mutations in *KRAS* [178]. In several clinical trials, evaluation of target inhibition was assessed with serial tumor biopsies and was associated with only modest inhibition of RAS signaling even at the maximum tolerated doses. It is therefore currently unclear whether FTIs would constitute effective RAS mutation-specific therapies even if appropriate dose levels could be reached. One FTI in particular, tipifarnib, was evaluated in a single-agent, single-arm phase II trial among patients with metastatic melanoma [179]. The lack of response among the first 14 patients enrolled led to closure of the trial. Since these patients were unselected with regards to their *NRAS* mutation status, it is unlikely that more than 1–2 patients on the trial harbored an *NRAS* mutation. Another phase II trial was conducted combining tipifarnib and sorafenib in genetically unselected patients, to test whether this combination would inhibit two points within the MAPK pathway. This regimen was associated with minimal clinical activity and was abandoned after the first stage of accrual [180].

The current strategies being considered instead involve targeting the pathways downstream of Ras activation. There is now good preclinical evidence that simultaneous blockade of the MEK and PI3K pathways leads to the regression of Ras-driven tumors in animal models [181, 182]. Other studies have shown that dual inhibition of BRAF and CRAF or BRAF and PI3K (using shRNA knockdown) was effective at reducing the growth and survival of *NRAS*-mutated human melanoma xenografts [183]. Although *NRAS*-mutated melanomas are known to rely upon CRAF for their MAPK signaling, there is little evidence that sorafenib is any more effective on the *NRAS* mutants than melanoma cell lines with *BRAF* mutations [132]. MEK inhibition has been evaluated in *NRAS* mutant melanoma with mixed results. In vitro, panels of *NRAS* mutant melanoma show variable sensitivity to MEK inhibition with such agents, with inhibition of proliferation rather than induction of apoptosis being the most prevalent response. The factors underlying the level of response of *NRAS* mutant melanoma cell lines to MEK inhibitors are currently unknown [140, 141]. Several potent and selective inhibitors of MEK have emerged from phase I clinical trials. The most active of the new

generation of these compounds, GSK2110212, is associated with tumor regression in a subset of patients with *BRAF* wild-type melanoma at least some of whom were likely to be *NRAS* mutant [184]. As we look to the future, the new generation of MEK inhibitors will be combined with potent and selective inhibitors of PI3K, AKT, and mTOR. The first combination regimen of a MEK inhibitor (AZD6244) with an AKT inhibitor (MK-2206) will begin phase II evaluation in 2011. This represents the first of what is anticipated to be a growing array of combination regimens targeting RAF/MEK/ERK and PI3K/AKT pathway signaling in *NRAS* mutant tumors.

The importance of matching the correct targeted therapy to the requisite melanoma genotype is illustrated by recent preclinical studies showing that inhibitors of BRAF paradoxically activate MAPK signaling in tumors that lacked activating *BRAF* mutations. Reports from at least six independent groups have shown that BRAF inhibition activates MAPK in cell lines with *NRAS* and *KRAS* mutations as well as those cell lines where the MAPK pathway is activated through other oncogenes such as *HER2* [147, 165, 166, 185–187]. Mechanistic studies showed that PLX4032 and other BRAF inhibitors were able to prevent the formation of BRAF–CRAF complexes and instead promoted the formation of CRAF–CRAF dimers, leading in turn to MEK activation [147, 187]. There is also evidence that PLX4032 increases the invasive potential of *NRAS*-mutated melanoma cells through the activation of ERK and FAK signaling [165]. Additional studies demonstrated that BRAF inhibitors may even contribute to the progression of *NRAS*-mutated melanomas in part by suppressing apoptosis through the modulation of Mcl-1 expression [186].

c-KIT

A number of small molecule RTK inhibitors have been developed that target KIT activity, the best studied of which is imatinib mesylate, an RTK inhibitor with activity against Bcr Abl, PDGFR, and c-KIT [79, 188]. It is becoming apparent *KIT* mutational status, rather than genomic amplification, is most predictive of response to small molecule KIT inhibitors [113]. The available evidence also suggests that the nature of the *KIT* mutation dictates which KIT inhibitor should be used [113, 189]. To date, only a few relevant preclinical studies have been published on melanoma cell lines derived from either acral or mucosal melanomas [190, 191]. The first of these characterized three primary mucosal melanoma cell lines, of which one was noted to have an exon 11 V559D mutation in *c-KIT* [190]. Treatment of this cell line with imatinib led to cell-cycle arrest and apoptosis induction and was associated with inhibition of JAK/STAT, PI3K/ AKT, and MAPK signaling and the inhibition of Bcl-2, survivin, and Mcl-1 expression [190] (Fig. 17.4). The second study reported the identification of a mucosal melanoma cell line with a D820Y exon 17 mutation in *c-KIT* (the mutation often associated with imatinib resistance in GIST) that showed sensitivity to sunitinib [191]. One other recent publication reported the identification of a nonacral/nonmucosal melanoma cell lines harboring an L576P *KIT* mutation [192]. In this instance, the cell line was found to be resistant to imatinib, nilotinib, and sorafenib but sensitive to dasatanib [192]. There is also some evidence suggesting that the presence of constitutive KIT activity (as shown by phospho-KIT) may be predictive of KIT inhibitor response [116].

Although imatinib is now routinely used in the treatment of patients with CML and GIST, its activity in nonselected groups of melanoma patients has been very disappointing [193]. Phase II clinical trials of imatinib in patients with metastatic melanoma revealed no objective responses and were associated with poor survival rates and significant toxicity [193]. Another phase II trial of melanoma patients selected on the basis of their tumors expressing one of the molecular targets of the inhibitor by immunohistochemistry (PDGFR, c-KIT, c-abl, or abl-related gene) was also negative [194]. In this trial, however, one significant response was observed in a patient with acral lentiginous melanoma. Analysis of the patient's tumor showed it to have the highest c-KIT expression of the entire cohort, albeit lacking a c-KIT receptor mutation. It was also shown that imatinib

treatment induced a significant level of apoptosis in this tumor and in the surrounding endothelial cells [194]. In recent years, there have been a number of cases reported where KIT mutant melanoma patients have responded to a variety of KIT inhibitors. The first patient to be reported was a 79-year-old woman with metastatic mucosal melanoma. Immunohistochemical staining revealed the tumor to have very strong staining for c-KIT, and mutational analysis demonstrated the presence of a seven-codon duplication in exon 11 [195]. After 4 weeks of treatment with imatinib (400 mg daily), regression of the metastatic lesions was noted on a PET/CT scan. Another recent case report described a patient with a mucosal melanoma that stained strongly for c-KIT, harbored an activating exon 13 (K642E) mutation, and showed increased copy number [196]. Following surgical removal of the primary tumor, the patient developed metastatic spread and was then put on imatinib therapy, which ultimately led to a resolution of the metastatic nodules [196]. Two further case studies have also reported significant imatinib responses in the metastatic setting for patients with acrolentiginous and mucosal melanomas harboring L576P and V559A *KIT* mutations, respectively, [189, 197]. Interestingly, not all *KIT*-mutant melanoma patients show responses to imatinib, and there is evidence that other kinase inhibitors may also be effective. One report details a case of a mucosal melanoma patient harboring a V560D mutation in *c-KIT* showing a complete response to sorafenib [198] and another case of a KIT mutation-positive (L576P) vaginal mucosal melanoma patient who responded to dasatanib [192]. Although the initial round of clinical studies on imatinib in melanoma were negative, studies involving selection of melanoma patients with activating mutations in *c-KIT* are now underway. The preliminary results from the phase II multi-institutional trial of imatinib patients with mucosal, acral lentiginous melanoma, or melanoma arising on chronically sun-damaged skin demonstrated responses in zero out of ten patients with amplified/wild-type c-KIT but partial responses in five out of ten patients with *c-KIT* mutations [113]. The final results of this trial are still awaited.

Nonmelanoma Skin Cancers: Epidemiology and Incidence of Basal Cell Carcinoma

BCC is the most common of the keratinocyte skin cancers and is so named because of its resemblance to the basal cells of the epidermis [199]. Based upon immunohistochemical studies, BCC is considered to be a malignancy of follicular germinitive cells. It accounts for the vast majority of all skin cancers (~75%), with an incidence predicted to be 100 per 100,000 [199]. BCC is the most prevalent of all cancers in Caucasians, who have an average lifetime risk of 30% for developing this tumor [200]. The highest incidence of BCC is in Australia, where 1,383 new cases are identified yearly per 100,000 [201]. BCCs occur more frequently in men compared to women (at a ratio of 2:1), and the average age of disease onset is 60 years [199]. Interestingly, women <40 years of age have an increased risk of BCC compared to their male counterparts, a fact probably attributable to increased sun tanning behavior (such as use of tanning salons) in young females [199]. Risk factors for BCC development include sun/UV exposure (mainly intermittent), severe childhood sunburns, fair skin, a history of ionizing radiation exposure, and exposure to oral psoralens and arsenic. Like melanoma, there is evidence that age at time of sun exposure is an important determinant of BCC development, with individuals born in Australia showing a greater risk for BCC than those who migrated to Australia when older than 10 years of age [201]. The exact etiology and even the precise incidence of BCC are difficult to describe, as the occurrence of this cancer is not routinely recorded in cancer registries because of the large numbers of cases [199].

BCCs are generally slow growing, infiltrative lesions that normally arise on sun-exposed areas such as the face and neck, as palpable, translucent tumors with wispy telangiectasias on their surface. There are many histological subtypes that may also be distinguished by their clinical characteristics. Nodular BCC, the most common form (70% of all cases), has a pearly appearance with a rolled border and central crusting with ulceration. Superficial BCC (10–15% prevalence) has a scaly, erythematous plaque-like appearance. Although BCCs rarely metastasize (~0.5% of cases), they are often locally invasive and can cause significant levels of tissue damage when they infiltrate the cartilage, muscle, and bone. Metastasis of BCC is associated with significant mortality (3.6 year median survival) with the most common sites of spread being the lung, liver, and bone [202].

The Molecular Basis of BCC: Hedgehog Signaling

For many years, the underlying molecular causes of BCC remained obscure. A significant breakthrough was made with the discovery of genetic mutations in the hedgehog signaling (HH) pathway in patients with a rare condition known as Gorlin syndrome or basal cell nevus syndrome (BCNS) in which susceptible patients are noted to form hundreds of BCC-like lesions [203]. Family-based linkage studies of BCNS kindreds identified the causative factor to be mutations in the patched gene (PTCH-1), a key negative regulator of the HH signaling pathway (Fig. 17.6a) [204]. Under physiological conditions, the HH pathway plays a key role in development and influences embryogenesis, epithelial and mesenchymal tissue interactions, and cell differentiation. When PTCH-1 is mutated, its suppressive effects upon the related transmembrane protein smoothened (SMO) are relieved, allowing for the activation of the downstream GLI family of transcription factors (so-named because they were first identified in GLIoblastoma) [205] (Fig. 17.6b). GLI family transcription factors control the expression of many genes involved in aberrant tissue differentiation, proliferation, survival, and ultimately the development of BCC [205] (Fig. 17.6).

There is now good experimental evidence that upregulated HH signaling is the key event underlying the development of most BCC and that little other signaling activity aside from HH is required for BCC initiation [204]. In agreement with this idea, ~90% of all sporadic BCC harbor mutations

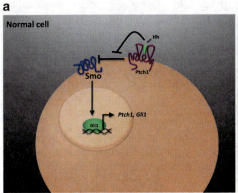 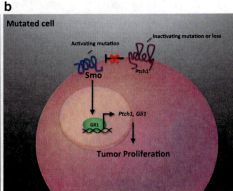

Fig. 17.6 (a) Hedgehog signaling in normal development. Under physiological conditions, patched (PTCH1) suppresses signaling through smoothened (SMO), which in turn represses the transcription of GLI1 target genes. (b) Hedgehog signaling in BCC. Inactivating mutations found in the majority of BCC prevents the repression of smoothened (SMO) leading to constitutive expression of GLI-1 family target genes

in one allele of PTCH-1, with a further 10% of all BCC showing activating mutations in SMO [205]. Mechanistically, genome-wide association studies of keratinocytes with constitutive HH signaling revealed a role for platelet-derived growth factor-α (PDGF-α), an upregulation of Bcl-2, caspase 8, and a FADD-like apoptosis regulator CFLAR in HH-mediated tumorigenesis [205].

Treatment of BCC: Surgery and Topical Therapy

The gold standard for BCC treatment is complete surgical excision. This has been further refined by the use of Mohs surgery, which decreases recurrence rates to ~1.4% (5-year follow-up). Indications for Mohs surgery include recurrent tumor at a previously excised site, an aggressive BCC subtype, poorly defined tumor margins, and the presence of a tumor at an anatomically restrictive site [201, 202, 206]. Patients who are poor surgical candidates can be treated by the application of topical therapies including cryotherapy, radiotherapy (particularly in patients with large tumors), photodynamic therapy using the photosensitizer aminolevulinic acid, and topical chemotherapy drugs, such as 5-fluorouracil (5-FU) [200]. One of the most promising topical treatments for BCC is imiquimod, which belongs to the imidazoquinolone class of drugs [207]. It exerts its antitumor effects by binding to toll-like receptors (TLR) 7 and 8 of macrophages and plasmacytoid dendritic cells resulting in the activation of the innate immune response [208, 209]. Monocytic activation in turn leads to the production of several pro-inflammatory cytokines such as interferon-alpha (IFN-α), tumor necrosis factor-alpha (TNF-α), and interleukin-12 (IL-12), and it is the secretion of these and other cytokines that leads to a cell-mediated cytotoxic Th1 response. In addition, imiquimod has been shown to induce pro-apoptotic factors such as Fas receptor (FasR), also known as CD95, Bax, and caspases 9 and 3 [207–209]. Five percent imiquimod cream (Aldara®, 3M Corporation) has been FDA approved for treatment of superficial BCC, with trials underway to measure its efficacy in other subtypes of BCC such as nodular BCC.

Targeted Therapy of Nonmelanoma Skin Cancers: Inhibition of HH Signaling

Although most cases of BCC are treated by surgical excision, there is currently no standard of care for the treatment of more advanced forms of BCC, such as locally extensively invasive or metastatic BCC. Current strategies for advanced BCC have centered upon the targeting of constitutive HH signaling using SMO antagonists. Of these, the SMO inhibitor furthest along in clinical development is GDC-0449 (vismodegib; Genentech/Roche), which is currently undergoing phase II clinical evaluation. The results of the multicenter phase I trial of GDC-0449 for the treatment of locally advanced and metastatic BCC were reported in September of 2009 in The New England Journal of Medicine [210]. In this study, a total of 33 patients received oral GDC-0449. The median duration of study treatment was 9.8 months with 18 patients showing an objective response assessed by RECIST criteria, physical examination, or both [210]. Of these, two individuals showed a complete response, and 16 had a partial response. Stable disease was observed in 11 patients, and 4 patients had progressive disease. Among the 18 patients with metastatic BCC and 15 patients with locally advanced BCC, the overall response rates were 50% and 60%, respectively. Correlative studies showed GLI1 mRNA levels to be elevated in the majority of BCC patients enrolled on study and that PTCH1 gene mutations were observed in nine out of ten patient specimens analyzed [210]. Two of the four patients who progressed on SMO inhibitor therapy were noted to have increased levels of HH signaling, suggesting the existence of novel resistance mechanisms [210]. At this time, a number of other SMO antagonists, including BMS-833923 (Bristol-Myers Squibb/Exelixis), IPI-926 (Infinity), LDE-225 (Novartis), and PF-04449913 (Pfizer), are currently in phase Ib trials for advanced solid tumors including BCC [211].

Squamous Cell Carcinoma: Incidence, Epidemiology, and Risk Factors

SCC is the second most common skin malignancy. Overall prevalence is at least 200,000 cases a year, with a mortality rate of 2,000 cases a year. The incidence of SCC has been steadily rising over the last 30 years, especially in the 40-year-old or less age group, with rates now standing at 3.9 cases per 100,000 and a cumulative lifetime risk of 7–11% [212]. The increase in SCC incidence has been linked to sun exposure, especially in tropical areas, and to sun tanning behavior. Identifiable predisposing risk factors include older age, male gender, Celtic ancestry, oral psoralens (used to treat psoriasis), UVA therapy, coal-tar products (found in some dandruff shampoos), high cumulative dose ionizing radiation, and chronic epidermal damage [212]. Of these, UV exposure is thought to be the major causative factor for SCC [213]. The UV spectrum is divided into two major carcinogenic wavelengths: UVA (320–400 nm) and UVB (290–320 nm). UV photon absorption by DNA leads to mutation through the dimerization of adjacent pyrimidine bases. The two major photoproducts induced by UV are cyclobutane pyrimidine dimers (CPD) and the pyrimidine–pyrimidone photoproduct (6-4PP) [214]. UVB is ~1,000 times more potent at inducing photodimerizations than UVA [215]. The failure to repair CPDs leads to DNA mutations that typically manifest themselves as C to T and CC to TT transitions in a number of key genes implicated in cancer development including p53, PTCH1, p16, and RAS [216]. The fact that SCC, BCC, and melanoma commonly show mutations and aberrant activity of p53, p16, and *RAS* is taken as strong evidence for the causative role of UV radiation in the development of these cancers. Recent studies have also implicated human papilloma virus (HPV) (genus beta) infection in the initiation and development of SCC [217]. In a population-based case control study, 62% of cutaneous SCC patients ($n=252$) were found to be seropositive for HPV as compared 53% seropositivity (odds ratio of 1.6, confidence interval of 1.2–2.3) in a matched control population [217]. The two specific HPV serotypes implicated in this study were HPV-5 and HPV-20 [217]. Further studies have shown the presence of HPV-38 in ~50% of skin carcinomas but only 10% of normal skin samples. Similarly, HPV-38 was also identified in 43% of actinic keratoses as well as 13% of SCC and 16% of BCC [218]. HPV infection is known to introduce a number of viral genes, such as *E6*, which facilitate oncogenic transformation by affecting the stability of p53 and *E7* which disrupts the activity of the retinoblastoma protein, an important cell-cycle regulator.

Immunosuppression has also been demonstrated to be an etiological factor for aggressive forms of SCC. Organ transplant patients, such as those undergoing renal, cardiac, and pulmonary transplants, have 60–100-fold risk of developing a subtype of SCC that shows an increased risk for metastasis (>20%) [219]. Immunosuppresive drug regimens implicated in SCC development include calcineurin inhibitors, mTOR inhibitors, antimetabolites, and oral glucocorticoids. Sites of chronic wounds, including burn wounds, stasis wounds, and osteomyeletic sinus tracts, have also been implicated as risk sites for future SCC development. The cardinal feature is a persistent inflammatory reaction with increased proteolytic activity.

SCCs can be stratified on the basis of their malignant potential. Low-risk subtypes occur in the setting of precursor actinic keratoses (AK) lesions and HPV-associated verrucous lesions. HPV-associated lesions produce exophytic growths that show invasion into the dermis. Intermediate-risk subtypes including adenoid and lymphoepithelioloma-like carcinoma that show increasing levels of atypia, loss of adhesion, and increased frequency of mitoses. High-risk lesions include adenosquamous carcinoma and desmoplastic SCC [220, 221]. Clinically, SCC lesions most often present as a shallow-based ulcer with a surrounding indurated, raised border. At times, the lesion can be hidden beneath a thin, dry scale or at the base of a cutaneous horn. Overall, the majority of SCC lesions occur on sun-exposed sites. SCCs contain malignant keratinocytes with varying degrees of keratinization that can invade into the dermis. The potential for SCC to metastasize is minimal, estimated to be 0.3–3.7% [222], but when metastasis occurs, significant mortality results and 5-year survival rates for metastatic SCC are ~30%. There is an increased tendency toward local recurrence and metastasis when the SCC arises at certain anatomic sites such as on the lips (14%) and the external ear (9%). Primary SCCs with a diameter >2 cm (30.3%), a depth greater than 4 mm (45.7%), and perineural involvement are at greatest risk of metastatic spread [223].

Treatment of SCC

Surgical excision is the primary modality for removing SCC localized to the skin. In more cosmetically sensitive areas such as the face, Moh's micrographic surgery has proven useful and spares uninvolved tissue. In patients who are poor surgical candidates, smaller lesions may be amenable to cryotherapy, using topically applied liquid nitrogen or electrodessication and curettage. Another useful technique involves using aminolevulinic acid applied topically onto the lesion leading to the production of localized oxygen radicals, followed by photodynamic therapy. 5-FU is a nucleotide analogue that inhibits tumor proliferation by blocking DNA synthesis. Its use as a topical therapy for SCC is limited by its inability to penetrate to deeper skin layers and side effects that range from severe pruritus to pain and severe inflammation. Although topical imiquimod treatment is FDA-approved for BCC, it is not currently approved for use in SCC. There is evidence from short-term trials (maximum 16 weeks) that imiquimod has some efficacy against cutaneous and invasive SCC [224–226], and investigations are underway to determine the safety and efficacy of long-term treatment.

The Molecular Basis of SCC

Although both BCC and SCC are keratinocyte tumors, the mechanisms of initiation are very different. Whereas BCC arises de novo as the result of a defined molecular event (activation of HH signaling), SCC instead follows a more complex, stepwise path to malignancy. To date, one of the major genetic changes implicated in SCC development is the acquisition of *p53* mutations, which are found in >90% of all SCC [227, 228].

Under normal physiological conditions, p53 activation protects against tumor development by initiating cell-cycle checkpoints and apoptosis in cells following either DNA damage or oncogene activation. As discussed previously, *p53* is susceptible to UV-induced signature mutations, which can lead to impaired p53–DNA binding, an abrogation of the apoptotic response and increased tumor cell invasion and motility [229]. Convincing evidence for the role of p53 inactivation in SCC development comes from transgenic animal studies, with *p53* knockout out mice showing a much earlier onset of UV-induced skin cancer than their wild-type counterparts [230]. Although the acquisition of *p53* mutations occurs early in the development of SCC, there is controversy as to whether the nature of the *p53* mutation acquired predicts for the eventual aggressiveness of the tumor. One other possible molecular candidate for SCC initiation and progression is the epidermal growth factor receptor (EGFR). Upon exposure to UV radiation, ROS generation leads to EGFR signaling in keratinocytes, which in turn stimulates p38 MAPK and JNK resulting in increased cell proliferation and an escape from apoptosis [231, 232]. Further evidence for the role of EGFR signaling in SCC development comes from preclinical studies showing that pharmacological inhibition of EGFR abrogates UV-induced skin tumor formation in mice [233]. A role for persistent JNK signaling in SCC progression has also been suggested, with studies showing that >70% of all SCCs have constitutive activity in this pathway [234]. One of the hallmarks of cancer is resistance to apoptosis. Overexpression of antiapoptotic members of the Bcl-2 protein family, particularly Bcl-XL, has been implicated in SCC development [235]. In vitro studies have shown that increased Bcl-XL expression protects immortalized keratinocytes from UV-induced apoptosis and that Bcl-XL knockdown sensitizes cells to UV-induced apoptosis. In a similar vein, transgenic mice with targeted Bcl-XL overexpression in their epidermal keratinocytes are more likely to develop UV-induced skin cancers [236, 237]. Continued research is expected to lead to important new insights into the molecular basis of SCC initiation and progression.

Future Perspectives

We are only at the beginning of understanding the molecular events underlying skin cancer development and progression. As both basic and clinical researches into the biology of melanoma, SCC, and BCC progress, a future can be envisaged where highly personalized, patient-specific therapy regimens are developed. It is hoped that disseminated melanoma, rather than continuing to represent a dismal diagnosis, can be 1 day reduced to the level of a manageable, chronic disease. It is also hoped that effective targeted therapies for both BCC and SCC will reduce and prevent the mortality associated with the development of metastases.

Acknowledgments Work in the Smalley lab was supported by The Melanoma Research Foundation, The Bankhead-Coley Research Program (09BN-14), The American Cancer Society (#93-032-13), and the NIH/National Cancer Institute (U54 CA143970-01). The authors thank Drs. Vernon Sondak and Jane Messina for useful discussions and their constructive criticism of the manuscript.

References

1. Jemal A, Bray F, Center MM, Ferlay J, Ward E, Forman D. Global cancer statistics. CA Cancer J Clin. 2011;61(2):69–90.
2. Lachiewicz AM, Berwick M, Wiggins CL, Thomas NE. Epidemiologic support for melanoma heterogeneity using the surveillance, epidemiology, and end results program. J Invest Dermatol. 2008;128(5):1340–2.
3. Rigel DS. Epidemiology of melanoma. Semin Cutan Med Surg. 2010;29(4):204–9.
4. Fisher DE, James WD. Indoor tanning-science, behavior, and policy. N Engl J Med. 2010;363(10):901–3.
5. Moan J, Dahlback A, Setlow RB. Epidemiological support for an hypothesis for melanoma induction indicating a role for UVA radiation. Photochem Photobiol. 1999;70(2):243–7.
6. Holman CD, Armstrong BK. Cutaneous malignant melanoma and indicators of total accumulated exposure to the sun: an analysis separating histogenetic types. J Natl Cancer Inst. 1984;73(1):75–82.
7. Pfahlberg A, Kolmel KF, Gefeller O. Timing of excessive ultraviolet radiation and melanoma: epidemiology does not support the existence of a critical period of high susceptibility to solar ultraviolet radiation-induced melanoma. Br J Dermatol. 2001;144(3):471–5.

8. Pleasance ED, Cheetham RK, Stephens PJ, et al. A comprehensive catalogue of somatic mutations from a human cancer genome. Nature. 2010;463(7278): 191–6.

9. Green AC, Williams GM, Logan V, Strutton GM. Reduced melanoma after regular sunscreen use: randomized trial follow-up. J Clin Oncol. 2011;29(3): 257–63.

10. Meyle KD, Guldberg P. Genetic risk factors for melanoma. Hum Genet. 2009;126(4):499–510.

11. Begg CB, Orlow I, Hummer AJ, et al. Lifetime risk of melanoma in CDKN2A mutation carriers in a population-based sample. J Natl Cancer Inst. 2005; 97(20):1507–15.

12. Arumi-Uria M, McNutt NS, Finnerty B. Grading of atypia in nevi: correlation with melanoma risk. Mod Pathol. 2003;16(8):764–71.

13. MacKie RM, English J, Aitchison TC, Fitzsimons CP, Wilson P. The number and distribution of benign pigmented moles (melanocytic naevi) in a healthy British population. Br J Dermatol. 1985;113(2): 167–74.

14. Newton-Bishop JA, Chang YM, Iles MM, et al. Melanocytic nevi, nevus genes, and melanoma risk in a large case-control study in the United Kingdom. Cancer Epidemiol Biomarkers Prev. 2010;19(8): 2043–54.

15. Balch CM, Soong SJ, Gershenwald JE, et al. Prognostic factors analysis of 17,600 melanoma patients: validation of the American Joint Committee on Cancer melanoma staging system. J Clin Oncol. 2001;19(16):3622–34.

16. Breslow A. Thickness, cross-sectional areas and depth of invasion in the prognosis of cutaneous melanoma. Ann Surg. 1970;172(5):902–8.

17. Clark Jr WH, From L, Bernardino EA, Mihm MC. The histogenesis and biologic behavior of primary human malignant melanomas of the skin. Cancer Res. 1969;29(3):705–27.

18. Balch CM, Gershenwald JE, Soong SJ, et al. Final version of 2009 AJCC melanoma staging and classification. J Clin Oncol. 2009;27(36):6199–206.

19. Lens MB, Dawes M, Newton-Bishop JA, Goodacre T. Tumour thickness as a predictor of occult lymph node metastases in patients with stage I and II melanoma undergoing sentinel lymph node biopsy. Br J Surg. 2002;89(10):1223–7.

20. Sondak VK, Taylor JM, Sabel MS, et al. Mitotic rate and younger age are predictors of sentinel lymph node positivity: lessons learned from the generation of a probabilistic model. Ann Surg Oncol. 2004; 11(3):247–58.

21. Gonzalez U. Cloud over sentinel node biopsy: unlikely survival benefit in melanoma. Arch Dermatol. 2007;143(6):775–6.

22. Kanzler MH. The current status of evaluation and treatment of high-risk cutaneous melanoma: therapeutic breakthroughs remain elusive. Arch Dermatol. 2007;143(6):785–7.

23. Morton DL, Thompson JF, Cochran AJ, et al. Sentinel-node biopsy or nodal observation in melanoma. N Engl J Med. 2006;355(13):1307–17.

24. Ohsie SJ, Sarantopoulos GP, Cochran AJ, Binder SW. Immunohistochemical characteristics of melanoma. J Cutan Pathol. 2008;35(5):433–44.

25. Prieto VG, Shea CR. Use of immunohistochemistry in melanocytic lesions. J Cutan Pathol. 2008;35 Suppl 2:1–10.

26. Thies A, Berlin A, Brunner G, et al. Glycoconjugate profiling of primary melanoma and its sentinel node and distant metastases: implications for diagnosis and pathophysiology of metastases. Cancer Lett. 2007;248(1):68–80.

27. Kashani-Sabet M, Rangel J, Torabian S, et al. A multi-marker assay to distinguish malignant melanomas from benign nevi. Proc Natl Acad Sci U S A. 2009;106(15):6268–72.

28. Carlson JA, Ross JS, Slominski A, et al. Molecular diagnostics in melanoma. J Am Acad Dermatol. 2005;52(5):743–75. quiz 775-748.

29. Gould Rothberg BE, Bracken MB, Rimm DL. Tissue biomarkers for prognosis in cutaneous melanoma: a systematic review and meta-analysis. J Natl Cancer Inst. 2009;101(7):452–74.

30. Larson AR, Konat E, Alani RM. Melanoma biomarkers: current status and vision for the future. Nat Clin Pract Oncol. 2009;6(2):105–17.

31. Bosserhoff AK. Novel biomarkers in malignant melanoma. Clin Chim Acta. 2006;367(1–2):28–35.

32. Gimotty PA, Van Belle P, Elder DE, et al. Biologic and prognostic significance of dermal Ki67 expression, mitoses, and tumorigenicity in thin invasive cutaneous melanoma. J Clin Oncol. 2005;23(31): 8048–56.

33. Haass NK, Smalley KS, Li L, Herlyn M. Adhesion, migration and communication in melanocytes and melanoma. Pigment Cell Res. 2005;18(3):150–9.

34. Shih IM, Speicher D, Hsu MY, Levine E, Herlyn M. Melanoma cell–cell interactions are mediated through heterophilic Mel-CAM/ligand adhesion. Cancer Res. 1997;57(17):3835–40.

35. Johnson JP, Bar-Eli M, Jansen B, Markhof E. Melanoma progression-associated glycoprotein MUC18/MCAM mediates homotypic cell adhesion through interaction with a heterophilic ligand. Int J Cancer. 1997;73(5):769–74.

36. Shih LM, Hsu MY, Palazzo JP, Herlyn M. The cell–cell adhesion receptor Mel-CAM acts as a tumor suppressor in breast carcinoma. Am J Pathol. 1997;151(3):745–51.

37. Shih IM, Elder DE, Speicher D, Johnson JP, Herlyn M. Isolation and functional characterization of the A32 melanoma-associated antigen. Cancer Res. 1994;54(9):2514–20.

38. Kraus A, Masat L, Johnson JP. Analysis of the expression of intercellular adhesion molecule-1 and MUC18 on benign and malignant melanocytic lesions using monoclonal antibodies directed

against distinct epitopes and recognizing denatured, non-glycosylated antigen. Melanoma Res. 1997;7 Suppl 2:S75–81.

39. Xie S, Luca M, Huang S, et al. Expression of MCAM/MUC18 by human melanoma cells leads to increased tumor growth and metastasis. Cancer Res. 1997;57(11):2295–303.

40. Johnson JP, Rummel MM, Rothbacher U, Sers C. MUC18: a cell adhesion molecule with a potential role in tumor growth and tumor cell dissemination. Curr Top Microbiol Immunol. 1996;213(Pt 1): 95–105.

41. Lehmann JM, Holzmann B, Breitbart EW, Schmiegelow P, Riethmuller G, Johnson JP. Discrimination between benign and malignant cells of melanocytic lineage by two novel antigens, a glycoprotein with a molecular weight of 113,000 and a protein with a molecular weight of 76,000. Cancer Res. 1987;47(3):841–5.

42. Lehmann JM, Riethmuller G, Johnson JP. MUC18, a marker of tumor progression in human melanoma, shows sequence similarity to the neural cell adhesion molecules of the immunoglobulin superfamily. Proc Natl Acad Sci U S A. 1989;86(24):9891–5.

43. Pearl RA, Pacifico MD, Richman PI, Wilson GD, Grover R. Stratification of patients by melanoma cell adhesion molecule (MCAM) expression on the basis of risk: implications for sentinel lymph node biopsy. J Plast Reconstr Aesthet Surg. 2008;61(3):265–71.

44. Pacifico MD, Grover R, Richman PI, Daley FM, Buffa F, Wilson GD. Development of a tissue array for primary melanoma with long-term follow-up: discovering melanoma cell adhesion molecule as an important prognostic marker. Plast Reconstr Surg. 2005;115(2):367–75.

45. Ostmeier H, Fuchs B, Otto F, et al. Prognostic immunohistochemical markers of primary human melanomas. Br J Dermatol. 2001;145(2):203–9.

46. Nolte C, Moos M, Schachner M. Immunolocalization of the neural cell adhesion molecule L1 in epithelia of rodents. Cell Tissue Res. 1999;298(2):261–73.

47. Thies A, Schachner M, Moll I, et al. Overexpression of the cell adhesion molecule L1 is associated with metastasis in cutaneous malignant melanoma. Eur J Cancer. 2002;38(13):1708–16.

48. Hortsch M. The L1 family of neural cell adhesion molecules: old proteins performing new tricks. Neuron. 1996;17(4):587–93.

49. Montgomery AM, Becker JC, Siu CH, et al. Human neural cell adhesion molecule L1 and rat homologue NILE are ligands for integrin alpha v beta 3. J Cell Biol. 1996;132(3):475–85.

50. Voura EB, Ramjeesingh RA, Montgomery AM, Siu CH. Involvement of integrin alpha(v)beta(3) and cell adhesion molecule L1 in transendothelial migration of melanoma cells. Mol Biol Cell. 2001;12(9): 2699–710.

51. Meier F, Busch S, Gast D, et al. The adhesion molecule L1 (CD171) promotes melanoma progression. Int J Cancer. 2006;119(3):549–55.

52. Fogel M, Mechtersheimer S, Huszar M, et al. L1 adhesion molecule (CD 171) in development and progression of human malignant melanoma. Cancer Lett. 2003;189(2):237–47.

53. Talantov D, Mazumder A, Yu JX, et al. Novel genes associated with malignant melanoma but not benign melanocytic lesions. Clin Cancer Res. 2005;11(20): 7234–42.

54. van de Stolpe A, van der Saag PT. Intercellular adhesion molecule-1. J Mol Med. 1996;74(1):13–33.

55. Johnson JP, Stade BG, Holzmann B, Schwable W, Riethmuller G. De novo expression of intercellular-adhesion molecule 1 in melanoma correlates with increased risk of metastasis. Proc Natl Acad Sci U S A. 1989;86(2):641–4.

56. Natali P, Nicotra MR, Cavaliere R, et al. Differential expression of intercellular adhesion molecule 1 in primary and metastatic melanoma lesions. Cancer Res. 1990;50(4):1271–8.

57. Natali PG, Hamby CV, Felding-Habermann B, et al. Clinical significance of alpha(v)beta3 integrin and intercellular adhesion molecule-1 expression in cutaneous malignant melanoma lesions. Cancer Res. 1997;57(8):1554–60.

58. Schadendorf D, Gawlik C, Haney U, Ostmeier H, Suter L, Czarnetzki BM. Tumour progression and metastatic behaviour in vivo correlates with integrin expression on melanocytic tumours. J Pathol. 1993;170(4):429–34.

59. Schadendorf D, Heidel J, Gawlik C, Suter L, Czarnetzki BM. Association with clinical outcome of expression of VLA-4 in primary cutaneous malignant melanoma as well as P-selectin and E-selectin on intratumoral vessels. J Natl Cancer Inst. 1995; 87(5):366–71.

60. Miele ME, Bennett CF, Miller BE, Welch DR. Enhanced metastatic ability of TNF-alpha-treated malignant melanoma cells is reduced by intercellular adhesion molecule-1 (ICAM-1, CD54) antisense oligonucleotides. Exp Cell Res. 1994;214(1):231–41.

61. Aeed PA, Nakajima M, Welch DR. The role of polymorphonuclear leukocytes (PMN) on the growth and metastatic potential of 13762NF mammary adenocarcinoma cells. Int J Cancer. 1988;42(5):748–59.

62. Giavazzi R, Chirivi RG, Garofalo A, et al. Soluble intercellular adhesion molecule 1 is released by human melanoma cells and is associated with tumor growth in nude mice. Cancer Res. 1992;52(9):2628–30.

63. Becker JC, Termeer C, Schmidt RE, Brocker EB. Soluble intercellular adhesion molecule-1 inhibits MHC-restricted specific T cell/tumor interaction. J Immunol. 1993;151(12):7224–32.

64. Brummer J, Ebrahimnejad A, Flayeh R, et al. cis Interaction of the cell adhesion molecule CEACAM1 with integrin beta(3). Am J Pathol. 2001;159(2): 537–46.

65. Thies A, Moll I, Berger J, et al. CEACAM1 expression in cutaneous malignant melanoma predicts the development of metastatic disease. J Clin Oncol. 2002;20(10):2530–6.

66. Ebrahimnejad A, Streichert T, Nollau P, et al. CEACAM1 enhances invasion and migration of melanocytic and melanoma cells. Am J Pathol. 2004;165(5):1781–7.

67. Hsu MY, Wheelock MJ, Johnson KR, Herlyn M. Shifts in cadherin profiles between human normal melanocytes and melanomas. J Investig Dermatol Symp Proc. 1996;1(2):188–94.

68. Tang A, Eller MS, Hara M, Yaar M, Hirohashi S, Gilchrest BA. E-cadherin is the major mediator of human melanocyte adhesion to keratinocytes in vitro. J Cell Sci. 1994;107(Pt 4):983–92.

69. Haass NK, Smalley KS, Herlyn M. The role of altered cell–cell communication in melanoma progression. J Mol Histol. 2004;35(3):309–18.

70. Haass NK, Herlyn M. Normal human melanocyte homeostasis as a paradigm for understanding melanoma. J Investig Dermatol Symp Proc. 2005;10(2): 153–63.

71. Danen EH, de Vries TJ, Morandini R, Ghanem GG, Ruiter DJ, van Muijen GN. E-cadherin expression in human melanoma. Melanoma Res. 1996;6(2):127–31.

72. Sanders DS, Blessing K, Hassan GA, Bruton R, Marsden JR, Jankowski J. Alterations in cadherin and catenin expression during the biological progression of melanocytic tumours. Mol Pathol. 1999;52(3):151–7.

73. Krengel S, Groteluschen F, Bartsch S, Tronnier M. Cadherin expression pattern in melanocytic tumors more likely depends on the melanocyte environment than on tumor cell progression. J Cutan Pathol. 2004;31(1):1–7.

74. Andersen K, Nesland JM, Holm R, Florenes VA, Fodstad O, Maelandsmo GM. Expression of S100A4 combined with reduced E-cadherin expression predicts patient outcome in malignant melanoma. Mod Pathol. 2004;17(8):990–7.

75. Nishizawa A, Nakanishi Y, Yoshimura K, et al. Clinicopathologic significance of dysadherin expression in cutaneous malignant melanoma: immunohistochemical analysis of 115 patients. Cancer. 2005;103(8):1693–700.

76. Atkins MB. The role of cytotoxic chemotherapeutic agents either alone or in combination with biologic response modifiers. In: Kirkwood JK, ed. Molecular Diagnosis, Prevention and Therapy of Melanoma. New York: Marcel Dekker; 2007. p. 1–2

77. Sawyers C. Targeted cancer therapy. Nature. 2004; 432(7015):294–7.

78. Bauer S, Duensing A, Demetri GD, Fletcher JA. KIT oncogenic signaling mechanisms in imatinib-resistant gastrointestinal stromal tumor: PI3-kinase/AKT is a crucial survival pathway. Oncogene. 2007; 26(54):7560–8.

79. Druker BJ, Talpaz M, Resta DJ, et al. Efficacy and safety of a specific inhibitor of the BCR-ABL tyrosine kinase in chronic myeloid leukemia. N Engl J Med. 2001;344(14):1031–7.

80. Curtin JA, Busam K, Pinkel D, Bastian BC. Somatic activation of KIT in distinct subtypes of melanoma. J Clin Oncol. 2006;24(26):4340–6.

81. Curtin JA, Fridlyand J, Kageshita T, et al. Distinct sets of genetic alterations in melanoma. N Engl J Med. 2005;353(20):2135–47.

82. Smalley KS, Nathanson KL, Flaherty KT. Genetic subgrouping of melanoma reveals new opportunities for targeted therapy. Cancer Res. 2009;69(8): 3241–4.

83. Davies H, Bignell GR, Cox C, et al. Mutations of the BRAF gene in human cancer. Nature. 2002;417 (6892):949–54.

84. Dhomen N, Marais R. BRAF signaling and targeted therapies in melanoma. Hematol Oncol Clin North Am. 2009;23(3):529–45. ix.

85. Wellbrock C, Karasarides M, Marais R. The RAF proteins take centre stage. Nat Rev Mol Cell Biol. 2004;5(11):875–85.

86. Garnett MJ, Marais R. Guilty as charged: B-RAF is a human oncogene. Cancer Cell. 2004;6(4):313–9.

87. Wan PT, Garnett MJ, Roe SM, et al. Mechanism of activation of the RAF-ERK signaling pathway by oncogenic mutations of B-RAF. Cell. 2004;116(6): 855–67.

88. Smalley KSM. A pivotal role for ERK in the oncogenic behaviour of malignant melanoma? Int J Cancer. 2003;104(5):527–32.

89. Sherr CJ. G1 phase progression: cycling on cue. Cell. 1994;79(4):551–5.

90. Bhatt KV, Spofford LS, Aram G, McMullen M, Pumiglia K, Aplin AE. Adhesion control of cyclin D1 and p27Kip1 levels is deregulated in melanoma cells through BRAF-MEK-ERK signaling. Oncogene. 2005;24(21):3459–71.

91. Wellbrock C, Ogilvie L, Hedley D, et al. V599EB-RAF is an oncogene in melanocytes. Cancer Res. 2004;64(7):2338–42.

92. Hingorani SR, Jacobetz MA, Robertson GP, Herlyn M, Tuveson DA. Suppression of BRAF(V599E) in human melanoma abrogates transformation. Cancer Res. 2003;63(17):5198–202.

93. Wellbrock C, Marais R. Elevated expression of MITF counteracts B-RAF-stimulated melanocyte and melanoma cell proliferation. J Cell Biol. 2005;170(5):703–8.

94. Pollock PM, Harper UL, Hansen KS, et al. High frequency of BRAF mutations in nevi. Nat Genet. 2003;33(1):19–20.

95. Michaloglou C, Vredeveld LC, Soengas MS, et al. BRAFE600-associated senescence-like cell cycle arrest of human naevi. Nature. 2005;436(7051):720–4.

96. Sharpless NE, DePinho RA. Cancer: crime and punishment. Nature. 2005;436(7051):636–7.

97. Hayward NK. Genetics of melanoma predisposition. Oncogene. 2003;22(20):3053–62.

98. Tsao H, Goel V, Wu H, Yang G, Haluska FG. Genetic interaction between NRAS and BRAF mutations and PTEN/MMAC1 inactivation in melanoma. J Invest Dermatol. 2004;122(2):337–41.

99. Stahl JM, Sharma A, Cheung M, et al. Deregulated Akt3 activity promotes development of malignant melanoma. Cancer Res. 2004;64(19):7002–10.

100. Davies MA, Stemke-Hale K, Tellez C, et al. A novel AKT3 mutation in melanoma tumours and cell lines. Br J Cancer. 2008;99(8):1265–8.

101. Dankort D, Curley DP, Cartlidge RA, et al. Braf(V600E) cooperates with Pten loss to induce metastatic melanoma. Nat Genet. 2009;41(5):544–52.

102. Padua RA, Barrass N, Currie GA. A novel transforming gene in a human malignant melanoma cell line. Nature. 1984;311(5987):671–3.

103. Padua RA, Barrass NC, Currie GA. Activation of N-ras in a human melanoma cell line. Mol Cell Biol. 1985;5(3):582–5.

104. Downward J. Targeting RAS signalling pathways in cancer therapy. Nat Rev Cancer. 2003;3(1):11–22.

105. Brose MS, Volpe P, Feldman M, et al. BRAF and RAS mutations in human lung cancer and melanoma. Cancer Res. 2002;62(23):6997–7000.

106. Lin WM, Baker AC, Beroukhim R, et al. Modeling genomic diversity and tumor dependency in malignant melanoma. Cancer Res. 2008;68(3):664–73.

107. Milagre C, Dhomen N, Geyer FC, et al. A mouse model of melanoma driven by oncogenic KRAS. Cancer Res. 2010;70(13):5549–57.

108. Whitwam T, Vanbrocklin MW, Russo ME, et al. Differential oncogenic potential of activated RAS isoforms in melanocytes. Oncogene. 2007;26(31): 4563–70.

109. Dhomen N, Marais R. New insight into BRAF mutations in cancer. Curr Opin Genet Dev. 2007;17(1): 31–9.

110. Sahai E, Marshall CJ. RHO-GTPases and cancer. Nat Rev Cancer. 2002;2(2):133–42.

111. Mishra PJ, Ha L, Rieker J, et al. Dissection of RAS downstream pathways in melanomagenesis: a role for Ral in transformation. Oncogene. 2010;29(16): 2449–56.

112. Dumaz N, Hayward R, Martin J, et al. In melanoma, RAS mutations are accompanied by switching signaling from BRAF to CRAF and disrupted cyclic AMP signaling. Cancer Res. 2006;66(19):9483–91.

113. Woodman SE, Davies MA. Targeting KIT in melanoma: a paradigm of molecular medicine and targeted therapeutics. Biochem Pharmacol. 2010;80(5):568–74.

114. Rivera RS, Nagatsuka H, Gunduz M, et al. C-kit protein expression correlated with activating mutations in KIT gene in oral mucosal melanoma. Virchows Arch. 2008;452(1):27–32.

115. Antonescu CR, Busam KJ, Francone TD, et al. L576P KIT mutation in anal melanomas correlates with KIT protein expression and is sensitive to specific kinase inhibition. Int J Cancer. 2007;121(2): 257–64.

116. Smalley KS, Contractor R, Nguyen TK, et al. Identification of a novel subgroup of melanomas with KIT/cyclin-dependent kinase-4 overexpression. Cancer Res. 2008;68(14):5743–52.

117. Zandi R, Larsen AB, Andersen P, Stockhausen MT, Poulsen HS. Mechanisms for oncogenic activation of the epidermal growth factor receptor. Cell Signal. 2007;19(10):2013–23.

118. Scott G, Ewing J, Ryan D, Abboud C. Stem cell factor regulates human melanocyte-matrix interactions. Pigment Cell Res. 1994;7(1):44–51.

119. Scott G, Liang H, Luthra D. Stem cell factor regulates the melanocyte cytoskeleton. Pigment Cell Res. 1996;9(3):134–41.

120. Chabot B, Stephenson DA, Chapman VM, Besmer P, Bernstein A. The proto-oncogene c-kit encoding a transmembrane tyrosine kinase receptor maps to the mouse W locus. Nature. 1988;335(6185):88–9.

121. Witte ON. Steel locus defines new multipotent growth factor. Cell. 1990;63(1):5–6.

122. Spritz RA, Giebel LB, Holmes SA. Dominant negative and loss of function mutations of the c-kit (mast/stem cell growth factor receptor) proto-oncogene in human piebaldism. Am J Hum Genet. 1992;50(2): 261–9.

123. Kawa Y, Ito M, Ono H, et al. Stem cell factor and/or endothelin-3 dependent immortal melanoblast and melanocyte populations derived from mouse neural crest cells. Pigment Cell Res. 2000;13 Suppl 8:73–80.

124. Alexeev V, Yoon K. Distinctive role of the cKit receptor tyrosine kinase signaling in mammalian melanocytes. J Invest Dermatol. 2006;126(5): 1102–10.

125. Hemesath TJ, Price ER, Takemoto C, Badalian T, Fisher DE. MAP kinase links the transcription factor Microphthalmia to c-Kit signalling in melanocytes. Nature. 1998;391(6664):298–301.

126. Li G, Satyamoorthy K, Herlyn M. N-cadherin-mediated intercellular interactions promote survival and migration of melanoma cells. Cancer Res. 2001;61(9):3819–25.

127. Monsel G, Ortonne N, Bagot M, Bensussan A, Dumaz N. c-Kit mutants require hypoxia-inducible factor 1alpha to transform melanocytes. Oncogene. 2010;29(2):227–36.

128. Natali PG, Nicotra MR, Winkler AB, Cavaliere R, Bigotti A, Ullrich A. Progression of human cutaneous melanoma is associated with loss of expression of c-kit proto-oncogene receptor. Int J Cancer. 1992;52(2):197–201.

129. Lassam N, Bickford S. Loss of c-kit expression in cultured melanoma cells. Oncogene. 1992;7(1):51–6.

130. Huang S, Luca M, Gutman M, et al. Enforced c-KIT expression renders highly metastatic human melanoma cells susceptible to stem cell factor-induced apoptosis and inhibits their tumorigenic and metastatic potential. Oncogene. 1996;13(11):2339–47.

131. Huang S, Jean D, Luca M, Tainsky MA, Bar-Eli M. Loss of AP-2 results in downregulation of c-KIT and enhancement of melanoma tumorigenicity and metastasis. EMBO J. 1998;17(15):4358–69.

132. Smalley KS, Xiao M, Villanueva J, et al. CRAF inhibition induces apoptosis in melanoma cells with non-V600E BRAF mutations. Oncogene. 2009; 28(1):85–94.

133. Jilaveanu L, Zito C, Lee SJ, et al. Expression of sorafenib targets in melanoma patients treated with carboplatin, paclitaxel and sorafenib. Clin Cancer Res. 2009;15(3):1076–85.

134. Edwards RH, Ward MR, Wu H, et al. Absence of BRAF mutations in UV-protected mucosal melanomas. J Med Genet. 2004;41(4):270–2.
135. Bauer J, Buttner P, Murali R, et al. BRAF mutations in cutaneous melanoma are independently associated with age, anatomic site of the primary tumor and the degree of solar elastosis at the primary tumor site. Pigment Cell Melanoma Res. 2011;24(2):345–51.
136. Viros A, Fridlyand J, Bauer J, et al. Improving melanoma classification by integrating genetic and morphologic features. PLoS Med. 2008;5(6):e120.
137. Ellerhorst JA, Greene VR, Ekmekcioglu S, et al. Clinical correlates of NRAS and BRAF mutations in primary human melanoma. Clin Cancer Res. 2011;17(2):229–35.
138. King AJ, Patrick DR, Batorsky RS, et al. Demonstration of a genetic therapeutic index for tumors expressing oncogenic BRAF by the kinase inhibitor SB-590885. Cancer Res. 2006;66(23):11100–5.
139. Tsai J, Lee JT, Wang W, et al. Discovery of a selective inhibitor of oncogenic B-Raf kinase with potent antimelanoma activity. Proc Natl Acad Sci U S A. 2008;105(8):3041–6.
140. Haass NK, Sproesser K, Nguyen TK, et al. The mitogen-activated protein/extracellular signal-regulated kinase kinase inhibitor AZD6244 (ARRY-142886) induces growth arrest in melanoma cells and tumor regression when combined with docetaxel. Clin Cancer Res. 2008;14(1):230–9.
141. Solit DB, Garraway LA, Pratilas CA, et al. BRAF mutation predicts sensitivity to MEK inhibition. Nature. 2006;439(7074):358–62.
142. Wilhelm SM, Carter C, Tang L, et al. BAY 43-9006 exhibits broad spectrum oral antitumor activity and targets the RAF/MEK/ERK pathway and receptor tyrosine kinases involved in tumor progression and angiogenesis. Cancer Res. 2004;64(19):7099–109.
143. Sharma A, Trivedi NR, Zimmerman MA, Tuveson DA, Smith CD, Robertson GP. Mutant V599EB-Raf regulates growth and vascular development of malignant melanoma tumors. Cancer Res. 2005;65(6):2412–21.
144. Hauschild A, Agarwala SS, Trefzer U, et al. Results of a phase III, randomized, placebo-controlled study of sorafenib in combination with carboplatin and paclitaxel as second-line treatment in patients with unresectable stage III or stage IV melanoma. J Clin Oncol. 2009;27(17):2823–30.
145. Whittaker S, Kirk R, Hayward R, et al. Gatekeeper mutations mediate resistance to BRAF-targeted therapies. Sci Transl Med. 2010;2(35):35ra41.
146. Paraiso KH, Fedorenko IV, Cantini LP, et al. Recovery of phospho-ERK activity allows melanoma cells to escape from BRAF inhibitor therapy. Br J Cancer. 2010;102(12):1724–30.
147. Poulikakos PI, Zhang C, Bollag G, Shokat KM, Rosen N. RAF inhibitors transactivate RAF dimers and ERK signalling in cells with wild-type BRAF. Nature. 2010;464(7287):427–30.
148. Montagut C, Sharma SV, Shioda T, et al. Elevated CRAF as a potential mechanism of acquired resistance to BRAF inhibition in melanoma. Cancer Res. 2008;68(12):4853–61.
149. Sondergaard JN, Nazarian R, Wang Q, et al. Differential sensitivity of melanoma cell lines with BRAFV600E mutation to the specific Raf inhibitor PLX4032. J Transl Med. 2010;8:39.
150. Tap WD, Gong KW, Dering J, et al. Pharmacodynamic characterization of the efficacy signals due to selective BRAF inhibition with PLX4032 in malignant melanoma. Neoplasia. 2010;12(8):637–49.
151. Yang H, Higgins B, Kolinsky K, et al. RG7204 (PLX4032), a selective BRAFV600E inhibitor, displays potent antitumor activity in preclinical melanoma models. Cancer Res. 2010;70(13):5518–27.
152. Schwartz GK, Robertson S, Shen A, et al. A phase I study of XL281, a selective oral RAF kinase in patients with advanced solid tumors. J Clin Oncol. 2009;27(15s):3513.
153. Bollag G, Hirth P, Tsai J, et al. Clinical efficacy of a RAF inhibitor needs broad target blockade in BRAF-mutant melanoma. Nature. 2009;467:596–9.
154. Villanueva J, Cipolla A, Kong J, et al. A kinase switch underlies acquired resistance to BRAF inhibitors. Pigment Cell Melanoma Res. 2009;22(6):136.
155. Kefford R, Arkenau H, Brown MP, et al. Phase I/II study of GSK2118436, a selective inhibitor of oncogenic mutant BRAF kinase, in patients with metastatic melanoma and other solid tumors. J Clin Oncol. 2010;28(15s):8503.
156. Smalley KS, Lioni M, Palma MD, et al. Increased cyclin D1 expression can mediate BRAF inhibitor resistance in BRAF V600E-mutated melanomas. Mol Cancer Ther. 2008;7(9):2876–83.
157. Lazar V, Ecsedi S, Szollosi AG, et al. Characterization of candidate gene copy number alterations in the 11q13 region along with BRAF and NRAS mutations in human melanoma. Mod Pathol. 2009;22(10):1367–78.
158. Paraiso KH, Xiang Y, Rebecca VW, et al. PTEN loss confers BRAF inhibitor resistance to melanoma cells through the suppression of BIM expression. Cancer Res. 2011;71:2750–60 doi: 10.1158/0008-5472.
159. Nathanson KL. Using genetics and genomics strategies to personalize therapy for cancer: focus on melanoma. Biochem Pharmacol. 2010;80(5):755–61.
160. Smalley KS, Contractor R, Haass NK, et al. Ki67 expression levels are a better marker of reduced melanoma growth following MEK inhibitor treatment than phospho-ERK levels. Br J Cancer. 2007;96(3):445–9.
161. Cartlidge RA, Thomas GR, Cagnol S, et al. Oncogenic BRAF(V600E) inhibits BIM expression to promote melanoma cell survival. Pigment Cell Melanoma Res. 2008;21(5):534–44.
162. Boisvert-Adamo K, Longmate W, Abel EV, Aplin AE. Mcl-1 is required for melanoma cell resistance to anoikis. Mol Cancer Res. 2009;7(4):549–56.
163. Boisvert-Adamo K, Aplin AE. Mutant B-RAF mediates resistance to anoikis via Bad and Bim. Oncogene. 2008;27(23):3301–12.

164. Flaherty KT, Puzanov I, Kim KB, et al. Inhibition of mutated, activated BRAF in metastatic melanoma. N Engl J Med. 2010;363(9):809–19.

165. Halaban R, Zhang W, Bacchiocchi A, et al. PLX4032, a selective BRAF(V600E) kinase inhibitor, activates the ERK pathway and enhances cell migration and proliferation of BRAF melanoma cells. Pigment Cell Melanoma Res. 2010;23(2):190–200.

166. Heidorn SJ, Milagre C, Whittaker S, et al. Kinase-dead BRAF and oncogenic RAS cooperate to drive tumor progression through CRAF. Cell. 2010; 140(2):209–21.

167. Rudin CM, Hann CL, Laterra J, et al. Treatment of medulloblastoma with hedgehog pathway inhibitor GDC-0449. N Engl J Med. 2009;361(12):1173–8.

168. Yauch RL, Dijkgraaf GJ, Alicke B, et al. Smoothened mutation confers resistance to a hedgehog pathway inhibitor in medulloblastoma. Science. 2009;326: 572–4.

169. O'Hare T, Shakespeare WC, Zhu X, et al. AP24534, a pan-BCR-ABL inhibitor for chronic myeloid leukemia, potently inhibits the T315I mutant and overcomes mutation-based resistance. Cancer Cell. 2009;16(5):401–12.

170. Michor F, Hughes TP, Iwasa Y, et al. Dynamics of chronic myeloid leukaemia. Nature. 2005;435(7046): 1267–70.

171. Nazarian R, Shi H, Wang Q, et al. Melanomas acquire resistance to B-RAF(V600E) inhibition by RTK or N-RAS upregulation. Nature. 2010;468:973–7.

172. Emery CM, Vijayendran KG, Zipser MC, et al. MEK1 mutations confer resistance to MEK and B-RAF inhibition. Proc Natl Acad Sci U S A. 2009;106(48):20411–6.

173. Jiang CC, Lai F, Thorne RF, et al. MEK-Independent survival of B-RAFV600E melanoma cells selected for resistance to apoptosis induced by the RAF inhibitor PLX4720. Clin Cancer Res. 2011;17(4): 721–30 doi: 10.1158/1078-0432.

174. Johannessen CM, Boehm JS, Kim SY, et al. COT drives resistance to RAF inhibition through MAP kinase pathway reactivation. Nature. 2010;468:968–72.

175. Christensen C, Guldberg P. Growth factors rescue cutaneous melanoma cells from apoptosis induced by knockdown of mutated (V 600 E) B-RAF. Oncogene. 2005;24(41):6292–302.

176. Gray-Schopfer VC, Karasarides M, Hayward R, Marais R. Tumor necrosis factor-alpha blocks apoptosis in melanoma cells when BRAF signaling is inhibited. Cancer Res. 2007;67(1):122–9.

177. Corcoran RB, Dias-Santagata D, Bergethon K, Iafrate AJ, Settleman J, Engelman JA. BRAF gene amplification can promote acquired resistance to MEK inhibitors in cancer cells harboring the BRAF V600E mutation. Sci Signal. 2010;3(149):ra84.

178. Konstantinopoulos PA, Karamouzis MV, Papavassiliou AG. Post-translational modifications and regulation of the RAS superfamily of GTPases as anticancer targets. Nat Rev Drug Discov. 2007; 6(7):541–55.

179. Gajewski TK ND, Johnson J, Linette G, Bucher C, Blaskovich M, Sebti S, Haluska F. Phase II study of the farnesyltransferase inhibitor R115777 in advanced melanoma: CALGB 500104. J Clin Oncol. 2006;24(18S)

180. Margolin KA, Moon J, Flaherty LE, Lao CD, Akerley WL, Sosman JA, Kirkwood JM, Sondak VK. Randomized phase II trial of sorafenib (SO) with temsirolimus (TEM) or tipifarnib (TIPI) in metastatic melanoma: Southwest Oncology Group Trial S0438. J Clin Oncol. 2010;28:15s.

181. Hoeflich KP, O'Brien C, Boyd Z, et al. In vivo anti-tumor activity of MEK and phosphatidylinositol 3-kinase inhibitors in basal-like breast cancer models. Clin Cancer Res. 2009;15(14):4649–64.

182. Engelman JA, Chen L, Tan X, et al. Effective use of PI3K and MEK inhibitors to treat mutant Kras G12D and PIK3CA H1047R murine lung cancers. Nat Med. 2008;14(12):1351–6.

183. Jaiswal BS, Janakiraman V, Kljavin NM, et al. Combined targeting of BRAF and CRAF or BRAF and PI3K effector pathways is required for efficacy in NRAS mutant tumors. PLoS One. 2009;4(5):e5717.

184. Infante JR, Fecher LA, Nallapareddy S, Gordon MS, Flaherty KT, Cox DS, DeMarini DJ, Morris SR, Burris HA, Messersmith WA. Safety and efficacy results from the first-in-human study of the oral MEK 1/2 inhibitor GSK1120212. J Clin Oncol. 2010;28:7.

185. Carnahan J, Beltran PJ, Babij C, et al. Selective and potent Raf inhibitors paradoxically stimulate normal cell proliferation and tumor growth. Mol Cancer Ther. 2010;9(8):2399–410.

186. Kaplan FM, Shao Y, Mayberry MM, Aplin AE. Hyperactivation of MEK-ERK1/2 signaling and resistance to apoptosis induced by the ongenic B-RAF inhibitor, PLX4720, in mutant N-Ras melanoma cell lines. Oncogene. 2010;30:366–71.

187. Hatzivassiliou G, Song K, Yen I, et al. RAF inhibitors prime wild-type RAF to activate the MAPK pathway and enhance growth. Nature. 2010;464(7287):431–5.

188. Heinrich MC, Griffith DJ, Druker BJ, Wait CL, Ott KA, Zigler AJ. Inhibition of c-kit receptor tyrosine kinase activity by STI 571, a selective tyrosine kinase inhibitor. Blood. 2000;96(3):925–32.

189. Terheyden P, Houben R, Pajouh P, Thorns C, Zillikens D, Becker JC. Response to imatinib mesylate depends on the presence of the V559A-mutated KIT oncogene. J Invest Dermatol. 2010;130(1): 314–6.

190. Jiang X, Zhou J, Yuen NK, et al. Imatinib targeting of KIT-mutant oncoprotein in melanoma. Clin Cancer Res. 2008;14(23):7726–32.

191. Ashida A, Takata M, Murata H, Kido K, Saida T. Pathological activation of KIT in metastatic tumors of acral and mucosal melanomas. Int J Cancer. 2009;124(4):862–8.

192. Woodman SE, Trent JC, Stemke-Hale K, et al. Activity of dasatinib against L576P KIT mutant

melanoma: molecular, cellular, and clinical correlates. Mol Cancer Ther. 2009;8(8):2079–85.

193. Ugurel S, Hildenbrand R, Zimpfer A, et al. Lack of clinical efficacy of imatinib in metastatic melanoma. Br J Cancer. 2005;92(8):1398–405.

194. Kim KB, Eton O, Davis DW, et al. Phase II trial of imatinib mesylate in patients with metastatic melanoma. Br J Cancer. 2008;99(5):734–40.

195. Hodi FS, Friedlander P, Corless CL, et al. Major response to imatinib mesylate in KIT-mutated melanoma. J Clin Oncol. 2008;26(12):2046–51.

196. Lutzky J, Bauer J, Bastian BC. Dose-dependent, complete response to imatinib of a metastatic mucosal melanoma with a K642E KIT mutation. Pigment Cell Melanoma Res. 2008;21(4):492–3.

197. Satzger I, Kuttler U, Volker B, Schenck F, Kapp A, Gutzmer R. Anal mucosal melanoma with KIT-activating mutation and response to imatinib therapy–case report and review of the literature. Dermatology. 2010;220(1):77–81.

198. Quintas-Cardama A, Lazar AJ, Woodman SE, Kim K, Ross M, Hwu P. Complete response of stage IV anal mucosal melanoma expressing KIT Val560Asp to the multikinase inhibitor sorafenib. Nat Clin Pract Oncol. 2008;5(12):737–40.

199. Dessinioti C, Antoniou C, Katsambas A, Stratigos AJ. Basal cell carcinoma: what's new under the sun. Photochem Photobiol. 2010;86(3):481–91.

200. Goppner D, Leverkus M. Basal cell carcinoma: from the molecular understanding of the pathogenesis to targeted therapy of progressive disease. J Skin Cancer. 2011;2011:650258.

201. Leibovitch I, Huilgol SC, Selva D, Richards S, Paver R. Basal cell carcinoma treated with Mohs surgery in Australia I. Experience over 10 years. J Am Acad Dermatol. 2005;53(3):445–51.

202. Leibovitch I, Huilgol SC, Selva D, Richards S, Paver R. Basal cell carcinoma treated with Mohs surgery in Australia II. Outcome at 5-year follow-up. J Am Acad Dermatol. 2005;53(3):452–7.

203. Hahn H, Wicking C, Zaphiropoulous PG, et al. Mutations of the human homolog of drosophila patched in the nevoid basal cell carcinoma syndrome. Cell. 1996;85(6):841–51.

204. Johnson RL, Rothman AL, Xie J, et al. Human homolog of patched, a candidate gene for the basal cell nevus syndrome. Science. 1996;272(5268):1668–71.

205. Epstein EH. Basal cell carcinomas: attack of the hedgehog. Nat Rev Cancer. 2008;8(10):743–54.

206. Leibovitch I, Huilgol SC, Selva D, Richards S, Paver R. Basal cell carcinoma treated with Mohs surgery in Australia III. Perineural invasion. J Am Acad Dermatol. 2005;53(3):458–63.

207. Navi D, Huntley A. Imiquimod 5 percent cream and the treatment of cutaneous malignancy. Dermatol Online J. 2004;10(1):4.

208. Stanley MA. Imiquimod and the imidazoquinolones: mechanism of action and therapeutic potential. Clin Exp Dermatol. 2002;27(7):571–7.

209. Amini S, Viera MH, Valins W, Berman B. Nonsurgical innovations in the treatment of nonmelanoma skin cancer. J Clin Aesthet Dermatol. 2010;3(6):20–34.

210. Von Hoff DD, LoRusso PM, Rudin CM, et al. Inhibition of the hedgehog pathway in advanced basal-cell carcinoma. N Engl J Med. 2009; 361(12):1164–72.

211. Caro I, Low JA. The role of the hedgehog signaling pathway in the development of basal cell carcinoma and opportunities for treatment. Clin Cancer Res. 2010;16(13):3335–9.

212. Greinert R. Skin cancer: new markers for better prevention. Pathobiology. 2009;76(2):64–81.

213. Armstrong BK, Kricker A. The epidemiology of UV induced skin cancer. J Photochem Photobiol B. 2001;63(1–3):8–18.

214. de Gruijl FR, van Kranen HJ, Mullenders LH. UV-induced DNA damage, repair, mutations and oncogenic pathways in skin cancer. J Photochem Photobiol B. 2001;63(1–3):19–27.

215. Lai LW, Ducore JM, Rosenstein BS. DNA-protein crosslinking in normal human skin fibroblasts exposed to solar ultraviolet wavelengths. Photochem Photobiol. 1987;46(1):143–6.

216. Matsumura Y, Ananthaswamy HN. Molecular mechanisms of photocarcinogenesis. Front Biosci. 2002;7:d765–83.

217. Karagas MR, Nelson HH, Sehr P, et al. Human papillomavirus infection and incidence of squamous cell and basal cell carcinomas of the skin. J Natl Cancer Inst. 2006;98(6):389–95.

218. Meyer T, Arndt R, Christophers E, Nindl I, Stockfleth E. Importance of human papillomaviruses for the development of skin cancer. Cancer Detect Prev. 2001;25(6):533–47.

219. Kosmidis M, Dziunycz P, Suarez-Farinas M, et al. Immunosuppression affects CD4+ mRNA expression and induces Th2 dominance in the microenvironment of cutaneous squamous cell carcinoma in organ transplant recipients. J Immunother. 2010; 33(5):538–46.

220. Cassarino DS, Derienzo DP, Barr RJ. Cutaneous squamous cell carcinoma: a comprehensive clinicopathologic classification–part two. J Cutan Pathol. 2006;33(4):261–79.

221. Cassarino DS, Derienzo DP, Barr RJ. Cutaneous squamous cell carcinoma: a comprehensive clinicopathologic classification. Part one. J Cutan Pathol. 2006;33(3):191–206.

222. Jensen V, Prasad AR, Smith A, et al. Prognostic criteria for squamous cell cancer of the skin. J Surg Res. 2010;159(1):509–16.

223. Farasat S, Yu SS, Neel VA, et al. A new American Joint Committee on Cancer staging system for cutaneous squamous cell carcinoma: creation and rationale for inclusion of tumor (T) characteristics. J Am Acad Dermatol. 2011;64(6):1051–9.

224. Brown VL, Atkins CL, Ghali L, Cerio R, Harwood CA, Proby CM. Safety and efficacy of 5% imiquimod cream for the treatment of skin dysplasia

225. Peris K, Micantonio T, Fargnoli MC, Lozzi GP, Chimenti S. Imiquimod 5% cream in the treatment of Bowen's disease and invasive squamous cell carcinoma. J Am Acad Dermatol. 2006;55(2):324–7.
226. Patel GK, Goodwin R, Chawla M, et al. Imiquimod 5% cream monotherapy for cutaneous squamous cell carcinoma in situ (Bowen's disease): a randomized, double-blind, placebo-controlled trial. J Am Acad Dermatol. 2006;54(6):1025–32.
227. Nindl I, Gottschling M, Krawtchenko N, et al. Low prevalence of p53, p16(INK4a) and Ha-ras tumour-specific mutations in low-graded actinic keratosis. Br J Dermatol. 2007;156 Suppl 3:34–9.
228. Ortonne JP. From actinic keratosis to squamous cell carcinoma. Br J Dermatol. 2002;146 Suppl 61:20–3.
229. Muller PA, Vousden KH, Norman JC. p53 and its mutants in tumor cell migration and invasion. J Cell Biol. 2011;192(2):209–18.
230. Ziegler A, Jonason AS, Leffell DJ, et al. Sunburn and p53 in the onset of skin cancer. Nature. 1994;372(6508):773–6.
231. Xu Y, Voorhees JJ, Fisher GJ. Epidermal growth factor receptor is a critical mediator of ultraviolet B irradiation-induced signal transduction in immortalized human keratinocyte HaCaT cells. Am J Pathol. 2006;169(3):823–30.
232. Bachelor MA, Cooper SJ, Sikorski ET, Bowden GT. Inhibition of p38 mitogen-activated protein kinase and phosphatidylinositol 3-kinase decreases UVB-induced activator protein-1 and cyclooxygenase-2 in a SKH-1 hairless mouse model. Mol Cancer Res. 2005;3(2):90–9.
233. El-Abaseri TB, Fuhrman J, Trempus C, Shendrik I, Tennant RW, Hansen LA. Chemoprevention of UV light-induced skin tumorigenesis by inhibition of the epidermal growth factor receptor. Cancer Res. 2005;65(9):3958–65.
234. Ke H, Harris R, Coloff JL, et al. The c-Jun NH2-terminal kinase 2 plays a dominant role in human epidermal neoplasia. Cancer Res. 2010;70(8):3080–8.
235. Delehedde M, Cho SH, Sarkiss M, et al. Altered expression of bcl-2 family member proteins in non-melanoma skin cancer. Cancer. 1999;85(7):1514–22.
236. Pena JC, Rudin CM, Thompson CB. A Bcl-xL transgene promotes malignant conversion of chemically initiated skin papillomas. Cancer Res. 1998;58(10):2111–6.
237. Taylor JK, Zhang QQ, Monia BP, Marcusson EG, Dean NM. Inhibition of Bcl-xL expression sensitizes normal human keratinocytes and epithelial cells to apoptotic stimuli. Oncogene. 1999;18(31):4495–504.

Molecular Pathology of Cancer Metastasis: Suggestions for Future Therapy

18

Adriano Angelucci and Edoardo Alesse

Abbreviations

ADAMs	A disintegrin and metalloproteinases
ADAMTS	ADAM with thrombospondin motifs
BMPs	Bone morphogenetic proteins
CTCs	Circulating tumor cells
DTCs	Disseminated tumor cells
ECM	Extracellular matrix
EGF	Epidermal growth factor
EMMPRIN	Extracellular matrix proteinase inducer
FAK	Focal adhesion kinase
FGF	Fibroblast growth factor
HS	Heparan sulfate
ICAM-1	Intercellular adhesion molecule-1
IGF-1	Insulin-like growth factor-1
IgSF	Immunoglobulin gene superfamily
IL	Interleukin
LMWHs	Low-molecular-weight heparins
MCF-1	Macrophage chemotactic factor-1
MEI	Metastatic efficiency index
MMP	Metalloproteinase
MT-MMP	Membrane-type MMP
OPG	Osteoprotegerin
OPN	Osteopontin
PA	Plasminogen activation
PAR	Protease-activated receptor
PDGF	Platelet-derived growth factor

PECAM-1	Platelet endothelial cell adhesion molecule-1
PSGL-1	P-selectin glycoprotein ligand-1
RANKL	Receptor activator of nuclear factor κB ligand
RECK	Reversion-inducing cysteine-rich protein with Kazal motifs
RT-PCR	Reverse-transcriptase polymerase chain reaction techniques
SLeA	Sialyl-Lewis(A)
SLeX	Sialyl-Lewis(X)
TEM	Transendothelial migration
TF	Tissue factor
TFG	Transforming growth factor
TFPI	Tissue factor pathway inhibitor
TIMP	Tissue inhibitors of metalloprotease
TNF	Tumor necrosis factor
tPA	Tissue-type plasminogen activator
UFH	Unfractioned heparin
uPA	Urokinase-type plasminogen activator
VCAM-1	Vascular cell adhesion molecule-1
VEGF	Vascular endothelial growth factor
vWF	von Willebrand factor

A Brief Historical Introduction

Metastasis is a cancer disseminated from the primary lesion to a non-contiguous anatomic localization. The use of the term "metastasis" in medicine, since the middle of seventeenth century, was not confined only to oncology. Metastasis means "the transfer of disease from one organ or part to another not directly connected with it" and

---

A. Angelucci, Ph.D. (✉) • E. Alesse, M.D., Ph.D.
Department of Experimental Medicine,
University of L'Aquila, Via Vetoio, Coppito 2,
L'Aquila 67100, Italy
e-mail: adriano.angelucci@univaq.it

M. Bologna (ed.), *Biotargets of Cancer in Current Clinical Practice*, Current Clinical Pathology,
DOI 10.1007/978-1-61779-615-9_18, © Springer Science+Business Media, LLC 2012

may refer to the transfer of pathogenic microorganism [1]. When we intend the transfer of cells, the term metastasis is widely accepted as referring to the diffusion of malignant tumor cells. The concept of metastatic dissemination is much more recent than that of cancer. The surgeon LeDran (1685–1770) was among the first to describe the ability of cancer to colonize lymph nodes, and he associated this condition with poor prognosis [2]. However, the basic metastatic relationship and the clinic importance of metastasis were well recognized only by physicians of the early nineteenth century. Travers (1829) indicated the possibility of hematogenous and lymphogenous dissemination of cancer that may colonize many different organs at the same time [3]. Joseph Claude Anthelme Recamier, in his 1829 treatise about tumors, used for the first time the term metastasis to indicate the propagation of cancer from the primary site [4].

To observe the first theories about metastasis formation, we have to wait the end of the nineteenth century and the establishment of two important processes: the application of the "cell theory" to metastasis and the systematic autopsy records for cancer death [5]. The concept of "particles of primary growth" disseminating through the body and forming emboli in smaller vessels is present in publications of the second half of ninententh century by various authors, including Stephen Paget [6]. An early mechanical approach to arrest in the vessels was raised, and this hypothesis was initially prevalent. In fact, in 1858, Virchow suggested that metastasis could be explained simply by the arrest of tumor cell emboli in the vasculature [7]. However, autopsy data frequently did not fit with the mechanical hypothesis, and some valid criticisms were raised as early as the end of nineteenth century. It was supposed that remote organs were not all alike passive and that a variable susceptibility of tissues to develop secondary tumors had to exist.

The importance of metastases in clinical progression of cancer emerged early as metastatic pattern at autopsy in patients dying of cancer. Since the middle of eighteenth century, accumulating data have clearly demonstrated that metastases, also in the form of clinically undetectable micrometastases, are present in the large majority of patients who died for cancer, and frequently, they involve more than one organ in the same patient. For example, Walshe reported that in about 60% of the cases at autopsy, the cancer invaded two or more locations [8]. In the twentieth century, increasingly effective animal models for the study of metastatic process have been developed, and the use of immunodeficient mice has permitted the evaluation of the metastatic potential of human cancer cell lines in intact organisms. Such models have contributed significantly to our understanding of the pathological aspects of metastatic process and have permitted to strengthen the hypothesis about the molecular basis of cancer metastasis. In the early 1990s, molecular methods were first used to detect circulating cancer cells using reverse-transcriptase polymerase chain reaction (RT-PCR) techniques [9]. Thanks to novel techniques to detect circulating tumor cells (CTCs) in peripheral blood and disseminated tumor cells (DTCs) in bone marrow, new diagnostic opportunities and improvements in the biological understanding of the metastatic process have been realized. DNA chip technology has represented one of the most recent remarkable advances in cancer research. The possibility to analyze simultaneously the expression of all known genes has offered new hopes in determining the "metastatic signature." The identification of a metastatic gene signature in the primary tumor will help to clarify the molecular bases of the metastatic process and to direct the future therapy.

Incidence of Metastasis

Despite the improvement in therapeutic approach, cancer is becoming the first cause of death in western countries. This is due to an increased lifetime expectancy and to a lower percentage decrease in death rates respect to other high prevalent diseases, as heart disease [10]. In addition, we have to consider that the malignancy as cause of death is probably underestimated. Most deaths for cancer are the consequence of the presence of metastases. The metastasis is a common outcome of cancer progression. In fact, as revealed by autopsy, unexpected metastases are frequently found in multiple organs of cancer patients, suggesting that the presence of metastasis is the rule and not the exception. Autopsy records based on 647 breast cancers were negative for metastases in only 14% of cases [11], and 27.5% was the total percentage of cases without metastases in 1,885 autopsy cases of prostatic cancer [12]. In two distinct autopsy series comprising 1,038 and 2,088 cases of several malignant tumors, including sarcomas, carcinomas, and melanoma, metastases were present in 73% and 68% of all cases, respectively [13, 14].

Autopsy rates have declined drastically in the second half of the twentieth century representing at present less than 20% of all hospital deaths [15]. The reasons for this decline are probably diverse and include modification in the health-care delivery system, an increased trust in advanced diagnostic technology, and a reduced apparent role of necropsy as a source of new knowledge. Although palpation, in the case of liver, spleen, and ascites, and direct observation, for skin, were used in the past to detect metastatic enlargement, the autopsy has represented for a long period the only method to detect metastasis. Autopsy represents, also today, the principal diagnostic tool for the secondary neoplasms. In fact, despite technological advances, the number of inaccurate clinical diagnoses of malignant tumor is about the 40% of cases, and the real underlying cause of death in the majority of these undiagnosed patients was directly related to the malignancy [16]. Inaccuracy in diagnosis regards not only the primary tumor but also metastases. In a 10-year retrospective study of all autopsies performed at the Medical Center of Louisiana, 54% of 100 undiagnosed cancers had tumor metastases, with 15% of them locally invasive and 39% with distant metastases [16]. The records of the Autopsy Service of the Yale-New Haven Hospital from 1953 through 1982 revealed the presence of 29% of undiagnosed lung cancer at necropsy, and, of these cases, the 29% had distant metastases [17]. This indicates that autopsy records can add valuable information about incidence and pattern of metastases also in modern

medicine. In addition, we have to consider that autopsy procedures themselves have inherent limitations, particularly with respect to false-negative report and that the pattern of metastasis is expected to change across different periods also because the patients progressively tend to live longer with their cancers, potentially permitting the development of more advanced patterns.

In many patients, metastases have occurred by the time of diagnosis, although this was not always clinically apparent. In certain cancer types, such as those of lung, ovary, pancreas, and stomach, the presence of distant metastases at diagnosis represents the most common clinical situation [18]. The current diagnostic tools, in fact, allow the identification of tumor with a long precedent history. For example, a 1-cm tumor has undergone at least 30 doublings since tumor initiation to diagnosis [19]. This time frame represents three-quarters of tumor's life history, a sufficient long interval that can explain the high incidence of metastasis at diagnosis [20]. However, also in absence of detectable distant metastases, a significant number of malignancies are at high risk for this complication at the time of diagnosis (Table 18.1). In colorectal cancer, once liver metastases are discovered, the median survival time is from 5 to 12 months. Surgical resection is the most effective primary treatment for carcinoma of the colon and rectum; however, recurrence rates for these diseases are high. These recurrences were dependent on the development of distant metastases in 40–80% of cases [21, 22]. The presence of distant metastases in these patients is associated with liver failure, pneumonia, or malnutrition [23]. When death occurs in the immediate postoperative period in lung cancer patients, autopsy sometimes shows that metastases to distant organs are already present. Some authors reported that 73% of patients who died for lung cancer within 1 month of operation had metastases, while up to 86% of patients who died later had metastases [24]. A large study evaluating the time appearance of metastases after surgical removal of the primary tumor demonstrated that in 20–45% of all cases of prostate, breast, and colon carcinoma, metastases became clinically detectable 2

Table 18.1 Frequency of metastases for selected cancers at three different times of investigation: at diagnosis of primary tumor, 2 or more years after surgical resection of primary cancer and in absence of metastases, and at autopsy

	Frequency of metastasis (%)		
Primary site	At diagnosis of primary tumor	Two or more years postresection of primary tumor	At autopsy in patients who died of cancer
Breast	6	34	93
Colorectal	19	20	84
Prostate	5	45	61

Based on data from [14] and Table 18.2

or more years after the removal of the primary tumor [13].

Recent improvement in immunocytochemical and molecular assays is clarifying the reasons for the high incidence of recurrence. Very sensitive assays have been developed that now allow the specific detection of "occult" metastatic tumor cells at the single-cell stage in the lymph nodes, peripheral blood, and bone marrow before the diagnosis of metastasis. Results obtained by this kind of analysis were frequently surprising. In patients with stage I, II, or III breast cancer, DTCs were found in 31% of the subjects [25]. In addition, CTCs were revealed up to 60% of primary breast and prostate cancer patients with no clinical signs of overt metastases [26, 27]. These data indicate that the metastatic process probably starts long before we are able to diagnose both the metastasis itself and even the primary tumor. Coherently, the presence of DTCs is accompanied by a substantially worse prognosis, with a significantly decreased overall survival, when compared to patients without DTCs [28].

The progresses in treatment and patient management are progressively warranting an overall improvement in survival. Therefore, the incidence of metastasis is expected to increase because the patients tend to live longer with their cancer permitting the achievement of more advanced steps in cancer progression. Moreover, conventional therapies are able to prolong the survival of patients with cancer but are not sufficiently effective in inhibiting metastatic growth. In fact, most cancer types are associated with disseminated disease that after treatment might persist as minimal residual disease. Studies of patterns of failure in inoperable primary pulmonary carcinoma treated with thoracic irradiation

and chemotherapy have shown at autopsy that 70% of patients with small cell carcinoma had carcinomatosis and that 55% of patients with adenocarcinoma and large cell carcinoma had distant metastases [29].

Metastatic Pattern

The prediction of metastatic pattern may have important therapeutic implications. The major problem in analyzing human metastatic pattern is the limitation in the current diagnostic techniques. In fact, imaging analysis does not permit the unequivocal detection of metastases less than 0.5 cm in diameter. Thus, the main theories about pathogenesis of metastasis have been formulated on the basis of autopsy data. From 1950 to 1982, there were seven autopsy series of breast cancer reporting the analysis of 2,147 patients. These studies reported similar findings, and the seven leading sites of metastatic involvement resulted lymph node, lung, bone, liver, pleura, adrenal gland, and brain (Table 18.2). Many other organs were involved but each one in a small number of patients [42]. Younger patients seem to develop a more generalized disease with a higher median number and a wider distribution of metastases. Younger breast cancer women (below 50 years of age) had a significantly higher incidence of metastasis than older women, both in the bone (81% vs 65%) and liver (80% vs 56%) [11]. The ability of different types of tumor to colonize one of the leading sites of metastasis is not the same. For example, prostate cancer has a higher tropism for bone with respect to colorectal cancer, and lung cancer colonizes kidney more frequently than colorectal cancer (Table 18.2).

Table 18.2 Frequency of metastases at autopsy in patients died for cancer in each of the four most common sites of primary cancers

Primary site	No metastasis (%)	Frequency of metastasis at autopsy (%)										
		Lymph node	Lungs	Liver	Bone	Pleura	Adrenals	Peritoneum	Kidney	Brain	Thyroid	Refs.
Lung	12–37	83–93	40–47	33–55	15–41	28	20–36	9	15–23	17–50	3–4	[13, 30–33]
Breast	0–14	39–67[a]	60–77	54–66	54–73	36–65	27–54	24–28	13–18	16–29	5–24	[11, 13, 33–35]
Colorectal	10–14	31–59	15–45	40–65	1–13	14	3–17	19–33	8	1–8	2	[13, 33, 36–39]
Prostate	28–51	63–87	46–50	15–66	67–91	13–21	13–23	10	11	2–13	[c]	[12, 13, 32, 40, 41]
Mean[b]	27	64	52	52	46	33	28	22	21	21	10	

When frequency was two or more, the minimum and the maximum values are indicated. Metastatic sites considered are the most frequently cited in literature

[a]Thorax and abdomen lymph nodes

[b]Mean is calculated considering all the values in the reported references

[c]This value was not indicated in the reported references

The autopsy frequently revealed the involvement of multiple organs in metastatic patients. Viadana found that the median number of metastases at autopsy in breast cancer patients was seven [11]. On the contrary, the chance of having isolated metastasis is low. In breast cancer patients, the incidence of having isolated metastasis in lung is 4–6%, bone 5%, and liver 2–12%, while the chance of involving lung, bone, and liver simultaneously is 42% [11, 43]. In 1,885 autopsy cases of prostatic cancer, from 1958 through 1979, the number of cases with metastasis to one organ was 87 (4.6%), those with metastases to two organs 139 (7.4%), and those with metastases to three or more organs 1,141 (60.5%) [12]. The lungs, liver, and bones were considered to be potential sources of further metastatic dissemination; in fact, metastases in various sites are very rare, with the exception of the central nervous system, when the three major sites are not seeded [11]. Androgen-independent prostate adenocarcinoma generates a widely disseminated pattern in most cases, and although bone was almost always affected, cases with only bone involvement are very rare [40]. However, autopsy findings cannot indicate any time sequence related to the appearance of metastases in different organs. Analyses of metastatic patterns with respect to metastatic cascade, instead, can be based upon the correlation in the involvement of different sites. In breast cancer, it appears that the lungs tend to release metastases to the central nervous system, pancreas, pituitary, and thyroid, while liver metastasis tends to be associated to pancreas and thyroid metastases [11]. The cascade pattern can be frequently interpreted either in terms of an anatomical proximity (e.g., liver and pancreas) or in terms of hematogenous dissemination (e.g., lungs and brain). A statistical association analysis revealed that in gastrointestinal carcinomas, metastases first occurred in the liver, then cancer cells disseminated from liver to lungs which in turn acted as generalizing sites for arterial metastases [44]. The sequential involvement of liver, lungs, and other organs in the formation of metastatic patterns has been confirmed in later analyses of large series of autopsy from primary carcinoma of the colon [45, 46].

The presence of cascades in the formation of metastases fits to a metachronous model in which a specific sequential seeding of target organs for each primary cancer exists. This is expected when circulating cancer cells are trapped in the first encountered capillary bed where they are, in the most part, killed. Animal studies have demonstrated that only a very small fraction of viable cancer cells originally delivered to the liver, via the portal vein, will pass through it to directly and synchronously seed the lungs [47]. As a result, the metachronous model, in agreement with the hematogenous theory, postulates that the anatomical localization of the capillary beds encountered along the spreading of metastatic cells from the primary sites determines not only the metastatic selectivity but also the pattern. The cascade process hypothesis has important therapeutic implications, suggesting that the antitumoral therapy directed to a key metastatic organ could avoid the formation of secondary metastases.

Clinical Outcome of Metastasis

There are more than 2.2 million deaths from cancer in North America and Europe each year, and it was estimated that distant metastases contribute in 90% of these deaths [48–50]. A strong positive correlation between metastasis diagnosis and reduction in survival exists. The 5-year relative survival rates among patients diagnosed with cancer decrease dramatically in presence of distant metastases. Considering only the four most frequent cancer types (lung, prostate, breast, and colon), the mean percent reduction in 5-year relative survival rates of metastatic patients with respect to locally diagnosed cancer patients is 82% (from 66%, prostate, to 96%, lung) [10, 48].

Although the causes of death associated to cancer are rarely delineated, terminally ill cancer patients report frequently symptoms that may justify the lethal outcome. Autopsy analysis revealed that death in cancer patients resulted, in decreasing order of frequency, from infection, organ failure, infarction, carcinomatosis, and

18 Molecular Pathology of Cancer Metastasis: Suggestions for Future Therapy

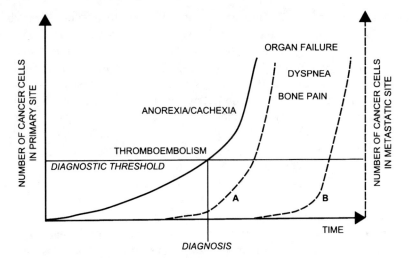

Fig. 18.1 Schematic representation of cancer progression with more frequent associated clinical outcome. There is a strong correlation between proliferation of cancer cells in primary site (*continuous line*) and metastatic sites (*broken line*) and increasing fatal clinical conditions. In the scheme, a diagnostic threshold fitting the usual clinic expectation and two possible metastatic situations are indicated. In the situation A, the metastasis is associated with cancer diagnosis, while in the situation B, the metastasis appears after the diagnosis. Condition B represents the more favorable situation in which it can be applied a preventive antimetastatic therapy avoiding possibly the lethal phenotype

hemorrhage [51]. The presence of metastasis is frequently the direct cause of these clinical outcomes, or it contributes to the aggravation of the symptoms.

The high clinical impact of metastases may be explained considering that incurable cancers are associated to important physiological alterations that contribute to produce those cancer syndromes that kill patients. Carcinomatosis, which is defined as widespread cancer dissemination, represents a peculiar cause of death in those patients having a severe metabolic or nutritional abnormality which precipitated death. Organ invasion by neoplastic cells determines death-associated organ failure in 25% of cancer patients and causes respiratory failure, cardiac insufficiency, hepatic coma, and central nervous system and renal failure [51]. Hepatic failure alone was the major cause of death in 10% and was a contributory factor in 5% of cancers [52]. Organ failure is associated to tumor size, and it has been suggested that survival time is determined by the speed needed to reach a total tumor mass of about 1 kg [32]. A direct role of metastatic growth can be associated to other common symptoms of patients with cancer, including dyspnea and bone complications (Fig. 18.1).

Dyspnea, or difficult breathing, occurs in 20–80% of patients with cancer, and it is experienced, in an increasingly severe form, in the time period just prior to death. The cause of dyspnea is variable in a single patient, but it is usually multifactorial, originating from both the direct action of cancer (primary or metastatic pulmonary parenchymal involvement, pulmonary lymphatic spread, malignant pleural effusion) and indirect factors (cachexia, emboli, infection) [53]. The presence of metastasis affects ventilation efficiency by both direct destruction of pulmonary tissue (lung metastasis) and indirect influence on physiological mechanism of respiration. Examples of the latter situation are rib metastases, causing pain during the full inspiration, and mediastinal metastases, compromising the activity of receptors in the bronchi and controlling the physiology of ventilation [53].

Skeletal involvement is associated with pain, fractures, and spinal cord compression. Although bone metastasis is not considered a relevant cause of death in cancer patients, a significant proportion of these patients require higher and higher doses of analgesics, risking concurrent aspiration pneumonia and coma-associated death [32].

Hemorrhage and thromboembolism are common complications of cancer causing morbidity and death in 43% of cancer patients. Clinical manifestations vary from venous thromboembolism to disseminated intravascular coagulation and arterial embolism. Metastatic cancer is most commonly associated to disseminated intravascular coagulation. Hypercoagulable state is a well-known clinical characteristic of cancer patients, and it has a role not only in thrombogenesis but also in the effective dissemination of cancer cells. The hypercoagulable state is realized in patients with cancer by several factors. Prothrombotic mechanisms are related both to the host response to cancer (inflammation, necrosis) and to direct cancer cell activity. Circulating malignant cells can activate blood coagulation in several ways: by damaging endothelial cells; by inducing hemodynamic perturbations; by releasing procoagulant, fibrinolytic, and proaggregating factors; by producing pro-inflammatory cytokines; and by interacting directly with host vascular and blood cells [54]. Cancer cell in blood can interact with activated platelets and leukocytes, and this characteristic, in conjunction with cancer-associated hypercoagulability, may account for the highly increased risk of venous thromboembolism in the first few months after diagnosis and in the presence of distant metastases [55].

Loss of appetite with weight loss is common among cancer patients. However, the profound weight loss suffered by patients with cachexia cannot be entirely attributed to poor caloric intake. Insufficient oral intake is superimposed upon complex metabolic aberrations that lead to an increase in basal energy expenditure and culminate in a loss of lean body mass from skeletal muscle wasting (sarcopenia) [56]. An impressive weight loss is associated with death in about 20% of cancer deaths. In cancer, cachexia is a multiorgan syndrome characterized by weight loss (at least 5%), muscle and adipose tissue

wasting and inflammation. The abnormalities associated with cachexia include alterations in carbohydrate, lipid, and protein metabolism [57]. Cachexia occurs in 30–90% of cancer patients with the highest frequency in patients with pancreatic and gastric cancer [58]. Although these metabolic abnormalities are not correlated to cancer staging, they are significant clinical complications in widespread malignancy in absence of other signs.

Pro-inflammatory cytokines, produced also by tumor cells, are responsible for most severe metabolic abnormalities associated to metastatic disease, including cachexia and coagulopathy. The maintaining of a chronic state of inflammation is frequently associated to cancer progression [59]. Cancer cachexia has been associated with elevated expression of key pro-inflammatory cytokines, including tumor necrosis factor (TNF), Interleukin-1 (IL-1), and IL-6. Similarly, IL-1 has a role in thrombosis [32]. Small molecule inhibitors and antibodies directed against these cytokines are currently in clinical development for inflammatory diseases. An indirect evidence from the use of monoclonal antibody against TNF-alpha has demonstrated a dose-dependent increased risk of malignancies in patients with rheumatoid arthritis [60]. However, the analysis of metastatic signatures has suggested that not a single cytokine or a small subset of cytokines was upregulated in all advanced signatures [32]. Because of the overlapping functions exerted by pro-inflammatory cytokines, it is probable that a single-agent therapy is inappropriate for the treatment of the metastatic disease.

Routes of Cancer Cell Dissemination

Cancer cells can leave the primary site of growth by anatomical contiguity or by utilizing the physiological drainage for that organ, the lymphatic and the blood vasculature. The traditional belief indicates that carcinomas tend to metastasize by lymphatics and sarcomas by bloodstream. However, today, there is a substantial agreement in considering this hypothesis a generalization without an absolute impact on clinical approach.

Cancer cell diffusion through body cavities may play an important role in metastatic process in some cancers. Gastrointestinal and gynecological cancers can invade peritoneal cavity. The formation of ascites may render clinically indistinguishable primary and metastatic tumors in the ovaries because of the diffusion through the peritoneal cavity. This process may generate peritoneal metastasis or guide distinct patterns of disease spread. Peritoneal metastases are determined by molecular properties of the peritoneal surfaces and by the hydrodynamics of peritoneal fluid. The Pouch of Douglas, right paracolic gutter, and ileocaecal valve are more common sites of metastasis because in these localizations, the peritoneal fluid flow is arrested. Following the peritoneal fluid flow, cancer cells sloughed from the ovarian surface initially reach the rectouterine and lateral paravesical recesses by way of gravity, and then flow cranially, mainly via the right paracolic gutter into the right subdiaphragmatic space [61].

In the history of the medicine, the practice to remove axillary lymph nodes in patients with breast cancer is an earlier concept with respect to that of lymphogenous metastasis. Only by the nineteenth century it became clear that cancer disseminates via the lymphatics and that it is able to grow macroscopically in lymph nodes [5]. Since the end of nineteenth century, unambiguous data have been accumulated, demonstrating that the pattern of lymphogenous metastasis could be largely accounted by lymphatic anatomy. It is well known that many cancers spread via the lymphatics to regional lymph nodes, and this peculiar characteristic is at present frequently used in clinical practice for diagnosis. Pelvic lymph nodes are involved in metastatic spread from gynecologic and colorectum cancers. Lymph node metastases are frequent in patients with advanced prostate cancer. Inguinal, pelvic, and retroperitoneal lymph nodes are affected in 53% of total cases of prostate cancer [12]. Tumor cells in abdominal and pelvic regions can spread along multiple lymphatic directions. Rectal cancers can colonize posterior pelvic, presacral, lateral pelvic, and hypogastric lymph nodes, and this contributes to the high local recurrence rate of these cancers [23]. A good example of the importance of circulatory anatomy in lymphogenous dissemination is seen in patients with carcinoma of the stomach with involvement of the left subclavicular lymph nodes [62]. Also prostate cancer cells, following the lymphatic roads, can metastasize frequently in distant localizations, including para-aortic (22% of total metastatic lymph nodes) and in neck and clavicle (18%) lymph nodes [12]. The rare unusual pattern in lymph node metastasis may be explained by the concept of "retrograde lymphatic embolism." In presence of obstruction of some lymphatics, it is possible that the direction of lymphatic flow in collateral vessels is reversed, permitting the dissemination toward unusual lymph nodes [63].

The prognostic value of lymph nodes metastasis has been studied in detail in different cancers. Although the staging of tumors takes on as fundamental element the involvement of nodes, the prognostic significance is generally high but variable according to the tumor type. Lymph node metastasis has been shown to be the single most important adverse prognostic factor in head and neck cancer. In prostate cancer, for instance, 75% of patients bearing lymph node metastases at the time of diagnosis will possess bone metastases within 5 years, regardless of treatment [64]. However, recent results in lung adenocarcinoma have demonstrated that the detection of tumor cells in bone marrow has a higher predictive value than metastatic involvement of regional lymph nodes, supporting the view that hematogenous spread of lung cancer cells is not directly correlated to the spread through lymphatics [65]. Hematogenous metastases in the absence of lymphatic spread, as detected in patients harboring bone marrow micrometastases in the absence of other detectable signs of spread, have been reported to occur in 20–40% of carcinomas [66]. For these reasons, it is debated whether lymphadenectomy and local radiation therapy may be a useful strategy in controlling local recurrence and metastatic spreading. For example, present concerns in breast cancer include the identification of a group of about 25% of women with small breast cancer, without demonstrable axillary node involvement, who develop metastases after mastectomy [67]. A recent randomized trial comprising 1,408 women with endometrial cancer found no evidence of a clinical benefit for systematic lymphadenectomy [68]. An initial point of view suggested that cancer spreads in a stepwise manner from primary tumor to the regional lymphatics and systematically to distant organs [69]. An opposite more recent theory suggests that hematogenous dissemination is independent from the lymph node involvement [70]. The current hypothesis, validated by recent clinical trials, affirms that lymph node involvement is both of prognostic importance, because it indicates a more malignant tumor, and of biological importance because persistent disease in lymph nodes can be the source of subsequent metastases [71].

Distant metastases are for the most part seeded via arteries having as starting point the left ventricle. Entry of cancer cells into blood vessels is usually confined to veins and microvasculature. On the contrary, arterial invasion occurs rarely. According to anatomy of blood circulation, there are three important sites that may be seeded via veins: lung by pulmonary circulation, liver by the portal vein, and spines by the paravertebral venous plexus of Batson. However, mainly in advanced disease, it is at present impossible to discriminate between arterial and venous metastases in these organs. The clinical course of patients with cancer of the colon and rectum offers a good example of the different possibilities of diffusion of cancer cells from the primary site (Fig. 18.2). Pathological examination reported the venous invasion by colorectum carcinoma in about the 50% of the cases [72]. Once tumor has entered veins, colorectal cancer cells spread to the liver and lungs through the low pressure abdominal venous drainage system. In addition, the vertebral plexus of veins described by Batson represents a pathway by which pelvic tumor spread can take place. By this "third circulation," colorectum cancer cells bypass lungs and can reach directly spine and central nervous system. Cerebrospinal spread may be enhanced by a partial obstruction of the low venous pressure system as the tumor volume increases [73].

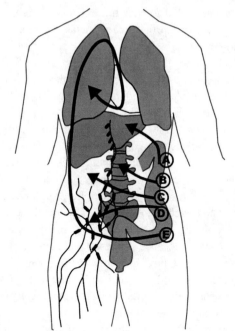

Route	Modality	Primary targets
A	Portal mesenteric spread	Liver
B	Vertebral venous spread	Spine, CNS
C	Peritoneal spread	Peritoneum
D	Lymphatic spread	Regional LN
E	Caval system spread	Lungs

Fig. 18.2 Pathways of spread of colorectal carcinoma

The Pathogenesis of Metastasis

The development of metastasis is dependent on a coevolutive process involving cancer and host cells. Although the events required for metastasis are the same for all tumors, the outcome of the metastatic process is dependent on the intrinsic properties of the tumor cells and the accidental interactions with different microenvironments and anatomical districts. Therefore, the time course and the outcome of cancer cell dissemination can vary considerably between different types of primary tumor and also between different patients with the same tumor. However, results from the whole genome expression and the computational analyses have revealed that only a small number of genes are differentially expressed between tumor and metastasis or between different metastases in the same patients. This is a recent surprising indication that challenges the traditional view of the metastatic as a very specialized phenotype acquired by few cells in the primary tumor. In fact, the process of cancer metastasis consists of sequential steps, and it is supposed that each step represents a selective challenge for cancer cells [74] (Fig. 18.3). Because of the complexity of this progression, the metastatic process is retained to be inefficient, and each step is rate limiting. A clear evidence of this inefficiency derives from in vivo models. In fact, even using highly metastatic cells, obtained in vitro by clonal selection, only a small percentage of cells present in the initial inoculum is able to form metastases [75].

The initial necessary, but not sufficient, events in the formation of a metastasis occur in the primary site: the formation of a neocapillary network supporting an appropriate number of tumor cell divisions, and the acquisition by cancer cells of an invasive phenotype. Both these events permit to cancer cells to reach a way of escape from primary site. Venules and lymphatics offer very little resistance to penetration by tumor cells entry into the circulation. Moreover, tumor-induced angiogenesis also offers to malignant cells an easy port of entry into the circulation. In fact, endothelium of tumor-associated vessels is often defective, mainly in those zones with reduced oxygenation and necrosis.

Loss of cell–cell adhesion within the primary tumor mass aids initial dissemination. Compared with normal epithelial cells, carcinoma cells show a diminished expression of the adhesion molecules cadherins involved in maintaining tight intercellular interactions. Cadherins are a superfamily of calcium-binding membrane glycoproteins capable of forming intercellular homotypic adhesive complexes that are essential for the maintenance of tissue integrity. Downmodulation of E-cadherin has been shown to be a very frequent event in carcinoma progression associated with the metastatic phenotype [76]. The loss of tight intercellular interactions is one of the events in the epithelial–mesenchymal transition (EMT) which determines the appearance of an invasive phenotype. Also other members of cadherin family are involved in

the metastatic process and may permit homotypic interaction or confer new interaction ability with normal cells encountered along the metastatic diffusion. N-cadherin has been shown to increase metastasis from mouse mammary tumors [76]. N-cadherin may regulate the interaction between cancer cells and normal cells which express N-cadherin, including endothelial and stromal cells [77, 78]. Aberrant expression of N-cadherin seems to have a dominant effect in cell–cell interaction since even in the presence of E-cadherin, it enhances the motility of tumor cells. OB-cadherin is expressed by metastatic prostate cancer cells and bone osteoblasts, and for this reason, it has been proposed to play a key role in the homing of prostate cancer cells in bone [79]. Preclinical observation confirmed this hypothesis [80]. Recently, the first N-cadherin antagonist (exherin) has been evaluated in clinical trials with cancer patients [81].

Cancer cells in order to reach distant organs must intravasate in lymphatics or venules. In general, the intravasation requires basement membrane breakdown by extracellular proteases. However, there are situations in which degradation of basement membrane is not so important: the presence of vascular clefts, which are lined by cancer cells; when basement membrane is very thin and leaky, e.g., in the lung; in presence of neovasculature that tends to be fenestrated; and an inflammatory state that renders endothelium more permeable.

Metastasis along lymphatics is described as occurring in successive stages: approach to lymphatic endothelium, intravasation, dissemination, intranodal arrest, and growth in the lymph node. Cancer cells can approach lymphatic capillary during the progressive growth of the tumor mass because the invasion of the connective. Moreover, the hydrostatic pressure of edema fluid in the tumor may be important in carrying tumor cells toward the lymphatic capillary [82]. Recently, it has become apparent that also lymphangiogenesis, the formation of new lymphatics, can contribute to the metastatic spreading [83–85]. In addition, tumor lymphangiogenesis has been proposed as a new prognostic parameter for the risk of lymph node metastasis [86].

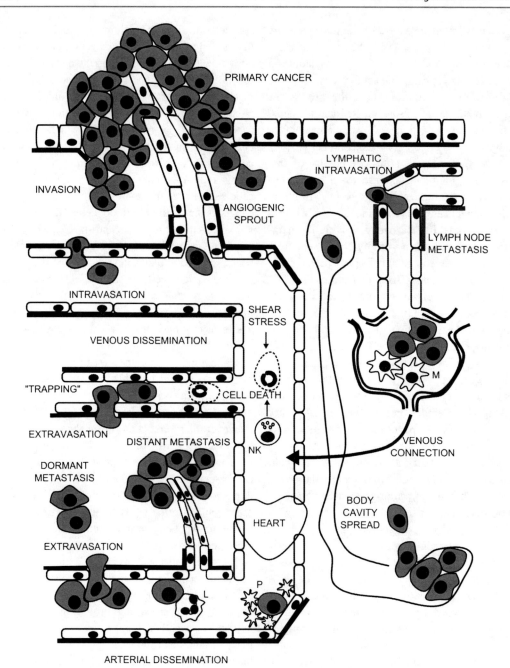

Fig. 18.3 Schematic representation of the metastatic cascade. Cancer cells (*grey cells*) evade from primary site of growth by invading the stroma and intravasating in lymphatics, venules, or body cavities. The blood circulation can be reached also through the new vessels associated with tumor-induced angiogenesis. Lymphatic dissemination generates a secondary growth in lymph nodes where cancer cells can interact with immune cells, including macrophages (M). From lymph node, cancer cells can reach blood circulation by venous connection. Once in bloodstream, cancer cells undergo apoptosis induced by shear stress, physical restriction in capillaries, and NK cells. Cancer cells can survive in blood interacting with platelets (P) and leukocytes (L), and this event favors also the extravasation. The target organ is reached or by venous route, utilizing an anatomic shunt, or by arterial route after the passage through the heart. The passage through capillaries determines the trapping of cancer cells and can force the transendothelial migration. The fate of cancer cells in the metastatic site is dependent on the development of a microenvironment permissive for the survival and that stimulates the growth of dormant cells. The induction of a pro-angiogenic environment is one of the key factors in sustaining metastatic growth

Progressive seeding to several lymph nodes is a common feature, and it may occur at a relatively early stage.

Lymph node is deeply modified by the growth of tumor cells, changing its anatomy until the complete replacement and destruction of the node. However, also a node containing a small metastasis may show marked reactive changes, including the presence of polymorphs, macrophages, and giant cells. Macrophages may be seen in abundance in the sinus, in a condition called sinus histiocytosis [87]. Both T and B cells may take place in this reaction and undergo to the normal process of antigenic response. Occasionally, nodal enlargement is due to reactive change rather than to the growth of tumor cell within it. The size of a nodal metastasis affects its prognostic significance. Small metastases, detected only by serial sectioning of nodes, are of little prognostic importance [88]. In general, the presence of a metastasis in a lymph node is not a cause of serious upset. Clinical relevance may derive by dangerous enlargement of specific lymph nodes, as in the case of bronchial carcinoma with the risk for the block of the superior vena cava. However, nodal metastasis increases the risk for hematogenous spreading by penetration of lymphaticovenous connections in or around the node. In fact, cancer cells disseminated in lymphatics can penetrate the bloodstream in two ways: by venous connection in lymph node or by passage up the lymphatic chain to thoracic duct.

Once in the bloodstream, to survive, cancer cells have to avoid several menaces: apoptosis (or anoikis) due to the loss of survival stimuli (growth factors or anchorage); shear stress; mechanical damages inflicted by passage through narrow vessels; attack by immune cells. Fidler demonstrated in a murine model that, after intravenous injection of melanoma cells, only 0.1% or less of the cells were viable at 24 h and only 0.01% of tumor cells produced experimental lung metastases [89]. However, several findings suggest the existence of effective mechanisms permitting the survival of tumor cells in the bloodstream. Metastatic cancer cells can travel in the bloodstream surrounded by other cancer cells, platelets, or fibrin [90]. Interaction with platelets protects blood-borne neoplastic cells from damaging mechanical factors present in the circulation and, probably, from immunological attack [91]. In addition, they lead to the activation of both tumor cells and platelets and in turn facilitate the extravasation [92]. A clear molecular link between thrombosis and tumor metastasis exists. Clinical statistics showed that half of cancer patients have accompanying platelet activation and thrombosis. Platelet-tumor aggregates further embolize, leading to ischemia and endothelial cell damage. As a result, tumor cells and platelets can bind to the subendothelial basement membrane and matrix. In addition, it has been shown that CTCs can lodge passively in precapillary vessels and capillaries, suggesting that mechanical entrapment is one of the main causes of metastatic cell arrest in distant organs. However, several data indicate that the intercellular adhesive interaction between cancer cells and endothelium is necessary for tumor cell arrest in microcirculation [93]. Thus, adherence of cancer cells to organ microvasculature endothelial cells is a critical step in the metastatic cascade because it determines the site of metastasis and it is a necessary step in tumor cell extravasation.

The mechanism of adhesion of cancer cells to endothelium is similar to that documented for binding of circulating leukocytes upon inflammatory response, and it involves two major steps: rolling and firm adhesion. In the case of cancer cells, this phenomenon has been described as "Docking and Locking" model [94]. Tumor cells express in vitro a preferential capacity to adhere to endothelial cells derived from a specific anatomic localization, and this can explain the pattern of metastasis observed in vivo. For example, prostate cancer cells preferentially adhere to human bone-marrow-derived endothelial cells compared to human endothelial cells isolated from different tissues, such as umbilical cord or derma [95].

Once cancer cell has arrested in microvasculature, it must break through the endothelial barrier and migrate through the underlying microenvironment. The presence of an aggregate of tumor cells may damage the endothelial layer and facilitates the migration. Alternatively, the hypercoagulability state associated to tumor cell spreading may create locally the favorable conditions to increase invasive potential of cancer cells. The inflammatory microenvironment that is generated by tumor embolus formation activates the adjacent endothelium and recruitment of leukocytes. Markers of endothelial cell activation, including adhesive proteins, and inflammation are upregulated during the first hours after microvascular arrest of cancer cells in models of experimental liver and lung metastasis [96, 97]. This situation facilitates cancer cell extravasation and colonization of the new microenvironment. The capacity by adhered cancer cells to penetrate the endothelial barrier is a key element in determining the efficiency and the pattern of metastasis. Although it was demonstrated that cancer cells can utilize the same molecular mechanism adopted by leukocytes, experimental data indicate that transendothelial migration (TEM) of cancer cells is realized with minor efficiency. In fact, whereas leukocytes complete TEM within 2 h of contact with endothelial cells in vitro, cancer cells appear to take significantly longer [98, 99]. The pattern of metastasis may be explained by a different efficiency in TEM for different sites. In vivo study has demonstrated that lung carcinoma cells extravasated into the liver and adrenals faster than in the brain [100]. In contrast to leukocytes that transmigrate the endothelium without damaging endothelial cells, tumor cells can induce endothelial cell retraction, apoptosis, or necrosis [101]. It has been previously reported in a preclinical model that surgical trauma may stimulate tumor malignant cell adhesion within the liver. Most interestingly, it was concluded that this surgical procedure, probably the abdominal trauma, impairs the hepatic blood supply, leading to ECM exposure and subsequent tumor cell adhesion and liver metastases [102].

When arrived in the new organ, malignant cells can die, grow further, or remain in a dormant state for a long time (dormant metastasis). The phenomenon of metastatic dormancy in the secondary site was thought to be due to the time necessary for tumor cells to mutate and select traits that permit them to initiate a new proliferative phase. We may keep in mind that the current data support a clonal origin for metastases, such that different metastases originate from different single cells [103, 104]. In fact, several preclinical models have indicated that a single metastatic lesion has a unicellular origin even when heterogeneous clumps of cancer cells are injected intravenously [105, 106]. For this reason, it is plausible that after the colonization of the new microenvironment, single cancer cells take time before to become clinically manifest metastases. This pause in progression is the explanation for the discrepancy between the estimated and observed disease-free periods and offers important therapeutic opportunities [107]. In fact, by understanding molecular mechanisms underlying survival of dormant cells, it is possible to prolong this phase or to induce cell death. The mechanisms that can explain metastatic dormancy include the lack of fitness for the new microenvironment, the inability to induce angiogenesis, and the host defense through immunosurveillance [108]. It is frequently used the term "niche" to indentify a new metastatic microenvironment permissive for cancer growth.

Once a metastasis is established, it can produce secondary metastases ("metastases of metastasis"). The increment in the frequency for other metastases as soon as one or more organs are seeded by the primary cancer may be explained either in terms of acquisition by cancer cells of a generalized pro-metastatic ability or in terms of hematogenous dissemination. It was supposed that secondary metastases are generated through a cascade process rather than a direct dissemination from primary. Liver and lung may play a principal role in this cascade process [109].

Preclinical studies have recently suggested that primary tumor may act on distant organs favoring the implantation of metastatic cells. In the resulting model, called "premetastatic niche," tumor cells in the primary site by the release of systemic cytokines, including VEGF, can modify the metastatic organ prior the arrival of tumor cells. These modifications stimulate an increase in vascular permeability in the target organ and include the deposition of ECM proteins, as fibronectin, in the subendothelial matrix and the release of chemotactic factors that may recall tumor cells or bone-marrow-derived hematopoietic progenitor cells [110]. Moreover, the increase in metalloproteinases expression observed in the premetastatic niche could promote vascular remodeling, thus favoring tumor cell arrival [111].

Models of Metastatic Progression

The molecular processes underlying the incidence and the pattern of metastases remain largely obscure. In this background, models of the metastatic process become important, as they permit to generate therapeutic hypotheses and contribute to the design of clinical trials. The key unanswered questions concern the mechanisms allowing the dispersion of tumor cells and the starting time of diffusion of tumor cells from the primary site.

The mechanical theory, better known as "hemodynamic theory," assesses that the chance to colonize a remote organ is dependent on anatomical and physical clues. Once in the bloodstream, cancer cells can arrest in capillaries in reason of their size. The formation of multicellular clumps of tumor cells can facilitate the arrest in small capillaries, and, as postulated in mechanical trapping theory, the ability to form homotypic aggregates may represent an important characteristic of metastatic cells [112]. Moreover, the hemodynamic theory implies that an organ is preferentially affected in reason of the amount of blood received. For this reason, those organs representing effective blood filters are more susceptible to metastasis. Several doubtless examples can be offered to demonstrate the value of the hemodynamic mechanism. In colorectal cancer, portal venous spread of disease to the liver is very common, particularly from cancers of the right colon. Other clear examples are represented by some specific vascular connections existing between primary and metastatic sites. Vertebral and brain metastases are frequently associated with primary cancers of pelvic organs, also in absence of pulmonary metastasis. The dissemination of tumor cells in this case may be explained

by the presence of Batson's plexus. Vascular shunt has been indicated as the principal explanation because cancer cells can avoid arrest in a target organ, thereby seeding in the next in-line organ. Portacaval venous shunts could account for the dissemination of gastrointestinal cancers to the lungs, completely bypassing the liver. In a similar manner, a porta-ovarian shunt between the mesenteric and right ovarian venous plexus could permit direct spread of gastrointestinal tract cancers to the ovaries [5].

The hemodynamic theory implies that the extravasated cancer cells have the same ability to growth in all secondary organs. Paget was the first to perceive that organs with the same hemodynamic probability to develop metastasis are not always equally affected. Such findings prompted Paget to develop the theory of "seed and soil," in which he suggested that malignant cells, although "carried in all directions" (like seeds), grow only in those distant organs (soil) with a "congenial" environment. Evidence supporting the seed and soil theory has derived from autopsies until the middle of twentieth century when the first experimental data tested Paget's hypothesis [113, 114].

The pattern of metastasis may be explained by an interplay between mechanical and molecular factors. The same fathers of the two theories, Ewing and Paget, demonstrated to be skeptic about the exclusivity of their own hypothesis. Ewing frequently referred in his works of a "Genius loci" or a predilection of metastases for particular organs in contrast to the mechanism of circulation [115]. However, Ewing did not give explanation about the underlying mechanisms of this phenomenon. In order to solve this conflict, Weiss reconsidered the major patterns of involvement of eight common target organs, in 16 frequent types of primary cancer, as recorded at autopsy [46]. In this analysis, he considered only those target organs in which metastases may be explained by arterial but not venous dissemination, and he utilized as normalizing value the measurements of blood flow in those organs. In particular, Weiss calculated for each target organ a metastatic efficiency index (MEI) as the result of percentage involvement divided by blood flow (ml/min). In accordance with mechanical theory, the MEI should be equal for all organs, because the metastatic incidence is postulated as directly proportional to blood flow. However, Weiss observed that MEIs had a large range of variability, and for this reason, he suggested that high MEIs were associated to "friendly" seed-and-soil interactions while low MEIs indicated "hostile" seed-and-soil interactions. In the new landscape suggested by Weiss, known as the "theory of the synthesis," we find evidence for seed and soil effects for one-third of the target sites, while for the other sites, the probability of metastasis appears linked to the blood flow. The majority of target organs represent a good soil only for some primary tumors. The thyroid is frequently metastasized by breast, uterus, esophagus, ovary, and bladder cancer. Bone represents a good soil mostly for breast and prostate cancer. On the contrary, adrenal glands are frequently colonized by several primary tumors indicating a favorable soil effect, regardless of the seed. Moreover, Weiss analysis indicated that in the 40% of the cases explainable by the seed and soil effects, the target organ represents a "hostile" soil for a variable number of primary tumors. Skin represents a very improbable metastatic localization for primary cancer of cervix uteri, colorectum, esophagus, kidney, and prostate. Thus, at present, it is thought that the exclusivity of the two theories is only apparent and that both of them do contribute, with a peculiar weight, to metastases according to different combinations of primary/secondary growth sites. Nowadays, in the majority of the cases, it is difficult to assess the relative importance of the mechanical and molecular events.

A second unsolved problem in the modeling of metastatic process is about the moment in which metastatic cells originate from the primary site and colonize distant organs. In the linear progression model, the metastatic potential is gained by tumor cells only after an adequate accumulation of genetic and epigenetic alterations. According to this model, the acquisition by tumor cells of the full metastatic potential is dependent on the tumor size and a sufficient number of cell divisions. In agreement with this hypothesis, the chance of metastasis increases with the growth of the primary tumor. For this reason, the surgical

excision of smaller lesions in many cases, as for melanoma, is thought to be curative. The linear progression model constitutes the basis of the routinely used TNM classification system. However, many data suggest that a causal role between primary tumor size and metastatic risk does not exist. On the contrary, the parallel progression model states that metastasis can be initiated long before clinically detectable disease. Recently, highly sensitive methods, including PCR based ones, has permitted to detect the presence of few DTCs also in clinically localized malignancies supporting the parallel progression model. It is probable that the dissemination phase of the metastatic process may be realized, in some cases, earlier than it was previously supposed. Bone marrow DTCs can be detected in a substantial proportion of patients with the earliest stage of disease. However, also the presence of bone marrow DTCs was significantly associated with higher tumor stage, worse differentiation, and lymph node metastasis, indicating that distant metastases is dependent on the progression of the primary tumor. In fact, the rate of detection of bone marrow DTCs was clearly associated with stage of disease. In lung cancer, the rate of detection of bone marrow DTCs is 29% in patients with stage I or II disease and 46% in patients with stage III disease. Moreover, the low incidence, 5% of all cases, of cancer detected by metastasis rather than by primary lesion suggests that the dissemination of tumor cells in absence of the full malignant progression of primary tumor is a very improbable event.

A clear clinical confirmation about the value of these models is currently lacking [116]. However, also in this context, an intermediate interpretation is plausible. Combining the recent data from microarray and genetic analysis with the consolidated suggestions from animal models, it is probable that although the metastatic phenotype takes origin from the natural evolution of cancer cell populations in the primary tumor, significant differences exist between metastatic cells and the majority of the tumor cells in the primary site. These differences may account for a relatively small number of genes that can be targeted for blocking the metastatic process.

In addition, it is also probable that metastases can occur at different moments during the natural history of the cancer in dependence of tumor type, individual genetic background and chance.

Molecular Basis for Therapy of Metastatic Disease

Available therapies for metastatic cancer are similar to those used for primary tumors. However, surgical excision, when possible, localized radiotherapy and systemic chemotherapy offer, at best of the current clinical practice, a little improvement in survival expectation. Supportive care is usually the only treatment available for clinically evident, widely disseminated disease. The presence of multiple metastatic lesions renders ineffective the surgical approach. The 5-year survival after hepatic resection in metastatic patients with colorectum, breast, kidney, and ovary carcinoma is less than 10% [117]. Systemic chemotherapy may offer benefit in lung metastasis from chemosensitive tumors, such as germinal cell tumors and osteosarcoma. Targeted therapy is expected to improve our therapeutic efficacy, but, as the recent experience from clinical trials suggests, an improvement in the knowledge of the molecular basis of metastatic process is needed. Two basic questions remain to be answered: when does metastatic process start? and how much complex is the metastatic phenotype? These two aspects are strictly interconnected. In fact, more complex is the metastatic phenotype, later is the metastatic dissemination.

It is well known that metastasis-free periods in patients can last few months, several years, or even as much as 25 years [118]. The longer is the time window necessary to form clinical detectable metastasis, the greater is the possibility for prevention. DNA-sequence-based studies are yielding new insights into the evolution of cancer and confirm a high variability in the clinical situations. Analysis of tumor-DNA sequence data in pancreatic cancer suggests that the subclones with metastatic potential develop over an additional 5 years from the birth of the founder tumor cell of the non-metastatic clone [119]. Thus, also in an aggressive malignancy, the early detection of the primary tumor offers a broad time window of opportunity for prevention of deaths from metastatic disease. Comparative analysis of the number and type of mutations in tumor cells from the same patient permits to determine the time intervals required for the progression from benign to malignant tumor and from advanced tumor to metastasis. This approach has demonstrated that the average time interval between the birth of a large adenoma founder cell and the birth of an advanced colorectal carcinoma founder is 17 years, while the average interval between the birth of the advanced carcinoma founder cell and the liver metastasis founder cell is only 1.8 years. These data have threatening implications for our attempts to find curative therapies for metastatic disease and in particular suggest a model in which the metastatic phenotype is largely selected in primary clonal expansion [120].

The current knowledge suggests that the tumor cells within a malignant tumor are not all metastatic, and only acquired genetic variability within developing clones of tumors permits the emergence of new tumor cell variants that display increased malignancy [121]. Primary cancers, in fact, contain a mix of distinct subclones, each containing several hundreds of millions of cells that are present within the primary tumor for years before the metastases become clinically evident. Direct evidence that individual cancer cells differ in their metastatic capabilities was offered by several studies involving clonal cell lines derived from advanced cancer [122–124]. Moreover, recent data confirm that both initial biological heterogeneity and the natural selection during the progression of metastasis play a role [104, 125, 126]. Biological heterogeneity in the primary tumors was observed also for markers associated to invasion and metastasis. Immunohistochemical studies have shown that the expression of proteins associated to invasive phenotype varies among different regions of neoplasms [127].

During the metastatic progression, cancer cells may become phenotypically less stable, and this process can facilitate their biological diversification. In experimental models, highly metastatic cells demonstrated a severalfold higher spontaneous mutation rate than poorly metastatic clones [128]. This genetic instability is fundamental in generating tumor clones resistant to host defense and environmental restraints [129]. At the same time, the high biological heterogeneity of metastatic cells has important implication in the selection for clones resistant to drugs commonly used to treat tumors. Although clinical confirmation has been challenging, probably due to methodological obstacles, the hypothesis of clonal selection has been confirmed by several preclinical studies [130]. These studies indicated that metastases originate from a single proliferating cell. Tumor cell proliferation coupled with selective pressure in target metastatic site determines the outcome of new phenotypic diversification of single clonal metastatic lesions. Importantly, this biological heterogeneity is found both within a single metastasis and among different metastases [104].

Microarray technology has offered new insights in interpreting the genetic basis of different aspects of metastatic process. A first approach was oriented to reveal the presence of a "metastatic signature" in primary tumor. This approach is based on the hypothesis of heterogeneity and infers that metastatic propensity is expressed early by a relatively small subpopulation of cells within the tumor. It has also been proposed that a set of genes expressed in primary tumor may permit the selective organ tropism [131, 132]. Surprisingly, results from different expression profiling have revealed that a small number of genes are differentially expressed between tumors and metastases, and they are able to predict the clinical outcome [133–135]. This prediction is highly accurate but not perfect. However, these data imply that the majority of genes that determine a metastatic phenotype yield a selective growth advantage also within the primary tumor and that they are not limited to a small subpopulation of cells. Although the genes in these signatures have been inconsistent, they belong to important biological processes and pathways involved in metastasis, including angiogenesis, invasiveness, and apoptosis. These data are in agreement with genetic analysis of metastatic subclones that revealed several mutated genes present in metastatic lesions but not in primary cancer. These genes include those that may have a role in invasive or metastatic ability through heterotypic cell adhesion, motility, and proteolysis [119].

A second approach utilized in microarray analysis examined the expression profile of primary cancers and paired metastases. These analyses revealed that metastases generally share a high degree of clonality with matched primary tumor, but at the same time, there were statistically significant differences [136, 137]. Moreover, these studies also suggested that the heterogeneity both within and between metastases was the result of a genetic program developed over a long time. The time needed for developing clinical detectable metastases may be also the reason underlying the genetic differences observed in asynchronous metastases with respect to matched primary tumor [126].

Numerous are the potential therapeutic targets that have been investigated to date, and new targets will be certainly discovered in the future. Metastases are formed by cells with well-established cancer phenotype, and for this reason, some of the potential targets are shared by primary tumors, including angiogenic factors, growth factor receptors, signaling molecules, and apoptosis modulators. However, successful invasion and metastasis depend upon additional cellular changes enabling the expression by cancer cell of new biological characteristics. Cancer cells in their metastatic progression do not invent new abilities but express cellular function typical of other differentiated cells. During metastatic dissemination, cancer cells mimic frequently the behavior of activated immune cells. In particular, they use the same molecular strategies of leukocytes in reaching an inflammatory site. Several evidences indicate that an inflammatory response may, in some cases, facilitate carcinogenesis and cancer progression. Paradoxically, the production of pro-inflammatory cytokines by the host immune cells can stimulate cancer cell growth and facilitate invasion and metastasis. The stimulation of a chronic inflammatory state by immune cells may be important also during the carcinogenesis and the first phase of tumor growth.

During metastatic progression, cancer cells acquire themselves the capacity to produce inflammatory cytokines in a self-activating feedback loop. These cytokines can induce the formation of a favorable metastatic microenvironment and cause morbidity and mortality through the induction of cancer-associated clinical syndromes.

In the following chapters, we recapitulate the most updated knowledge about the molecular processes that have been successfully targeted or that appear to be the most plausible present and future targets in metastatic patients. These processes involve especially the capacity of cancer cells to interact with and to modify the changeable microenvironments.

Targeting the Adhesive Interactions

The expression by cancer cells of an adhesive phenotype specific for different microenvironment is important in several steps of the metastatic cascade. Interaction with ECM components sustains proliferation, modulates differentiation, and promotes survival, migration, and invasion. Interactions with normal cells are fundamental in the TEM and in the formation of protective cell complex with platelets and leukocytes in the blood.

Adhesive contacts between cells and ECM components are mediated by integrins, the most widely distributed protein superfamily of adhesion receptors [138]. Integrins are transmembrane heterodimers assembled through the non-covalent association between an α and a β subunit. Twenty-four heterodimers have been identified as the result of the combinations of 18 different α subunits and 8 different β subunits. Each integrin is a receptor for one or several ECM ligands, and different integrins can bind the same ligand. Their ligands include the widely expressed collagen, fibronectin, laminin, and vitronectin. Nearly half of the integrins, including αvβ3, α5β1, αIIbβ3, αvβ6, and α3β1, recognize the tripeptide Arg–Gly–Asp (RGD) in their ligands [139]. Other integrins recognize alternative short peptide sequences; for example, integrin α4β1 recognizes Glu–Ile–Leu–Asp–Val (EILDV) and Arg–Glu–Asp–Val (REDV) [140].

Some integrins can also mediate cell–cell interactions, binding to members of the family of intercellular adhesion molecule (ICAM) and vascular cell adhesion molecule (VCAM), expressed on target cells. Integrin α4β1 binds cell surface receptors, such as VCAM-1, and integrin β2 plays a central role in the firm adhesion of inflammatory cells on endothelium [141]. The binding to ECM ligands is possible only when integrins are expressed in their active form. Integrin activation comprises the conformational modification of the extracellular domains which changes the integrin's affinity for their ligands. By interacting with the ECM, integrins form clusters on cell membrane and transfer signal inside the cells modulating many cellular functions, such as migration, survival, proliferation, differentiation, and gene expression. This mechanism is called "outside-in signaling." The intracellular signaling is due mainly to the formation of focal adhesion complex containing kinases and adaptor proteins. Focal adhesion kinase (FAK), once localized to focal adhesions, is thought to be one of the principal effectors in linking signals initiated by integrins to cytoskeleton, thus controlling migration [142]. Integrins mediate also synthesis of cyclins and inositol lipids and activation of mitogen-activated protein kinase (MAPK) [143]. On the other hand, intracellular signaling activated by other receptors on the cell membrane could induce conformational changes in integrins, thus altering their functional activity, a process called "inside-out signaling" [144]. Therefore, integrins and growth factor receptors can exchange or amplify their signaling pathways via both "outside-in" and "inside-out" signaling.

The role of integrins in tumor progression and their ability to crosstalk with growth factor receptors has made them appealing therapeutic targets. Cancer frequently shows an abnormal pattern of integrin with respect to the initial normal phenotype, and during its progression, cancer cells express a predominant integrin pattern. For example, αvβ1 and αvβ3 are expressed in carcinoma cells and rarely in normal epithelial cells [145, 146]. Changes in integrin expression facilitate the migration and survival in changing tissue microenvironment during the metastatic process. As the tumor cell makes its way toward the endothelial basement membrane, the adhesive phenotype has to undergo a switch from cell–cell adhesion to cell–ECM adhesion. For example, in the progression toward the invasive phenotype, cancer cells alter expression or location of laminin-binding integrins, such as α6β4 [147]. This switch can be realized by both conformational activation of existing integrins and the expression of entirely new integrins [148, 149].

It is thought that the altered expression of integrins in carcinomas is involved in several steps of the metastatic process: (a) detachment and migration in the primary tumor; (b) secretion of ECM proteases; (c) adhesive interactions in blood with leukocytes, platelets, and endothelial cells; (d) adhesive interaction with the target ECM; and (e) angiogenesis and lymphangiogenesis. The blockade of integrins expressed by tumor cells can cause a reduction of proliferation, and, in some experimental models, it can induce also apoptosis. αvβ3 and αvβ5 integrin activation is important in maintaining a high growth rate in colorectal carcinoma [150]. In addition, suppression of αvβ6 in colorectal carcinoma downmodulates the ECM proteolytic capacity by cancer cells, thus inhibiting their invasiveness [151].

Basic and clinical studies have indicated that antagonists of several integrins can be particularly effective in suppressing tumor-associated angiogenesis either alone or in combination with current cancer therapeutics. To date, the integrins αvβ3 and αvβ5 appear to be the ones most closely associated with tumor angiogenesis [152]. As demonstrated firstly for αvβ3, angiogenic growth factors, including basic fibroblast growth factor (bFGF), TNF, and IL-8, are able to induce the expression of several integrins on blood vessels [153]. The upregulation of integrins α1β1, α2β1, α4β1, α5β1, α6β1, α6β4, α9β1, αvβ3, and αvβ5 is a physiological response in endothelial cells associated to wounds and inflammation. However, the same molecules also regulate pathological angiogenesis. Integrins expressed in endothelial cells have a key role in cell survival and migration

during angiogenesis. Recent evidence shows that integrins, different from those involved in angiogenesis, may have a role also in lymphangiogenesis, and thus, antagonists of these integrins might be useful also in preventing lymph node metastasis. Integrins α1β1 and α2β1 are expressed on lymphatic endothelium in healing wounds in response to VEGF and may be involved in the metastatic process [154].

Integrin antagonists currently in preclinical and clinical developments include monoclonal antibodies targeting the extracellular domain of the integrin heterodimer (e.g., etaracizumab), peptide mimetics which are orally bioavailable, non-peptidic molecules mimicking the RGD sequence (e.g., cilengitide), and synthetic peptides containing an RGD sequence (e.g., S247) [155]. Inhibitors of integrin αvβ3, αvβ5, and α5β1 are currently in clinical trials for the treatment of cancer. Of these integrin antagonists, all have proved nontoxic, probably because the targeted integrins are only expressed in angiogenic endothelial cells and in tumor cells. S247 is a potent antagonist of αvβ3 in vitro, and its oral administration reduced dramatically in animal models lung and hepatic metastasis from breast and colon cancer, respectively [156, 157]. Paradoxically low concentrations of RGD-mimetic integrin inhibitors can enhance the tumor growth and angiogenesis [158]. At the same time, several antiangiogenic agents, including ATN-161, have demonstrated a hormetic (i.e., bell-shaped curves) dose–responses. For this reason, in the future, it will be of fundamental importance the identification of biomarkers of angiogenesis that should allow to identify the active dose of integrin antagonists [159]. Etaracizumab (MEDI-522, Vitaxin, Abegrin), a humanized monoclonal antibody, which has specificity for the integrin αvβ3, is currently in phase II trial for treatment of invasive or metastatic solid tumors. Etaracizumab demonstrated an acceptable safety profile and had an effective biological outcome as demonstrated by suppression of FAK activation, in melanoma cells and in blood vessels [160, 161]. Recent results from trials on clinical efficacy of etaracizumab in advanced melanoma demonstrated no apparent effects [160, 162]. $\alpha v \beta 3$ is also the predominant integrin on osteoclasts, the cells responsible for bone resorption in metastatic osteolytic lesions. The use of an $\alpha v \beta 3$ antagonist was able to impair osteoclast attachment, without affecting osteoclast formation [163]. However, it is not yet clear whether targeting αv expressed on osteoclasts would have a significant effect on bone metastases.

In order to achieve better efficacy targeting simultaneously more sensible integrins, antagonists directed against αv integrins have been developed. Intetumumab (human antibody, CNTO95) is under evaluation in phase I/II clinical trials for different advanced solid tumors. Cilengitide (cyclic RGD peptide, EMD121974, NSC707544) was the first integrin inhibitor to reach phase 3 development. Also for these integrin antagonists, the expected results based upon preclinical studies are far to be reached, and, to date, a significant interest is limited to specific tumor types, as cilengitide for glioblastoma [164].

Antagonists of $\alpha 5 \beta 1$ are undergoing clinical testing in several solid tumors. A chimeric mouse-human anti-$\alpha 5 \beta 1$ antibody, volociximab (M200), and ATN-161, a five-amino-acid peptide derived from the synergy region of fibronectin, demonstrated an encouraging efficacy, when combined with chemotherapy, in preclinical model of metastasis. ATN-161 reduced colorectal liver metastases, breast cancer metastases, and improved survival in mice [165, 166].

Several preclinical experiments, using different approaches, have demonstrated that inhibition of tumor cell–platelet interactions reduced metastasis in vivo. Interactions with platelets are complex and involve multiple proteins, including integrins, thrombin, and von Willebrand factor (vWF). Integrin $\alpha v \beta 3$ expressed on tumor cell binds through the bridges of fibronectin, fibrinogen, or vWF, integrin $\alpha II(b)\beta 3(a)$ expressed on platelet. This binding stimulates the activation of platelets and tumor cells resulting in the enhancement of adhesion to endothelial cells and transmigration [167]. Also soluble fibrin significantly increased platelet adherence to tumor cells. This effect was primarily mediated by the integrins $\alpha II(b)\beta 3$ on the platelet and ICAM-1 (CD54) on the tumor cells [168]. The use of the blocking Fab against $\alpha II(b)\beta 3$, abciximab, an antiplatelet drug, significantly reduced platelet adherence to tumor cells and VEGF release by platelets [169]. vWF is a multimeric plasma glycoprotein that interacts with $\alpha II\beta 3$ and $\alpha v \beta 3$ integrins. The vWF plays an important role in tumor metastasis and hemostasis. In particular, the expression of vWF in ECM modifies cancer cell adhesion [170, 171].

Targeting the Prothrombotic Condition

Thromboembolism is a common complication of advanced cancers. The prothrombotic state is determined by two events: aberrant activation of the coagulation system and interaction between cancer cells and blood cells, including platelets and leukocytes (Fig. 18.4). In addition, also homotypic tumor cell aggregation may play a role in metastasis-associated thrombosis. A recent study suggests that the cancer cells may form thrombi as a result of an intravascular proliferation following the adhesion to the endothelium [172]. Although in vitro studies have correlated the ability to form homotypic aggregates with higher metastatic potential, there is no experimental evidence showing the presence of floating aggregates of tumor cells in blood [173]. Therefore, it is more plausible that cell–cell aggregation is initiated by a single cancer cell stably adhered to the vessel wall.

Hypercoagulability is a frequent clinical sign in cancer patients. According to the classic model, fibrin can coat tumor cells and leads to the formation of thrombi in the microvasculature. Many components of the coagulation and fibrinolytic systems contribute directly or indirectly to cancer progression. Overexpression of tissue factor (TF), a cysteine protease that activates factor X, is thought to be one of the key factors for coagulopathy in malignant disorders. TF is a transmembrane receptor that is constitutively expressed in cancer cells, and it contributes to tumor metastasis [174, 175]. Clinical case series have reported

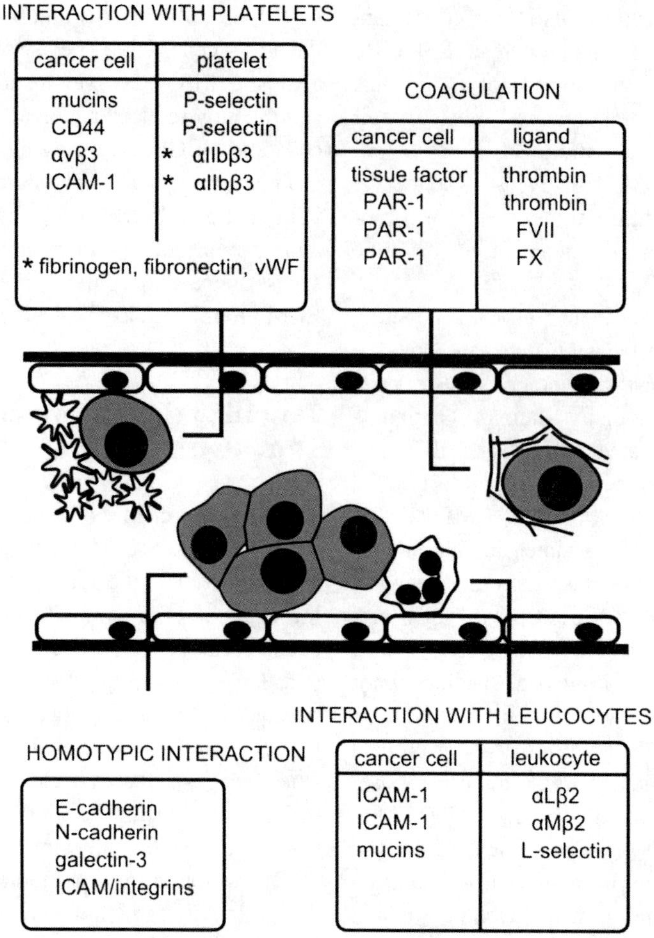

INTERACTION WITH PLATELETS

cancer cell	platelet
mucins	P-selectin
CD44	P-selectin
αvβ3	* αIIbβ3
ICAM-1	* αIIbβ3

* fibrinogen, fibronectin, vWF

COAGULATION

cancer cell	ligand
tissue factor	thrombin
PAR-1	thrombin
PAR-1	FVII
PAR-1	FX

INTERACTION WITH LEUCOCYTES

cancer cell	leukocyte
ICAM-1	αLβ2
ICAM-1	αMβ2
mucins	L-selectin

HOMOTYPIC INTERACTION

E-cadherin
N-cadherin
galectin-3
ICAM/integrins

Fig. 18.4 Molecular targets associated with survival of cancer cells in blood. The main functional events are the interaction of cancer cells with platelets and leukocytes, and the induction of a pro-coagulation state. Homophilic interaction of cancer cells is supposed to play a role but only after adhesion to endothelium

a correlation between TF expression and tumor metastasis in patients with colorectal and lung cancers [176]. TF is absent from endothelial cells surface, but its expression can be stimulated by pro-inflammatory cytokine, e.g., TNF. TF plays a direct role in the generation of thrombin and fibrin. The only known endogenous modulator of blood coagulation initiated by TF is tissue factor pathway inhibitor (TFPI)—a plasma Kunitz-type serine protease inhibitor [177]. Together, upregulation of TF and downregulation of thrombomodulin lead to a prothrombotic condition in the vascular wall. Tumor-derived VEGF also induces the expression of TF by endothelial cells, which implies the involvement of TF in tumor neovascularization [178].

Aberrant platelet activation and aggregation are associated to severe forms of thrombosis, including disseminated intravascular coagulation and pulmonary embolism. Metastatic patients frequently present with signs of thrombosis, and this provides a rationale for the use of antithrombotic agents as preventive strategy against metastatic syndromes. In addition, several clinical observations indicate a relationship between the activation of platelet or coagulation system and the metastatic spreading via the bloodstream. Thrombin plays a key role in stimulating tumor-platelet aggregation. In the circulation, thrombin activates platelets to express P-selectin on their surface allowing the binding to tumor cells expressing the P-selectin ligand. This binding determines the production of thrombin at a more rapid rate on the catalytic surface of platelets, and it leads to a firmer bond between platelets and tumor cells. In turn, thrombin, through the activity of the receptor protease-activated receptor-1 (PAR-1), may activate tumor cells. PARs belong to a family of G-protein-coupled receptors that are proteolytically activated by a variety of proteases. PAR-1 is cleaved, at its N-terminus, by thrombin and thus activated. The activation of PAR-1 contributes to the acquisition of the metastatic phenotype, upregulating gene products involved in adhesion, invasion, and angiogenesis.

Anticoagulant therapy for prevention and treatment of venous thromboembolism has consisted of unfractionated heparin (UFH), low-molecular-weight heparins (LMWHs), and vitamin K antagonists. Recently, compounds that specifically block activated coagulation factor X (e.g., fondaparinux, idraparinux, rivaroxaban, apixaban) and thrombin (e.g., dabigatran, etexilate) have been developed [179]. Heparin is a glycosaminoglycan exclusively expressed and stored in mast cells and consists of N- and O-sulfated alternating galactosamine/glucosamine and glucuronic acid/iduronic acid moieties [180]. A number of studies in mouse models have shown heparin and chemically modified heparin to reduce the number of metastases from different types of cancer [181, 182]. Recently, LMWHs have replaced heparin in most indications. In experimental model of hematogenous dissemination, LMWHs, including tinzaparin, dalteparin, nadroparin, and enoxaparin, have shown potent inhibition of lung and liver metastases from melanoma, colon, and breast cancer [183–186]. Some clinical trials, originally not targeted at assessing the anticancer properties of heparins, have shown an improvement in survival in patients with malignancies [187]. In a more recent trial, the use of dalteparin in a large cohort of patients with advanced malignancy did not significantly improve 1-year survival rates. An improved sur-

vival was reported only in a subgroup of patients with a better prognosis and a metastatic disease secondary to administration of heparin [188]. However, the satisfactory safety and tolerability profile of LMWH could contribute to suggest the use of these drugs as adjuvant therapy for localized diseases with a high risk of metastasis.

Surprisingly, the antimetastatic effects of LMWH appeared to be dependent mainly on their ability to interfere with selectins (P- and L-selectins) and integrins ($\alpha 4\beta 1$) binding rather than on their anticoagulant properties [185, 189]. Inhibition of the interaction between platelets and tumor cells through P-selectin leads to attenuation of metastasis in vitro [190]. For this reason, the ability to inhibit selectin binding ability could be an important parameter in the selection of the more effective LMWH in the future clinical trials. Because LMWHs also retain some anticoagulant activity, non-anticoagulant heparins are preferable for potential clinical use because they could be administered at high doses.

Targeting the Transendothelial Migration

The adhesion of cancer cells to endothelium utilizes the same adhesion molecules normally used in the homing of immune cells: selectins, immunoglobulin gene superfamily (IgSF) members, and integrins (Fig. 18.5). The IgSF receptors involved in adhesion to endothelium are ICAM-1, VCAM-1, and platelet endothelial cell adhesion molecule-1 (PECAM-1). These adhesion molecules have a sequential, but frequently overlapping, function during the adhesion and extravasation of leucocytes and tumor cells. Schematically, selectins are involved in the early phase of rolling, IgSF receptors and integrins permit the cell arrest on the endothelium and in collaboration with PECAM-1 facilitate the diapedesis or TEM. The expression of most of these adhesion molecules is not constitutive but is dependent on inflammatory stimuli. In the same way, it is plausible that the adhesion of tumor cells is dependent upon the aberrant activation of endothelial cells. For example, it has been

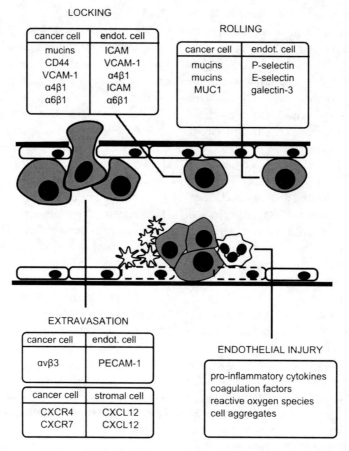

Fig. 18.5 Molecular targets associated with adhesion to endothelium and transendothelial migration of cancer cells. Cancer cells take contact with endothelium in two steps: a reversible interaction with endothelial cells, called docking, and a following firm adhesion to endothelium, called locking phase. The extravasation is realized by a paracellular transmigration or after direct injury of endothelial cells

demonstrated that thrombus formation in the microvasculature may induce in endothelial cells the expression of adhesion molecules that facilitate tumor cell migration into the extravascular space. It was found that there was a marked increase in adhesion of cancer cells to endothelial cells in the presence of cytokines such as IL-1 and TNF that are known to induce the expression of adhesion molecules [191–193]. Cytokines produced by tumor cells can attract leukocytes which can be used by tumor cells to enhance binding and invasion of endothelium. αLβ2 and αMβ2 expressed on neutrophils may adhere to ICAM-1 on both vascular endothelial cells and tumor cells, and the formation of these heterotypic cell aggregates on endothelium aids extravasation [194]. The expression of VCAM-1 and ICAM-1 is also induced by pro-inflammatory cytokines. Colorectal cancer cells trigger TNF production by liver macrophages in sinusoidal vessels surrounding metastatic tumor cells, which induces expression of VCAM-1 and ICAM-1 [195].

Selectins are type-I transmembrane glycoproteins consisting of an extracellular C-type lectin domain, an epidermal growth factor (EGF) domain, two to nine consensus repeats, a transmembrane domain, and a cytoplasmic tail [196]. Expression of P- and E-selectin is tightly regulated during homeostasis, thereby ensuring spatial and temporal adhesion/recruitment of leukocytes. E-selectin is expressed exclusively by endothelial cells, P-selectin is expressed also by platelets, and L-selectin is found only on leukocytes. Selectins recognize clusters of a repetitive carbohydrates motif: sialyl-Lewis(X) (SLeX) and the isomer sialyl-Lewis(A) (SLeA). The presence of E-selectin ligands on cancer cells correlates with enhanced adhesion to activated endothelium [197, 198]. Selectin-mediated interactions not only facilitate in cell adhesion but may also participate in signal transduction, thereby affecting cell migration and activation of other adhesion molecules including integrins [199]. The transgenic overexpression of E-selectin in the mouse liver is able to redirect metastases to this organ [200]. The role of selectins has been well documented for colon cancer cell arrest in hepatic sinusoids [201]. The contribution of L-selectin to metastasis was analyzed in L-selectin-deficient mice. The absence of L-selectin led to attenuation of metastasis. This finding actively implicates leukocytes to the process of metastasis, since L-selectin expression is restricted to leukocytes [202]. Furthermore, an emerging body of experimental evidence suggests that cancer cell homing to target organs may be regulated by other specific adhesive proteins. CD44, a hyaluronan receptor normally involved in the hematopoietic stem cell homing to bone marrow, mediates myeloma, breast, and prostate cancer cell adhesion to bone marrow endothelium. CD44 is one of the several ligands of E-selectin. Other ligands potentially involved in metastasis are P-selectin glycoprotein ligand-1 (PSGL-1), E-selectin ligand 1(ESL-1), CD43 (sialophorin), and $\beta2$-integrins [203].

The adhesion of cancer cells to endothelium is made possible also by altered cell surface expression of glycosylation. The activation of endothelium of metastasis-prone tissues may occur in response to desialylated carbohydrate structure expressed on circulating cancer cells. This activation is manifested by increase in endothelial cell surface galectin-3 expression that induces the rolling of human breast and prostate carcinoma cells in target organ microvasculature [204]. The major ligand of galectin-3 on cancer cells is thought to be the terminal β-galactosides expressed by the transmembrane mucin protein MUC1 [205]. Galectin-3, also called MAC-2 antigen, is the only known member of the chimera-type group constituted of a non-lectin domain connected to a typical carbohydrate-recognition domain. Galectin-3 is involved in many immunoregulatory processes, such as cell–cell adhesion and adhesion of cells to matrix glycoproteins [206]. As a multifunctional protein with multiple cellular localizations, galectin-3 is overexpressed in many types of human cancers, and its suppression in metastatic human colon cancer cells before inoculation of the cells into nude mice results in significant reduction of tumor growth and metastasis [207]. A proposed mechanism for the role of galectin-3 in cancer cell hematogenous dissemination involves cancer cell homotypic aggregation and heterotypic adhesion to endothelium [208]. Moreover, galectin-3 interacts with basement matrix glycans (e.g., laminin and fibronectin) and can promote tumor cell extravasation.

Reduction of endothelial cell activation in experimental models was associated with decreased metastasis [209]. Moreover, the expression of specific pattern of glycosylation on cancer cells has been associated with poor prognosis and high rate of metastasis. Overexpression of SLeX and SLeA has frequently been identified on tumor cell-derived mucins. Mucins are major carriers of altered glycosylation that occur during progression of carcinomas. Mucins are high-molecular-weight molecules containing a protein core substituted with a large number of O-linked glycan structures characterized by the expression of SLeX/A structures [210]. In particular, the expression of sialylated fucosylated glycan SLeX/A permits the interaction with platelets, leukocytes, and endothelium through the binding of all the three selectins. However, the expression of SLeX on cancer cells is not sufficient to explain the adhesive properties in all the models studied [211]. Selectin inhibitors are currently in development phase for a possible application as anti-inflammatory and immunomodulating drugs. Inhibitors tested in preclinical studies include glycan-based molecules, small molecules including glycomimetics, soluble forms of ligands, and antibodies either targeting selectins or their ligands [212]. Disaccharide-based inhibitor in preclinical models led to reduction of metastatic incidence through the decrease in the synthesis of SLeX structures by cancer cells [213, 214].

ICAMs and VCAMs are IgSF members expressed on endothelial cells. ICAM-1 and VCAM-1 are involved in leukocyte arrest and traverse the endothelium through the binding to integrins. VCAM-1 expressed on endothelial cells was found to bind to $\alpha 4$ integrins expressed on renal cell carcinoma and melanoma [192, 215]. The activation of the integrins that permits the binding to VCAM-1 and ICAM-1 is induced by chemokines such as CXCL12. The expression of VCAM-1 on bone marrow endothelium can mediate bone metastasis [215]. Integrin $\beta 2$ is involved in the adhesion of tumor cells to endothelium. Interestingly melanoma cells expressing ICAM formed aggregates with neutrophils which facilitate the extravasation of tumor cells [194]. High metastatic murine breast cancer, selected in vivo by serial intravenous inoculation, demonstrated a significant increment in the expression of ICAM-1 [216]. Several investigations with monoclonal antibodies against ICAM-1 and VCAM-1 demonstrated anti-inflammatory properties with tremendous therapeutic potential in heart and kidney transplant as well as in rheumatoid arthritis [217, 218]. To date, an anti-ICAM-1 antibody is tested in clinical trials as anti-inflammatory therapy to ischemic stroke [219].

PECAM-1 can participate directly in tight binding of leukocytes to vascular endothelium by interacting with $\alpha v\beta 3$ or another PECAM-1 molecule and subsequently by mediating diapedesis [220]. PECAM-1 is expressed on endothelium, platelets, and most leukocytes. The importance of PECAM-1 was demonstrated by specific antibodies neutralizing PECAM-1 that are able to selectively block leukocytes transmigration [221]. Anti-PECAM-1 mAb therapy suppressed both end-stage metastatic progression and tumor-induced cachexia in tumor-bearing mice. Importantly, this antimetastatic effect was independent from tumor type [222].

The activation of integrins, necessary for the arrest of cancer cells on endothelium, is induced by chemokines. Chemokines are members of a superfamily of chemotactic cytokines. They are defined on the basis of a conserved tetra-cysteine motif, and the relative position of the first two cysteine (separated or not by a non-conserved amino acid, X) defines two major subclasses, CXC and CC chemokines. Of the about 50 known chemokines, only three cannot be classified in these subclasses: CX3CL1, XCL1, and XCL2. Chemokines are secreted factors that bind G-coupled receptors with seven transmembrane domains denominated CC chemokine receptors (CCR) or CXC chemokine receptors (CXCR). There is a high redundancy in chemokine family as multiple chemokines bind to the same receptor and some chemokines bind to multiple receptors [223]. Chemokine function is not restricted to stimulation of chemotaxis, but it is known that they also play roles in proliferation, hematopoiesis, angiogenesis, and neovascularization. The response of tumor cells to specific chemokines can be within the microenvironment, or in regional or distal organ sites. Effects of chemokine signals can be both short- and long-distance and are important in the formation of a concentration gradient which can attract cancer cells.

Several CXC chemokines have enhanced expression in metastatic sites, including CXCL1, 2, 3, 5, 6, 8, and 12 [224]. The ability of tumor cell lines to transmigrate in endothelial co-culture system is correlated with the expression of chemokine receptors. It could be envisioned that chemokines might affect the overall expression of surface molecules such as integrins or selectins, which in turn will control the rolling capacity of cancer cells and enable extravasation to specific organs [225]. To date, the most promising candidates for targeted therapy are CXCR4 and CCR7 and the respective ligands CXCL12 and CCL19/21. Recently, another receptor, CX3CR1, has been associated to the ability of pancreatic ductal adenocarcinoma to infiltrate nerves. In this study, CX3CL1, produced by neurons and nerve fibers, created a gradient that attracted pancreatic cancer cells [226].

CXCR4 expression in the primary breast cancer has been correlated with the degree of metastasis in several sites, including lymph node, lung, liver, and bone [131, 227–229]. CXCL12 also known as stromal cell-derived factor-1alpha, SDF-1alpha, is expressed by fibroblasts within tissues involved in the spread of breast cancer cells such as the lymph nodes, lung, liver, and bone marrow [230]. CXCL12 also binds to CXCR7, and interestingly, it has been reported that expression of CXCR7 on breast and lung cancer cells correlates with metastasis [231].

CCR7 expression has been associated with lymph node metastasis in several cancers, including breast and colorectal cancer [232]. The ligands CCL19 and CCL21 are secreted by lymph nodes and are normally involved in the chemoattraction of T lymphocytes and dendritic cells. Recent findings suggest that the gradient of CCL19/CCL21 chemokines is generated not only by lymphatic vessels but also by the tumor cells themselves. This phenomenon suggests the existence of a mechanism of progressive self-recruitment (or "autologous chemotaxis") of cancer cells in the metastatic site [233].

Targeting chemokines and chemokine receptors will likely allow limiting metastasis. The observation that upregulation of chemokines is an event associated to few physiological situations but to advanced cancer, offers a potential way to target specifically metastatic cells. This strategy has been tested in preclinical studies, and for some of the most promising inhibitors, clinical trials are running or in planning. Chemokines may be antagonized by blocking antibody and the structure of chemokines receptors makes them attractive targets for small molecules inhibitors. A third class of antagonists includes peptide inhibitors that bind to chemokine receptors. Blocking the CXCL12/CXCR4 axis by different targeting strategies has demonstrated to be a successful approach for decreasing breast cancer metastasis in preclinical models [234, 235]. Plerixafor (AMD3100, BKT140) is a small molecule inhibitor that binds to CXCR4, thus inhibiting CXCL12 binding and downstream signaling events [236]. A peptide designed to the amino-terminal region of CXCR4, TN14003, significantly reduced pulmonary metastasis [237].

Targeting the ECM Remodeling

Expression of an invasive phenotype is an essential prerequisite of the metastatic process. Metastatic cells have the ability to degrade the ECM through the expression of membrane-associated and secreted proteases (Fig. 18.6). The progression to malignancy is often associated with deregulation of the normal mechanisms regulating proteolysis, resulting in numerous proteases having altered and upregulated activity in cancer. As a result, many different extracellular proteases have been proposed as potential therapeutic targets. These include enzymes belonging to different classes: zinc-based proteases containing metalloproteinases (MMPs), a disintegrin and metalloproteinases (ADAMs), and ADAM with thrombospondin motifs (ADAMTS); serine proteases including plasmin and plasminogen activators; and cysteine and aspartic proteases including cathepsins. There is a functional overlap between different ECM proteases, and a similar redundancy must be taken into account in the design of antiproteolytic therapies. Moreover, cancer-promoting proteases function as part of an extensive multidirectional network of proteolytic interactions [238]. Beside the traditional view of a role in the invasion of ECM, these proteases interact significantly with important signaling pathways in tumor biology, involving chemokines, cytokines, and kinases. In fact, MMPs are also able to cleave non-ECM molecules, including growth factors, cytokines, and chemokines from their membrane-anchored proforms [239].

Metalloproteinases

MMPs can be classified according to their tissue localization in secreted-type and membrane-type MMPs (MT-MMPs), or according to their substrate in collagenases (MMP-1, -8, and -13), gelatinases (MMP-2 and -9), stromelysins (MMP-3, -10, and -11), and a heterogeneous group containing matrilysin (MMP-7), metalloelastase (MMP-12), enamelysin (MMP-20), endometase (MMP-26), and epilysin (MMP-28). The group of MT-MMPs

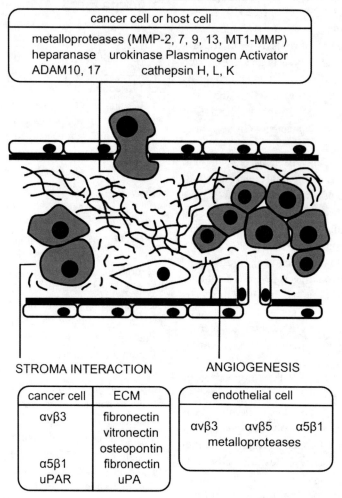

Fig. 18.6 Molecular targets associated with growth of cancer cells in the secondary site. The scheme is a simplified representation of the main functional events supporting the metastatic growth as discussed in the text. After the invasion of the tissue, a permissive environment is created by ECM remodeling. Host cells play a central role in this step by interacting with cancer cells and by releasing extracellular proteases. The cancer-induced expression of metalloproteinases and integrins by endothelial cells permits the angiogenesis and sustains cancer growth

includes four type-I transmembrane enzymes (MMP-14, MMP-15, MMP-16, and MMP-24) and two glycosylphosphatidylinositol (GPI)-anchored proteases (MMP-17 and MMP-25).

Different growth factors and cytokines enhance MMP gene expression, including TNF and IL-1 [240], while transforming growth factor-β (TFG-β) and glucocorticoids suppressed it [241, 242]. EMMPRIN is a transmembrane glycoprotein belonging to the immunoglobulin superfamily [243], expressed in many tumors, including breast cancer, lymphoma, oral squamous cell carcinoma, glioma, melanoma, and lung, bladder, and kidney carcinomas [244, 245]. The action of EMMPRIN in tumor progression was initially linked to the stimulation of several MMPs, including MMP-1, 2, 3, 9, 11, MT1-MMP, and MT2-MMP [243, 246]. EMMPRIN is also able to induce MMP production in tumor cells in an autocrine fashion [246] and to enhance in vivo tumor angiogenesis by upregulating VEGF [247].

MMPs are synthesized as inactive proenzymes in which the prodomain, interacting with the catalytic zinc (II) ion, does not permit the enzymatic activity. Pro-MMPs activation is due to the removal of the prodomain by several proteases including endopeptidase furin, plasmin, and other members of MMP family. For example, with the exception of MMP-17 and MMP-23, MT-MMPs are capable of activating pro-MMP-2. The activity of MMPs is the result of a complex balance between activators and inhibitors activity. Tissue inhibitors of metalloproteinases (TIMPs) are the best known selective inhibitors for MMPs. TIMPs include four members (TIMP-1–4) that are expressed in most tissues, cells, and in body fluids and whose transcription is regulated by cytokines and growth factors [248]. In addition, MMP-2, MMP-9, and MT1-MMP are inhibited by RECK (reversion-inducing cysteine-rich protein with Kazal motifs) which is a GPI-linked glycoprotein [239]. RECK has been reported to inhibit also ADAM10 [249].

Several MMPs have been detected in human specimens from metastatic sites, and their expression in these sites is frequently higher with respect to corresponding primary tumors. MMP-9 is a hallmark of liver metastases from colorectal cancer [250] and of bone metastasis from various carcinomas [251, 252], MMP-2 and MT1-MMP have been detected in bone lesions from metastatic prostatic cancer, and MT1-MMP immunostaining was detected in 80% of brain metastases from lung adenocarcinoma [253]. Thus, it is thought that MMPs play a central role also in the progression of secondary lesions. Interestingly, a microarray study aimed to identify bone-specific breast cancer metastasis genes revealed that the majority of bone-associated genes were involved in ECM remodeling, including MMP-2 and MMP-13 [254]. In particular, upregulation of MMP-13 at the tumor-bone interface leads to osteoclast activation and increases active MMP-9 and receptor activator of nuclear factor κB ligand (RANKL) levels [255, 256]. Other MMPs, including MMP-1, determine the release of EGF-like growth factors, including amphiregulin (AREG), heparin-binding EGF (HB-EGF), and TGF-α, thus suppressing osteoblast production of osteoprotegerin (OPG), a decoy receptor for RANKL which inhibits osteoclast differentiation [257]. A critical event in the development of bone lytic lesions is the stimulation of osteoclastogenesis by aberrant high level of RANKL. MMP-7 is able to cleave RANKL, which is predominantly present as a transmembrane receptor on osteoblast surface, to a soluble form (sRANKL) that is critical for widespread osteoclast activation. The main contribution to MMP expression and formation of metastatic niche may be offered by non-tumoral cells. The expression of MMP-2 by stellate-shaped cells in the perisinusoidal space adjacent to liver tumors suggests that hepatic stellate cells, upon differentiation to myofibroblasts, may contribute to the dissemination of liver metastases through the sinusoidal network [258]. MMP-2 and MMP-9 overexpression by pulmonary cells is able to increment the number of lung metastasis in experimental models [259, 260]. Similarly, osteoblasts, in presence of breast cancer cells, produce more MMP-1, thus stimulating osteolysis [261].

The range of proteases targeted by pharmacological inhibitors in the past and current clinical trials is quite broad. Early attempts to target ECM-degrading enzymes were realized having as target MMPs. However, clinical trials using broad-spectrum MMP inhibitors have failed to show any significant impact on cancer progression [262]. This was probably owing to a lack of understanding of the extensive roles of these proteins in cell biology. Moreover, trials were frequently carried out without information on the activity of MMP acting locally in the cancer tissue of individual patients. The lack of efficacy of broad-spectrum MMP inhibitors has been attributed also to the inhibition of non-desired MMPs. In fact, there are several instances in which expression of MMPs provides protective effects by suppressing tumor growth. The antitumor activities of MMPs are associated to their expression not in tumor cells but in tumor-associated cells, mainly in macrophages. This is the case of MMP-8 and MMP-12 [263]. Moreover, it is possible that clinical trials have been conducted with inappropriate timing and dosing regimens. It is plausible, according to the current experience, that MMP inhibitors result more active in early, rather than in late stage cancer. Advancement in the therapeutic use of MMP inhibitors is probably dependent on the ability to selectively target cancer-associated activities in the correct stage of tumor progression. For this reason, presently, it is preferred a strategy based on the use of high selective MMP inhibitors. Commercial development of the third generation of MMP inhibitors has been recently initiated.

Serine Proteases

The activity of the serine protease plasmin is the result of the proteolytic cascade reactions of the plasminogen activation (PA) system. This complex system controls the activation of the proenzyme plasminogen and involves, as late effectors, the proteolytic enzymes urokinase-type plasminogen activator (uPA) and the tissue-type plasminogen activator (tPA). The plasmin formation or activation may be blocked by three serine protease inhibitors belonging to the family called serpins, PAI-1 and PAI-2, that inhibit plasminogen activators, and alpha2-antiplasmin that forms inactive complex with plasmin. Plasmin has a great impact on tissue remodeling. In fact, it can directly or indirectly cleave several ECM components including laminin, fibronectin, fibrin, vitronectin, and collagen. In addition, plasmin can activate elastase and MMPs [264]. Plasmin has been also involved in the release of ECM-bound growth factors such as VEGF and bFGF either directly or indirectly through the activation of pro-MMPs [265, 266].

The principal PA activator during physiological and pathological tissue remodeling processes is uPA, whereas tPA is involved primarily in thrombolysis [267]. uPA is secreted as a single polypeptide chain proenzyme, pro-uPA, which is activated by plasmin. Pro-uPA and uPA bind with high affinity to a cell surface uPA receptor, uPAR, a glycolipid-anchored three-finger fold protein [268], and this binding both confines and enhances uPA-catalyzed plasminogen activation at the cell surface. uPAR has also been reported to have a variety of biological func-

tions independent of its role in uPA-mediated proteolysis. It also mediates cell signaling, proliferation, migration, and survival. This phenomenon is quite surprising because being a GPI-anchored receptor with no transmembrane domain, uPAR could not be capable of mediating intracellular signaling. It is now apparent that uPAR can exist in dynamic signaling complexes on the cell surface that include integrins, EGFR, platelet-derived growth factor receptor (PDGFR), and possibly other cellular components able to activate an intracellular signaling pathway [269]. uPAR expression is restricted quite tightly to tumor tissue, and it is rarely expressed in adjacent normal tissue. However, uPAR expression may be upregulated during wound healing and inflammatory response. uPAR levels have been strongly correlated with metastatic potential and advanced disease, which has been demonstrated in tumor samples obtained from patients with colon and breast cancer [270]. uPAR expression appears to increase with grade or stage of the tumor and may be enriched in metastatic lesions [271].

Potential uPA/uPAR targeting strategies include selective inhibitors of uPA activity, antagonist peptides, monoclonal antibody, and gene therapy techniques. The anti-uPA inhibitor WX-UK1 has been tested for toxicity in phase I clinical trial in combination with capecitabine in advanced malignancies. The antibody ATN-658 inhibited the growth and invasion in a pancreatic carcinoma murine model [244]. Interestingly, in this model, because the antibody is specific for human uPAR, the antiproliferative activity was due to a direct antagonistic effect on tumor cells. ATN-658 inhibited also the growth of human colon and prostate carcinoma cells when implanted in the murine liver and tibia, respectively [272, 273]. A therapeutic strategy involving the blockade of uPA/uPAR system was successful in different experimental models of metastasis [274, 275]. Despite the preclinical success, the importance of uPA/uPAR in human therapy has yet to be fully demonstrated. To date, few uPA inhibitors entered clinical trials. Moreover, because plasminogen gene deficiency is the cause of severe human disease, the toxicity associated to a complete and specific inhibition of the uPA system is expected to be an important clinical aspect [276]. However, a capped 8 amino acid peptide derived from human single chain uPA has been studied in cancer patients and was well tolerated and safe [277].

ADAM/ADAMTS

The evidence that ADAM and ADAMTS have more critical biological functions in metastatic process than expected suggests to consider also these targets in the future clinical trials. Hence, the development of ADAM inhibitors is an area of fertile preclinical activity [278, 279]. Human ADAMs are 21 transmembrane proteins classified within the reprolysin family. There are many examples of the upregulation of proteolytic ADAMs in tumor tissues, and studies have localized their expression at the invasive front of tumor, both in cancer cells and in stromal cells [280]. ADAMTS include 19 members and possess one or several thrombospondin-like motif. ADAMTS do not have a transmembrane domain, and cleave ECM substrates, including procollagens and fibronectin, or specific Glu-X bonds of aggregan, brevican, and versican. For this reason, ADAMTS4 and ADAMTS5 are also called aggreganase-1 and -2, respectively [281]. ADAMTS13 is a vWF-cleaving protease [282].

The majority of ADAMs have intact metalloproteinase domains with the capacity to degrade fibronectin, collagen IV, and gelatin. A definitive correlation with more aggressive disease or metastatic phenotype has not yet documented. However, an important implication in cancer progression derives from their capacity of cleaving transmembrane protein ectodomains adjacent to the cell membrane. Several cytokines, chemokines, and growth factors are solubilized by ADAM sheddase activities. This could be necessary for the creation of the metastatic niche through both paracrine and autocrine signaling [283]. ADAM17, also called TNF-converting enzyme (TACE), has been most extensively studied, and it is known to release soluble TNF, pro-TGF-α, pro-HB-EGF, pro-amphiregulin, and pro-epiregulin

from their membrane precursors [284]. The release of growth factors by ADAM, as indicated for EGFR family ligands, may abrogate the effectiveness of targeted therapy against these receptors [285]. Therefore, the use of ADAM inhibitors finds a strong rationale as therapy in combination with anti-EGFR family receptor inhibitors. In this respect, particular interest is focused on ADAM10 and ADAM17 that have been implicated in EGFR transactivation activities [283]. Reduced expression of TIMP3, the main physiological inhibitor of ADAM10 and 17, was found to correlate with an aggressive tumor phenotype in a number of human tumors [286].

Cathepsins

Today, cathepsins are classified based on their structure and catalytic type into serine (cathepsins A and G), aspartic (cathepsins D and E), and cysteine cathepsins. The cysteine cathepsins are 11 proteases which have a protein-degrading function in the lysosomes of the majority of cell types. Because of specific molecular mechanisms occurring frequently in malignant cells, cathepsins can be shunted to the cell surface and secreted into the extracellular space, where they degrade components of the ECM [287, 288]. Despite this, during the past decade, important and specific functions of cathepsins have been discovered to occur also in other locations inside cells, such as secretory vesicles, the cytosol, and the nucleus [289]. All cathepsins are synthesized as inactive precursors which can be activated by autolysis at acidic pH, in the case of endopeptidases cathepsins, or by endopeptidases, in the case of exopeptidases cathepsins. Cathepsins are normally controlled by interactions with their endogenous inhibitors, members of the cystatin superfamily of protease inhibitors [290]. Cathepsins B, C, H, L, S, and X/Z have been found to play a role in cancer [291]. Cathepsins function as part of an extensive multidirectional network of proteolytic interactions. However, it is thought that cathepsin B is one of the key proteases which plays a central role in modulating proteolytic signal. In fact, cathepsin B can be activated by several proteases, including cathepsin D, G, uPA, tPA, and elastase, and it can cleave a wide variety of targets depending on its subcellular localization. Cathepsin B can activate MMP-2, MMP-3, uPA, and inactivate TIMPs [241].

Cathepsins H and L are promising targets for anticancer therapy also because they are overexpressed only in cancer cells. Using genetic ablation or specific inhibitors of cathepsin L, it is possible to reduce metastasis in animal models of human melanoma [292]. Similar results were obtained also for murine lung and colon carcinoma [293, 294]. In these studies, broad-spectrum cathepsin inhibitors (E-64, JPM-OEt) have been frequently used, and they seem to have higher therapeutic potential than inhibitors specific for cathepsin L (CLIK-148, Z-FF-FMK). This may due to the compensatory activities by other cathepsins. However, the improvement in our knowledge about the role of cathepsins may render suitable also the use of specific inhibitors. In fact, interestingly, the inhibition of cathepsin L by a selective inhibitor determined a reduction of bone metastases from melanoma but not a reduction of metastases in other localizations [294]. A specific role in bone metastasis has been suggested also for cathepsin K. Cathepsin K is a lysosomal cysteine proteinase that is highly expressed in osteoclasts and has been identified as the crucial enzyme in collagen breakdown during bone resorption. Preclinical studies have demonstrated that cathepsin K inhibitors are effective in reducing skeletal tumor burden [295]. An inhibitor of cathepsin K, odanacatib, suppressed bone resorption similarly to zoledronic acid in women with breast cancer and metastatic bone disease [296]. Several companies have developed inhibitors of cathepsin K (e.g., balicatib, relacatib) with some of these inhibitors reaching clinical trials for osteoporosis [297].

Heparanase

Although animal studies using non-anticoagulant species of heparin indicate that it is possible to separate the antimetastatic and anticoagulant activities of heparin, the two activities have a common molecular basis. Unfractionated heparin and other sulfated polysaccharides have been suggested to exert antimetastatic activity by maintaining the integrity of heparan sulfate (HS) side chains and in particular by inhibiting heparanase [298]. HS is a common constituent in glucidic chains of proteoglycans on ECM and cell surfaces. Anticoagulant activities of cell surfaces have been predominantly attributed to HS. The anticoagulant activities are realized by different mechanisms: catalyzing function for antithrombin, facilitating catabolism of coagulant factors, and association with TFPI. In addition, HSs have important structural function. In fact, they cross-link various components of the subendothelial basement membrane, including laminin and collagens, thereby contributing to the integrity of the blood vessel wall. Heparanase is an endo-beta-D-glucuronidase able to degrade heparin and heparan sulfate side chains to fragments of similar size (5–7 kDa) and is thought to be important in migrating leucocytes to extravasate through the vascular basal lamina. Heparanase activity is correlated with the metastatic potential of cancer cells, and it contributes to enhanced remodeling of ECM. On the contrary, expression of heparanase in normal tissues is restricted primarily to the placenta, keratinocytes, platelets, and activated cells of the immune system, with little or no expression in connective tissue cells and most normal epithelia. Upregulation of heparanase was reported in inflammation and wound healing [299]. The heparanase is preferentially expressed in metastatic cell lines [300], and high expression was also found in colon carcinoma cells metastasized to lung, liver, and lymph nodes [301]. When heparanase expression was induced by transfection in low-metastasizing murine cancer cells, it made them able to massively colonize the lung and liver [302].

Heparanase inhibitors have demonstrated to be effective in reducing incidence of metastasis in preclinical models. The heparan sulfate mimetic inhibitor PI-88 is a mixture of natural highly sulfated oligosaccharides and is a potent inhibitor of heparanase. PI-88 inhibited rat mammary metastasis but also the primary tumor growth [303]. It is likely that PI-88 may have such a broad anticancer activity because it targets angiogenesis. In fact, HS is thought to play an important role in regulating accessibility of growth factors and pro-angiogenic factors. Growth factors more extensively studied in this context are FGF-2 and VEGF. These factors are sequestered by HS chains of proteoglycans and are released upon cleavage by heparanase [304]. In clinical trials of advanced and metastatic carcinomas, PI-88 has demonstrated to ameliorate disease outcome, but it was associated with significant hematologic toxicity, including neutropenia, thrombocytopenia, and hemorrhage. For this reason, further evaluation may be warranted to obtain a more manageable safety profile with such agents [305, 306].

Targeting the Metastatic Growth

Once extravasated, the fate of cancer cell, proliferation or growth arrest/death, is decided by the cell fitness for the new environment. A major role in this step is played by the presence of a permissive microenvironment. Different metastatic sites can be (or become) permissive in a peculiar way. First, metastatic cell proliferation is dependent on the net balance of positive and negative signals present at the arrival of tumor cells in the new microenvironment. These signals derive from paracrine and endocrine pathways. The ability of metastatic cell to interpret these signals determines its fate [108]. The undifferentiated proliferating phenotype of a single cancer cell reaching the metastatic site may be dependent on one or few specific growth factors. Thus, the presence of suitable local growth factors may play a key role in stimulating a new proliferative phase for metastatic cells. Nerve growth factor and neurotrophin-3 produced in central nervous system are able to sustain the proliferation of melanoma cells. Insulin-like growth factor-1 (IGF-1) has a high concentration in the liver, and it is able to control cell cycle progression in those tumor cells expressing IGF-1 receptor [307]. The redundancy in signaling pathways can help cancer cells to proliferate in the early phase of

metastatic growth. An example is offered by EGFR axis activation. Different carcinomas are maintained in an undifferentiated state by chronic and aberrant EGFR activation. Blocking EGFR in lung, breast, prostate, and head and neck carcinoma resulted in tumor suppression in vivo. Thus, it is plausible that a metastatic microenvironment lacking EGFR ligands can favor dormancy. However, by using different experimental models, it was demonstrated that EGFR activation can be achieved also by the formation of complexes with uPAR and integrin β1, two molecular markers frequently associated to tumor progression [308, 309]. This is in agreement with the evidence that DTCs lacking uPAR expression predicted better overall survival [310]. Therefore, it seems reasonable to suggest that strategies aimed at inducing and/or maintaining tumor cell dormancy should include concomitantly blocking EGFR and uPAR, and/or integrin complexes [108].

Remodeling of ECM may play a key role in the growth of metastatic cells (Fig. 18.6). Alteration in ECM homeostasis may lead to a permissive soil that enables tumor cells to escape from dormancy [311]. For example, increased fibronectin expression by mesenchymal cells was reported to be important in the formation of the premetastatic niche [110]. Fibrotic breast cancer displays an unusually dense collagenous stroma and is associated with a higher risk of developing bone and lymph node metastasis [312]. Moreover, clinical studies have shown elevated plasma concentration of small integrin-binding ligand, N-linked glycoprotein (SIBLING) proteins, including bone sialoprotein and osteopontin (OPN), in patients with metastatic disease compared to normal samples [313]. Several studies have demonstrated that OPN promotes metastasis [314]. OPN is produced by tumor cells but also by numerous normal cell types, including osteoblasts, osteoclasts, endothelial cells, and activated immune cells. OPN, upon binding to integrins, can induce cell survival, migration, and release of ECM-degrading enzymes. Blocking antibodies against OPN demonstrated efficacy in the inhibition of lung metastases induced by the injection of human hepatocellular carcinoma

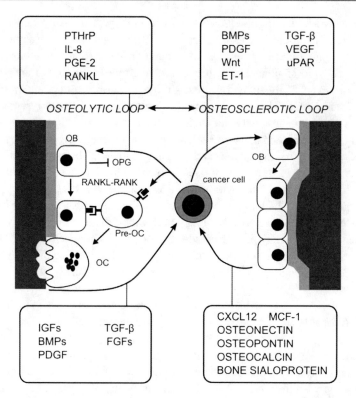

Fig. 18.7 Molecular and cellular network underlying the growth of metastatic cells in bone. Cancer cells can induce a prevalent bone lesion, osteolytic or osteosclerotic, and in both situations, a positive feedback can sustain cancer growth. Osteoblasts (OB) are stimulated to release new matrix in osteosclerotic lesion and to induce osteoclastogenesis in osteolytic lesion. Differentiation of osteoclasts is due mainly to an increased ratio RANKL/OPG. The mineralized matrix is degraded by mature osteoclasts (OC), and this event is associated to the release of growth factors. The activities of osteoclasts and osteoblasts are tightly interconnected, and this determines the development of mixed lesions

cells in nude mice [315]. Alternatively, OPN-induced metastasis can be blocked by inhibitors of integrins αvβ3 and β1.

MMPs play a central role in the creation of the metastatic niche. Generally, MMPs in the metastatic sites are expressed at higher levels with respect to corresponding primary tumors. The production of MMPs by tumor or stromal cells can (1) modify the ECM, (2) release cytokines and growth factors that are sequestered to ECM, and (3) drive angiogenesis. ECM has in all tissues an important role in maintaining organ homeostasis. Several studies have indicated that components of the ECM are able to modulate the phenotype of various cells, including metastatic cancer cells [316]. The modification of the ECM by MMPs may determine the shift from a protective and homeostatic to a growth-promoting microenvironment. MMPs are expressed in metastases according to a specific pattern, and this may represent an important element in designing new clinical trials. The pattern of MMPs may be very dissimilar in different metastatic environments [254]. For example, brain-seeking clones of breast cancer cell line express significantly higher mRNA levels of MMP-1 and -9 in comparison to bone-seeking and parental cells [317].

It is well known that cancer progression is driven also by tumor-associated normal cells. The most impressive interaction is that realized by bone-seeking tumors and bone cells (Fig. 18.7). In bone metastasis, the homeostasis of the mineralized matrix, which is controlled by osteoclasts and osteoblasts, is dramatically perturbed by metastatic cells. In turn, the aberrant activity of bone cells can generate a positive feedback loop, referred to as the "vicious cycle," that represents the driving force for the development of bone metastases [318]. The increased osteoclastogenesis, which is the prevalent cellular event associated to osteolytic bone metastasis, typical of breast and lung cancer, determines the bone resorption and the release of growth factors immobilized in the bone matrix [319]. These growth factors, including IGFs, TGF-β, bone morphogenetic proteins (BMPs), FGFs, and PDGF, act back on the tumor cells and the other cells within the bone to potentiate the vicious cycle [318]. According to the "vicious cycle" model, the osteoclast differentiation from monocytes is induced by the RANKL produced by osteoblasts which in turn are stimulated by cancer-derived factors. Breast cancer cells can produce several osteoclastogenic factors, including parathyroid hormone-related protein (PTHrP), IL-8, and prostaglandin E2 (PGE2) [320–322].

RANKL, together with its receptor, RANK, represents a suitable target in the therapy for bone metastasis. The operative role of osteoclasts in the full spectrum of bone lesions (lytic, blastic, "mixed") supports the use of inhibitor of osteoclasts in all types of bone lesion. Denosumab, a fully human monoclonal antibody against RANKL, has been shown to inhibit osteoclast-mediated bone resorption, and in clinical trial performed in patients with bone metastases, it has demonstrated a better efficacy in suppressing bone resorption with respect to zoledronic acid [257]. Further clinical trials are necessary to clarify whether denosumab can effectively block bone metastasis growth. Other inhibitors targeting osteoclast function are currently in preclinical or clinical development. Antagonists of the αvβ3 integrin suppressed the development of osteolytic breast cancer metastases. In fact, αvβ3 is the most abundant integrin in osteoclasts, and it permits the adhesion of the osteoclasts to bony surfaces mediating bone resorption [323].

Bone metastases may be associated also to a prevalent bone formation, and in this case, they are referred to as "osteoblastic" or "sclerotic." Osteoblastic lesions are a typical feature of bone metastasis from prostate cancer; however, the continuous increase in osteoblast number stimulates the consequent high bone turnover determining an excess also in bone resorption [324]. Osteoblasts are activated by BMPs, TGF-β, PDGF, VEGF, Wnt, uPAR, and endothelin 1. Patients with metastatic prostate cancer have elevated levels of plasma endothelin 1 compared with patients with organ-confined cancer [325]. Endothelin A, the receptor for endothelin 1, can be targeted by highly selective inhibitors, including atrasentan (ABT-627) and zibotentan (ZD4054). Clinical trials conducted up to now demonstrated that endothelin 1 inhibitors were effective in reducing bone remodeling, as indicated by serum bone turnover markers, but had no effect in the clinical progression of the metastatic disease [326, 327]. In future clinical trials, it should be evaluated whether endothelin A inhibitors can be effective in combination therapy with chemotherapeutic drugs. Additional factors isolated from prostate cancer cell lines and serum samples from patients are candidates for playing a role in activation of osteoblasts. Prostate cancer cells secrete BMPs which recruit osteoblast precursors and activate the promoter of VEGF. VEGF itself stimulates osteoblast migration and differentiation, amplifying the signal [328]. uPA stimulates osteoblast mitogenesis either directly or perhaps by activating TGF-β [328, 329]. In osteosclerotic lesions, osteoblasts can secrete factors that support the growth of cancer cells in bone. The newly formed bone may secrete chemoattractants, including CXCL12, and macrophage chemotactic factor-1 (MCF-1), that favor migration and enhance the invasion capability of cancer cells. Moreover, bone matrix proteins osteonectin, OPN, osteocalcin, and bone sialoprotein produced by osteoblasts are able to enhance the metastatic potential of breast and prostate cancer cells [330–332]

Conclusions

Distant metastases are the most advanced stage in cancer progression and are associated with high rate of mortality. Significant improvements in our knowledge about the pathogenesis of metastasis have been achieved in the last years; however, several unanswered questions remain. The present curative therapies have demonstrated to be ineffective, while on the other side, the the possibility for an effective preventive action has not been yet defined. Moreover, there are some aspects of the metastatic cascade that are not easily targetable. Once cancer cells have diffused through the circulation, hydrodynamic features can determine their metastatic fate at least in 50% of cases. In addition, cancer is frequently diagnosed when it has already acquired the full metastatic potential, and this determines the involvement of multiple organs in terminal cancer patients. For this reason, and because the high frequency in detecting CTCs, a therapeutic strategy aimed to control the metastasis in a single site cannot reach curative success. On the other hand, a variety of novel molecular targets have been found, and the blockade of general functional processes associated to metastatic dissemination has been successfully tested in preclinical models. These include the molecular events that permit the survival of cancer cells in blood, the adhesion to endothelium, the ability to modify the ECM, and the interaction with normal cells in the metastatic site.

Today, it is clear that the evolutive process that regulates the metastatic diffusion frequently favors the phenotypic convergence between metastatic and normal circulating cells, such as immune cells. However, we have to remember two important features that characterize cancer cells and that can limit our therapeutic opportunities: the expression of a high redundancy in signaling pathways and a large phenotypic heterogeneity. For these reasons, the future therapeutic decisions should be taken with a major attention about the molecular interactions expressed by the targeted molecule and about the specific evolutive history of cancer in the single patient.

References

1. Dorland WAN. Dorland's illustrated medical dictionary. 25th ed. Philadelphia: Saunders; 1974.
2. LeDran H. Observations in surgery. 3rd ed. London: Crowther; 1758.
3. Travers B. Observations on the local diseases termed malignant. Med Chir Trans. 1829;15:195–262.
4. Récamier J. Recherches sur le traitement du cancer. Paris: Gabon; 1829.

5. Weiss L. Metastasis of cancer: a conceptual history from antiquity to the 1990s. Cancer Metastasis Rev. 2000;19(3–4):I–XI, 193–383.
6. Paget S. The distribution of secondary growths in cancer of the breast. 1889. Cancer Metastasis Rev. 1989;8(2):98–101.
7. Virchow R. Cellular pathology. As based upon physiological and pathological histology. Lecture XVI–Atheromatous affection of arteries. 1858. Nutr Rev. 1989;47(1):23–5.
8. Walshe W. The nature and treatment of cancer. London: Taylor & Walton; 1846.
9. Smith B, Selby P, Southgate J, Pittman K, Bradley C, Blair GE. Detection of melanoma cells in peripheral blood by means of reverse transcriptase and polymerase chain reaction. Lancet. 1991;338(8777): 1227–9.
10. Jemal A, Ward E, Hao Y, Thun M. Trends in the leading causes of death in the United States, 1970–2002. JAMA. 2005;294(10):1255–9.
11. Viadana E, Bross ID, Pickren JW. An autopsy study of some routes of dissemination of cancer of the breast. Br J Cancer. 1973;27(4):336–40.
12. Saitoh H, Hida M, Shimbo T, Nakamura K, Yamagata J, Satoh T. Metastatic patterns of prostatic cancer. Correlation between sites and number of organs involved. Cancer. 1984;54(12):3078–84.
13. Henneford J, Baserga R, Wartman WB. The time of appearance of metastases after surgical removal of the primary tumor. Br J Cancer. 1962;16:599–607.
14. Walther H. Krebsmetastasen. Basel: Schwabe; 1948.
15. Marwick C. Pathologists request autopsy revival. JAMA. 1995;273(24):1889, 1891.
16. Burton EC, Troxclair DA, Newman 3rd WP. Autopsy diagnoses of malignant neoplasms: how often are clinical diagnoses incorrect? JAMA. 1998;280(14): 1245–8.
17. Chan CK, Wells CK, McFarlane MJ, Feinstein AR. More lung cancer but better survival. Implications of secular trends in "necropsy surprise" rates. Chest. 1989;96(2):291–6.
18. Jemal A, Murray T, Ward E, et al. Cancer statistics, 2005. CA Cancer J Clin. 2005;55(1):10–30.
19. Del Monte U. Does the cell number 10(9) still really fit one gram of tumor tissue? Cell Cycle. 2009;8(3):505–6.
20. Fidler IJ, Balch CM. The biology of cancer metastasis and implications for therapy. Curr Probl Surg. 1987;24(3):129–209.
21. Cass AW, Million RR, Pfaff WW. Patterns of recurrence following surgery alone for adenocarcinoma of the colon and rectum. Cancer. 1976;37(6): 2861–5.
22. Morson BC, Vaughan EG, Bussey HJ. Pelvic recurrence after excision of rectum for carcinoma. Br Med J. 1963;2(5348):13–8.
23. Welch JP, Donaldson GA. The clinical correlation of an autopsy study of recurrent colorectal cancer. Ann Surg. 1979;189(4):496–502.

24. Weiss W, Gillick JS. The metastatic spread of bronchogenic carcinoma in relation to the interval between resection and death. Chest. 1977;71(6):725–9.
25. Braun S, Vogl FD, Naume B, et al. A pooled analysis of bone marrow micrometastasis in breast cancer. N Engl J Med. 2005;353(8):793–802.
26. Kraeft SK, Sutherland R, Gravelin L, et al. Detection and analysis of cancer cells in blood and bone marrow using a rare event imaging system. Clin Cancer Res. 2000;6(2):434–42.
27. Weckermann D, Muller P, Wawroschek F, Harzmann R, Riethmuller G, Schlimok G. Disseminated cytokeratin positive tumor cells in the bone marrow of patients with prostate cancer: detection and prognostic value. J Urol. 2001;166(2):699–703.
28. Braun S, Pantel K, Muller P, et al. Cytokeratin-positive cells in the bone marrow and survival of patients with stage I, II, or III breast cancer. N Engl J Med. 2000;342(8):525–33.
29. Cox JD, Yesner RA. Causes of treatment failure and death in carcinoma of the lung. Yale J Biol Med. 1981;54(3):201–7.
30. Galluzzi S, Payne PM. Bronchial carcinoma: a statistical study of 741 necropsies with special reference to the distribution of blood-borne metastases. Br J Cancer. 1955;9(4):511–27.
31. Ochsner A, DeBakey M. Significance of metastasis in primary carcinoma of the lungs: report of 2 cases with unusual site of metastasis. J Thorac Surg. 1942;11:357–87.
32. Loberg RD, Bradley DA, Tomlins SA, Chinnaiyan AM, Pienta KJ. The lethal phenotype of cancer: the molecular basis of death due to malignancy. CA Cancer J Clin. 2007;57(4):225–41.
33. Abrams HL, Spiro R, Goldstein N. Metastases in carcinoma; analysis of 1000 autopsied cases. Cancer. 1950;3(1):74–85.
34. Viadana E, Cotter R, Pickren JW, Bross ID. An autopsy study of metastatic sites of breast cancer. Cancer Res. 1973;33(1):179–81.
35. Cho SY, Choi HY. Causes of death and metastatic patterns in patients with mammary cancer. Ten-year autopsy study. Am J Clin Pathol. 1980;73(2):232–4.
36. Abrams MS, Lerner HJ. Survival of patients at Pennsylvania Hospital with hepatic metastases from carcinoma of the colon and rectum. Dis Colon Rectum. 1971;14(6):431–4.
37. Bacon H, Gilbert P. Sites of metastases from carcinoma of the anus, rectum and sigmoid colon. JAMA. 1938;111:219–21.
38. Buirge R. Carcinoma of the large intestine; review of 416 autopsy records. Arch Surg. 1941;42:801–18.
39. Cedermark BJ, Blumenson LE, Pickren JW, Elias EG. The significance of metastases to the adrenal gland from carcinoma of the stomach and esophagus. Surg Gynecol Obstet. 1977;145(1):41–8.
40. Shah RB, Mehra R, Chinnaiyan AM, et al. Androgen-independent prostate cancer is a heterogeneous group of diseases: lessons from a rapid autopsy program. Cancer Res. 2004;64(24):9209–16.

41. Bubendorf L, Schopfer A, Wagner U, et al. Metastatic patterns of prostate cancer: an autopsy study of 1,589 patients. Hum Pathol. 2000;31(5):578–83.
42. Lee YT. Patterns of metastasis and natural courses of breast carcinoma. Cancer Metastasis Rev. 1985;4(2):153–72.
43. Viadana E, Au KL. Patterns of metastases in adenocarcinomas of man. An autopsy study of 4,728 cases. J Med. 1975;6(1):1–14.
44. Viadana E, Bross ID, Pickren JW. The metastatic spread of cancers of the digestive system in man. Oncology. 1978;35(3):114–26.
45. Weiss L, Grundmann E, Torhorst J, et al. Haematogenous metastatic patterns in colonic carcinoma: an analysis of 1541 necropsies. J Pathol. 1986;150(3):195–203.
46. Weiss L. Comments on hematogenous metastatic patterns in humans as revealed by autopsy. Clin Exp Metastasis. 1992;10(3):191–9.
47. Weiss L, Ward PM, Holmes JC. Liver-to-lung traffic of cancer cells. Int J Cancer. 1983;32(1):79–83.
48. Society AC. Cancer facts & figures 2010. Atlanta: American Cancer Society; 2010.
49. Higginson IJ, Costantini M. Dying with cancer, living well with advanced cancer. Eur J Cancer. 2008;44(10):1414–24.
50. Hanahan D, Weinberg RA. The hallmarks of cancer. Cell. 2000;100(1):57–70.
51. Inagaki J, Rodriguez V, Bodey GP. Proceedings: causes of death in cancer patients. Cancer. 1974;33(2):568–73.
52. Ambrus JL, Ambrus CM, Mink IB, Pickren JW. Causes of death in cancer patients. J Med. 1975;6(1):61–4.
53. Dudgeon DJ, Lertzman M, Askew GR. Physiological changes and clinical correlations of dyspnea in cancer outpatients. J Pain Symptom Manage. 2001;21(5):373–9.
54. Prandoni P, Falanga A, Piccioli A. Cancer and venous thromboembolism. Lancet Oncol. 2005;6(6):401–10.
55. Blom JW, Doggen CJ, Osanto S, Rosendaal FR. Malignancies, prothrombotic mutations, and the risk of venous thrombosis. JAMA. 2005;293(6):715–22.
56. Tisdale MJ. Cachexia in cancer patients. Nat Rev Cancer. 2002;2(11):862–71.
57. Argiles JM, Alvarez B, Lopez-Soriano FJ. The metabolic basis of cancer cachexia. Med Res Rev. 1997;17(5):477–98.
58. Muscaritoli M, Bossola M, Aversa Z, Bellantone R, Rossi Fanelli F. Prevention and treatment of cancer cachexia: new insights into an old problem. Eur J Cancer. 2006;42(1):31–41.
59. Balkwill F, Mantovani A. Inflammation and cancer: back to Virchow? Lancet. 2001;357(9255):539–45.
60. Bongartz T, Sutton AJ, Sweeting MJ, Buchan I, Matteson EL, Montori V. Anti-TNF antibody therapy in rheumatoid arthritis and the risk of serious infections and malignancies: systematic review and meta-analysis of rare harmful effects in randomized controlled trials. JAMA. 2006;295(19):2275–85.

61. Pannu HK, Bristow RE, Montz FJ, Fishman EK. Multidetector CT of peritoneal carcinomatosis from ovarian cancer. Radiographics. 2003;23(3):687–701.
62. Zeidman I. Experimental studies on the spread of cancer in the lymphatic system. III. Tumor emboli in thoracic duct; the pathogenesis of Virchow's node. Cancer Res. 1955;15(11):719–21.
63. Zeidman I. Experimental studies on the spread of cancer in the lymphatic system. IV. Retrograde spread. Cancer Res. 1959;19:1114–7.
64. Middleton RG, Smith Jr JA. Radical prostatectomy for stage B2 prostatic cancer. J Urol. 1982;127(4): 702–3.
65. Passlick B, Kubuschok B, Izbicki JR, Thetter O, Pantel K. Isolated tumor cells in bone marrow predict reduced survival in node-negative non-small cell lung cancer. Ann Thorac Surg. 1999;68(6):2053–8.
66. Pantel K, Cote RJ, Fodstad O. Detection and clinical importance of micrometastatic disease. J Natl Cancer Inst. 1999;91(13):1113–24.
67. Veronesi U, Banfi A, Salvadori B, et al. Breast conservation is the treatment of choice in small breast cancer: long-term results of a randomized trial. Eur J Cancer. 1990;26(6):668–70.
68. Kitchener H, Swart AM, Qian Q, Amos C, Parmar MK. Efficacy of systematic pelvic lymphadenectomy in endometrial cancer (MRC ASTEC trial): a randomised study. Lancet. 2009;373(9658):125–36.
69. Halsted WS. I. The results of radical operations for the cure of carcinoma of the breast. Ann Surg. 1907;46(1):1–19.
70. Fisher B. Laboratory and clinical research in breast cancer–a personal adventure: the David A. Karnofsky memorial lecture. Cancer Res. 1980;40(11):3863–74.
71. Kawada K, Taketo MM. Significance and mechanism of lymph node metastasis in cancer progression. Cancer Res. 2011;71(4):1214–8.
72. Burns FJ, Pfaff Jr J. Vascular invasion in carcinoma of the colon and rectum. Am J Surg. 1956;92(5): 704–9.
73. Vider M, Maruyama Y, Narvaez R. Significance of the vertebral venous (Batson's) plexus in metastatic spread in colorectal carcinoma. Cancer. 1977;40(1): 67–71.
74. Poste G, Fidler IJ. The pathogenesis of cancer metastasis. Nature. 1980;283(5743):139–46.
75. Price JE, Aukerman SL, Fidler IJ. Evidence that the process of murine melanoma metastasis is sequential and selective and contains stochastic elements. Cancer Res. 1986;46(10):5172–8.
76. Perl AK, Wilgenbus P, Dahl U, Semb H, Christofori G. A causal role for E-cadherin in the transition from adenoma to carcinoma. Nature. 1998;392(6672): 190–3.
77. Qi J, Chen N, Wang J, Siu CH. Transendothelial migration of melanoma cells involves N-cadherin-mediated adhesion and activation of the beta-catenin signaling pathway. Mol Biol Cell. 2005;16(9):4386–97.
78. Hazan RB, Kang L, Whooley BP, Borgen PI. N-cadherin promotes adhesion between invasive breast cancer cells and the stroma. Cell Adhes Commun. 1997;4(6):399–411.
79. Tomita K, van Bokhoven A, van Leenders GJ, et al. Cadherin switching in human prostate cancer progression. Cancer Res. 2000;60(13):3650–4.
80. Chu K, Cheng CJ, Ye X, et al. Cadherin-11 promotes the metastasis of prostate cancer cells to bone. Mol Cancer Res. 2008;6(8):1259–67.
81. Perotti A, Sessa C, Mancuso A, et al. Clinical and pharmacological phase I evaluation of Exherin (ADH-1), a selective anti-N-cadherin peptide in patients with N-cadherin-expressing solid tumours. Ann Oncol. 2009;20(4):741–5.
82. Butler TP, Grantham FH, Gullino PM. Bulk transfer of fluid in the interstitial compartment of mammary tumors. Cancer Res. 1975;35(11 Pt 1):3084–8.
83. Roma AA, Magi-Galluzzi C, Kral MA, Jin TT, Klein EA, Zhou M. Peritumoral lymphatic invasion is associated with regional lymph node metastases in prostate adenocarcinoma. Mod Pathol. 2006;19(3):392–8.
84. Dadras SS, Lange-Asschenfeldt B, Velasco P, et al. Tumor lymphangiogenesis predicts melanoma metastasis to sentinel lymph nodes. Mod Pathol. 2005;18(9):1232–42.
85. Hirakawa S, Kodama S, Kunstfeld R, Kajiya K, Brown LF, Detmar M. VEGF-A induces tumor and sentinel lymph node lymphangiogenesis and promotes lymphatic metastasis. J Exp Med. 2005; 201(7):1089–99.
86. Ji RC. Lymphatic endothelial cells, tumor lymphangiogenesis and metastasis: new insights into intratumoral and peritumoral lymphatics. Cancer Metastasis Rev. 2006;25(4):677–94.
87. Tsakraklides V, Olson P, Kersey JH, Good RA. Prognostic significance of the regional lymph node histology in cancer of the breast. Cancer. 1974;34(4):1259–67.
88. Pickren JW. Significance of occult metastases. A study of breast cancer. Cancer. 1961;14:1266–71.
89. Fidler IJ. Metastasis: quantitative analysis of distribution and fate of tumor embolilabeled with 125 I-5-iodo-2′-deoxyuridine. J Natl Cancer Inst. 1970; 45(4):773–82.
90. Glinsky VV. Intravascular cell-to-cell adhesive interactions and bone metastases. Cancer Metastasis Rev. 2006;25(4):531–40.
91. Nieswandt B, Hafner M, Echtenacher B, Mannel DN. Lysis of tumor cells by natural killer cells in mice is impeded by platelets. Cancer Res. 1999;59(6):1295–300.
92. Im JH, Fu W, Wang H, et al. Coagulation facilitates tumor cell spreading in the pulmonary vasculature during early metastatic colony formation. Cancer Res. 2004;64(23):8613–9.
93. Glinskii OV, Huxley VH, Glinsky GV, Pienta KJ, Raz A, Glinsky VV. Mechanical entrapment is insufficient and intercellular adhesion is essential for metastatic cell arrest in distant organs. Neoplasia. 2005;7(5):522–7.

94. Honn KV, Tang DG. Adhesion molecules and tumor cell interaction with endothelium and subendothelial matrix. Cancer Metastasis Rev. 1992;11(3–4): 353–75.

95. Lehr JE, Pienta KJ. Preferential adhesion of prostate cancer cells to a human bone marrow endothelial cell line. J Natl Cancer Inst. 1998;90(2):118–23.

96. Khatib AM, Kontogiannea M, Fallavollita L, Jamison B, Meterissian S, Brodt P. Rapid induction of cytokine and E-selectin expression in the liver in response to metastatic tumor cells. Cancer Res. 1999;59(6):1356–61.

97. Vidal-Vanaclocha F, Fantuzzi G, Mendoza L, et al. IL-18 regulates IL-1beta-dependent hepatic melanoma metastasis via vascular cell adhesion molecule-1. Proc Natl Acad Sci USA. 2000;97(2): 734–9.

98. Voura EB, Sandig M, Kalnins VI, Siu C. Cell shape changes and cytoskeleton reorganization during transendothelial migration of human melanoma cells. Cell Tissue Res. 1998;293(3):375–87.

99. Naumov GN, Wilson SM, MacDonald IC, et al. Cellular expression of green fluorescent protein, coupled with high-resolution in vivo videomicroscopy, to monitor steps in tumor metastasis. J Cell Sci. 1999;112(Pt 12):1835–42.

100. Paku S, Dome B, Toth R, Timar J. Organ-specificity of the extravasation process: an ultrastructural study. Clin Exp Metastasis. 2000;18(6):481–92.

101. Nicolson GL. Organ specificity of tumor metastasis: role of preferential adhesion, invasion and growth of malignant cells at specific secondary sites. Cancer Metastasis Rev. 1988;7(2):143–88.

102. van der Bij GJ, Oosterling SJ, Bogels M, et al. Blocking alpha2 integrins on rat CC531s colon carcinoma cells prevents operation-induced augmentation of liver metastases outgrowth. Hepatology. 2008;47(2):532–43.

103. Fidler IJ. Critical factors in the biology of human cancer metastasis: twenty-eighth G.H.A. Clowes memorial award lecture. Cancer Res. 1990;50(19):6130–8.

104. Campbell PJ, Yachida S, Mudie LJ, et al. The patterns and dynamics of genomic instability in metastatic pancreatic cancer. Nature. 2010;467(7319):1109–13.

105. Talmadge JE, Fidler IJ. Enhanced metastatic potential of tumor cells harvested from spontaneous metastases of heterogeneous murine tumors. J Natl Cancer Inst. 1982;69(4):975–80.

106. Fidler IJ, Talmadge JE. Evidence that intravenously derived murine pulmonary melanoma metastases can originate from the expansion of a single tumor cell. Cancer Res. 1986;46(10):5167–71.

107. Demicheli R. Tumour dormancy: findings and hypotheses from clinical research on breast cancer. Semin Cancer Biol. 2001;11(4):297–306.

108. Aguirre-Ghiso JA. Models, mechanisms and clinical evidence for cancer dormancy. Nat Rev Cancer. 2007;7(11):834–46.

109. Bross ID, Viadana E, Pickren J. Do generalized metastases occur directly from the primary? J Chronic Dis. 1975;28(3):149–59.

110. Kaplan RN, Riba RD, Zacharoulis S, et al. VEGFR1-positive haematopoietic bone marrow progenitors initiate the pre-metastatic niche. Nature. 2005; 438(7069):820–7.

111. Yan HH, Pickup M, Pang Y, et al. Gr-1+CD11b+ myeloid cells tip the balance of immune protection to tumor promotion in the premetastatic lung. Cancer Res. 2010;70(15):6139–49.

112. Fidler IJ. Biological behavior of malignant melanoma cells correlated to their survival in vivo. Cancer Res. 1975;35(1):218–24.

113. Sugarbaker ED. The organ selectivity of experimentally induced metastases in rats. Cancer. 1952;5(3): 606–12.

114. Kinsey DL. An experimental study of preferential metastasis. Cancer. 1960;13:674–6.

115. Ewing J. Neoplastic diseases: a treatise on tumors. 3rd ed. Philadelphia: Saunders; 1919.

116. Klein CA. Parallel progression of primary tumours and metastases. Nat Rev Cancer. 2009;9(4):302–12.

117. McCarter MD, Fong Y. Metastatic liver tumors. Semin Surg Oncol. 2000;19(2):177–88.

118. Karrison TG, Ferguson DJ, Meier P. Dormancy of mammary carcinoma after mastectomy. J Natl Cancer Inst. 1999;91(1):80–5.

119. Yachida S, Jones S, Bozic I, et al. Distant metastasis occurs late during the genetic evolution of pancreatic cancer. Nature. 2010;467(7319):1114–7.

120. Jones S, Chen WD, Parmigiani G, et al. Comparative lesion sequencing provides insights into tumor evolution. Proc Natl Acad Sci USA. 2008;105(11): 4283–8.

121. Nowell PC. The clonal evolution of tumor cell populations. Science. 1976;194(4260):23–8.

122. Fidler IJ, Kripke ML. Metastasis results from preexisting variant cells within a malignant tumor. Science. 1977;197(4306):893–5.

123. Nicolson GL, Brunson KW, Fidler IJ. Specificity of arrest, survival, and growth of selected metastatic variant cell lines. Cancer Res. 1978;38(11 Pt 2):4105–11.

124. Kozlowski JM, Hart IR, Fidler IJ, Hanna N. A human melanoma line heterogeneous with respect to metastatic capacity in athymic nude mice. J Natl Cancer Inst. 1984;72(4):913–7.

125. Waghorne C, Thomas M, Lagarde A, Kerbel RS, Breitman ML. Genetic evidence for progressive selection and overgrowth of primary tumors by metastatic cell subpopulations. Cancer Res. 1988; 48(21):6109–14.

126. Kuukasjarvi T, Karhu R, Tanner M, et al. Genetic heterogeneity and clonal evolution underlying development of asynchronous metastasis in human breast cancer. Cancer Res. 1997;57(8):1597–604.

127. Fidler IJ. The organ microenvironment and cancer metastasis. Differentiation. 2002;70(9–10):498–505.

128. Cifone MA, Fidler IJ. Increasing metastatic potential is associated with increasing genetic instability of

128. clones isolated from murine neoplasms. Proc Natl Acad Sci USA. 1981;78(11):6949–52.

129. Welch DR, Tomasovic SP. Implications of tumor progression on clinical oncology. Clin Exp Metastasis. 1985;3(3):151–88.

130. Talmadge JE, Fidler IJ. AACR centennial series: the biology of cancer metastasis: historical perspective. Cancer Res. 2010;70(14):5649–69.

131. Kang Y, Siegel PM, Shu W, et al. A multigenic program mediating breast cancer metastasis to bone. Cancer Cell. 2003;3(6):537–49.

132. Minn AJ, Gupta GP, Siegel PM, et al. Genes that mediate breast cancer metastasis to lung. Nature. 2005;436(7050):518–24.

133. Wang Y, Klijn JG, Zhang Y, et al. Gene-expression profiles to predict distant metastasis of lymph-node-negative primary breast cancer. Lancet. 2005; 365(9460):671–9.

134. Sorlie T, Tibshirani R, Parker J, et al. Repeated observation of breast tumor subtypes in independent gene expression data sets. Proc Natl Acad Sci USA. 2003;100(14):8418–23.

135. van de Vijver MJ, He YD, Van't Veer LJ, et al. A gene-expression signature as a predictor of survival in breast cancer. N Engl J Med. 2002;347(25): 1999–2009.

136. Suzuki M, Tarin D. Gene expression profiling of human lymph node metastases and matched primary breast carcinomas: clinical implications. Mol Oncol. 2007;1(2):172–80.

137. Gancberg D, Di Leo A, Cardoso F, et al. Comparison of HER-2 status between primary breast cancer and corresponding distant metastatic sites. Ann Oncol. 2002;13(7):1036–43.

138. Hynes RO. Cell adhesion: old and new questions. Trends Cell Biol. 1999;9(12):M33–7.

139. Plow EF, Haas TA, Zhang L, Loftus J, Smith JW. Ligand binding to integrins. J Biol Chem. 2000;275(29):21785–8.

140. Komoriya A, Green LJ, Mervic M, Yamada SS, Yamada KM, Humphries MJ. The minimal essential sequence for a major cell type-specific adhesion site (CS1) within the alternatively spliced type III connecting segment domain of fibronectin is leucine-aspartic acid-valine. J Biol Chem. 1991;266(23):15075–9.

141. Jin H, Varner J. Integrins: roles in cancer development and as treatment targets. Br J Cancer. 2004;90(3):561–5.

142. Angelucci A, Bologna M. Targeting vascular cell migration as a strategy for blocking angiogenesis: the central role of focal adhesion protein tyrosine kinase family. Curr Pharm Des. 2007;13(21): 2129–45.

143. Schlaepfer DD, Jones KC, Hunter T. Multiple Grb2-mediated integrin-stimulated signaling pathways to ERK2/mitogen-activated protein kinase: summation of both c-Src- and focal adhesion kinase-initiated tyrosine phosphorylation events. Mol Cell Biol. 1998;18(5):2571–85.

144. Luo BH, Carman CV, Springer TA. Structural basis of integrin regulation and signaling. Annu Rev Immunol. 2007;25:619–47.

145. Varner JA, Cheresh DA. Integrins and cancer. Curr Opin Cell Biol. 1996;8(5):724–30.

146. Lukashev ME, Werb Z. ECM signalling: orchestrating cell behaviour and misbehaviour. Trends Cell Biol. 1998;8(11):437–41.

147. Folgiero V, Bachelder RE, Bon G, Sacchi A, Falcioni R, Mercurio AM. The alpha6beta4 integrin can regulate ErbB-3 expression: implications for alpha6beta4 signaling and function. Cancer Res. 2007; 67(4):1645–52.

148. Stewart DA, Cooper CR, Sikes RA. Changes in extracellular matrix (ECM) and ECM-associated proteins in the metastatic progression of prostate cancer. Reprod Biol Endocrinol. 2004;2:2.

149. Heino J, Ignotz RA, Hemler ME, Crouse C, Massague J. Regulation of cell adhesion receptors by transforming growth factor-beta. Concomitant regulation of integrins that share a common beta 1 subunit. J Biol Chem. 1989;264(1):380–8.

150. Conti JA, Kendall TJ, Bateman A, et al. The desmoplastic reaction surrounding hepatic colorectal adenocarcinoma metastases aids tumor growth and survival via alphav integrin ligation. Clin Cancer Res. 2008;14(20):6405–13.

151. Wang J, Zhang Z, Xu K, et al. Suppression of integrin alphaupsilonbeta6 by RNA interference in colon cancer cells inhibits extracellular matrix degradation through the MAPK pathway. Int J Cancer. 2008;123(6):1311–7.

152. Friedlander M, Theesfeld CL, Sugita M, et al. Involvement of integrins alpha v beta 3 and alpha v beta 5 in ocular neovascular diseases. Proc Natl Acad Sci USA. 1996;93(18):9764–9.

153. Brooks PC, Clark RA, Cheresh DA. Requirement of vascular integrin alpha v beta 3 for angiogenesis. Science. 1994;264(5158):569–71.

154. Hong YK, Lange-Asschenfeldt B, Velasco P, et al. VEGF-A promotes tissue repair-associated lymphatic vessel formation via VEGFR-2 and the alpha-1beta1 and alpha2beta1 integrins. FASEB J. 2004; 18(10):1111–3.

155. Avraamides CJ, Garmy-Susini B, Varner JA. Integrins in angiogenesis and lymphangiogenesis. Nat Rev Cancer. 2008;8(8):604–17.

156. Shannon KE, Keene JL, Settle SL, et al. Antimetastatic properties of RGD-peptidomimetic agents S137 and S247. Clin Exp Metastasis. 2004;21(2): 129–38.

157. Reinmuth N, Liu W, Ahmad SA, et al. Alphavbeta3 integrin antagonist S247 decreases colon cancer metastasis and angiogenesis and improves survival in mice. Cancer Res. 2003;63(9):2079–87.

158. Reynolds AR, Hart IR, Watson AR, et al. Stimulation of tumor growth and angiogenesis by low concentrations of RGD-mimetic integrin inhibitors. Nat Med. 2009;15(4):392–400.

159. Reynolds AR. Potential relevance of bell-shaped and u-shaped dose-responses for the therapeutic targeting of angiogenesis in cancer. Dose Response. 2009;8(3):253–84.

160. Moschos SJ, Sander CA, Wang W, et al. Pharmacodynamic (phase 0) study using etaracizumab in advanced melanoma. J Immunother. 2010;33(3):316–25.

161. Zhang D, Pier T, McNeel DG, Wilding G, Friedl A. Effects of a monoclonal anti-alphavbeta3 integrin antibody on blood vessels - a pharmacodynamic study. Invest New Drugs. 2007;25(1):49–55.

162. Hersey P, Sosman J, O'Day S, et al. A randomized phase 2 study of etaracizumab, a monoclonal antibody against integrin alpha(v)beta(3), + or - dacarbazine in patients with stage IV metastatic melanoma. Cancer. 2010;116(6):1526–34.

163. Gramoun A, Shorey S, Bashutski JD, et al. Effects of Vitaxin, a novel therapeutic in trial for metastatic bone tumors, on osteoclast functions in vitro. J Cell Biochem. 2007;102(2):341–52.

164. Nabors LB, Mikkelsen T, Rosenfeld SS, et al. Phase I and correlative biology study of cilengitide in patients with recurrent malignant glioma. J Clin Oncol. 2007;25(13):1651–7.

165. Stoeltzing O, Liu W, Reinmuth N, et al. Inhibition of integrin alpha5beta1 function with a small peptide (ATN-161) plus continuous 5-FU infusion reduces colorectal liver metastases and improves survival in mice. Int J Cancer. 2003;104(4):496–503.

166. Khalili P, Arakelian A, Chen G, et al. A non-RGD-based integrin binding peptide (ATN-161) blocks breast cancer growth and metastasis in vivo. Mol Cancer Ther. 2006;5(9):2271–80.

167. Karpatkin S, Pearlstein E, Ambrogio C, Coller BS. Role of adhesive proteins in platelet tumor interaction in vitro and metastasis formation in vivo. J Clin Invest. 1988;81(4):1012–9.

168. Biggerstaff JP, Seth N, Amirkhosravi A, et al. Soluble fibrin augments platelet/tumor cell adherence in vitro and in vivo, and enhances experimental metastasis. Clin Exp Metastasis. 1999;17(8): 723–30.

169. Amirkhosravi A, Amaya M, Siddiqui F, Biggerstaff JP, Meyer TV, Francis JL. Blockade of GpIIb/IIIa inhibits the release of vascular endothelial growth factor (VEGF) from tumor cell-activated platelets and experimental metastasis. Platelets. 1999;10(5): 285–92.

170. Terraube V, Marx I, Denis CV. Role of von Willebrand factor in tumor metastasis. Thromb Res. 2007;120 Suppl 2:S64–70.

171. Gomes N, Legrand C, Fauvel-Lafeve F. Shear stress induced release of von Willebrand factor and thrombospondin-1 in HUVEC extracellular matrix enhances breast tumour cell adhesion. Clin Exp Metastasis. 2005;22(3):215–23.

172. Al-Mehdi AB, Tozawa K, Fisher AB, Shientag L, Lee A, Muschel RJ. Intravascular origin of metastasis from the proliferation of endothelium-attached tumor cells: a new model for metastasis. Nat Med. 2000;6(1):100–2.

173. Glinsky VV, Glinsky GV, Glinskii OV, et al. Intravascular metastatic cancer cell homotypic aggregation at the sites of primary attachment to the endothelium. Cancer Res. 2003;63(13):3805–11.

174. Rao LV, Pendurthi UR. Tissue factor-factor VIIa signaling. Arterioscler Thromb Vasc Biol. 2005; 25(1):47–56.

175. Versteeg HH, Ruf W. Emerging insights in tissue factor-dependent signaling events. Semin Thromb Hemost. 2006;32(1):24–32.

176. Seto S, Onodera H, Kaido T, et al. Tissue factor expression in human colorectal carcinoma: correlation with hepatic metastasis and impact on prognosis. Cancer. 2000;88(2):295–301.

177. Lwaleed BA, Bass PS. Tissue factor pathway inhibitor: structure, biology and involvement in disease. J Pathol. 2006;208(3):327–39.

178. Contrino J, Hair G, Kreutzer DL, Rickles FR. In situ detection of tissue factor in vascular endothelial cells: correlation with the malignant phenotype of human breast disease. Nat Med. 1996;2(2): 209–15.

179. Bounameaux H. The novel anticoagulants: entering a new era. Swiss Med Wkly. 2009;139(5–6):60–4.

180. Lever R, Page CP. Novel drug development opportunities for heparin. Nat Rev Drug Discov. 2002; 1(2):140–8.

181. Niers TM, Klerk CP, DiNisio M, et al. Mechanisms of heparin induced anti-cancer activity in experimental cancer models. Crit Rev Oncol Hematol. 2007;61(3):195–207.

182. Smorenburg SM, Van Noorden CJ. The complex effects of heparins on cancer progression and metastasis in experimental studies. Pharmacol Rev. 2001;53(1):93–105.

183. Harvey JR, Mellor P, Eldaly H, Lennard TW, Kirby JA, Ali S. Inhibition of CXCR4-mediated breast cancer metastasis: a potential role for heparinoids? Clin Cancer Res. 2007;13(5):1562–70.

184. Stevenson JL, Choi SH, Varki A. Differential metastasis inhibition by clinically relevant levels of heparins–correlation with selectin inhibition, not antithrombotic activity. Clin Cancer Res. 2005;11(19 Pt 1):7003–11.

185. Amirkhosravi A, Mousa SA, Amaya M, Francis JL. Antimetastatic effect of tinzaparin, a low-molecular-weight heparin. J Thromb Haemost. 2003;1(9): 1972–6.

186. Bereczky B, Gilly R, Raso E, Vago A, Timar J, Tovari J. Selective antimetastatic effect of heparins in preclinical human melanoma models is based on inhibition of migration and microvascular arrest. Clin Exp Metastasis. 2005;22(1):69–76.

187. Hettiarachchi RJ, Smorenburg SM, Ginsberg J, Levine M, Prins MH, Buller HR. Do heparins do more than just treat thrombosis? The influence of

heparins on cancer spread. Thromb Haemost. 1999;82(2):947–52.

188. Kakkar AK, Levine MN, Kadziola Z, et al. Low molecular weight heparin, therapy with dalteparin, and survival in advanced cancer: the fragmin advanced malignancy outcome study (FAMOUS). J Clin Oncol. 2004;22(10):1944–8.

189. Schlesinger M, Simonis D, Schmitz P, Fritzsche J, Bendas G. Binding between heparin and the integrin VLA-4. Thromb Haemost. 2009;102(5):816–22.

190. Borsig L, Wong R, Feramisco J, Nadeau DR, Varki NM, Varki A. Heparin and cancer revisited: mechanistic connections involving platelets, P-selectin, carcinoma mucins, and tumor metastasis. Proc Natl Acad Sci USA. 2001;98(6):3352–7.

191. Okada T, Okuno H, Mitsui Y. A novel in vitro assay system for transendothelial tumor cell invasion: significance of E-selectin and alpha 3 integrin in the transendothelial invasion by HT1080 fibrosarcoma cells. Clin Exp Metastasis. 1994;12(4):305–14.

192. Lafrenie RM, Gallo S, Podor TJ, Buchanan MR, Orr FW. The relative roles of vitronectin receptor, E-selectin and alpha 4 beta 1 in cancer cell adhesion to interleukin-1-treated endothelial cells. Eur J Cancer. 1994;30A(14):2151–8.

193. Sheski FD, Natarajan V, Pottratz ST. Tumor necrosis factor-alpha stimulates attachment of small cell lung carcinoma to endothelial cells. J Lab Clin Med. 1999;133(3):265–73.

194. Liang S, Slattery MJ, Dong C. Shear stress and shear rate differentially affect the multi-step process of leukocyte-facilitated melanoma adhesion. Exp Cell Res. 2005;310(2):282–92.

195. Khatib AM, Auguste P, Fallavollita L, et al. Characterization of the host proinflammatory response to tumor cells during the initial stages of liver metastasis. Am J Pathol. 2005;167(3):749–59.

196. Kansas GS. Selectins and their ligands: current concepts and controversies. Blood. 1996;88(9):3259–87.

197. Mannori G, Crottet P, Cecconi O, et al. Differential colon cancer cell adhesion to E-, P-, and L-selectin: role of mucin-type glycoproteins. Cancer Res. 1995;55(19):4425–31.

198. Barthel SR, Wiese GK, Cho J, et al. Alpha 1,3 fucosyltransferases are master regulators of prostate cancer cell trafficking. Proc Natl Acad Sci USA. 2009;106(46):19491–6.

199. Crockett-Torabi E. Selectins and mechanisms of signal transduction. J Leukoc Biol. 1998;63(1):1–14.

200. Biancone L, Araki M, Araki K, Vassalli P, Stamenkovic I. Redirection of tumor metastasis by expression of E-selectin in vivo. J Exp Med. 1996;183(2):581–7.

201. Krause T, Turner GA. Are selectins involved in metastasis? Clin Exp Metastasis. 1999;17(3):183–92.

202. Borsig L, Wong R, Hynes RO, Varki NM, Varki A. Synergistic effects of L- and P-selectin in facilitating tumor metastasis can involve non-mucin ligands and implicate leukocytes as enhancers of metastasis. Proc Natl Acad Sci USA. 2002;99(4):2193–8.

203. Laubli H, Borsig L. Selectins promote tumor metastasis. Semin Cancer Biol. 2010;20(3):169–77.

204. Glinskii OV, Turk JR, Pienta KJ, Huxley VH, Glinsky VV. Evidence of porcine and human endothelium activation by cancer-associated carbohydrates expressed on glycoproteins and tumour cells. J Physiol. 2004;554(Pt 1):89–99.

205. Yu LG, Andrews N, Zhao Q, et al. Galectin-3 interaction with Thomsen-Friedenreich disaccharide on cancer-associated MUC1 causes increased cancer cell endothelial adhesion. J Biol Chem. 2007;282(1):773–81.

206. Kaltner H, Stierstorfer B. Animal lectins as cell adhesion molecules. Acta Anat (Basel). 1998;161(1–4):162–79.

207. Bresalier RS, Mazurek N, Sternberg LR, et al. Metastasis of human colon cancer is altered by modifying expression of the beta-galactoside-binding protein galectin 3. Gastroenterology. 1998;115(2):287–96.

208. Khaldoyanidi SK, Glinsky VV, Sikora L, et al. MDA-MB-435 human breast carcinoma cell homo- and heterotypic adhesion under flow conditions is mediated in part by Thomsen-Friedenreich antigen-galectin-3 interactions. J Biol Chem. 2003;278(6):4127–34.

209. Kobayashi K, Matsumoto S, Morishima T, Kawabe T, Okamoto T. Cimetidine inhibits cancer cell adhesion to endothelial cells and prevents metastasis by blocking E-selectin expression. Cancer Res. 2000;60(14):3978–84.

210. Hollingsworth MA, Swanson BJ. Mucins in cancer: protection and control of the cell surface. Nat Rev Cancer. 2004;4(1):45–60.

211. Satoh M, Numahata K, Kawamura S, Saito S, Orikasa S. Lack of selectin-dependent adhesion in prostate cancer cells expressing sialyl Le(x). Int J Urol. 1998;5(1):86–91.

212. Ley K. The role of selectins in inflammation and disease. Trends Mol Med. 2003;9(6):263–8.

213. Fuster MM, Brown JR, Wang L, Esko JD. A disaccharide precursor of sialyl Lewis X inhibits metastatic potential of tumor cells. Cancer Res. 2003;63(11):2775–81.

214. Brown JR, Fuster MM, Li R, Varki N, Glass CA, Esko JD. A disaccharide-based inhibitor of glycosylation attenuates metastatic tumor cell dissemination. Clin Cancer Res. 2006;12(9):2894–901.

215. Garofalo A, Chirivi RG, Foglieni C, et al. Involvement of the very late antigen 4 integrin on melanoma in interleukin 1-augmented experimental metastases. Cancer Res. 1995;55(2):414–9.

216. Takahashi M, Furihata M, Akimitsu N, et al. A highly bone marrow metastatic murine breast cancer model established through in vivo selection exhibits enhanced anchorage-independent growth and cell

216. migration mediated by ICAM-1. Clin Exp Metastasis. 2008;25(5):517–29.
217. Flavin T, Ivens K, Rothlein R, et al. Monoclonal antibodies against intercellular adhesion molecule 1 prolong cardiac allograft survival in cynomolgus monkeys. Transplant Proc. 1991;23(1 Pt 1):533–4.
218. Haug CE, Colvin RB, Delmonico FL, et al. A phase I trial of immunosuppression with anti-ICAM-1 (CD54) mAb in renal allograft recipients. Transplantation. 1993;55(4):766–72. discussion 772–763.
219. del Zoppo GJ. Acute anti-inflammatory approaches to ischemic stroke. Ann NY Acad Sci. 2010;1207: 143–8.
220. Dunon D, Piali L, Imhof BA. To stick or not to stick: the new leukocyte homing paradigm. Curr Opin Cell Biol. 1996;8(5):714–23.
221. Rosenblum WI, Nelson GH, Wormley B, Werner P, Wang J, Shih CC. Role of platelet-endothelial cell adhesion molecule (PECAM) in platelet adhesion/aggregation over injured but not denuded endothelium in vivo and ex vivo. Stroke. 1996;27(4): 709–11.
222. DeLisser H, Liu Y, Desprez PY, et al. Vascular endothelial platelet endothelial cell adhesion molecule 1 (PECAM-1) regulates advanced metastatic progression. Proc Natl Acad Sci USA. 2010; 107(43):18616–21.
223. Zlotnik A, Yoshie O. Chemokines: a new classification system and their role in immunity. Immunity. 2000;12(2):121–7.
224. Bieche I, Chavey C, Andrieu C, et al. CXC chemokines located in the 4q21 region are up-regulated in breast cancer. Endocr Relat Cancer. 2007;14(4): 1039–52.
225. Miles FL, Pruitt FL, van Golen KL, Cooper CR. Stepping out of the flow: capillary extravasation in cancer metastasis. Clin Exp Metastasis. 2008;25(4): 305–24.
226. Marchesi F, Piemonti L, Fedele G, et al. The chemokine receptor CX3CR1 is involved in the neural tropism and malignant behavior of pancreatic ductal adenocarcinoma. Cancer Res. 2008;68(21):9060–9.
227. Kato M, Kitayama J, Kazama S, Nagawa H. Expression pattern of CXC chemokine receptor-4 is correlated with lymph node metastasis in human invasive ductal carcinoma. Breast Cancer Res. 2003;5(5):R144–50.
228. Helbig G, Christopherson 2nd KW, Bhat-Nakshatri P, et al. NF-kappaB promotes breast cancer cell migration and metastasis by inducing the expression of the chemokine receptor CXCR4. J Biol Chem. 2003;278(24):21631–8.
229. Andre F, Cabioglu N, Assi H, et al. Expression of chemokine receptors predicts the site of metastatic relapse in patients with axillary node positive primary breast cancer. Ann Oncol. 2006;17(6):945–51.
230. Allinen M, Beroukhim R, Cai L, et al. Molecular characterization of the tumor microenvironment in breast cancer. Cancer Cell. 2004;6(1):17–32.
231. Miao Z, Luker KE, Summers BC, et al. CXCR7 (RDC1) promotes breast and lung tumor growth in vivo and is expressed on tumor-associated vasculature. Proc Natl Acad Sci USA. 2007;104(40): 15735–40.
232. Gunther K, Leier J, Henning G, et al. Prediction of lymph node metastasis in colorectal carcinoma by expression of chemokine receptor CCR7. Int J Cancer. 2005;116(5):726–33.
233. Shields JD, Fleury ME, Yong C, Tomei AA, Randolph GJ, Swartz MA. Autologous chemotaxis as a mechanism of tumor cell homing to lymphatics via interstitial flow and autocrine CCR7 signaling. Cancer Cell. 2007;11(6):526–38.
234. Smith MC, Luker KE, Garbow JR, et al. CXCR4 regulates growth of both primary and metastatic breast cancer. Cancer Res. 2004;64(23):8604–12.
235. Liang Z, Wu T, Lou H, et al. Inhibition of breast cancer metastasis by selective synthetic polypeptide against CXCR4. Cancer Res. 2004;64(12):4302–8.
236. Fricker SP, Anastassov V, Cox J, et al. Characterization of the molecular pharmacology of AMD3100: a specific antagonist of the G-protein coupled chemokine receptor, CXCR4. Biochem Pharmacol. 2006; 72(5):588–96.
237. Takenaga M, Tamamura H, Hiramatsu K, et al. A single treatment with microcapsules containing a CXCR4 antagonist suppresses pulmonary metastasis of murine melanoma. Biochem Biophys Res Commun. 2004;320(1):226–32.
238. Mason SD, Joyce JA. Proteolytic networks in cancer. Trends Cell Biol. 2011;21(4):228–37.
239. Nagase H, Visse R, Murphy G. Structure and function of matrix metalloproteinases and TIMPs. Cardiovasc Res. 2006;69(3):562–73.
240. Westermarck J, Kahari VM. Regulation of matrix metalloproteinase expression in tumor invasion. FASEB J. 1999;13(8):781–92.
241. Kostoulas G, Lang A, Nagase H, Baici A. Stimulation of angiogenesis through cathepsin B inactivation of the tissue inhibitors of matrix metalloproteinases. FEBS Lett. 1999;455(3):286–90.
242. Vincenti MP. The matrix metalloproteinase (MMP) and tissue inhibitor of metalloproteinase (TIMP) genes. Transcriptional and posttranscriptional regulation, signal transduction and cell-type-specific expression. Methods Mol Biol. 2001;151:121–48.
243. Biswas C, Zhang Y, DeCastro R, et al. The human tumor cell-derived collagenase stimulatory factor (renamed EMMPRIN) is a member of the immunoglobulin superfamily. Cancer Res. 1995;55(2): 434–9.
244. Bauer TW, Liu W, Fan F, et al. Targeting of urokinase plasminogen activator receptor in human pancreatic carcinoma cells inhibits c-Met- and insulin-like growth factor-I receptor-mediated migration and invasion and orthotopic tumor growth in mice. Cancer Res. 2005;65(17):7775–81.
245. Reimers N, Zafrakas K, Assmann V, et al. Expression of extracellular matrix metalloproteases inducer on

245. micrometastatic and primary mammary carcinoma cells. Clin Cancer Res. 2004;10(10):3422–8.

246. Sun J, Hemler ME. Regulation of MMP-1 and MMP-2 production through CD147/extracellular matrix metalloproteinase inducer interactions. Cancer Res. 2001;61(5):2276–81.

247. Tang Y, Nakada MT, Kesavan P, et al. Extracellular matrix metalloproteinase inducer stimulates tumor angiogenesis by elevating vascular endothelial cell growth factor and matrix metalloproteinases. Cancer Res. 2005;65(8):3193–9.

248. Welgus HG, Stricklin GP. Human skin fibroblast collagenase inhibitor. Comparative studies in human connective tissues, serum, and amniotic fluid. J Biol Chem. 1983;258(20):12259–64.

249. Muraguchi T, Takegami Y, Ohtsuka T, et al. RECK modulates Notch signaling during cortical neurogenesis by regulating ADAM10 activity. Nat Neurosci. 2007;10(7):838–45.

250. Zeng ZS, Guillem JG. Distinct pattern of matrix metalloproteinase 9 and tissue inhibitor of metalloproteinase 1 mRNA expression in human colorectal cancer and liver metastases. Br J Cancer. 1995; 72(3):575–82.

251. Arkona C, Wiederanders B. Expression, subcellular distribution and plasma membrane binding of cathepsin B and gelatinases in bone metastatic tissue. Biol Chem. 1996;377(11):695–702.

252. Nemeth JA, Yousif R, Herzog M, et al. Matrix metalloproteinase activity, bone matrix turnover, and tumor cell proliferation in prostate cancer bone metastasis. J Natl Cancer Inst. 2002;94(1):17–25.

253. Yoshida S, Takahashi H. Expression of extracellular matrix molecules in brain metastasis. J Surg Oncol. 2009;100(1):65–8.

254. Klein A, Olendrowitz C, Schmutzler R, et al. Identification of brain- and bone-specific breast cancer metastasis genes. Cancer Lett. 2009;276(2): 212–20.

255. Wilson TJ, Nannuru KC, Futakuchi M, Sadanandam A, Singh RK. Cathepsin G enhances mammary tumor-induced osteolysis by generating soluble receptor activator of nuclear factor-kappaB ligand. Cancer Res. 2008;68(14):5803–11.

256. Nannuru KC, Futakuchi M, Varney ML, Vincent TM, Marcusson EG, Singh RK. Matrix metalloproteinase (MMP)-13 regulates mammary tumor-induced osteolysis by activating MMP9 and transforming growth factor-beta signaling at the tumor-bone interface. Cancer Res. 2010;70(9): 3494–504.

257. Fizazi K, Bosserman L, Gao G, Skacel T, Markus R. Denosumab treatment of prostate cancer with bone metastases and increased urine N-telopeptide levels after therapy with intravenous bisphosphonates: results of a randomized phase II trial. J Urol. 2009;182(2):509–15. discussion 515–506.

258. Musso O, Theret N, Campion JP, et al. In situ detection of matrix metalloproteinase-2 (MMP2) and the metalloproteinase inhibitor TIMP2 transcripts in human primary hepatocellular carcinoma and in liver metastasis. J Hepatol. 1997;26(3):593–605.

259. Itoh T, Tanioka M, Yoshida H, Yoshioka T, Nishimoto H, Itohara S. Reduced angiogenesis and tumor progression in gelatinase A-deficient mice. Cancer Res. 1998;58(5):1048–51.

260. Itoh T, Tanioka M, Matsuda H, et al. Experimental metastasis is suppressed in MMP-9-deficient mice. Clin Exp Metastasis. 1999;17(2):177–81.

261. Ohishi K, Fujita N, Morinaga Y, Tsuruo T. H-31 human breast cancer cells stimulate type I collagenase production in osteoblast-like cells and induce bone resorption. Clin Exp Metastasis. 1995; 13(4):287–95.

262. Overall CM, Kleifeld O. Tumour microenvironment - opinion: validating matrix metalloproteinases as drug targets and anti-targets for cancer therapy. Nat Rev Cancer. 2006;6(3):227–39.

263. Martin MD, Matrisian LM. The other side of MMPs: protective roles in tumor progression. Cancer Metastasis Rev. 2007;26(3–4):717–24.

264. Morgan H, Hill PA. Human breast cancer cell-mediated bone collagen degradation requires plasminogen activation and matrix metalloproteinase activity. Cancer Cell Inst. 2005;5(1):1.

265. Roth D, Piekarek M, Paulsson M, et al. Plasmin modulates vascular endothelial growth factor-A-mediated angiogenesis during wound repair. Am J Pathol. 2006;168(2):670–84.

266. Kim MH. Flavonoids inhibit VEGF/bFGF-induced angiogenesis in vitro by inhibiting the matrix-degrading proteases. J Cell Biochem. 2003;89(3): 529–38.

267. Dano K, Romer J, Nielsen BS, et al. Cancer invasion and tissue remodeling–cooperation of protease systems and cell types. APMIS. 1999;107(1):120–7.

268. Roldan AL, Cubellis MV, Masucci MT, et al. Cloning and expression of the receptor for human urokinase plasminogen activator, a central molecule in cell surface, plasmin dependent proteolysis. EMBO J. 1990;9(2):467–74.

269. Mazar AP. Urokinase plasminogen activator receptor choreographs multiple ligand interactions: implications for tumor progression and therapy. Clin Cancer Res. 2008;14(18):5649–55.

270. Wang Y. The role and regulation of urokinase-type plasminogen activator receptor gene expression in cancer invasion and metastasis. Med Res Rev. 2001;21(2):146–70.

271. Suzuki S, Hayashi Y, Wang Y, et al. Urokinase type plasminogen activator receptor expression in colorectal neoplasms. Gut. 1998;43(6):798–805.

272. Van Buren G, Gray MJ, Dallas NA, et al. Targeting the urokinase plasminogen activator receptor with a monoclonal antibody impairs the growth of human colorectal cancer in the liver. Cancer. 2009; 115(14):3360–8.

273. Rabbani SA, Ateeq B, Arakelian A, et al. An anti-urokinase plasminogen activator receptor antibody (ATN-658) blocks prostate cancer invasion,

273. migration, growth, and experimental skeletal metastasis in vitro and in vivo. Neoplasia. 2010;12(10): 778–88.

274. Ossowski L, Reich E. Antibodies to plasminogen activator inhibit human tumor metastasis. Cell. 1983;35(3 Pt 2):611–9.

275. Margheri F, D'Alessio S, Serrati S, et al. Effects of blocking urokinase receptor signaling by antisense oligonucleotides in a mouse model of experimental prostate cancer bone metastases. Gene Ther. 2005;12(8):702–14.

276. Schuster V, Mingers AM, Seidenspinner S, Nussgens Z, Pukrop T, Kreth HW. Homozygous mutations in the plasminogen gene of two unrelated girls with ligneous conjunctivitis. Blood. 1997;90(3):958–66.

277. Berkenblit A, Matulonis UA, Kroener JF, et al. A6, a urokinase plasminogen activator (uPA)-derived peptide in patients with advanced gynecologic cancer: a phase I trial. Gynecol Oncol. 2005;99(1):50–7.

278. Fridman JS, Caulder E, Hansbury M, et al. Selective inhibition of ADAM metalloproteases as a novel approach for modulating ErbB pathways in cancer. Clin Cancer Res. 2007;13(6):1892–902.

279. Kenny PA, Bissell MJ. Targeting TACE-dependent EGFR ligand shedding in breast cancer. J Clin Invest. 2007;117(2):337–45.

280. Mazzocca A, Coppari R, De Franco R, et al. A secreted form of ADAM9 promotes carcinoma invasion through tumor-stromal interactions. Cancer Res. 2005;65(11):4728–38.

281. Tortorella M, Pratta M, Liu RQ, et al. The thrombospondin motif of aggrecanase-1 (ADAMTS-4) is critical for aggrecan substrate recognition and cleavage. J Biol Chem. 2000;275(33):25791–7.

282. Levy GG, Nichols WC, Lian EC, et al. Mutations in a member of the ADAMTS gene family cause thrombotic thrombocytopenic purpura. Nature. 2001; 413(6855):488–94.

283. Murphy G. The ADAMs: signalling scissors in the tumour microenvironment. Nat Rev Cancer. 2008;8(12):929–41.

284. Sahin U, Weskamp G, Kelly K, et al. Distinct roles for ADAM10 and ADAM17 in ectodomain shedding of six EGFR ligands. J Cell Biol. 2004; 164(5):769–79.

285. Liu PC, Liu X, Li Y, et al. Identification of ADAM10 as a major source of HER2 ectodomain sheddase activity in HER2 overexpressing breast cancer cells. Cancer Biol Ther. 2006;5(6):657–64.

286. Cruz-Munoz W, Kim I, Khokha R. TIMP-3 deficiency in the host, but not in the tumor, enhances tumor growth and angiogenesis. Oncogene. 2006; 25(4):650–5.

287. Gocheva V, Joyce JA. Cysteine cathepsins and the cutting edge of cancer invasion. Cell Cycle. 2007;6(1):60–4.

288. Joyce JA, Baruch A, Chehade K, et al. Cathepsin cysteine proteases are effectors of invasive growth and angiogenesis during multistage tumorigenesis. Cancer Cell. 2004;5(5):443–53.

289. Reiser J, Adair B, Reinheckel T. Specialized roles for cysteine cathepsins in health and disease. J Clin Invest. 2010;120(10):3421–31.

290. Calkins CC, Sloane BF. Mammalian cysteine protease inhibitors: biochemical properties and possible roles in tumor progression. Biol Chem Hoppe Seyler. 1995;376(2):71–80.

291. Hazen LG, Bleeker FE, Lauritzen B, et al. Comparative localization of cathepsin B protein and activity in colorectal cancer. J Histochem Cytochem. 2000;48(10):1421–30.

292. Rofstad EK, Mathiesen B, Kindem K, Galappathi K. Acidic extracellular pH promotes experimental metastasis of human melanoma cells in athymic nude mice. Cancer Res. 2006;66(13):6699–707.

293. Navab R, Pedraza C, Fallavollita L, et al. Loss of responsiveness to IGF-I in cells with reduced cathepsin L expression levels. Oncogene. 2008; 27(37):4973–85.

294. Katunuma N, Tsuge H, Nukatsuka M, Fukushima M. Structure-based development of cathepsin L inhibitors and therapeutic applications for prevention of cancer metastasis and cancer-induced osteoporosis. Adv Enzyme Regul. 2002;42:159–72.

295. Le Gall C, Bellahcene A, Bonnelye E, et al. A cathepsin K inhibitor reduces breast cancer induced osteolysis and skeletal tumor burden. Cancer Res. 2007;67(20):9894–902.

296. Jensen AB, Wynne C, Ramirez G, et al. The cathepsin K inhibitor odanacatib suppresses bone resorption in women with breast cancer and established bone metastases: results of a 4-week, double-blind, randomized, controlled trial. Clin Breast Cancer. 2010;10(6):452–8.

297. Bone HG, McClung MR, Roux C, et al. Odanacatib, a cathepsin-K inhibitor for osteoporosis: a two-year study in postmenopausal women with low bone density. J Bone Miner Res. 2010;25(5):937–47.

298. Naggi A, Casu B, Perez M, et al. Modulation of the heparanase-inhibiting activity of heparin through selective desulfation, graded N-acetylation, and glycol splitting. J Biol Chem. 2005;280(13):12103–13.

299. Vlodavsky I, Friedmann Y. Molecular properties and involvement of heparanase in cancer metastasis and angiogenesis. J Clin Invest. 2001;108(3):341–7.

300. Hulett MD, Freeman C, Hamdorf BJ, Baker RT, Harris MJ, Parish CR. Cloning of mammalian heparanase, an important enzyme in tumor invasion and metastasis. Nat Med. 1999;5(7):803–9.

301. Friedmann Y, Vlodavsky I, Aingorn H, et al. Expression of heparanase in normal, dysplastic, and neoplastic human colonic mucosa and stroma. Evidence for its role in colonic tumorigenesis. Am J Pathol. 2000;157(4):1167–75.

302. Vlodavsky I, Friedmann Y, Elkin M, et al. Mammalian heparanase: gene cloning, expression and function in tumor progression and metastasis. Nat Med. 1999;5(7):793–802.

303. Parish CR, Freeman C, Brown KJ, Francis DJ, Cowden WB. Identification of sulfated oligosaccharide-based

303. inhibitors of tumor growth and metastasis using novel in vitro assays for angiogenesis and heparanase activity. Cancer Res. 1999;59(14):3433–41.

304. Ilan N, Elkin M, Vlodavsky I. Regulation, function and clinical significance of heparanase in cancer metastasis and angiogenesis. Int J Biochem Cell Biol. 2006;38(12):2018–39.

305. Khasraw M, Pavlakis N, McCowatt S, et al. Multicentre phase I/II study of PI-88, a heparanase inhibitor in combination with docetaxel in patients with metastatic castrate-resistant prostate cancer. Ann Oncol. 2010;21(6):1302–7.

306. Liu CJ, Lee PH, Lin DY, et al. Heparanase inhibitor PI-88 as adjuvant therapy for hepatocellular carcinoma after curative resection: a randomized phase II trial for safety and optimal dosage. J Hepatol. 2009;50(5):958–68.

307. Long L, Nip J, Brodt P. Paracrine growth stimulation by hepatocyte-derived insulin-like growth factor-1: a regulatory mechanism for carcinoma cells metastatic to the liver. Cancer Res. 1994;54(14):3732–7.

308. Aguirre Ghiso JA, Kovalski K, Ossowski L. Tumor dormancy induced by downregulation of urokinase receptor in human carcinoma involves integrin and MAPK signaling. J Cell Biol. 1999;147(1):89–104.

309. Angelucci A, Gravina GL, Rucci N, et al. Suppression of EGF-R signaling reduces the incidence of prostate cancer metastasis in nude mice. Endocr Relat Cancer. 2006;13(1):197–210.

310. Heiss MM, Allgayer H, Gruetzner KU, et al. Individual development and uPA-receptor expression of disseminated tumour cells in bone marrow: a reference to early systemic disease in solid cancer. Nat Med. 1995;1(10):1035–9.

311. Barkan D, Green JE, Chambers AF. Extracellular matrix: a gatekeeper in the transition from dormancy to metastatic growth. Eur J Cancer. 2010;46(7):1181–8.

312. Hasebe T, Sasaki S, Imoto S, Mukai K, Yokose T, Ochiai A. Prognostic significance of fibrotic focus in invasive ductal carcinoma of the breast: a prospective observational study. Mod Pathol. 2002;15(5):502–16.

313. Fedarko NS, Jain A, Karadag A, Van Eman MR, Fisher LW. Elevated serum bone sialoprotein and osteopontin in colon, breast, prostate, and lung cancer. Clin Cancer Res. 2001;7(12):4060–6.

314. Bellahcene A, Castronovo V, Ogbureke KU, Fisher LW, Fedarko NS. Small integrin-binding ligand N-linked glycoproteins (SIBLINGs): multifunctional proteins in cancer. Nat Rev Cancer. 2008;8(3):212–26.

315. Ye QH, Qin LX, Forgues M, et al. Predicting hepatitis B virus-positive metastatic hepatocellular carcinomas using gene expression profiling and supervised machine learning. Nat Med. 2003;9(4):416–23.

316. Hendrix MJ, Seftor EA, Seftor RE, Kasemeier-Kulesa J, Kulesa PM, Postovit LM. Reprogramming

317. metastatic tumour cells with embryonic microenvironments. Nat Rev Cancer. 2007;7(4):246–55.

317. Stark AM, Anuszkiewicz B, Mentlein R, Yoneda T, Mehdorn HM, Held-Feindt J. Differential expression of matrix metalloproteinases in brain- and bone-seeking clones of metastatic MDA-MB-231 breast cancer cells. J Neurooncol. 2007;81(1):39–48.

318. Guise TA, Kozlow WM, Heras-Herzig A, Padalecki SS, Yin JJ, Chirgwin JM. Molecular mechanisms of breast cancer metastases to bone. Clin Breast Cancer. 2005;5 Suppl(2):S46–53.

319. Hauschka PV, Mavrakos AE, Iafrati MD, Doleman SE, Klagsbrun M. Growth factors in bone matrix. Isolation of multiple types by affinity chromatography on heparin-Sepharose. J Biol Chem. 1986;261(27):12665–74.

320. Mastro AM, Gay CV, Welch DR, et al. Breast cancer cells induce osteoblast apoptosis: a possible contributor to bone degradation. J Cell Biochem. 2004;91(2):265–76.

321. Bendre MS, Gaddy-Kurten D, Mon-Foote T, et al. Expression of interleukin 8 and not parathyroid hormone-related protein by human breast cancer cells correlates with bone metastasis in vivo. Cancer Res. 2002;62(19):5571–9.

322. Kundu N, Yang Q, Dorsey R, Fulton AM. Increased cyclooxygenase-2 (cox-2) expression and activity in a murine model of metastatic breast cancer. Int J Cancer. 2001;93(5):681–6.

323. Nakamura I, le Duong T, Rodan SB, Rodan GA. Involvement of alpha(v)beta3 integrins in osteoclast function. J Bone Miner Metab. 2007;25(6):337–44.

324. Zheng Y, Zhou H, Fong-Yee C, Modzelewski JR, Seibel MJ, Dunstan CR. Bone resorption increases tumour growth in a mouse model of osteosclerotic breast cancer metastasis. Clin Exp Metastasis. 2008;25(5):559–67.

325. Nelson JB, Hedican SP, George DJ, et al. Identification of endothelin-1 in the pathophysiology of metastatic adenocarcinoma of the prostate. Nat Med. 1995;1(9):944–9.

326. Carducci MA, Saad F, Abrahamsson PA, et al. A phase 3 randomized controlled trial of the efficacy and safety of atrasentan in men with metastatic hormone-refractory prostate cancer. Cancer. 2007;110(9):1959–66.

327. Schelman WR, Liu G, Wilding G, Morris T, Phung D, Dreicer R. A phase I study of zibotentan (ZD4054) in patients with metastatic, castrate-resistant prostate cancer. Invest New Drugs. 2011;29(1):118–25.

328. Maes C, Goossens S, Bartunkova S, et al. Increased skeletal VEGF enhances beta-catenin activity and results in excessively ossified bones. EMBO J. 2010;29(2):424–41.

329. Koeneman KS, Yeung F, Chung LW. Osteomimetic properties of prostate cancer cells: a hypothesis

supporting the predilection of prostate cancer metastasis and growth in the bone environment. Prostate. 1999;39(4):246–61.

330. Angelucci A, Festuccia C, D'Andrea G, Teti A, Bologna M. Osteopontin modulates prostate carcinoma invasive capacity through RGD-dependent upregulation of plasminogen activators. Biol Chem. 2002;383(1):229–34.

331. Jacob K, Webber M, Benayahu D, Kleinman HK. Osteonectin promotes prostate cancer cell migration and invasion: a possible mechanism for metastasis to bone. Cancer Res. 1999;59(17):4453–7.

332. Tuck AB, Chambers AF, Allan AL. Osteopontin overexpression in breast cancer: knowledge gained and possible implications for clinical management. J Cell Biochem. 2007;102(4):859–68.

Current and Future Developments in Cancer Therapy Research: miRNAs as New Promising Targets or Tools

19

Marilena V. Iorio, Patrizia Casalini,
Claudia Piovan, Luca Braccioli, and Elda Tagliabue

Abbreviation

3′-UTR	3′-Untranslated region
AML	Acute lymphocytic leukemia
CLL	Chronic lymphocytic leukemia
EMT	Epithelial–mesenchymal transition
HCC	Hepatocellular carcinoma
MM	Multiple myeloma
Pol II	Polymerase II
Pre-miR	Precursor miRNA molecule
Pre-mRNA	Precursor mRNA molecule
Pri-miR	Primary miRNA transcript

Definition and Biogenesis

After the initial discovery in 1993, when a small RNA encoded by the lin-4 locus was associated to the developmental timing of the nematode *Caenorhabditis elegans* by modulating the protein lin-14 [1], microRNAs have undergone a long period of silence. It took indeed several more years to realize that these small (19–22 nucleotides) RNA molecules are actually expressed in several organisms, including *Homo sapiens*, highly conserved across different species, highly specific for tissue and developmental stage, and playing crucial functions in the regulation of important processes, such as development, proliferation, differentiation, apoptosis, and stress response. In the last few years, microRNAs have indeed taken their place in the complex circuitry of cell biology, revealing a key role as regulators of gene expression.

MicroRNA genes represent approximately 1% of the genome of different species, and each of them has hundreds of different conserved or non-conserved targets: it has been estimated that about 30% of the genes are regulated by at least one microRNA [2].

MicroRNAs are transcribed for the most part by RNA polymerase II as long primary transcripts (pri-microRNAs) characterized by hairpin structures and containing typical eukaryotic mRNA features such as cap structures and poly(A) tail.

Most microRNAs localize in intergenic regions; however, some of them are located in intronic regions of known genes, in sense or antisense orientation. This finding supports the notion that at least a part of them is transcribed as distinct transcriptional units. Fifty percent of known microRNA genes are located nearby other microRNAs, supporting the hypothesis that clustered microRNAs can be transcribed from their own promoters as polycistronic pri-microRNAs [3].

MicroRNAs are mostly transcribed by RNA polymerase II (Pol II), although the possibility that a small number of miRNA genes might be transcribed by other RNA polymerases cannot be excluded. Pol II produces mRNAs and some of

M.V. Iorio, Ph.D. • P. Casalini, Ph.D. • C. Piovan, Ph.D.
• L. Braccioli, Ph.D. • E. Tagliabue, Ph.D. (✉)
Department of Experimental Oncology,
Fondazione IRCCS Istituto Nazionale dei Tumori,
AmadeoLab, via Amadeo 42, Milan 20133, Italy
e-mail: elda.tagliabue@istitutotumori.mi.it

the noncoding RNAs, such as *small nucleolar RNAs* and some of the *small nuclear RNAs* present in the spliceosoma, the complex of specialized RNA and protein subunits that removes introns from a transcribed pre-mRNA.

Many microRNAs are differentially expressed during the development, as frequently observed with genes transcribed by Pol II.

According to their genomic localization, microRNAs can be classified in (a) exonic microRNAs located in noncoding transcripts, (b) intronic microRNAs located in noncoding transcripts, and (c) intronic microRNA located in protein-coding transcripts. Mixed miRNA genes can be assigned to one of the above groups depending on the given splicing pattern. Intronic microRNAs are transcribed within the mRNA of the host gene generating a hairpin structure, recognized and cleaved by the spliceosome machinery [4]. Exonic microRNAs are transcribed within the pri-miR (up to 1 kb long) containing both the 5'-cap and the 3'-poly(A) tail.

Processing of a microRNA consists of two phases, one taking place into the nucleus and operated by RNAse III Drosha and the second one in the cytoplasm, by RNAse III Dicer. Drosha is a highly conserved 160 kDa protein containing two RNAse III domains and one double-strand RNA-binding domain. Drosha forms a huge complex, 500 kDa in *D. melanogaster* and 650 kDa in *H. sapiens*, called microprocessor and containing the cofactor DiGeorge syndrome critical region 8 (DGCR8), also known as Pasha in *D. melanogaster* and *C. elegans*.

The hairpin structure present in the pri-miRNA (primary transcript) is recognized and cleaved by RNAse III Drosha into 70-nts-long pre-microRNAs (precursor molecule).

These precursor molecules are actively exported by a Ran-GTP and exportin 5-mediated mechanism to the cytoplasm, where an additional step is mediated by the RNAse III Dicer, which acts in complex with the transactivating response RNA-binding protein (TRBP) generating a dsRNA of approximately 22 nucleotides, named miRNA/miRNA*. Dicer is an extremely conserved protein through eukaryotes, first identified

for its involvement in siRNA (*small interfering RNAs*) generation.

Dicer is a very large enzyme (~200 kDa) conserved among the species and containing different domains: a double-strand RNA-binding domain (dsRBD), two RNAse III catalytic domains, one PAZ domain, which binds the 3'-end of small RNAs, and other domains with ATPasic and RNA-helicasic activity. Dicer recognizes the double-strand region of the pre-miR in association with different proteins: RDE-4 (RNAi *defective* 4) in *C. elegans*, R2D2 e FMR1 (fragile X mental retardation syndrome 1 homolog) in *D. melanogaster*, and members of the Argonaute family in other species. In particular, these proteins are not needed for the endonucleasic activity of Dicer, but they play a role in stabilizing the complex Dicer-miR [5]. In mammalians, the Argonaute 2 (AGO2) protein complex, characterized by RNAse H activity, cooperates in the Dicer-mediated processing of some pre-miRs, yielding to another intermediate processing product, called AGO2-cleaved precursor miR (ac-pre-miR) [4].

The mature single-stranded microRNA product is then incorporated in the complex known as *miRNA-containing ribonucleoprotein complex* (miRNP), miRgonaute, or *miRNA-containing RNA-induced silencing complex* (miRISC), which generally selects one of the two strands as guide strand (mature miR) according to thermodynamic properties, whereas the other strand is likely subjected to degradation. miRISC is a ribonucleoproteic complex containing Argonaute proteins, the mature miR, the star miR, and several additional factors, some of them necessary for the enzymatic activity. Argonaute proteins are conserved among species and containing the PAZ and PIWI domains. The PAZ domain is involved in the recognition of the microRNA [6], whereas the PIWI domain seems to be involved in releasing the mature microRNA through an interaction with Dicer [7]. In *H. sapiens,* miRISC complex is formed by the Argonaute homologue eIF2C2 protein, the glycine–tryptophan protein of 182 kDa (GW182), and the helicases Gemin3 and Gemin4 [8]. The choice of the pre-miR strand that will

19 Current and Future Developments in Cancer Therapy Research…

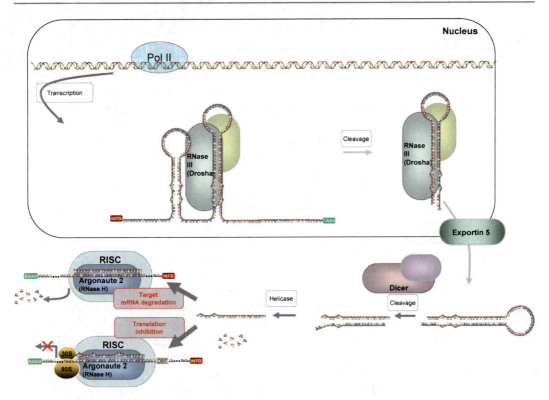

Fig. 19.1 Biogenesis, processing, and maturation of miRNAs. miRNAs are transcribed mainly by RNA polymerase II as long primary transcripts characterized by hairpin structures (pri-miRNAs) and processed in the nucleus by RNAse III Drosha in a 70-nucleotide-long pre-miRNA. This precursor molecule is exported by the exportin 5 to the cytoplasm, where RNAse III Dicer generates a dsRNA of approximately 22 nucleotides, named miRNA/miRNA*. The mature miRNA product is then incorporated in the complex known as miRISC, whereas the other strand is usually subjected to degradation. As part of this complex, the mature miRNA is able to regulate gene expression binding through partial homology the 3′-UTR of target mRNAs and leading to mRNA degradation in case of perfect matching or translation inhibition when there is partial complementarity. *RISC* RNA-induced silencing complex

generate the active complex resides in the relative thermodynamic stability of the two strands forming the duplex: the strand with a more unstable 5′-end is included in the miRISC complex.

As part of this complex, the mature microRNA is able to regulate gene expression at posttranscriptional level, binding through partial complementarity to the 3′-UTR of target mRNAs, and leading to some degree of mRNA degradation and translation inhibition (Fig. 19.1).

MicroRNAs exert their function mostly binding a specific sequence within the 3′-UTR of target mRNAs. The 5′-end of microRNAs (seed site) is important in the target recognition mechanism [2]: nucleotides 2–8 (seed sites) of many miRNAs present a perfect match with the 3′-UTR seed regions involved in translational block and are also well conserved in homologue microRNAs.

MicroRNAs can regulate gene expression through the degradation of target mRNAs, concordantly with the evidence that mRNA levels can be reduced in presence of elevated levels of miRNAs. It has been demonstrated that a high complementary match between the microRNA and the target mRNA can lead to an Ago 2-mediated mRNA degradation. Recent studies suggested that also other processes are involved, like deadenylation, 5′-uncapping, and exonuclease activity. Indeed, mRNA degradation mechanism requires Ago 2 complex, GW182, and deadenylating and decapping enzymes [9].

Furthermore, the cleavage site does not depend on the match between miR and its target, but it is due to microRNA sequence only: the cleavage takes place between the corresponding mRNA residues of the 10th and the 11th nucleotide of the microRNA.

After the cleavage process, the microRNA remains intact and can drive the functioning of another miRISC complex [10]. However, the mechanisms underlying the mRNA target selection remain still unclear.

MicroRNAs can also inhibit gene expression blocking the translation of mRNAs target. The first evidence of this mechanism is the observation that many miR-targeted mRNAs maintain their level in presence of an abundance of the respective microRNAs, whereas the levels of the encoded protein are decreased [9]. The exact mechanism underlying the miRISC-mediated translational blockade remains still unknown: it is unclear whether the block overcomes at the beginning or in the next phases of the translational process. However, current models see the involvement of eIF4F, formed by eIF4A, eIF4E, and eIF4G. This proteic complex binds the 5'-cap of mRNAs and starts the translation initiation process. The translation initiation factor eIF3, interacting with eIF4G, contributes to the assembly of the ribosomal subunit 40S at the 5'-end of mRNAs and leads to the formation of the preinitiation complex. The elongation phase takes place when the ribosomal subunit 60S is assembled at the preinitiation complex in correspondence to the start codon AUG. eIF4G and eIF3 interact with the poly(A)-binding protein (PAPB1) resulting in mRNA circularization, phenomenon that leads to a higher translation efficiency [9]. A controversial body of evidence shows that microRNAs are able to inhibit both the preinitiation and the elongation phase. In 2006, Petersen et al. proposed a model in which miRISC acts as a repressor of the elongation phase, suggesting that miRISC can promote an early dissociation of the ribosome from the mRNA [11].

Controversially, three different models have been proposed to explain the initiation phase inhibition operated by miRISC:

In the first model, miRISC competes with eIF4E for the binding to the 5'-cap of the target mRNA, thus leading to the inhibition of the translational start; in the second model, miRISC blocks the mRNA circularization through the inhibition of the assembly of the 60S subunit with the 40S subunit, located on the target mRNA at the preinitiation complex.

The synergic action of multiple miRISC complexes leads to an efficient block of the translation process [12] explaining the presence of multiple seed regions within the same target.

MicroRNAs can also act through a different mechanism mediated by miRISC: the target mRNAs are seized into cytoplasmic foci called processing bodies (P-bodies), formed by mRNA and proteins [13]; since P-bodies lack of the translational machinery, this mechanism leads to a translational blockade of the sequestered mRNAs. In some instance, a deadenylation process coupled with the translational inhibition has been reported [9]. The deadenylation process is mediated by GW182 and Ago proteins. Whereas GW182 interacts with Ago through its glycine- and tryptophan-rich domains, it is also able to recruit through his C-terminus PAPB and the deadenylating enzymes CCR4 and CAF1 [4]. Furthermore, it has been observed that the number, the position, and the kind of nucleotide mismatches between the microRNA and the mRNA can play a role in the repression mechanism selection, deciding if the target mRNA would be degraded or translationally repressed.

MicroRNAs in Human Cancer: From Profiling Studies to Definition of a Functional Role as Oncogenes and Tumor Suppressors

Profiling of different cell types and tissues indicated that the pattern of miRNA expression is cell type and tissue specific, suggesting that the program regulating expression of miRNAs is exquisitely cell type dependent and tightly associated with cellular differentiation and development. Some of the most important miRNAs which are aberrantly expressed in tumors are listed in Table 19.1.

The first evidence of the involvement of microRNAs in human cancer derived from studies on chronic lymphocytic leukemia (CLL), the most common human leukemia in the Western world, particularly in an attempt to identify tumor suppressors at chromosome 13q14. Cytogenetic studies indicate deletions at chr.13q14 in approximately 50% of CLLs and loss of heterozygosity

19 Current and Future Developments in Cancer Therapy Research...

Table 19.1 MicroRNAs aberrantly expressed in tumors

Tumor type	Upregulated miRNA	Downregulated miRNA	Target
CLL		miR-29, miR-181	TCL1
	miR-155		
		miR-15a, miR-16-1	BCL2
AML		miR-29	MCL1
			DNMT
Lymphoma	miR-155		
	miR-17-92		PTEN, BIM,E2F1
	miR-106b-25		E2F1
MM	miR-21		
	miR-19a, miR-19b		SOCS1
Breast cancer	miR-21		PTEN, PDCD4, TPM1
		miR-125b	HER2, HER3
		miR-205	HER3
		miR-10b (associated with metastasis)	HOXD10
	miR-373		
		miR-200	ZEB
Lung cancer		let-7	RAS, HMGA2, C-MYC
	miR-155		
HCC		miR-122a	Cyclin G1
	miR-221		p27
		miR-34a	MET

(LOH) in approximately 70% of CLLs. By taking advantage of chromosome translocations and small deletions, Dr. Croce's group found that the critical region of 13q14 does not contain a protein-coding tumor suppressor gene but two microRNA genes, miR-15a and miR-16-1, that are expressed in the same polycistronic RNA. This result indicated that the deletion of chromosome 13q14 caused the loss of these two microRNAs, first evidence that microRNAs could be involved in the pathogenesis of human cancer [14]. Study of a large collection of CLLs showed knock down or knock out of miR-15a and miR-16-1 in approximately 69% of CLLs. Since such alteration is present in most indolent CLLs, they speculated that loss of miR-15a and miR-16-1 could be the initiating event or a very early event in the pathogenesis of this disease [14]. Immediately after these initial observations, they mapped all the known microRNA genes and found that many of them are located in regions of the genome involved in chromosomal alterations, such as deletion or amplification, in many different human tumors, in which the presumed tumor suppressor genes or oncogenes, respectively, failed to be discovered after many years of investigation [15]. Indeed, in cancer development chromosomal regions that encompass microRNAs involved in the negative regulation of a transcript encoding a known tumor suppressor may be amplified. This amplification would result in the increased expression of the microRNA and the consequent silencing of the tumor suppressor gene. Vice versa, microRNAs able to inhibit oncogenes are often located in fragile regions of the genome, where deletions or mutations can be responsible for their reduced levels and the resulting overexpression of the target oncogene (Fig. 19.2).

We can certainly affirm that alterations in microRNAs expression are not isolated, but the rule in human cancer. After these early studies indicating the role of microRNA genes in the pathogenesis of human cancer, Dr. Croce's group and others have developed platforms to assess the global expression of microRNA genes in normal and diseased tissues, and have carried out profiling studies to assess microRNA dysregulation in

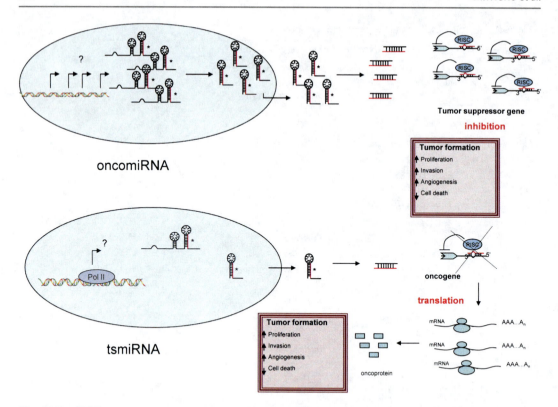

Fig. 19.2 miRNAs as oncogenes or tumor suppressor genes. miRNAs can have oncogenic effects (oncomiRNA) when they target tumor suppressor genes. When an oncomiRNA is overexpressed, for example, because the encoding gene is located in an amplified region of the genome, this will lead to downregulation of the targets and to tumor formation (*upper panel*). Conversely, a miRNA can be characterized by tumor suppressor properties if the main target in that specific cellular context is an oncogene; in this case, if the miRNA expression is lost, for example, because the encoding gene is located in a deleted region of the genome, the resulting effect will be tumorigenic (*lower panel*). In summary, what usually happens in a tumor is the overexpression of an oncogenic miRNA and/or the loss of a miRNA with oncosuppressive properties

human cancer. This was an attempt to establish whether microRNA profiling could be used for tumor classification, diagnosis, and prognosis [16].

Indeed, the predictive values of such microRNA signature have been validated for several types of tumors. Furthermore, the small size of miRNAs certainly contributes to a higher stability in comparison with mRNAs, allowing the study of their expression in fixed tissues or other biological material, and thus supporting their possible use as novel, minimally invasive, and robust biomarkers: indeed, it has been recently described how miRNAs can be reliably extracted and detected from paraffin-embedded tissues, from blood (either total blood, plasma, or serum) [17] and from circulating exosomes [18]. Moreover, it has been reported that the profile of circulating miRNA of individuals affected by different neoplasias can reflect the pattern observed in the tumor tissues, evidence suggesting the fascinating possibility of using circulating miRNAs as easily detectable tumor biomarkers [19], especially for early diagnosis: very recently, Sozzi's group [20] has identified microRNA-expression signatures with strong predictive, diagnostic, and prognostic potential, analyzing plasma samples of lung cancer patients collected 1–2 years before the onset of disease.

Concerning breast cancer, for example, a pilot study performed by Roth et al. [21] provided the first evidence that tumor-associated circulating microRNAs are elevated in the blood of breast cancer patients and associated with tumor progression. In particular, the authors evaluated the relative concentrations of breast cancer-associated miR-10b, miR-34a, miR-141, and miR-155 in the blood serum of 89 patients with primary breast cancer and metastatic disease and 29 healthy women, finding that miR-10b, miR-34a, and miR-155 discriminated M1-patients from healthy controls.

Heneghan et al. [22] surveyed a panel of seven candidate miRNAs in whole blood RNAs from 148 breast cancer patients and 44 age-matched and disease-free controls. They found that the expression of miR-195 was significantly elevated in breast cancer patients and reduced in postoperative whole blood compared to the preoperative samples of the same patients. Zhao et al. [23] performed a microarray-based microRNA profiling in plasma samples from 20 women with early stage breast cancer (10 Caucasian American (CA) and 10 African American (AA) and 20 matched healthy controls (10 CAs and 10 AAs), demonstrating that the altered levels of circulating miRNAs might have great potential to serve as novel, noninvasive biomarkers for early detection of breast cancer.

Switching then from profiling studies to the definition of a functional role of microRNAs, it has been demonstrated that their aberrant expression in cancer is not just a random association, but the indication of a causal role exerted by these small RNA molecules in the tumorigenic process. Indeed, due to the role of microRNAs in regulating the expression of signaling molecules, such as cytokine, growth factors, proapoptotic and antiapoptotic genes, it has been demonstrated that miRNAs can act either as oncogenes or tumor suppressor, and more recently, it has been demonstrated that a microRNA can exploit both functions according to the cellular context of its target genes. Another important issue concerns the role of miRNAs in regulating the interaction between cancer cells and the microenvironment, particularly concerning neo-angiogenesis or tissue invasion and metastasis.

Leukemia/Lymphoma

Chronic Lymphocytic Leukemia

As mentioned, the first evidence of alterations of microRNA genes in human cancer came from studies of CLL. In a large study of indolent versus aggressive CLL, Calin et al. discovered a signature of 13 microRNAs capable of distinguishing between indolent and aggressive CLL [24]. Interestingly, it was found that miR-155, overexpressed in different lymphomas including the ABC type of diffuse large B-cell lymphoma, is also upregulated in aggressive CLLs (where it is induced by MYB, [25], whereas members of the miR-29 family and miR-181 were found to be underexpressed and later demonstrated to directly regulate the TCL1 oncogene, overexpressed in the aggressive form of CLL [26].

More recently, a prognostic signature has been identified in CLL patients with chromosome 17p deletions (who develop a more aggressive disease), revealing that miR-15a, miR-21, miR-34a, miR-155, and miR-181b are differentially expressed in comparison with normal 17p and normal karyotype. Moreover, miR-21 expression levels were significantly higher in patients with poor prognosis and predicted overall survival (OS), and miR-181b expression levels significantly predicted treatment-free survival [27].

Because of the "wait and watch" approach to the treatment of CLL, a signature able to distinguish between CLL with good and bad prognosis was also found. Sequencing of many microRNAs, including those in the signature, allowed the identification of germ line and somatic mutations of microRNA genes, including miR-15 and miR-16-1 and miR-29 family members. Interestingly, mutations in the miR-15/16 precursor were also identified, affecting the processing of the pri-miR into the pre-miR. In two cases, the mutant was in homozygosity in the leukemic cells, while normal cells of the two patients were heterozygous for this abnormality, indicating a loss of the normal miR-15/16 allele in the leukemic cell [24]. Thus miR-15a and miR-16-1 behave like typical tumor suppressors in CLL. Interestingly, Raveche et al. [28] mapped a gene responsible for an indolent form of CLL in the New Zealand Black (NZB) mouse strain on chromosome 14, in a region homologous to 13q14 in humans. Sequence analysis of this region showed a mutation in the precursor of miR-15/16 in the NZB mouse strain 6 nts 3′ to miR-16-1 (in the human cases, the mutation was 7 nts 3′ to miR-16-1), that also affected the processing of the miR-15/16 precursor. Thus, germline mutation of miR-15/16 can cause the indolent form of CLL both in human and mouse. By using different algorithms to identify targets of miR-15a and miR-16-1, it was found that BCL2, an oncogene protecting cells from apoptosis, was a putative target of both miR-15a and miR-16-1. Knock-down experiments showed this to be the case [29]. Thus, loss of miR-15a and miR-16-1 leads to high constitutive level of the oncogene BCL2, contributing to the development of an indolent B-cell leukemia. In follicular lymphoma, another common indolent B-cell malignancy, BCL2 gene becomes dysregulated as result of a t(14; 18) chromosome translocation, because of its juxtaposition to immunoglobulin enhancers, indicating that constitutive overexpression of BCL2 causes an indolent B-cell tumor. Moreover, it was also found that loss of miR-15a and miR-16-1 causes, although indirectly, overexpression of MCL1, another oncogene of the BCL2 family of inhibitors of apoptosis [30]. Interestingly, a recent clinical trial of CLL patients with ABT737, an inhibitor of BCL2 developed by Abbott, showed partial resistance of the leukemic cells to the drug, because ABT737 is specific for BCL2 but not for MCL1. Thus, treatment with either miR-15a or miR-16-1 may abrogate the resistance to the drug and improve the responsiveness. Additional experiments in vitro and in vivo also showed that miR-15a or miR-16-1 can be exploited to cause death of leukemic cells, suggesting the possibility of a microRNA-based therapeutic intervention [30].

To further demonstrate a causal role of miR-15a and miR-16-1 loss in the occurrence of CLL, Klein et al. [31] have applied a genetic approach generating sophisticated mouse models that have either deletion of DLEU2 (a noncoding RNA gene including the miR-15a and miR-16-1 cluster in its intron 4) together with both miRNA genes (MDR deleted) or deletion of the two miRNA genes only. After 15–18 months, about 5% of the animals displayed monoclonal B-cell lymphocytosis, which is a possible precursor to CLL. More importantly, 1/5 of the MDR-deleted and 1/8 of the miR-15a/16-1 deleted mice developed CLL or the related small cell lymphocytic

leukemia. In addition, 9% of the MDR-deleted and 2% of the miR-15a/16-1-deleted animals developed a phenotype reminiscent of human diffuse large B-cell lymphoma, a disease known to progress from CLL at low frequency. Thus, the deletion of the MDR caused B-cell lymphoproliferative disorders, nicely recapitulating the spectrum of human CLL phenotypes.

More recently, Fabbri et al. [32] have shed more light into the molecular mechanisms behind the involvement of miR-15a and miR-16-1 in the biology of CLL, describing a feedback regulatory loop connecting miR-15a and miR-16-1, p53 and miR-34b/34c cluster, which critically influences the pathogenesis of CLL. The oncosuppressor p53 is indeed at the same time directly targeted by miR-15a and miR-16-1 and able to induce the expression of these microRNAs and of miR-34b/34c, which in turn directly regulate ZAP70. In this model, the loss of miR-15a/miR-16-1 expression, represented by CLLs with 13q deletions, not only shifts the balance toward higher levels of the antiapoptotic proteins BCL2 and myeloid cell leukemia sequence 1 (BCL2-related) (MCL1), as previously demonstrated, but also toward higher levels of the tumor suppressor protein TP53. Consequently, in patients with CLLs with 13q deletions, while the number of apoptotic cells may decrease because of the increased levels of antiapoptotic proteins, the TP53 tumor suppressor pathway remains intact, thus keeping the increase in tumor burden relatively low. This novel finding explains how 13q deletions are associated with the indolent form of CLL. Moreover, increased TP53 levels, as found in patients with CLLs with 13q deletions, are associated with transactivation of miR-34b/miR-34c and reduced levels of ZAP70, a tyrosine kinase relevant in the initial step of T-cell receptor-mediated signal transduction. Low expression levels of ZAP70 have been found to be positively correlated with survival in patients with CLL, further explaining the indolent course of CLL carrying 13q deletions.

Acute Myelocytic Leukemia

Acute myelocytic leukemia (AML) is a heterogeneous disease that includes several entities with different genetic abnormalities and clinical features. Garzon et al. have reported unique microRNA profiles in the main molecular and cytogenetic subgroups of AML. In addition, a subset of these microRNAs was associated with overall and disease-free survival [33]. Another study identified a microRNA-expression signature with prognostic significance in patients with AML belonging to the molecular high-risk group, including 12 microRNAs associated with event-free survival [34]. Five probes represented miR-181a and miR-181b; their increased expression was associated with a decreased risk of an event (failure to achieve CR, relapse, or death). This result was confirmed by a subsequent study showing that upregulated miR-181a predicted favorable outcome in CN-AML (AML with normal cytogenetics) [35].

Members of the miR-29 family are located in two clusters on two human chromosomes: miR-29b1/29a is located on chromosome 7q32, while miR-29b2/c is located on chromosome 1q23. Importantly, chromosome 7q is the region frequently deleted in myelodysplastic syndrome (MDS) and therapy-related AML [36]. Members of the miR-29 family have been shown to be downregulated in aggressive CLL [24], invasive breast cancer [37], lung cancer [38], and cholangiocarcinoma [39]. Transfection of miR-29b induces apoptosis in cholangiocarcinoma cell lines and reduces the tumorigenicity of lung cancer cells in nude mice. Moreover, it was shown that rhabdomyosarcoma looses miR-29 expression because of an elevation of NFkB and YY1 levels, and introduction of miR-29s into the tumor delays rhabdomyosarcoma progression in mice [40]. MiR-29s were also found to directly target MCL1 [39], an oncogene overexpressed in AMLs, and the de novo DNA methyltransferases DNMT-3A and -3B, while indirectly, through regulation of the transactivator Sp1, the maintenance DNA methyltransferase DNMT1 [35, 38]. Thus loss of miR-29 family members results in the constitutive overexpression of MCL1 and of DNMT, causing epigenetic changes characteristic of AML. These recent results suggest that loss of miR-29s may be important, perhaps critical, for the pathogenesis of a major group of MDSs and AMLs (Fig. 19.3).

Lymphoma

Early studies have shown that miR-155 is upregulated in a subgroup of Burkitt's lymphoma, diffuse large B-cell lymphoma (DLBCL), primary mediastinal B-cell lymphoma (PMBL), and Hodgkin's lymphoma [41, 42]. This microRNA is encoded by the terminal portion of the BIC (B-cell integration cluster) gene, which was originally identified as a common retroviral integration site in avian-leukosis-virus-induced B-cell lymphomas [43]. Dr. Croce's group demonstrated that mice overexpressing miR-155 in B lymphocytes develop polyclonal preleukemic pre-B-cell proliferation followed by full-blown B-cell malignancy [44]. Moreover, two knock-out mice models have demonstrated a critical role of miR-155 in immunity by showing that BIC/miR-155$^{-/-}$ have defective dendritic cell functions, impaired cytokine secretion, and T_H cells intrinsically biased toward T_H2 differentiation [45, 46]. Moreover, miR-155 could represent the connection between inflammation, immunity, and cancer since its expression can be induced by mediators of inflammation and is involved in response to endotoxic shock [47].

He et al. [48] reported that miR-17-92 polycistron was upregulated in 65% of B-cell lymphoma patients and demonstrated in a mouse model that this miR cluster cooperates with the oncogene MYC in accelerating tumor development. More recently, a different group observed that the overexpression of miR-17-92 in lymphocytes caused a lymphoproliferative disease, autoimmunity, and premature death [49]. The enhanced proliferation of the transgenic lymphocytes was mediated by direct regulation of proapoptotic PTEN and Bim. O'Donnell et al. [50] investigated the regulation of miR-17-92 in lymphoma, demonstrating that the expression of this cluster is directly activated by the oncogene c-Myc. Moreover, miR-17-92 cluster, as well as its paralog, miR-106b-25 [51], establishes with the transcription factor E2F1, a downstream target of c-Myc, a negative feedback loop: E2F1 represents indeed a direct target of the two microRNA clusters, but it also induces their expression. Thus, MYC simultaneously activates E2F1 transcription and limits its expression, allowing a tightly controlled proliferative signal.

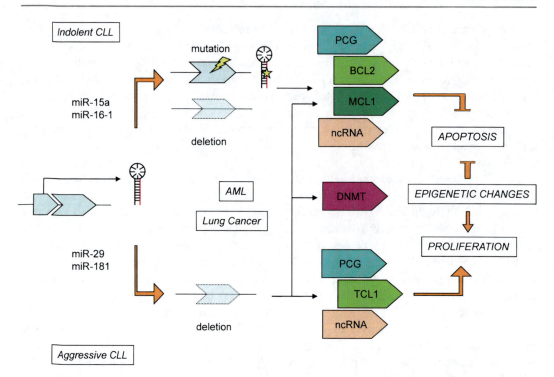

Fig. 19.3 Molecular alterations in CLL and AML. Deletion or downregulation of *miR-15a/miR-16-1* cluster, located at chromosome 13q14.3 and directly involved in the regulation of *BCL2* and *MCL1* expression, represents an early event in the pathogenesis of CLL. During the evolution of malignant clones, other miRNAs (miRs) can be deleted (such as *miR-29*) or overexpressed (such as *miR-155*), contributing to the aggressiveness of B-CLL. Such abnormalities can influence the expression of other protein-coding genes (PCGs), such as the *TCL1* oncogene, directly regulated by *miR-29* and *miR-181*, or affect other noncoding RNAs (ncRNAs). The consequences of this steady accumulation of abnormalities are represented by the reduction of apoptosis and the induction of survival and proliferation of malignant B cells, leading to the evolution of more aggressive clones. Members of the *miR-29* family, lost in AML and in other tumor types as lung cancer, have also been shown to directly target *MCL1* and *DNMT3A* and *B* (adapted from Iorio MV, Croce CM. MicroRNAs in cancer: small molecules with a huge impact. J Clin Oncol. 2009;27(34):5848–56. Reprinted with permission. © 2008 American Society of Clinical Oncology. All rights reserved)

Multiple Myeloma

Few recent reports have linked microRNAs to this plasma cell malignancy, as the aberrant expression of miR-335, miR-342-3p, and miR-561 in comparison to normal plasma cells [52] or the Stat3-mediated activation of the oncogenic miR-21 in response to IL-6 [53]. Mir-15a and miR-16-1 have been described as oncosuppressor microRNAs also in this tumor subtype [54–56]. Pichiorri et al. [57] described a microRNA signature characteristic of this neoplasia. They evaluated by both microarray analysis and real-time PCR the expression of microRNAs in MM-derived cell lines, CD138+ bone marrow PCs from subjects with MM or monoclonal gammopathy of undetermined significance (MGUS), and normal donors, identifying the oncogenic miR-21 and miR-181 among the microRNAs aberrantly expressed. Two miRNAs, miR-19a and 19b, part of the miR-17-92 cluster, were also shown to downregulate expression of SOCS-1, a gene frequently silenced in MM that plays a critical role inhibiting IL-6 growth signaling. Moreover, xenograft studies using human MM cell lines treated with miR-19a and b precursors or miR-181a and b antagonists resulted in significant suppression of tumor growth in nude mice, confirming the involvement of these microRNAs in the development of multiple myeloma (MM). More recently, the same group [58] have demonstrated that miR-192, 194, and 215, which are downregulated in a subset of newly diagnosed MMs, can be

19 Current and Future Developments in Cancer Therapy Research...   527

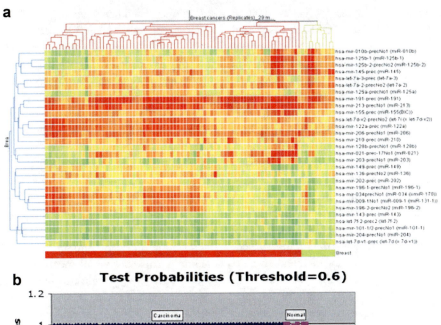

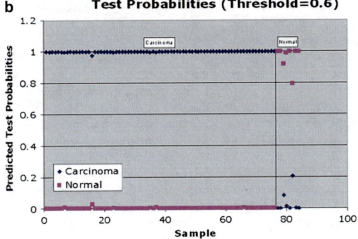

Fig. 19.4 Cluster analysis and PAM prediction in breast cancer and normal breast tissues. (**a**) Tree generated by a cluster analysis showing the separation of breast cancer from normal tissues on the basis of miRNA differentially expressed ($P<0.05$) between breast cancer and normal tissue. The *bar* at the bottom indicates the group of cancer samples (*red*) or the group of normal breast tissues (*yellow*). (**b**) PAM analysis displaying the graphical representation of the probabilities (0.0–1.0) of each sample for being a cancerous or a normal tissue (adapted from Iorio MV, Ferracin M, Liu CG, et al. MicroRNA gene expression deregulation in human breast cancer. Cancer Res. 2005;65:7065–70)

transcriptionally activated by p53 and modulate MDM2 expression. In addition, miR-192 and 215 target the IGF pathway, preventing enhanced migration of plasma cells into bone marrow.

MicroRNAs in Solid Malignancies

MicroRNAs in Breast Cancer

One of the first solid tumors to be profiled for microRNAs expression was, in 2005, breast cancer. Iorio et al. [37] described indeed the first microRNA signature characteristic of breast carcinoma, identifying 13 microRNAs able to discriminate tumors and normal tissues with an accuracy of 100% (Fig. 19.4). Among the most significant microRNAs differentially expressed, some were extensively studied since their initial discovery and revealed an important role on the biology of breast cancer: miR-21, overexpressed in breast carcinoma, has been demonstrated to mediate cell survival and proliferation directly targeting the oncosuppressor genes PTEN, PDCD4, and TPM1, and it has been associated with advanced clinical stage, lymph node metastasis, and patient poor prognosis [59, 60] also in PABC (pregnancy-associated breast cancer) [61]. miR-21 has been also detected as circulating microRNA, freely present in the circulation [62, 63] or in exosomes, as described in ovarian cancer [64]. Very recently, Ota et al. [65] have interestingly demonstrated that increased expression of miR-21 can be found in bone marrow of breast cancer patients, and that the level of this microRNA and its target PDCD4 have a prognostic value.

Moreover, miR-21, one of the first cancer microRNAs described, has been found overexpressed in a variety of other malignancies: glioblastoma [66, 67], ovary [68], lung [69, 70], and more [71]. In colorectal cancer and pancreas endocrine and exocrine tumor, miR-21 overexpression is also associated with poor survival and poor therapeutic outcome [72–74].

Conversely, downregulated microRNAs, as miR-125a and b and miR-205, regulate oncogenes as tyrosine kinase receptors HER2 and HER3, respectively [75, 76].

Let-7, tumor suppressor miR initially discovered in *C. elegans*, where it induces cell cycle exit and terminal differentiation, has been described as a new regulator of self-renewal and tumorigenicity of breast cancer cells [77], targeting molecules originally described in lung cancer: RAS [78] as well as the oncogene HMGA2 [79], and even MYC itself [80]. Overexpression of let-7 miRNA family can suppress tumor development in mouse models of breast and lung cancer [77, 81].

In the signature published in 2005, we could also identify miRNAs differentially expressed according to specific biopathological features, such as grade and stage of the disease, vascular invasion, proliferation index, and expression of hormone receptors [37]. In particular, we could identify a panel of miRNAs differentially expressed in estrogen receptor (ER)+ *versus* ER− breast carcinoma patients, being miR-191 and miR-26, the most significantly overexpressed, and *miR-206*, the most significantly downmodulated.

miR-206 has been lately demonstrated by another group to directly target ERα [82]. Moreover, Foekens et al. described a subset of miRNAs significantly associated with ER + luminal signature, identifying in particular four miRNAs associated with breast cancer aggressiveness [83]. Among them, miR-128a has also been implicated in the resistance to AI (aromatase inhibitor) letrozole [84]. In a recent study performed in Dr. Croce's laboratory, we demonstrated [85] that miR-221 and miR-222 are involved in a negative feedback regulation with ERalpha, been able to directly target the receptor (as demonstrated also by Zhao et al. [86], which in turn represses the transcription of the two miRNAs through direct binding to responsive elements on their promoter sequences. Moreover, other groups have demonstrated that overexpression of *miR-221* and *miR-222* is responsible for resistance to antiestrogenic therapies, such as tamoxifen [86, 87] and fulvestrant [88].

Our group particularly focused on the study of miR-205 involvement in breast cancer biology. Previous studies showed that miR-205 expression is significantly underexpressed in human breast cancer [89, 90] and associated with absence of vascular invasion [37], although it has also been shown to be upregulated in other tumors types, as ovarian cancer [68]. We recently demonstrated [89] that miR-205 is able to interfere with the HER receptor family-mediated survival pathway by directly targeting HER3 receptor and thus inhibiting its downstream mediator Akt. In addition, other studies indicated that miR-205 is a negative regulator of the epithelial–mesenchymal transition (EMT), an early phase of the process of metastasis, targeting the transcription factors ZEB1 and ZEB2, and that expression of miR-205 is lost in mesenchymal breast cancer cell lines [91] and triple-negative breast cancer [92]. Moreover, miR-205 also targets VEGF-A, a factor which plays a key role in the process of invasion and metastasis [90]. Finally, in a very recent study, silencing of miR-200 family and miR-205 has been associated with EMT and acquisition of stem-like properties in carcinogen-induced transformation of human lung epithelial cells [93].

19 Current and Future Developments in Cancer Therapy Research...

Table 19.2 miRNAs in human breast cancer

Name	Localization	Expression and role	Targets
miR-21	17q23.2	Overexpressed Amplified Oncogenic role	*BCL2* *TPM1* *PDCD4*
miR-155	21p21.3	Overexpressed	
miR-206	6p12.2	Overexpressed	*ERα*
miR-125a	19q13.41	Downmodulated Oncosuppressor Downmodulated	*ERBB2, ERBB3*
miR-125b	11q24.1	Deleted Oncosuppressor	*ERBB2, ERBB3*
miR-145	5q32	Downmodulated	
miR-10b	2q31.1	Downmodulated but associated with metastatic potential	*Homeobox D10*
miR-9-1	1q22	Downmodulated, hypermethylated	
miR-27a	19p13.12	Oncogenic role in MDA-MB-231 cells	*ZBTB10*
miR-17-5p	13q31.3	Oncosuppressor in breast cells lines	*AIB1*
Let-7	[a]	Downmodulated Reduced in BT-ICs	*RAS* *HMGA2*

Modified from Iorio MV, Casalini P, Tagliabue E, et al. MicroRNA profiling as a tool to understand prognosis, therapy response and resistance in breast cancer. Eur J Cancer. 44(18):2753–9. ©2008. With permission from Elsevier
[a]Members of *Let-7* family have different chromosomal localization

Table 19.2 summarizes the information available to date about some of the most important miRNAs involved in human breast cancer, and the cartoon reported in Fig. 19.5 illustrates the involvement of microRNAs in the complicated network of molecules regulating breast cancer biology.

Lung Cancer

One of the first oncosuppressor microRNAs identified is let-7a, which regulates RAS [78] as well as the oncogene HMGA2 [78, 79], and even MYC itself [80]. Overexpression of let-7 microRNA family can suppress tumor development in mouse models of breast and lung cancer [77, 81]. In the two most common forms of non-small cell lung cancers (adenocarcinomas and squamous cell carcinomas), high expression of miR-155 and low expression of oncosuppressor let-7 correlate with poor prognosis [69]. The association of let-7a with survival was also confirmed by an independent study performed by Yu et al. [94], who identified a miR signature as independent predictor of cancer relapse and survival of NSCLC (non-small cell lung cancers) patients.

As in other tumor types, also in lung cancer, microRNAs can represent accurate diagnostic markers. However, data are not always consistent: whereas in 2009, it has been described that squamous and nonsquamous NSCLCs can be distinguished according to the expression of miR-205 [95]; more recently, another group [96] underlines how, despite the relative quantification of miR-205 and miR-21 seems to be a promising diagnostic tool to discriminate adenocarcinomas (ADCs) compared with squamous cell carcinomas (SQCCs), the molecular approach is still not completely satisfactory as it may misclassify a nonnegligible percentage of cases. Therefore, the authors state that it cannot represent a substitute of accurate morphologic and immunophenotypical characterization of tumors, but it could be used as an adjunctive diagnostic criterion in selected cases.

MicroRNAs have also been found in the circulation in lung cancer patients, either free or associated with exosomes: Rabinowits et al. [97] found a similarity between the circulating exosomal miRNA and the tumor-derived miRNA patterns; in addition Hu et al. [98] found that

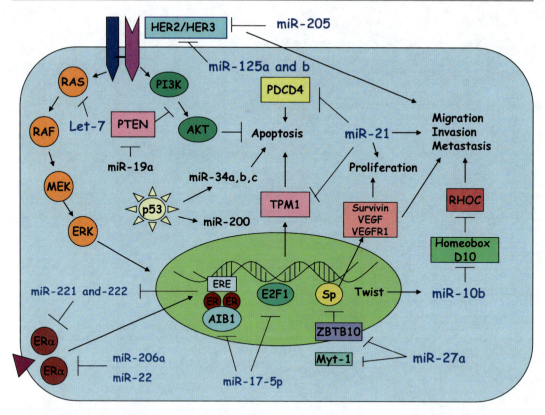

Fig. 19.5 miRNAs take their place in breast cancer biology. Summary of the interconnections between miRNAs and tumor suppressor genes and oncogenes in breast cancer (adapted from Iorio MV, Casalini P, Tagliabue E, et al. MicroRNA profiling as a tool to understand prognosis, therapy response and resistance in breast cancer. Eur J Cancer. 44(18):2753–9. ©2008. With permission from Elsevier)

levels of four miRNAs (i.e., miR-486, miR-30d, miR-1, and miR-499) present in the serum of lung cancer patients were significantly associated with overall survival. More recently, Sozzi's group [20] has identified microRNA-expression signatures with strong predictive, diagnostic, and prognostic potential analyzing plasma samples of lung cancer patients collected 1–2 years before the onset of disease, thus suggesting their possible use as noninvasive biomarkers for early diagnosis.

Notably, microRNAs are also stably present in sputum and can be used as highly sensitive and specific markers for early detection of lung adenocarcinoma, in particular, a panel of four microRNAs (miR-21, miR-486, miR-375, and miR-200b) [99].

miR-200c, demonstrated to inhibit the EMT process in breast cancer [91], is lost in more aggressive and invasive NSCLC (non-small cell lung cancer) cell lines and associated with chemoresistance [100].

MiR-21, known onco-microRNA in several human tumors, seems to play an important role also in lung carcinogenesis, both in smokers and in never-smokers, being overexpressed and further enhanced by the activated EGFR signaling pathway [101]. Moreover, it has been associated with disease progression and survival [102], also in stage I lung tumors, as recently reported [103].

Among the microRNAs acting as oncogenes, Garofalo et al. [104] have shown that miR-221 and 222 are overexpressed in aggressive non-small cell lung cancer and hepatocarcinoma cells, and that they induce TRAIL resistance and enhanced cellular migration by targeting PTEN and TIMP3 tumor suppressors and activation of AKT pathway and metallopeptidases. Moreover, they demonstrated that the MET oncogene is involved in miR-221 and 222 activation through the c-Jun transcription factor.

Focusing on *(c) hepatocellular carcinoma (HCC)*, Murakami et al. [105] reported that miR-222, miR-106a, and miR-17-92 clusters are associated with the degree of tumor differentiation, while high levels of the oncosuppressor miR-125b correlate with good survival [106]. MiR-125b has also been shown to induce growth inhibition in vitro in a model of human thyroid anaplastic carcinoma [107]. Other studies focused on the identification of molecules targeted by microRNAs deregulated in HCC: miR-122a, downmodulated in HCC, directly regulates Cyclin G1 [108], and miR-221, upregulated in this neoplasia, directly targets p27 [109], as also shown in thyroid cancer [107], and contributes to liver tumorigenesis [110], glioblastoma [111], prostate cancer [112], and melanoma [113]. One of the first evidences proving miR alteration in human melanoma is a genomic study performed by Zhang et al. [114], who reported DNA copy abnormalities in microRNA genes also in two other epithelial tumors, breast, and ovary. Interestingly, the results obtained by this genomic analysis were largely overlapping with the expression profiles on the same tumor types [37, 68].

Interestingly, the downregulation of miR-26 has been associated to poor prognosis but better response to interferon therapy [115].

Ovarian Cancer

The first report of a putative involvement of miR-NAs in the biology of human ovarian cancer was the genomic study performed by Zhang et al., who used an array comparative genomic hybridization (aCGH) approach to identify miRNA loci gained/lost in ovarian cancer, breast cancer, and melanoma [114]. Many of the miRNAs resulting from this study were later confirmed to be differentially expressed in the miRNA expression profiling performed by our group in 2007 [68].

After this initial evidence, several groups have investigated the role of miRNAs in the pathogenesis of ovarian cancer, either as biomarkers, potential research tools, or targets for specific therapies. miRNA let-7i was recently found to be

a tumor suppressor significantly downregulated in platinum-resistant ovarian tumors, and let-7i gain of function restored drug sensitivity of chemoresistant ovarian cancer cells, thus representing a candidate biomarker and therapeutic target [116]. An oncosuppressive role for miR-15/16 has been described also in ovarian cancer, where these two miRNAs regulate the expression of the oncogenic protein Bmi1 [117].

In another study, 27 miRNAs significantly associated with chemotherapy response, showing that (similar to DNA methylation) miRNAs represent possible prognostic and diagnostic biomarkers for ovarian cancer [118]. miR-214 has been reported to target PTEN, thus contributing to cisplatin resistance [119]. Interestingly, levels of *Dicer* and *Drosha* mRNA in ovarian cancer cells have been associated with clinical outcome [120].

Circulating microRNAs have been found in sera of ovarian cancer patients: levels of eight microRNAs (miR-21, miR-141, miR-200a, miR-200c, miR-200b, miR-203, miR-205, and miR-214), previously demonstrated as diagnostic, were compared in exosomes isolated from sera specimens of women with benign disease and various stages of ovarian cancer, and the expression profile resulted similar between tumor cells and tumor-derived exosomes in comparison with respective controls [120].

Interestingly, miR-200c, downregulated in breast cancer, where it inhibits the EMT process [121], is overexpressed in ovarian cancer [68], where the targeting of ZEB1 and 2 mediates the opposite phenomenon, the mesenchymal to epithelial transition (MET) [122].

MicroRNAs in Invasion, Angiogenesis, and Metastasis

MicroRNAs have been demonstrated to exert a crucial role not only in controlling the primary tumor growth by regulating pathways involved in cell cycle and proliferation, but also to be determinant in modulating migration, invasion, and the interaction with the microenvironment, mechanisms related to the acquisition of a more aggressive phenotype, and promoting the onset of the metastatic process: the scientific world has coined the definition "metastomiRs."

One of the first studies reporting a prometastatic role for a miRNA was published by Ma et al. [123]. They observed that miR-10b was downmodulated in all the breast carcinomas from metastasis-free patients, as previously reported [37], but surprisingly, 50% of metastasis-positive patients had elevated miR-10b levels in their primary tumors. Induced by transcription factor Twist, miR-10b inhibits the translation of mRNA encoding homeobox D10 (HOXD10), releasing the expression of the prometastatic gene *RHOC* and, thus, leading to tumor cell invasion and metastasis.

The same group has later identified miR-9 as a new "metastomiR": activated by MYC and MYCN and correlated with tumor grade and metastatic status, miR-9 directly targets CDH1, the E-cadherin-encoding messenger RNA, leading to increased cell motility and invasiveness, activation of beta-catenin signaling, and upregulation of VEGF. Moreover, overexpression of miR-9 in otherwise nonmetastatic breast tumor cells enables these cells to form pulmonary micrometastases in mice. Conversely, inhibiting miR-9 by using a "miRNA sponge" in highly malignant cells inhibits metastasis formation [124].

Through a functional screen aimed to discover miRNAs promoting cell migration in vitro, Huang et al. [125] identified miR-373 and validated its metastatic potential in tumor transplantation experiments using breast cancer cells.

MiR-34a, which is lost in several tumor types and involved into the network mediated by the well-known "genome guardian" p53 [126], inhibits migration and invasion by downregulation of MET expression in human HCC cells [127]. Oncosuppressive miR-145 inhibits not only tumor growth but also cell invasion and metastasis by direct targeting of mucin 1 [128].

EMT is thought to promote malignant tumor progression, and several groups have recently investigated whether miRNAs are involved in this process, and there are data to support this hypothesis. Indeed, members of the miR-200 family of miRNAs and miR-205 have been shown to reduce cell migration and invasiveness

targeting ZEB transcription factors, known inducers of EMT [91, 129], and PKCε, as demonstrated in prostate cancer [130]. In addition ZEB1, which promotes not only tumor cell dissemination but also the tumor-initiating capacity, has been shown to repress expression of miR-200 family [131, 132] and stemness-inhibiting miR-203 [133].

The oncogenic *miR-21* stimulates intravasation, extravasation, and metastasis in different tumor types, included colorectal cancer [134] and breast cancer [135], whereas oncosuppressor miR-205 has the opposite effects, reducing invasion in vitro and suppressing lung metastasis in vivo [90]. With the same aim of searching for regulators of breast cancer metastasis, Tavazoie et al. [136] identified miR-126 and miR-335 as metastasis suppressors: reduced levels of the two miRNAs are associated with poor metastasis-free survival of breast cancer patients, while their reexpression inhibits metastasis in a cell transplantation model.

Interestingly, it has been recently observed that primary tumors and metastases from the same tissue show a similar pattern of miRNAs expression [137]. Being a more accurate classifier than mRNA expression studies, miRNA profiling has thus revealed the potential to solve one of the most demanding issues in cancer diagnostics: the origin of metastasis of unknown primary tumors.

In the metastatic process, neo-angiogenesis is the crucial step allowing cells to reach and disseminate through the systemic circulation. miRNAs can control tumor progression also at this level, either promoting or inhibiting the proliferation of endothelial cells. miR-221 and miR-222 repress the proliferative and angiogenic properties of c-Kit in endothelial cells [138], and miR-221 downregulation has been recently linked to tumor progression and recurrence in a high-risk prostate cancer [116], whereas hypoxic reduction of miR-16, miR-15b, miR-20a, and miR-20b expression directly targets VEGF, supporting the angiogenic process [139]. On the other hand, VEGF levels can be indirectly increased by miR-27b, through reduction of the zinc finger protein ZBTB10 and the consequent activation of Sp transcription factor [140], and by miR-126, through repression of Sprouty-related protein SPRED1 and phosphoinositol 3-kinase regulatory subunit 2 (PIK3R2) [141]. Angiogenesis can be also promoted by miR-210, activated by hypoxia and directly represses endothelial ligand ephrin A3 [142], and by the miR-17-92 cluster, which sustains MYC angiogenic properties through repression of connective tissue growth factor (CTGF) and the antiangiogenic adhesive glycoprotein thrombospondin 1 (TSP1) [143], also targeted by miR-27b and let-7f [144].

Interestingly, Dicer expression seems to be associated with metastatic properties: a microRNA family, miR-103/107, which attenuates miRNA biosynthesis by targeting Dicer, a key component of the miRNA processing machinery, is associated with metastasis and poor outcome in human breast cancer. Functionally, miR-103/107 confers migratory capacities in vitro and empowers metastatic dissemination of otherwise nonaggressive cells in vivo. Inhibition of miR-103/107 opposes migration and metastasis of malignant cells. At the cellular level, a key event fostered by miR-103/107 is induction of epithelial-to-mesenchymal transition (EMT), attained by downregulating miR-200 levels [145]. Metastasis suppression is also mediated by TAp63, a p53 family member, which coordinately regulates Dicer and miR-130b [146].

MicroRNA Expression Regulation

General Principles of miRNA Genomic Organization

miRNAs are frequently expressed as polycistronic transcripts. To date, 1,048 human miRNA precursor sequences have been deposited in miRBase [147]. Approximately one-third (390) of these miRNAs are located in 113 clusters, each measuring ≤51 kb in the human genome (51 kb being the longest distance between miRNAs belonging to the same cluster). These miRNA clusters are coexpressed based on evidence from miRNA profiling data from a variety of tissues and cell lines [148, 149]. Presentation of miRNA profiles in the form of expression clusters provides a readily interpretable summary of expression data and stresses the importance of cistronic expression regulation; dysregulation of one member of the cluster should be accompanied by similar dysregulation of other cluster members. Since miRNA genes are frequently multicopy, determining the relative contribution of each genomic location to mature miRNA expression is challenging.

miRNA Expression Regulation: Genomic and Epigenetic Mechanisms

miRNA expression can be altered by several mechanisms in human cancer: chromosomal abnormalities, as suggested by the evidence that microRNAs are frequently located in regions of the genome involved in alterations in cancer [15], and recently confirmed by a genetic study in ovarian carcinoma, breast cancer, and melanoma [114]; mutations, as the inherited mutations in the primary transcripts of miR-15a and miR-16-1 responsible for reduced expression of the two microRNAs in vitro and in vivo in CLL [28]; polymorphisms (SNPs), as described in lung cancer [98]; defects in the miRNA biogenesis machinery, as supported by the changes in microRNA expression as a consequence of an altered Drosha or Dicer activity [120, 150–152], and epigenetic changes, as altered DNA methylation (Fig. 19.6).

Moreover, aberrant expression of Drosha or Dicer enzymes has been correlated with disease progression and outcome in different human tumors, even though results are still controversial: strong expression of the central microRNA biosynthesis enzyme Dicer predicts poor prognosis in patients with colorectal cancer [153] and prostate cancer, whereas in breast, lung, and ovarian cancer [120] and neuroblastoma [154], Dicer has been shown to be a marker of good prognosis. Thus further studies on the cellular functions of Dicer need to address these issues.

An extensive analysis of genomic sequences of miRNA genes have shown that approximately half of them are associated with CpG islands, suggesting that they could be subjected to this mechanism of regulation [155]. Several evidences

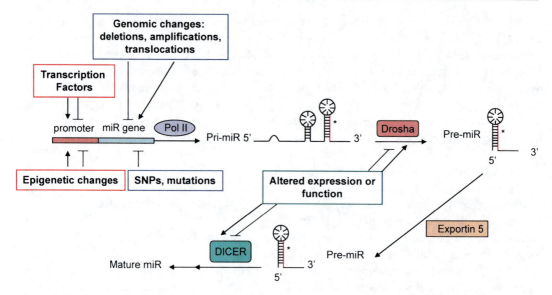

Fig. 19.6 Mechanisms of miRNA regulation. The deregulated miRNA expression observed in cancer can be caused by chromosomal abnormalities, mutations, polymorphisms (SNPs), transcriptional deregulation, defects in the miRNA biogenesis machinery, and epigenetic changes (adapted from Iorio MV, Croce CM. MicroRNAs in cancer: small molecules with a huge impact. J Clin Oncol. 2009;27(34):5848–56. Reprinted with permission. ©2008 American Society of Clinical Oncology. All rights reserved)

have indeed proved that an altered methylation status can be responsible for the deregulated expression of microRNAs in cancer, as the silencing of putative tumor suppressor microRNAs: treating T24 bladder cancer cells and human fibroblasts with DNA methyltransferase (DNMT) inhibitor 5-Aza-2′-deoxycytidine, Saito et al. [156] observed a strong upregulation of miR-127, microRNA characterized by a CpG island promoter, able to target the proto-oncogene BCL-6, and silenced in several cancer cells. With the same approach of unmask epigenetically silenced microRNAs inducing chromatin remodeling by drug treatment, it has been demonstrated that miR-9-1 is hypermethylated and consequently downmodulated in breast cancer [157], as well as the clustered miR-34b and miR-34c in colon cancer [158].

Conversely, the upmodulation of putative oncogenic microRNAs in cancer can be due to DNA hypomethylation, as shown in lung adenocarcinoma for let-7a-3 [159] or in epithelial ovarian cancer for miR-21 [68].

A different approach to identify epigenetically regulated microRNAs was represented by the miR profiling of DNMT1- and DNMT3b-deficient colorectal cancer cells: among the 18 microRNAs upmodulated in comparison to WT cells, the only one resulting unmethylated in normal tissue but hypermethylated, and thus silenced, in tumor was miR-124a, embedded in a large CpG island and able to target cyclin D kinase 6, which mediates the phosphorylation of RB tumor suppressor gene [160].

Methylation is not the only epigenetic mechanism that can affect microRNAs expression: Scott et al. [161] showed that in SKBR3 breast carcinoma cells histone deacetylase inhibition is followed by the extensive and rapid alteration of microRNAs levels.

The existence of epigenetic drugs, such as DNA demethylating agents and histone deacetylase inhibitors, able to reverse an aberrant methylation or acetylation status, raises the intriguing possibility to regulate microRNA levels, for example, to restore the expression of tumor suppressor microRNAs, thus reverting a tumoral phenotype.

To complicate the scenario connecting microRNAs and epigenetics, microRNAs themselves can regulate the expression of components of the epigenetic machinery, creating a highly controlled feedback mechanism: miR-29 family directly targets the de novo DNA methyltransferases DNMT-3A and -3B, while indirectly, through regulation of the transactivator Sp1, the maintenance DNA methyltransferase DNMT1. Interestingly, introduction of miR-29s into lung cancers and AMLs results in reactivation of silenced tumor suppressors and inhibition of tumorigenesis [35, 38]. Loss of miR-290 cluster in Dicer-deficient mouse ES cells leads to the downregulation of DNMT3a, DNMT3b, and DNMT1 through upmodulation of their repressor, RBL-2, proven target of miR-290 [162, 163]; miR-1, involved in myogenesis and related diseases, directly targets HDAC4 [164].

Alterations in miRNA Transcriptional Regulation

Some autonomously expressed miRNA genes have promoter regions that allow miRNAs to be highly expressed in a cell-type-specific manner and can even drive high levels of oncogenes in cases of chromosomal translocation. The miR-142 gene, a marker of hematopoietic cells, is located on chromosome 17 and was found at the breakpoint junction of a t(8;17) translocation, which causes an aggressive B-cell leukemia due to strong upregulation of a translocated *MYC* gene. The translocated *MYC* gene, which was also truncated at the first exon, was located only four nucleotides from the 3′-end of the miR-142 precursor, placing the translocated *MYC* under the control of the upstream miR-142 promoter. In an animal model for HCC, a similar event placed *MYC* downstream the miR-122a promoter active only in hepatocytes.

Many transcription factors regulate miRNA expression in a tissue-specific and disease state-specific fashion, and some miRNAs are regulated by well-established tumor suppressor or oncogene pathways, such as TP53, MYC, and RAS. The miRNA and its transcriptional regulators can participate in complex feedback regulation loops. Examples include the TP53-regulated miR-34a [165, 166], the RAS-regulated miR-21 [167], and the MYC-regulated miR-17-92 cluster [143].

MicroRNAs/Anti-microRNAs in Cancer Treatment

An increasing body of evidence collected up to date demonstrates how microRNAs could represent valid diagnostic, prognostic, and predictive markers in cancer. Indeed, the aberrant microRNA expression correlates with specific biopathological features, disease outcome, and response to specific therapies in different tumor types. Moreover, several indications in preclinical models underline the feasibility and the efficacy of a microRNA-based therapy in cancer, using these small molecules as both targets and tools (Fig. 19.7 and Table 19.3).

Reintroduction of miR-15a/16-1, for example, induces apoptosis in leukemic MEG01 cells and inhibits tumor growth in vivo in a xenograft model [30], whereas the inhibition of oncogenic miR-21 with antisense oligonucleotides generates a proapoptotic and antiproliferative response in vitro in different cellular models and reduces tumor development and metastatic potential in vivo [168].

Moreover, microRNAs involved in specific networks, as the apoptotic, proliferation, or receptor-driven pathways, could likely influence the response to targeted therapies or to chemotherapy: inhibition of miR-21 and miR-200b enhances sensitivity to gemcitabine in cholangiocytes, probably by modulation of CLOCK, PTEN, and PTPN12 [169], whereas reintroduction of miR-205 in breast cancer cells can improve the responsiveness to tyrosine kinase inhibitors through HER3 silencing [89], and enforced expression of miR-15b or miR-16 could sensitize multidrug-resistant gastric cells to vincristine-induced apoptosis [170].

Nevertheless, effective delivery into target tissues remains a major hurdle for microRNA-based therapy, including the applications of antagomirs and synthetic miRNA duplexes.

In the case of reduction in the levels of the mature microRNA (due to deletion present in the microRNA gene or to other mechanisms as defects in the processing machinery and aberrant transcription), the therapeutic approach could be

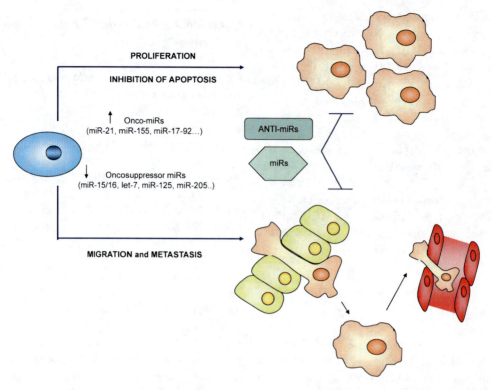

Fig. 19.7 miRNAs as therapeutic tools. The reintroduction by transfection of synthetic miRNAs lost during cancer development or progression or the inhibition of oncogenic miRs by using anti-miRNA oligonucleotides could help counteract tumor proliferation, extended survival, and the acquisition of a metastatic potential, thus representing potential therapeutic tools (adapted from Iorio MV, Croce CM. MicroRNAs in cancer: small molecules with a huge impact. J Clin Oncol. 2009;27(34):5848–56. Reprinted with permission. © 2008 American Society of Clinical Oncology. All rights reserved)

the exogenous delivery of synthetic double-stranded hairpin by complexing with lipids or delivery proteins. As reported by Tazawa et al. [171], miR-34a transiently inhibits human colon cancer tumor progression when administered subcutaneously in complexes with atelocollagen, recently shown to be a very useful system to efficiently deliver small interfering RNA molecules into tumors in vivo. Chen et al. have developed a liposome-polycation-hyaluronic acid (LPH) nanoparticle formulation modified with tumor-targeting single chain antibody fragment (scFv) for systemic delivery of miR-34a to lung metastasis of murine melanoma cells [172].

However, the vulnerability of unmodified dsRNAs to nucleases in vivo limits the use of this class of compound to privileged local environments where locally administration is feasible.

Using a conditional mouse lung cancer model, in which the expression of oncogenic *K-ras* could be conditionally activated, Esquela-Kerscher et al. showed that the intranasal administration of an adenovirus expressing *let-7a* RNA hairpin reduced tumor formation in vivo [173]. In 2009, Kota et al. [174] presented a study on therapeutic microRNA delivery suppressing tumor formation in a murine liver cancer model. The authors demonstrated that systemic administration of miR-26a in a mouse model of HCC using adeno-associated virus (AVV) resulted in inhibition of cancer cell proliferation, in the induction of tumor-specific apoptosis. These results are consistent with previous findings made by that same group, which demonstrated that MYC-induced liver tumors result in concomitant downregulation of various microRNAs [175].

Table 19.3 MicroRNA-based therapeutic approaches

Strategy	MicroRNA modulation	Advantages	Limitations	Experimental data	Clinical applications
Inhibition of mature miRNA by modified (2'-OME or 2'-MOE) AMOs or antagomiRNAs (AMOs conjugated with cholesterol)	Modified 2-OH residues of the ribose 2'-*O*-methyl/2'-*O*-methoxyethyl, or conjugation with cholesterol	High stability, good bioavailability and biodistribution	Toxicity, off-target effects, require high doses	In vitro and in vivo data (animals)	Silencing of oncomiRs
Inhibition of mature microRNAs by locked nucleic acid (LNA) antisense oligos	One or more nucleotide binding blocks; extramethylene bridge fixes ribose moiety	Good biodistribution, very effective	Off-target effects	In vitro and in vivo data, clinical trials ongoing	Silencing of oncomiRs
Inhibition of mature miRNAs with miRNA sponges	Sponge plasmid vector, encoding sequences complementary to the miRNA	Possibility to silence miRNA families	Limited stability, poor delivery, off-target effects	In vitro data	Silencing of oncomiRNA families
Replacement of mature miRNAs by partially double-stranded miRNA mimetics	Natural pre-miRNAs equivalent to endogenous products	Nanotechnology-based conjugations are very stable and effective	Toxicity, off-target effects	In vitro and in vivo (animals) data	Restoring tumor suppressor miRNAs
Replacement of mature miRNAs by transduction with adenovirus-associated vectors coding for miRNAs	To achieve persistent miRNA replacement	Very stable, very effective	Toxicity, off-target effects	In vitro and in vivo data	Restoring tumor suppressor miRNAs

In short-term experiments of cardiac hypertrophy, conducted by Carè et al., [176], overexpression of miR-133 by adenovirus delivery resulted in a significant reduction in the size of left ventricular cardiac myocytes and a significant decrease in the expression of fetal genes. To achieve stable miRNA reintroduction, the expression can be enforced by a viral vector with Pol III promoter upstream an artificial short hairpin RNA (shRNA) that bypasses Drosha processing, yet is cleaved and loaded into miRISC by Dicer. Most constructs have used Pol III promoters, including U6, H1, and tRNA [177–179]; however, these promoters have no cell specificity. Moreover, exceedingly, high levels of shRNA expression increase the probability of off-target silencing and elicit nonspecific effects such as interferon response, and they can also saturate exportin 5 pathway of endogenous miRNAs with fatal consequences [180]. Alternatively, the entire pri-miRNA can be expressed from an RNA Pol II promoter, leaving open the possibility for tissue-specific or induced ectopic miRNA expression. Furthermore, most miRNAs are known to be downstream Pol II promoters, within known protein-coding genes and expressed by Pol II activity [181]. Therefore, strategies using Pol II-directed synthesis of shRNA that mimic the natural miRNA synthesis could be an efficient therapeutic approach.

To achieve miRNA loss of function, chemically modified anti-miR oligonucleotides (AMOs) have been developed [182]. The most important property of such oligonucleotides is the specificity and high binding affinity to RNA, and a number of them have been pursued in clinical trials. miRNA downregulation has been achieved by using 2-O-methyl oligonucleotides [75, 76]. miR-122 inhibition was obtained by treating mice with AMOs containing 2-O-methoxyethyl groups resulted in reduced plasma cholesterol [183]. Intravenous administration of cholesterol-conjugated AMOs against miR-16, miR-122, miR-192, and miR-194 resulted in a marked reduction of corresponding miRNA levels in liver, lung, kidney, heart, intestine, fat, skin, bone marrow, muscle, ovaries, and adrenals [182, 184].

Very interestingly, Ma et al., after the demonstration of the crucial role of miR-10b as metastomiR in breast cancer, have exploited a possible therapeutic application, reporting that systemic treatment of tumor-bearing mice with miR-10b antagomirs suppresses breast cancer metastasis [124].

Other modified AMOs are represented by locked nucleic acid (LNA) oligonucleotides, able to inhibit exogenously introduced miRNAs with high specificity [185].

The first clinical trial in human of LNA-anti-miR (a placebo-controlled, double-blind, randomized, single-dose, dose-escalating safety study of SPC3649 in a total of 64 healthy male volunteers) has been conducted by Denmark's Santaris to study SPC3649 (LNA-anti-miR-122) (ClinicalTrials.gov Identifier: NCT00688012). *miR-122* is an abundant miRNA in the liver. The hepatitis C virus (HCV) genome harbors two closely spaced *miR-122* target sites in the 5′ noncoding region required for HCV replication. Kauppinen et al. showed that administration of LNA-anti-miR into mice resulted in a dose-dependent depletion of mature *miR-122* [186]. An efficacy study was later conducted by Elmen et al. on nonhuman primates [187], where they observed a dose-dependent sequestration of mature miR-122 and a long-lasting decrease of total plasma cholesterol. The same group has very recently developed tiny (8-mer) LNAs to obtain the simultaneous inhibition of miRNAs within families sharing the same seed, with concomitant upregulation of direct targets [188].

However, the same limitations encountered with the application of synthetic miRNA duplexes are encountered in the applications of antagomirs, namely, their effective delivery into target tissues.

An interesting approach to overcome these problems is to target miRNA by saturating them with target mRNAs. Ebert et al. [189] developed miRNA inhibitory transgenes, called "microRNA sponges," expressing an mRNA containing multiple tandem binding sites for an endogenous miRNA and thus able to stably interact with the corresponding miRNA and prevent its association with its endogenous targets. Both designed polymerase Pol II- and Pol III-driven miRNA sponges showed more efficiency for miRNA inhibition compared to standard 2'-*O*-Me antagomirs.

Lentiviral vectors have proven to be effective tool to ectopically express miRNAs using suitable transcriptional control units. It has been reported by Gentner et al. [179, 190] that stable miRNA-223 knockdown can be achieved in vivo by transducing bone marrow stem and progenitor cells with multiple target sequences from strong promoters and transplanting them into lethally irradiated congenic recipients. They demonstrated that overexpressing miR-targets specifically affects the targeted miRNA rather than saturating the effector pathway. However, the need for strong promoters and multiple vector integrations to obtain a high miR-target expression could increase the risk of insertional mutagenesis in target cells, potentially confounding the identification of miRNA knockdown phenotypes, and thus representing a potential limitation of this strategy.

Su et al. [191] have applied a nanotechnologic approach to the use of anti-miRNAs: systemic delivery of a chemically stabilized anti-miR-122 complexed with interfering nanoparticles (iNOPs) effectively silences the liver-expressed miR-122 in mice, thus resulting in lowering of plasma cholesterol.

Beside targeted therapies and chemotherapy, microRNAs could also alter the sensitivity to radiotherapy, as recently reported by Slack's group [192]: a potential therapeutic use for anti-miR-34 as a radiosensitizing agent in p53-mutant breast cancer could be considered; in lung cancer cells, let-7 family can suppress the resistance to anticancer radiation therapy, probably through RAS regulation.

Evidences described up to date provide the experimental bases for the use of microRNAs as both targets and tools in anticancer therapy, but there are at least two primary issues to address to translate these fundamental research advances into medical practice: the development of engineered animal models to study cancer-associated microRNAs and the improvement of the efficiency of miRNAs/anti-miRs delivery in vivo.

Concluding Remarks and Future Perspectives

Fifteen years ago, when microRNAs seemed just a peculiar discovery in *C. elegans*, the scientific world did not probably even imagine that those small noncoding molecules would have a large impact on our understanding of cellular biology and gene regulation.

MicroRNAs contribute to maintain the balance among genes regulating cells' fate, and their deregulation, a frequent hallmark in different human malignancies, can destabilize this equilibrium, thus contributing to cancer development and/or progression, from initiation to metastatic disease. However, despite the increasing and encouraging body of evidence linking microRNAs to cancer biology, many important questions remain to be addressed: in fact, although the identification and validation of microRNA targets greatly improved in the last few years, we still know very little about the cellular and molecular circuits where they are involved. The scenario is surely complicated by the ability of microRNAs to target multiple molecules, sometimes belonging to related pathways, and at the same time by the redundancy existing among microRNAs. This gives rise to a complex regulatory network where biological effects and properties of a particular microRNA do not always allow a linear explanation.

Improvement of computation programs of microRNA targets prediction and experimental methods of validation will certainly contribute to elucidate their mechanisms of action, and genetically modified murine models will likely help in determining the oncogenic and tumor suppressor potential of individual microRNAs.

Data available to date clearly support the involvement of microRNA in cancer etiology and strongly suggest a possible use of these molecules as markers of diagnosis and prognosis, and eventually, as new targets or tools for a specific therapy (Fig. 19.8): stepping from the bench to clinical applications would be the next great challenge in cancer research.

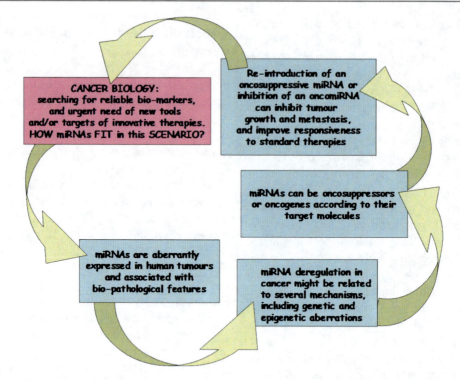

Fig. 19.8 Workflow summarizing the progressive steps and the different issues considered to investigate the hypothesis of a concrete role of miRNAs in cancer biology and to support their possible clinical applications

Acknowledgments This work was partially supported by Associazione Italiana per la Ricerca sul Cancro (AIRC).

Marilena V. Iorio is supported by a Start Up AIRC Grant.

References

1. Lee RC, Feinbaum RL, Ambros V. The C. elegans heterochronic gene lin-4 encodes small RNAs with antisense complementarity to lin-14. Cell. 1993; 75(5):843–54.
2. Bartel DP. MicroRNAs: genomics, biogenesis, mechanism, and function. Cell. 2004;116:281–97.
3. Kim VN. MicroRNA biogenesis: coordinated cropping and dicing. Nat Rev Mol Cell Biol. 2005;6(5):376–85.
4. Krol J, Loedige I, Filipowicz W. The widespread regulation of microRNA biogenesis, function and decay. Nat Rev Genet. 2010;11:597–610.
5. Yi R, Qin Y, Macara IG, Cullen BR. Exportin-5 mediates the nuclear export of pre-microRNAs and short hairpin RNAs. Genes Dev. 2003;17(24): 3011–6.
6. Lingel A, Simon B, Izaurralde E, Sattler M. Structure and nucleic-acid binding of the Drosophila Argonaute 2 PAZ domain. Nature. 2003;426(6965):465–9.
7. Tahbaz N, Kolb FA, Zhang H, Jaronczyk K, Filipowicz W, Hobman TC. Characterization of the interactions between mammalian PAZ PIWI domain proteins and Dicer. EMBO Rep. 2004;5(2):189–94.
8. Mourelatos Z, Dostie J, Paushkin S, et al. miRNPs: a novel class of ribonucleoproteins containing numerous microRNAs. Genes Dev. 2002;16:720–8.
9. Wahid F, Shehzad A, Khan T, Kim YY. MicroRNAs: synthesis, mechanism, function, and recent clinical trials. Biochim Biophys Acta. 2010;1803:1231–43.
10. Chen X. A microRNA as a translational repressor of APETALA2 in Arabidopsis flower development. Science. 2004;303(5666):2022–5.
11. Petersen CP, Bordeleau ME, Pelletier J, Sharp PA. Short RNAs repress translation after initiation in mammalian cells. Mol Cell. 2006;21:533–42.
12. Doench JG, Petersen CP, Sharp PA. siRNAs can function as miRNAs. Genes Dev. 2003;17(4):438–42.
13. Kulkarni M, Ozgur S, Stoecklin G. On track with P-bodies. Biochem Soc Trans. 2010;38:242–51.
14. Calin GA, Dumitru CD, Shimizu M, et al. Frequent deletions and down-regulation of micro- RNA genes miR15 and miR16 at 13q14 in chronic lymphocytic leukemia. Proc Natl Acad Sci USA. 2002;99:15524–9.
15. Calin GA, Sevignani C, Dumitru CD, et al. Human microRNA genes are frequently located at fragile sites and genomic regions involved in cancers. Proc Natl Acad Sci USA. 2004;101:2999–3004.

16. Calin GA, Croce CM. MicroRNA signatures in human cancers. Nat Rev Cancer. 2006;6(11): 857–66.
17. Mitchell PS, Parkin RK, Kroh EM, et al. Circulating microRNAs as stable blood-based markers for cancer detection. Proc Natl Acad Sci USA. 2008; 105(30):10513–8.
18. Valadi H, Ekstrom K, Bossios A, Sjostrand M, Lee JJ, Lotvall JO. Exosome-mediated transfer of mRNAs and microRNAs is a novel mechanism of genetic exchange between cells. Nat Cell Biol. 2007;9(6):654–9.
19. Lawrie CH, Gal S, Dunlop HM, et al. Detection of elevated levels of tumour-associated microRNAs in serum of patients with diffuse large B-cell lymphoma. Br J Haematol. 2008;141(5):672–5.
20. Boeri M, Verri C, Conte D, et al. MicroRNA signatures in tissues and plasma predict development and prognosis of computed tomography detected lung cancer. Proc Natl Acad Sci USA. 2011;108:3713–8.
21. Roth C, Rack B, Muller V, Janni W, Pantel K, Schwarzenbach H. Circulating microRNAs as blood-based markers for patients with primary and metastatic breast cancer. Breast Cancer Res. 2010;12(6):R90.
22. Heneghan HM, Miller N, Kerin MJ. Circulating miRNA signatures: promising prognostic tools for cancer. J Clin Oncol. 2010;28(29):e573–4.
23. Zhao H, Shen J, Medico L, Wang D, Ambrosone CB, Liu S. A pilot study of circulating miRNAs as potential biomarkers of early stage breast cancer. PLoS One. 2010;5(10):e13735.
24. Calin GA, Ferracin M, Cimmino A, et al. A MicroRNA signature associated with prognosis and progression in chronic lymphocytic leukemia. N Engl J Med. 2005;353:1793–801.
25. Vargova K, Curik N, Burda P, et al. MYB transcriptionally regulates the miR-155 host gene in chronic lymphocytic leukemia. Blood. 2011;117(14):3816–25.
26. Pekarsky Y, Santanam U, Cimmino A, et al. Tcl1 expression in chronic lymphocytic leukemia is regulated by miR-29 and miR-181. Cancer Res. 2006;66:11590–3.
27. Rossi S, Shimizu M, Barbarotto E, et al. microRNA fingerprinting of CLL patients with chromosome 17p deletion identify a miR-21 score that stratifies early survival. Blood. 2010;116(6):945–52.
28. Raveche ES, Salerno E, Scaglione BJ, et al. Abnormal microRNA-16 locus with synteny to human 13q14 linked to CLL in NZB mice. Blood. 2007;109: 5079–86.
29. Cimmino A, Calin GA, Fabbri M, et al. miR-15 and miR-16 induce apoptosis by targeting BCL2. Proc Natl Acad Sci USA. 2005;102:13944–9.
30. Calin GA, Cimmino A, Fabbri M, et al. MiR-15a and miR-16-1 cluster functions in human leukemia. Proc Natl Acad Sci USA. 2008;105:5166–71.
31. Klein U, Lia M, Crespo M, et al. The DLEU2/miR-15a/16-1 cluster controls B cell proliferation and its deletion leads to chronic lymphocytic leukemia. Cancer Cell. 2010;17(1):28–40.

32. Fabbri M, Bottoni A, Shimizu M, et al. Association of a microRNA/TP53 feedback circuitry with pathogenesis and outcome of B-cell chronic lymphocytic leukemia. JAMA. 2011;305(1):59–67.
33. Garzon R, Volinia S, Liu CG, et al. MicroRNA signatures associated with cytogenetics and prognosis in acute myeloid leukemia. Blood. 2008;111(6): 3183–9.
34. Marcucci G, Maharry K, Radmacher MD, et al. Prognostic significance of, and gene and microRNA expression signatures associated with, CEBPA mutations in cytogenetically normal acute myeloid leukemia with high-risk molecular features: a Cancer and Leukemia Group B Study. J Clin Oncol. 2008; 26(31):5078–87.
35. Garzon R, Liu S, Fabbri M, et al. MicroRNA -29b induces global DNA hypomethylation and tumor suppressor gene re-expression in acute myeloid leukemia by targeting directly DNMT3A and 3B and indirectly DNMT1. Blood. 2009;113:6411–8.
36. Le Beau MM, Albain KS, Larson RA, et al. Clinical and cytogenetic correlations in 63 patients with therapy-related myelodysplastic syndromes and acute nonlymphocytic leukemia: further evidence for characteristic abnormalities of chromosomes no. 5 and 7. J Clin Oncol. 1986;4:325–45.
37. Iorio MV, Ferracin M, Liu CG, et al. MicroRNA gene expression deregulation in human breast cancer. Cancer Res. 2005;65:7065–70.
38. Fabbri M, Garzon R, Cimmino A, et al. MicroRNA-29 family reverts aberrant methylation in lung cancer by targeting DNA methyltransferases 3A and 3B. Proc Natl Acad Sci USA. 2007;104:15805–10.
39. Mott JL, Kobayashi S, Bronk SF, Gores GJ. mir-29 regulates Mcl-1 protein expression and apoptosis. Oncogene. 2007;26:6133–40.
40. Wang H, Garzon R, Sun H, et al. NF-kappaB-YY1-miR-29 regulatory circuitry in skeletal myogenesis and rhabdomyosarcoma. Cancer Cell. 2008;14:369–81.
41. Metzler M, Wilda M, Busch K, Viehmann S, Borkhardt A. High expression of precursor microRNA-155/BIC RNA in children with Burkitt lymphoma. Genes Chromosomes Cancer. 2004;39:167–9.
42. Kluiver J, Poppema S, De Jong D, et al. BIC and miR-155 are highly expressed in Hodgkin, primary mediastinal and diffuse large B cell lymphomas. J Pathol. 2005;207:243–9.
43. Tam W, Hughes SH, Hayward WS, Besmer P. Avian bic, a gene isolated from a common retroviral site in avian leukosis virus-induced lymphomas that encodes a noncoding RNA, cooperates with c-myc in lymphomagenesis and erythroleukemogenesis. J Virol. 2002;76:4275–86.
44. Costinean S, Zanesi N, Pekarsky Y, et al. Pre-B cell proliferation and lymphoblastic leukemia/high-grade lymphoma in E(mu)-miR155 transgenic mice. Proc Natl Acad Sci USA. 2006;103:7024–9.
45. Thai TH, Calado DP, Casola S, et al. Regulation of the germinal center response by microRNA-155. Science. 2007;316:604–8.

46. Rodriguez A, Vigorito E, Clare S, et al. Requirement of bic/microRNA-155 for normal immune function. Science. 2007;316:608–11.

47. Tili E, Michaille JJ, Cimino A, et al. Modulation of miR-155 and miR-125b levels following lipopoly-saccharide/TNF-alpha stimulation and their possible roles in regulating the response to endotoxin shock. J Immunol. 2007;179:5082–9.

48. He L, Thomson JM, Hemann MT, et al. A microRNA polycistron as a potential human oncogene. Nature. 2005;435:828–33.

49. Xiao C, Srinivasan L, Calado DP, et al. Lymphoproliferative disease and autoimmunity in mice with increased miR-17-92 expression in lymphocytes. Nat Immunol. 2008;9:405–14.

50. O'Donnell KA, Wentzel EA, Zeller KI, Dang CV, Mendell JT. c-Myc-regulated microRNAs modulate E2F1 expression. Nature. 2005;435:839–43.

51. Petrocca F, Visone R, Onelli MR, et al. E2F1-regulated microRNAs impair TGFbeta-dependent cell-cycle arrest and apoptosis in gastric cancer. Cancer Cell. 2008;13:272–86.

52. Ronchetti D, Lionetti M, Mosca L, et al. An integrative genomic approach reveals coordinated expression of intronic miR-335, miR-342, and miR-561 with deregulated host genes in multiple myeloma. BMC Med Genomics. 2008;1:37.

53. Loffler D, Brocke-Heidrich K, Pfeifer G, et al. Interleukin-6 dependent survival of multiple myeloma cells involves the Stat3-mediated induction of microRNA-21 through a highly conserved enhancer. Blood. 2007;110:1330–3.

54. Roccaro AM, Sacco A, Thompson B, et al. MicroRNAs 15a and 16 regulate tumor proliferation in multiple myeloma. Blood. 2009;113(26): 6669–80.

55. Lerner M, Harada M, Loven J, et al. DLEU2, frequently deleted in malignancy, functions as a critical host gene of the cell cycle inhibitory microRNAs miR-15a and miR-16-1. Exp Cell Res. 2009; 315(17):2941–52.

56. Gatt ME, Zhao JJ, Ebert MS, et al. MicroRNAs 15a/16-1 function as tumor suppressor genes in multiple myeloma. Blood. 2010. doi:10.1182/blood-2009-11-253294.

57. Pichiorri F, Suh SS, Ladetto M, et al. MicroRNAs regulate critical genes associated with multiple myeloma pathogenesis. Proc Natl Acad Sci USA. 2008;105:12885–90.

58. Pichiorri F, Suh SS, Rocci A, et al. Downregulation of p53-inducible microRNAs 192, 194, and 215 impairs the p53/MDM2 autoregulatory loop in multiple myeloma development. Cancer Cell. 2010;18(4):367–81.

59. Yan LX, Huang XF, Shao Q, et al. MicroRNA miR-21 overexpression in human breast cancer is associated with advanced clinical stage, lymph node metastasis and patient poor prognosis. RNA. 2008;14:2348–60.

60. Qian B, Katsaros D, Lu L, et al. High miR-21 expression in breast cancer associated with poor disease-free survival in early stage disease and high TGF-beta1. Breast Cancer Res Treat. 2009;117(1): 131–40.

61. Walter BA, Gomez-Macias G, Valera VA, Sobel M, Merino MJ. miR-21 expression in pregnancy-associated breast cancer: a possible marker of poor prognosis. J Cancer. 2011;2:67–75.

62. Asaga S, Kuo C, Nguyen T, Terpenning M, Giuliano AE, Hoon DS. Direct serum assay for microRNA-21 concentrations in early and advanced breast cancer. Clin Chem. 2011;57:84–91.

63. Wang F, Zheng Z, Guo J, Ding X. Correlation and quantitation of microRNA aberrant expression in tissues and sera from patients with breast tumor. Gynecol Oncol. 2010;119:586–93.

64. Taylor DD, Gercel-Taylor C. MicroRNA signatures of tumor-derived exosomes as diagnostic biomarkers of ovarian cancer. Gynecol Oncol. 2008;110(1):13–21.

65. Ota D, Mimori K, Yokobori T, et al. Identification of recurrence-related microRNAs in the bone marrow of breast cancer patients. Int J Oncol. 2011;38: 955–62.

66. Chan JA, Krichevsky AM, Kosik KS. MicroRNA-21 is an antiapoptotic factor in human glioblastoma cells. Cancer Res. 2005;65:6029–33.

67. Ciafre SA, Galardi S, Mangiola A, et al. Extensive modulation of a set of microRNAs in primary glioblastoma. Biochem Biophys Res Commun. 2005;334:1351–8.

68. Iorio MV, Visone R, Di Leva G, et al. MicroRNA signatures in human ovarian cancer. Cancer Res. 2007;67:8699–707.

69. Yanaihara N, Caplen N, Bowman E, et al. Unique microRNA molecular profiles in lung cancer diagnosis and prognosis. Cancer Cell. 2006;9(3):189–98.

70. Markou A, Tsaroucha EG, Kaklamanis L, Fotinou M, Georgoulias V, Lianidou ES. Prognostic value of mature microRNA-21 and microRNA-205 overexpression in non-small cell lung cancer by quantitative real-time RT-PCR. Clin Chem. 2008;54:1696–704.

71. Volinia S, Calin GA, Liu CG, et al. A microRNA expression signature of human solid tumors defines cancer gene targets. Proc Natl Acad Sci USA. 2006;103(7):2257–61.

72. Schetter AJ, Leung SY, Sohn JJ, et al. MicroRNA expression profiles associated with prognosis and therapeutic outcome in colon adenocarcinoma. JAMA. 2008;299:425–36.

73. Roldo C, Missiaglia E, Hagan JP, et al. MicroRNA expression abnormalities in pancreatic endocrine and acinar tumors are associated with distinctive pathologic features and clinical behavior. J Clin Oncol. 2006;24:4677–84.

74. Bloomston M, Frankel WL, Petrocca F, et al. MicroRNA expression patterns to differentiate pancreatic adenocarcinoma from normal pancreas and chronic pancreatitis. JAMA. 2007;297:1901–8.

75. Meister G, Landthaler M, Dorsett Y, Tuschl T. Sequence-specific inhibition of microRNA- and siRNA-induced RNA silencing. RNA. 2004;10(3): 544–50.

76. Hutvagner G, Simard MJ, Mello CC, Zamore PD. Sequence-specific inhibition of small RNA function. PLoS Biol. 2004;2(4):E98.

77. Yu F, Yao H, Zhu P, et al. let-7 regulates self renewal and tumorigenicity of breast cancer cells. Cell. 2007;131:1109–23.

78. Johnson SM, Grosshans H, Shingara J, et al. RAS is regulated by the let-7 microRNA family. Cell. 2005;120(5):635–47.

79. Mayr C, Hemann MT, Bartel DP. Disrupting the pairing between let-7 and Hmga2 enhances oncogenic transformation. Science. 2007;315:1576–9.

80. Sampson VB, Rong NH, Han J, et al. MicroRNA let-7a down-regulates MYC and reverts MYC-induced growth in Burkitt lymphoma cells. Cancer Res. 2007;67:9762–70.

81. Kumar MS, Erkeland SJ, Pester RE, et al. Suppression of non-small cell lung tumor development by the let-7 microRNA family. Proc Natl Acad Sci USA. 2008;105:3903–8.

82. Adams BD, Furneaux H, White BA. The micro-ribonucleic acid (miRNA) miR-206 targets the human estrogen receptor-alpha (ERalpha) and represses ERalpha messenger RNA and protein expression in breast cancer cell lines. Mol Endocrinol. 2007;21(5): 1132–47.

83. Foekens JA, Sieuwerts AM, Smid M, et al. Four miRNAs associated with aggressiveness of lymph node-negative, estrogen receptor-positive human breast cancer. Proc Natl Acad Sci USA. 2008;105: 13021–6.

84. Masri S, Liu Z, Phung S, Wang E, Yuan YC, Chen S. The role of microRNA-128a in regulating TGFbeta signaling in letrozole-resistant breast cancer cells. Breast Cancer Res Treat. 2010;124:89–99.

85. Di Leva G, Gasparini G, Piovan C, et al. A regulatory "miRcircuitry" involving miR-221&222 and ERalpha determines ERalpha status of breast cancer cells. J Natl Cancer Inst. 2010;102:706–21.

86. Zhao JJ, Lin J, Yang H, et al. MicroRNA-221/222 negatively regulates estrogen receptor alpha and is associated with tamoxifen resistance in breast cancer. J Biol Chem. 2008;283(45):31079–86.

87. Miller TE, Ghoshal K, Ramaswamy B, et al. MicroRNA-221/222 confers tamoxifen resistance in breast cancer by targeting p27Kip1. J Biol Chem. 2008;283:29897–903.

88. Rao X, Di LG, Li M, et al. MicroRNA-221/222 confers breast cancer fulvestrant resistance by regulating multiple signaling pathways. Oncogene. 2011;30:1082–97.

89. Iorio MV, Casalini P, Piovan C, et al. microRNA-205 regulates HER3 in human breast cancer. Cancer Res. 2009;69:2195–200.

90. Wu H, Zhu S, Mo YY. Suppression of cell growth and invasion by miR-205 in breast cancer. Cell Res. 2009;19:439–48.

91. Gregory PA, Bracken CP, Bert AG, Goodall GJ. MicroRNAs as regulators of epithelial-mesenchymal transition. Cell Cycle. 2008;7(20):3112–8.

92. Radojicic J, Zaravinos A, Vrekoussis T, Kafousi M, Spandidos DA, Stathopoulos EN. MicroRNA expression analysis in triple-negative (ER, PR and Her2/neu) breast cancer. Cell Cycle. 2011;10: 507–17.

93. Png KJ, Yoshida M, Zhang XH, et al. MicroRNA-335 inhibits tumor reinitiation and is silenced through genetic and epigenetic mechanisms in human breast cancer. Genes Dev. 2011;25:226–31.

94. Yu SL, Chen HY, Chang GC, et al. MicroRNA signature predicts survival and relapse in lung cancer. Cancer Cell. 2008;13:48–57.

95. Lebanony D, Benjamin H, Gilad S, et al. Diagnostic assay based on hsa-miR-205 expression distinguishes squamous from non-squamous non-small-cell lung carcinoma. J Clin Oncol. 2009;27: 2030–7.

96. Del Vescovo V, Cantaloni C, Cucino A, et al. miR-205 Expression levels in nonsmall cell lung cancer do not always distinguish adenocarcinomas from squamous cell carcinomas. Am J Surg Pathol. 2011;35(2):268–75.

97. Rabinowits G, Gercel-Taylor C, Day JM, Taylor DD, Kloecker GH. Exosomal microRNA: a diagnostic marker for lung cancer. Clin Lung Cancer. 2009; 10(1):42–6.

98. Hu Z, Chen J, Tian T, et al. Genetic variants of miRNA sequences and non-small cell lung cancer survival. J Clin Invest. 2008;118:2600–8.

99. Yu L, Todd NW, Xing L, et al. Early detection of lung adenocarcinoma in sputum by a panel of microRNA markers. Int J Cancer. 2010;127(12):2870–8.

100. Ceppi P, Mudduluru G, Kumarswamy R, et al. Loss of miR-200c expression induces an aggressive, invasive, and chemoresistant phenotype in non-small cell lung cancer. Mol Cancer Res. 2010;8(9):1207–16.

101. Seike M, Goto A, Okano T, et al. MiR-21 is an EGFR-regulated anti-apoptotic factor in lung cancer in never-smokers. Proc Natl Acad Sci USA. 2009;106(29):12085–90.

102. Markou A, Tsaroucha EG, Kaklamanis L, Fotinou M, Georgoulias V, Lianidou ES. Prognostic value of mature microRNA-21 and microRNA-205 overexpression in non-small cell lung cancer by quantitative real-time RT-PCR. Clin Chem. 2008;54(10):1696–704.

103. Saito M, Schetter AJ, Mollerup S, et al. The association of microRNA expression with prognosis and progression in early stage, non small cell lung adenocarcinoma: a retrospective analysis of three cohorts. Clin Cancer Res. 2011. doi:10.1158/1078-0432.CCR-10-2961.

104. Garofalo M, Di LG, Romano G, et al. miR-221&222 regulate TRAIL resistance and enhance tumorigenicity through PTEN and TIMP3 downregulation. Cancer Cell. 2009;16(6):498–509.

105. Murakami Y, Yasuda T, Saigo K, et al. Comprehensive analysis of microRNA expression patterns in hepatocellular carcinoma and non-tumorous tissues. Oncogene. 2006;25:2537–45.

106. Li W, Xie L, He X, et al. Diagnostic and prognostic implications of microRNAs in human hepatocellular carcinoma. Int J Cancer. 2008;123:1616–22.
107. Visone R, Pallante P, Vecchione A, et al. Specific microRNAs are downregulated in human thyroid anaplastic carcinomas. Oncogene. 2007;26:7590–5.
108. Gramantieri L, Ferracin M, Fornari F, et al. Cyclin G1 is a target of miR-122a, a microRNA frequently down-regulated in human hepatocellular carcinoma. Cancer Res. 2007;67:6092–9.
109. Fornari F, Gramantieri L, Ferracin M, et al. MiR-221 controls CDKN1C/p57 and CDKN1B/p27 expression in human hepatocellular carcinoma. Oncogene. 2008;27:5651–61.
110. Pineau P, Volinia S, McJunkin K, et al. miR-221 overexpression contributes to liver tumorigenesis. Proc Natl Acad Sci USA. 2010;107(1):264–9.
111. Le Sage C, Nagel R, Egan DA, et al. Regulation of the p27(Kip1) tumor suppressor by miR-221 and miR-222 promotes cancer cell proliferation. EMBO J. 2007;26:3699–708.
112. Galardi S, Mercatelli N, Giorda E, et al. miR-221 and miR-222 expression affects the proliferation potential of human prostate carcinoma cell lines by targeting p27Kip1. J Biol Chem. 2007;282:23716–24.
113. Felicetti F, Errico MC, Bottero L, et al. The promyelocytic leukemia zinc finger-microRNA-221/-222 pathway controls melanoma progression through multiple oncogenic mechanisms. Cancer Res. 2008;68(8):2745–54.
114. Zhang L, Huang J, Yang N, et al. microRNAs exhibit high frequency genomic alterations in human cancer. Proc Natl Acad Sci USA. 2006;103:9136–41.
115. Ji J, Shi J, Budhu A, et al. MicroRNA expression, survival, and response to interferon in liver cancer. N Engl J Med. 2009;361(15):1437–47.
116. Yang N, Kaur S, Volinia S, et al. MicroRNA microarray identifies Let-7i as a novel biomarker and therapeutic target in human epithelial ovarian cancer. Cancer Res. 2008;68(24):10307–14.
117. Bhattacharya R, Nicoloso M, Arvizo R, et al. MiR-15a and MiR-16 control Bmi-1 expression in ovarian cancer. Cancer Res. 2009;69(23):9090–5.
118. Boren T, Xiong Y, Hakam A, et al. MicroRNAs and their target messenger RNAs associated with ovarian cancer response to chemotherapy. Gynecol Oncol. 2009;113(2):249–55.
119. Yang H, Kong W, He L, et al. MicroRNA expression profiling in human ovarian cancer: miR-214 induces cell survival and cisplatin resistance by targeting PTEN. Cancer Res. 2008;68(2):425–33.
120. Merritt WM, Lin YG, Han LY, et al. Dicer, Drosha, and outcomes in patients with ovarian cancer. N Engl J Med. 2008;359(25):2641–50.
121. Gregory PA, Bert AG, Paterson EL, et al. The miR-200 family and miR-205 regulate epithelial to mesenchymal transition by targeting ZEB1 and SIP1. Nat Cell Biol. 2008;10(5):593–601.
122. Bendoraite A, Knouf EC, Garg KS, et al. Regulation of miR-200 family microRNAs and ZEB transcription factors in ovarian cancer: evidence supporting a mesothelial-to-epithelial transition. Gynecol Oncol. 2010;116(1):117–25.
123. Ma L, Teruya-Feldstein J, Weinberg RA. Tumour invasion and metastasis initiated by microRNA-10b in breast cancer. Nature. 2007;449:682–8.
124. Ma L, Reinhardt F, Pan E, et al. Therapeutic silencing of miR-10b inhibits metastasis in a mouse mammary tumor model. Nat Biotechnol. 2010;28(4):341–7.
125. Huang Q, Gumireddy K, Schrier M, et al. The microRNAs miR-373 and miR-520c promote tumour invasion and metastasis. Nat Cell Biol. 2008;10:202–10.
126. He L, He X, Lim LP, et al. A microRNA component of the p53 tumour suppressor network. Nature. 2007;447:1130–4.
127. Li N, Fu H, Tie Y, et al. miR-34a inhibits migration and invasion by down-regulation of c-Met expression in human hepatocellular carcinoma cells. Cancer Lett. 2009;275:44–53.
128. Sachdeva M, Mo YY. MicroRNA-145 suppresses cell invasion and metastasis by directly targeting mucin 1. Cancer Res. 2010;70(1):378–87.
129. Park SM, Gaur AB, Lengyel E, Peter ME. The miR-200 family determines the epithelial phenotype of cancer cells by targeting the E-cadherin repressors ZEB1 and ZEB2. Genes Dev. 2008;22:894–907.
130. Gandellini P, Folini M, Longoni N, et al. miR-205 Exerts tumor-suppressive functions in human prostate through down-regulation of protein kinase Cepsilon. Cancer Res. 2009;69:2287–95.
131. Burk U, Schubert J, Wellner U, et al. A reciprocal repression between ZEB1 and members of the miR-200 family promotes EMT and invasion in cancer cells. EMBO Rep. 2008;9(6):582–9.
132. Bracken CP, Gregory PA, Kolesnikoff N, et al. A double-negative feedback loop between ZEB1-SIP1 and the microRNA-200 family regulates epithelial-mesenchymal transition. Cancer Res. 2008;68(19):7846–54.
133. Wellner U, Schubert J, Burk UC, et al. The EMT-activator ZEB1 promotes tumorigenicity by repressing stemness-inhibiting microRNAs. Nat Cell Biol. 2009;11(12):1487–95.
134. Asangani IA, Rasheed SA, Nikolova DA, et al. MicroRNA-21 (miR-21) post-transcriptionally downregulates tumor suppressor Pdcd4 and stimulates invasion, intravasation and metastasis in colorectal cancer. Oncogene. 2008;27:2128–36.
135. Zhu S, Wu H, Wu F, Nie D, Sheng S, Mo YY. MicroRNA-21 targets tumor suppressor genes in invasion and metastasis. Cell Res. 2008;18:350–9.
136. Tavazoie SF, Alarcon C, Oskarsson T, et al. Endogenous human microRNAs that suppress breast cancer metastasis. Nature. 2008;451:147–52.
137. Rosenfeld N, Aharonov R, Meiri E, et al. MicroRNAs accurately identify cancer tissue origin. Nat Biotechnol. 2008;26:462–9.
138. Poliseno L, Tuccoli A, Mariani L, et al. MicroRNAs modulate the angiogenic properties of HUVECs. Blood. 2006;108(9):3068–71.

139. Hua Z, Lv Q, Ye W, et al. MiRNA-directed regulation of VEGF and other angiogenic factors under hypoxia. PLoS One. 2006;1:e116.

140. Mertens-Talcott SU, Chintharlapalli S, Li X, Safe S. The oncogenic microRNA-27a targets genes that regulate specificity protein transcription factors and the G2-M checkpoint in MDA-MB-231 breast cancer cells. Cancer Res. 2007;67(22):11001–11.

141. Fish JE, Santoro MM, Morton SU, et al. miR-126 regulates angiogenic signaling and vascular integrity. Dev Cell. 2008;15:272–84.

142. Pulkkinen K, Malm T, Turunen M, Koistinaho J, Yla-Herttuala S. Hypoxia induces microRNA miR-210 in vitro and in vivo ephrin-A3 and neuronal pentraxin 1 are potentially regulated by miR-210. FEBS Lett. 2008;582(16):2397–401.

143. Dews M, Homayouni A, Yu D, et al. Augmentation of tumor angiogenesis by a Myc-activated microRNA cluster. Nat Genet. 2006;38(9):1060–5.

144. Kuehbacher A, Urbich C, Zeiher AM, Dimmeler S. Role of Dicer and Drosha for endothelial microRNA expression and angiogenesis. Circ Res. 2007; 101(1):59–68.

145. Martello G, Rosato A, Ferrari F, et al. A MicroRNA targeting dicer for metastasis control. Cell. 2010; 141(7):1195–207.

146. Su X, Chakravarti D, Cho MS, et al. TAp63 suppresses metastasis through coordinate regulation of Dicer and miRNAs. Nature. 2010;467(7318):986–90.

147. Griffiths-Jones S, Saini HK, van Dongen S, Enright AJ. miRBase: tools for microRNA genomics. Nucleic Acids Res. 2008;36(Database issue):D154–8.

148. Baskerville S, Bartel DP. Microarray profiling of microRNAs reveals frequent coexpression with neighboring miRNAs and host genes. RNA. 2005; 11(3):241–7.

149. Chiang HR, Schoenfeld LW, Ruby JG, et al. Mammalian microRNAs: experimental evaluation of novel and previously annotated genes. Genes Dev. 2010;24(10):992–1009.

150. Thomson JM, Newman M, Parker JS, Morin-Kensicki EM, Wright T, Hammond SM. Extensive post-transcriptional regulation of microRNAs and its implications for cancer. Genes Dev. 2006;20:2202–7.

151. Nakamura T, Canaani E, Croce CM. Oncogenic All1 fusion proteins target Drosha-mediated microRNA processing. Proc Natl Acad Sci USA. 2007;104: 10980–5.

152. Karube Y, Tanaka H, Osada H, et al. Reduced expression of Dicer associated with poor prognosis in lung cancer patients. Cancer Sci. 2005;96:111–5.

153. Faber C, Horst D, Hlubek F, Kirchner T. Overexpression of Dicer predicts poor survival in colorectal cancer. Eur J Cancer. 2011;47(9):1414–9.

154. Lin RJ, Lin YC, Chen J, et al. microRNA signature and expression of Dicer and Drosha can predict prognosis and delineate risk groups in neuroblastoma. Cancer Res. 2010;70(20):7841–50.

155. Weber B, Stresemann C, Brueckner B, Lyko F. Methylation of human microRNA genes in normal and neoplastic cells. Cell Cycle. 2007;6:1001–5.

156. Saito Y, Liang G, Egger G, et al. Specific activation of microRNA-127 with downregulation of the proto-oncogene BCL6 by chromatin-modifying drugs in human cancer cells. Cancer Cell. 2006;9:435–43.

157. Lehmann U, Hasemeier B, Christgen M, et al. Epigenetic inactivation of microRNA gene hsa-mir-9-1 in human breast cancer. J Pathol. 2008;214(1): 17–24.

158. Toyota M, Suzuki H, Sasaki Y, et al. Epigenetic silencing of microRNA-34b/c and B-cell translocation gene 4 is associated with CpG island methylation in colorectal cancer. Cancer Res. 2008;68: 4123–32.

159. Brueckner B, Stresemann C, Kuner R, et al. The human let-7a-3 locus contains an epigenetically regulated microRNA gene with oncogenic function. Cancer Res. 2007;67:1419–23.

160. Lujambio A, Ropero S, Ballestar E, et al. Genetic unmasking of an epigenetically silenced microRNA in human cancer cells. Cancer Res. 2007;67: 1424–9.

161. Scott GK, Mattie MD, Berger CE, Benz SC, Benz CC. Rapid alteration of microRNA levels by histone deacetylase inhibition. Cancer Res. 2006;66(3): 1277–81.

162. Benetti R, Gonzalo S, Jaco I, et al. A mammalian microRNA cluster controls DNA methylation and telomere recombination via Rbl2-dependent regulation of DNA methyltransferases. Nat Struct Mol Biol. 2008;15(3):268–79.

163. Sinkkonen L, Hugenschmidt T, Berninger P, et al. MicroRNAs control de novo DNA methylation through regulation of transcriptional repressors in mouse embryonic stem cells. Nat Struct Mol Biol. 2008;15:259–67.

164. Chen JF, Mandel EM, Thomson JM, et al. The role of microRNA-1 and microRNA-133 in skeletal muscle proliferation and differentiation. Nat Genet. 2006;38:228–33.

165. Chang TC, Wentzel EA, Kent OA, et al. Transactivation of miR-34a by p53 broadly influences gene expression and promotes apoptosis. Mol Cell. 2007;26(5):745–52.

166. Raver-Shapira N, Marciano E, Meiri E, et al. Transcriptional activation of miR-34a contributes to p53-mediated apoptosis. Mol Cell. 2007;26(5):731–43.

167. Frezzetti D, De MM, Zoppoli P, et al. Upregulation of miR-21 by Ras in vivo and its role in tumor growth. Oncogene. 2011;30(3):275–86.

168. Si ML, Zhu S, Wu H, Lu Z, Wu F, Mo YY. miR-21-mediated tumor growth. Oncogene. 2007;26: 2799–803.

169. Meng F, Henson R, Lang M, et al. Involvement of human micro-RNA in growth and response to chemotherapy in human cholangiocarcinoma cell lines. Gastroenterology. 2006;130:2113–29.

170. Xia L, Zhang D, Du R, et al. miR-15b and miR-16 modulate multidrug resistance by targeting BCL2 in human gastric cancer cells. Int J Cancer. 2008;123(2):372–9.

171. Tazawa H, Tsuchiya N, Izumiya M, Nakagama H. Tumor-suppressive miR-34a induces senescence-like growth arrest through modulation of the E2F pathway in human colon cancer cells. Proc Natl Acad Sci USA. 2007;104(39):15472–7.

172. Chen Y, Zhu X, Zhang X, Liu B, Huang L. Nanoparticles modified with tumor-targeting scFv deliver siRNA and miRNA for cancer therapy. Mol Ther. 2010;18(9):1650–6.

173. Esquela-Kerscher A, Trang P, Wiggins JF, et al. The let-7 microRNA reduces tumor growth in mouse models of lung cancer. Cell Cycle. 2008;7(6):759–64.

174. Kota J, Chivukula RR, O'Donnell KA, et al. Therapeutic microRNA delivery suppresses tumorigenesis in a murine liver cancer model. Cell. 2009;137(6):1005–17.

175. Chang TC, Yu D, Lee YS, et al. Widespread microRNA repression by Myc contributes to tumorigenesis. Nat Genet. 2008;40(1):43–50.

176. Care A, Catalucci D, Felicetti F, et al. MicroRNA-133 controls cardiac hypertrophy. Nat Med. 2007;13:613–8.

177. Tiscornia G, Singer O, Ikawa M, Verma IM. A general method for gene knockdown in mice by using lentiviral vectors expressing small interfering RNA. Proc Natl Acad Sci USA. 2003;100(4):1844–8.

178. Xia H, Mao Q, Eliason SL, et al. RNAi suppresses polyglutamine-induced neurodegeneration in a model of spinocerebellar ataxia. Nat Med. 2004;10(8):816–20.

179. Kawasaki H, Taira K. Short hairpin type of dsRNAs that are controlled by tRNA(Val) promoter significantly induce RNAi-mediated gene silencing in the cytoplasm of human cells. Nucleic Acids Res. 2003;31(2):700–7.

180. Grimm D, Streetz KL, Jopling CL, et al. Fatality in mice due to oversaturation of cellular microRNA/short hairpin RNA pathways. Nature. 2006;441(7092):537–41.

181. Lee Y, Kim M, Han J, et al. MicroRNA genes are transcribed by RNA polymerase II. EMBO J. 2004;23(20):4051–60.

182. Weiler J, Hunziker J, Hall J. Anti-miRNA oligonucleotides (AMOs): ammunition to target miRNAs implicated in human disease? Gene Ther. 2006;13:496–502.

183. Esau C, Davis S, Murray SF, et al. miR-122 regulation of lipid metabolism revealed by in vivo antisense targeting. Cell Metab. 2006;3(2):87–98.

184. Krutzfeldt J, Rajewsky N, Braich R, et al. Silencing of microRNAs in vivo with 'antagomirs'. Nature. 2005;438:685–9.

185. Orom UA, Kauppinen S, Lund AH. LNA-modified oligonucleotides mediate specific inhibition of microRNA function. Gene. 2006;372:137–41.

186. Elmen J, Lindow M, Silahtaroglu A, et al. Antagonism of microRNA-122 in mice by systemically administered LNA-antimiR leads to up-regulation of a large set of predicted target mRNAs in the liver. Nucleic Acids Res. 2008;36:1153–62.

187. Elmen J, Lindow M, Schutz S, et al. LNA-mediated microRNA silencing in non-human primates. Nature. 2008;452:896–9.

188. Obad S, Dos Santos CO, Petri A, et al. Silencing of microRNA families by seed-targeting tiny LNAs. Nat Genet. 2011;43(4):371–8.

189. Ebert MS, Neilson JR, Sharp PA. MicroRNA sponges: competitive inhibitors of small RNAs in mammalian cells. Nat Methods. 2007;4:721–6.

190. Gentner B, Schira G, Giustacchini A, et al. Stable knockdown of microRNA in vivo by lentiviral vectors. Nat Methods. 2009;6:63–6.

191. Su J, Baigude H, McCarroll J, Rana TM. Silencing microRNA by interfering nanoparticles in mice. Nucleic Acids Res. 2011. doi:10.1093/nar/gkq1307.

192. Weidhaas JB, Babar I, Nallur SM, et al. MicroRNAs as potential agents to alter resistance to cytotoxic anticancer therapy. Cancer Res. 2007;67:11111–6.

Index

A

Activated B-cell-like (ABC)
  lymphomas, 121
  subtype, 120
Activation induced cytidine deaminase (AID) enzyme, 116
Acute lymphoblastic leukemia (ALL)
  aberrant NOTCH signaling, 177–178
  B-lineage ALL, 176
  characterization, 176
  defined, 176
  PI3K/AKT/mTOR pattern, 178
  T-ALL, 177
Acute myeloid leukemia (AML)
  categorization, 173–174
  D-cyclins, 175–176
  description, 524–525
  FLT3, 174
  IDH1 and IDH2 mutants, 174
  immunophenotypes, 175
  KIT, 174
Acute promyelocytic leukemia (APL)
  defined, 178–179
  PML-RARα, 179–180
Adhesive interactions, cancer metastasis
  abciximab, 489
  ATN-161, 489
  α5β1 antagonists, 489
  integrins, 487, 488
  intetumumab, 489
  "outside-in" and "inside-out" signaling, 487
  S247, 488
  αvβ3 antagonist, 489
  vWF, 489
Afatinib role, NSCLC
  EGFR family receptors, 106
  EGFR-TKI, treatment of EGFR-mutation, 106, 107
  LUX-Lung 1 and LUX-Lung 2, 106
  reversible EGFR-TKI, 105
AFP-L3. *See* Alpha-fetoprotein Lens culinaris
      agglutinin 3 (AFP-L3)
AID enzyme. *See* Activation induced cytidine
      deaminase (AID) enzyme
AKT
  melanoma initiation and development, 446
  NRAS mutant tumors, 454
ALL. *See* Acute lymphoblastic leukemia (ALL)

Alpha-fetoprotein (AFP)
  HCC, 279
  measurements, 280
Alpha-fetoprotein Lens culinaris agglutinin 3 (AFP-L3)
  HCC, 280
  malignant liver cells, 280
AML. *See* Acute myeloid leukemia (AML)
Anaplastic thyroid carcinoma (ATC)
  AJCC classification, 65
  cytokeratin, 65
  PDTC, 64–65
Androgen levels, 360, 374
Androgen receptor (AR)
  gene mutations, 358
  NET, 376
Angiogenesis, 372, 374
Angiogenic markers, 395
Ann Arbor staging system, 118, 120
Anti-angiogenetic drugs, 372
Anti-angiogenic agents
  clinical application, 41, 42
  VEGF trap, 41
Anti-angiogenic therapy
  tumour vascularisation, 39–40
  VEGF signals, 40
Anti-EGFR agents
  cetuximab, 98–99
  family distinct receptors, 94
  homo/heterodimerization, 95
  pathway, 95
  protein, 94
  reversible EGFR-TKIs
    BR.21 trial, 95
    chemotherapy, 97–98
    clinical features, 95
    del19 and L858R, 96–97
    gefitinib and erlotinib, 95
    ORR and PFS, 95
    role, treatment mutation, 95, 96
Anti-EGFR therapy
  EGFR signalling, 32, 36
  markers, 39
  panitumumab, 38
  TKIs, 36
  validation status, 38
  zalutumumab, 38

Anti-microRNAs, cancer treatment
anti-miR oligonucleotides (AMOs), 538
lentiviral vectors, 539
liposome-polycation-hyaluronic acid (LPH), 536
LNA-antimiR, 538
microRNA sponges, 538
miR-15a/16-1, 535
therapeutic tools and approaches, 536, 537
APL. *See* Acute promyelocytic leukemia (APL)
AR. *See* Androgen receptor (AR)
Array comparative genomic hybridization (a-CGH), 448
ATC. *See* Anaplastic thyroid carcinoma (ATC)
Atrasentan, 372

B
Basal cell carcinoma (BCC)
epidemiology and incidence, 456
HH signaling, 456–457
keratinocyte skin cancers, 456
therapy, 457–458
treatment
5-fluorouracil (5-FU), 457
interferon-alpha (IFN-α), 457
Basal-like breast carcinoma (BLBC), 206
B-cell NHL
autocrine/paracrine mechanisms, 128
BAFF-R and mTOR kinase, 128
BCR signaling pathways, 126–127
in vitro and in vivo, 127
lymphoma cells and PKC-β, 128
phosphorylates tyrosines, 127
PIP3 complex, 128
B-cell receptor (BCR) signaling pathway, 129
Benign prostatic hyperplasia (BPH)
biopsy, 369
nodules, 361
therapeutic procedures, 363
Bevacizumab role, NSCLC
adverse events, phase III and IV trials, 100, 102
angiogenesis inhibitor, 99–100
anti-VEGF therapy, 102
AVAiL and SAiL, 100
ECOG, 100
E4599 trial, 100
phase III trials, plus chemotherapy, 100, 101
Biomarkers
clinical practice
categories, 251
LOE, 251
CRC, 252
current and emerging, 252
diagnosis
EBV (*see* Epstein–Barr virus (EBV))HNSCC, 21
HPV (*see* Human papillomavirus
(HPV))odontogenic tumours, 29
proteomic, serum, 24
salivary gland tumours, 29
serum markers, 24
tissue, 21–22

transcriptomic and proteomic, saliva, 23
validation status, 29
endometrial cancer, 383
genomic
saliva, 22–23
serum, 24
immunohistochemistry, 406
molecular and genomic, 390
prostate cancer (*see* Prostate cancer)
standard radio/chemotherapy treatment, 5
therapy
anti-angiogenic (*see* Anti-angiogenic therapy)
anti-angiogenic agents, 41
antibodies, 36
anti-EGFR (*see* Anti-EGFR therapy)
cetuximab, 37–38
HPV-positive OPC, 41–44
toxicity profile, 38
tyrosine kinase inhibitors, 39
validation status, 38
VEGF function, inhibition, 40–41
tumor blood vessels, 12
Biotarget
CA-125, 382–383
HE4, 383–384
proteomics, 385
screening, 382
ultrasound, 384–385
use
CA-125 and HE4, 387, 389
CA-125 and TVU, 386
ROCA, 386–387
screening performance, 385–386
UKCTOCS, 387, 388
Bispecific T-cell engager (BiTE) Abs, 141
Bladder cancer
angiogenesis
aflibercept, 342
bevacizumab, 341–342
pazopanib, 341
sorafenib, 341
sunitinib, 341
biomarkers, 338
chemotherapy, 335
cystoscopy, 328
diagnosis, 327
first-line combination chemotherapy, 337
follow-up, 342–343
imaging, 327
M-distant metastasis, 326
multiple modality bladder-sparing treatment
adjuvant chemotherapy, 336
metastatic disease, 336–337
muscle-invasive, treatment
bladder-sparing approach, 335
continent cutaneous diversions, 334
ileal conduit, 334
MIBC management, 334–335
neoadjuvant radiotherapy, 335
neoadjuvant treatment, 332–333

Index 549

orthotopic diversions, 334
radical surgery, 333
ureterocutaneostomy, 333–334
ureterosigmoidostomy, 334
N-lymph nodes, 326
non-muscle-invasive, treatment
adjuvant treatment, 330–332
CT/MRI imaging, 329–330
follow-up, TaT1 and CIS, 332
radical surgery, 332
TUR, 328–329
physical examination, 327
quality of life, 342
radiotherapy, 335
risk factors, 327
second-line chemotherapy, 337–338
synthesis, 343
targeting EGFR pathway
cetuximab, 339
erlotinib, 339
gefitnib, 339
lapatinib, 340
trastuzumab, 339–340
T-primary tumor, 326
TURB, 335
urine cytology, 327
urine markers, 328
BLBC. *See* Basal-like breast carcinoma (BLBC)
BNCT. *See* Boron neutron capture therapy (BNCT)
Bombesin, 372, 376
Bone tumors
adamantinoma, 427
cisplatin and methotrexate, 429
Boron neutron capture therapy (BNCT), 7
BPH. *See* Benign prostatic hyperplasia (BPH)
BRAF
CDK, 449
mutant melanoma
cell signaling scheme, pathways, 444, 445
MAPK signaling, 444, 446
mouse modeling studies, 446
solar elastosis, 447
Brain tumors, GBM, 12
BRCA 1/2, 393–394
Breast cancer
ancillary studies, 203
antioestrogen therapy
aromatase inhibitors, 209–210
SERDs, 208–209
SERMs, 208
chemotherapy, 210
classification
epithelial malignant lesions, 203, 204
gene expression profiling, 203
histological sections, 203, 204
diagnostic procedures
intraoperative, 202
operative, 202–203
preoperative, 201–202
histopathology, 203–206

mammary gland
branching ductal system, 195
human mammary gland, 195, 196
luminal and myoepithelial cells, 196
physiology and regulation, 196–197
mechanisms, tumourigenesis
defined, 198
and epigenetic factors, 199–200
genetic mutations, 200–201
and hormones, 198–199
microRNAs
interconnections, 530
Let-7, 528
miR-21, 527, 528
miR-205, 528
miR-206, 528
types, 529
progesterone role, 198
prognostic and predictive markers
human EGFR, 207
oestrogen and progesterone receptors, 206, 207
tumour proliferation rate, 206
sporadic clonal evolution mode, 197
targeted therapy, 210–213
therapeutic approaches classification, 207, 208

C
CA-125. *See* Cancer antigen 125 (CA-125)
Cachexia, 476
Cancer antigen 125 (CA-125)
description, 382
HE4, 387, 389
JANUS project, 382–383
ROCA, 386–387
serum bank, 382
TVU, 386
Cancer metastasis
adhesive interactions (*see* Adhesive interactions, cancer metastasis)
cell dissemination routes, 477–478
cell theory, 470
clinical outcome
autopsy analysis, 474–475
cachexia, 476
carcinomatosis, 475
dyspnea, 475
hemorrhage and thromboembolism, 476
pro-inflammatory cytokine, 476
skeletal involvement, 475–476
survival rate, 474
weight loss, 476
DNA chip technology, 470
ECM remodeling, 495–501
growth
ECM remodeling, 501
IGF-1, 501
MMPs, 502
molecular and cellular network, 502
osteoblastic lesions, 503

Cancer metastasis (*cont.*)
    osteosclerotic lesions, 503
    RANKL, 503
    vicious cycle, 502–503
  incidence
    autopsy rates, 471
    conventional therapies, 472
    death rate, 470
    DTCs, 472
    frequency, 472
    immunocytochemical and molecular assays, 472
  molecular basis, therapy
    biological heterogeneity, 485
    DNA-sequence-based studies, 485
    expression profile, primary cancer and paired
      metastases, 486
    genetic instability, 485–486
    microarray technology, 486
    pro-inflammatory cytokines, 486–487
    targeted therapy, 485
  pathogenesis
    cadherins, 479
    cell–cell adhesion, 479
    CTCs, 481
    "Docking and Locking" model, 481
    in vivo study, 482
    intrinsic properties, tumor cells, 478
    lymphangiogenesis, 479
    macrophages, 481
    metastatic cascade, 480
    premetastatic niche, 482–483
    TEM, 482
    tumor cells, bloodstream, 481
  pattern
    autopsy data, 472, 473
    breast cancer, 474
    isolated metastasis, 473
    metachronous model, 474
  progression models
    DTCs, 484
    hemodynamic theory, 483
    linear progression model, 484
    MEI, 483–484
    microarray and genetic analysis, 484–485
    vascular shunt, 483
  prothrombotic condition
    anticoagulant therapy, 491
    hypercoagulability, 489–490
    LMWHs, 491
    PAR-1, 491
    thrombin, 490–491
    tissue factor (TF), 489–490
  transendothelial migration, 491–495
Cancer of Prostate Strategic Urologic Research Endeavor
    (CaPSURE), 357–358
Cancer therapy research. *See* MicroRNAs, cancer therapy
CaPSURE. *See* Cancer of Prostate Strategic Urologic
    Research Endeavor (CaPSURE)
Carcinoembryonic antigen (CEA) levels, 252
CDK4. *See* Cyclin-dependent kinase 4 (CDK4)
CEA. *See* Carcinoembryonic antigen (CEA)

Cell dissemination routes, cancer metastasis
  breast cancer, 477–478
  colorectal carcinoma, 478
  hematogenous metastases, 477
  lymph node metastases, 477
  lymphogenous dissemination, 477
  peritoneal metastases, 477
Cell signaling pathway
  cell cycle genes, 409, 410
  IGFs, 412
  K-ras, 410
  MAPK, 412
  molecular alterations, 412–413
  molecular pathways and targets, 409, 411
  PI3K-Akt-mTOR, 412
  receptor tyrosine kinases, 409
  TP53 and PTEN, 410
Central nervous system (CNS) tumors
  biotargets
    GBMs, 5–10
    standard radio/chemotherapy treatment, 5
    targeted therapies, 11–15
  and childhood (ages 0–19) brain, 2, 3
  clinical presentation
    malignancies, 5
    principal groups, 4–5
    psychomotor asthenia, 5
  description, 1
  distribution and incidence rates, 1–3
  genetic/epigenetic pathways, 15
  incidence and mortality, 1–4
  SEER, 4
  survival rates, USA, 4
Cetuximab
  chemotherapy, 38
  clinical studies, anti-EGFR therapy, HNSCC, 37
  NSCLC
    anticancer activity, 99
    anti-EGFR antibody, 98
    BMS099, 98
    FLEX trial, 98
    KRAS oncogene, 99
    PFS and OS, 99
    potential predictors, OS, 99
    RMD, 37–38
  use, monotherapy, 37
CGH. *See* Comparative genomic hybridisation (CGH)
Chemotherapy
  and BCG, 331
  chloroethylating drugs and TMZ, 7
  cytotoxic agents, 7–8
  neoadjuvant, 332–333
Chromosomal instability (CIN), 253–254
Chronic lymphocytic leukemia (CLL)
  microRNAs
    BCL2, 524
    chromosome 17p deletions, 523
    germline mutation, miR-15/16, 524
    oncosuppressor p53, 524
    13q deletions, 524
    sequencing, 523

Index

objective, 171
oblimersen, 172
ofatumumab and lumiliximab, 172
rituxima, 171–172
SDF-1/CXCR4, 173
Chronic myeloid leukemia (CML)
    BCR-ABL1, 170
    dasatinib, nilotinib and bosutinib, 170
    imatinib, 170
    neoplasm, 168
CIN. *See* Chromosomal instability (CIN)
Circulating tumor cells (CTC)
    detection, 375
    PCa, 375
Cirrhosis
    child A or B, 282–283
    and HCC, 273
    hepatic, 279
CLL. *See* Chronic lymphocytic leukemia (CLL)
CML. *See* Chronic myeloid leukemia (CML)
CNS tumors. *See* Central nervous system (CNS) tumors
Colorectal. *See* Colorectal cancer (CRC)
Colorectal cancer (CRC)
    biology
        adenoma–carcinoma sequence, 246–247
        MAPK and PI3K pathway activation, 248–249
        MSI, 247
    biomarker-informed management, 262–263
    biomarkers, clinical practice, 251–252
    CEA, 252
    chemotherapy
        adjuvant therapy, 249–250
        metastatic, 249
    chromosome 18q deletion, 254
    CIN, 253–254
    description, 245
    dietary factors, 245
    EGFR, 250
    epidemiology, 245–246
    Ki67 proliferative index, 254
    LOE supporting biomarker, 262
    mismatch repair/MSI, 253
    multimodality management, 249
    P53, 254
    pharmacogenetics and therapeutic efficacy
        biomarker analysis, 259
        determinants of response/toxicity,
          targeted therapies, 259
        DPD, 258
        5-fluorouracil metabolism, 256–257
        gene-expression signatures, 259–261
        GWAS, 261
        high-throughput arrays, 259, 260
        irinotecan sensitivity, 259
        MTHFR, 258
        oxaliplatin sensitivity, 258–259
        proteomics, 261–262
        TP, 258
        TS, 257–258

PIK3CA, 250–251
staging, 246
tumour signalling transduction
    BRAF, 255–256
    EGFR, 254–255
    IGF2, 256
    KRAS, 255
    NRAS, 256
    PIK3CA, 256
    PTEN, 256
    VEGF, 250
Comparative genomic hybridisation (CGH), 33–34
Computed tomography (CT), HCC, 277–278
Crizotinib role, NSCLC
    EML4-ALK fusion, 102–103
    PROFILE 1007 and PROFILE 1005, 103
    TKI targeting, 103
    treatment, EML4-ALK-positive, 103, 104
CTCL. *See* Cutaneous T-cell lymphoma (CTCL)
Cutaneous T-cell lymphoma (CTCL), 134
Cyclin-dependent kinase 4 (CDK4), 440
Cycline
    angiogenesis markers and VEGF, 395
    EGF and HER signaling, 395–396
    maspin, 395
Cystectomy. *See* Radical cystectomy (RC)
Cytokine release syndrome, 163, 172
Cytotoxic drugs
    bendamustine, 126
    pixantrone and pralatrexate, 126

D

Dermatofibrosarcoma protuberans (DFSP), 424, 427
Des-gamma-carboxyprothrombin (DCP)
    description, 279
    level, 279
DFSP. *See* Dermatofibrosarcoma protuberans (DFSP)
Diffuse large B-cell lymphoma (DLBCL)
    ABC and PMBL, 121
    classification, 121
    lymphoid architecture, 120
    malignant clone, GCB, 120–121
    novel therapeutic strategies, 122
    prognostic factors, 121–122
    WHO classification, tumors, 120
Digital rectal exam (DRE)
    PCa screening programs, 363
    PSA, 370
Dihydropyrimidine dehydrogenase (DPD), 258
Disseminated tumor cells (DTCs), 470
DLBCL. *See* Diffuse large B-cell
        lymphoma (DLBCL)
DLI. *See* Donor lymphocyte infusion (DLI)
"Docking and Locking" model, 481
Donor lymphocyte infusion (DLI), 125
DPD. *See* Dihydropyrimidine dehydrogenase (DPD)
DRE. *See* Digital rectal exam (DRE)
Dyspnea, 475

E

EBV. *See* Epstein–Barr virus (EBV)
ECM remodeling, cancer metastasis
  ADAM/ADAMTS, 499
  cathepsins, 499–500
  heparanase, 500–501
  MMPs, 495–498
  serine proteases, 498–499
E-GC. *See* Oesophago-gastric cancer (E-GC)
EGFRs. *See* Epidermal growth factor receptors (EGFRs)
EMT. *See* Epithelial–mesenchymal transition (EMT)
Endometrial cancer
  categorization, 403–404
  cell signaling pathways, 409–413
  clinical characteristics
    description, 404
    dietary hypotheses, 404–405
    hormonal hypotheses, 404
    IGF, 405
    obesity and, 405
  description, 403
  family history, 406, 408
  gene mutations
    HNPCC, 408–409
    microarray technology, 409
    MSI, 408
  histology
    clear cell and serous histologies, 406, 407
    EIN and EIC, 406
    grades, 406, 407
    subtypes, 405–406
  immunohistochemistry, 406, 408
  surgical staging, 405
  symptoms, 404
  translational implications, therapy
    hormone therapy, 413
    metformin, 413
    PI3K pathway inhibitors, 413–414
    therapeutic targets, 413–414
Endometrial hyperplasia, 403
Endothelin receptor, 372
EpCAM
  description, 237
  expression, 237
  monoclonal antibodies, 237–238
Epidermal growth factor (EGF)
  EGFRs (*see* Epidermal growth factor receptors
    (EGFRs))and HER signaling, 395–396
Epidermal growth factor receptor 2 (EGFR 2), 223
Epidermal growth factor receptors (EGFRs)
  anti-EGFR agents
    cetuximab, 98–99
    reversible EGFR-TKIs, 95–98
  dual and HER2 inhibitors, 212
  family inhibitors
    gefitinib and erlotinib, 212
    HER2/neu overexpression, 211–212
    pathways, 210, 211
    pertuzumab, 212
  gastric cancer, 225–226
  gastro oesophageal cancer, 226

gene amplification and mutations, 33
HER2, 223
immunohistochemistry, 33
inhibitors
  description, 226
  gastric cancer, 227–228
  oesophageal and GEJ cancer, 226–227
MAPK and PI3K pathways, 250
oesophageal and GEJ adenocarcinoma, 225
oesophageal SCC, 224–225
pathways, 222–223
prognostic factors, GBM
  amplification and downstream lipid kinase, 9
  ErbB family, tyrosine kinase receptors, 8
  PKB/Akt and variant 3, 9
  STAT3 and MUC1, 8
protein subclasses, 223
signalling and action, anti-EGFR agents, 32
target therapy
  cetuximab treatment, 11
  gefitinib (ZD-1839) and erlotinib (OSI-774), 11
tyrosine kinase inhibitors, 224
Epigenetic drugs
  DNMTs, 135
  HDAC family members, 132–133
  HDACi, 133–135
Epithelial–mesenchymal transition (EMT), 479
Epstein–Barr virus (EBV)
  detection, diagnosis
    serum testing, 28
    VCA-p18, 29
  SNUC, 28
Erlotinib role, NSCLC
  gefitinib, 95
  PFS, 106
  platinum-based chemotherapy, 95
  TALENT and TRIBUTE, 97
  vandetanib, 107
Extracellular matrix (ECM) remodeling
  ADAM/ADAMTS, 499
  cathepsins
    cathepsin B, 499
    cathepsins H and L, 500
    cysteine, 499
  heparanase
    growth factors, 501
    heparan sulfate (HS), 500
    PI-88, 500–501
  MMPs, 495–498
  serine proteases
    ATN-658, 498
    capped 8 amino acid peptide, 499
    plasmin, 498
    plasminogen activation (PA) system, 498

F

Fine needle aspiration cytology (FNAC), 201–202
FL. *See* Follicular lymphoma (FL)
FLT3. *See* FMS-like tyrosine kinase 3 (FLT3)
FMS-like tyrosine kinase 3 (FLT3)

Index

AML patients, 161
mutations, 173, 174
FNAC. *See* Fine needle aspiration cytology (FNAC)
Follicular lymphoma (FL)
    characterization, 122
    GC B and stromal cells, 123
    Helicobacter pylori, hepatitis C virus and EBV, 122
    morphology, 122
    non-malignant microenvironment, 123
    tregs, 123
Follicular thyroid carcinomas (FTCs)
    HCC/oncocytic/oxyphilic, 64
    hematogenous diffusion, 64
    molecular genetics
        description, 69
        PAX8/PPARγ rearrangement, 69–70
        PI3K/AKT pathway, 70
        RAS oncogenes, 69
FTCs. *See* Follicular thyroid carcinomas (FTCs)

G

Galectin-3, 493
Gastric cancer
    EGFR, 225–226
    oesophagus (*see* Oesophago-gastric cancer)
Gastrin releasing peptide (GRP), 376
Gastrointestinal stromal tumor (GIST), 419
Gastro-oesophageal junction (GEJ)
    EGFR inhibitors, 226–227
    HER2 expression, 232–233
    oesophageal adenocarcinomas, 222, 225
GBM. *See* Glioblastoma multiforme (GBM)
GCB. *See* Germinal-center B-cell-like (GCB)
Gefitinib role, NSCLC
    erlotinib, 95
    EURTAC, 95
    MET proto-oncogene, 105
GEJ. *See* Gastro-oesophageal junction (GEJ)
Gene expression profiling, 35
Gene-expression signatures
    description, 259
    high-throughput platforms, 261
    RT-qPCR, 260
Gene fusions
    description, 373
    PCa cases, 373, 374
    PSA test, 365, 373
Genome-wide association studies (GWAS), 361
Genomic biomarkers
    saliva
        gene promoter methylation, 23
        mtDNA, 23
        p53 mutation, 22–23
    serum, 24
Genomics
    MAGP2, 397
    revolution, 396
Germinal-center B-cell-like (GCB)
    DLBCL, 131

PMBL cells, 121
    subtype, 120
GIST. *See* Gastrointestinal stromal tumor (GIST)
Gleason grading system, 362
Gleason score, 362, 363
Glioblastoma multiforme (GBM)
    CNS tumors and genetic disorders, 6
    genomics and prognostic factors
        EGFRs, 8–9
        epigenetic changes, 10–11
        LOH, 8
        p53/MDM2/p14^{ARF}, 10
        PTEN, 9–10
    glial cells, 5–6
    microarray technology, 8
    overall survival (OS), 6
    pathology
        corpus callosum, 6
        perineuronal and perivascular satellitosis, 6
    treatment
        chemotherapy, 7–8
        radiotherapy (RT), 7
        surgery, 7
GM-CSF. *See* Granulocyte/monocyte colony-stimulating factor (GM-CSF)
Granulocyte/monocyte colony-stimulating factor (GM-CSF), 142
Grouping, sarcomas
    group 1
        DFSP, 424, 427
        Ewing's sarcoma, 427
        gastrointestinal stromal tumors, 424
        pigmented villonodular synovitis, 427
        synovial sarcoma, 427
    group 2
        adamantinoma, 427
        chordoma, 427
    group 3
        dedifferentiated liposarcoma, 428
        MPNST, 428
    group 4
        angiosarcoma, 429
        current therapy, 429
        leiomyosarcoma, 428
        MFH, 428
        osteosarcoma, 429
        rhabdomyosarcomas, 428–429
        targeted therapy, sarcomas, 429–433
GRP. *See* Gastrin releasing peptide (GRP)
GWAS. *See* Genome-wide association studies (GWAS)

H

HBV. *See* Hepatitis B virus (HBV)
HCC. *See* Hepatocellular carcinoma (HCC)
HCV. *See* Hepatitis C virus (HCV)
HDT. *See* High-dose therapy (HDT)
Head and neck cancer. *See* Head and neck squamous cell carcinoma (HNSCC)

Head and neck squamous cell carcinoma (HNSCC)
  biomarkers (*see* Biomarkers)
  CGH, 33–34
  cyclooxygenase 2, 43
  description, 19
  EGFR, 32–33
  epidemiology
    malignant odontogenic tumours, 21
    malignant salivary gland tumours, 21
    oropharynx, 20
    sinonasal tract and nasopharynx, 20–21
    tobacco smoking and alcohol intake, 20
    worldwide incidence, 19, 20
  family, src kinases, 43
  gene expression profiling, 35
  genes, prognosis
    OPMLs, 30
    perineural/lymphovascular, 29–30
  global markers/patterns, 33
  HPV and prognosis, 33
  individual biomarkers, 31–32
  molecular analysis, 35–36
  molecular markers, 36
  odontogenic carcinomas, 44
  OPMLs, 30–31
  PI3K/AKT/mTOR pathway, 43
  salivary gland, 44
  sinonasal and nasopharynx, 44
  surgical margin analysis, 35
  TRAIL receptor, 43–44
  validation status, 36
Hedgehog (HH) signaling
  inhibition, targeted therapy, 457–458
  molecular basis, BCC, 456–457
Hematopoietic stem cells (HSCs)
  PML-RARα activation, 180
  propagation, leukemic growth, 165
Hematopoietic stem cell transplantation (HSCT), 125
Hemopoietic and nonhemopoietic diseases, 162
Hepatic angiography
  CTHA, 278
  description, 278, 280
Hepatic resection, 280, 485
Hepatitis B virus (HBV)
  HCC, 274
  vaccination programs, 274
Hepatitis C virus (HCV)
  HBV and, 275
  infection, 273, 279
  risk, 274
Hepatocellular carcinoma (HCC)
  description, 273
  diagnosis
    AFP, 279
    AFP-L3, 280
    CT, 277
    DCP, 279
    hepatic angiography, 278
    MRI, 278
    US, 277

pathology, 275–276
risk factors
  afatoxin, 274
  age, 274
  alcohol, 274
  description, 273
  HBV, 274
  HCV, 274
  hemochromatosis, 275
  male sex, 274
  NASH, 275
  obesity and diabetes, 274–275
staging systems, 280
surveillance, 275
treatment
  chemotherapy, 283
  liver transplantation, 281–282
  percutaneous local ablation, 282
  prevention, 283
  surgical resection, 280–281
  TACE, 282–283
Hepatocyte growth factor/mesenchymal-epithelial
    transition (HGF/MET), 428
HER2. *See* Human epidermal receptor 2 (HER 2)
Hereditary nonpolyposis colon cancer (HNPCC)
  histologic appearance, 406
  MSI, 408
  ovarian cancer, 408
  syndrome, 406
High-dose therapy (HDT), 124
HNSCC. *See* Head and neck squamous cell
    carcinoma (HNSCC)
HPV. *See* Human papillomavirus (HPV)
HPV-positive oropharyngeal carcinoma
    (HPV-positive OPC)
  management, 41, 42
  potential role, gene therapy, 43
  therapeutic vaccination, 43
HSCs. *See* Hematopoietic stem cells (HSCs)
HSCT. *See* Hematopoietic stem cell transplantation
    (HSCT)
Human cancer
  AML, 524–525
  breast, 527–529
  CLL (*see* Chronic lymphocytic leukemia (CLL))
  lungs, 529–531
  lymphoma, 525
  MM (*see* Multiple myeloma (MM))
  ovary, 531
Human epidermal receptor 2 (HER 2)
  expression, gastric cancer, 231
  expression, GEJ cancers, 232–233
  identification, 229–231
  inhibitors
    gastric and junctional cancers, 233
    oesophageal cancers, 233–234
  oesophageal adenocarcinoma, 232
  oesophageal SCC, 232
Human papillomavirus (HPV)
  detection methods

Index

GP5+/6+ PCR, 28
HNSCC, 26, 27
ISH, 26
PCR amplification, viral DNA, 26
p16 immunohistochemistry, 26–28
RTPCR amplification, viral E6/E7 mRNA, 26
double-stranded DNA virus, 24
head and neck tumours
positive oropharyngeal carcinoma, 26
specimens testing, 25
prognosis
immunomodulation, 33
infection, HNSCC, 33, 34
role, carcinogenesis
E6 and E7 act, 25
E2F, 25
mutational events, 24–25

I

ICAM-1. *See* Intercellular adhesion molecule (ICAM)-1
IGF1R. *See* Insulin-like growth factor 1 receptor (IGF1R)
IgVH. *See* Immunoglobulin heavy-chain variable gene (IgVH)
IMiD drugs. *See* Immunomodulatory (IMiD) drugs
Immunoglobulin gene superfamily (IgSF), 491
Immunoglobulin heavy-chain variable gene (IgVH)
CLL patients, somatic hypermutation, 171
molecular profile, 171
Immunomodulatory (IMiD) drugs
antineoplastic agents, 146
lenalidomide, 146
Immunotherapy
active
antitumor effect, Id-KLH, 142
B-cell tumor, 145–146
biovest study, 144
cocktail, maturation cytokines, 145
features and interpretation, clinical trials, 142, 143
GM-CSF, 142
Id protein, 141–142
in vivo transfection and antigen production, 144
indolent B-cell NHLs, 141
standard chemotherapy *vs.* vaccination protocol, 144
strategies, 141, 142
therapeutic cancer vaccine, 141
tolerance mechanisms, 146
vaccine, 145
mAb
anti-CD20, 137
B-cell antigen targets, 136
CD20, 136
CD70 and CD74, 140
clinical development B-cell malignancies, 138–139
131I-tositumomab, 140
ocrelizumab and valine/phenylalanine, 137
ofatumumab and veltuzumab, 137
retrospective analysis, 140
rituximab, 136–137

role, CD40, 140
SMIPs and BiTE Abs, 141
TRU-015 and TRU-016, 141
90Y-ibritumomab, 140–141
Insulin-like growth factor 1 receptor (IGF1R)
Ewing's sarcoma, 420
hormone system, 431
oncogenic gene product, 433
signaling pathway, 432
Integrin
activation, 494
antagonists, 488
cell–cell interactions, 487
description, 487
expression, 487–488
inhibitors, 488, 489
integrin $\alpha4\beta1$, 487
integrin $\beta2$, 494
"outside-in" and "inside-out" signaling, 487
upregulation, 488
$\alpha v\beta3$ and $\alpha v\beta5$ integrin activation, 488
Intercellular adhesion molecule (ICAM)-1, 443
International Prognostic Index (IPI), 123
Intetumumab, 489
Intravesical agents, 331–332
Invasion
arterial, 478
ECM, 495
neoplastic cells, 475
pancreatic carcinoma murine model, 498
Invasive lobular carcinoma (ILC), 205
IPI. *See* International Prognostic Index (IPI)

K

Keyhole limpet hemocyanin (KLH), 141, 142
KRAS
mutations, 255, 410
role, 255

L

Leukemias
ALL, 176–178
AML, 173–176
APL, 178–180
CLL, 171–173
CML, 168–171
identification, agents, 187
inhibitors, phosphatidylinositol 3-kinase, 187
JAK2+MPNs, 180–181
MDS, 182–184
microenvironment and LSCs, 184–185
MoAb, 161–168
molecular pathophysiology, BCR-ABL, 160
myeloid/lymphoid, 160
TP53 and apoptosis
inactivation mechanisms, p53 responses, 185, 186
MDM2, 185–186
treatment with nutlin-3, 186–187

Leukemic microenvironment and LSC
  CXCR4 levels, 185
  defined, 184
  NFkB and AKT pathways, 184
  NRP-1, 185
  survival and drug resistance, 184
Leukemic stem cells (LSCs)
  AML, 166, 175
  CD123, 166
  defined, 165
  and microenvironment, 184–185
Level of evidence (LOE), 251
LIN. *See* Lobular intraepithelial neoplasia (LIN)
Liver transplantation procedure, 281–282
Lobular intraepithelial neoplasia (LIN), 205
LOE. *See* Level of evidence (LOE)
LOH. *See* Loss of heterozygosity (LOH)
Loss of heterozygosity (LOH)
  genetic alteration, GBM, 8
  oncology, 8
LSCs. *See* Leukemic stem cells (LSCs)
Lung cancer, miRNA
  DNA copy abnormalities, 531
  HCC, 531
  let-7a, 529
  miR-21, 530
  miR-200c, 530
  sputum, 529
Lymphangiogenesis, 479, 488
Lymphoma, microRNAs, 525
Lynch syndrome. *See* Hereditary non polyposis
    colon cancer (HNPCC)

M
Macrophage colony-stimulating factor (M-CSF), 435
Magnetic resonance imaging (MRI)
  Gd-EOB-DTPA, 278
  SPIO, 278
MAGP2. *See* Microfibril-associated glycoprotein 2
    (MAGP2)
Malignant fibrous histiocytoma (MFH), 428
Malignant odontogenic tumours, 21
Malignant salivary gland tumours (ICD10 C07–08), 21
Mammalian target of rapamycin (mTOR)
  defined, 173
  hyperactivation, 412
  inhibitor, 173, 184
  inhibitors
  PI3K, 414
  regulation, 413
  role, 412
Mammary serine protease inhibitor (Maspin), 395
Mammary tumour model, 199
Maspin. *See* Mammary serine protease inhibitor (Maspin)
M-CSF. *See* Macrophage colony-stimulating
    factor (M-CSF)
MDS. *See* Myelodysplastic syndromes (MDS)
Medroxyprogesterone acetate (MPA)
  mice, synthetic progestin, 198
  tumourigenesis, 198–199

Medullary thyroid cancer (MTC)
  molecular genetics
    genetic lesions and RET mutations, 72
    involvement, RAS mutations, 72
    MEN 2 families, 71–72
    RET gene, 71
  neuroendocrine tumor, 65
  tumor diameter, 65
MEI. *See* Metastatic efficiency index (MEI)
Melanoma
  BRAF mutant melanoma
    cell signaling scheme, pathways, 444, 445
    constitutive MAPK signaling, 444, 446
    signaling pathways, 446
    signal transduction cascade, 446
  c-KIT mutant
    a-CGH, 448
    EGF receptor, 449
    imatinib mesylate, 454
    immunohistochemistry, 455
    MITF, 449
    PDGF, 448
    SCF, 448
    structure, signaling pathway, 447, 448
    tumor growth and suppression,
        metastasis, 450
  diagnosis and prognosis
    cell-cell and cell-matrix proteins, 442
    Clark level Breslow thickness and mitotic rate,
        440, 441
    E-cadherin, 444
    ICAM-1, 443
    lymph nodes, 440
    PCNA, 442
  HH signaling
    BCNS, 456
    -mediated tumorigenesis, 456, 457
  incidence, epidemiology, and risk factors
    CDK4, 440
    ultraviolet (UV) radiation exposure, 439
  malignant transformation, melanocytes, 439
  matching therapies, genotypes
    pharmacodynamic studies, 452
    putative mechanisms, 452, 453
    sorafenib, 451
  molecular subtypes
    CML, 444
    GIST, 444
  nonmelanoma skin cancers
  BCC (*see* Basal cell carcinoma (BCC))
  SCC (*see* Squamous cell carcinomas (SCC))
  NRAS mutant
    drug discovery, 453
    FTIs, 453
    intracellular signaling, 445, 447
    MAPK cascade, 447
    MAPK signaling, 454
    oncogenic mutation, 446
    protein kinase A (PKA) activity, 447
  pathological and prognostic features, 450
  subgroups, 450

Index 557

targeted therapy, nonmelanoma skin cancers
(*see* Targeted therapies)
Metalloproteinase (MMPs)
classification, 495–496
EMMPRIN, 496
inhibitors, 497–498
metastatic niche, creation, 502
RANKL, 497
synthesis, 497
TIMPs, 497
Metastatic efficiency index (MEI), 483–484
MetastomiRs, 532
Methyltetrahydrofolate reductase (MTHFR), 258
MFH. *See* Malignant fibrous histiocytoma (MFH)
Microfibril-associated glycoprotein 2 (MAGP2), 397
MicroRNAs, cancer therapy
anti-microRNAs (*see* Anti-microRNAs, cancer
treatment)classification, 518
cleavage process, 519–520
CLL, 520–521
deadenylation process, 520
Dicer, 518
expression regulation
genomic and epigenetic mechanisms, 533–535
principles, genomic organization, 533
transcriptional regulation, 535
gene expression, 519, 520
genes, 517
invasion, angiogenesis and metastasis
Dicer expression, 533
EMT, 532
metastomiRs, 531–532
miR-34a, 532
neo-angiogenesis, 532
oncogenic miR-21, 532
localization, 517
miRISC, 518–519
oncogenes and tumor suppressor
aberrant expression, 520, 521
AML, 524–525
breast cancer, 522–523, 527–529
CLL, 523–524
dysregulation, 521
lung cancer, 529–531
lymphoma, 525
microarray-based microRNA profiling, 523
MM, 526–527
ovarian cancer, 531
polymerase II (Pol II), 517–518
processing, 518
steps, hypothesis, 540
3'-UTR, 519
Microsatellite instability (MSI), 253
Microwave coagulation, 282
miRNA-containing RNA-induced silencing complex
(miRISC), 518–519
Mitogen-activated protein kinase (MAPK) cascade, 447
Mitogen-activated protein kinase (MAPK) pathway, 412
MMPs. *See* Metalloproteinase (MMPs)

moAbs. *See* Monoclonal antibodies (moAbs)
Monoclonal antibodies (MoAbs)
alemtuzumab, 164
CD52 expression, 161–162, 167, 168
CD19 expression, normal and leukemic B cells,
161, 165
CD20 expression patterns, B-cell leukemias, 161, 163
distribution, individual CD19 antigen concentration,
161, 166
distribution, individual CD20 antigen concentration,
161, 164
and epratuzumab, 166
GO, 164
lintuzumab, 164–165
ofatumumab, 163
potential effector mechanisms, 161, 162
rituximab, 162, 166
MPA. *See* Medroxyprogesterone acetate (MPA)
MPNs. *See* Myeloproliferative neoplasms (MPNs)
MSI. *See* Microsatellite instability (MSI)
MTC. *See* Medullary thyroid cancer (MTC)
MTHFR. *See* Methyltetrahydrofolate reductase (MTHFR)
mTOR. *See* Mammalian target of rapamycin (mTOR)
Multiple myeloma (MM)
microRNAs
mir-15a and miR-16-1, 526
miR-192 and 215, 527
xenograft studies, 526
preclinical lymphoma, 131
relapsed/refractory CLL, 172
and Waldenström macroglobulinemia, 129
Myelodysplastic syndromes (MDS)
categorization, patients, 184
defined, 182
DNA methyltransferases, 183
genetic abnormalities, 182–183
Myeloproliferative neoplasms (MPNs)
BCR–ABL-positive, 168
JAK2
defined, 180–181
JAK tyrosine inhibitors testing, 181
TKIs, 181

N
NASH. *See* Nonalcoholic steatohepatitis (NASH)
N-cadherin, 479
Needle core biopsy (NCB), 202
Neoplasia
and hesitate, 371
prostatic origin, 366
NET. *See* Neuroendocrine transdifferentiation (NET)
Neuroendocrine (NE) differentiation
NET process, 376
PCa, 376
VPA, 376
Neuroendocrine transdifferentiation (NET), 376
NHLs. *See* Non-Hodgkin's lymphoma (NHLs)
Nonalcoholic steatohepatitis (NASH), 273–274

Non-Hodgkin's lymphoma (NHLs)
  AID enzyme, 116
  Ann Arbor staging system, 118, 120
  anticancer agents, 147
  B-cell origin, 115
  cellular origins, human B-cell lymphomas., 117, 118
  description, 115
  development, B-cell, 116, 117
  DLBCL, 120–122
  FL, 122–123
  HSP90, 147
  lymphoma classification, B-cell, 117, 119
  molecular processes, remodel Igs, 115, 116
  novel antilymphoma therapies
    apoptotic pathway, 135–136
    cytotoxic drugs, 126
    epigenetic drugs, 132–135
    IMiD drugs, 146
    immunotherapy (*see* Immunotherapy)
    signal transduction inhibitor therapy, lymphoma, 126–132
  proteasome inhibitors, 146
  standard therapeutic approach
    algorithm, 123–125
    DLI and HSCT, 125
    IPI and mAbs, 123
    prognostic factors, 123
    R-CHOP, 123
    rituximab, 125–126
Non-small-cell lung cancer (NSCLC)
  chemotherapy
    cisplatin/carboplatin, 94
    cytotoxics, 93–94
    meta-analysis, 93
    pemetrexed, 94
  description, 93
  EGFR/VEGF, 93
  MET receptor signals, 105, 109
  never smokers
    HER2 insertions, 109
    multiple factors, 109
    peculiar clinicopathological features, 108–109
    reversible EGFR-TKIs, 109
  targeted therapies (*see* Targeted therapies)
  wild-type KRAS, 109
Novel antilymphoma therapy, NHLs
  apoptotic pathway
    ABT-263, 135
    Bcl-2 family members, 135
    extrinsic/death receptor-dependent, 136
    signals, tumor suppressor p53, 136
    survivin, 135–136
  cytotoxic drugs, 126
  epigenetic drugs, 132–135
  immunotherapy (*see* Immunotherapy)
  signal transduction inhibitor therapy, lymphoma
    (*see* Signal transduction inhibitor therapy)
NRAS
  drug discovery, 453
  FTIs, 453

MAPK signaling, 454
  mutant melanoma, 447
NSCLC. *See* Non-small-cell lung cancer (NSCLC)

O
Odontogenic tumours, 29
Oesophageal cancer. *See* Oesophago-Gastric Cancer
Oesophago-gastric cancer (E-GC)
  aetiology, 221–222
  description, 221
  EpCAM, 237–238
  HER 2 (*see* Human epidermal receptor 2 (HER 2))
  pathology spectrum
    Barrett's carcinoma, 222
    EGFRs (*see* Epidermal growth factor receptors (EGFRs))
    GEJ, 222
  VEGF (*see* Vascular endothelial growth factor (VEGF))
Oestrogen
  antagonists and deprivation, 208
  and progesterone receptors, 206
Oncogenes
  activation, 186
  MLL, 174
  RARα, 179
OPMLs. *See* Oral potentially malignant lesions (OPMLs)
Oral potentially malignant lesions (OPMLs)
  aneuploidy, 30–31
  hazard model, 30
  microsatellite analysis, LoH, 25, 30
  p53 expression and mutations, 30
  pre-malignant disease, 30
Ovarian cancer
  aurora-A, 396
  biotargets, 382–389
  CA-125, 391
  cycline, 394–396
  description, 381
  diagnostics, 389–390
  genomic profiles, 396–397
  miRNAs
    chemotherapy response, 531
    let-7i, 531
    miR-200c, 531
  molecular prognostic biotargets, 391–394
  prognostic biotargets, 390
  traditional prognostic biotargets, 390–391

P
Papillary thyroid carcinoma (PTC)
  BRAF oncogenes
    AKAP9-BRAF fusion protein, 69
    BRAFV600E mutation, 68–69
    downstream effectors, MAPK pathway, 68
    K601E point mutation, 69
    serine-threonine Raf kinase family, 68
  classification, 63
  fusion oncogenes, 65, 66

Index

lymphatic vessels, 63
MAPK signaling pathway, 65, 66
microcarcinoma, 63
RAS oncogenes, 69
RET oncogenes
  autophosphorylation and signaling., 67
  fusion genes, 67
  GDNF and GFRα1-4, 67
  pediatric patients, 67
  transcriptional program, 67–68
spatial genome topology, 65–66
TK domain, 66–67
TRK oncogenes, 68
variants, 64
PCa. *See* Prostate cancer (PCa)
PCA3. *See* Prostate cancer gene 3 (PCA3)
PDGFR. *See* Platelet-derived growth factor receptor
  (PDGFR)
PDTC. *See* Poorly differentiated thyroid carcinoma
  (PDTC)
Percutaneous ethanol injection, 282
Percutaneous local ablation therapies, 282
Peripheral T-cell lymphoma (PTCL), 126
Phase I trials
  monotherapy, 432
  novel targeted therapies, sarcoma patients, 436
  STS, 420
Phosphatase and tensin homolog (PTEN)
  BRAF, 446
  mutated melanoma, 446
  mutations, 410
  phosphatase activity, 410
  PI3K, 9, 410
  p53 mutations, 9–10
  role, 412
  TP53, 410
  tumor-suppressor gene, 9
Phosphatidylinositol 3-kinase (PI3K)
  amplification, 412
  apoptosis and cell proliferations, 410
  dysregulation, 412
  inhibitors, 413
  and mTOR, 414
  pathway inhibitors, 413
  signaling pathway, 410
PI3K/AKT/mTOR pathway inhibitors
  activity, mTORC2, 130
  everolimus, 130
  P101δ and CAL-101, 129
  perifosine, 129
  phosphorylation, 130
  rapamycin and rationale, 130
PIN. *See* Prostatic intraepithelial neoplasia (PIN)
PKC. *See* Protein kinase C (PKC)
PKC-β pathway. *See* Protein kinase C-beta (PKC-β)
  pathway
Platelet-derived growth factor receptor (PDGFR)
  imatinib (STI-571), 11–12
  open-label phase II trial, 12
  single-arm phase II clinical trial, 12

Plerixafor, 495
PMBL. *See* Primary mediastinal B-cell lymphoma
  (PMBL)
PML-RARα. *See* Promyelocytic leukemia-retinoic acid
  receptor-α (PML-RARα)
Poorly differentiated thyroid carcinoma (PDTC)
  and ATC
    BRAF mutations, 71
    characterization, 70–71
    point mutations, CTNNB1 and RAS genes, 71
    TP53 mutations and thyroidectomy, 71
  insular, trabecular, and solid, 64
Predictive biomarker, 251
Primary mediastinal B-cell lymphoma (PMBL), 121
Prognosis, 419, 428
Prognostic biomarker, 251
Prognostic biotargets
  description, 390
  molecular
    BRCA 1/2, 393–394
    P53 and MDM2, 392–393
    ploidy, 391
    TP53, 391–393
  traditional factors, 390–391
Prognostic factors, 8–11
Promyelocytic leukemia-retinoic acid receptor-α
  (PML-RARα)
  activation, 180
  description, 179
  heterotetramers, 180
Prostate cancer (PCa)
  biomarkers, 355–356
  clinical features
    DRE, 360, 363
    PSA, 364
    staging, 363–364
    symptoms, 364
  CTC, 375
  current research issues and new biomarkers
    discovery, 372–373
  cytology and grading
    Gleason grading system, 362
    Gleason score, 363
  diagnosis biomarkers
    CT and MRI, 365
    prostatic cytology, 364
    PSA test, 364–366
  epidemiology
    autopsy, 357
    CaPSURE, 357–358
    incidence rates, USA, 356
    PSA serum test, 356–357
  follow-up, biomarkers, 368–369
  gene fusions, 373
  genetics and causes
    AR, 358
    gene fusion, 359
    inflammation-related genes, 358
    onco-suppressor genes, 358
    PTEN-negative models, 358

Prostate cancer (PCa) (cont.)
  genetic studies
    description, 373
    SNPs, 374–375
  invasive carcinoma features, 361–362
  and metastatic spreading routes, 363
  morphology, 361
  NE, 376
  neoplasms, 363
  pathogenesis
    BPH, 361
    carcinogenesis experiments, 360–361
    PIN, 361
  pathology
    DRE, 360
    gland, 359
  PCA3, 373
  PIN, 361
  prognosis
    biomarkers, 369
    developments, 370
    pathological and clinical findings, 369
  progression and metastasis markers, 376
  PSA, 366–367
  PSP94, 375–376
  staging
    American AUC and TNM systems comparison, 367–368
    metastatic localization, 368
  therapy
    antiandrogenic, 371
    chemotherapy, 371
    concepts, 372
    hormone, 371
    radical prostatectomy, 370
  viruses and, 375
Prostate cancer gene 3 (PCA3)
  levels, therapy, 373
  PSA and, 373
  urinary test, 373
Prostate gland tumors
  anatomical limits, 369
  biopsy, 365
  growth and development, 360
  hormonal regulation, 371
  lesions, 361
  peripheral areas, 361
  proteins, 375
Prostate-specific antigen (PSA), 355
Prostatic intraepithelial neoplasia (PIN)
  characterization, 361
  foci, 361
  lesions, 361
  PCa, 361
Prostatic secretory protein-94 (PSP94), 375–376
Proteasome inhibitors
  carfilzomib and PR-047, 131–132
  IPSI-00 and NPI-0052, 132
  stabilization, IkB, 131
  ubiquitin and bortezomib, 131

Protein kinase C (PKC)
  cerebral irradiation, 13–14
  enzastaurin, 13
Protein kinase C-beta (PKC-β) pathway, 128
Proteomics
  SELDI-TOF, 385
  serum proteomic technology, 385
PSA. See Prostate-specific antigen (PSA)
PTC. See Papillary thyroid carcinoma (PTC)
PTCL. See Peripheral T-cell lymphoma (PTCL)
PTEN. See Phosphatase and tensin homolog (PTEN)

R
Radical cystectomy (RC), 333–335
Radiofrequency ablation, 282
Radiotherapy (RT)
  BNCT and stereotactic brachytherapy, 7
  CT scans and MRI, 7
Raf-MEK-ERK, 412
RANKL. See Receptor activator of nuclear factor kB ligand (RANKL)
RAS
  inhibitors
    prenylation (farnesylation), 130
    sorafenib (BAY 43-9006), 130–131
  mutant melanoma
    mitogen-activated protein kinase (MAPK) cascade, 447
    oncogenic mutation, 446
    protein kinase A (PKA) activity, 447
Receptor activator of nuclear factor kB ligand (RANKL), 497
Retrograde lymphatic embolism, 477
Risk of ovarian cancer algorithm (ROCA), 387
RT. See Radiotherapy (RT)

S
Salivary biomarkers, 22
Salivary gland carcinomas, 44
Salivary gland tumours, 29
Sarcomas
  anaplastic lymphoma kinase, 434
  bone and soft tissue, 419
  classification, soft tissue tumors, 420–422
  clinical, pathologic, molecular classes, 422, 423
  death receptor/TRAIL, 434
  genetic aberrations/translocations, 424–426
  group 1, 424, 427
  group 2, 427
  group 3, 428
  group 4, 428–433
  HGF, 435–436
  major subtype, 424
  M-CSF 1, 435
  molecular characterization, 437
  mTOR, 433–434
  the past, 419–420
  platelet-derived growth factor receptor pathway, 434

Index

p53 pathway/MDM2 pathway, 435
present and future
IGF1R, 420
STS, 420
receptor activator, NF-kB ligand, 435
targets and clinical trials, 436–437
TET-family genetic rearrangements, 424
VEGFR, 434–435
Sarcoma therapy, 429
SCC. *See* Squamous cell carcinomas (SCC)
SELDI-TOF. *See* Surface-enhanced laser desorption
and ionization time-of-flight
Selective oestrogen receptor downregulators (SERDs),
208–209
Selective oestrogen receptor modulators (SERMs), 208
SERDs. *See* Selective oestrogen receptor
downregulators (SERDs)
SERMs. *See* Selective oestrogen receptor modulators
(SERMs)
Signal transducer and activator of transcription-3
(STAT3), 8
Signal transduction inhibitor therapy
B-cell NHL (*see* B-cell NHL)
BCR, 129
PI3K/AKT/mTOR pathway, 129–130
proteasome, 131–132
Ras, 130–131
Sinonasal tract and nasopharynx (ICD10 C31 and C11),
20–21
Sinonasal undifferentiated carcinoma (SNUC), 28
Small-modular immunopharmaceuticals
(SMIPs), 141
SMIPs. *See* Small-modular immunopharmaceuticals
(SMIPs)
SNUC. *See* Sinonasal undifferentiated carcinoma
(SNUC)
Soft tissue sarcomas (STS)
ifosfamide and Adriamycin, 429
solid tumors, 429
Sorafenib, 283
Sporadic clonal evolution model, 197
Squamous cell carcinomas (SCC). *See also* Head and
neck squamous cell carcinoma (HNSCC)
incidence, epidemiology and risk factors
actinic keratoses (AK) lesions, 459
HPV, 458
molecular basis
acquisition, p53 mutations, 459
EGFR, 460
treatment, 459
STAT3. *See* Signal transducer and activator
of transcription-3 (STAT3)
Surface-enhanced laser desorption and ionization
time-of-flight (SELDI-TOF), 385

T

TACE. *See* Transcathether arterial chemoembolization
(TACE)
Targeted therapies

ALK, lung cancer, 102–103
antiangiogenic agents
different forms, VEGFR, 99
growth and survival, 99
monoclonal, bevacizumab, 99–102
antiangiogenic drugs, 213
antiangiogenic therapy
erlotinib, 107
sorafenib, 108
vandetanib, 107
anti-EGFR agents
monoclonal antibodies, 98–99
reversible EGFR-TKIs, 95–98
chemotherapy, 161
crizotinib, 102–103
CXCR4 and CCR7, 494–495
dual EGFR and HER2 inhibitors, 212
EGFR family inhibitors, 210–212
EGFRs, 11
endometrial cancer, 413
FLT3 inhibitors, 161
genotypes
pharmacodynamic studies, 452
putative mechanisms, 452, 453
sorafenib, 451
GIST, 419
HGF/MET autocrine loop, 428
histone deacetylase inhibitors, 15
identification, biological markers, 160
inhibitors, Ras pathway, 212–213
integrins, 15
leukemia, 162
ligand–toxin conjugates, 14–15
LSC-targeted therapies, 184
malignant glioma (MG), 11
mammalian, rapamycin, 13
nonmelanoma skin cancers, 457–458
PDGFR, 11–12
PKC, 13–14
RAS, 13
resistance, reversible EGFR-TKIs
D761Y and T854A mutations, 105
gefitinib/erlotinib, 103
irreversible EGFR-TKIs, 105–106
MET inhibitors, 106–107
MET receptor signals, 105
primary/acquired resistance, 103
T790M mutation, 103, 105
response rates approach, 414
rhabdomyosarcoma, 428
sarcoma
drug development, 429
fusion transcription factors, 430–431
imaging responses, 429, 433
insulin-like growth factor/Akt/mTOR, 431–433
pathways and specific targeted therapies, 431
tumor subclassification, 429, 432
TKIs, 176–177
VEGFR, 12–13
TC. *See* Thyroid cancer (TC)

TEM. *See* Transendothelial migration (TEM)
Temozolomide (TMZ), 7
Thalidomide, 83, 131, 146, 372
Thymidine phosphorylase (TP), 258
Thymidylate synthetase (TS), 257–258
Thyroid cancer (TC)
   agents
      17-AAG, 84
      antiangiogenic, 83
      bortezomib, 83–84
      redifferentiating, 83
   ATC, 64–65
   c cells, 62, 63
   classification, 62, 63
   description, 61
   doxorubicin, 62
   FTCs (*see* Follicular thyroid carcinomas (FTCs))
   gene defects
      aurora kinases, 73
      EGFR, 73
      VEGF expression, 72–73
   metastatic disease, 62
   MTC
      molecular genetics, 71–72
      neuroendocrine tumor, 65
   OS *vs.* PFS, 84
   pathogenesis and progression, 62
   PDTC
      and ATC, 70–71
      insular, trabecular and solid, 64
   PTC (*see* Papillary thyroid carcinoma (PTC))
   TKIs (*see* Tyrosine kinase inhibitors (TKIs))
   TSH suppression and RAI, 62
Tissue biomarkers
   cytological features *vs.* molecular analysis, 21
   FISH and AI, 22
   microRNA, 22
   MSI and p16 methylation, 21–22
   SELDI-TOF mass spectrometry, 22
TKIs. *See* Tyrosine kinase inhibitors (TKIs)
TNFR. *See* Tumor necrosis factor receptor (TNFR)
TNF-related apoptosis-inducing ligand (TRAIL), 434
TP. *See* Thymidine phosphorylase (TP)
TP53
   inactivation, 410
   mutations, 410
   p53 protein, 410
   and PTEN, 410
TRAIL. *See* TNF-related apoptosis-inducing ligand
      (TRAIL)
Transcathether arterial chemoembolization (TACE),
      282–283
Transendothelial migration (TEM)
   chemokines, 494
   disaccharide-based inhibitor, 494
   endothelium, 493
   expression
      CCR7, 495
      CXCR4, 494–495
      galectin-3, 493
   ICAMs and VCAMs, 494

   IgSF receptors, 491
   mucins, 493
   PECAM-1, 491, 494
   selectins, 492–493
   VCAM-1 and ICAM-1, 492
Transmembrane protease, serine 2 (TMPRSS2)
      gene fusion, 373
Transurethral resection (TUR), 328–329
Transvaginal ultrasound (TVU)
   CA-125, 386
   ROCA, 387
Treatment, SCC, 459
TS. *See* Thymidylate synthetase (TS)
Tumor necrosis factor receptor (TNFR), 136
Tumor suppressor gene
   TP53 and PTEN, 410
   TP53 inactivation, 410
Tumour stem cells
   development, 198
   identification, 197
TUR. *See* Transurethral resection (TUR)
Tyrosine kinase inhibitors (TKIs)
   activity
      levels, circulating biomarkers, 81
      motesanib, 80–81
      organ-specification, 80
      pazopanib, 80
      thyroglobulin, 81
      V804L, 80
   afatinib, 105–106
   BCR-ABL, 160
   biological targets and treatment
      BRAF, 79
      clinical trials, TC, 73–77
      molecular markers and pathways,
         TC pathogenesis, 79, 80
      motesanib and cabozantinib, 78
      NCCN and ATA, 79
      pazopanib, 78
      primary thyroid tumors, 79
      sorafenib and sunitinib, 78
      vandetanib, 78–79
      ZETA trial, 79
   chemotherapy, targeted therapies, 161
   FLT3 inhibitory activity, 174
   improvement, activity
      mTOR, 81–82
      RR range and tipifarnib, 81
      synergistic effect, 81
   resistance, EGFR, 103–105
   reversible EGFR, 95–98
   second-generation, 170
   targeted therapy, 176–177
   toxicities, 82

U
UKCTOCS. *See* United Kingdom collaborative
      trial of ovarian cancer screening
      (UKCTOCS)
Ultraviolet radiation

Index 563

acquisition, mutations, 439
cancer development, 458
EGFR signaling, 460
United Kingdom collaborative trial of ovarian cancer
screening (UKCTOCS), 387

V

Valproic acid (VPA)
HDACi, 134
NIS gene expression, 83
PCa cells, 376
Vascular endothelial growth factor (VEGF)
angiogenesis, 41
angiogenesis markers, 395
bevacizumab, 41
CRC, 250
inhibitors, 235–237, 413
and MMP-9, 199

NSCLC, 99–102
platelet-derived, 40–41
role, neovasculature, 213
Vascular endothelial growth factor
receptor (VEGFR)
AZD-2171, 12
bevacizumab (Avastin), 434
cediranib, 435
vatalanib, 12–13
VEGF. *See* Vascular endothelial growth factor (VEGF)
VEGFR. *See* Vascular endothelial growth factor receptor
(VEGFR)
Viruses and prostate cancer, 375
VPA. *See* Valproic acid (VPA)

X

Xenotropic murine leukemia virus-related virus
(XMRV), 375

Printed by Publishers' Graphics LLC
MO20120723